PRIMER ON
KIDNEY DISEASES

Second Edition

PRIMER ON KIDNEY DISEASES
Second Edition

EDITOR
ARTHUR GREENBERG

Division of Nephrology
Department of Medicine
Duke University
Durham, North Carolina

ASSOCIATE EDITORS

Alfred K. Cheung
Division of Nephrology and Hypertension
University of Utah School of Medicine
and Veterans Affairs Medical Center
Salt Lake City, Utah

Thomas M. Coffmann
Division of Nephrology
Department of Medicine
Duke University and Durham
Veterans Administration Medical Center
Durham, North Carolina

Ronald J. Falk
Department of Medicine
Division of Nephrology
University of North Carolina
Chapel Hill, North Carolina

J. Charles Jennette
Department of Pathology
and Laboratory Medicine
University of North Carolina
Chapel Hill, North Carolina

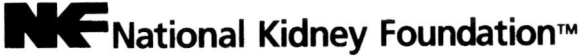 National Kidney Foundation™

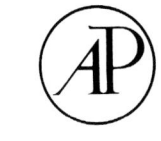

ACADEMIC PRESS

San Diego   London   New York   Boston   Sydney   Tokyo   Toronto

The opinions expressed and approaches recommended are those of
the authors and not those of the National Kidney Foundation or Academic
Press. Great care has been taken by the authors and editors to maintain
the accuracy of the information contained herein. However, neither
Academic Press nor the National Kidney Foundation nor the editors and
authors can be held responsible for errors or for any consequences arising
from the use of this information.

This book is printed on acid-free paper. ∞

Academic Press
a division of Harcourt Brace & Company
525 B Street, Suite 1900, San Diego, California 92101-4495
http://www.apnet.com

Academic Press Limited
24-28 Oval Road, London NW1 7DX
http://www.hbuk.co.uk/ap/

Library of Congress Cataloging-in-Publication Data

Primer on kidney diseases / edited by Arthur Greenberg ... {et al.}.
        p.   cm.
    Includes index.
    ISBN 0-12-299090-0
    1. Kidneys--Diseases.   2. Nephrology.   I. Greenberg, Arthur,
date.   II. National Kidney Foundation
    [DNLM: 1. Kidney Diseases.   2. Kidney--Pathology.   WJ 300 N2773
    1994]
    RC902.N28   1994
    616.6' 1--dc20
    DNLM/OLC
    for Library of Congress   94-26276
                                                                         CIP

PRINTED IN CANADA
97 98 99 00 01 02 FR 9 8 7 6 5 4 3 2 1

CONTENTS

SECTION 9
THE KIDNEY IN SPECIAL CIRCUMSTANCES

SECTION 10
CHRONIC RENAL FAILURE AND ITS THERAPY

SECTION 11
HYPERTENSION

CONTRIBUTORS

Numbers in parentheses indicate the pages on which the authors' contributions begin.

William T. Abraham, MD (183), Department of Medicine, University of Colorado School of Medicine, Denver, Colorado 80262

Sharon G. Adler, MD (164), Harbor–UCLA Medical Center, Division of Nephrology, Torrance, California 90509

Michael Allon, MD (98), Division of Nephrology, University of Alabama at Birmingham, Birmingham, Alabama 35233

Sharon Anderson, MD (42), Division of Nephrology and Hypertension, Oregon Health Sciences University, Portland, Oregon 97201

Gerald B. Appel, MD (160), Columbia Presbyterian Medical Center and Columbia University College of Physicians and Surgeons, New York, New York 10032

Arasb Ateshkadi, PhD (298), Department of Pharmacy Practice, College of Pharmacy, University of Utah, Salt Lake City, Utah 84112

Ellis D. Avner, MD (323,343), Department of Pediatrics, Case Western Reserve University School of Medicine and Rainbow Babies and Childrens Hospital of University Hospitals of Cleveland, Cleveland, Ohio 44106

Arvind Bagga, MD (193), Department of Pediatric Nephrology, Cedars–Sinai Medical Center, Los Angeles, California 90048

Robert R. Bahnson, MD (371), Division of Urology, Ohio State University Medical Center, Columbus, Ohio 43201

James E. Balow, MD (208), NIDDK, National Institutes of Health, Bethesda, Maryland 20892

Daniel Batlle, MD (71), Division of Nephrology/Hypertension, Department of Medicine, Northwestern University Medical School, Chicago, Illinois 60611

Wendy E. Bloembergen, MD (422), University of Michigan, Ann Arbor, Michigan 48103

Gregory L. Braden, MD (332), Renal Division, Baystate Medical Center, Springfield, Massachusetts 01199

Julia Breyer, MD (215), Division of Nephrology, Vanderbilt University Medical Center, Nashville, Tennessee 37232

Josephine P. Briggs, MD (3), NIDDK, National Institutes of Health, Bethesda Maryland 20892

Vardaman M. Buckalew, Jr., MD (291), Department of Internal Medicine, Section on Nephrology, Bowman Gray School of Medicine, Winston–Salem, North Carolina 27157

David A. Bushinsky, MD (106), University of Rochester School of Medicine and Dentistry and Nephrology Unit, Strong Memorial Hospital, Rochester, New York 14642

Alfred K. Cheung, MD (408), Division of Nephrology and Hypertension, University of Utah School of Medicine, Salt Lake City, Utah 84112

Diane M. Cibrik, MD (141), Department of Medicine, School of Medicine, Case Western Reserve University, Cleveland, Ohio 44109

Thomas M. Coffman, MD (260), Division of Nephrology, Department of Medicine, Duke University and Durham Veterans Affairs Medical Center, Durham, North Carolina 27705

Vivette D'Agati, MD (153), Columbia University College of Physicians and Surgeons, New York, New York 10032

James A. Delmez, MD (448), Renal Division, Washington University School of Medicine, St. Louis, Missouri 63110

Garabed Eknoyan, MD (345), Department of Medicine, Baylor College of Medicine, Houston, Texas 77030

David H. Ellison, MD (114), Section of Nephrology, Yale University School of Medicine, New Haven, Connecticut 06510

Murray Epstein, MD (188), University of Miami School of Medicine, Miami, Florida 33125

Jonathan T. Fairbank, MD (47), College of Medicine, University of Vermont and Division of Nuclear Medicine, Fletcher Allen Health Care, Burlington, Vermont 05401

Ronald J. Falk, MD (127,200), Department of Medicine, Division of Nephrology, University of North Carolina, Chapel, Hill, North Carolina 27599

William F. Finn, MD (329,335), Division of Nephrology and Hypertension, Department of Medicine, University of North Carolina School of Medicine, Chapel Hill, North Carolina 27599

John M. Flack, MD (506), Department of Medicine, Wayne State University Medical School, Harper Hospital, Detroit, Michigan 48201

Robert N. Foley, MD (455), Division of Nephrology, Memorial University of Newfoundland, St. John's, Newfoundland, Canada A1B 3V6

Cosmo L. Fraser, MD (459), Department of Medicine, University of California, San Francisco, and Geriatric Nephrol-

ix

ogy, Veterans Affairs Medical Center, San Francisco, California 94121

Ragini Fredrich, MD (193), Department of Pediatric Nephrology, Cedars–Sinai Medical Center, Los Angeles, California 90048

Patricia A. Gabow, MD (313), PKD Research, University of Colorado Health Sciences Center, Denver, Colorado 80262

Marc B. Garnick, MD (227), Harvard Medical School, Brookline, Massachusetts 02146

Martin Goldberg, MD (92), Temple University School of Medicine, Philadelphia, Pennsylvania 19140

R. Ariel Gomez, MD (383), Department of Pediatrics, University of Virginia, Charlottesville, Virginia 22908

Arthur Greenberg, MD (27,269), Division of Nephrology, Department of Medicine, Duke University, Durham, North Carolina 27705

Martin C. Gregory, MD (318), University of Wasatch Clinics, Salt Lake City, Utah 84112

Jonathan Himmelfarb, MD (465), Division of Nephrology, Maine Medical Center, Portland, Maine 04102

Thomas H. Hostetter, MD (429), Renal Division, University of Minnesota, Minneapolis, Minnesota 55455

Susan H. Hou, MD (388), Section of Nephrology, Rush Medical College, Chicago, Illinois 60612

Florence N. Hutchison, MD (282), Medical University of South Carolina and Ralph H. Johnson Department of Veterans Affairs Medical Center, Charleston, South Carolina 29403

J. Charles Jennette, MD (127,200), Department of Pathology and Laboratory Medicine, University of North Carolina, Chapel Hill, North Carolina 27599

Edward R. Jones, MD (80), The Germantown Hospital and Medical Center, Philadelphia, Pennsylvania 19144

Stanley C. Jordan, MD (193), Department of Pediatric Nephrology, Cedars–Sinai Medical Center, Los Angeles, California 90048

Bruce A. Julian, MD (170), Department of Medicine, Division of Nephrology, University of Alabama at Birmingham, Birmingham, Alabama 35294

Clifford E. Kashtan, MD (36), Division of Pediatric Nephrology, Department of Pediatrics, University of Minnesota Medical School, Minneapolis, Minnesota 55455

Bertram L. Kasiske, MD (477), Division of Nephrology, Department of Medicine, University of Minnesota School of Medicine, Minneapolis, Minnesota 55415

Paul L. Kimmel, MD (433), Department of Medicine, George Washington University Medical Center, Washington, DC 20037

James P. Knochel, MD (273), Department of Internal Medicine, Presbyterian Hospital, Dallas, Texas 75231

Stephen M. Korbet, MD (348), Section of Nephrology, Rush Medical College, Chicago, Illinois 60612

Eugene C. Kovalik, MD (472), Division of Nephrology, Duke University Medical Center and Veterans Affairs Medical Center, Durham, North Carolina 27710

Wilhelm Kriz, MD (3) Institute for Anatomy and Cell Biology, University of Heidelberg, Heidelberg 1, Germany

Andrew S. Levey, MD (20), Tufts University School of Medicine and New England Medical Center, Boston, Massachusetts 02111

Nicolaos E. Madias, MD (86), Tufts University School of Medicine and Division of Nephrology, New England Medical Center, Boston, Massachusetts 02111

Bradley J. Maroni, MD (440), Renal Division, Department of Medicine, Emory University School of Medicine, Atlanta, Georgia 30322

Catherine M. Meyers, MD (277), Renal-Electrolyte Division, Department of Medicine, University of Pennsylvania School of Medicine, Philadelphia, Pennsylvania 19104

Dawn S. Milliner, MD (337), Division of Nephrology, Mayo Clinic, Rochester, Minnesota 55905

Howard J. Mindell, MD (47), College of Medicine, University of Vermont and Division of Diagnostic Radiology, Fletcher Allen Health Care, Burlington, Vermont 05401

Asha Moudgil, MD (193), Department of Pediatric Nephrology, Cedars–Sinai Medical Center, Los Angeles, California 90048

Joseph V. Nally Jr., MD (496), Department of Nephrology and Hypertension, The Cleveland Clinic Foundation, Cleveland, Ohio 44195

Cynthia C. Nast, MD (164), University of California at Los Angeles and Cedars–Sinai Medical Center, Los Angeles, California 90509

Douglas J. Norman, MD (482), Oregon Health Sciences University, Portland, Oregon 97201

Paul M. Palevsky, MD (64), University of Pittsburgh School of Medicine and Veterans Affairs Pittsburgh, Healthcare System, Pittsburgh, Pennsylvania 15204

Patrick S. Parfrey, MD (455), Division of Nephrology, Memorial University of Newfoundland, St. John's, Newfoundland, Canada A1B 3V6

Beth Piraino, MD (416), Renal-Electrolyte Division, Department of Medicine, University of Pittsburgh Medical Center, Pittsburgh, Pennsylvania 15213

Jerome G. Porush, MD (395), Division of Nephrology and Hypertension, Brookdale University Hospital and Medical Center 11212

Robert Safirstein, MD (247), Division of Nephrology, University of Texas Medical Branch, Galveston, Texas 77555

Paul W. Sanders, MD (220), Division of Nephrology, University of Alabama at Birmingham, Birmingham, Alabama 35233

Caroline O.S. Savage, MD (175), Renal Unit, The Queen Elizabeth Hospital, Edgbaston, Birmingham B15 2TH, United Kingdom

Jon I. Scheinman, MD (309), Pediatric Nephrology, Medical College of Virginia, Richmond, Virginia 23298

Jurgen B. Schnermann, MD (3), Department of Physiology, University of Michigan Medical School, Ann Arbor, Michigan 48103

Patricia Y. Schoenfeld, MD (237), University of California Renal Center at San Francisco General Hospital, San Francisco, California 94110

Robert W. Schrier, MD (183), Department of Medicine, University of Colorado School of Medicine, Denver, Colorado 80262

John R. Sedor, MD (141), Department of Medicine, School of Medicine, Case Western Reserve University, Metro-Health Medical Center, Cleveland, Ohio 44109

Norman J. Siegel, MD (149), Department of Pediatrics, Yale University School of Medicine, New Haven, Connecticut 06520

Richard L. Siegler, MD (232), University of Utah School of Medicine, Salt Lake City, Utah 84132

Walter E. Stamm, MD (366), Division of Allergy and Infectious Diseases, University of Washington, Seattle, Washington 98195

Laura P. Svetkey, MD (501), Duke University Medical Center, Durham, North Carolina 27705

Stephen C. Textor, MD (491), Mayo Medical School and Division of Hypertension, Mayo Clinic, Rochester, Minnesota 55905

Robert D. Toto, MD (253), Department of Internal Medicine, Division of Nephrology, Vanderbilt University Medical Center, Nashville, Tennessee 37232

Prof. Dr. R. Vanholder (403), Department of Internal Medicine, Nephrology Unit, University Hospital, Gent, B-9000 Belgium

Jorge A. Velosa, MD (356), Division of Nephrology, Mayo Clinic, Rochester, Minnesota 55905

Joseph G. Verbalis, MD (57), Division of Endocrinology and Metabolism, Georgetown University, Washington, DC 20007

Alan G. Wasserstein, MD (360), Renal Electrolyte and Hypertension Division, Hospital of the University of Pennsylvania, Philadelphia, Pennsylvania 19104

Christof Westenfelder, MD (266), Division of Nephrology, University of Utah and Veterans Affairs Medical Center, Salt Lake City, Utah 84148

FOREWORD TO THE FIRST EDITION

On more than one occasion the possibility of publishing a primer on kidney diseases has been entertained by the professional membership of the National Kidney Foundation. On none of those occasions did the project progress beyond a consideration of such a notion. It was only some three years ago, when Dr. Arthur Greenberg submitted a written proposal for a nephrology primer to the Scientific Advisory Board of the National Kidney Foundation that action on this project was initiated. That it got into motion is entirely due to his perseverance and dedication. That the primer is now a reality is due to the commitment and leadership provided by its Editor, Arthur Greenberg, and his Associate Editors: Alfred K. Cheung, Thomas M. Coffman, Ronald J. Falk, and J. Charles Jennette. The work of the Consulting Editors: Joel D. Kopple, Neil Kurtzman, Manuel Martinez-Maldonado, and Shaul G. Massry has been relatively easier, but nevertheless demanding and extremely important to providing an independent external review process to the text. On behalf of the National Kidney Foundation I thank the Editors and Consulting Editors for their time and effort in making the *Primer on Kidney Diseases* a reality. A debt of gratitude is due to all the authors for their valuable contributions to the *Primer*. For bringing everyone's effort to its final fruition we are grateful to our publishers, Academic Press, Inc., and especially to Jasna Markovac, Editor-in-Chief, who was kind enough to act as our Biomedical Editor throughout the developmental phase of the *Primer*.

A word of explanation concerning the cover design: the frame is based on the symbols for the elements developed by John Dalton at the beginning of the nineteenth century. The four corner symbols, clockwise, beginning in the upper left corner represent sodium, phosphorus, potassium, and magnesium. The symbols in the boxes framing the cover, beginning from each corner, are those of hydrogen, oxygen, ammonia, carbon dioxide, and carbon. The figures on the cover are reproductions from the drawings of Leonardo da Vinci. The background is his classic drawing of man in equilibrium, befitting for a text on the kidney whose ultimate function is to maintain equilibrium in man by maintaining the "milieu interieur." Superimposed is a drawing of a scarred left kidney and atrophied right kidney from Leonardo's *Anatomical Notebooks,* yet another befitting diagram for a text on kidney diseases.

Garabed Eknoyan
1994

FOREWORD TO THE SECOND EDITION

The reservation with which work on the First Edition of the *Primer on Kidney Diseases* was begun is now history. The successful reception it received has been a rewarding experience for everyone involved in its production. Thus, it was with greater confidence and enthusiasm that work on the Second Edition was undertaken. The Editors were gracious enough to accept the challenge for a revised and updated *Primer.* They are the only constants of this new edition. To provide continuity, while at the same time allowing for new input, it was decided from the outset to invite new contributors to author at least one third of the chapters. The same rule was applied to the Consulting Editors. The change was deemed necessary to maintain the vitality of the *Primer,* and this policy will be continued in the future. A very special note of thanks is due to the former authors and Consulting Editors who contributed so much to the success of the First Edition.

All of the improved features of the Second Edition reflect the creativity and commitment of the Editor, Arthur Greenberg, and his Associate Editors: Alfred K. Cheung, Thomas M. Coffman, Ronald J. Falk, and J. Charles Jennette. As with the First Edition, each of the chapters was reviewed by the Editors, as well as one of the Consulting Editors: James V. Donadio, Garabed Eknoyan, Shaul G. Massry, William E. Mitch, and Sandra Sabatini. On behalf of the National Kidney Foundation, I thank the Editors and Consulting Editors for their diligent effort in bringing the Second Edition to fruition. A special thanks goes to returning and new authors of the *Primer.* Without their contributions, the revision would not have been possible. The support received from the Publishers, and particularly that of Jasna Markovac, has been invaluable. They have been as understanding, cooperative, and responsive as anyone could wish from a publisher.

Garabed Eknoyan

PREFACE TO THE FIRST EDITION

During the past twenty years, at least a half dozen excellent multivolume texts in nephrology or renal physiology have appeared, testifying to the expansion of clinical and basic science information in renal medicine. Many books covering fluid and electrolyte disorders, dialysis, or renal transplantation have also been published during this time. Collectively, they function superbly as reference works for nephrologists and nephrology fellows. They are less useful students or busy clinicians. The purpose of this book is different. Like any primer, it is an introductory textbook. It is targeted at medical students, house officers, and primary care physicians. For them, we hope to provide a fresh, succinct, and accessible but comprehensive overview of clinical nephrology.

The *Primer* begins with a description of the normal kidney and of techniques used to evaluate kidney function and anatomy. Subsequent sections cover the glomerular diseases, tubulointerstitial diseases, acute renal failure, chronic renal failure, and hypertension. Reviews of dialysis and renal transplantation offer information useful to the non-nephrologist called upon to care for patients approaching end-stage renal disease or patients with stable functioning renal allografts. The final chapters consist of practical discussions of acid–base and electrolyte disorders, stressing the pragmatic application of renal physiology to clinical problems.

Contributors to the *Primer* were asked to adhere to strict page limits, chosen to reflect the relative importance of the topic and the depth of the pertinent medical literature. Determining the proper length was an imprecise business. Some chapters may appear longer than warranted by the prevalence of the disease condition they describe, because we did not want to substitute brevity for clarity. Additional details may be obtained from the suggested readings that follow each chapter. These sources are just that; we thought recent reviews and key primary articles would be more valuable than a detailed listing of potentially obscure or overly technical citations. Reference to these reviews and the multivolume nephrology texts will direct the interested reader to primary sources.

Chapters were thoroughly reviewed before acceptance. Each was read by a member of the Editorial Board, by the Editor, and then by a member of the National Kidney Foundation Scientific Advisory Board serving as a Consulting Editor. Authors were then asked to revise their manuscripts and the review process was repeated. We are grateful for the authors' efforts to distill the essential content into the smallest possible space and for their unfailing cooperation with the entire editorial process. Although a general consensus was not always achievable, we believe that the chapters all reflect views accepted by a broad range of nephrologists.

In keeping with its overall goals, the National Kidney Foundation has a specific educational mission: to encourage "dissemination of both existing and newly acquired knowledge to the professional community." The editors hope that in serving this purpose, the *Primer* will facilitate the care of patients with kidney disease. Perhaps it will also serve as an invitation to students and medical residents to look more closely at the specialty that focuses on kidney disease, nephrology.

I am most grateful to the Consulting Editors and, especially, to the Co-Editors for their enthusiasm and commitment at every stage of this project. Finally, imitation is the sincerest form of flattery. As a student and house officer, I found the *Primer on the Rheumatic Diseases* (now in its tenth edition) an excellent summary of that field. Drs. H. Ralph Schumacher, Jr., and Arthur Grayzell of the Arthritis Foundation generously provided many suggestions that were very helpful in initiating work on this first *Primer on Kidney Diseases*. The Editors and the National Kidney Foundation hope this new book will prove equally handy, and they welcome your suggestions for improvement of future editions.

Arthur Greenberg
1994

PREFACE TO THE SECOND EDITION

The Editors are gratified by the warm response to the first edition of the *Primer*. The book is too big to fit in the pocket of a white coat, but many more students and house officers than expected are carrying it and reading it while rotating on nephrology services. Our goals for this new edition, which appears 3 years after the original, have not changed. The book is still targeted at students, house staff, and practitioners, for whom we have tried to provide a comprehensive, accessible, and pragmatic summary of the management of renal diseases and fluid and electrolyte disorders.

Readers of the first edition will notice some modifications. The book is now divided into 11 sections, covering renal function and its assessment, electrolyte disorders, glomerular disease, the kidney in systemic disease, acute renal failure, drugs and the kidney, hereditary renal diseases, tubulointerstitial diseases, the kidney in special circumstances, chronic renal disease, and hypertension. Two chapters dealing with the characteristics of kidney function in the very young and the very old have been added, along with a separate chapter introducing the tubulointerstitial diseases. The chapter serving as an overview of glomerular diseases now includes an outstanding series of schematic diagrams of glomerular pathology contributed by Charles Jennette. Analgesic abuse nephropathy and the effects of NSAIDs on the kidney are now covered together. With the cooperation of Jasna Markovac and Tari Paschall at Academic Press, we have been able to render the photomicrographs of the urine sediment and renal pathology in color.

To keep the *Primer* fresh, it was our original intent to rotate authors periodically. Accordingly, roughly one third of the chapters have new authors. The Editors gratefully acknowledge the hard work of these new contributors and the efforts of returning authors, all of whom have updated the text and references of their chapters. All authors, old and new, cooperated patiently and graciously with the *Primer's* editorial process, which is also unchanged. Each chapter was read by the Editor, an Associate Editor, and a member of the NKF Scientific Advisory Board acting as a Consulting Editor. Requests for revision were solicited, and the review process was repeated before chapters were accepted.

I want to acknowledge the support of Gary Eknoyan, who this year serves as NKF President. With Shaul Massry, he was instrumental in launching the first edition and guided this revision as well. The assistance of three new Consulting Editors, Sandra Sabatini, James Donadio, and William Mitch, was invaluable, as was the assistance of both veterans. I am again indebted to Alfred Cheung, Tom Coffman, Ron Falk, and Charles Jennette for their critical insights, estimable advice, and hard work.

Arthur Greenberg

SECTION I

STRUCTURE AND FUNCTION OF THE KIDNEY AND THEIR CLINICAL ASSESSMENT

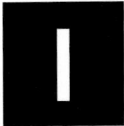

OVERVIEW OF RENAL FUNCTION AND STRUCTURE

JOSEPHINE P. BRIGGS, WILHELM KRIZ, AND JURGEN B. SCHNERMANN

BASIC CONCEPTS

Functions of the Kidney

The main functions of the kidneys can be categorized as follows:

1. Maintenance of body composition. The volume of fluid in the body, its osmolarity, electrolyte content and concentration, and its acidity are all regulated by the kidney by variation in urine excretion of water and ions. Electrolytes regulated by changes in urinary excretion include Na^+, K^+, Cl^+, Ca^+, Mg^{2+}, and PO^+_4.
2. Excretion of metabolic endproducts and foreign substances. The kidney excretes a number of products of metabolism, most notably urea, and a number of toxins and drugs.
3. Production and secretion of enzymes and hormones.
   a. Renin is an enzyme produced by the granular cells of the juxtaglomerular apparatus and catalyzes the formation of angiotensin from a plasma globulin, angiotensinogen. Angiotensin is a potent vasoconstrictor peptide and contributes importantly to salt balance and blood pressure regulation.
   b. Erythropoietin, a glycosylated, 165-amino-acid protein produced by renal cortical interstitial cells, stimulates the maturation of erythrocytes in the bone marrow.
   c. 1,25-Dihydroxyvitamin D_3, the most active form of vitamin D_3, is formed by proximal tubule cells. This steroid hormone plays an important role in the regulation of body calcium and phosphate balance.

In later chapters of this *Primer*, the pathophysiological mechanisms and consequences of derangements in kidney function are discussed in detail. This chapter reviews the basic anatomy of the kidney and the normal mechanisms for urine formation—glomerular filtration and tubular transport.

The Kidney and Homeostasis

Numerous functions of the body proceed optimally only when body fluid composition and volume are maintained within an appropriate range. For example:

- Cardiac output and blood pressure are dependent on optimum plasma volume.
- Most enzymes function best over rather narrow ranges of pH or ion concentration.
- Cell membrane potentials depend on K^+ concentration.
- Membrane excitability depends on Ca^+ concentration.

The principal job of the kidneys is the correction of perturbations in the composition and volume of body fluids that occur as a consequence of food intake, metabolism, environmental factors, and exercise. Typically, in healthy people, such perturbations are corrected within a matter of hours, so that in the long term, body fluid volume and the concentration of most ions do not deviate much from normal set points. In many disease states, however, these regulatory processes are disturbed, resulting in persistent deviations in body fluid volumes or ionic concentrations. Understanding these disorders requires an understanding of the normal regulatory processes.

The Balance Concept

The maintenance of stable body fluid composition requires that appearance and disappearance rates of any substance in the body balance each other. Balance is achieved when:

Ingested amount + Produced amount = Excreted amount + Consumed amount.

For a large number of organic compounds, balance is the result of metabolic production and consumption. However, electrolytes are not produced or consumed by the body; balance is achieved by adjusting excretion to match intake. Therefore, when a person is in balance for sodium, potassium, and other ions, the amount excreted must equal the amount ingested. Since the kidneys are the principal organs where *regulated* excretion takes place, urinary excretion of such solutes closely follows the dietary intake. A central theme of physiology of the kidneys is understanding the mechanisms by which urine composition is altered to maintain the body in balance.

Body Fluid Composition

To a large extent, humans are composed of water. Adipose tissue is low in water content; thus, in obese people, the fraction of body weight that is water is lower than that in lean individuals. As a consequence of slightly greater fat content, women, on the average, contain less water than men, about 55% instead of 60%. Useful round numbers to remember for bedside estimates of body fluid volumes are given in Table 1. Typical ionic compositions of the intracellular and extracellular fluid compartments are given in Table 2.

KIDNEY STRUCTURE

The kidneys are two bean-shaped organs lying in the retroperitoneal space, each weighing about 150 g. The kidney is an anatomically complex organ, consisting of many different types of highly specialized cells, arranged in a highly organized three-dimensional pattern. The functional unit of the kidney is called a *nephron* (there are approximately 1 million nephrons in one human kidney); each nephron consists of a *glomerulus* and a long tubule which is made of a single layer of epithelial cells (the nephron is depicted schematically in Fig. 1). The nephron is segmented into distinct parts—proximal tubule, loop of Henle, distal tubule, collecting duct—each with a typical cellular appearance and special functional characteristics.

The nephrons are packed tightly together to make up the kidney parenchyma, which can be divided into regions. The outer layer of the kidney is called the *cortex;* it contains all the glomeruli, much of the proximal tubule, and some of the more distal portions as well. The inner section, called the *medulla,* consists largely of the parallel arrays of the loops of Henle and collecting ducts. The medulla is formed into cone-shaped regions, called *pyramids* (the human kid-

TABLE 2

Typical Ionic Composition of Plasma and Intracellular Fluid

	Plasma (mEq/L)	Intracellular fluid (mEq/L)
Cations		
K^+	4	140
Na^+	143	12
Ca^{2+}		
(ionized)	2	0.001
Mg^{2+}	1	38
Total cations	150 mEq/L	190 mEq/L
Anions		
Cl^-	104	4
HCO_3^-	24	12
Phosphates	2	40
Protein	14	50
Other	6	88
Total anions	150 mEq/L	190 mEq/L

ney typically has 7 to 9), which extend into the renal pelvis. The tips of the medullary pyramids are called *papillae.* The medulla is important for concentration of the urine; the extracellular fluid in this region of the kidney has much higher solute concentration than plasma—as much as four times higher, with highest solute concentrations reached at the papillary tips.

The process of urine formation begins in the *glomerular capillary tuft,* where an ultrafiltrate of plasma is formed. The filtered fluid is collected in *Bowman's capsule* and enters the renal tubule to be carried over a circuitous course, successively modified by exposure to the sequence of specialized tubular epithelial segments with different transport functions. The *proximal convoluted tubule,* which is located entirely in the renal cortex, absorbs approximately two-thirds of the glomerular filtrate. Fluid remaining at the end of the proximal convoluted tubule enters the *loop of Henle,* which dips down in a hairpin configuration into the medulla. Returning to the cortex, the tubular fluid passes close by its parent glomerulus at the *juxtaglomerular apparatus,* then enters the *distal convoluted tubule* and finally the *collecting duct,* which courses back through the medulla, to empty into the renal pelvis at the tip of the renal papilla. Along the tubule, most of the glomerular filtrate is absorbed, but some additional substances are secreted. The final product, the urine, enters the renal pelvis and then the ureter, collects in the bladder, and is finally excreted from the body.

RENAL CIRCULATION

Anatomy of the Circulation

The renal artery, which enters the kidney at the renal hilum, carries about one-fifth of the cardiac output; this represents the highest tissue-specific blood flow of all larger organs in the body (about 350 mL/min 100 g tissue). As a

TABLE I

Bedside Estimates of Body Fluid Compartment Volumes

Remember	Example for 60-kg patient
Total body water = 60% × body wt	60% × 60 kg = 36 L
Intracellular water = 2/3 total body water	2/3 × 36 L = 24 L
Extracellular water = 1/3 total body water	1/3 × 36 L = 12 L
Plasma water = 1/4 extracellular water	1/4 × 12 L = 3 L
Blood volume = $\dfrac{\text{Plasma water}}{1\text{-Hct}}$	3 L ÷ (1–0.40) = 6.6 L

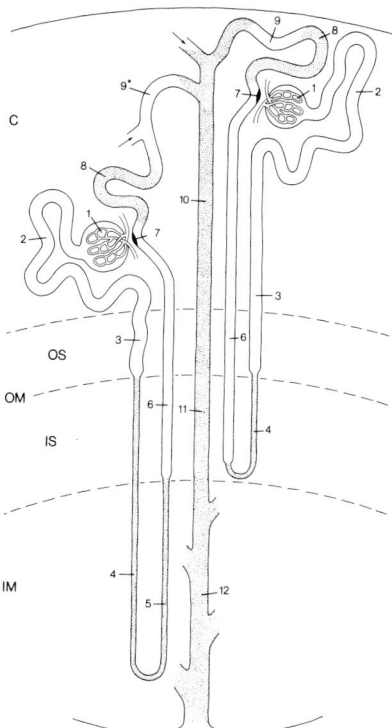

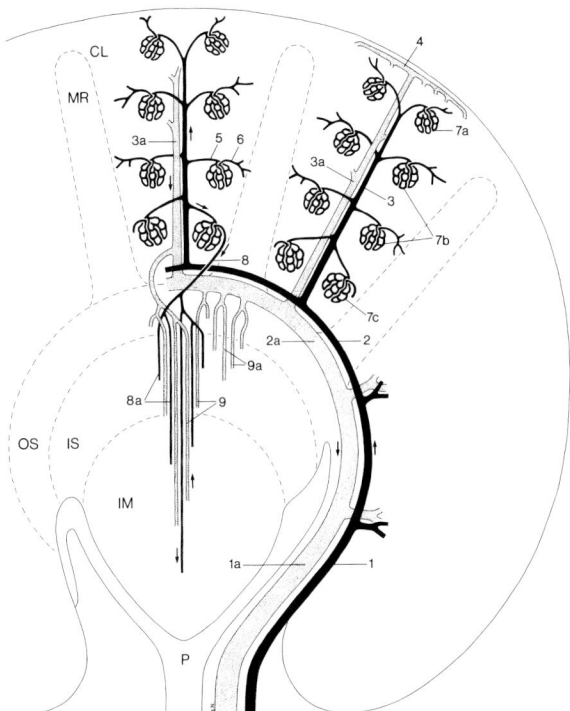

FIGURE 1 Organization of the nephron. The human kidney is made up of a million nephrons, two of which are shown schematically here. Each nephron consists of the following parts: glomerulus (1), proximal convoluted tubule (2), proximal straight tubule (3), thin descending limb of the loop of Henle (4), thin ascending limb (5), thick ascending limb (6), macula densa (7), distal convoluted tubule (8), and connecting tubule (9). Several nephrons coalesce to empty into a collecting duct, which has three distinct regions: the cortical collecting duct (10), the outer medullary collecting duct (11), and the inner medullary collecting duct (12). As shown, the deeper glomeruli give rise to nephrons with loops of Henle which descend all the way to the papillary tips, while the more superficial glomeruli have loops of Henle that bend at the junction between the inner and outer medulla.

FIGURE 2 Organization of the renal vascular system. The renal artery bifurcates soon after entering the kidney parenchyma and gives rise to a system of arched-shaped vessels that run along the border betweeen the cortex and the medulla. In this diagram, the vascular elements surrounding a single renal pyramid are shown. The human kidney typically has seven to nine renal pyramids. Here the arterial supply and glomeruli are shown in black, and the venous system is shown in grey. The peritubular capillary network which arises from the efferent arterioles is omitted, for simplicity. The vascular elements are named as follows: interlobar artery and vein (1 and 1a), arcuate artery and vein (2 and 2a), interlobular artery and vein (3 and 3a), stellate vein (4), afferent arteriole (5), efferent arteriole (6), glomerular capillaries (7), juxtamedullary efferent arteriole, supplying descending vasa recti (8), and ascending vasa recti (9).

consequence of this generous perfusion, the renal arteriovenous O_2 difference is much lower than that of most other tissues (and blood in the renal vein is noticeably redder in color than that in other veins). The renal artery bifurcates several times after it enters the kidney and then breaks into the *arcuate arteries,* which run, in an arch-like fashion, along the border between the cortex and the outer medulla. As shown in Fig. 2, the arcuate vessels give rise, typically at right angles, to *interlobular arteries,* which run to the surface of the kidney. The *afferent arterioles* supplying the glomeruli come off the interlobular vessels.

Two Capillary Beds

The renal circulation is unusual in that it breaks into two separate capillary beds: the glomerular bed and the peritubular capillary bed. These two capillary networks are

arranged in series so that all the renal blood flow passes through both. As blood leaves the glomerulus, the capillaries coalesce into the *efferent arteriole,* but almost immediately the vessels bifurcate again to form the peritubular capillary network. This second network of capillaries is the site where tubular reabsorbate is returned to the circulation. Pressure in the first capillary bed, that of the glomerulus, is rather high (about 40 to 50 mm Hg), while pressure in the peritubular capillaries is similar to that in capillary beds elsewhere in the body (about 5 to 10 mm Hg).

About 25% of the plasma that arrives at the glomerulus passes through the filtration barrier to become the filtrate. Blood cells, most of the proteins, and about 75% of the fluid and small solutes stay in the capillary and leave the glomerulus via the efferent arteriole. This postglomerular blood, which has a relatively high concentration of protein and red cells, enters the peritubular capillaries, where the high oncotic pressure from the high protein concentration facilitates the reabsorption of fluid. The peritubular capillaries coalesce to form venules and eventually the renal vein.

Medullary Blood Supply

The blood supplying the medulla is also postglomerular: specialized peritubular vessels, called *vasa recta*, arise from the efferent arterioles of the glomeruli nearest the medulla (the *juxtamedullary glomeruli*). Like medullary renal tubules, these vasa recta form hairpin loops dipping into the medulla.

GLOMERULUS

Structure

The structure of the glomerulus is shown schematically in Fig. 3 and in the photomicrographs in Fig. 4. The glomer-

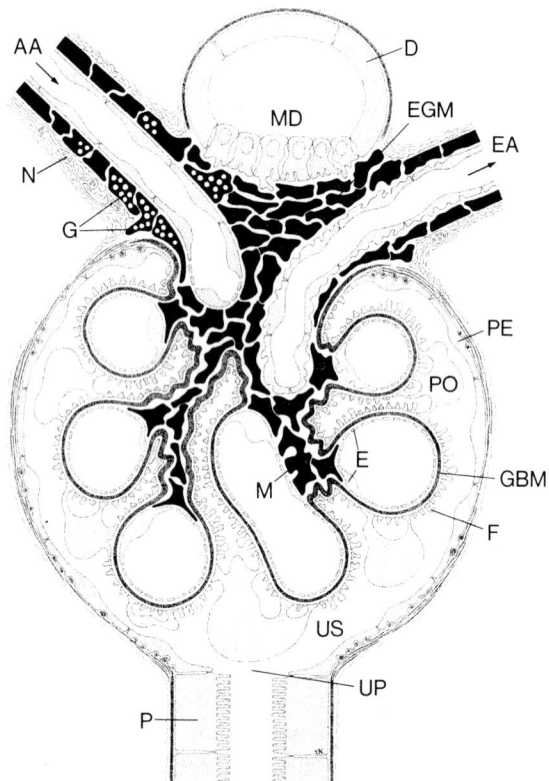

FIGURE 3 Anatomy of the glomerulus and juxtaglomerular apparatus. Schematic diagram of a section of a glomerulus and its juxtaglomerular apparatus. Structures shown are as follows: afferent arteriole (AA), efferent arteriole (EA), macula densa (MD), distal tubule (D), juxtaglomerular granular cell (G), sympathetic nerve endings (N), mesangial cell (M), extraglomerular mesangial cell (EGM), endothelial cell (E), epithelial podocyte (PO), with foot process (F), parietal epithelial cell (PE), glomerular basement membrane (GBM), urinary space (US), urinary pole (UP), and proximal tubule (P).

ulus is a ball of capillaries, consisting of endothelial cells, and surrounded by specialized epithelial cells. Directly adherent to the basement membrane that surrounds the capillary loops is an inner layer of epithelial cells called the *glomerular podocytes*. These are large, highly differentiated cells that form an array of lace-like foot processes over the outer layer of these capillaries. An outer epithelial capsule, called *Bowman's capsule,* acts as a pouch to capture the filtrate and direct it into the beginning of the proximal tubule. As shown in the accompanying figures, the capillaries are held together by a stalk of cells, called the *glomerular mesangium.*

Glomerular Filtration Barrier

Urine formation begins at the glomerular filtration barrier. The glomerular filter through which the ultrafiltrate has to pass consists of three layers: the fenestrated endothelium, the intervening glomerular basement membrane, and the podocyte layer (Fig. 5). This complex "membrane" is freely permeable to water and small dissolved solutes, but retains most of the proteins and other larger molecules, as well as all blood particles. The main determinant of passage through the glomerular filter is molecular size. A molecule like inulin (5 kDa) passes freely through the filter, and even a small protein like myoglobin (16.9 kDa) is filtered to a large extent. Substances of increasing size are retained with increasing efficiency until at a size about 60 to 70 kDa the amount filtered becomes very small. Filtration also depends on ionic charge, and negatively charged proteins, such as albumin, are retained to a greater extent than would be predicted by size alone. In certain glomerular diseases, proteinuria develops because of loss of this charge selectivity.

Ultrafiltration in the Glomerulus

Filtrate formation in the glomerulus is governed by the same forces, often called Starling forces, which determine fluid transport across blood capillaries in general. The glomerular filtration rate (GFR) is equal to the product of the net filtration pressure, the hydraulic permeability, and the filtration area,

$$\text{GFR} = L_\text{p} \times \text{Area} \times P_\text{net},$$

where L_p is the hydraulic permeability, and P_net is the net ultrafiltration pressure. Net ultrafiltration pressure or effective filtration pressure is the difference between the hydrostatic and oncotic pressure difference across the capillary loop,

$$P_\text{net} = \Delta P - \Delta \pi = (P_\text{GC} - P_\text{B}) - \Pi_\text{GC} - \Pi_\text{B}),$$

where P is hydrostatic pressure, Π is oncotic pressure, and the subscripts GC and B refer to the glomerular capillaries and Bowman's space.

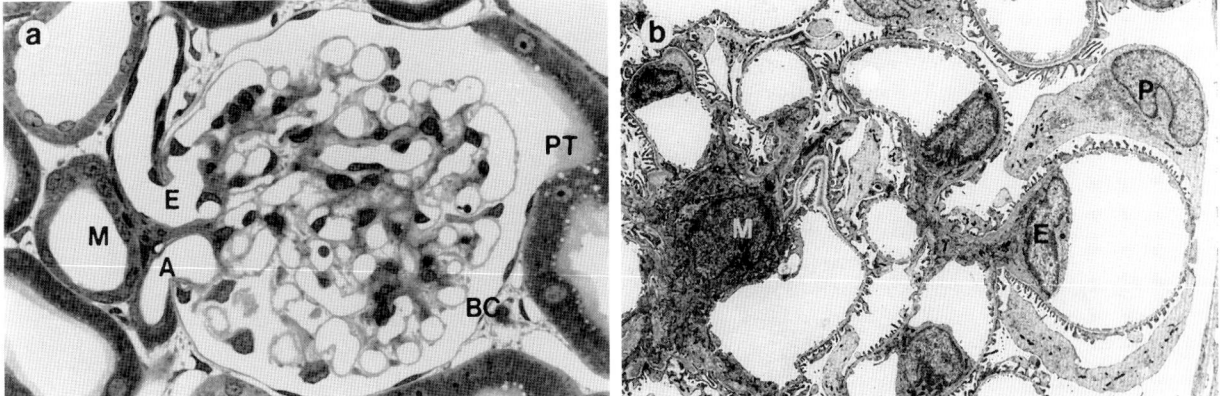

FIGURE 4 Structure of the glomerulus. (a) A light micrograph of a glomerulus, showing the afferent arteriole (A), efferent arteriole (E), macula densa (M), Bowman's capsule (BC), and beginning of the proximal tubule (PT). The typical diameter of a glomerulus is about 100 to 150 μm, which is just barely visible to the naked eye. (b) Higher power view of glomerular capillary loops, showing the epithelial podocyte (P), endothelial cells (E) and mesangial cells (M).

Changes in GFR can result from changes in the permeability/surface area product ($L_p \times$ Area) or from changes in net ultrafiltration pressure. One factor influencing P_{net} is the resistance in the afferent and efferent arterioles. An increase in resistance in the afferent arteriolar (before blood gets to the glomerulus) will *decrease* P_{GC} and GFR. However an increase in resistance as blood exits through the efferent arteriole will tend to *increase* P_{GC} and GFR. Changes in P_{net} can also occur as a result of an increase in renal arterial pressure, which will tend to increase P_{GC} and GFR. Obstruction of the tubule will increase P_B and decrease GFR, and a decrease in plasma protein concentration will tend to increase GFR.

Determination of GFR

GFR is measured by determining the urinary excretion of a marker substance that must fulfill the key requirement that the amount filtered per minute is equal to the amount excreted in the urine per minute. This requirement is met if this substance (1) is neither absorbed nor secreted by the renal tubules, (2) is freely filterable across the glomerular membranes, and (3) is not metabolized or produced by the kidneys. These critical properties are ideally met by *inulin,* a large sugar molecule with a molecular weight of about 5000. Inulin is often infused in experimental studies to measure GFR. An endogenous substance that has similar properties and is used in the clinical setting is creatinine. As shown in Table 3, the formula for GFR derives from a simple rearrangement of the statement indicating that the amount filtered per minute equals the amount excreted per minute. A formula of this general form, called the clearance formula, denotes the volume of plasma (mL/ min) cleared of a particular substance by excretion into the urine—its clearance rate. In the case of inulin, the clearance of inulin is equal to GFR. The clearance of creatinine is slightly greater than GFR (15 to 20%) because the excreted amount exceeds the amount filtered as a result of some tubular secretion of creatinine. GFR is typically about 100 mL/min for women and 120 mL/min for men.

Juxtaglomerular Apparatus

Tightly adherent to every glomerulus, in between the entry and the exit of the arterioles, is a plaque of distal tubular cells called the *macula densa,* which is part of the juxtaglomerular apparatus. This cell plaque is in the distal tubule, at the very terminal end of the thick ascending limb of the loop of Henle, right before the transition to the distal convoluted tubule. This is a special position along the nephron, because at this site NaCl concentration is quite variable. Low rates of flow result in a very low salt concentration at this site, 15 mEq/L or less, while at higher flow rates salt concentration rises to 40 to 60 mEq/L. NaCl concentration at this site regulates glomerular blood flow, through a mechanism called tubuloglomerular feedback; increases in salt concentration cause a decrease in glomerular blood flow.

The other unique cells that make up the juxtaglomerular apparatus are the renin-containing juxtaglomerular granular cells. Renin secretion is also regulated locally by salt concentration in the tubule at the macula densa. In addition, the granular cells have extensive sympathetic innervation, and renin secretion is controlled by the sympathetic nervous system.

TUBULAR FUNCTION: BASIC PRINCIPLES

Absorption and Secretion in the Renal Tubules

The glomerular filtrate undergoes a series of modifications before becoming the final urine. These changes consist of removal or absorption and addition or secretion of sol-

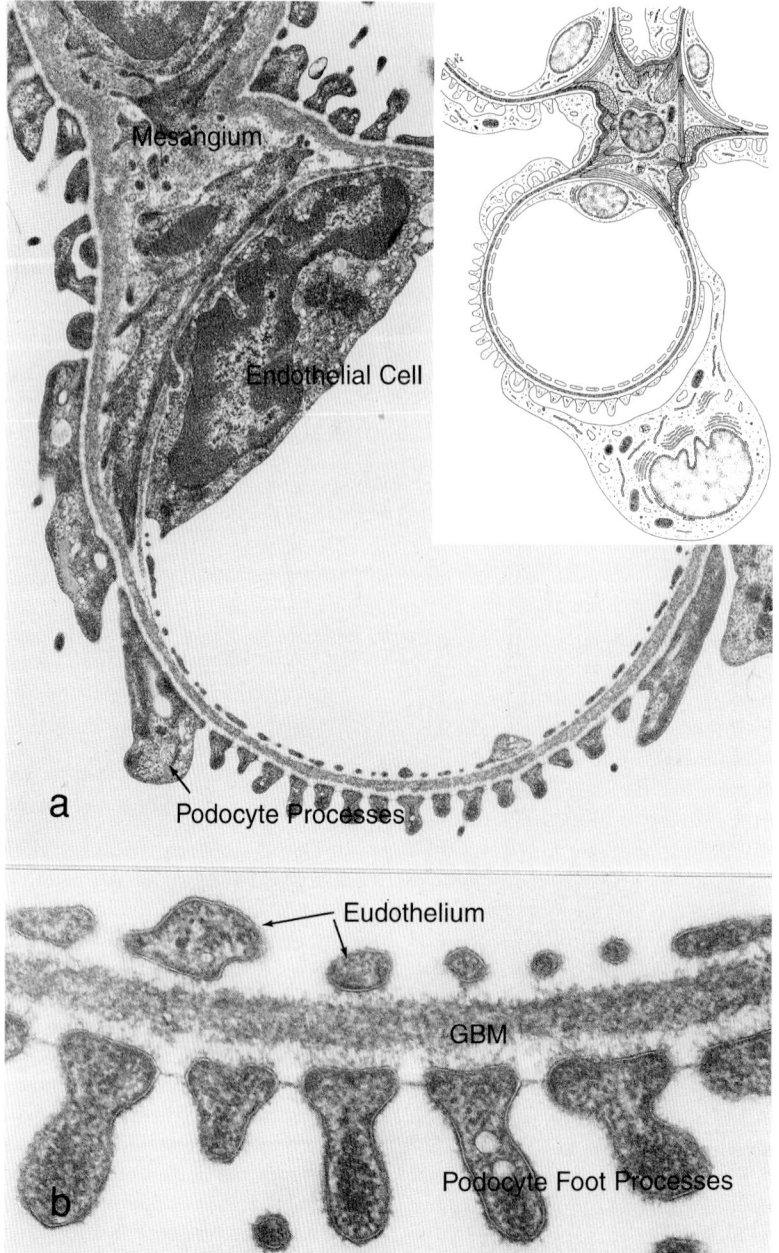

FIGURE 5 Structure of the glomerular capillary loop and the filtration barrier. (a) A single capillary loop showing the endothelial and foot process layers and the attachments of the basement membrane to the mesangium. Pressure in the glomerular capillary bed is substantially higher than in other capillaries. As shown in the diagrammatic insert, the mesangium provides the structural supports which permit these cells to withstand these high pressures. (b) The glomerular filtration barrier.

utes and fluid. absorption and secretion indicate directions of transport, not mechanisms.

1. *Absorption.* Absorption, the movement of solute or water from tubular lumen to blood, is the predominant process in the renal handling of Na^+, Cl^-, H_2O, HCO_3^- glucose, amino acids, protein, PO_4^+, Ca^+, Mg^{2+}, urea, uric acid, and others.

2. *Secretion.* Secretion, the movement of solute from blood or cell interior to tubular lumen, is important in the renal handling of H^+, K^+, NH_4^+, and a number of organic acids and bases.

    Substances can move into or out of the tubule either by the transcellular pathway, which requires traversing the luminal and the basolateral cell membranes, or by the para-

TABLE 3
Derivation of the Formula for GFR

Step 1: Filtered amount of inulin = Excreted amount of inulin
$$(GFR \cdot GFR_{in}) = (U_{in} \cdot V)$$
where   GFR is glomerular filtration rate,
GFR$_{in}$ is the concentration of inulin in the filtrate
U_{in} is the concentration of inulin in urine
V is the urine flow rate

Step 2: Inulin is freely filterable, so its concentrations in plasma and filtrate are identical. Hence
$$\text{Filtered amount of inulin} = GFR \cdot P_{in}$$
where P_{in} is the concentration of inulin in plasma.

Step 3: Rearranging, this produces
$$GFR \cdot P_{in} = U_{in} \cdot V$$
and hence
$$GFR = \frac{U_{in} \times V}{P_{in}}$$

cellular pathway between cells (Fig. 6). Many specialized membrane proteins participate in the movement of substances across cell membranes along the renal tubule. Some of the important membrane transport mechanisms, together with examples of substances that use these mechanisms, and proteins that are important for these processes are given in Table 4.

Segmentation of the Nephron

One of the more striking characteristics of the renal tubule is dramatic cellular heterogeneity. Early renal anatomists recognized that there are marked differences in the appearance of the cells of the proximal tubule, loops of Henle, and distal tubule. These different nephron segments also differ markedly in function, distribution of important transport proteins, and responsiveness to drugs such as diuretics that inhibit transport.

Proximal Tubule

The proximal tubules absorb the bulk of filtered small solutes. These solutes are present in proximal tubular fluid at the same concentration as in plasma. Approximately 60% of the filtered Na$^+$, Cl$^-$, K$^+$, Ca$^+$, and water and more than 90% of the filtered HCO$_3^-$ are absorbed along the proximal tubule. This is also the segment that normally reabsorbs virtually all the filtered glucose and amino acids by Na-dependent cotransport. An additional function of the proximal tubule is phosphate transport, which is regulated by parathyroid hormone. In addition to these reabsorption functions, secretion of solutes also occurs along the proximal tubule. The terminal portion of the proximal tubule, the S3 or pars recta, is the site of secretion of numerous organic anions and cations, a mechanism used by the body for eliminating a number of drugs and toxins. The proximal tubule, as shown in Fig. 7, has a prominent brush border, extensive interdigitated foot basolateral in-

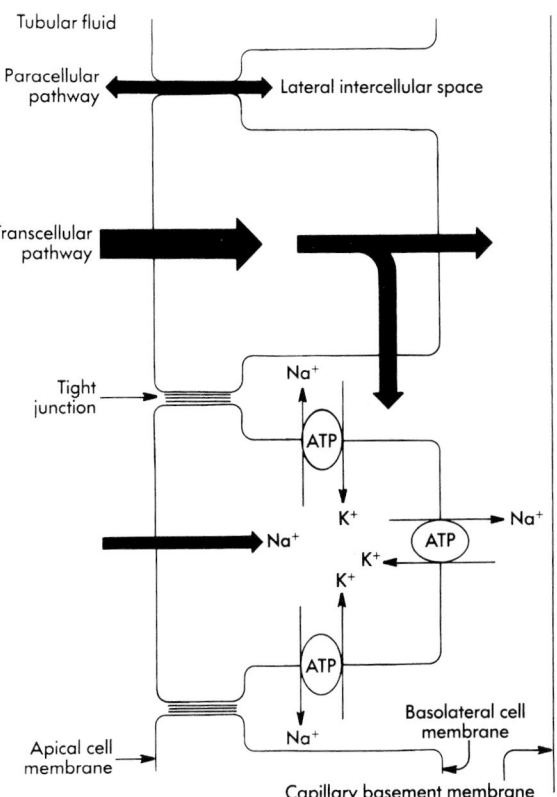

FIGURE 6 General scheme for epithelial transport. The driving force for solute movement is primarily generated by the action of the Na,K-ATPase in the basolateral membrane. Solute and water can move through either a paracellular pathway between cells or a transcellular transport pathway, which requires movement across both luminal and basolateral membranes. From BM Koeppen, BA Stanton, *Renal Physiology,* Mosby, St. Louis, 1992. With permission.

foldings, and large prominent mitochondria, which supply the energy for Na,K = ATPase.

Loop of Henle

The loop of Henle consists of the terminal or straight portion of the proximal tubule, thin descending and ascending limbs, and the thick ascending limb and is important for generation of a concentrated medulla and for dilution of the urine. The thick ascending limb is often called the diluting segment, since transport along this water impermeant segment results in development of a dilute tubular fluid. The thick ascending limb is also a major site of Mg^{2+} reabsorption along the nephron. The principal luminal transporter expressed in this segment is the Na$^+$–K$^+$–2Cl cotransporter, which is the target of diuretics such as furosemide. The morphology of loop of Henle epithelia is illustrated in Fig. 8.

Distal Nephron

The distal nephron, which includes the distal convoluted tubule, the connecting tubule, and the cortical and medul-

TABLE 4
Types of Membrane Transport Mechanisms Used in the Kidney

Mechanism	Examples of substances	Examples of transport protein
Facilitated or carrier mediated	Glucose, urea	GLUT1 carrier, urea carrier
Active transport (pumps)	Na^+, K^+, H^+, Ca^{2+}	Na,K-ATPase, H-ATPase, Ca ATPase
Coupled transport		
Cotransport	Cl^-, glucose, amino acids, formate, phosphate	Na–K–Cl cotransporter
Countertransport	Bicarbonate, H^+	Cl/HCO_3 exchanger, Na/H antiporter
Osmosis	H_2O	Water channels (aquaporins)

lary collecting duct, is the portion of the nephron where final adjustments in urine composition, tonicity, and volume are made. Distal segments are the sites where the most critical regulatory hormones, like aldosterone and vasopressin, regulate acid and potassium excretion and to determine final urinary concentrations of potassium, sodium, and chloride.

Both distal convoluted tubule and connecting tubule have well-developed basolateral infoldings with abundant mitochondria, like the proximal tubule, although they are easily distinguished from proximal tubule by the lack of brush border (Fig. 9). The distal convoluted tubule is the principal site of action of thiazide diuretics.

The collecting duct cells are cuboidal, and their basolateral folds do not interdigitate extensively. When there is a sizable osmotic gradient, and water moves across this epithelium, the spaces between cells become wide. The collecting duct changes in its appearance as it travels from the cortex to the papillary tip (Fig. 10). In the cortex there are two different cell types in the collecting duct: principal cells and intercalated cells. Principal cells are the main site of salt and water transport, and intercalated cells are the

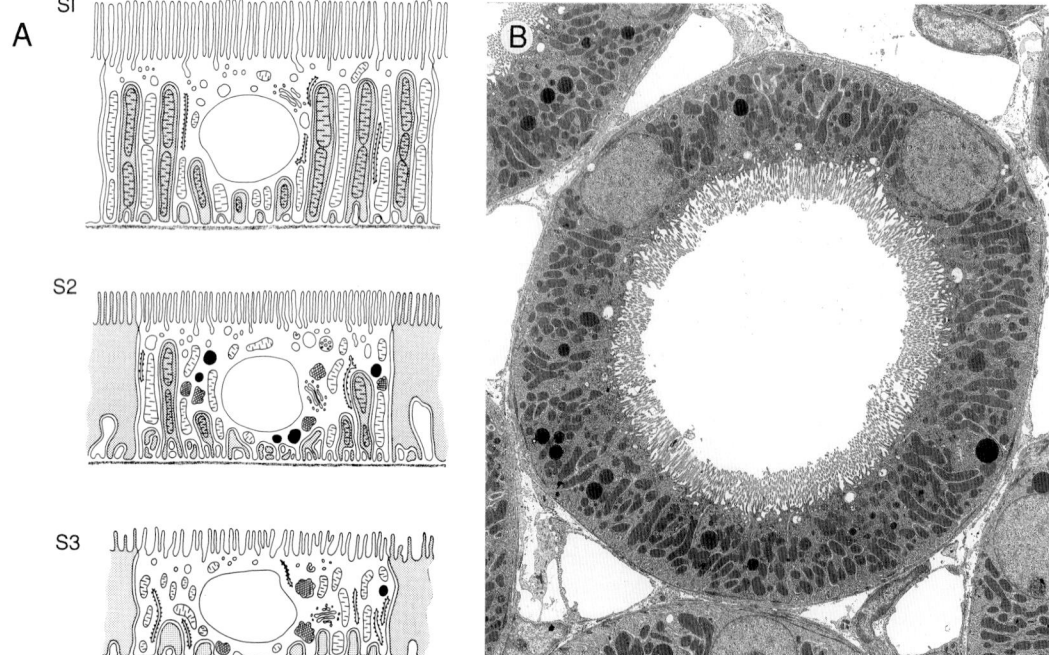

FIGURE 7 Proximal tubule. The proximal tubule consists of three segments: S1, S2, and S3. The left panel shows schematic diagrams of the typical cells from these three segments, the right panel shows a cross section of the S1 segment. The S1 begins at the glomerulus, and extends several millimeters, before the transition to the S2 segment. The S3 segment, which is also called the proximal straight tubule, descends into the renal medulla to the inner medulla. The proximal tubule is characterized by a prominent brush border, which increases the membrane surface area by a factor of about 40-fold. The basolateral infoldings, which are lined with mitochondria, are interdigitated with the basolateral infoldings of adjacent cells (in these diagrams, processes that come from adjacent cells are shaded). These adaptations are most prominent in the first parts of the proximal tubule, and are less well developed later along the proximal tubule.

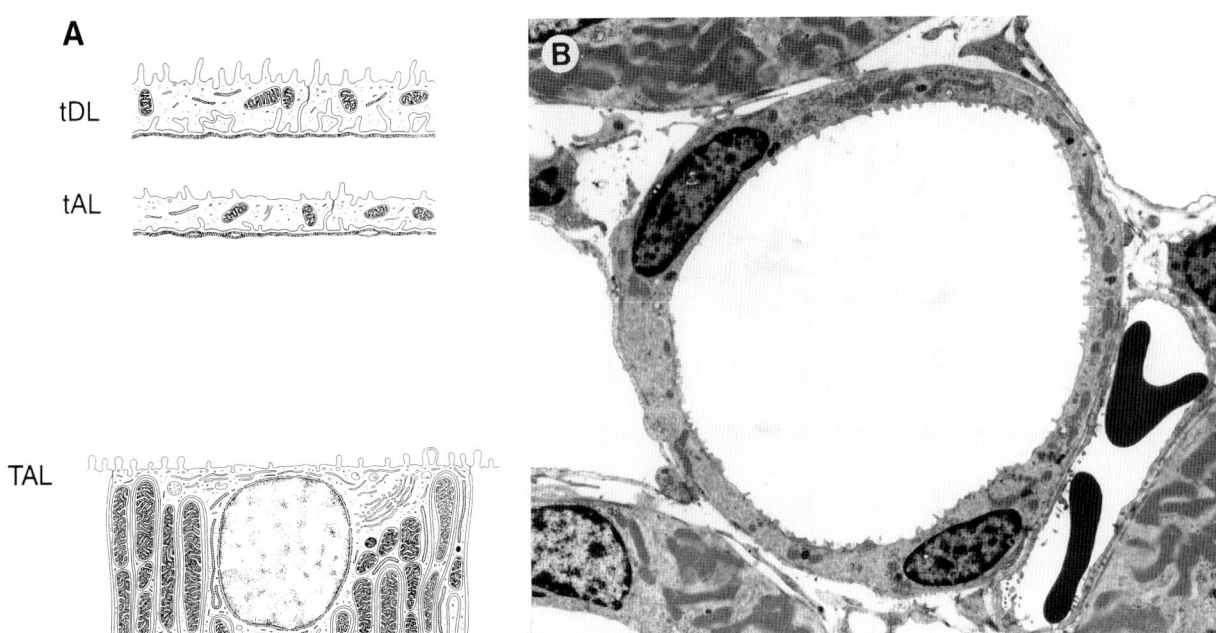

FIGURE 8 Loop of Henle. The loop of Henle makes a hairpin loop into the medulla. Segments included in the loop are terminal portion of the proximal tubule, the thin descending (tDL), and ascending limbs (tAL), as well as the thick ascending limb (TAL). The left panel shows schematic drawings of cell morphology, the right panel shows a cross-section through the thin descending limb in the outer medulla. The thin limbs, as their names suggest, are shallow epithelia without the prominent mitochondria of more proximal segments. The thick limb, in contrast, is a taller epithelium with basolateral infoldings and well-developed mitochondria. This segment is water impermeable, and transport along this segment is important for generation of interstitial solute gradients, and a low salt concentration and dilute fluid in the tubular lumen.

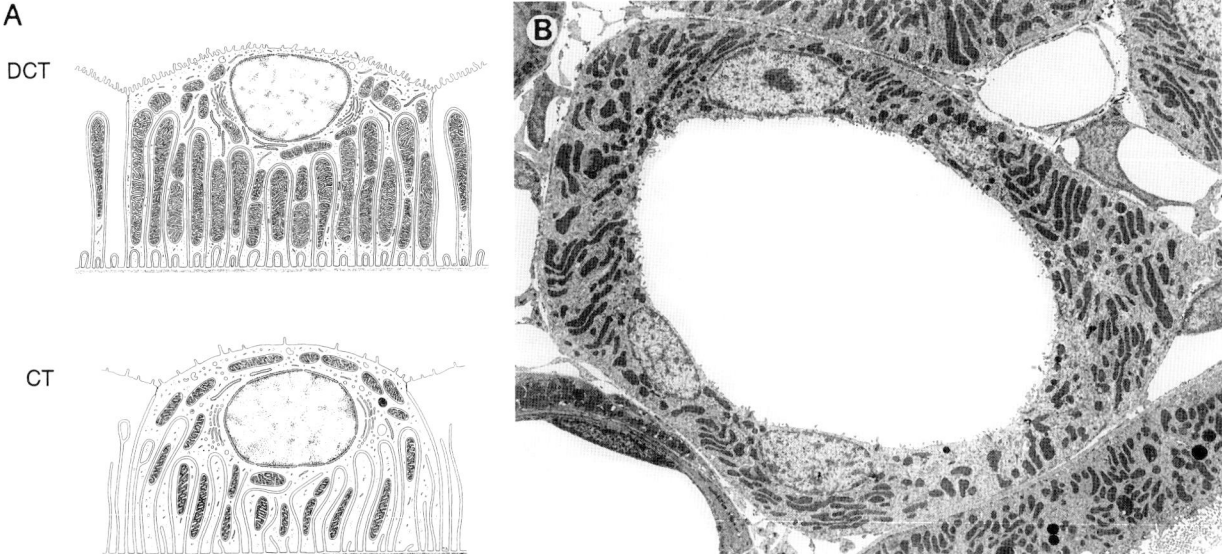

FIGURE 9 Distal convoluted tubule. The distal convoluted tubule is customarily divided into two parts: the true distal convoluted tubule (DCT, shown schematically on the left, and in cross-section on the right) and the connecting tubule (CT), where cell morphology is somewhat more similar to collecting duct.

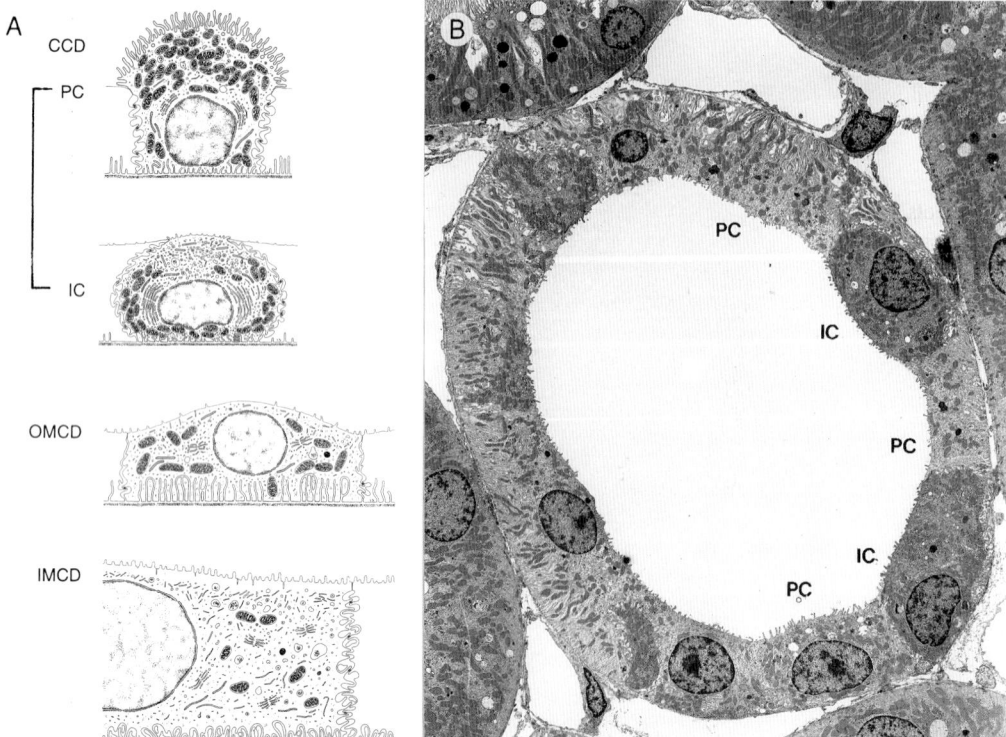

FIGURE 10 Collecting duct. The collecting duct changes its morphology as it travels from cortex to medulla. In the cortex there are two cell types—principal cells (PC) and intercalated cells (IC). Appearance is shown schematically on the left and in a cross-section on the right.

key sites for acid–base regulation. The medullary collecting duct in its most terminal portions comes increasingly to resemble the tall cells typical of transitional epithelium.

SALT AND VOLUME REGULATION

Absorption of Sodium

Because of its high extracellular concentration, large amounts of Na^+ and its accompanying anions are present in the glomerular filtrate, and the absorption of this filtered Na^+ is in a quantitative sense the dominant work performed by the renal tubules. The amount of Na^+ absorbed by the tubules is the difference between the amount of Na^+ filtered and the amount of Na^+ excreted,

$$Na^+ \text{ absorption} = \text{Filtered } Na^+ - Na^+ \text{ Excretion}$$

or

$$Na^+ \text{ absorption} = (GFR \times P_{Na}) - (V \times U_{Na}),$$

where U_{Na} is the urinary Na^+ concentration and P_{Na} is the plasma Na^+ concentration. With a GFR of 120 mL/min and a plasma Na^+ concentration of 145 mEq/L, 17.4 mEq of Na^+ is filtered every minute or about 25,000 mEq or 575 g of Na per day. Since only about 100 to 250 mEq of Na is excreted per day (this reflects the average intake provided by a typical Western diet), or can estimate that the tubule reabsorbs somewhat more than 99% of the fil-

tered Na. The fractional excretion of Na^+ (FE_{Na}) is defined as the fraction of filtered Na^+ excreted in the urine. Using creatinine as a GFR estimate, FE_{Na} is calculated from

$$FE_{Na} = \frac{\text{Excreted Na}}{\text{Filtered Na}} = \frac{U_{Na} \times V}{P_{Na} \times GFR}$$

$$= \frac{U_{Na} \times V}{P_{Na} \times \left(\frac{U_{Cr}}{P_{Cr}}\right) \cdot V} = \frac{U_{Na}/P_{Na}}{U_{Cr}/P_{Cr}}.$$

FE_{Na} is usually less than 1%. However, this value depends on Na intake and can vary physiologically from nearly 0% at extremely low intakes to about 2% at extremely high intakes. FE_{Na} can also exceed 1% in disease states where tubular transport of Na is impaired (for example, in most cases of acute renal failure).

Mechanisms of Na^+ Absorption

Tubular Na^+ absorption is a primary active transport process driven by the enzyme Na,K-ATPase. In renal epithelial cells, as in most cells of the body, this pump translocates Na^+ out of cells (and K^+ into cells) and thereby lowers intracellular Na concentration (and elevates intracellular K^+ concentration). A key for the generation of net Na^+ movement from tubular lumen to blood is the asymmetrical distribution of this enzyme: it is present exclusively in the basolateral membrane (the blood side) of all nephron segments, but not in their luminal membranes. Delivery of Na to the pump sites is maintained by Na entry into the luminal side of the cells along a favorable electrochemical gradient. Since Na permeability of the luminal membrane is much higher than that of the basolateral membrane, Na entry is fed from the luminal Na pool. The asymmetric permeability is due to the presence of a variety of different transport proteins or channels exclusively in the luminal membrane.

A number of these luminal transporters are the target molecules for diuretic action. Principal entry mechanisms for Na^+ and Cl^- in the different nephron segments (and effective diuretics) are:

1. Early proximal: Na^+-dependent cotransporter, Na^+/H^+ exchanger
2. Late proximal: Na^+/H^+ exchanger, Cl^-/anion exchanger
3. Thick ascending limb of the loop of Henle: $Na^+–K^+–2Cl^-$ cotransporter (furosemide-sensitive carrier)
4. Distal convoluted tubule: Na^+/Cl^- cotransporter (thiazide-sensitive carrier)
5. Collecting duct: Na^+ channel (amiloride-sensitive channel)

Regulation of NaCl Excretion

Because Na^+ salts are the most abundant extracellular solutes, the amount of sodium in the body (the total body sodium) determines extracellular fluid volume. Therefore, excretion or retention of Na^+ salts by the kidneys is critical for the regulation of extracellular fluid volume.[1] A disturbance in volume regulation, particularly enhanced salt retention, is common in disease states. The sympathetic, nervous system, the renin–angiotensin–aldosterone system (RAS), atrial natriuretic peptide (ANP), and vasopressin represent the four main regulatory systems that change their activity in response to changes in body fluid volume. These changes in activity mediate the effects of body fluid volume on urinary Na excretion.

Sympathetic Nervous System

A change in extracellular fluid volume is sensed by stretch receptors on blood vessels, principally those located on the low pressure side of the circulation in the thorax, for example, in the vena cava, cardiac atria, and pulmonary vessels. A decreased firing rate in the afferent nerves from these volume receptors enhances sympathetic outflow from cardiovascular medullary centers. Increased renal sympathetic tone enhances renal salt reabsorption and can decrease renal blood flow at higher frequencies. In addition to its direct effects on renal function, increased sympathetic

outflow promotes the activation of another salt retaining system: the RAS.

Renin–Angiotensin System

Renin is an enzyme that is formed by and released from granular cells in the wall of renal afferent arterioles near the entrance to the glomerulus. These granular cells are part of the juxtaglomerular apparatus (see Fig. 3). Renin is an enzyme that cleaves angiotensin I from angiotensinogen, a large circulating protein made principally in the liver. Angiotensin I, a decapeptide, is converted by angiotensin-converting enzyme to the biologically active angiotensin II. Renin is the rate-limiting step in the production of angiotensin II and it is therefore the plasma level of renin that determines plasma angiotensin II. The three principal mechanisms in control of renin release are:

1. *Macula densa mechanism.* Macula densa refers to a group of distinct epithelial cells in the wall of the thick ascending limb of the loop of Henle, where it makes contact with its own glomerulus. At this location, NaCl concentration is between 30 and 40 mEq/L, and it varies as a direct function of tubular fluid flow rate; i.e., it increases when flow rate is high and decreases when flow rate is low. A decrease in NaCl concentration at the macula densa strongly stimulates renin secretion, whereas an increase inhibits it. The connection to the regulation of body fluid volume is the dependence of the flow rate past the macula densa cells upon body Na content: flow. It is high in states of Na excess and low in Na depletion.

2. *Baroreceptor mechanism.* Renin secretion is stimulated by a decrease in arterial pressure, an effect believed to be mediated by a "baroreceptor" in the wall of the afferent arteriole responding to pressure, stretch, or shear stress.

3. *β-adrenergic stimulation.* An increase in renal sympathetic activity or in circulating catecholamines stimulates renin release through β-adrenergic receptors on the juxtaglomerular granular cells.

Angiotensin II has direct and indirect effects to promote salt retention. It enhances Na^+ reabsorption in the proximal tubule (stimulation of Na/H exchange) and, because it is a potent renal vasoconstrictor, it may reduce GFR by reducing glomerular capillary pressure or plasma flow. Angiotensin II affects salt balance indirectly by stimulating the production and release of the steroid hormone aldosterone from the zona glomerulosa of the adrenal gland. Aldosterone acts on the collecting duct to augment salt reabsorption (and K^+ secretion).

Atrial Natriuretic Factor

Atrial natriuretic factor (ANF) is a peptide hormone that is synthesized by atrial myocytes and released in response to increased atrial distension. Thus, ANF secretion is increased in volume expansion and inhibited in volume depletion. The main cause of the ANF-induced natriuresis is an inhibition of Na^+ reabsorption along the collecting duct, but an increase in GFR may sometimes play a contributory role.

---

[1] Plasma Na concentration does not correlate at all with total body sodium or the fullness of the extracellular fluid spaces. In fact, a low serum Na can be observed in states in which there is either excess total body sodium or deficiency of total body sodium. However, plasma Na concentration is the principal determinant of extracellular fluid osmolarity. In general, abnormalities in Na concentration arise from defects in tonicity regulation, not volume regulation.

Vasopressin or Antidiuretic Hormone (ADH)

Vasopressin is regulated primarily by body fluid osmolarity. However, in states in which intravascular volume is depleted, the set point for vasopressin release is shifted, so that for any given plasma osmolarity, vasopressin levels are higher than they would be normally. This shift promotes water retention to aid in restoration of body fluid volumes.

WATER AND OSMOREGULATION

Regulation of Body Fluid Osmolarity

When water intake is low or water is lost from the body (in hypotonic fluids such as sweat, for example), the kidneys conserve water by producing a small volume of concentrated urine. In dehydration, urine production is less than a liter per day (less than 0.5 mL/min) and the osmotic concentration may reach 1200 mOsm/kg H_2O. When water intake is high, urine flow may increase to as much as 14 L/day (10 mL/min) with an osmolality substantially lower than that of plasma (75 to 100 mOsm/kg). These wide variations in urine volume and osmotic concentration do not obligatorily affect the excretion of the daily solute load. Thus, the daily solute excess of about 1200 mOsm/day may be excreted in 12 L of urine (with a U_{osm} of 100 mOsm/L) or in 1 L (with a U_{osm} of 1200 mOsm/L). The hormone responsible for the regulatory changes in urine volume and tonicity is ADH (synonym: vasopressin).

Role of ADH in Osmolarity Regulation

ADH is a nine-amino-acid peptide produced by neurons located in the supraoptic and pareventricular nuclei of the hypothalamus. It is stored in and released from granules in nerve terminals that are located in the posterior pituitary (neurohypophysis). The release of ADH is exquisitely sensitive to changes in plasma osmolarity, with increases in P_{osm} above a threshold of about 285 mOsm/kg leading to increases in ADH secretion and plasma ADH concentrations. As has been pointed out, the actual set point for release depends on body fluid volume as well.

The most important function of ADH is the regulation of water permeability of the distal portions of the nephron, particularly the collecting duct. As shown schematically in Fig. 11, ADH binds to receptors (R) in the basolateral membrane of collecting duct cells. This activates adenylate cyclase (AC) to form cAMP. cAMP activates a protein kinase, which leads to the phosphorylation of undefined proteins. This phosphorylation causes membrane fusion of vesicles that contain preformed water channels. The result is an up to 20-fold increase in water permeability of the apical (luminal) membrane of collecting duct cells. Upon removal of ADH, water channels are rapidly removed from the apical membrane by endocytosis.

Tubular Water Absorption

At each point along the nephron, the osmotic pressure of the tubular fluid is lower than that in the interstitial space. This transtubular osmotic pressure difference provides the

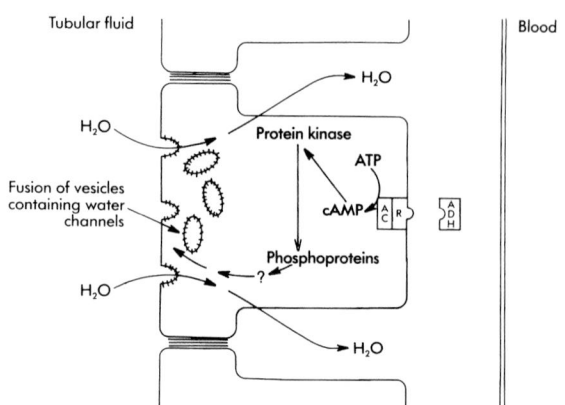

FIGURE 11 Mechanism of action of ADH on the collecting duct. ADH combines with a basolateral receptor (R) which is coupled to adenyl cyclase (AC). Generation of cyclic AMP leads to activation of protein kinase A, and phosphorylation of target proteins. Preformed water channels contained in vesicles located under the luminal membrane are inserted into the luminal membrane, resulting in a tenfold increase in its water permeability. From BM Koeppen, BA Stanton, *Renal Physiology,* Mosby, St. Louis, 1992. With permission.

driving force for tubular water reabsorption. The rate of fluid absorption in a given nephron segment is determined by the magnitude of this gradient and the osmotic water permeability of the segment. Even though the osmotic pressure difference across the proximal tubule epithelium is very small (3 to 4 mOsm/L), the rate of fluid absorption is very high because this segment has a very high water permeability. In contrast, osmotic gradients across the thick ascending limb may be as high as 250 mOsm/L, and yet virtually no water flows across this segment because it is highly water impermeable. This segment dilutes the urine because it absorbs Na^+ and Cl^- without water.

In contrast to the invariability of water conductivity in the proximal tubule and the thick ascending limb, water permeability in the collecting duct can be altered under the influence of ADH. If ADH is absent, water permeability and water absorption are low, and the hypotonicity generated in the thick ascending limb persists along the collecting duct. As a consequence, a dilute urine is excreted. If ADH is present, the collecting duct becomes quite water permeable, and water is reabsorbed until the tubular fluid in the collecting duct equilibrates with the hypertonic interstitium. The final urine in this case is osmotically concentrated and has a low volume.

Medullary Hypertonicity

To allow osmotically driven water absorption, the osmotic concentration in the medullary interstitium must be slightly higher than that in the collecting duct lumen. Thus, when a final urine with an osmolarity of 1200 mOsm/kg is excreted, the medullary interstitium at the tips of the papillae must be a little higher than 1200 mOsm/kg. The generation of such a unique extracellular environment is achieved by a countercurrent multiplication system that exists in the renal medulla in the form of the countercurrent arrangement of descending and ascending limbs of the loops of Henle.

Countercurrent Multiplication

In two adjacent tubes with flow in opposite directions, the fluid can attain an osmotic concentration difference in the system's longitudinal axis that can by far exceed that seen at each level along it. This principle of countercurrent multiplication requires energy expenditure and the presence of unique differences in membrane characteristics between the two limbs of the system.

The countercurrent multiplier represented by the loops of Henle is believed to generate an osmotic gradient because:

1. Active NaCl transport across the ascending limb (the so-called single effect of the countercurrent system) generates an osmotic difference between tubular fluid and surrounding local interstitium.
2. A low water permeability of the ascending limb prevents dissipation of this gradient.
3. A high water permeability of the descending limb permits equilibration of descending limb contents with the surrounding local interstitium.

How such a system can result in progressive increases in osmotic concentration along the corticopapillary axis is shown in Fig. 12. In Step 1 (time zero), the fluid in the descending and ascending limbs and the interstitium is isoosmotic to plasma. In Step 2, NaCl is absorbed from the ascending limb into the interstitium until a gradient of 200 mOsm/kg is reached. In Step 3, the fluid in the descending limb equilibrates osmotically with the interstitium by water movement out of the tubule. In Step 4, the hypertonic fluid is presented to the TAL with an increased solute concentration in the region near the tip of the system. Again active NaCl transport along the ascending limb establishes a 200 mOsm/kg gradient increasing interstitial concentrations and by water abstraction descending limb contents. Note that concentrations near the tip begin to be higher than those near the base. Continued operation of such a mechanism will gradually result in generation of a gradient of hypertonicity, with the highest osmolarities at the papillary tip.

The tubular fluid leaving the ascending limb of the loop of Henle countercurrent multiplier is hypotonic. However, the medullary interstitium has been osmotically "charged." Since the collecting ducts on their way to the papillary tip return into the hypertonic medullary environment, their content can now be concentrated by water flow along an osmotic gradient.

Role of Urea in the Countercurrent Mechanism

In addition to Na^+ and Cl^-, urea is the other major solute present in the renal medulla in an osmotically concentrated form. Urea enters the medulla by reabsorption across the collecting duct. Marked differences in the permeability to urea allow reabsorption to proceed only across the terminal portions of the medullary collecting duct. In the early por-

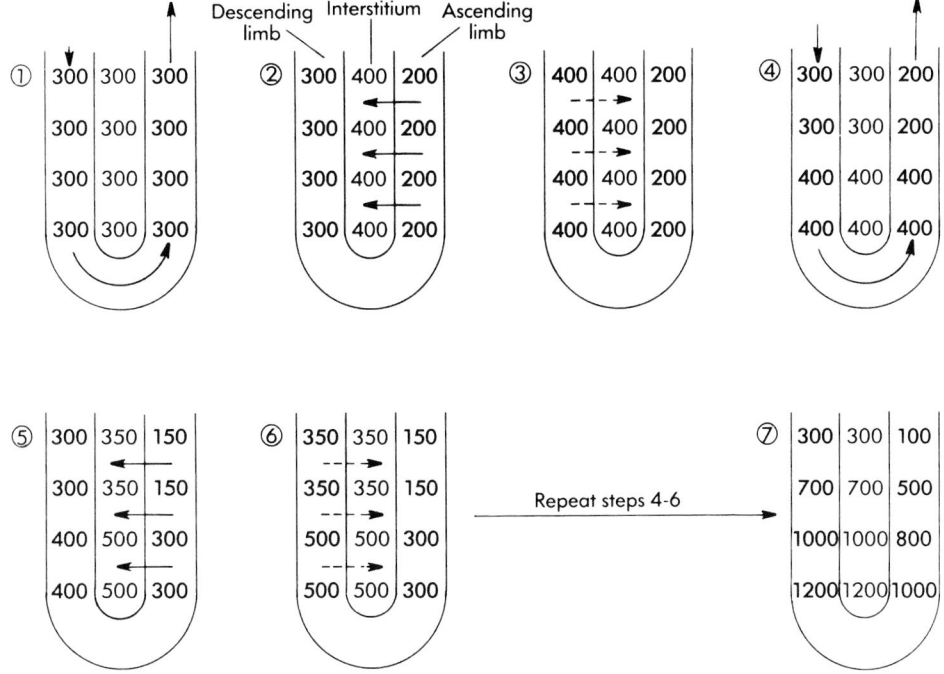

FIGURE 12 The process of countercurrent multiplication. See text for details. From BM Koeppen, BA Stanton, *Renal Physiology*, Mosby, St. Louis, 1992. With permission.

tions of the collecting duct, urea permeability is low and reabsorption of urea cannot occur. Since water leaves the tubule under the influence of ADH, the urea staying behind is progressively concentrated. As a consequence, a substantial urea gradient develops, providing the driving force for urea reabsorption when the permeability to urea permits it. The contribution of urea accumulation to osmotic water absorption along the inner medullary collecting duct must be sizable since about half of inner medullary tonicity is accounted for by urea. Therefore, a reduction in urea synthesis by reducing protein intake markedly impairs the concentrating ability of the kidneys.

Comparison between Volume Regulation and Osmoregulation

Osmoregulation is under control of a single hormonal system, ADH, whereas volume regulation is under control of a set of redundant and overlapping control mechanisms. Lack or excess of ADH results in defined and rather dramatic clinical syndromes of excess water loss or water retention. In contrast, a defect in a single volume regulatory mechanism generally results in more subtle abnormalities, because of the redundant regulatory capacity from the other mechanisms. Thus, excess aldosterone results in a mild volume retention followed by "escape" and return to normal Na^+ excretion, due to the action of the other mechanisms. Similarly, excess ANF probably produces only a modest decrement in volume, with no persistent abnormality in Na^+ excretion. Severe salt-retaining states, such as liver cirrhosis and congestive heart failure, are characterized by activation of all the volume regulatory mechanisms. Finally, the symptoms characteristic of disorders of osmoregulation and of volume regulation are different, with hypo- and hypernatremia being the hallmark of deranged osmoregulation, and edema or hypovolemia resulting from deranged volume regulation.

REGULATION OF BODY FLUID POTASSIUM AND ACIDITY

Both potassium and hydrogen ions are present in body fluids at low concentrations, about 4 to 4.5 mEq/L for K^+ and about 40 nEq/L for H^+. Both ions show a number of features:

1. Relatively small deviations in either K^+ or H^+ concentrations can be life threatening, and therefore the regulation of K^+ and H^+ concentration requires control systems with high sensitivity and precision.
2. Constancy of both K^+ and H^+ ion concentration over the long term is achieved by regulated excretion of these ions in the urine. However, in both cases, other mechanisms exist that provide immediate protection against excessive deviations of plasma concentrations from normal.
3. Regulation in the renal excretion of both K^+ and H^+ is caused to a large extent by variation in the secretion of these ions by collecting ducts. The principal cell of the collecting duct is the cell type responsible for regulated K^+

secretion; the intercalated cell is the cell type responsible for H^+ secretion (see Fig. 10).
4. The rate of both K^+ and H^+ secretion is increased by aldosterone.
5. A primary derangement of K^+ balance can cause an acidity disturbance and a primary acidity disturbance can derange K^+ homeostasis.

Regulation of Body Fluid Potassium

Distribution of Body K^+

Due to the presence of Na,K-ATPase in virtually all cell membranes, K^+ is mostly in the intracellular space. Of the 3500 mEq of body potassium, only about 1 to 2% is present in the extracellular space, where it has a concentration of 4 to 5 mEq/L. The remainder (about 98%) is stored in cells.

The distribution has the potential risk in that the release of even a small amount of K^+ from intracellular stores can elevate plasma K^+ concentration substantially (for example, in insulin deficiency, cell lysis, severe exercise). On the other hand, the distribution of K^+ between the extracellular and intracellular space is utilized as a means to buffer acute changes in plasma K^+ concentrations. For example, the administration of an acute oral K^+ load induces much smaller changes in plasma K^+ concentration than would occur if all absorbed K^+ were to remain in the extracellular space. K^+ ions are shifted into cells under the stimulatory influence of insulin and epinephrine. The effect of both hormones reflects mainly an activation of the Na,K-ATPase. Another important factor determining K^+ distribution is plasma H^+ concentration. An increase in H^+ ions causes uptake of H^+ into cells and intracellular buffering and this uptake to some extent occurs in exchange for K^+. Thus, acidosis will tend to increase plasma K^+, and alkalosis will tend to decrease it.

Renal Handling of K^+

K^+ homeostasis in the long term requires the excretion of an amount equivalent to the daily K^+ intake (50 to 150 mEq). This represents a fractional K^+ excretion (FE_{K+}) of about 10%, much higher than FE_{Na}^+. About 60 to 70% of filtered K^+ is absorbed along the proximal tubule and further reabsorption of K^+ takes place in the thick ascending limb of the loop of Henle, so that only about 10% of filtered K^+ enters the distal tubule. Along the collecting duct, K^+ is both secreted and absorbed. Collecting duct K^+ secretion increases when dietary K^+ intake is elevated. On the other hand, when intake is low, collecting duct K^+ secretion virtually ceases and absorption is dominant. Thus, while K^+ absorption along the proximal tubule and the loop of Henle does not change very much depending on intake, collecting duct K secretion is variable, and this variability accounts almost completely for the variation in urinary K^+ excretion.

Mechanisms of K^+ Secretion

K^+ secretion across the collecting duct epithelium utilizes the transcellular route. K^+ uptake across the basolateral membrane is driven by Na,K-ATPase, which elevates intracellular K^+ concentration to a level above electrochemical equilibrium. K^+ can then move along a favorable gradient from cell interior to tubule lumen utilizing potassium channels in the luminal membrane.

Three major variables determine the rate at which K^+ is secreted by collecting duct cells:

1. Changes in the activity of Na,K-ATPase affect uptake and thereby intracellular K^+ concentration. An increase in pump activity will increase intracellular K^+ levels and will tend to stimulate K^+ secretion.

2. Changes in the electrochemical gradient affect the driving force for K^+ movement across the luminal membrane. Both an increase in intracellular K^+ concentration and in the lumen negative transepithelial potential difference will increase the driving force and will tend to increase K^+ secretion.

3. Changes in the permeability of the luminal membrane determine the amount of K^+ that can be secreted for a given driving force. Thus, an increase in luminal K^+ conductance will increase K^+ secretion.

Regulation of K^+ Excretion

1. *Plasma K^+ concentration.* One important determinant of K^+ excretion is plasma K^+ concentration. For example, the change in K^+ excretion following a change in dietary K^+ intake is mediated by an increase in plasma K^+. The effect of plasma K^+ on secretion is induced partly by a direct effect on intracellular K^+ concentration.

2. *Aldosterone.* At any level of plasma K^+, K^+ secretion will also depend upon plasma aldosterone levels. Aldosterone enhances K^+ secretion by activation of Na,K-ATPase and by an increase in K^+ permeability of the luminal membrane. Aldosterone is partly responsible for the diet-induced increase in K^+ excretion since its production and secretion are directly stimulated by plasma K^+ concentration. This effect is independent of angiotensin.

3. *Tubular flow rate.* An increase in tubular flow rate past the K^+-secreting cells stimulates, and a decrease reduces, K^+ secretion. This effect is the consequence of flow-dependent changes in the K^+ gradient across the apical membrane. K^+ secretion causes an increase in K^+ concentration in the tubular fluid, which eventually decreases the K^+ gradient and the rate of K^+ secretion. An increase in flow diminishes the rate of rise of luminal K^+ concentration so that a more favorable K^+ gradient for K^+ secretion is maintained.

4. *Distal sodium delivery.* When more Na^+ is delivered to the distal nephron, if reabsorption increases, the net electrical charge in the lumen will become more negative. This favorable electrochemical gradient will tend to increase urinary K^+ secretion.

5. *Hydrogen ions.* A decrease in H^+ ion concentration in alkalotic states causes a stimulation of K^+ secretion. This effect is mediated by the rise in intracellular K^+ concentration that occurs in alkalosis.

Diuretics and K^+ Excretion

Diuretics increase tubular flow rate. Agents such as loop diuretics and thiazides that inhibit NaCl and water absorp-tion in segments prior to the collecting duct (in the loop of Henle and in the distal tubule respectively) increase the flow of fluid past the collecting duct cells which causes increased K^+ secretion. In addition, the diuretics cause volume depletion, which stimulates aldosterone secretion.

Regulation of Body Fluid Acidity

Basic Considerations

Maintenance of the extracellular pH around 7.4 depends on the operation of buffer systems that accept H^+ when it is produced and liberate H^+ when it is consumed. The state of the demand on total body buffering can be determined by assessing the behavior of the HCO_3/CO_2 system, which is the major extracellular buffer. The law of mass action for this buffer system states that

$$pH = 6.1 + \log \frac{[HCO_3]}{[CO_2]}$$

Since $[CO_2]$ equals the solubility coefficient times the P_{CO2}, this can be rewritten

$$pH = 6.1 + \log \frac{[HCO_3^-]}{0.03 \times P_{CO_2}}$$

This, the familiar Henderson-Hasselbach equation tells us that pH constancy depends on a constant ratio in the concentration between the two buffer components. If this ratio increases because either HCO_3^- increases or CO_2 decreases, pH will increase (alkalosis). If the ratio decreases, because either HCO_3^- decreases or CO_2 increases, pH decreases (acidosis). Regulation of HCO_3^- is mainly a function of the kidneys, and regulation of CO_2 is a respiratory function.

The regulation of HCO_3^- concentration by the kidneys consists of two main components:

1. *Absorption of HCO_3^-.* Because of the high GFR and because plasma HCO_3^- concentrations are also relatively high (24 mEq/L), large amounts of HCO_3^- are filtered. Retrieval of this filtered HCO_3^- is absolutely essential for acid-base balance. It is important to note that this process of renal HCO_3^- absorption does not add new HCO_3^- to the blood, but merely prevents a loss of filtered HCO_3^- into the urine. Therefore, renal HCO_3^- absorption cannot correct an existing metabolic acidosis.

2. *Excretion of H^+ ions.* Under normal dietary conditions, approximately 40 to 80 mmol H^+ ions are generated daily (mostly sulfuric acid from the metabolism of sulfur-containing amino acids). These H^+ ions are buffered and therefore consume HCO_3^-. The kidneys must excrete these H^+ ions to regenerate the HCO_3^- pool (this second task can therefore also be labeled as generation of "new" HCO_3^-).

Mechanisms of Bicarbonate Absorption

Filtered HCO_3^- (about 4300 mEq/day) is efficiently absorbed by renal tubules, predominantly the proximal tubules, so that under normal acid-base conditions very little HCO_3 is found in the urine. As a rule, all tubular HCO_3^- absorption is the consequence of H^+ ion secretion, and not of direct absorption of HCO_3^- ions. H^+ ions are continuously generated inside the cells from the dissociation of H_2O (or by CO_2 reacting with H_2O) and transported into the lumen. In the lumen, secreted H^+ ions combine with filtered HCO_3^- to form carbonic acid, which is broken down to CO_2 and H_2O in a reaction that is catalyzed by a carbonic anhydrase located in the apical brush border membrane. CO_2 and H_2O are then absorbed passively. The OH- ions which are generated in the cell during this process combine with CO_2 to form HCO_3^-, a reaction catalyzed by a cytosolic carbonic anhydrase. HCO_3^- exits across the basolateral side of the cell and returns to the blood in association with Na^+. The net balance of this process can be expressed as

$$H_2O + CO_2 \leftarrow H_2CO_3 \leftarrow HCO_3^- + \overset{|}{H^+} \leftarrow H_2O \rightarrow OH^- + CO_2 \rightarrow \overset{|}{H}CO_3^- + Na^+$$

(tubular lumen)   (cell interior)   (blood)

Specific transport proteins in renal epithelial cells cause the H^+ and HCO_3^- to move in the right directions. Two different mechanisms, both located in the apical membrane, are responsible for the movement of protons into the tubular fluid:

1. The first is a Na^+/H^+ exchanger that is driven by the Na^+ gradient and is found in the proximal tubule. In terms of mEq transported, it contributes most to HCO_3^- absorption.

2. The second is a primary active transport of H^+ ions. An H^+-ATPase has been found in the luminal membrane of one class of intercalated collecting duct cells. There is also some evidence for the presence of an H,K-ATPase similar to that found in parietal cells of the gastric mucosa. Active H^+ ion transport is responsible for the secretion of smaller amounts of H^+ than Na^+/H^+ exchange, but it can proceed against a steeper gradient.

There are also at least two mechanisms for the transport of HCO_3^- across the basolateral membrane. The movement of HCO_3^- can be coupled to the movement of Na ions and this is the major exit mechanism in the proximal tubule. In the collecting duct, HCO_3^- exit occurs predominantly through a basolateral Cl/HCO_3 exchanger (equivalent to the band 3 protein of red cells).

Bicarbonate Secretion

While net HCO_3^- transport for the whole kidney is always in the reabsorptive direction, certain intercalated cells in the cortical portion of the collecting duct can actually secrete HCO_3^-. The HCO_3^--secreting cells have a polarity that is the reverse of the H^+-secreting cells; i.e., they possess a basolateral H^+-ATPase and probably a luminal Cl/HCO_3 exchanger. HCO_3^- secretion may be important during consumption of a diet providing base equivalents and for the correction of metabolic alkalosis.

Excretion of H^+ Ions (Formation of New HCO_3^-)

Urinary acid excretion cannot to any significant extent occur as free H^+ ions. The absolute minimum urinary pH in humans is about 4.5, corresponding to an H^+ concentra-

tion of only 0.03 mEq/L. Since about 40 to 80 mEq of H^+ must be excreted per day, it is clear that most H^+ ions must be excreted in a bound or buffered form. Excretion of bound H^+ is achieved by: (1) the titration of luminal nonbicarbonate buffers and (2) by the renal synthesis and excretion of ammonium ions.

Titratable Acidity

Binding of secreted H^+ ions to filtered nonbicarbonate buffer anions leads to the formation and excretion of urinary titratable acidity (titratable acidity is defined as the number of moles NaOH that has to be added to bring urine pH back to 7.4). The ability to buffer H^+ ions depends on its dissociation constant (pK) and the quantity of buffer. Under normal conditions only the $HPO_4^{-2}/H_2PO_4^-$ buffer is present in amounts sufficient to act as intratubular H^+ acceptor. This buffer pair has a pK of 6.8 and is excreted at a daily rate of about 50 mmol. Using the Henderson-Hasselbach equation for the phosphate buffer (pH 6.8 + log $[HPO_4^{-2}]/[H_2PO_4^-]$) the following relations can be calculated (considering only that fraction of total PO_4^- that is actually excreted, about 25 to 30% of the filtered PO_4 load):

	pH	HPO_4^{-2} (mmol/day)	$H_2PO_4^-$ (mmol/day)	H^+ buffered (mmol/day)
Filtrate	7.4	40	10	0
End proximal	6.8	25	25	15
Urine	4.8	0.5	49.5	39.5

This table shows that the buffer capacity of HPO_4^{-2} can be fully utilized if the intratubular pH is lowered sufficiently. In some situations other urinary buffers become important. In diabetic ketoacidosis large amounts of β-hydroxybutyrate are excreted (e.g., 300 mmol/L). Even though this buffer has a pK of 4.8 it will carry up to 150 mmol H^+ ions per liter.

Ammonium Excretion

The second form of bound H^+ ions in the urine is ammonium. The excretion of NH_4^+ is equivalent to the generation of HCO_3^- or excretion of H^+. Glutamine, formed in the liver from glutamate and extracted from the blood by uptake mechanisms in the luminal and basolateral membranes of renal proximal tubule cells, is the major source of urinary ammonium. Ammonium is generated in the proximal tubule by a metabolic pathway in which the degradation of glutamine to glutamate and further to α-ketoglutarate yields 2 NH_4^+ ions and 2 HCO_3^- ions (rather than NH_3, CO_2, and H_2O). While the NH_4^+ ions are secreted through distinct transport pathways into the lumen of the proximal tubule, the new HCO_3^- ions are added to the blood HCO_3^- pool.

It is essential that the NH_4^+ that is formed by renal proximal tubules is preferentially secreted into the tubular lumen and then excreted in the urine. If the generated NH_4^+ was absorbed by the renal tubular epithelium (or secreted preferentially into the blood), it would be used to form urea. Ureagenesis forms H^+ ions which would consume the produced HCO_3^- and thereby negate net base production. This is shown in the following reactions:

$$2NH_4 + 2CO_2 \rightarrow urea + H_2O + 2H^+$$

or

$$2NH_4 + 2HCO_3^- \rightarrow urea + CO_2 + 3H_2O$$
$$(urea: H_2NCONH_2).$$

Urinary H^+ excretion in the form of NH_4^+ is on the order of 40 to 50 mmol/day. Renal NH_4 formation and excretion are greatly enhanced in metabolic acidosis. Failure of proximal tubules to generate NH_4 is the main reason that chronic renal failure leads to metabolic acidosis.

Regulation of H^+ Ion Secretion

1. *Intracellular pH.* Systemic pH changes, whether caused by changes in plasma HCO_3^- (metabolic) or by changes in P_{CO_2} (respiratory), alter H^+ secretion (and therefore HCO_3^- absorption). Intracellular acidification, as occurs in acidosis, stimulates H^+ secretion and intracellular alkalinization (alkalosis) inhibits it.

2. *Aldosterone.* In addition to affecting $Na+$ absorption and K^+ secretion, aldosterone stimulates H^+ secretion by collecting ducts.

3. *Potassium.* Changes in plasma K^+ concentration can affect H^+ secretion, in part by changing intracellular pH. Thus, hypokalemia increases intracellular acidity and stimulates H^+ ion secretion. While the effect of hypokalemia alone is relatively small, a marked stimulation of H^+ secretion results when hypokalemia occurs with high plasma aldosterone levels. In this situation, which can occur in primary hyperaldosteronism or with administration of diuretics, metabolic alkalosis may be generated by the kidneys.

RENAL HANDLING OF GLUCOSE AND AMINO ACIDS

An important function of the renal tubule is retrieval of the glucose and amino acids that are present in glomerular filtrate and which would be lost to the body if they were not reabsorbed. To a large extent, this is a proximal tubule function, and disordered glucose and amino acid transport is characteristic of diseases that disturb proximal tubular function.

Glucose transport by the proximal tubule occurs via a transport protein present in the luminal membrane that carries a glucose molecule together with a sodium ion, the glucose–sodium cotransporter. This transporter uses the sodium concentration gradient (sodium concentration is, of course, higher outside the cell than in) to drive the movement of glucose into the cell. Glucose then diffuses out of the cell across the basolateral membrane, a process facilitated by a second carrier protein. The resulting reabsorption process is highly efficient, and in normal circumstances practically all the filtered glucose is removed from the proximal tubule fluid and glucose is virtually absent from urine.

When plasma glucose concentration rises, increasing amounts of glucose are filtered, and at a certain point the filtered load of glucose exceeds the capacity of the proximal

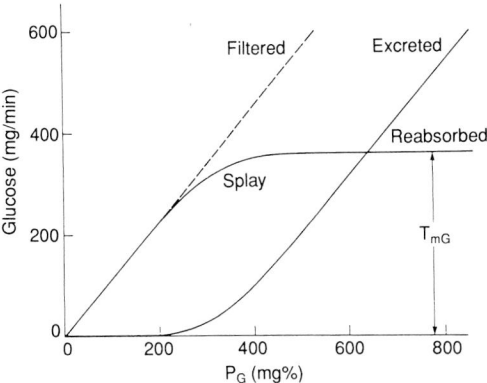

FIGURE 13 Glucose reabsorption. Shown is a typical titration curve for renal glucose reabsorption. At plasma glucose concentrations less than approximately 200 mg%, the filtered glucose is completely reabsorbed, and no glucose is excreted in the urine. When plasma glucose exceeds this level, the filtered load of glucose exceeds the transport capacity of the tubule, and glucose apears in the urine.

transport mechanisms. This maximum reabsorption rate is called the tubular transport maximum for glucose (T_{mG}; Fig. 13). When glucose delivery exceeds the T_{mG}, the excess glucose is excreted in the urine.

Many of the same principles apply to the reabsorption of amino acids. Also a function of the proximal tubule, amino acid absorption is also highly effective. For most amino acids, less than 1% of the amount filtered escapes into the urine. A number of different luminal and basolateral transport proteins are needed to remove the amino acids from the glomerular filtrate. A specific transporter carries the dibasic amino acids, L-arginine and L-lysine, and another carrier is responsible for removal of the acidic amino acids from the tubular fluid. There also are luminal transporters which, like the sodium–glucose cotransporter, exploit the sodium concentration gradient for cotransport of certain amino acids together with sodium. Other carrier molecules in the basement membrane facilitate the exit of the amino acids from the cell.

Bibliography

For a more thorough introduction to normal kidney function:

Berne RM, Levy MN: *Physiology*, 3rd ed. Chapters 41–43, Mosby-Year Book Inc., St. Louis, 1993.

Koeppen B, Stanton B: *Renal Physiology.* Mosby-Year Book, St. Louis, 1992.

Guyton AC: *Textbook of Medical Physiology*, 8th ed. Saunders, New York, Chapters 25–31, 1991.

Rose BD: *Clinical Physiology of Acid-Base and Electrolyte Disorders*, 4th ed. McGraw-Hill, New York, 1994.

Vander A: *Renal Physiology*, 4th ed. McGraw-Hill, New York, 1991.

Shayman JA: *Renal Physiology*, Lippincott, Philadelphia, 1995.

For more detail on topics covered in this chapter:

Adrogue HJ, Madias NE: Changes in plasma potassium concentration during acute acid-base disturbances. *Am J Med* 71:456–467, 1981.

Baylis C: Glomerular filtration dynamics. In: Lote CJ (ed) *Advances in Renal Physiology.* Grune & Stratton, London, pp. 33–83, 1986.

Beauwkes R, Bonventre JV: Tubular organization and vascular-tubular relations in the dog kidney. *Am J Physiol* 229:695–703, 1975.

Debnam ES, Unwin RJ: Hyperglycemia and intestinal and renal glucose transport: implications for diabetic renal injury. *Kidney Int* 50:1101–1109, 1996.

Kaplan B, Batlle DC: Regulation of potassium balance and metabolism. In: Jacobsen HR, Striker GE, Klahr S (eds). *Principles and Practice of Nephrology.* Mosby, St. Louis, 1995.

Levine SD: Diuretics. *Med Clin North Am* 73:271–282, 1989.

Levey AS: Measurement of renal function in chronic renal disease. *Kidney Int* 38:167–184, 1990.

Lifton RP: Genetic determinants of human hypertension. *Proc Natl Acad Sci USA* 92:8545–8551, 1995.

Robertson GL: Physiology of ADH Secretion. *Kidney Int* 32(Suppl 21):S-20, 1987.

Schrier RW: The edematous patient. In Schrier RW (ed) *Manual of Nephrology.* Little Brown, Boston, 1990.

2

CLINICAL EVALUATION OF RENAL FUNCTION

ANDREW S. LEVEY

INTRODUCTION

This chapter focuses on the clinical assessment of the glomerular filtration rate (GFR) because it is generally considered the best index of overall renal function in health and disease. A brief consideration of other renal functions is important before discussing the pathophysiology and clinical evaluation of the GFR in detail.

Glomerular Function

Abnormalities in glomerular function may be classified into three general categories: alterations in the filtration of water and small solutes (assessed as the GFR); alterations in the filtration barrier to macromolecules, manifested as proteinuria; and alterations in the continuity of the glomerular capillary wall, manifested as hematuria. Proteinuria and glomerular diseases causing hematuria are discussed in Chapters 4 and 5.

Tubular Function

Because of the diverse functions of the tubules, abnormalities in tubular function are more difficult to classify. In general, abnormalities are due to defects in the reabsorption of water or solutes or the secretion of solutes in local-

ized nephron segments. They may occur in isolation or in combination, with or without glomerular abnormalities. When they occur in combination and with glomerular abnormalities, there is usually widespread renal parenchymal injury. The severity of the impairment in some tubular functions, for example, ammonia excretion and urinary concentration, may correlate better with the severity of structural damage than does the impairment in GFR. When abnormalities in tubular function occur in isolation, they give rise to a number of diverse syndromes, such as renal tubular acidosis and nephrogenic diabetes insipidus.

GLOMERULAR FILTRATION RATE

Virtues of the GFR as an index of renal function are that it is a direct measure of renal function, it is reduced prior to the onset of symptoms of renal failure, the impairment in GFR correlates with the severity of some of the structural abnormalities observed in chronic renal diseases, and signs and symptoms of uremia occur when GFR falls below 5–10 ml/min. Nonetheless, it is not an ideal index. The GFR is difficult to measure, and the measurements can be insensitive for detecting renal disease, estimating its severity, and monitoring its progression.

Normal Range for GFR

Because GFR varies directly with renal size, which in turn varies with body size, GFR is conventionally factored by body surface area. In normal humans, GFR is approximately 125 ml · min^{-1} · 1.73 m^{-2} or 180 L · day^{-1} · 1.73 m^{-2}. The value of 1.73 m^2 reflects the average value for young men and women. Despite adjustment for body surface area, however, the normal GFR for women is approximately 8% lower than that for men. GFR declines with age; in men, the decrement is approximately 10 ml · min^{-1} · 1.73 m^{-2} per decade after the age of 40 years (Chapter 61). Hence, the normal GFR in 80-year-old men is approximately 80 ml · min^{-1} · 1.73 m^{-2}. Cross-sectional studies in normal women indicate roughly similar results. In children, normal adult values are obtained after 2 years of age (see Chapter 59).

Determinants of GFR

As described in Chapter 1, glomerular filtration is a passive process of ultrafiltration of plasma across the semipermeable glomerular capillary wall. In principle, the level of GFR is the sum of the filtration rates of each of the approximately two million nephrons

$$GFR = N \times SNGFR, \qquad (1)$$

where N is the number of nephrons and SNGFR is single nephron GFR. The determinants of SNGFR are expressed in the equation

$$SNGFR = L_p \times area \times P_{net}, \qquad (2)$$

where L_p is hydraulic permeability, area is filtration area, and P_{net} is net ultrafiltration pressure, the difference between the mean transcapillary hydrostatic (ΔP) and oncotic ($\Delta \pi$) pressure gradients. Although not explicit in this equation, SNGFR varies directly with the renal plasma flow, because of the relationship among renal plasma flow, ΔP, and $\Delta \pi$.

It is not possible to measure the number of nephrons, SNGFR, or its determinants in humans. These factors have been quantitated in animals with experimentally induced renal diseases. In many conditions, ΔP is increased, thereby sustaining SNGFR and GFR at a level higher than would be expected from the decline in $L_p \times$ area and the number of nephrons. As a result, the GFR may not accurately reflect the extent of renal injury. GFR is also affected by conditions other than renal disease (Table 1). These

conditions affect SNGFR rather than the number of nephrons and may alter the level of GFR in healthy individuals and in patients with renal disease.

Measurement of GFR from Renal Clearance

GFR cannot be measured directly; it is assessed from renal clearance. The renal clearance of a substance x is given by the equation

$$C_x = U_x V / P_x, \qquad (3)$$

where C_x is the clearance of x, U_x is the urinary concentration of x, V is the urine flow rate, and P_x is the average plasma concentration of x during the interval of urine collection. The term $U_x V$ is thus the urinary excretion rate of x. The value for clearance is related to the efficiency of excretion; the greater the excretion per unit concentration in plasma, the higher the clearance.

If substance x is freely filtered across the glomerular capillary wall and excreted only by glomerular filtration, its rate of glomerular filtration is equal to its rate of urinary excretion,

$$GFR \times P_x = U_x V, \qquad (4)$$

where the term $GFR \times P_x$ is the filtered load of x. By substitution into Eq. (3),

$$C_x = GFR. \qquad (5)$$

Hence, substance x would be defined as an "ideal filtration marker" whose renal clearance could be used to assess GFR.

If substance x also undergoes tubular reabsorption or secretion, then clearance does not equal GFR. The value for the renal clearance of x would depend not only on the level of renal function, but also on the mechanism of renal excretion. Because $U_x V$ is the algebraic sum of the rates of excretion of substance x by glomerular filtration, tubular reabsorption, and tubular secretion, the clearance of x would exceed GFR for substances that are filtered and secreted and would be less than GFR for substances that are filtered and reabsorbed. Much investigation has been directed to identifying exogenous and endogenous substances, termed filtration markers, which fulfill the criteria for an ideal filtration marker and permit accurate, precise, and convenient assessment of GFR from measurement of renal clearance.

Relation of GFR to Plasma Solute Concentrations

An important concept for the following discussion is the steady state of solute balance. A steady state with regard to substance x is achieved when its rate of generation in body fluids (from either endogenous production or exogenous intake) is constant and equal to its rate of disappearance from body fluids (from either excretion or metabolism). In these circumstances, the plasma concentration of x is constant. In the steady state, if substance x is excreted only in the urine, its generation and urinary excretion are equal, as depicted in the equation

TABLE I
Conditions Other Than Renal Disease That Affect GFR

Pregnancy
Reduced renal perfusion
Marked surfeit or deficit of extracellular fluid volume
Nonsteroidal anti-inflammatory drugs
Acute protein load and habitual protein intake
Blood glucose control (in diabetics)
Level of arterial blood pressure and class of antihypertensive agent used for therapy

$$G_x = U_x V, \qquad (6)$$

where G_x is the generation rate of x. An important corollary is that, in the steady state, the rate of generation of solutes excreted in the urine can be assessed from their rate of urinary excretion.

From rearrangement of Eq. (3) and substitution of Eq. (5), it becomes clear that the steady state plasma concentration of an ideal filtration marker is determined by its rate of production and its excretion by glomerular filtration.

$$P_x = \frac{U_x V}{\text{GFR}} = \frac{G_x}{\text{GFR}}. \qquad (7)$$

Thus, P_x is inversely related to GFR, and GFR can be assessed from the level of P_x.

COMMON CLINICAL MEASUREMENTS TO ASSESS GFR

In clinical practice, GFR is usually estimated from the serum level or renal clearances of the endogenous filtration markers, creatinine and urea.

Estimation of GFR from Serum Creatinine

The use of serum creatinine as an index of GFR is based on two assumptions: (1) creatinine is an ideal filtration marker whose clearance (C_{cr}), therefore, equals GFR; and (2) creatinine balance is in the steady state with constant generation (G_{cr}) and excretion ($U_{cr}V$). Under these conditions, the serum level (P_{cr}) would be inversely related to GFR.

$$P_{cr} = U_{cr}V/\text{GFR} = G_{cr}/\text{GFR}. \qquad (8)$$

Neither assumption is entirely correct. Nonetheless, the level of serum creatinine concentration is generally an adequate index of GFR for clinical decision making. However, in some circumstances, serious errors can result from estimation of GFR from serum creatinine. These are discussed in a later section.

The magnitude of GFR is sufficient to maintain a low serum concentration of creatinine. The normal value is approximately 0.8 to 1.2 mg/dl, with slightly lower values in women than in men. Figure 1 shows hypothetical changes in creatinine production, excretion, balance, and serum creatinine concentration following a 50% decrement in GFR. A new steady state is reached when the serum creatinine concentration rises sufficiently so that the filtered load of creatinine, and hence its urinary excretion, again equals its generation. In the new steady state, the reduced level of GFR is reflected by a reciprocal increase in the steady-state plasma concentration (Fig. 2).

Thus, in the steady state, changes in serum creatinine reflect changes in GFR. Because of their reciprocal relationship, a large change in GFR is required to raise serum creatinine from the normal to the elevated range. However, once serum creatinine is elevated, even small changes in GFR raise it substantially more. Expression of the serum creatinine level as its reciprocal ($1/P_{cr}$) allows the magnitude of decline in GFR to be more clearly appreciated.

Estimation of GFR from Creatinine Clearance

Because of differences among individuals in creatinine generation and excretion, creatinine clearance provides a

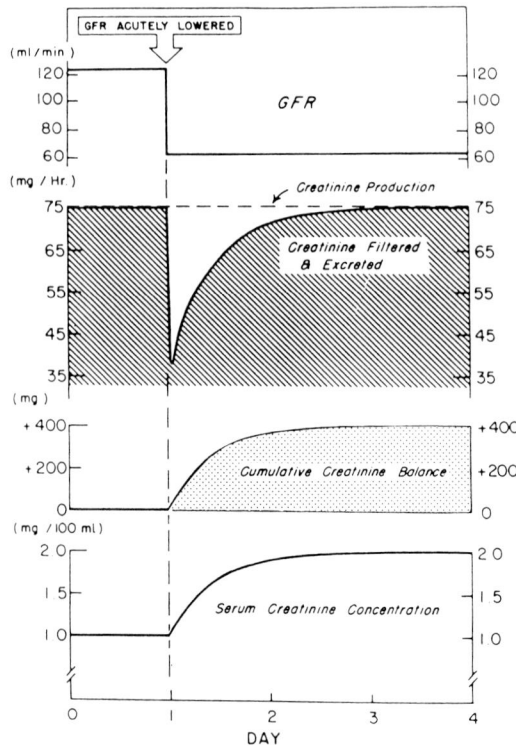

FIGURE 1 Effect of a sudden decrease in GFR on creatinine excretion, production, balance, and serum creatinine concentration. Reprinted with permission from Kassirer JP: *N Engl J Med* 285:385–389, 1971.

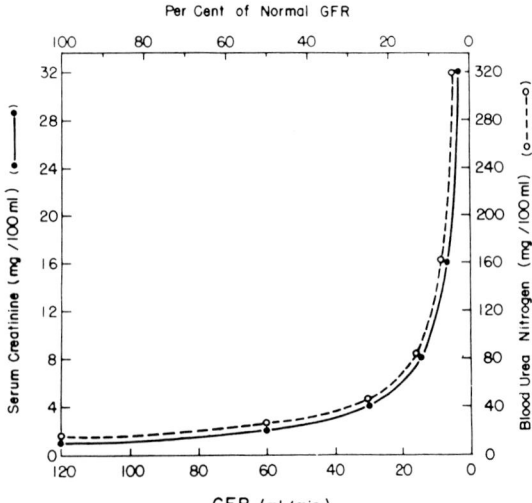

FIGURE 2 Relationship of GFR to steady-state levels of serum creatinine and BUN. Reprinted with permission from Kassirer JP: *N Engl J Med* 285:385–389, 1971.

more accurate estimate of GFR than serum creatinine. Most commonly, creatinine clearance is calculated from a 24-hour urine collection for creatinine and a single measurement of serum creatinine, assuming a steady state:

$$C_{cr} = U_{cr}V/P_{cr}. \qquad (9)$$

A shorter timed urine specimen collection under supervision reduces inaccuracy due to errors in timing and completeness of collection.

Another advantage of estimating GFR from creatinine clearance rather than from serum creatinine is that a steady state is not required. Additional serum measurements can be obtained to estimate the average serum concentration during the urine collection. Measurements can be made either at the midpoint of the urine collection or at the beginning and end of the urine collection and averaged.

Estimation of Creatinine Clearance from Serum Creatinine

As discussed later, creatinine generation can be approximated from age, gender, and body size. Therefore, in the steady state, creatinine clearance can be estimated from these factors and the serum level, without urine collection. The formula derived by Cockcroft and Gault (1976) is particularly simple to use,

$$C_{cr} = ((140 - age) \times weight)/(P_{cr} \times 72) \\ (men) \qquad (10)$$

$$C_{cr} = (((140 - age) \times weight)/(P_{cr} \times 72)) \times 0.85, \\ (women) \qquad (11)$$

where C_{cr} is in milliliters per minute, age is in years, weight is in kilograms, and P_{cr} is in milligrams per deciliter. These formulas were derived from individuals without renal disease. In patients with renal disease, however, there is a wide range of differences between the estimates of creatinine clearance and simultaneously measured GFR.

Estimation of GFR from BUN and Urea Clearance

Urea is also excreted principally by glomerular filtration; hence, the steady-state urea level also varies inversely with GFR (Fig. 2). However, due to the renal tubular reabsorption of urea and the many factors that affect urea generation, the serum level and renal clearance of urea are poor indexes of GFR. Nonetheless, there are special circumstances in which it is useful to measure them.

Urea is usually measured as urea nitrogen, and for historical reasons, the serum level is commonly referred to as the blood urea nitrogen (BUN). The normal value is approximately 8 to 12 mg/dl; thus, the normal ratio of BUN to creatinine is approximately 10:1. In principle, a reduction in GFR would lead to a rise in BUN but would not alter the BUN:creatinine ratio. As discussed later, deviations in the ratio may indicate alterations in urea reabsorption or generation.

Most important is the well-recognized relationship of the level of renal function, the BUN level, and clinical features of uremia. A useful "rule of thumb" is that a BUN level greater than 100 mg/dl is associated with a higher risk of complications in both acute and chronic renal failure and may indicate the need to initiate dialysis. However, as discussed below, if urea generation is reduced, the BUN may remain below this level even if GFR declines to very low levels and uremic symptoms arise.

Measurement of GFR Using Exogenous Filtration Markers

Inulin, a 5200-Da polymer of fructose, meets the criteria for an ideal filtration marker, and its renal clearance is regarded as the "gold standard" for the measurement of GFR. However, the classic method of inulin clearance requires a continuous intravenous infusion and bladder catheterization and the chemical assay for inulin is difficult.

TABLE 2

Clinical Conditions That Cause Errors in the Estimation of GFR from Measurement of Creatinine Clearance or Serum Creatinine[a]

Condition	Effect on C_{cr}	Effect on P_{cr}	Comment
Plasma ketosis	None	Increase	Interference with the picric acid assay for creatinine.
Therapy with certain cephalosporins or fluctyosine	None	Increase	Interference with the picric acid and iminohydrolase assays for creatinine, respectively.
Therapy with cimetidine or trimethoprim trimethoprim	Decrease	Increase	Inhibition of tubular secretion of creatinine.
Ingesting cooked meat	Increase	Increase	Transient increase in GFR and creatinine generation.
Restriction of dietary protein	Decrease	Decrease	Sustained decrease in GFR and creatinine generation.
Vigorous prolonged exercise	None	Increase	Increase in muscle creatinine generation.
Muscle wasting	None	Decrease	Decrease in muscle creatinine generation.
Muscle growth	None	Increase	Increase in muscle creatinine generation.
Renal disease[b]	Increase	Decrease	Decrease in GFR, but stimulation of tubular secretion of creatinine, and possible decrease in creatinine generation.

[a] C_{cr}, creatinine clearance; P_{cr}, serum creatinine; GFR, glomerular filtration rate. Modified from Levey AS: Assessing the effectiveness of therapy to prevent the progression of renal disease. *Am J Kidney Dis* 22:207–214, 1993.

[b] Effects on C_{cr} and P_{cr} relative to effects on GFR (i.e., C_{cr} is higher than expected and P_{cr} is lower than expected for the reduction in GFR, see text).

Hence, this method is not suitable in practice and remains largely a research tool.

To simplify the assessment of GFR, investigators have studied other clearance methods, using a bolus injection and alternative filtration markers, such as low-molecular-weight compounds chelated to radioisotopes. Urine is collected after voiding or the urine collection is omitted and plasma clearance is measured. In the United States, the two most frequently used markers are [^{125}I]iothalamate and [^{99m}Tc]DTPA. Simultaneous measurements of renal clearance of these markers, by alternative methods, and of inulin, by classic techniques, reveal similar although not identical results. These alternative methods for measuring GFR have become popular in clinical research in recent years and can be used in practice when estimates of GFR from endogenous filtration markers are likely to be inaccurate, as discussed below.

LIMITATIONS TO CLINICAL ASSESSMENT OF GFR

The following sections describe the renal handling and metabolism of creatinine and urea and the measurement of creatinine. The purpose is to highlight clinical conditions in which errors may occur in the interpretation of the serum level or renal clearance of creatinine or urea as an index of GFR (Tables 2 and 3). With appropriate awareness of these limitations, the careful practitioner can usually make a satisfactory assessment of the level of renal function from these measurements.

Renal Handling of Creatinine

Creatinine (molecular mass, 113 Da) is both freely filtered by the glomerulus and also secreted by the proximal tubule. In normal individuals, creatinine secretion accounts for 5 to 10% of excreted creatinine; hence, clearance exceeds GFR by approximately 10 ml $\cdot$ min^{-1} $\cdot$ 1.73 m^{-2}. In contrast, creatinine secretion is enhanced in patients with reduced GFR, leading to a greater disparity between creatinine clearance and GFR (Fig. 3). Moreover, the magnitude of creatinine secretion is variable among individuals and over time. Therefore, the value for creatinine clearance overestimates the GFR, and the magnitude of the overestimation is not predictable. The most serious errors occur within the range of GFR from 40 to 80 ml $\cdot$ min^{-1} $\cdot$ 1.73 m^{-2}, where creatinine clearance can remain normal. Consequently, it can be difficult to detect the onset or early progression of the decline in GFR from measurements of creatinine clearance.

Some drugs, notably trimethoprim and cimetidine, competitively inhibit creatinine secretion, thereby reducing creatinine clearance and raising the serum creatinine concentration, despite no effect on GFR. Indeed, some investigators have recommended assessing GFR from measurements of creatinine clearance during high-dose cimetidine treatment. Clinically, it can be difficult to determine whether the serum creatinine has risen because of a drug-induced inhibition of secretion or a decline in GFR. A clue that inhibition of creatinine secretion is responsible is an unchanged blood urea nitrogen concentration, since urea clearance is unaffected by these drugs.

Creatinine Metabolism

Creatinine is derived largely from the metabolism of creatine in muscle, which originates in part from dietary creatine contained in meat. Cooking meat converts a variable fraction of creatine to creatinine which is absorbed and

TABLE 3
Clinical Conditions That Cause Errors in the Estimation of GFR from Measurement of Urea Clearance or BUN[a]

Condition	Effect on		Comment
	C_{urea}	BUN	
Dehydration	Decrease	Increase	Increased urea reabsorption
Reduced renal perfusion (volume depletion, congestive heart failure)	Decrease	Increase	Reduced GFR, increased urea reabsorption, increased urea generation
Overhydration	Increase	Decrease	Reduced urea reabsorption
Increased renal perfusion (volume expansion, pregnancy, syndrome of inappropriate ADH secretion)	Increase	Decrease	Increased GFR, reduced urea reabsorption
Restriction of dietary protein	None	Decrease	Reduced urea generation
Increased dietary protein	None	Increase	Increased urea generation
Accelerated catabolism (fever, trauma, GI bleeding, cell lysis, therapy with tetracycline or corticosteroids)	None	Increase	Increased urea generation
Liver disease	Decrease[b]	Variable[b]	Decreased GFR, increased urea reabsorption, decreased urea generation.
Renal disease	None[b]	Decrease[b]	Decreased GFR, no change in urea reabsorption, decreased urea generation (if dietary protein is restricted).

[a] C_{urea}, urea clearance; BUN, blood (serum) urea nitrogen; GFR, glomerular filtration rate.
[b] Effects on C_{urea} and BUN relative to effects on GFR (e.g., C_{urea} is lower than expected for the reduction in GFR).

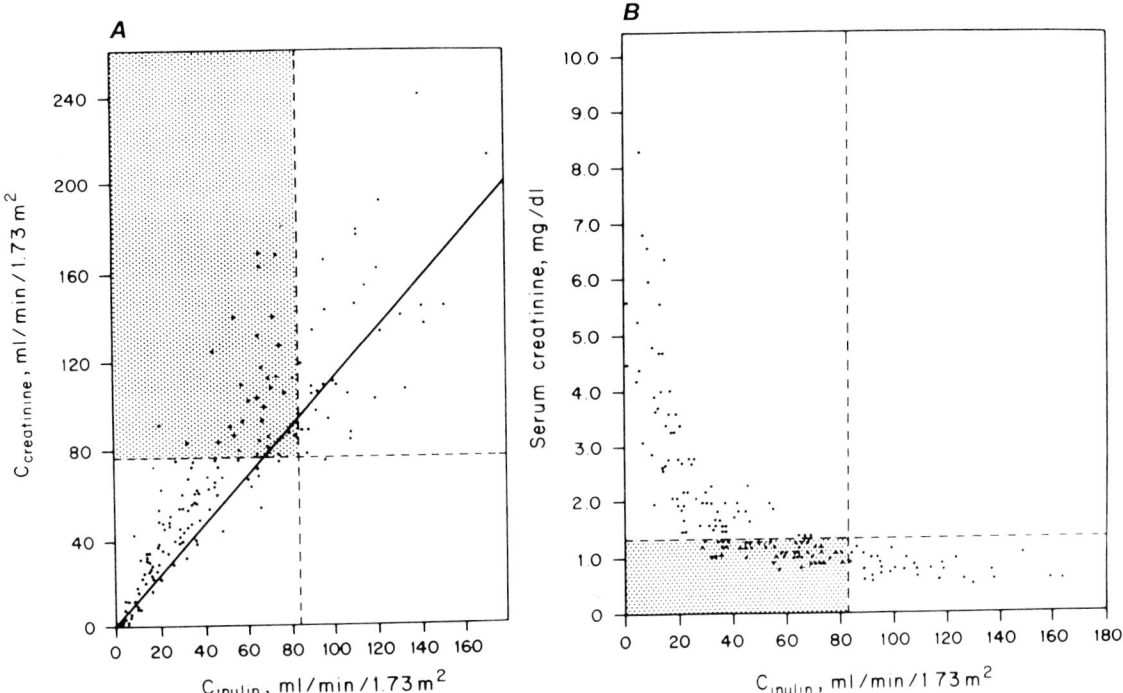

FIGURE 3 Relationship of creatinine clearance (left) and serum creatinine (right) to GFR (inulin clearance) in patients with renal disease. Horizontal lines indicate lower limit of normal for creatinine clearance (left) and upper limit of normal for serum creatinine (right). Vertical lines indicate lower limit of normal for GFR. Diagonal line (left) is the line of identity. Shaded areas indicate the proportion of patients in whom the level of creatinine clearance or serum creatinine is normal despite reduced GFR. Reprinted with permission from Shemesh *et al.: Kidney Int* 28:830–838, 1985, and Levey *et al.: Annu Rev Med* 39:469–490, 1988.

enters the creatinine pool. Hence, creatinine generation parallels total muscle mass, and to a lesser extent, meat intake. Lower values are found in women, children, the elderly, malnourished individuals, and those with restricted meat intake, leading to lower serum creatinine levels. As a corollary, in these groups, serum creatinine may remain normal despite a reduction in creatinine clearance. Therefore, in detecting a reduction in GFR, an elevated serum creatinine is an even less-sensitive indicator than a reduced creatinine clearance. Indeed, GFR can be reduced to as low as 20 ml $\cdot$ min^{-1} $\cdot$ 1.73 m^{-2}, despite normal serum creatinine concentration (Fig. 3).

Factors affecting creatinine generation are especially important in patients with chronic renal disease. Meat intake is often restricted in conjunction with a low-protein diet, and malnutrition and muscle wasting are common. These factors tend to blunt the rise in serum creatinine as creatinine clearance declines. In addition, extrarenal elimination of creatinine can occur, contributing to maintenance of serum creatinine at a lower level. For these reasons, the serum creatinine level tends to overestimate the creatinine clearance, which, as discussed above, tends to overestimate the level of GFR. Hence, it can be difficult to assess the level of GFR from the serum creatinine concentration or changes in GFR from changes in serum creatinine.

Creatinine Measurement

The most important technical difficulty is the imprecision in serum creatinine assays at low values that are characteristic of the normal range, especially in women and children. Hence, it can be difficult to determine whether changes in the serum level within the normal range represent analytical variability or changes in GFR. In addition, various substances can interfere with the serum assays, leading to spurious elevations in the serum level (Table 2).

Renal Handling of Urea

Urea (molecular mass, 60 Da) is freely filtered by the glomerulus. However, 35 to 65% of the filtered load is reabsorbed by the proximal and distal tubules. Hence, urea clearance is less than GFR. Urea reabsorption varies inversely with renal blood flow and the state of hydration (Table 3). Dehydration, reduced renal perfusion, or the early phase of obstruction of the urinary tract causes increased urea reabsorption, decreased urea clearance, and a high BUN:creatinine ratio. Conversely, overhydration or increased renal perfusion causes decreased urea reabsorption, increased urea clearance, and a reduced BUN:creatinine ratio. The BUN:creatinine ratio is useful in the differential diagnosis of acute or chronic renal insufficiency. Reduced renal perfusion (e.g., extracellular volume contraction or congestive heart failure) or recent-onset urinary tract obstruction usually causes the BUN:creatinine ratio to rise to >20:1. In contrast, in acute tubular necrosis and most causes of chronic renal disease, the BUN:creatinine ratio remains normal (approximately 10:1). As discussed below, the BUN:creatinine ratio also can be elevated in states of increased urea generation associated with acute or chronic renal insufficiency.

Another useful application of the measurement of urea clearance is to assess the overall level of renal function in patients with advanced chronic renal disease. As GFR declines, urea reabsorption is reduced and affected less by the state of hydration. By coincidence, the proportion of the filtered load of urea that is reabsorbed approximates the proportion of excreted creatinine that is secreted. In patients with GFR <15 ml $\cdot$ min^{-1} $\cdot$ 1.73 m^{-2}, the average of the values for urea and creatinine clearance approximates the GFR. In patients with chronic renal failure treated by dialysis, residual renal function is generally measured by urea clearance. Values for urea clearance <1 ml/min indicate negligible residual renal function.

Urea Metabolism

Urea is the end product of protein catabolism and is synthesized primarily by the liver. Approximately one quarter of synthesized urea is metabolized in the intestine to carbon dioxide and ammonia. The ammonia thus generated returns to the liver where it is reconverted to urea. In the steady state, the level of BUN is an index of urea generation. Dietary protein intake is the principal determinant of urea generation (Table 3). A high dietary protein intake raises the BUN and consequently the BUN:creatinine ratio. Other factors that increase urea generation in-

clude accelerated catabolism of endogenous protein, as occurs during febrile illnesses, trauma, gastrointestinal bleeding, tumor lysis or therapy with tetracyclines or corticosteroids (Table 3). On the other hand, urea generation may be reduced in liver disease leading to a BUN:creatinine ratio $<10:1$.

Bibliography

Cockcroft DW, Gault MH: Prediction of creatinine clearance from serum creatinine. *Nephron* 16:31–41, 1976.

Kassirer JP: Clinical evaluation of kidney function: Glomerular function. *N Engl J Med* 285:385–389, 1971.

Levey AS: Use of measurements of GFR to assess the progression of renal disease. *Semin Nephrol* 9:370–379, 1989.

Levey AS: Nephrology forum: Measurement of renal function in chronic renal disease. *Kidney Int* 38:167–184, 1990.

Luke RG: Uremia and the BUN. *N Engl J Med* 305:1213–1215, 1981.

Miller TR, Anderson RJ, Linas SL, Henrich WL, Berns AS, Gabow PA, Schrier RW: Urinary diagnostic indices in acute renal failure: A prospective study. *Ann Int Med* 89:47–50, 1978.

Perrone RD, Madias NE, Levey AS: Serum creatinine as an index of renal function: New insights into old concepts. *Clin Chem* 38:1933–1953, 1992.

Rolin HA, Hall PM, Wei R: Inaccuracy of estimated creatinine clearance for prediction of iothalamate glomerular filtration rate. *Am J Kidney Dis* 4:48–54, 1984.

Roubenoff R, Drew H, Moyer M, Petri M, Whiting-O'Keefe Q, Hellmann DB: Oral cimetidine improves the accuracy and precision of creatinine clearance. *Ann Intern Med* 113:501–506, 1990.

Shemesh O, Golbetz H, Kriss JP, Myers BD: Limitations of creatinine as a filtration marker in glomerulopathic patients. *Kidney Int* 28:830–838, 1985.

Smith HW: Diseases of the kidney and urinary tract. In: *The Kidney: Structure and Function in Health and Disease.* Oxford University Press, New York, Chap. 26, pp. 836–887, 1951.

Walser M: Progression of chronic renal failure in man. *Kidney Int* 37:1195–1210, 1990.

3

URINALYSIS

ARTHUR GREENBERG

The microscopic examination of the urine sediment is an indispensable part of the evaluation of patients with renal insufficiency, proteinuria, hematuria, urinary tract infection, or nephrolithiasis. This task must not be delegated; it should be performed personally. The relatively simple chemical tests performed in the routine urinalysis provide important information about a number of primary renal and systemic disorders. Examination of the urine sediment gives valuable clues about the renal parenchyma. The features of a complete urinalysis are listed in Table 1.

SPECIMEN COLLECTION AND HANDLING

Urine should be collected with a minimum of contamination. A clean catch midstream collection is preferred. If this is not feasible, bladder catheterization is appropriate in adults; the risk of a urinary tract infection following a single catheterization is insignificant. Suprapubic aspiration is employed in infants. In the uncooperative male patient, a clean, freshly applied condom catheter and urinary collection bag may be used. Urine in the collection bag of a patient with an indwelling bladder catheter is subject to stasis. Fresh urine may be collected by withdrawing urine from above a clamp placed on the drainage tube.

The chemical composition of the urine changes with standing and the formed elements degenerate over time. The urine is best examined fresh; a brief period of refrigeration is acceptable. Because bacteria multiply at room temperature, bacterial counts from unrefrigerated urine are unreliable. High urine osmolality and low pH favor cellular preservation. These two characteristics of the first voided morning urine give it particular value in evaluating for suspected glomerulonephritis.

PHYSICAL AND CHEMICAL PROPERTIES OF THE URINE

Appearance

Normal urine is clear, with a faint yellow tinge due to the presence of urochromes. As the urine becomes more concentrated, its color deepens. Bilirubin, other pathologic metabolites, and a variety of drugs may discolor the urine or change its smell. Suspended erythrocytes, leukocytes, or crystals may render the urine turbid. Conditions associated with a change in the appearance of the urine are listed in Table 2.

Specific Gravity

The specific gravity of a fluid is the ratio of its weight to the weight of an equal volume of distilled water. The urine specific gravity is a conveniently determined but inaccurate surrogate for osmolality. Specific gravities of 1.001 to 1.035 correspond to an osmolality range of 50 to 1000 mOsm/kg. A specific gravity near 1.010 connotes isosthenuria, with a urine osmolality matching that of plasma. Relative to osmolality, the specific gravity is elevated when dense solutes such as protein, glucose, or radiographic contrast are present. Formulas that correct specific gravity for glycosuria or proteinuria are available but of little practical utility. It is better to measure osmolality directly.

Three methods are available for specific gravity measurement. The hydrometer is most accurate, but it requires a sufficient volume of urine to float the hydrometer as well as equilibration of the specimen to the hydrometer calibration temperature. The second method is based on the well-characterized relationship between urine specific gravity and refractive index. Refractometers calibrated in specific gravity units are commercially available; they require only a drop of urine. Finally, the specific gravity may also be estimated by dipstick.

The specific gravity is used to determine whether the urine is or can be concentrated. During a solute diuresis accompanying hyperglycemia, diuretic therapy, or relief of obstruction, the urine is isosthenuric. In contrast, with a water diuresis due to overhydration or diabetes insipidus, the specific gravity is typically 1.004 or lower. In the absence of proteinuria, glycosuria, or iodinated contrast administration, a specific gravity of more than 1.018 implies preserved concentrating ability. Measurement of specific gravity is useful in differentiating between prerenal azotemia and acute tubular necrosis (ATN) and in assessing the import of proteinuria observed in a randomly voided urine.

Chemical Composition of the Urine—Dipstick Methodology

Tedious individual assays of protein, glucose (or other reducing substances), or ketones have been supplanted by more convenient dipstick methods. The urine dipstick is a plastic strip to which paper tabs impregnated with chemical reagents have been glued. The reagents in each strip are chromogenic. After timed development, the color on the paper segment is compared to a chart. Some reactions

TABLE 1

The Routine Urinalysis

Appearance

Specific gravity

Chemical tests (Dipstick)
  pH
  Protein
  Glucose
  Ketones
  Blood
  Urobilinogen
  Bilirubin
  Nitrites
  Leukocyte esterase

Microscopic examination (formed elements)
  Crystals: Urate; calcium phosphate, oxalate, or carbonate,
    triple phosphate; cystine; drugs
  Cells: Leukocytes, erythrocytes, renal tubular cells, oval fat
    bodies, transitional epithelium, squamous
  Casts: Hyaline, granular, RBC, WBC, tubular cell,
    degenerating cellular, broad, waxy, lipid-laden
  Infecting organisms: Bacteria, yeast, trichomonas, nematodes
  Miscellaneous: spermatozoa, mucous threads, fibers, starch,
    hair, and other contaminants

TABLE 2

Selected Substances That May Alter the Physical Appearance
or Odor of the Urine

Color change	Substances
White	Chyle, pus, phosphate crystals
Pink/red/brown	Erythrocytes, hemoglobin, myoglobin, porphyrins, beets, senna, cascara, levodopa, methyldopa, deferoxamine, phenolphthalein and congeners, food colorings, metronidazole, phenacetin
Yellow/orange/brown	Bilirubin, urobilin, phenazopyridine urinary analgesics, senna, cascara, mepacrine, iron compounds, nitrofurantoin, riboflavin, rhubarb, sulfasalazine, rifampin, fluorescein, phenytoin
Brown/black	Methemoglobin, homogentisic acid (alcaptonuria), melanin (melanoma), levodopa, methyldopa
Blue or green green/brown	Biliverdin, *Pseudomonas* infection, dyes (methylene blue and indigo carmine), triamterene, vitamin B complex, methocarbamol, indican, phenol, chlorophyll

Odor	Substance or condition
Sweet or fruity	Ketones
Ammoniacal	Urea-splitting bacterial infection
Maple syrup	Maple syrup urine disease
Musty or mousy	Phenylketonuria
Sweaty feet	Isovaleric or glutaric acidemia or excess butyric or hexanoic acid
Rancid	Hypermethioninemia, tyrosinemia

are highly specific. Others are sensitive to the presence of interfering substances or extremes of pH. Heavy discoloration of the urine with bilirubin or blood may obscure the color changes.

pH

The pH test pads employ indicator dyes that change color with pH. The physiologic urine pH ranges from 4.5 to 8.0. The determination is most accurate if done promptly, because growth of urea-splitting bacteria and loss of CO_2 raise pH. In addition, bacterial metabolism of glucose may produce organic acids and lower pH. These strips are not sufficiently accurate to be used for the diagnosis of renal tubular acidosis.

Protein

Protein measurement uses the protein-error-of-indicators principle. The pH at which some indicators change color varies with the protein concentration of the bathing solution. Protein indicator strips are buffered at an acid pH near their color change point. Wetting them with a protein containing specimen induces a color change. The protein reaction may be scored from trace to 4+ or by concentration. Their equivalence is as follows: trace, 5 to 20 mg/dL; 1+, 30 mg/dL; 2+, 100 mg/dL; 3+, 300 mg/dL; 4+, greater than 2000 mg/dL. Highly alkaline urine, especially after contamination with quaternary ammonium skin cleansers, may produce false-positive reactions. Protein strips are highly sensitive to albumin but less so to globulins, hemoglobin, or light chains. When light-chain proteinuria is suspected, an acid precipitation assay must be employed. An acid that denatures protein is added to the urine specimen and the density of precipitate is related to the protein concentration. Urine negative by dipstick but positive with sulfosalicyclic acid is highly suspicious for light chains. Tolbutamide, high-dose penicillin, sulfonamides, and radiographic contrast may give false-positive turbimetric reactions. If the urine is very concentrated, the presence of a modest amount of protein is less likely to correspond to significant proteinuria on a 24-hour basis. The protein indicator used for routine dipstick analysis is not sensitive enough to detect microalbuminuria. Special dipsticks are available for screening for microalbuminuria in incipient diabetic nephropathy (see Chapters 5 and 29).

Blood

Reagent strips for blood rely on the peroxidase activity of hemoglobin to catalyze an organic peroxide with subsequent oxidation of an indicator dye. Free hemoglobin produces a homogeneous color. Intact red cells cause punctate staining. False-positive reactions occur if the urine is contaminated with other oxidants such as povidone–iodine, hypochlorite, or bacterial peroxidase. Ascorbate causes false negatives. Myoglobin is also detected, because it has intrinsic peroxidase activity. A urine that is positive for blood by dipstick but shows no red cells on microscopic examination is suspect for myoglobinuria or hemoglobinuria. Pink discoloration of serum may occur with hemolysis, but free myoglobin is seldom present in a concentration sufficient to change the color of plasma. A specific assay for urine myoglobin will confirm the diagnosis.

Specific Gravity

Specific gravity reagents strips actually measure ionic strength using indicator dyes with ionic-strength-dependent pK_a's. They do not detect glucose or nonionic radiographic contrast.

Glucose

In contrast to the obsolete copper sulfate-based tablet tests that detected any reducing substances, modern dipstick reagent strips are specific for glucose. They rely on glucose oxidase to catalyze the formation of hydrogen peroxide which reacts with peroxidase and a chromogen to produce a color change. High concentrations of ascorbate or ketoacids reduce test sensitivity. However, the degree of glycosuria occurring in diabetic ketoacidosis is sufficient to prevent false negatives despite ketonuria.

Ketones

Ketone reagent strips depend on the development of a purple color after acetoacetate reacts with nitroprusside. They do not detect acetone or β-hydroxybutyrate. False positives may occur in patients taking levodopa.

Urobilinogen

Urobilinogen is a colorless substance produced in the gut from metabolism of bilirubin. Some is excreted in feces and the rest reabsorbed and excreted in the urine. In obstructive jaundice, bilirubin does not reach the bowel, and urinary excretion of urobilinogen is diminished. In other forms of jaundice, urobilinogen is increased. The urobilinogen test is based on the Ehrlich reaction in which diethylaminobenzaldehyde reacts with urobilinogen in acid medium to produce a pink color. Sulfonamides may produce false positives and degradation of urobilinogen to urobilin false negatives.

Bilirubin

Bilirubin reagent strips rely on the chromogenic reaction of bilirubin with diazonium salts. Conjugated bilirubin is not normally present in the urine. False positives may be observed in patients receiving chlorpromazine or phenazopyridine. False negatives occur in the presence of ascorbate.

Nitrite

This screening test for bacteriuria relies on the ability of gram negative bacteria to convert urinary nitrate to nitrite which activates a chromogen. False-negative results occur with infection with enterococcus or other organisms that do not produce nitrite, when ascorbate is present, or when urine has not been retained in the bladder long enough (approximately 4 hours) to permit sufficient production of nitrite from nitrate.

Leukocytes

Granulocyte esterases can cleave pyrrole amino acid esters, producing free pyrrole that subsequently reacts with a chromogen. The test threshold is 5 to 15 WBC/HPF. False negatives occur with glycosuria, high specific gravity, cephalexin or tetracycline therapy, or excessive oxalate excretion. Contamination with vaginal debris may give a positive test result without true urinary tract infection.

MICROSCOPIC EXAMINATION OF THE SPUN URINARY SEDIMENT

Specimen Preparation and Viewing

Standardization of procedure ensures comparability of serial urine specimens. Twelve milliliters of urine should be spun in a conical centrifuge tube for 5 minutes at 1500 to 2000 rpm (450g). After centrifugation, the tube is inverted and drained. The pellet is resuspended in the few drops of urine that remain in the tube after inversion by flicking the base of the tube gently with a finger or with the use of a pipette. Care should be taken to fully suspend the pellet without excessive agitation. A drop of urine is poured onto a microscope slide or transferred with the pipette. The drop should be sufficient in size that a standard 22×22-mm coverslip just floats on the urine. If too little is used, the specimen rapidly dries out. If an excess of urine is applied, it will spill onto the microscope objective or stream distractingly under the coverslip. Rapid commercial urine stains or the Papanicolaou stain may be used to enhance detail. Most nephrologists prefer the convenience of viewing unstained urine. Subdued light is necessary. The condenser and diaphragm are adjusted to maximize contrast and definition. When the urine is dilute and few formed elements are present, detection of motion of objects suspended in the urine ensures that the focal plane is correct. One should scan the urine at low power (100$\times$) to obtain a general impression of its contents before moving to high power (400$\times$) to look at individual fields. It is useful to scan large areas at low power and move to high power when a structure of interest is identified. Cellular elements should be quantitated by counting or estimating the number in at least ten representative high power fields. Casts may be quantitated by counting the number per low power field, although most observers use less specific terms such as rare, occasional, few, frequent, and numerous.

Cellular Elements

The principal formed elements of the urine are listed in Table 1. The figures constitute an atlas of selected formed elements.

Erythrocytes

Red blood cells (RBC; Figs. 1A and 1B) may find their way into the urine from any source between the glomerulus and the urethral meatus. The presence of more than two or three erythrocytes per HPF is usually pathologic. Erythrocytes are biconcave discs 7 μm in diameter. They become

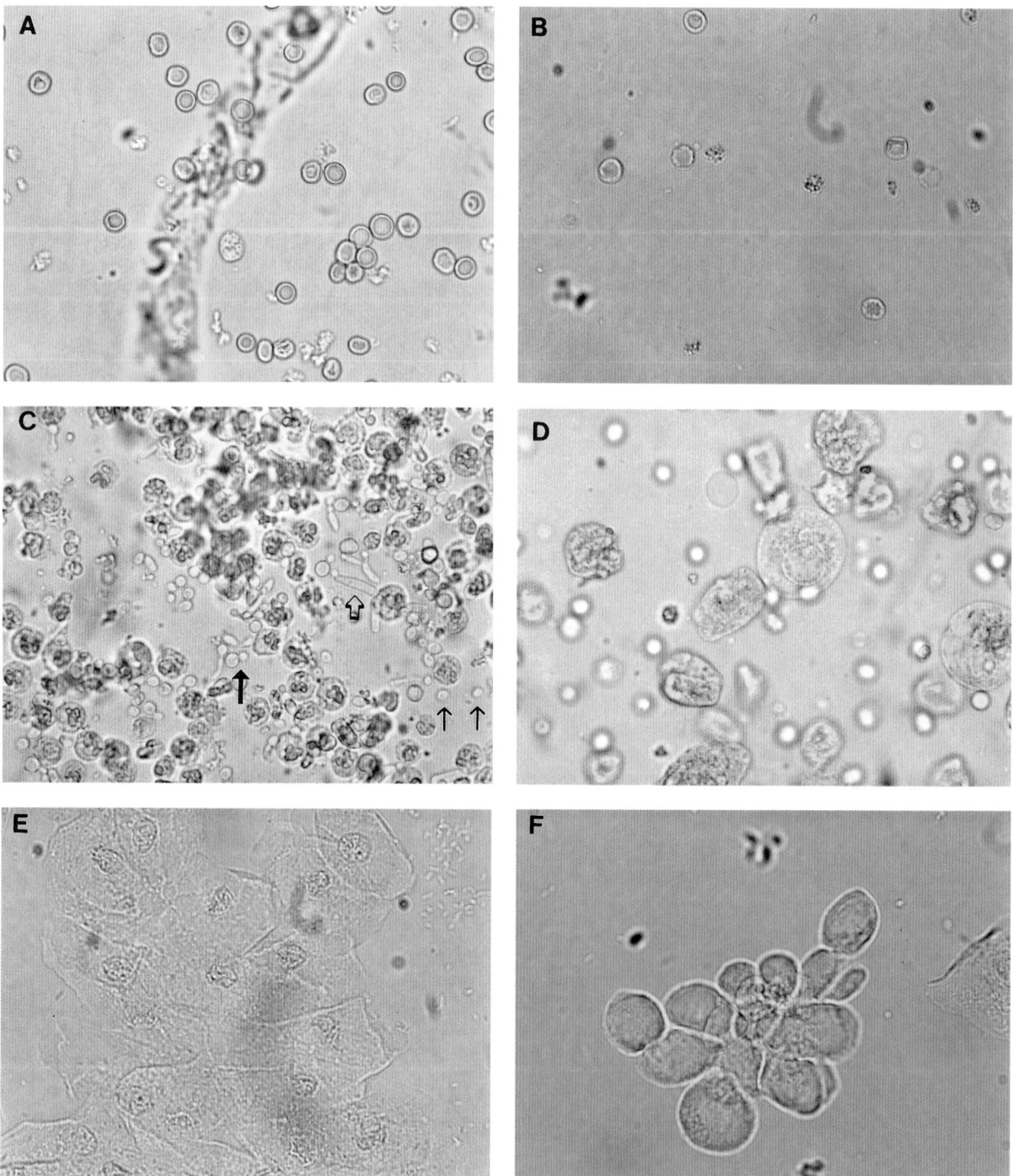

FIGURE I   Cellular elements in the urine. In this and subsequent figures (Figs. 2–4), all photographs were made from unstained sediments and, except as specified, photographed at 400× original magnification. (A) Nondysmorphic red blood cells. Note that they appear as uniform, biconcave disks. (B) Dysmorphic red blood cells from a patient with IgA nephropathy. Their shape is irregular, with membrane blebs and spicules. (C) White blood cells from a patient with an indwelling bladder catheter. Numerous individual (small arrows) and budding yeast (single thick arrow) as well as hyphal forms (open arrow) are present. (D) Renal tubular epithelial cells. Note the variability of shape. The erythrocytes in the background are much smaller. (E) Squamous epithelial cells. (F) Transitional epithelial cells in a characteristic clump.

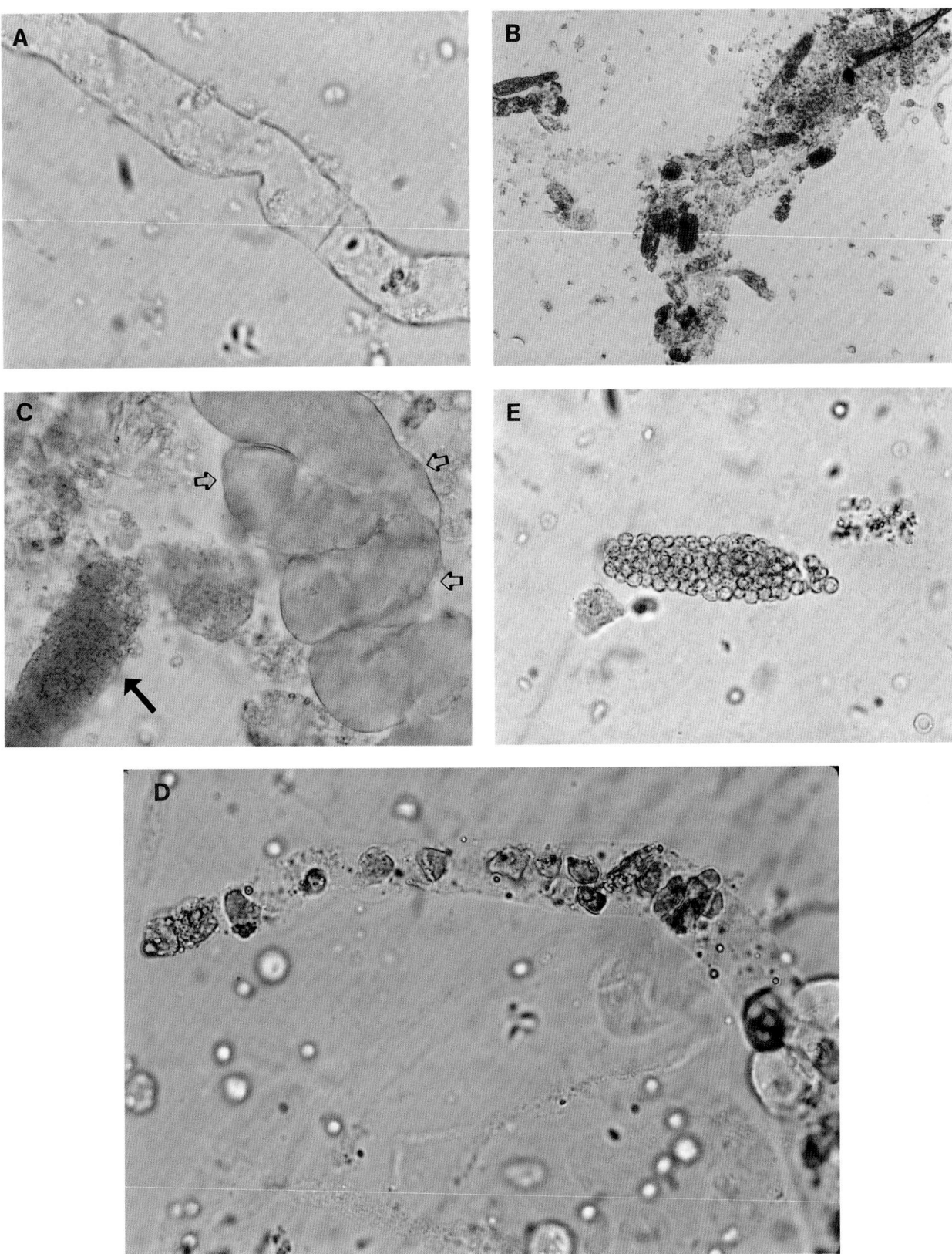

FIGURE 2   Casts. (A) Hyaline cast. (B) "Muddy brown" granular casts and amorphous debris from a patient with ATN (original magnification, 100×). (C) Waxy cast (open arrows) and granular cast (solid arrow) from a patient with lupus nephritis and a telescoped sediment. Note the background hematuria. (D) Tubular cell cast. Note the hyaline cast matrix. (E) Red blood cell cast. Background hematuria is also present.

crenated in hypertonic urine. In hypotonic urine, they swell or burst, leaving ghosts. Erythrocytes originating in the renal parenchyma are dysmorphic, with spicules, blebs, submembrane cytoplasmic precipitation, membrane folding, and vesicles. Those originating in the collecting system retain their uniform shape. Some experienced observers report success differentiating renal parenchymal from collecting system bleeding by systematic examination of erythrocytes using phase contrast microscopy.

Leukocytes

Polymorphonuclear leukocytes (PMN; Fig. 1C) are approximately 12 μm in diameter and are most readily recognized in a fresh urine before their multilobed nuclei or granules have degenerated. Swollen PMNs with prominent granules displaying Brownian motion are termed "glitter" cells. PMNs indicate urinary tract inflammation. They may occur with intraparenchymal diseases such as glomerulonephritis or interstitial nephritis. They are a prominent feature of upper or lower urinary tract infection. In addition, they may appear with periureteral inflammation as in regional ileitis or acute appendicitis.

Renal Tubular Epithelial Cells

Tubular cells (Fig. 1D) are larger than PMNs, ranging from 12 to 20 μm. Proximal tubular cells are oval- or egg-shaped and tend to be larger than the cuboidal distal tubular cells, but since their size varies with urine osmolality, they cannot be reliably differentiated. In hypotonic urine, it may be difficult to distinguish tubular cells from swollen PMNs. A few tubular cells may be seen in a normal urine. More commonly, they indicate tubular damage or inflammation from ATN or interstitial nephritis.

Other Cells

Squamous cells (Fig. 1E) of urethral, vaginal, or cutaneous origin are large, flat cells with small nuclei. Transitional epithelial cells (Fig. 1F) line the renal pelvis, ureter, bladder, and early urethra. They are rounded cells several times the size of leukocytes and often occur in clumps. In hypo-

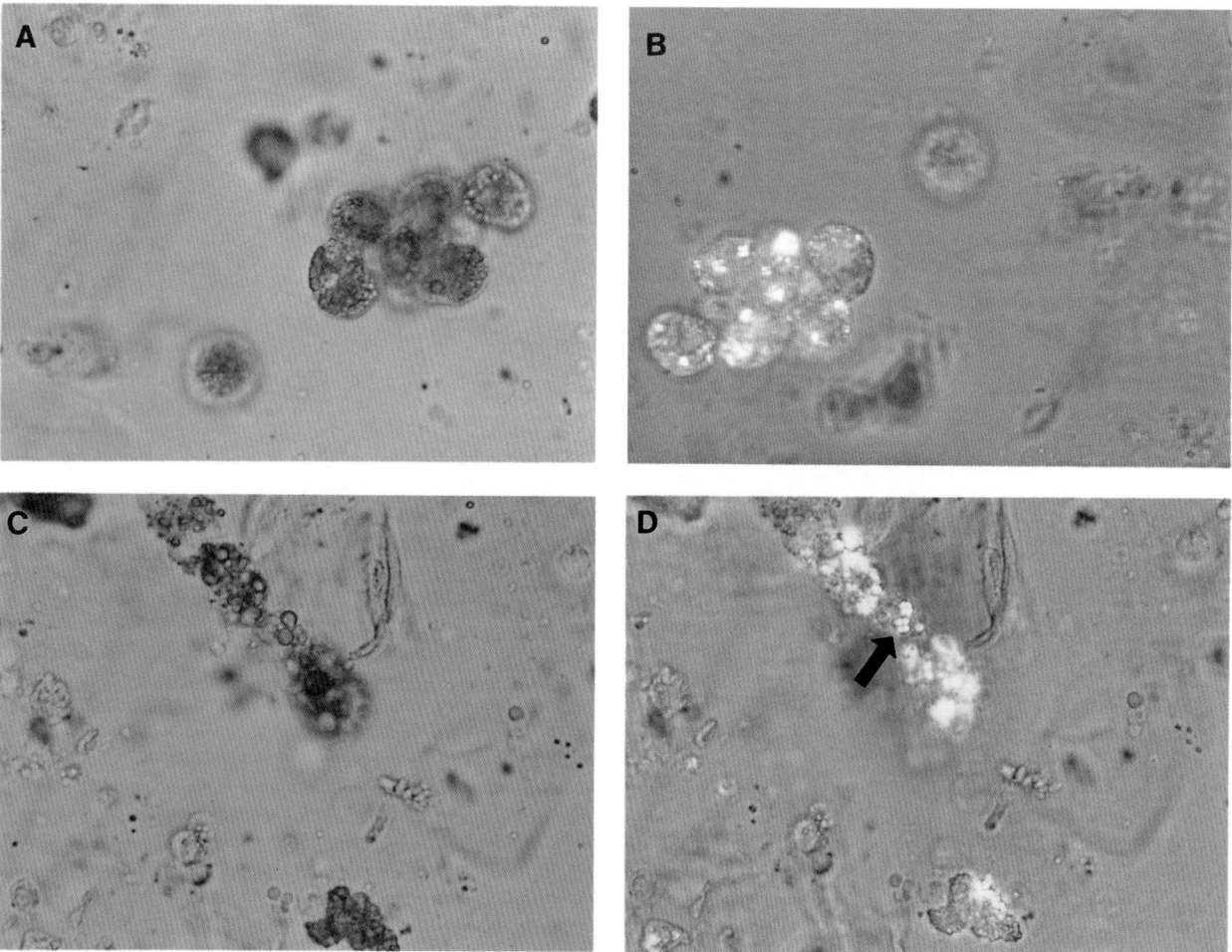

FIGURE 3 Lipid. (A) Oval fat bodies, bright field illumination. (B) Same field under polarized light. Characteristic Maltese cross shown at arrow. (C) Lipid-laden cast, bright field illumination. (D) Same field under polarized light. Characteristic Maltese cross shown at arrow.

tonic urine, they may be confused with swollen tubular epithelial cells.

Casts and Other Formed Elements

Casts are appropriately named. As demonstrated by immunofluorescence studies, they consist of a matrix of Tamm–Horsfall urinary mucoprotein in the shape of the distal tubular or collecting duct segment in which they were formed. The matrix has a straight margin helpful in differentiating casts from clumps of cells or debris.

Hyaline Casts

Hyaline casts consist of mucoprotein alone. Because their refractive index is very close to that of urine, they may be difficult to see, thus requiring subdued light and careful manipulation of the iris diaphragm. Hyaline casts are nonspecific. They occur in concentrated normal urine as well as numerous pathologic conditions (Fig. 2A).

Granular Casts

Granular casts consist of finely or coarsely granular material. Immunofluorescence studies show that fine granules derive from altered serum proteins. Coarse granules may result from degeneration of embedded cells. Granular casts are nonspecific but usually pathologic. They may be seen after exercise or with simple volume depletion and as a finding in ATN, glomerulonephritis, or tubulointerstitial disease (Figs. 2B and 2C).

Waxy Casts

Waxy casts or broad casts are made of hyaline material with a much higher refractive index than hyaline casts,

hence their waxy appearance. They behave as though they are more brittle than hyaline casts and frequently have fissures along their edge. Broad casts form in tubules that have become dilated and atrophic due to chronic parenchymal disease (Fig. 2C).

Red Blood Cell Casts

RBC casts indicate intraparenchymal bleeding. The hallmark of glomerulonephritis, they are less frequently seen with tubulointerstitial disease. RBC casts have been described along with hematuria in normal individuals after exercise. Fresh RBC casts retain their brown pigment and consist of readily discernible erythrocytes in a tubular-shaped cast matrix (Fig. 2D). Over time, the heme color is lost along with the distinct cellular outline. With further degeneration, RBC casts are hard to distinguish from coarsely granular casts. RBC casts may be diagnosed by the company they keep. They appear in a background of hematuria with dysmorphic red cells, granular casts, and proteinuria. Occasionally, the evidence for intraparenchymal bleeding is a hyaline cast with embedded red cells. These have the same pathophysiologic implication as RBC casts.

White Blood Cell Casts

WBC casts consist of white cells in a protein matrix. They are characteristic of pyelonephritis and are useful in distinguishing this disorder from lower tract infection. They may also be seen with interstitial nephritis and other tubulointerstitial disorders.

Tubular Cell Casts

These casts consist of a dense agglomeration of sloughed tubular cells or just a few tubular cells in a hyaline matrix.

TABLE 3
Common Urinary Crystals

Description	Composition	Comment
Crystals found in acid urine		
Amorphous	Uric acid	Cannot be distinguished from amorphous
	Sodium urate	phosphates except by urine pH, may be orange tinted by urochromes
Rhomboid prisms	Uric acid	
Rosettes	Uric acid	
Bipyramidal	Calcium oxalate	Also termed "envelope-shaped"
Dumbbell shaped	Calcium oxalate	
Needles	Uric acid, sulfa drugs, radiographic contrast	Clinical history provides useful confirmation. Sulfa may resemble sheaves of wheat; urate and contrast crystals are thicker.
Hexagonal plates	Cystine	Presence may be confirmed with nitroprusside test
Crystals found in alkaline urine		
Amorphous	Phosphates	Indistinguishable from urates except by pH
Coffin-lid (beveled rectangular prisms)	Triple (magnesium ammonium) phosphate	Seen with urea-splitting infection and bacteriuria
Granular masses or dumbbells	Calcium carbonate	Larger than amorphous phosphates
Yellow-brown masses with or without spicules	Ammonium biurate	

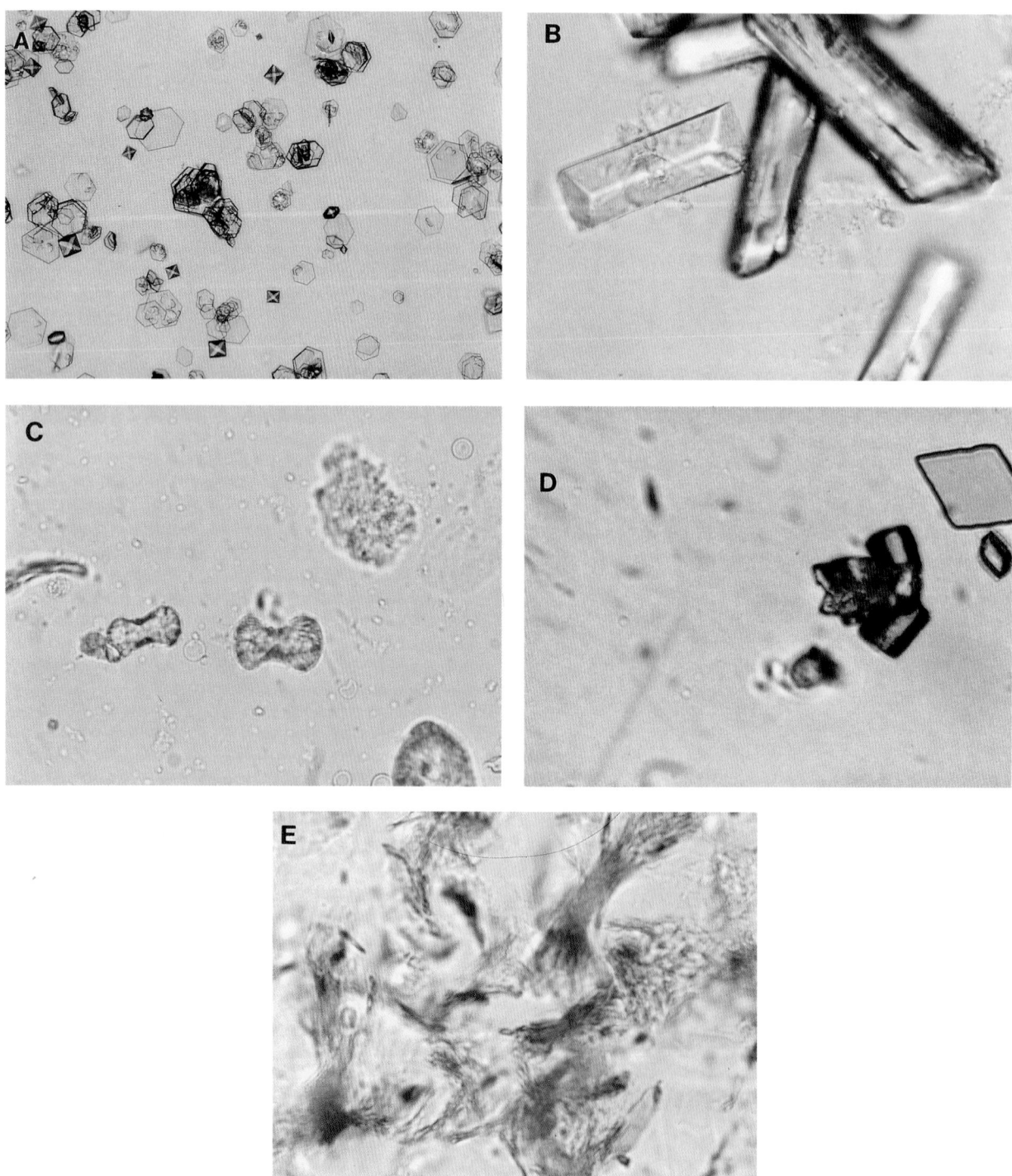

FIGURE 4 Crystals. (A) Hexagonal cystine and bipyramidal or "envelope-shaped" oxalate (arrows). Photo courtesy of Dr. Thomas O. Pitts. (B) "Coffin-lid"-shaped triple phosphate. (C) Dumbell-shaped oxalate. (D) Rhomboid urate. (E) Needle-shaped urate.

They occur in concentrated urine, but are more characteristically seen with the sloughing of tubular cells that occurs with ATN (Fig. 2E).

Bacteria, Yeast, and Other Infectious Agents

Bacillary or coccal forms of bacteria may be discerned even on an unstained urine. Examination of a gram stain preparation of unspun urine allows estimation of the bacterial count. One organism per HPF of unspun urine corresponds to 20,000 organisms/mm^3. Individual and budding yeasts and hyphal forms occur with candida infection or colonization. *Candida* organisms are similar in size to red cells but they are greenish spheres, not biconcave discs. When budding forms or hyphae are present, yeast are obvious (Fig. 1C). *Trichomonas* organisms are identified by their teardrop shape and motile flagellum.

Lipiduria

In the nephrotic syndrome with lipiduria, tubular cells reabsorb luminal fat. Sloughed tubular cells containing fat droplets are called oval fat bodies. Fatty casts contain lipid laden tubular cells or free lipid droplets. By light microscopy, lipid droplets appear round and clear with a green tinge. Cholesterol esters are anisotropic; cholesterol-containing droplets rotate polarized light, producing a Maltese cross appearance under polarized light. Triglycerides appear similar by light microscopy, but they are isotropic. Crystals, starch granules, mineral oil, and other urinary contaminants are also anisotropic. Before concluding that anisotropic structures are lipid, the observer must compare polarized and bright field views of the same object (Fig. 3).

Crystals

Crystals may be present spontaneously or precipitate with refrigeration of a specimen. They may be difficult to identify because of similar shapes; the common urinary crystals are described in Table 3. The pH is an important clue to identity, because solubility of a number of urinary constituents is pH dependent. The three most distinctive crystal forms are cystine, calcium oxalate, and magnesium ammonium (triple) phosphate. Cystine crystals are hexagonal plates resembling benzene rings. Calcium oxalate crystals are classically described as envelope shaped, but when viewed as they rotate in the urine under the microscope, they appear bipyramidal (Fig. 4A). "Coffin lid"-shaped triple phosphates are rectangular with beveled ends (Fig. 4B). Oxalate may also occur in dumbell-shaped crystals (Fig. 4C). Urate may have several forms, including rhomboids (Fig. 4D) or needles (Fig. 4E).

Characteristic Urine Sediments

The urine sediment is a rich source of diagnostic information. Occasionally, a single finding, e.g., cystine crystals, is pathognomonic. More often, the sediment must be considered as a whole and interpreted in conjunction with clinical and other laboratory findings. Several patterns bear emphasis.

In the acute nephritic syndrome, the urine may be pink or pale brown and turbid. Blood and moderate proteinuria are present by dipstick. The microscopic examination shows RBCs and RBC casts as well as granular and hyaline casts. WBC casts are rare. In the nephrotic syndrome, the urine is clear or yellow. Increased foaming may be noted because of the elevated protein content. In comparison to the sediment of nephritic patients, the nephrotic sediment is bland. Hyaline casts and lipiduria with oval fat bodies or lipid-laden casts predominate. Granular casts and a few tubular cells may also be present along with a few RBCs. With some forms of chronic glomerulonephritis, a telescoped sediment is observed. This term refers to the presence of the elements of a nephritic sediment together with broad or waxy casts indicative of tubular atrophy and dipstick findings of heavy proteinuria (Fig. 2C). In pyelonephritis, WBC casts and innumerable WBCs are present along with bacteria. In lower tract infection, WBC casts are absent. The sediment in ATN shows tubular cells, tubular cell casts, and muddy brown granular casts (Fig. 2B). The typical urinary findings in individual renal disorders are discussed in their respective chapters.

Bibliography

Birch DF, Fairley KF, Becker GJ, Kincaid-Smith P: *A Color Atlas of Urine Microscopy.* New York, Chapman & Hall, 1994.
Braden GL, Sanchez PG, Fitzgibbons JP, Stupak WJ, Germain MJ: Urinary doubly refractile lipid bodies in nonglomerular renal disease. *Am J Kidney Dis* 11:332–337, 1988.
Fairley KF, Birch DF: Hematuria: a simple method for identifying glomerular bleeding. *Kidney Int* 21:105–108, 1982.
Fassett RG, Owen JE, Fairley J, Birch DF, Fairley KF: Urinary red-cell morphology during exercise. *Br Med J* 285:1455–1457, 1982.
Graff L: *A Handbook of Routine Urinalysis.* Lippincott, Philadelphia, 1983.
Kincaid-Smith P: Haematuria and exercise-related haematuria. *Br Med J* 285:1595–1597, 1982.
McQueen EG: Composition of urinary casts. *Lancet* 2:397–398, 1966.
Raymond JR, Yarger WE: Abnormal urine color: differential diagnosis. *Southern Med J* 81:837–841, 1988.
Rutecki GJ, Goldsmith C, Schreiner GE: Characterization of proteins in urinary casts. Fluorescent-antibody identification of Tamm-Horsfall mucoprotein in matrix and serum proteins in granules. *N Engl J Med* 284:1049–1052, 1971.
Schumann GB, Harris S, Henry JB: An improved technique for examining urinary casts and a review of their significance. *Am J Clin Pathol* 69:18–23, 1978.
Schumann GB, Schweitzer SC: Examination of the urine. In: Henry JB (ed) *Clinical Diagnosis and Management by Laboratory Methods.* 18th ed. Saunders, Philadelphia, pp. 387–444, 1991.
Stamey TA, Kindrachuk RW: *Urinary Sediment and Urinalysis. A Practical Guide for the Health Professional.* Saunders, Philadelphia, 1985.
Voswinckel P: A marvel of colors and ingredients. The story of urine test strips. *Kidney Int* 46:S3–S7, 1994.
Zimmer JG, Dewey R, Waterhouse C, Terry R: The origin and nature of anisotropic urinary lipids in the nephrotic syndrome. *Ann Intern Med* 54:205–214, 1961.

4

HEMATURIA

CLIFFORD E. KASHTAN

INTRODUCTION

Hematuria, while potentially benign, is frequently a harbinger of disease in the kidneys or urinary tract. As such it requires the conscientious attention of the clinician. In this section the causes of hematuria will be reviewed, and an approach to its diagnostic evaluation presented. Differences between the pediatric and adult populations will be stressed, as will easily avoided pitfalls that may trap the unwary. The reader is encouraged to consult relevant chapters for detailed descriptions of the various entities mentioned herein.

EPIDEMIOLOGY

Hematuria, the presence of excessive numbers of red blood cells (RBCs) in the urine, may be *macroscopic (gross),* in which the urine is pink, red, or cola-colored, or *microscopic,* i.e., visible only with aid of a microscope. Normal individuals may excrete as many as 10^4 to 10^5 RBCs in the urine during a 12-hour period, corresponding to several RBCs in the sediment of a randomly collected, centrifuged urine specimen examined with a high-power objective. Thus, a working definition of hematuria is the presence of greater than 4 RBCs per high-power field (HPF) of urine sediment.

Studies of school children have indicated that the prevalence of microhematuria is high (about 4%). In the majority of children with a urine specimen showing microhematuria, follow-up urinalyses are normal, and these children do not develop urinary tract pathology. For this reason, in a child with isolated microhematuria, a second specimen should be obtained before an extensive evaluation.

Among an unselected population of adults over 35 years of age, the prevalence of asymptomatic microhematuria (>1 RBC/HPF of sediment) was found to be about 13%. The positive predictive value of microhematuria for serious urologic disease was low overall, being most useful in elderly men. As in the pediatric population, patients with excessive numbers of RBCs in several urine samples are more likely to have significant underlying urinary tract pathology.

The causes of hematuria (Tables 1 to 3) are age-dependent. Although glomerular causes predominate in children and young adults, fewer than 5% of cases of hematuria in patients over 40 years of age result from glomerular lesions.

Neoplasms of the urinary tract account for 15 to 20% of patients with hematuria after 40 years of age, and approximately two-thirds of these are carcinomas of the bladder. In children, the neoplastic disorders that cause hematuria are Wilms tumors and rhabdomyosarcomas of the bladder, and make up only a small fraction of cases of hematuria. However, because early recognition and treatment of Wilms tumor result in excellent outcomes, prompt imaging of the upper urinary tract is imperative in the child younger than 3 years of age with hematuria. Urinary tract calculi are a common cause of hematuria in adults. While calculi may cause hematuria in children, their incidence is low except in certain defined populations (see below). The neonate with hematuria is much more likely to have renal vein thrombosis or renal cortical infarction (associated with umbilical arterial catheters) than are older children or adults. Urinary tract infection (UTI) is a frequent cause of hematuria in children and adults, with prostate disease being particularly important in older males.

The epidemiologic characteristics of hematuria clearly affect the approach to evaluation. Although the yield from cystoscopy is relatively high in the adult patient with hematuria, cystoscopy is rarely indicated in the child. Children with hematuria should be evaluated by a pediatrician or nephrologist, with referral to a urologist if initial evaluation suggests cystoscopy will aid in localizing the source of hematuria.

It should be recalled that urine dipsticks identify myoglobin and filtered free hemoglobin as well as hemoglobin released by RBCs undergoing lysis on the reagent strip (see Chapter 3). For this reason, dipsticks may be used to screen patients for hematuria but results need to be validated by microscopic examination of the urine. Similarly, a variety of synthetic and natural products can alter the appearance of the urine, and urine microscopy will quickly determine whether the change in color is due to the presence of RBCs. In infants, urates can cause brownish diaper stains that may be mistaken for hematuria.

EVALUATION (Fig. 1)

Level I: History, Physical Examination, and Urinalysis (Table 4)

The initial evaluation of the patient with hematuria consists of a careful history and physical examination,

TABLE 1
Hematuria: Glomerular Causes

Proliferative glomerulonephritis
  Primary
    IgA nephropathy
    Postinfectious glomerulonephritis
    Membranoproliferative glomerulonephritis
    Idiopathic rapidly progressive (crescentic)
      glomerulonephritis
    Fibrillary glomerulonephritis
  Secondary (associated with systemic diseases)
    Nephritis of anaphylactoid (Henoch-Schönlein) purpura
    Systemic lupus erythematosus
    Antiglomerular basement membrane nephritis (including
      Goodpasture syndrome)
    Systemic vasculitis
    Chronic bacteremia (subacute bacterial endocarditis,
      "shunt nephritis")
    Essential mixed cryoglobulinemia
    Nephritis associated with hepatitis B or C
Nonproliferative glomerulopathies
  Minimal change nephrotic syndrome
  Focal (global or segmental) glomerulosclerosis
  Membranous nephropathy
  Hemolytic uremic syndrome
Familial glomerular diseases
  Alport syndrome
  Thin glomerular basement membrane disease ("benign"
    familial hematuria)
  Fabry disease
  Nail-patella syndrome

TABLE 2
Hematuria: Nonglomerular Renal Causes

Neoplasms	Renal cell carcinoma
	Wilms tumor
	Benign cysts
	Angiomyolipoma (tuberous sclerosis)
	Multiple myeloma
Vascular	Renal infarct
	Renal vein thrombosis
	Malignant hypertension
	Arteriovenous malformation
	Loin-pain hematuria syndrome
Metabolic	Hypercalciuria
	Idiopathic
	Hyperparathyroidism
	Hyperoxaluria
	Hyperuricosuria
	Cystinuria
Familial	Polycystic kidney disease (autosomal dominant)
	Medullary cystic disease/familial juvenile nephronophthisis
	Medullary sponge kidney
Papillary necrosis	Analgesic abuse
	Sickle cell disease and trait
	Renal tuberculosis
	Diabetes mellitus
	Obstructive uropathy
	Alcoholism
	Ankylosing spondylitis
Hydronephrosis	Any cause
Drugs	Drug-induced acute interstitial nephritis (especially semisynthetic penicillins)
Trauma	Renal contusion or laceration
	Exercise-induced hematuria

as well as analysis of the urine. It is the aim of the history and physical to establish whether the hematuria is isolated or associated with findings that may indicate its origin and the likelihood that it represents significant urinary tract disease.

History

Increased frequency of urination and dysuria (pain or burning with urination) often accompany UTI. Hesitancy (difficulty in initiating the urine stream), a weak stream, and dribbling are suggestive of bladder obstruction from a calculus, tumor, or enlarged prostate. Loin pain is associated with the loin-pain hematuria syndrome, while colicky flank pain that radiates into the groin is a frequent complaint in patients with a ureteral calculus and in some patients with papillary necrosis. Arthralgia/arthritis and rashes suggest a systemic inflammatory disorder such as anaphylactoid (Henoch-Schönlein) purpura (in which crampy abdominal pain and melena may also be present), systemic lupus erythematosus (SLE) or systemic vasculitis. Hematuria following a prodrome of bloody diarrhea suggests the hemolytic-uremic syndrome. A history of pharyngitis or skin infection 1 to 2 weeks prior to the onset of gross hematuria suggests poststreptococcal glomerulonephritis. Hematuria may occur in patients with an inherited or drug-induced coagulopathy, but is rarely the presenting complaint. A history of deafness may be present in the patient

with Alport syndrome (hereditary nephritis), as may a family history of hematuria, renal failure, or deafness. Because transient (24 to 48 hours) hematuria may be seen in individuals who exert themselves strenuously (exercise-induced hematuria), a history of exercise and physical activity should be obtained. Travel to tropical areas may expose an individual to *Schistosoma haematobium*. Children from some areas of Southeast Asia are prone to the development of calcium oxalate stones of the urinary tract, perhaps due to dietary factors. A family history of urinary tract stones should also be sought.

In the patient referred for evaluation of hematuria, characterization of the pattern of hematuria is useful. Patients with persistent microhematuria *and* episodic gross hematuria frequently have glomerular disease, while those with intermittent or continuous asymptomatic microhematuria, or episodic gross hematuria with complete clearing of the urine between episodes, are less likely to have significant renal pathology. Episodic gross hematuria provoked by mild upper respiratory infections is not unusual in patients with glomerular disease, particularly IgA nephropathy.

TABLE 3
Hematuria: Extrarenal Causes

Calculi	Ureter, bladder, prostate
Neoplasms	Transitional cell carcinoma (renal pelvis, ureter, bladder)
	Adenocarcinoma, benign hypertrophy (prostate)
	Squamous cell carcinoma (urethra)
Infections	Acute cystitis, prostatitis, urethritis
	Bacterial
	Chlamydia trachomatis
	Tuberculosis
	Schistosomiasis
Drugs	Cyclophosphamide (hemorrhagic cystitis)
	Anticoagulants (heparin, coumadin)
Trauma	Contusion or laceration
	Exercise-induced hematuria
	Foreign body of urethra or bladder
	Decompression of severely distended bladder
Genital or anal bleeding	Vulvovaginitis
	Vaginal foreign body
	Anal fissure

Brown or cola-colored urine suggests hematuria arising in the kidney, while pink or red urine suggests extrarenal hematuria. Blood clots usually, but not invariably, indicate bleeding from an extrarenal source.

Physical Examination

Elevated blood pressure and/or peripheral edema in the patient with hematuria indicates glomerular pathology. A rash may accompany anaphylactoid purpura nephritis, systemic vasculitis, mixed cryoglobulinemia, or SLE. Swollen, inflamed joints in hematuric patients suggest anaphylactoid purpura nephritis, SLE, vasculitis, or cryoglobulinemia.

RBCs arising in the vagina or vulva may mix with urine in girls with vulvovaginitis or a vaginal foreign body, or girls who have been the victims of sexual abuse, giving the appearance of hematuria. Similarly, bleeding from an anal fissure can present as apparent hematuria in children who wear diapers. Prostatitis, benign prostatic hypertrophy (BPH) and carcinoma of the prostate, each of which may be associated with hematuria, can be detected by rectal examination. Because BPH is such a frequent finding in elderly men, it should not be assumed to be the cause of hematuria until other causes are excluded. In adolescents and adults with hematuria, sexually transmitted diseases (STDs) need to be considered. Examination of the penis or vulva for discharge may be indicated.

Urinalysis

Proteinuria accompanying hematuria strongly indicates glomerular disease. Proteinuria may be detected by dipstick (1+ or greater) or timed collection (greater than 4 mg · $m^{-2} \cdot h^{-1}$ in the child and 150 mg/24 h in the adult). In the patient with hematuria and proteinuria, evaluation should start with the glomerular causes of hematuria (Table 1).

Patients with gross hematuria may excrete up to 500 mg protein/24 h, due to the blood in the urine. Like proteinuria, RBC casts are indicative of glomerular disease, but are more difficult to document. Pyuria (the presence of white blood cells in the urine) is frequently present in patients with UTI or STD. Crystals with typical morphologic characteristics are frequently visible in the urine of patients with hematuria due to calculi composed of cystine or oxalate.

Some clinicians employ phase-contrast microscopy of the urine to assess RBC morphology. The presence of dysmorphic RBCs suggests renal parenchymal disease, while their absence indicates bleeding from an extrarenal site (see Chapter 3).

Level II: Other Studies

A patient's history, physical examination, and urinalysis will often provide the clinician with a strong suspicion regarding the origin of the hematuria. This suspicion will direct the ensuing evaluation, leading to the correct diagnosis quickly while avoiding unnecessary procedures.

Glomerular Hematuria (Table 1)

As noted above, the presence of proteinuria and/or RBC casts in the patient with hematuria indicates glomerular disease. Similarly, persistent microhematuria with episodic gross hematuria suggests a glomerular process. While renal biopsy is the definitive diagnostic procedure in this clinical situation, it is not without risk and should be reserved for select patients.

Once hematuria has been localized to the glomerulus, levels of serum complement, antistreptococcal antibodies, antinuclear antibodies, creatinine, and blood urea nitrogen (BUN) should be measured. Other blood studies should be obtained in selected patients, e.g., antineutrophil cytoplasmic antibodies in patients suspected of systemic vasculitis; antiglomerular basement membrane antibodies in patients with a rapidly progressive acute nephritic syndrome, with or without pulmonary hemorrhage; and cryoglobulins when mixed cryoglobulinemia is suspected.

A negative family history for renal disease or hematuria does not rule out a diagnosis of hereditary nephropathy, such as Alport syndrome, thin glomerular basement membrane disease (also known, somewhat misleadingly, as benign familial hematuria), or autosomal dominant polycystic kidney disease, because some patients with these diseases represent new mutations or the offspring of asymptomatic disease carriers. Complete evaluation of the family of a patient with hematuria requires obtaining urinalyses on all accessible family members. Patients suspected of having Alport syndrome should undergo audiologic examination and ophthalmologic evaluation, since certain ocular abnormalities (anterior lenticonus, yellowish perimacular flecks, posterior polymorphous dystrophy) are diagnostic or very suggestive of this disease.

Poststreptococcal glomerulonephritis remains an important cause of the acute nephritic syndrome (hematuria and two or more of the following: proteinuria, edema, hy-

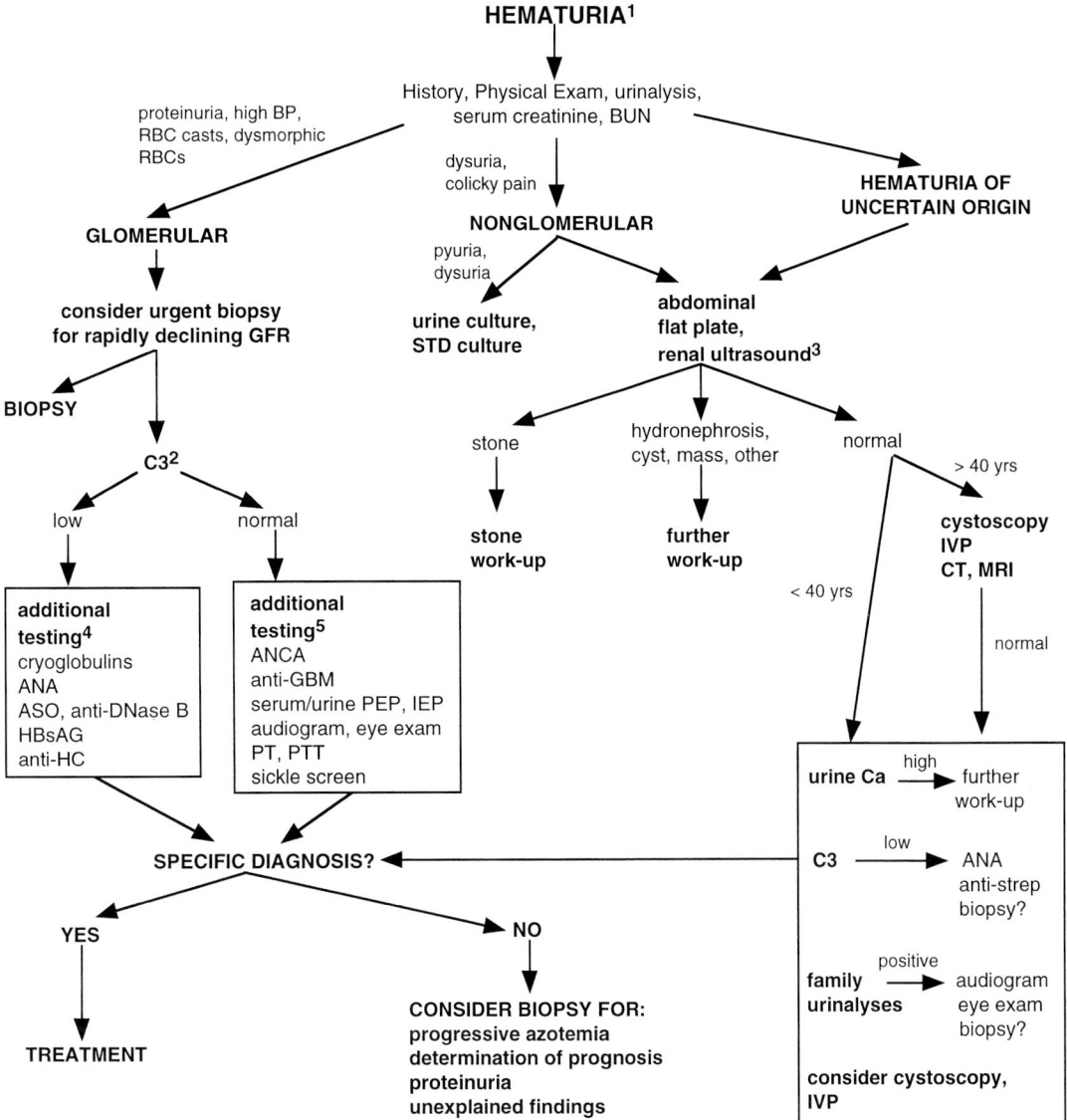

FIGURE I   (1) This algorithm's design is based on two questions: (a) Is the hematuria glomerular or nonglomerular? (b) Given the patient's age, what conditions must be promptly identified/excluded [e.g., Wilms tumor in child <3 yr, urinary tract malignancy in adult >40 yr, rapidly progressive glomerulonephritis (RPGN)]? (2) In practice, C3, antinuclear antibodies (ANA), and antistrep antibodies are often obtained at presentation. (3) This is the first imaging test to obtain in the child <3 yr. (4) Nonstreptococcal infections may provoke a proliferative glomerulonephritis (GN) similar to poststreptococcal disease. Biopsy may not be needed in the patient with typical features of postinfectious GN if C3 and urinalysis normalize appropriately. Some patients with low C3 and positive antistrep antibodies have features atypical of poststreptococcal GN (e.g., nephrotic syndrome, progressive azotemia) and need a biopsy to confirm the diagnosis. Biopsy is indicated in patients with systemic lupus erythematosus and evidence of clinically significant GN, in order to establish the type and severity of lupus nephritis. Children with features typical of anaphylactoid purpura usually do not need a biopsy unless they have nephrotic-range proteinuria or reduced creatinine clearance. (5) These studies are indicated in selected patients, e.g., anti-GBM antibodies in the patient with RPGN or pulmonary hemorrhage, ANCA and CRP in patients with suspected vasculitis, serum/urine protein and immunoelectrophoresis for suspected multiple myeloma, audiogram and eye exam for suspected Alport syndrome.

pertension, and reduced glomerular filtration rate). Kidney biopsy is usually not indicated in the patient with acute nephritic syndrome, hypocomplementemia, and evidence of recent streptococcal infection. Kidney biopsy *is* usually indicated in the patient with the acute nephritic syndrome who does not have evidence of streptococcal infection or hypocomplementemia, and in the great majority of patients in whom hematuria is accompanied by proteinuria. In pa-

TABLE 4
Hematuria: Initial Evaluation

History	Frequency, hesitancy	Bleeding tendency
	Force of stream	Deafness
	Dysuria	Family history
	Loin pain	Exercise history
	Renal colic	Travel history
	Arthralgia	Medications
	Rash	
Physical	Blood pressure	Flank mass
	Edema	Genital or anal bleeding
	Rash	Deafness
	Purpura	Prostatic enlargement or
	Arthritis	tenderness
Urine	Proteinuria	Bacteriuria
	Casts	Crystals
	Pyuria	

tients with isolated hematuria, the clinical utility of kidney biopsy must be considered on a case-by-case basis. Diagnostic accuracy requires the performance of immunofluorescence and electron microscopy as well as light microscopy on all renal biopsy specimens from patients with glomerular hematuria.

Up to 20% of children with steroid-responsive, minimal change nephrotic syndrome present with microscopic hematuria. Therefore, the presence of hematuria in the child of appropriate age (6 months to 6 years) with nephrotic syndrome should not change the initial approach (a trial of oral prednisone).

Nonglomerular Hematuria (Tables 2 and 3)

The history, physical examination, and urinalysis may suggest the likely source of bleeding in the patient with isolated hematuria and may direct the subsequent evaluation. For example, a history of renal colic suggests a urinary tract calculus. Since more than 90% of calculi contain calcium, most will be revealed by a plain film of the abdomen. Intravenous pyelography (IVP) may be used to precisely localize radiopaque stones in the urinary tract, or to discover radiolucent calculi. Suspicion of a urinary tract calculus should increase if the patient has a history of diffuse bowel disease or bowel resection (secondary hyperoxaluria) or a family history of urolithiasis (see Chapter 56).

The presence of pyuria, with or without dysuria, suggests UTI or STD. In the patient with suspected UTI, a sterilely collected urine specimen should be sent for routine bacterial culture and expectant antibiotic therapy should be initiated. Specific cultures for agents causing STD (e.g., chlamydia, *Neisseria gonorrhea*) may be indicated.

Individuals of African ancestry with hematuria should be evaluated for sickle hemoglobinopathy, which accounts for about one-third of cases of hematuria in this population. Sickle cell trait frequently first presents as hematuria (see Chapter 44).

Loin pain-hematuria syndrome is characterized by recurrent episodes of loin/lumbar pain, which is usually unilat-

eral and may be quite severe, associated with gross or microscopic hematuria. Most patients are women, 20 to 40 years of age. Renal biopsy findings are essentially normal, while renal angiographic findings are variable.

The medication history may be revealing in patients with hematuria. Administration of oral or intravenous cyclophosphamide may be associated with hemorrhagic cystitis, ureteritis, and pyelitis, either acutely or as a late event. This complication of cyclophosphamide therapy is seen most commonly now in patients undergoing bone marrow transplantation, but may also complicate treatment of systemic vasculitis and SLE. Diagnosis of hemorrhagic cystitis is made by cystoscopy. Certain drugs, especially the semisynthetic penicillins, may produce acute interstitial nephritis; pyuria and acute renal failure are the two main features, but hematuria may also be observed (Chapter 40). Diagnosis of this condition may require renal biopsy. The long-term, excessive use of phenacetin- or acetaminophen-containing analgesics may result in analgesic-abuse nephropathy, one manifestation of which may be hematuria due to papillary necrosis. Patients with diabetes mellitus or urinary tract obstruction are also susceptible to papillary necrosis (see Chapter 53). Chronic administration of furosemide to premature infants with bronchopulmonary dysplasia may be associated with urolithiasis.

When the history, physical examination, and urinalysis provide no clues to the origin of hematuria, a renal ultrasound serves as a useful screening procedure. Kidneys that are hydronephrotic for any reason may bleed after minimal trauma. Autosomal dominant polycystic kidney disease can usually be diagnosed by ultrasound by the third decade of life. Renal ultrasound will also identify simple renal cysts which, in the absence of other causes, may be the source of hematuria. Some renal tumors will be visible by ultrasound. Renal vein thrombosis often produces substantial renal enlargement; this condition should be suspected in the neonate with hematuria, or the nephrotic patient who presents with the new onset of gross hematuria and unilateral flank pain. Renal ultrasound will also frequently identify the patient with nephrocalcinosis, although care must be taken in the interpretation of hyperechoic renal pyramids in the neonate.

Further evaluation when history, physical examination, urinalysis, and renal ultrasound fail to provide a diagnosis depends heavily on the age of the patient. Because of the higher incidence of urinary tract malignancy in older individuals, patients over 40 years of age should undergo intravenous pyelography (see Chapter 6) and cystoscopy, and urinary cytology should be performed. These studies have a lower yield in younger patients, in whom urinary tract malignancies are infrequent. However, prompt imaging by ultrasound is mandatory in children younger than 3 years with hematuria, in order to detect Wilms tumor. Renal ultrasound will also detect renal vein thrombosis or hydronephrosis in the neonate with hematuria.

In children and young adults, asymptomatic gross or microscopic hematuria is frequently due to idiopathic hypercalciuria. This condition may be associated with hematuria in the absence of any radiographically detectable calculi, although the risk of developing a stone is high. There is frequently a family history of urolithiasis. Idiopathic hypercalciuria may reflect excessive intestinal uptake of calcium (absorptive hypercalciuria) or insufficient tubular reabsorption of calcium (renal hypercalciuria). Hypercalciuria is present when the urinary calcium excretion is greater than 4 mg $\cdot$ kg^{-1} $\cdot$ day^{-1} (0.1 mmol $\cdot$ kg^{-1} $\cdot$ day^{-1}).

Renal biopsy should be considered in the patient with persistent microhematuria (>6 to 12 months) in whom other evaluations are unrevealing. A variety of glomerular disorders, including many of those listed in Table 2, may present as isolated hematuria. The degree of parental or patient anxiety may influence the timing of biopsy in these cases.

On occasion, hematuria occurs secondary to a vascular anomaly, such as arteriovenous fistula, hemangioma, or varices of the kidney or ureter. Renal arteriography may be revealing in such cases. The yield of renal arteriography is probably highest when cystoscopy documents unilateral upper urinary tract bleeding in a patient with a normal renal ultrasound and CT scan.

Bibliography

Andres A, Praga M, Bello I, Diaz-Rolón JA, Gutierrez-Millet V, Morales JM, Rodicio JL: Hematuria due to hypercalciuria and hyperuricosuria in adult patients. *Kidney Int* 36:96–99, 1989.

Blumenthal SS, Fritsche C, Lemann J: Establishing the diagnosis of benign familial hematuria: The importance of examining the urine sediment of family members. *JAMA* 259:2263–2266, 1988.

Burden RP, Dathan JR, Etherington MD, Guyer PB, MacIver AG: The loin-pain/hematuria syndrome. *Lancet* 1:897–900, 1979.

Copley JB: Isolated asymptomatic hematuria in the adult. *Am J Med Sci* 291:101–111, 1986.

Copley JB, Hasbasrgen JA: "Idiopathic" hematuria: A prospective evaluation. *Arch Intern Med* 147:434–437, 1987.

Dodge WF, West EF, Smith EH, Bunce H: Proteinuria and hematuria in schoolchildren: epidemiology and early natural history. *J Pediatr* 88:327–347, 1976.

Fairley KF, Birch DF. Hematuria: a simple method for identifying glomerular bleeding. *Kidney Int* 21:105–108, 1982.

Froom P, Ribak J, Benbassat J. Significance of microhaematuria in young adults. *Br Med J* 288:20–22, 1984.

Garcia CD, Miller LA, Stapleton FB. Natural history of hematuria associated with hypercalciuria in children. *Am J Dis Child* 145:1204–1207, 1991.

Hayashi M, Kume T, Nihira H: Abnormalities of renal venous system and unexplained renal hematuria. *J Urol* 124:12–16, 1979.

Ingelfinger JR, Davis AE, Grupe WE: Frequency and etiology of gross hematuria in a general pediatric setting. *Pediatrics* 59:557–561, 1977.

Jones DJ, Langstaff RJ, Holt SD, Morgans BT: The value of cystourethroscopy in the investigation of microscopic haematuria in adult males under 40 years: A prospective study of 100 patients. *Br J Urol* 62:541–545, 1988.

Mohr DN, Offord KP, Owen RA, Melton LJ: Asymptomatic microhematuria and urologic disease: A population-based study. *JAMA* 256:224–229, 1986.

Schuster GA, Lewis GA: Clinical significance of hematuria in patients on anti-coagulant therapy. *J Urol* 137:923–925, 1987.

Siegel AJ, Hennekens CH, Solomon HS, Boeckel BV: Exercise-related hematuria: Findings in a group of marathon runners. *JAMA* 241:391–392, 1979.

Tiebosch ATMG, Frederick PM, van Breda Vriesman PJC, et al: Thin-basement-membrane nephropathy in adults with persistent hematuria. *N Engl J Med* 320:14–18, 1989.

Trachtman H, Weiss RA, Bennett B, Griefer I: Isolated hematuria in children: Indications for a renal biopsy. *Kidney Int* 25:94–99, 1984.

Vehaskari VM, Rapola J, Koskimies O, Savilahti E, Vilska J, Hallman N: Microscopic hematuria in schoolchildren: Epidemiology and clinicopathologic evaluation. *J Pediatr* 95:676–684, 1979.

5

PROTEINURIA

SHARON ANDERSON

Proteinuria characterizes almost every form of glomerular disease and contributes to all of the complications of the nephrotic syndrome. Indeed, proteinuria or one of its complications is often the first indication that renal disease is present.

RENAL PROTEIN HANDLING

To understand the pathogenesis of proteinuria, it is first important to review the handling of protein by the normal kidney. There are three major components of proteinuria. The first is the amount of protein being presented to the glomerular capillary (the filtered load), which is dependent both on the protein concentration in the plasma and on the glomerular filtration rate (GFR). The second major determinant relates to permeability (ability to traverse the glomerular capillary barrier), which is dependent both on the integrity of the glomerular capillary wall and on specific attributes of the particular protein molecule. The glomerular capillary barrier normally presents a formidable barrier to protein. The glomerular capillary wall consists of three layers (Fig. 1): the fenestrated endothelium, the glomerular basement membrane (GBM), and the epithelial cells which are attached to the basement membrane by foot processes. The primary barrier to filtration is the GBM.

Experiments using test macromolecules, such as dextran, have shown that factors determining the ability of a given protein molecule to pass through the GBM are molecular size, charge, and shape. The glomerular capillary wall is highly permeable to small solutes and water, but limits passage of larger molecules. Inulin (MW 5200, 16 Å) is completely filtered, while albumin (MW 69,000, 36 Å) is filtered only to a small degree. Below MW 60,000, there is a progressive increase in filtration. The inverse relationship between molecular size and degree of filtration suggests that "pores" (functional, not structural) may exist within the GBM through which only molecules of a certain size may pass. Molecular charge is another important determinant. Anionic dextrans are filtered to a very limited degree; by comparison, filtration of neutral and cationic dextrans is much higher. The glomerular capillary wall contains sialoproteins and proteoglycans (such as heparan sulfate) that are negatively charged. Most circulating macromolecules are anionic within the physiologic pH range. Thus, filtration of albumin and other macromolecules is limited in part by electrostatic repulsion. Though molecular shape also appears to be important, less is known about this parameter.

Finally, the third component is the proximal tubule. Some proteins are in fact filtered, but are then catabolized and reabsorbed in the proximal tubule. Thus, the amount of protein in the urine depends on how much gets there, how well it passes through the glomerular barrier, and whether or not the proximal tubule degrades it if the protein does get into the glomerular filtrate.

CLINICAL PROTEINURIA: DEFINITION AND MEASUREMENT

In normal kidneys, low-molecular-weight proteins and small amounts of albumin (about 500 to 1500 mg/day) are filtered. These proteins enter the proximal tubule, where they are almost completely reabsorbed and catabolized by proximal tubular cells. The net result is daily protein excretion of about 40 to 80 mg. Of this amount, about 30 to 50 mg consists of Tamm-Horsfall protein, a mucoprotein secreted by tubular cells in the thick ascending loop of Henle. Abnormal proteinuria is defined as excretion of >150 mg/day.

Presence or absence of abnormal proteinuria is first detected by dipstick, which is read as 0 to 4+, corresponding to concentrations of 0 to >500 mg/dL. The most accurate quantitation is performed on a 24-hour urine collection. For this purpose, urinary protein concentration (mg/dL) is determined [for example, by precipitation with sulfosalicylic acid (SSA)], and then multiplied by total volume (dL/day) to obtain 24-hour protein excretion (in mg/day). In most situations, the results obtained with dipstick and with quantitative methods correlate fairly well. However, there is one important clinical situation in which the two methods differ. The dipstick is most sensitive to albumin, whereas quantitative methods detect all proteins. The dipstick may be negative when low-molecular-weight proteins, rather than albumin, are present in the urine. This occurs in certain tubular diseases, where proximal tubule catabolism of filtered proteins is impaired; or in diseases where there is excessive production and filtration of low-molecular-weight proteins, exceeding the proximal tubule's capacity to catabolize filtered proteins. The most important clinical example of this situation is multiple myeloma; the urine may contain large amounts of protein (detectable by quan-

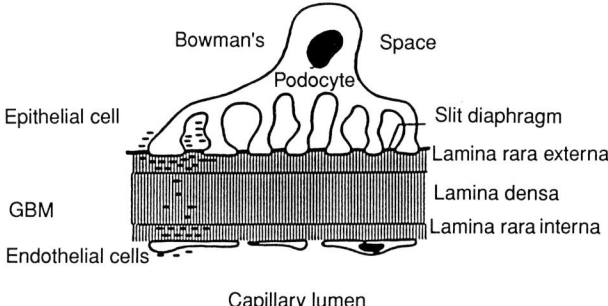

FIGURE 1   The glomerular barrier consists of the capillary endothelium, glomerular basement membrane, and glomerular epithelial cell.

titative methods) and yet be negative or only trace positive by dipstick. Such a condition should be suspected when the amount of protein determined quantitatively is disproportionately elevated, compared to the dipstick element. The diagnosis may be confirmed by urinary and serum electrophoreses, as described below.

An convenient alternative to 24-hour urine collection is to compare the concentrations (in mg/dL) of protein and creatinine (U_{prot}/U_{Cr} ratio) on a random spot urine specimen. Since urinary creatinine excretion is relatively constant (20 to 25 $mg \cdot kg^{-1} \cdot day^{-1}$ for men, 15 to 20 for women) an increase in the ratio indicates an increase in urinary protein excretion. The urinary protein/creatinine ratio is a fairly accurate estimate of total daily protein excretion and can be useful when used serially in a given patient. The normal ratio is <0.2 (less than 200 mg/day); values of 1.0 and 3.5 represent total protein excretion of 1.0 and 3.5 g/day, respectively.

Recently, it has been recognized that diabetes, essential hypertension, and some other diseases may manifest "microalbuminuria," which is defined as daily urinary albumin excretion of 30 to 300 mg/day. This level of albuminuria is above the normal range, yet below the limits of detectability by dipstick. Microalbuminuria is thought to be the earliest sign of nephropathy in Type I diabetes mellitus, and a powerful predictor of cardiovascular risk in Types I and II diabetes and other conditions. Microalbuminuria can be detected using sensitive laboratory techniques, when specifically requested. It is recommended that patients with Type I diabetes be screened annually, starting at 5 to 10 years after diagnosis of diabetes. Patients with Type II diabetes should be screened at the time of diagnosis, and then annually thereafter. While a 24-hour urine collection remains the gold standard, many clinicians have opted for the more easily obtainable spot urine microalbumin/creatinine ratio, with a value ≥30 μg albumin/mg creatinine representing clinical microalbuminuria. (See Chapter 29.)

MECHANISMS OF PROTEINURIA

Proteinuria can be usefully classified according to four major mechanisms: (1) functional proteinuria, (2) overpro-

duction (prerenal) proteinuria, (3) glomerular proteinuria, and (4) tubular proteinuria.

Functional proteinuria is the term used for a transient increase in protein excretion which occurs in various physiologic and experimental situations, in the absence of renal disease. For example, fever, emotional stress, acute medical illness, and infusions of norepinephrine or angiotensin II can all cause significant but transient increases in urinary protein excretion. Urinary protein excretion is increased two- to threefold during and immediately after heavy exercise. The mechanism for these forms of proteinuria most likely relates to glomerular hemodynamic changes, or possibly to changes in glomerular pore size, rather than to alterations in the GBM.

Some normal subjects also exhibit "orthostatic proteinuria," defined as protein excretion which is abnormally elevated in the upright position, but normal with recumbency. This benign condition is found in 2 to 5% of adolescents, but only rarely over the age of 30 years. Orthostatic proteinuria is usually less than 1 g/day and may be detected using split (16-hour day, 8-hour night) urine collections. Patients with postural or orthostatic proteinuria will have increased excretion while upright, and a normal level (<150 mg/day when extrapolated to 24 hours) in the recumbent specimen. If protein excretion is increased in both specimens, the patient is considered to have persistent, rather than orthostatic, proteinuria.

Overproduction (prerenal) proteinuria occurs when there is an increased plasma concentration of one or more filterable proteins, thereby increasing the filtered protein load, thus increasing excretion. There may be enhanced excretion of heavy chains, light chains, or other immunoglobulin fragments. The differential diagnosis includes Bence Jones proteinuria, myoglobinuria, hemoglobinuria, lysozymuria (myelomonocytic leukemias), and β_2-microglobulinuria (neoplasia).

Glomerular loss of proteins may result from several different mechanisms. The most important are: (1) loss of the negative charges in the GBM; (2) an increase in effective pore size or number, due to direct damage to the GBM or change in GBM structure due to loss of anionic proteins; or (3) disease-related changes in glomerular hemodynamics, particularly glomerular capillary pressure (P_{GC}). Studies in various experimental models have confirmed that diseases such as glomerulonephritis may be associated with abnormalities in the synthesis, composition, and negative charge density of the GBM, including changes in heparan sulfate content or incorporation into the GBM.

Hemodynamic factors also influence the ultrafiltration of macromolecules. Infusion of vasoactive hormones such as angiotensin II and norepinephrine, which increase P_{GC}, increase proteinuria in experimental animals. In addition, glomerular diseases which are characterized by glomerular capillary hypertension (increased P_{GC}) are regularly associated with proteinuria, while pharmacologic or dietary maneuvers like ACE inhibition or protein restriction that reduce P_{GC} reduce proteinuria.

The differential diagnosis of glomerular proteinuria includes all glomerular diseases (e.g., focal glomerulonephritis, poststreptococcal glomerulonephritis, minimal change disease, focal sclerosis, membranous glomerulonephritis, diabetic nephropathy).

Tubular proteinuria occurs when there is impaired tubular reabsorption of normally filtered proteins. The differential diagnosis includes hereditary diseases (e.g., Wilson's disease), toxic injury (cadmium, lead, gentamicin), metabolic causes (hypokalemia), Fanconi syndrome, chronic interstitial nephritis, and miscellaneous other causes (diuretic phase of acute tubular necrosis and amylase excretion in acute pancreatitis).

LABORATORY EVALUATION OF PROTEINURIA

Proteinuria is usually first detected by dipstick on a routine screening urinalysis. In occasional patients, proteinuria will be intermittent (present on some urinalyses, but not on others). This pattern may represent any of a number of minor glomerular or tubular lesions, and prognosis is often favorable if the patient does not progress to persistent proteinuria. Once proteinuria is persistent, further evaluation is indicated.

The next step is to quantify the amount. In general, >3 g/day is virtually always glomerular. Proteinuria <3 g/day is nondiagnostic and could represent a prerenal, glomerular, or tubular origin. If the origin of the proteinuria is unclear, the source of the urinary protein may next be evaluated by urine protein electrophoresis (Fig. 2). If the protein is >70% albumin, the source is glomerular. A tubular source will cause excretion of globulins more than albumin, with multiple peaks (representing a number of different proteins). A prerenal source usually reveals a single globulin peak, representing the protein whose plasma concentration is unusually high.

Once the origin of the proteinuria (prerenal, glomerular, or tubular) is determined, subsequent evaluation can begin.

For prerenal sources, the next steps may include a serum protein electrophoresis and/or serum and urine immunoelectrophoreses to further characterize the individual protein being excreted. The diagnosis can then usually be made, for example, by bone marrow or lymph node biopsy; further renal evaluation may not be necessary. For tubular sources, the clinical scenario usually indicates the etiology.

More extensive evaluation, often including a renal biopsy, is needed when the urinary protein is glomerular in origin. Almost every form of glomerular disease (including both nephritic and nephrotic syndromes) is characterized by proteinuria. Though a biopsy is frequently needed, occasional patients with relatively low amounts of proteinuria and stable renal function may be followed, and biopsy deferred until evidence of progression or complications arises. Again, the clinical setting, and other laboratory tests, may be useful. Determining the presence of a nephritic syndrome, a nephrotic syndrome, or a systemic illness helps to begin the differential diagnosis. Longstanding diabetes, together with presence of diabetic retinopathy and absence of signs of acute renal injury (e.g., red cell casts, active sediment), usually indicates diabetic nephropathy. Presence of other systemic diseases known to involve the glomerulus (e.g., systemic lupus erythematosus) can also indicate the diagnosis. Longstanding hypertension, with hypertensive nephrosclerosis, may be associated with proteinuria which is usually below the nephrotic range. Presence of pulmonary involvement suggests one of the pulmonary–renal syndromes (e.g., Goodpasture syndrome, small vessel vasculitis), while measurement of serum complement levels, antineutrophil cytoplasmic antibodies (ANCA), and cryoglobulin levels can all be helpful in narrowing the differential diagnosis. In many cases, however, if these tests are negative or nonspecific, a renal biopsy is required for definitive diagnosis.

CLINICAL CONSEQUENCES OF PROTEINURIA

Loss of albumin and other plasma proteins into the urine is the hallmark of the nephrotic syndrome, and contributes to virtually all of the systemic complications of this disorder. "Subnephrotic proteinuria" refers to urinary protein excretion of <3.5 g/day; the source may be prerenal, glomerular, or tubular. Severe clinical signs and symptoms are rare with this lower grade of proteinuria. However, in patients with the nephrotic syndrome (>3.5 g/day), the complications of proteinuria can be severe and even life-threatening.

Proteins are essential for all body processes, and excessive loss of these various proteins damages numerous systems, resulting in diverse complications (Table 1; Fig. 3). Some hormones, trace metals, and vitamins are lost in the urine. Alterations in coagulation factors, such as loss of antithrombin III, lead to problems with spontaneous thromboemboli. Loss of immunoglobulins and parts of the complement cascade can lead to problems with immunity and increased rates of infection. Massive urinary albumin losses create many of the most critical complications of the nephrotic syndrome. Though not yet proven, it has been suggested that the excessive load of albumin going through

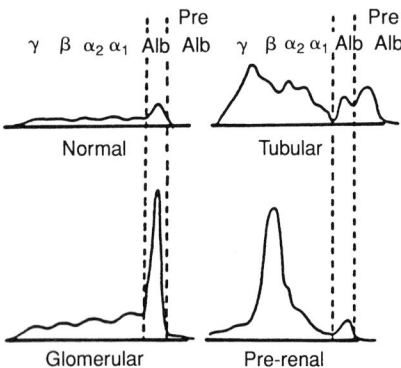

FIGURE 2 Schematic examples of urinary electrophoresis. The normal pattern (upper left) consists of a number of peaks, with albumin being the largest. In tubular proteinuria (upper right), a broad band representing multiple proteins is seen in the globulin range. In glomerular proteinuria (lower left), a large albumin peak is seen. When proteinuria is prerenal in origin, a single large monoclonal globulin peak (reflecting the circulating paraprotein) will be found.

TABLE I
Clinical Complications of Proteinuria

Hypoalbuminemia
   Edema
   Increased hepatic lipoprotein synthesis, hyperlipoproteinemia
   Increased platelet aggregability
Increased tubular protein reabsorption
   Possible tubular dysfunction, tubular damage
Loss of proteins carrying vitamins, hormones, and minerals
   Trace mineral deficiencies
   Hypocalcemia, Vitamin D deficiency
Loss of immunoglobulins
   Reduced cellular immunity, increased susceptibility to
     infection
Alterations in coagulation factors
   Spontaneous thromboembolism, renal vein thrombosis
Negative nitrogen balance, malnutrition
Alterations in drug metabolism (due to reduced protein
   binding)
   Diuretic resistance

the proximal tubule may lead to eventual tubular damage and dysfunction. Hypoalbuminemia contributes to massive edema formation, since albumin is the primary oncotic force keeping fluid inside the vascular space. Hypoalbuminemia also leads to hyperlipoproteinemia, with very high (>400 g/dL) serum cholesterol levels, since hypoalbuminemia stimulates hepatic synthesis of lipoproteins.

THERAPY OF PROTEINURIA

Successful treatment of the underlying glomerular disorder is, of course, the primary therapeutic goal, as this will both preserve renal function and reduce or eliminate proteinuria. However, some forms of glomerular disease have no specific therapy available, and other forms are not always successfully treated. In such cases, the presence of severe and symptomatic proteinuria may necessitate therapy aimed at reducing proteinuria specifically. Several therapeutic interventions have been successfully used to lower urinary protein excretion.

Dietary protein restriction may lower proteinuria in some, though not all, patients. This intervention works, in part, by reducing both GFR and P_{GC}, as well as by effects on glomerular permselectivity. For this purpose, the lowest allowable level of protein restriction is $0.6 \text{ g} \cdot \text{kg}^{-1} \cdot \text{day}^{-1}$, *plus* protein added to match urinary losses. Thus, a 70-kg patient with 10 g of proteinuria per day would receive a daily allotment of 52 g of protein, representing $0.6 \text{ g} \cdot \text{kg}^{-1} \cdot \text{day}^{-1}$, plus 10 additional grams to compensate for urinary losses. This therapy, which may also help to slow the progression of renal disease, should be used only in close collaboration with a renal dietician to avoid problems with negative nitrogen balance.

Angiotensin-converting enzyme (ACE) inhibitors have also proven useful in some cases. While effective reduction in blood pressure with any agent may offer some benefit, ACE inhibitors appear to be the most consistently effective. They reduce proteinuria, in part, by lowering efferent arteriolar resistance, thereby reducing P_{GC}. Other mechanisms

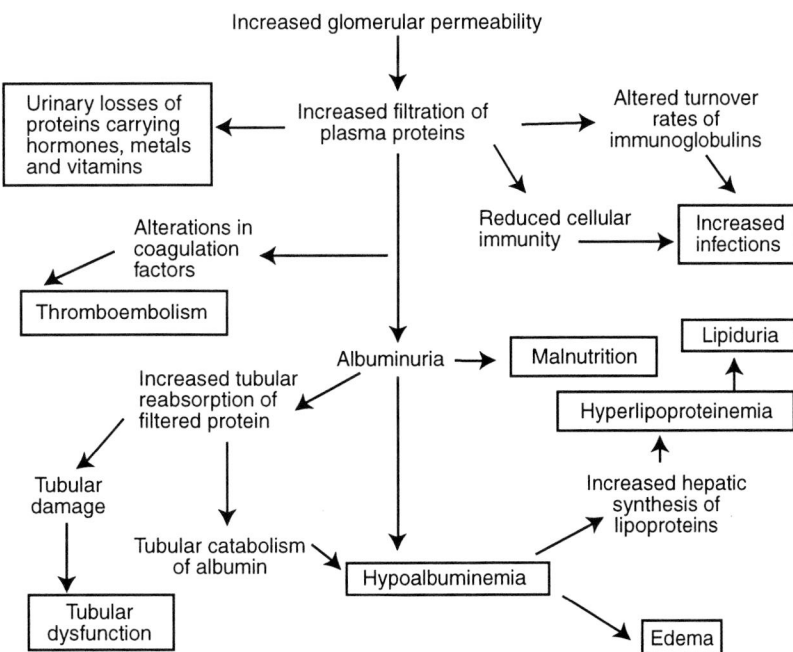

FIGURE 3 Major complications of the nephrotic syndrome. See text for discussion. Reproduced from Bernard DB: *Kidney Int* 33:1184–1202, 1988.

appear to be involved as well, including a direct effect on glomerular permselectivity. For maximum benefit, they should be given in conjunction with diuretic therapy and/or a low sodium diet, since continuation of liberal sodium intake may abolish the antiproteinuric efficacy of these drugs. However, ACE inhibition should be instituted cautiously. Patients with moderate to severe renal insufficiency may develop a rise in the serum creatinine, acute renal failure, or hyperkalemia with ACE inhibitors, and therefore this therapy should be avoided in patients at risk for these complications. ACE inhibitors are used most safely when GFR is not severely impaired. Other antihypertensive drugs have been less consistent in effect, but could certainly be tried if ACE inhibition is not possible. Limited, short-term studies suggest that angiotensin II receptor antagonists may also be effective in reducing proteinuria. Though less likely to cause cough, these drugs probably will have a side effect profile similar to ACE inhibitors.

Nonsteroidal anti-inflammatory drugs in high doses are also effective in reducing proteinuria, probably because they also tend to reduce GFR. While they can be useful, they can be used only when GFR is not severely impaired, to avoid the risks of acute renal failure and hyperkalemia. Because of the risk of lowering GFR, and the high incidence of gastrointestinal side effects at high doses, these agents are not as widely used to lower proteinuria, but may be considered in severe cases.

Bibliography

Anderson S, Kennefick TM, Brenner BM: Systemic and renal manifestations of glomerular disease. In: Brenner BM, Rector FC, Jr (eds) *The Kidney,* 5th ed. Philadelphia, Saunders, pp. 1981–2010, 1996.

Bennett PH, Haffner S, Kasiske BL, et al: Screening and management of microalbuminuria in patients with diabetes mellitus: Recommendations to the Scientific Advisory Board of the National Kidney Foundation from an ad hoc committee of the Council on Diabetes Mellitus of the National Kidney Foundation. *Am J Kidney Dis* 25:107–112, 1995.

Bernard DB. Extrarenal complications of the nephrotic syndrome. *Kidney Int* 33:1184–1202, 1988.

Bernard DB, Salant DJ: Clinical approach to the patient with proteinuria and the nephrotic syndrome. In: Jacobson H, Striker G, Klahr S (eds) *Principles and Practice of Nephrology,* 2nd ed. St. Louis, Mosby-Year Book, pp. 110–121, 1995.

Brenner BM, Hostetter TH, Humes DH: Molecular basis of proteinuria of glomerular origin. *N Engl J Med* 298:826–833, 1978.

Carlson JA, Harrington JT: Laboratory evaluation of renal function. In: Schrier RW, Gottschalk CW (eds) *Diseases of the Kidney,* 5th ed. Little, Brown, Boston, pp. 361–405, 1993.

Deen WM, Myers BD, Brenner BM: The glomerular barrier to macromolecules: Theoretical and experimental considerations. In: Brenner BM, Stein JH (eds) *Nephrotic Syndrome.* Churchill Livingstone, New York, pp. 1–29, 1982.

Ginsberg JSM, Chang BS, Matarese RA, Garella S: Use of single voided urine samples to estimate quantitative proteinuria. *N Engl J Med* 309:1543–1546, 1983.

Kanwar YS, Liu ZZ, Kashihara N, Wallner EI: Current status of the structural and functional basis of glomerular filtration and proteinuria. *Semin Nephrol* 11:390–413, 1991.

Kaplan NM. Microalbuminuria: A risk factor for vascular and renal complications. *Am J Med* 92(Suppl. 4B):4B-8S–4B-12S, 1992.

Kaysen GA. Hyperlipidemia in the nephrotic syndrome. *Am J Kidney Dis* 12:548–551, 1988.

Kaysen GA, Myers BD, Couser WG, Rabkin R, Felts JM: Mechanisms and consequences of proteinuria. *Lab Invest* 54:479–498, 1986.

Llach F: Hypercoagulability, renal vein thrombosis, and other thrombotic complications of nephrotic syndrome. *Kidney Int* 28:429–439, 1985.

Morrison G, Audet PR, Singer I: Clinically important drug interactions for the nephrologist. In: Bennett WM, McCarron DA, Brenner BM, Stein JH (eds) *Pharmacotherapy of renal disease and hypertension.* Churchill Livingstone, New York, pp. 49–97, 1987.

6

RENAL IMAGING TECHNIQUES

HOWARD J. MINDELL AND JONATHAN FAIRBANK

GENERAL CONSIDERATIONS

Investigation of patients with renal disorders often requires obtaining images of the kidneys and urinary tract. Although more helpful in evaluating renal masses or disorders of the urinary outflow tract than intrinsic renal parenchymal disease, imaging studies can either establish the general pathway for further investigation or lead to a specific diagnosis. In general, the choice of studies proceeds from less to more invasive or expensive studies, unless the expensive or invasive study is much more likely to be definitive. The current medical–economic environment favors the use of the simplest, safest, and cheapest approach that can answer the question at hand.

ULTRASONOGRAPHY

Ultrasonography (US) is entirely safe, independent of renal function, capable of multiplanar display, and does not require contrast agents or prior patient preparation. However, it lacks specificity in many instances (for example, in differentiating among renal parenchymal diseases), and technical problems may arise in large patients in whom tissue degrades the interrogating sound waves or when intestinal gas reflects sound, and prevents delineation of the underlying structure. Although US can exquisitely demonstrate vascular occlusive disease, in many patients it is inapplicable because of the technical reasons cited above. Doppler US, even with the use of color to show flow direction, has not enjoyed wide or universal success in screening for renovascular hypertension. In addition to the limitations noted, multiple renal arteries may be impossible to sort out by US alone. Nevertheless, US is a mainstay of renal imaging and is frequently the first study chosen. US can easily differentiate hydronephrosis (Fig. 1) from intrinsic renal parenchymal disease and renal cysts from solid tumors. It is also a useful method for delineating perinephric collections, pyelonephritic scars, and nephrocalcinosis. US can assist in evaluating renal transplants and can guide a variety of interventional approaches to the kidney, including biopsy, aspiration, and percutaneous nephrostomy.

EXCRETORY (INTRAVENOUS) UROGRAPHY

Intravenous urography (IVU) can noninvasively show the entire urinary tract. While other imaging modalities, such as US, may provide more detail regarding the renal parenchyma, the IVU remains an inexpensive, widely available, "low tech" test that gives excellent detail of the entire urinary tract, especially of the collecting system. The IVU remains the first choice in most patients with hematuria, pyuria, or flank pain. Other indications for IVU include urothelial malignancy, tuberculosis, papillary necrosis, and a variety of congenital anomalies. When the collecting system must be examined but IVU is inadequate because renal failure limits excretion of radiographic contrast and urinary tract visualization, retrograde urography or percutaneous antegrade urography may be needed. The former requires cystoscopy and ureteral catheter placement; the latter is performed after imaging guided puncture of the calyceal system. The IVU is used to evaluate renal donors and in the pre- and postoperative assessment of patients with nephrolithiasis and other lesions that can be treated with endoscopic manipulation of the ureter.

The contrast medium employed for intravenous urography and other studies is subject to two classes of reactions: idiosyncratic and toxic, such as acute renal failure. Approximately 0.1 to 0.2% of patients develop an idiosyncratic reaction characterized by urticaria, wheezing, dyspnea, or chest pain which may be followed by hypotension. The case fatality rate is estimated to be 1 in 85,000. Pretreatment with glucocorticoids or the use of low osmolality contrast media may reduce the incidence of this reaction. Substitution of the latter for conventional media is restricted because these agents are 10 times as costly. Low osmolarity agents are therefore typically restricted to patients with a history of prior contrast reaction, a strong generalized allergic history, or asthma. The second, toxic reactions, include acute renal failure. This occurs independent of the idiosyncratic reaction just described.

The risk of contrast nephropathy is highest in patients with diabetic nephropathy, intermediate in patients with renal insufficiency due to other causes, and low or normal for diabetics without renal disease. There are no absolute contraindications to the use of IV contrast, but it should be used with circumspection in such settings as advanced age, debility, congestive heart failure, and multiple myeloma. Patients with volume depletion are at greatest risk. Intravascular volume should be restored by fluid administration before contrast is given. A recent study suggested that overnight expansion with 0.5% saline affords protec-

47

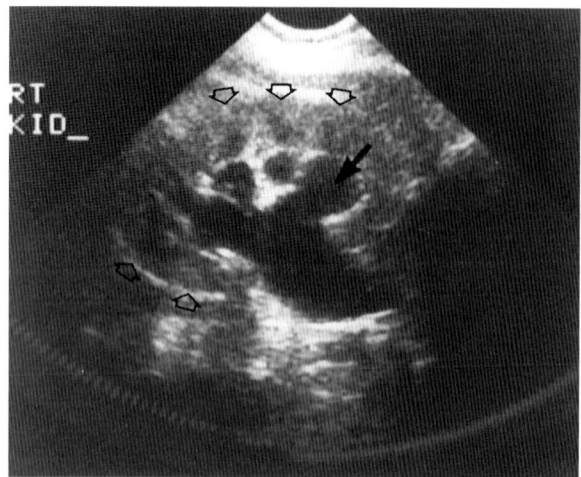

FIGURE 1   Ultrasound showing a sagittal section through the right kidney. The single black arrow indicates a dilated calyx in the lower pole. Note how the calyx connects to the dilated renal pelvis (black, fluid filled). Multiple open arrows indicate the margin of the renal cortex.

tion in patients who are not volume depleted (see Chapter 36).

It also bears emphasis that these comments about side effects of administration of radiographic contrast apply no matter what the procedure for which contrast is employed. They are not specific to IVU and concern about contrast administration must be taken into account when a CT with contrast or angiogram is ordered. Finally, the visualization of the urinary tract is diminished when the serum creatinine exceeds 2 to 3 mg/dL; the IVU is unlikely to successfully visualize the collecting system when the serum creatinine exceeds 4 mg/dL. Therefore, the risk of increased contrast administration should be weighed against its diminished potential benefit in these patients.

PLAIN ABDOMINAL RADIOGRAPH

The plain abdominal radiograph (KUB), while a standard prelude (scout film) for the IVU, may be requested alone or in conjunction with US. Renal or ureteric calculi may be visible on the KUB, although the former may require oblique views to confirm an intrarenal location (as opposed to the more anterior gallbladder, etc.), and the latter may require IVU to differentiate from pelvic phleboliths.

COMPUTED TOMOGRAPHY

Computed tomography (CT) offers far greater contrast resolution than conventional radiography, with detailed anatomic cross-sectional anatomic imaging unaffected by overlying structures such as bone or gas. Virtually the entire urinary system and retroperitoneum are well visualized on CT. CT plays the main role in staging renal neoplasms and has superseded IVU in trauma. CT may be useful in

pyelonephritis and its complications and in renal cystic disorders. With arterial occlusive disease, CT can show perfusion defects, where contrast fails to opacify segments of the renal parenchyma, and recent work has found that 3D reconstruction with helical CT may show the renal arterial vessels directly. With venous occlusive disease, CT can show flow abnormalities and stasis in the affected kidney and can directly demonstrate thrombus in the renal vein. CT can show urinary calculi that are not visible by radiography (urates) and unenhanced helical CT is a promising new technique in the diagnosis of renal colic.

MAGNETIC RESONANCE IMAGING

Magnetic resonance imaging (MRI) depends on first aligning the hydrogen nuclei (protons) of body tissues with a powerful magnetic field and then applying radiofrequency (RF) pulses. Energy released in these circumstances can be measured and used to create anatomic images dependent on characteristics of the tissues and the introduced magnetic and RF energy sources. MRI offers superb tissue contrast, with multiplanar imaging capabilities, although calcification is not well shown. MRI is safe, with no ionizing radiation, although MR contrast agents such as gadolinium may rarely induce patient reactivity. MR may not be suitable for use in claustrophobic patients or those with implanted ferromagnetic devices, such as pacemakers. MRI has a limited role in defining specific parenchymal lesions at present, although its sensitivity to iron in hemoglobin permits its use to image the kidneys in patients with paroxysmal nocturnal hemoglobinuria, myoglobinuria, and epidemic Korean fever. MRI can beautifully show the renal vasculature, and magnetic resonance angiography (MRA) is being evaluated as a potential replacement for conventional angiography or a rival to computed tomographic angiography (CTA) in assessing various arterial lesion, such as renal artery stenosis). MRI has the following main roles in renal imaging:

1. Delineating complex renal masses, where CT is not definitive.
2. Staging renal neoplasms, particularly in evaluating for renal vein or inferior vena caval extension of tumor.
3. Diagnosing renovascular lesions.
4. Where renal failure or contrast media reactivity preclude the use of other modalities. Magnetic resonance urography (MRU) has been recently introduced as an alternative to the IVU in highly selected circumstances.

RADIONUCLIDE IMAGING

For nuclear medicine studies, radiopharmaceutical agents with specific renal handling characteristics are employed (see Table 1). These agents are administered and then the patient is imaged with a gamma camera that can record the number of counts emitted and the location of their source. This permits quantitation of function in a

TABLE I
Most Commonly Used Radiopharmaceuticals in
Renal Imaging

Radionuclide	Mechanism of renal action	Major clinical usefulness
^{99m}Tc-DTPA	Glomerular filtration	Perfusion Parenchymal Imaging Estimate GFR Excretion
^{99m}Tc-DMSA	Tubular binding and tubular secretion	Pyelonephritis Estimation of tubular mass (i.e., cortical scar)
^{99m}Tc-GHP	Glomerular filtration and tubular secretion and tubular binding	Perfusion Excretion Estimation of tubular mass
^{99m}Tc-MAG 3	Tubular secretion and glomerular filtration	High renal extraction and useful images even with moderate renal dysfunction Estimate ERPF
^{67}Ga-citrate	N/A	Pyelonephritis Interstitial nephritis Renal abscess
^{99m}Tc-, ^{111}In-labeled WBCs	N/A	Renal abscess

region as well as anatomic delineation. Nuclear medicine techniques are particularly useful in assessing the adequacy of renal perfusion and in determining whether the outflow tract is intact. Renal parenchymal integrity may also be assessed.

The scanning method is varied according to the nature of the information sought. When anatomic information is desired, the scanning interval for each image typically encompasses several minutes. Late views may be obtained after a delay of hours or even 1 to 2 days. In contrast, when flow is being studied, images are typically of only a few seconds in duration. The resolution of nuclear medicine studies is poor. Anatomic information is of limited quality. Flow studies are, therefore, the major use of nuclear medicine techniques. Single-photon emission computed tomography (SPECT) is utilized at some centers to afford greater detail. The most common uses of nuclear medicine studies are listed below.

1. Measurement of renal function. Radionuclide studies permit calculation of glomerular filtration rate (GFR) and effective renal plasma flow (ERPF), even in cases of renal impairment. Appropriate radionuclides are injected intravenously and images obtained. The most accurate calculations of GFR and EPFR are obtained by withdrawing blood samples at predetermined intervals and using standard clearance calculations, but strictly count-based computer

imaging methods now closely rival this method, without requiring blood samples.

2. Measurement of "split" renal function. To determine whether nephrectomy is warranted or safe, it is often important for the surgeon to know the relative contribution to total renal function of each kidney. Computer-enhanced scan techniques can determine the contribution of each kidney to ERPF or GFR. Split renal function measurements are also helpful in follow up of surgical procedures that relieve unilateral obstruction.

3. Renovascular hypertension. Differential renal blood flow studies using ^{99m}Tc-DPTA or ^{99m}Tc-MAG3 pre- and postadministration of an ACE inhibitor such as captopril in an appropriately screened hypertensive patient with intact renal function will detect renovascular disease with a sensitivity and specificity exceeding 90%. (see chapter 78, Fig. 3.)

4. Contraindication to contrast media. While radionuclide methods do not provide the anatomic detail of other imaging methods, they may provide information regarding arterial perfusion, differential renal function, and urinary tract obstruction. Radionuclide methods may be particularly suitable for patients with renal failure or severe contrast media sensitivity.

Aside from pregnancy, there are no contraindications to the use of radionuclides for diagnostic purposes.

5. Evaluation of renal transplants. Radionuclide imaging may detect impaired blood flow at the renal arterial anastomotic site, urinary tract obstruction, and extravasation of urine due to disruption at the ureteric anastomosis. This modality complements US for these purposes.

6. Obstructive uropathy. The diuretic renogram (Fig. 2) is very helpful, particularly in children, who demonstrate an

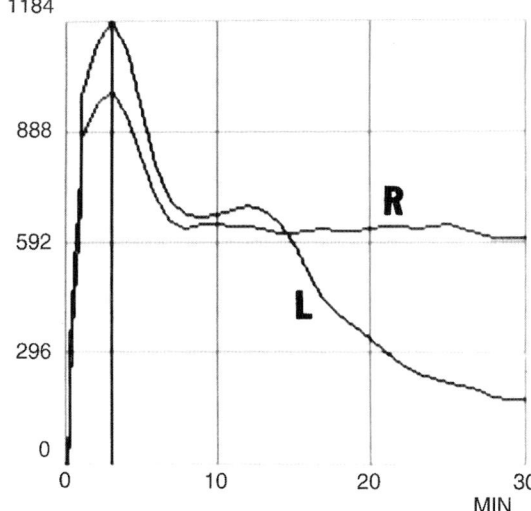

FIGURE 2 Radionuclide, diuretic renography. The plate shows an accumulation of counts over the kidneys, 30 minutes after intravenous injection, of furasemide and the tracer MAG3. The left kidney (left) is normal. Note the flat curve on the right, indicating that pooled isotope remains in the kidney, without a normal fall off as on the left side; the right side is partially obstructed.

enlarged renal pelvis by US or IVU. This test distinguishes between true obstruction at the ureteropelvic junction and nonobstructive hydronephrosis. Furosemide is injected before or after administration of ^{99m}Tc DTPA or MAG 3, renal images are obtained, and a renogram curve of activity in each kidney is constructed. Dilatation without significant obstruction is suggested when radionuclide accumulation in the dilated area is reduced at high urine flow rates.

7. Renal infection or scar. The IVU may appear normal in patients with pyelonephritis, and the differentiation between this and cystitis may be difficult. ^{99m}Tc-DMSA and glucoheptonate (GHP) are renal cortical scanning agents. Areas of inflammation or scar will demonstrate no uptake. The agents are also helpful in determining the amount of remaining renal cortex in children with chronic urinary tract infections and vesicoureteric reflux. ^{99m}Tc- or ^{111}In-labeled WBCs may be used to identify renal abscesses. In patients with low WBC counts, gallium-67 may be used.

ANGIOGRAPHY

Intravenous administration of contrast medium has not proved suitable for renal angiography, and direct intraarterial injections, either into the main renal arteries or selectively into smaller branches, are generally necessary in this modality.

Renal angiography can be used for diagnostic and/or therapeutic purposes.

Diagnostic Angiography

1. Suspected renal artery lesions. Renal angiography is the definitive imaging procedure where renovascular hypertension is suspected. It is indicated when medical therapy for hypertension is ineffective and the patient is a candidate for surgical or angioplastic therapy. As stated earlier, CTA and MRA are under investigation as replacements for conventional angiography in this area. Renal vein sampling for renin levels may assist selecting patients for treatment. Patients with acute occlusion or thrombosis of the renal arteries, embolic processes, or posttraumatic renal vascular injury may be candidates for renal angiography. In patients with polyarteritis nodosa, selective renal angiography is the only method with sufficient resolution to detect the characteristic tiny peripheral aneurysms.

2. Unexplained hematuria. Angiography may be required to investigate the cause for unexplained hematuria. Vascular malformations may be suspected on US or CT but generally will require angiography for definitive delineation, especially if therapy is planned.

3. Renal transplantation. Angiography may be needed to map the renal arterial system in prospective renal donors, where multiple renal arteries or vascular anomalies may complicate transplant surgery. CTA is used for this purpose at some transplant centers. Angiography is required to diagnose posttransplant renal artery stenoses or occlusions.

5. Renal vein disorders. Although renal vein thrombosis or occlusion can be shown by CT or MRI, rarely direct renal venography may be required, for instance if other modalities are not diagnostic.

6. Miscellaneous. Complex renal masses, or complications of polycystic disease or trauma, may require angiography.

Interventional Angiography

Angiography has become increasingly important as a therapeutic maneuver rather than a simple diagnostic technique. Balloon angioplasty may be used to dilate renal artery stenosis, both in the native and in the transplanted kidney (Fig. 3). Ostial lesions, previously thought to be refractory to this method, may be amenable to treatment with endovascular stinting. Further details on the use of

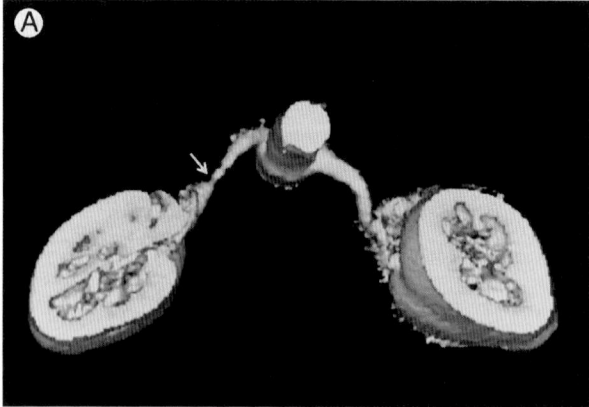
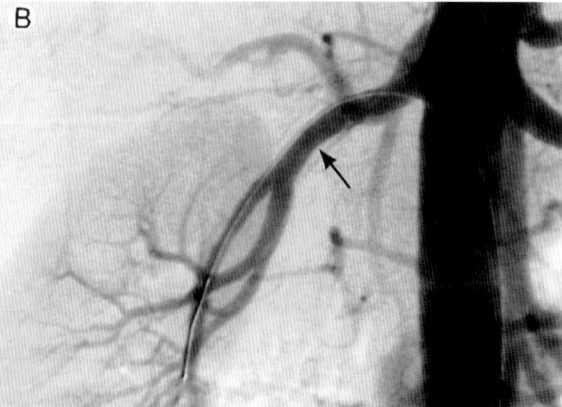

FIGURE 3   (a) Computed tomographic angiography (CTA) showing the computer-generated 3D reconstruction of the aorta and the main renal arteries, possible after a simple IV injection of contrast media. The arrow indicates a significant stenosis in the main right renal artery. (b) Selective right renal angiogram after successful angioplasty, in the same patient as (a), with an arrow showing the now patent right main renal artery. Figures courtesy of Dr. Ken Najarian, FAHC, Burlington, Vt.

angioplasty in renal artery stenosis are provided in Chapter 78. Angiography may also be used to embolize bleeding sites within the kidney that may have resulted from trauma or as a complication of interventional procedures such as a percutaneous biopsy. Angiography may also be used for selected infusion of a thrombolytic agent for treatment of renal artery or renal vein thrombosis.

Voiding Cystourethrography

This study is useful in demonstrating vesicoureteric reflux. Voiding cystourethrography (VCU) can be performed with fluoroscopic or radionuclide technique, depending on local preferences.

CHOICE OF IMAGING PROCEDURE FOR SPECIFIC CLINICAL SITUATIONS

Arterial Disease

US can readily diagnose aortic aneurysm, but CT is more accurate where aneurysmal bleeding is suspect, and CT or CTA are better for surgical planning, especially to show the exact levels of the renal arteries. CT can diagnose acute renal infarction by showing parenchymal perfusion defects with a peripheral "rim sign" of collateral flow. As previously suggested, although color Doppler US can demonstrate renovascular disease such as renal artery stenosis in individual patients, it is not recommended as a screening tool for renovascular hypertension. In selected patients where significant hypertension is not amenable to medical control, and where surgical or angioplastic therapy is contemplated, a combination of captopril renography and/or renal angiography is required. Because of the frequent occurrence of double, or even triple, renal arteries, US cannot reliably rule out significant renal artery stenosis. On the other hand, even where US clearly shows a renovascular lesion, angiography is always needed as a precursor to angioplasty or surgical intervention.

Congenital Disorders

The most common congenital renal anomalies for which imaging is used are the various forms of renal ectopia, fusion anomalies such as horseshoe kidney (Fig. 4), and obstructive processes of the ureteropelvic junction (UPJ) or distal ureter. US and IVU are the primary imaging tools in evaluating these lesions, although occasionally a as horseshoe kidney presents as an incidental finding at CT or with a radionuclide study, even a bone scan. UPJ obstruction can be further evaluated by diuretic urography or radionuclide renography.

Inflammatory Diseases

In acute pyelonephritis, the IVU is usually not indicated and in any case ordinarily not diagnostic. In selected patients, CT can diagnose acute pyelonephritis by showing characteristic peripheral radiolucent perfusion defects in

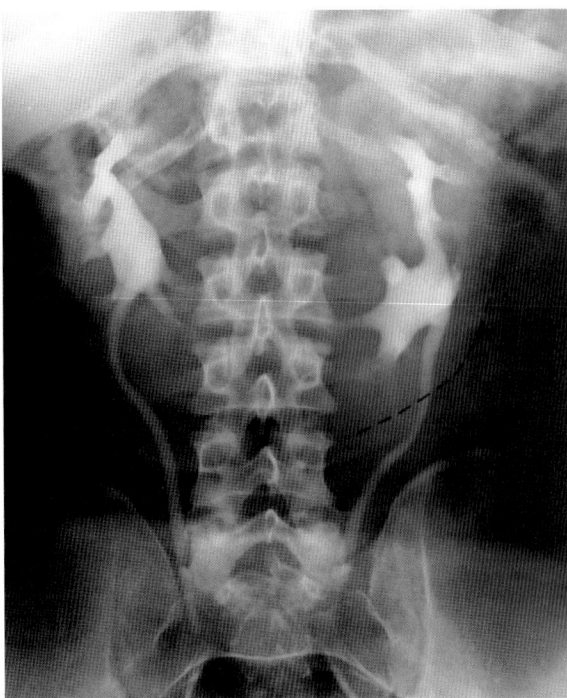

FIGURE 4 IVU demonstrating a horseshoe kidney. A black dashed line has been drawn to show the lower margin of the renal parechyma as it crosses the mid line to fuse with the opposite kidney.

the renal parenchyma, frequently with edema in the perinephric fat. When urinary tract infections follow an atypical or protracted course, US, and with better specificity CT, can delineate infected renal cysts, renal abcesses, or infected perirenal collections. Either US or CT can guide interventional procedures for diagnosing and treating these lesions. Tuberculosis causes strictures of the renal collecting systems or ureters, and the diagnosis may be suggested by IVU. Chronic pyelonephritis, frequently associated with reflux nephropathy, produces scarred, and in advanced disease, shrunken kidneys readily shown on IVU or cross sectional imaging.

Neoplasia

The main grouping of renal tumors divides renal parenchymal masses from urothelial lesions (see Chapter 58). Although cystic or solid renal parenchymal masses may be first detected by IVU, they require US and/or CT for further differentiation and staging (Fig. 5). MRI is available in some instances where more conventional imaging is not definitive, where the patient is sensitive to iodinated intravascular contrast media, or where a question about renal vasculature is unresolved. Urothelial tumors, nearly always transitional cell carcinoma (TCC), are best shown on IVU or retrograde pyelography—the latter serving as a guide for brush biopsy. In selected patients, cross sectional im-

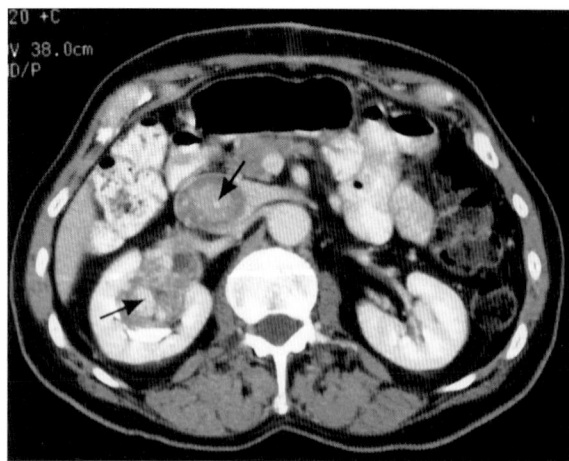

FIGURE 5 CT showing renal carcinoma. This cross section through the level of the kidneys was obtained using oral and IV contrast media. The lower black arrow points to the irregulary radiolucent, necrotic tumor mass. The second black arrow, higher in position as the reader views the illustration, points to a filling defect in the inferior vena cava, representing tumor thrombus. A normal cava would be homogeneously bright with enhancing blood, like the aorta.

aging such as CT may be needed to diagnose or confirm TCC of the renal pelvis or ureter.

Cystic Disorders

Benign renal cysts occur in up to 30% of normal adults and can nearly always be readily differentiated from solid neoplasm by US. Complex cysts may require CT for definitive evaluation. Both infantile autosomal recessive and adult autosomal dominant polycystic renal disease are readily diagnosed by US; the former may be detected in utero, and the latter lends itself to US for screening where indicated (see Chapter 45). Medullary sponge kidney (tubular ectasia) is diagnosed by IVU (see Fig. 1, Chapter 52).

Trauma

Helical (spiral) CT, where very rapid CT of the entire upper abdomen can be done in a single breath hold, has largely supplanted the IVU for evaluating renal trauma, because of its speed and accuracy, and its multiorgan sweep. CT also assesses the renal vascular supply, although angiography is needed in selected cases or major vascular trauma, where diagnosis and/or angiographic therapy is required.

Parenchymal disorders

Renal parenchymal disease consists of a broad range of processes, from inflammatory or immunologic disorders to toxic or ischemic lesions. Imaging can show small kidneys, and US may demonstrate echogenic, abnormal paren-

chyma, but rarely pinpoints the diagnosis, which may require renal biopsy, the latter amenable to US guidance. The main goal of imaging is to rule out obstruction, polycystic kidney disease, renal papillary necrosis, vascular disease, or reflux nephropathy. For patients presenting in renal failure, US is an excellent noninvasive method to differentiate intrinsic parenchymal disease from obstructive uropathy.

UROLITHIASIS

Most urinary calculi are calcified and therefore readily detectable by KUB. Radiolucent stones appear as filling defects in the contrast opacified area on IVU. These techniques are the main imaging studies employed for nephrolithiasis. Recently, helical unenhanced CT has shown promise in the diagnosis of renal colic due to ureteric calculi. CT can also demonstrate radiolucent calculi such as uric acid stones that are not seen on KUB. As the IVU can precisely locate the position of a ureteral calculus, it is used to plan therapy for renal or urinary calculi, although retrograde pyelography may be needed, especially during the course of stent placement or extracorporeal shock wave lithotripsy (ESWL). The role of ultrasound in patients with nephrolithiasis is limited. It is very sensitive in showing tiny intrarenal calculi or nephrocalcinosis but of only limited applicability in diagnosing ureteric stones as the mid and distal ureter are only rarely visualized by US.

Renal Transplantation

Renal transplantation donors need at least an IVU preoperatively, and as previously indicated, depending on institutional preferences, angiography or CTA to assess vascular anatomy. In recipients posttransplantation, color flow Doppler US documents the status of vascular perfusion to the transplanted kidney, and US can document hydronephrosis, renal volumes, and extrarenal collections such as lymphocele, but cannot reliably differentiate rejection from acute tubular necrosis. Radionuclide studies can also assess perfusion or obstruction, and rarely retrograde or even percutaneous antegrade pyelography is required to assess ureteral patency. Angiography may be needed to show renal artery stenoses to the transplant.

Ureteral Obstruction

Bilateral ureteric obstruction causing renal failure is rare in adults in the absence of malignancy. Although specific lesions such as retroperitoneal fibrosis must be considered, US can show hydronephrosis, but ureteric assessment will require IVU, or cross-sectional imaging such as CT or MRI to demonstrate the retroperitoneum, or retrograde pyelography. Acute unilateral ureteric obstruction, commonly due to renal colic with passage of a ureteric calculus is usually readily diagnosed by IVU (Fig. 6) although as previously suggested unenhanced CT is emerging as an effective technique in this area.

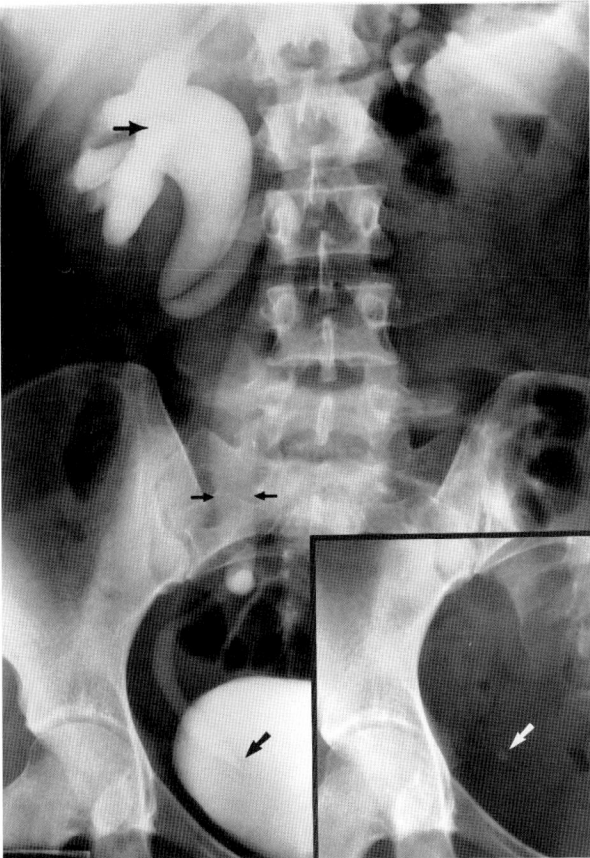

FIGURE 6 IVU shows acute obstruction from a ureteral calculus. The inset is a section from the "scout" KUB, showing a 5 mm opaque ureteric calculus (white arrow). The 30-minute film after IV contrast injection shows right hydronephrosis above (black arrow with slender tail), with hydroureter (paired black arrows) tapering to the calculus seen on the KUB (black arrow with thick tail).

Renal Vein Lesions

The renal vein can be evaluated as part of the cross-sectional imaging procedure used to study the primary lesion—i.e., if US is done to delineate a renal tumor, the renal vein may be also shown by color flow Doppler US. CT and MRI can also show the renal veins, as well as the IVC. Where isolated renal vein thrombosis is suspected, contrast CT can be definitive, both in showing the enlarged renal vein and collateral circulation that may develop and in showing the actual thrombus as a filling defect in the opacified renal vein. Again, where CT is suboptimal for technical reasons or the patient is reactive to iodinated contrast media, MRI can be diagnostic of disorders of the IVC or renal veins.

Bibliography

Blaufox MD, ed: *Evaluation of Renal Function and Disease with Radionuclides.* 2nd ed. Karger, Basel, 1989.

Bude RO, Rubin JA: Detection of renal artery stenosis with Doppler sonography: It is more complicated than originally thought. *Radiology* 196:612–613, 1995.

Dodd GD, Tublin ME, Shah A, Zajko AB: Review. Imaging of vascular complications associated with renal transplants. *AJR* 157:449–459, 1991.

Dunnick NR, Cohan RH: Commentary. Cost, corticosteroids, and contrast media. *AJR* 162:527–529, 1994.

Mindell HJ, Cochran ST: Commentary. Current perspectives in the diagnosis and treatment of urinary stone disease. *AJR* 163:1314–1315, 1994.

Pollack HM, ed: *Clinical Urography.* Saunders, Philadelphia, 1990.

Pollack HM, Wein AJ: State of the art imaging of renal trauma. *Radiology* 172:297–308, 1989.

Resnick MI, Rifkin MD: *Ultrasonography of the Urinary Tract.* 3rd ed. Williams and Wilkins, Baltimore, 1991.

Rubin GD, Dake MD, Napel S, McDonnell CH, Jeffrey RB: Three-dimensional spiral CT angiography of the abdomen: Initial clinical experience. *Radiology* 186:147–152, 1993.

Solomon R, Warner C, Mann D, D'Elia J, Silva P. Effects of saline, mannitol and furosemide on acute decreases in renal function produced by radiocontrast agents. *N Engl J Med* 331:1416–1420, 1994.

Steinberg EP, Moore RD, Powe NR, et al: Safety and cost effectiveness of high-osmolality as compared with low-osmolality contrast material in patients undergoing cardiac angiography. *N Engl J Med* 326:425–430, 1992.

Zagoria RJ, Berchtold RE, Dyer RB: Staging of renal adenocarcinoma: Role of various imaging procedures. *AJR* 164:363–370, 1995.

SECTION 2

ACID–BASE, FLUID, AND ELECTROLYTE DISORDERS

7

HYPONATREMIA AND HYPOOSMOLAR DISORDERS

JOSEPH G. VERBALIS

The incidence of hyponatremia depends on the nature of the patient population and also the criteria used to establish the diagnosis. Hospital incidences of 15 to 22% are common if hyponatremia is defined as plasma $[Na^+]$ <135 mEq/L, but only 1 to 4% of patients have a plasma $[Na^+] \leq 130$. Although most cases are mild, hyponatremia is important clinically because: (1) acute severe hyponatremia can cause substantial morbidity and mortality; (2) mild hyponatremia can progress to more dangerous levels during management of other disorders; (3) general mortality appears to be higher in patients with even asymptomatic hyponatremia; and (4) overly rapid correction of chronic hyponatremia can produce severe neurological deficits and death.

Definitions

Hyponatremia is of clinical significance only when it reflects corresponding hypoosmolality of the plasma. Plasma osmolality can be measured directly by osmometry, or calculated as

$$P_{osm} \text{ (mOsm/kg } H_2O) = 2 \times \text{plasma } [Na^+] \text{ (mEq/L)} + \text{glucose (mg/dL)}/18 + \text{BUN (mg/dL)}/2.8.$$

Both methods produce comparable results under most conditions, as does simply doubling the plasma $[Na^+]$. However, total osmolality is not always equivalent to "effective" osmolality, sometimes referred to as the "tonicity" of the plasma. Solutes compartmentalized to the extracellular fluid (ECF) are effective solutes, because they create osmotic gradients across cell membranes leading to osmotic movement of water from the intracellular fluid (ICF) to ECF compartments. Solutes that freely permeate cell membranes (urea, ethanol, methanol) are not effective solutes, since they do not create osmotic gradients across cell membranes and therefore are not associated with secondary water shifts. Only the concentration of effective solutes in plasma should be used to determine whether clinically significant hypoosmolality is present.

Hyponatremia and hypoosmolality are usually synonymous, but with two important exceptions. First, pseudohyponatremia can be produced by marked elevation of plasma lipids and/or proteins. In such cases the concentration of Na^+ per liter of plasma water is unchanged, but the concentration of Na^+ per liter of plasma is artifactually decreased because of the increased relative proportion occupied by lipid or protein. Fortunately, measurement of plasma $[Na^+]$ by ion-specific electrodes, which is now commonly employed by most clinical laboratories, is much less influenced by high concentrations of lipids or proteins than is measurement of plasma $[Na^+]$ by flame photometry, although such errors can nonetheless still occur. However, because direct measurement of plasma osmolality is based on the colligative properties of solute particles in solution, measured plasma osmolality will not be affected by the increased lipids or proteins. Second, high concentrations of effective solutes other than Na^+ can cause relative decreases in plasma $[Na^+]$ despite an unchanged plasma osmolality; this commonly occurs with hyperglycemia. Misdiagnosis can be avoided again by direct measurement of plasma osmolality, or by correcting the plasma $[Na^+]$ by 1.6 mEq/L for each 100 mg/dL increase in plasma glucose concentration above 100 mg/dL.

PATHOGENESIS

The presence of significant hypoosmolality always indicates excess water relative to solute in the ECF. Because water moves freely between the ICF and ECF, this also indicates an excess of total body water relative to total body solute. Imbalances between water and solute can be generated initially either by *depletion* of body solute more than body water or by *dilution* of body solute from increases in body water more than body solute (Table 1). It should be recognized, however, that this distinction represents an oversimplification, because most hypoosmolar states include components of both solute depletion and water retention (e.g., isotonic solute losses, as occurs during an acute hemorrhage, do not produce hypoosmolality until the subsequent retention of water from ingested or infused hypotonic fluids causes a secondary dilution of the remaining ECF solute). Nonetheless, this concept has proven useful because it provides a simple framework for understanding the diagnosis and therapy of hypoosmolar disorders.

DIFFERENTIAL DIAGNOSIS

The diagnostic approach to hypoosmolar patients should include a careful history (especially concerning medica-

TABLE I
Pathogenesis of Hypoosmolar Disorders[a]

Depletion (primary decreases in total body solute + secondary water retention)[b]:

1. Renal solute loss
   Diuretic use
   Solute diuresis (glucose, mannitol)
   Salt-wasting nephropathy
   Mineralocorticoid deficiency

2. Nonrenal solute loss
   Gastrointestinal (diarrhea, vomiting, pancreatitis, bowel obstruction)
   Cutaneous (sweating, burns)
   Blood loss

Dilution (primary increases in total body water ± secondary solute depletion)[c]:

1. Impaired renal free water excretion
   A. Increased proximal reabsorption
      Hypothyroidism
   B. Impaired distal dilution
      Syndrome of inappropriate antidiuresis (SIAD)
      Glucocorticoid deficiency
   C. Combined increased proximal reabsorption and impaired distal dilution
      Congestive heart failure
      Cirrhosis
      Nephrotic syndrome
   D. Decreased urinary solute excretion
      Beer potomania

2. Excess water intake
   Primary polydipsia
   Dilute infant formula

[a] Modified from Verbalis (1995).

[b] Virtually all disorders of solute depletion are accompanied by some degree of secondary retention of water by the kidneys in response to the resulting intravascular hypovolemia; this mechanism can lead to hypoosmolality even when the solute depletion occurs via hypotonic or isotonic body fluid losses.

[c] Disorders of water retention primarily cause hypoosmolality in the absence of any solute losses, but in some cases of SIAD secondary solute losses occur in response to the resulting intravascular hypervolemia and this can then further aggravate the dilutional hypoosmolality in the plasma (but note that this pathophysiology does not likely contribute to the hyponatremia of edema-forming states such as congestive heart failure and cirrhosis, since in these cases multiple factors favoring sodium retention will result in an increased total body sodium).

tions), clinical assessment of the ECF volume status, a thorough neurological evaluation, plasma electrolytes, glucose, BUN and creatinine, uric acid, calculated and/or directly measured plasma osmolality, and simultaneous urine electrolytes and osmolality. A definitive diagnosis is not always possible at the time of presentation, but an initial categorization according to the patient's clinical ECF volume status will allow a determination of the appropriate initial therapy in the majority of cases (Fig. 1).

Decreased ECF Volume (Hypovolemia)

Clinically detectable hypovolemia, generally determined most sensitively by careful measurement of orthostatic changes in blood pressure and pulse rate, always indicates some degree of solute depletion. Elevation of plasma BUN is a useful laboratory correlate of decreased ECF volume. Even isotonic or hypotonic volume losses can lead to hypoosmolality if water or hypotonic fluids are ingested or infused as replacement. A low urine Na^+ concentration (U_{Na}) in such cases suggests a nonrenal cause of the solute depletion, whereas a high U_{Na} suggests renal causes of solute depletion (Table 1). Diuretic use is the most common cause of hypovolemic hypoosmolality, and thiazides are more commonly associated with severe hyponatremia than are loop diuretics such as furosemide. Although this represents a prime example of solute depletion, the pathophysiological mechanisms underlying the hypoosmolality are complex and are composed of multiple potential components including free water retention. Furthermore, many such patients do not present with clinical evidence of marked hypovolemia, mainly because ingested water has been retained in response to nonosmotically stimulated vasopressin (AVP) secretion, as is often true for all disorders of solute depletion. To further complicate diagnosis, the U_{Na} may be high or low depending on when the last diuretic dose was taken. Consequently, almost any suspicion of diuretic use mandates careful consideration of this diagnosis. A low plasma $[K^+]$ is an important clue to diuretic use, because few other disorders that cause hyponatremia and hypoosmolality also cause appreciable hypokalemia. Whenever the possibility of diuretic use is suspected in the absence of a positive history, a urine screen for diuretics should be performed. Most other etiologies of renal or nonrenal solute losses causing hypovolemic hypoosmolality will be clinically apparent, although some cases of salt-wasting nephropathies (chronic interstitial nephropathy, polycystic kidney disease, obstructive uropathy, or Bartter's syndrome) or mineralocorticoid deficiency (Addison's disease) may be challenging to diagnose during early phases of these diseases.

Normal ECF Volume (Euvolemia)

Virtually any disorder associated with hypoosmolality can potentially present with a volume status that appears normal by standard methods of clinical evaluation. Because clinical assessment of volume status is not very sensitive, normal or low levels of plasma BUN and uric acid are very helpful laboratory correlates of relatively normal, or even slightly expanded, ECF volume. In these cases a low U_{Na} suggests a depletional hypoosmolality secondary to ECF losses with subsequent volume replacement by water or other hypotonic fluids. As discussed earlier, such patients may appear euvolemic by all the usual clinical parameters used to assess hydrational status. Primary dilutional disorders are less likely in the presence of a low U_{Na} ($\leq$30 mEq/L), although this pattern can occur in hypothyroidism. A high U_{Na} (>30 mEq/L) generally indicates a dilutional hypoosmolality such as syndrome of inappropriate antidiure-

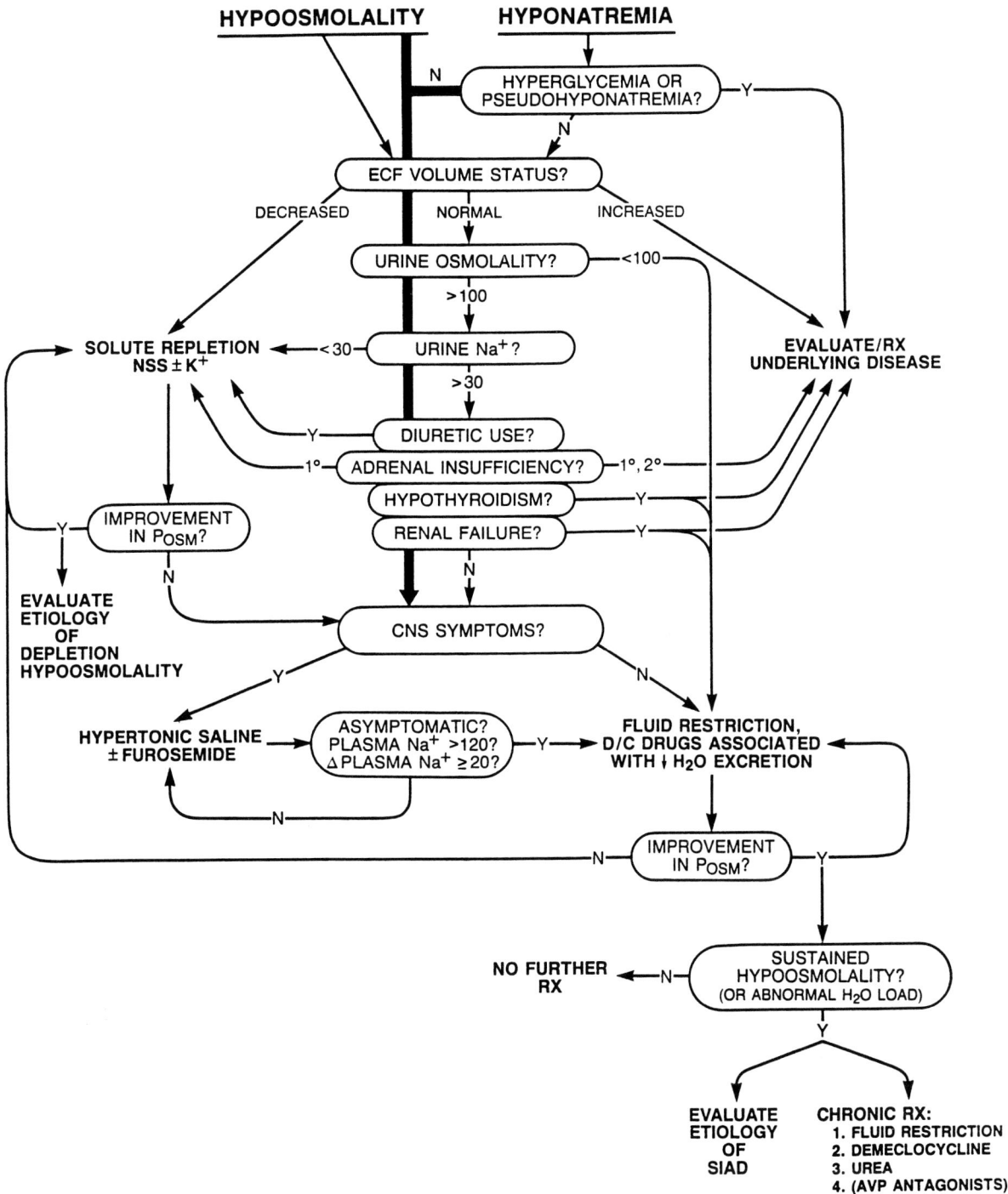

FIGURE I Schematic summary of the evaluation and therapy of hypoosmolar patients. The dark arrow in the center emphasizes that the presence of central nervous system dysfunction due to hyponatremia should always be assessed immediately, so that appropriate therapy can be started as soon as possible in symptomatic patients while the outlined diagnostic evaluation is proceeding. N, no; Y, yes; ECF, extracellular fluid volume; NSS, normal (isotonic) saline; Rx, treat; 1°, primary; 2°, secondary; P_{osm}, plasma osmolality; d/c, discontinue; SIAD, syndrome of inappropriate antidiuresis. Numbers referring to osmolality are in mOsm/kg H_2O, numbers referring to plasma Na^+ concentration are in mEq/L. Modified from Verbalis, 1995.

TABLE 2
Criteria for the Diagnosis of SIAD

Essential
1. Decreased effective osmolality of the extracellular fluid (P_{osm} < 275 mOsm/kg H_2O).
2. Inappropriate urinary concentration (U_{osm} > 100 mOsm/kg H_2O with normal renal function) at some level of hypoosmolality.
3. Clinical euvolemia, as defined by the absence of signs of hypovolemia (orthostasis, tachycardia, decreased skin turgor, dry mucous membranes) or hypervolemia (subcutaneous edema, ascites).
4. Elevated urinary sodium excretion while on a normal salt and water intake.
5. Absence of other potential causes of euvolemic hypoosmolality: hypothyroidism, hypocortisolism (Addison's disease or pituitary ACTH insufficiency) and diuretic use.

Supplemental
6. Abnormal water load test (inability to excrete at least 90% of a 20 mL/kg water load in 4 h and/or failure to dilute U_{osm} to < 100 mOsm/kg H_2O).
7. Plasma AVP level inappropriately elevated relative to plasma osmolality.
8. No significant correction of plasma [Na^+] with volume expansion but improvement after fluid restriction.

Note. Modified from Verbalis (1995).

sis (SIAD) (Table 1). SIAD is the most common cause of euvolemic hypoosmolality. Although originally described as the syndrome of inappropriate antidiuretic hormone secretion (SIADH), approximately 10 to 20% of patients who meet all established criteria for SIADH do not have measurably elevated plasma AVP levels, so it is actually more accurate to use the term SIAD rather than SIADH to describe this entire group of disorders. The clinical criteria necessary for a diagnosis of SIAD remain as defined by Bartter and Schwartz in 1967 (Table 2), but several points deserve emphasis. First, true ECF hypoosmolality must be present and hyponatremia secondary to pseudohyponatremia or hyperglycemia excluded. Second, urinary osmolality must be inappropriate for plasma hypoosmolality. This does not require a U_{osm} > P_{osm}, but simply that the urine osmolality is greater than maximally dilute (i.e., U_{osm} > 100 mOsm/kg H_2O). Furthermore, urine osmolality need not be inappropriately elevated at all levels of P_{osm} but simply at some level under 275 mOsm/kg H_2O, since in patients with a reset osmostat AVP secretion can be suppressed at some level of osmolality resulting in maximal urinary dilution and free water excretion at plasma osmolalities below this level. Although some consider a reset osmostat to be a separate disorder rather than a variant of SIAD, such cases nonetheless illustrate that some hypoosmolar patients can exhibit an appropriately dilute urine at some, though not all, plasma osmolalities. Third, clinical euvolemia must be present to diagnose SIAD, and this diagnosis cannot be made in a hypovolemic or edematous patient. This does not mean that patients with SIAD cannot become hypovolemic for other reasons, but in such cases

it is impossible to diagnose the underlying SIAD until the patient is rendered euvolemic. The fourth criterion, renal salt wasting, has probably caused the most confusion regarding SIAD. The importance of this criterion lies in its usefulness in differentiating hypoosmolality caused by a decreased relative intravascular volume in which case renal Na^+ conservation occurs, from dilutional disorders in which urinary Na^+ excretion is normal or increased due to ECF volume expansion. However, U_{Na} can also be high in renal causes of solute depletion such as diuretic use or Addison's disease, and conversely patients with SIAD can have a low urinary Na^+ excretion if they subsequently become hypovolemic or solute depleted—conditions sometimes produced by imposed salt and water restriction. Consequently, although high urinary Na^+ excretion is the rule in most patients with SIAD, its presence does not confirm this diagnosis nor does its absence rule out the diagnosis. The final criterion emphasizes that SIAD remains a diagnosis of exclusion, and the absence of other potential causes of hypoosmolality must always be verified. Glucocorticoid deficiency and SIAD can be especially difficult to distinguish, because hypocortisolism can cause elevated plasma AVP levels and also has direct renal effects to prevent maximal urinary dilution. No patient should be diagnosed as having SIAD without a thorough evaluation of adrenal function, preferably via a rapid ACTH stimulation test. Many different disorders have been associated with SIAD, and these can be divided into several major etiologic groups (Table 3).

Some cases of euvolemic hyponatremia do not fit particularly well into either the dilutional or depletional catego-

TABLE 3
Common Etiologies of SIAD

Tumors
  Pulmonary/mediastinal (bronchogenic carcinoma, mesothelioma, thymoma)
  Nonchest (duodenal carcinoma, pancreatic carcinoma, ureteral/prostate carcinoma, uterine carcinoma, nasopharyngeal carcinoma, leukemia)

Central nervous system disorders
  Mass lesions (tumors, brain abscesses, subdural hematoma)
  Inflammatory diseases (encephalitis, meningitis, lupus)
  Degenerative/demyelinative diseases (Guillain-Barré; spinal cord lesions)
  Miscellaneous (subarachnoid hemorrhage, head trauma, acute psychosis, delirium tremens, pituitary stalk section)

Drug induced
  Stimulated AVP release (nicotine, phenothiazines, tricyclics, serotonin reuptake inhibitors)
  Direct renal effects and/or potentiation of AVP effects (desmopressin, oxytocin, prostaglandin synthesis inhibitors)
  Mixed or uncertain actions (chlorpropamide, clofibrate, carbamazepine, cyclophosphamide, vincristine)

Pulmonary diseases
  Infections (tuberculosis, aspergillosis, pneumonia, empyema)
  Mechanical/ventilatory (acute respiratory failure, COPD, positive pressure ventilation)

ries. Chief among these is the hyponatremia that sometimes occurs in patients who ingest large volumes of beer with little food intake for prolonged periods, frequently called "beer potomania." Even though the volume of fluid ingested may not seem sufficiently excessive to overwhelm renal diluting mechanisms, in these cases free water excretion is limited by very low urinary solute excretion thereby causing water retention and dilutional hyponatremia. However, because such patients have very low Na^+ intakes as well, it is likely that relative depletion of body Na^+ stores also is a contributing factor to the hypoosmolality in some cases.

Increased ECF Volume (Edema, Ascites)

The presence of hypervolemia, as detected clinically by the presence of edema and/or ascites, indicates whole body sodium excess and hypoosmolality in these patients suggests a relatively decreased intravascular volume and/or pressure leading to water retention as a result of both elevated plasma AVP levels and decreased distal delivery of glomerular filtrate. Such patients usually have a low U_{Na} because of secondary hyperaldosteronism, but under certain conditions the U_{Na} may be elevated (e.g., glucosuria in diabetics, diuretic therapy). Hyponatremia generally does not occur until fairly advanced stages of diseases such as congestive heart failure, cirrhosis, and nephrotic syndrome, so diagnosis is usually not difficult. Renal failure can also cause retention of both sodium and water, but in this case the factor limiting excretion of excess body fluid is not decreased effective circulating volume but rather decreased glomerular filtration. It should be remembered that even though many edema-forming states have *secondary* increases in plasma AVP levels as a result of decreased effective arterial blood volume, they are not classified as cases of SIAD, since they fail to meet the criterion of clinical euvolemia (Table 2, point 3). Although it can be argued that this represents a semantic distinction, it is important with regard to segregating identifiable etiologies of hyponatremia that are associated with different methods of evaluation and therapy. Primary polydipsia also can cause hypoosmolality in a small subset of patients with underlying SIAD, particularly psychiatric patients with long-standing schizophrenia on neuroleptic drugs, or even more rarely in patients with normal kidney function if the volumes ingested exceed the maximum renal free water excretory rate of approximately 1000 mL/h. However, these patients rarely manifest overt signs of volume excess since water retention alone without sodium excess does not cause clinically apparent hypervolemia.

Although incidences will vary according to the population being studied, sequential analysis of hyponatremic patients admitted to a large university teaching hospital revealed that approximately 20% were hypovolemic, 20% had edema-forming states, 33% were euvolemic, 15% had hyperglycemia-induced hyponatremia, and 10% had renal failure. Consequently, euvolemic hyponatremia generally constitutes the largest single group of hyponatremic patients found in this setting.

CLINICAL MANIFESTATIONS OF HYPONATREMIA

The clinical manifestations of hyponatremia are largely neurological and primarily reflect brain edema resulting from osmotic water shifts into the brain. Significant symptoms generally do not occur until plasma $[Na^+]$ falls below 125 mEq/L, and the severity of symptoms can be roughly correlated with the degree of hypoosmolality. However, individual variability is marked, and, for any single patient, the level of plasma $[Na^+]$ at which symptoms will appear cannot be predicted. Furthermore, several factors other than the severity of the hypoosmolality also affect the degree of neurological dysfunction. Most important is the period during which hypoosmolality develops. Rapid development of severe hypoosmolality is frequently associated with marked neurologic symptoms, whereas gradual development over several days or weeks is often associated with relatively mild symptomatology despite profound degrees of hypoosmolality. This is because the brain can counteract osmotic swelling by excreting intracellular solutes (including potassium and organic osmolytes). Because this is a time-dependent process, rapid development of hypoosmolality can result in brain edema before this adaptation occurs, but with slower development of the same degree of hypoosmolality brain cells can lose solute sufficiently rapidly to prevent brain edema and neurological dysfunction. Underlying neurological disease also affects the level of hypoosmolality at which CNS symptoms appear; moderate hypoosmolality is of little concern in an otherwise healthy patient, but can cause morbidity in a patient with an underlying seizure disorder. Nonneurological metabolic disorders (hypoxia, hypercapnia, acidosis, hypercalcemia, etc.) similarly can affect the level of plasma osmolality at which CNS symptoms occur. Recent clinical studies have suggested that menstruating females and young children may be particularly susceptible to the development of neurological morbidity and mortality during hyponatremia, especially in the acute postoperative setting. The true clinical incidence as well as the underlying mechanisms responsible for these sometimes catastrophic cases remains to be determined.

THERAPY

Despite some continuing controversy regarding the optimal speed of correction of osmolality in hyponatremic patients, there is now a relatively uniform consensus about appropriate therapy in most cases (Fig. 1). If any degree of clinical hypovolemia is present, the patient should be considered to have a solute depletion-induced hypoosmolality and treated with isotonic (0.9%) NaCl at a rate appropriate for the estimated volume depletion. If diuretic use is known or suspected, saline should be supplemented with potassium (30 to 40 mEq/L) even if plasma $[K^+]$ is not low because of the propensity of such patients to have total body potassium depletion. Most often the hypoosmolar patient will be clinically euvolemic, but several situations will dictate a reconsideration of potential solute depletion even in the patient without clinically apparent hypovolemia: a decreased U_{Na}, any history of recent diuretic use, and any suggestion of primary adrenal insufficiency. Whenever a reasonable likelihood of depletional rather than dilutional hypoosmolality exists, it is appropriate to treat initially with a trial of isotonic NaCl. If the patient has SIAD, no harm will have been done with a limited (1 to 2 L) saline infusion, because such patients will simply excrete excess NaCl without significantly changing their P_{osm}. However, this therapy should be abandoned if plasma [Na$^+$] does not improve, because longer periods of continued isotonic NaCl infusion can worsen the hyponatremia by virtue of gradual water retention. The treatment of euvolemic hypoosmolar patients will vary depending on their presentation. A patient meeting all criteria for SIAD except that U_{osm} is low should simply be observed since this may represent spontaneous reversal of a transient form of SIAD. If there is any suspicion of either primary or secondary adrenal insufficiency, glucocorticoid replacement should be started immediately after completion of a rapid ACTH stimulation test. Prompt water diuresis following initiation of glucocorticoid treatment strongly supports glucocorticoid deficiency, but the absence of a quick response does not negate this diagnosis since several days of glucocorticoids are sometimes required for normalization of P_{osm}. Hypervolemic hypoosmolar patients are generally treated initially by diuresis and other measures directed at their underlying disorder. Such patients rarely require any therapy to increase plasma osmolality acutely, but often benefit from varying degrees of sodium and water restriction to reduce body fluid retention.

In any significantly hyponatremic patient one is faced with the question of how quickly the plasma osmolality should be corrected. Although hyponatremia is associated with a broad spectrum of neurological symptoms, sometimes leading to death in severe cases, too rapid correction of severe hyponatremia can produce pontine and extrapontine myelinolysis—a brain demyelinating disease that also can cause substantial neurological morbidity and mortality. Recent clinical and experimental results suggest that optimal treatment of hyponatremic patients entails balancing the risks of hyponatremia against the risks of correction for each patient. Several factors should therefore be considered in making a treatment decision in hyponatremic patients: the severity of the hyponatremia, the duration of the hyponatremia, and the patient's symptomatology. Neither sequelae from hyponatremia itself nor myelinolysis after therapy is very likely in patients whose serum [Na$^+$] remains $\geq$120mEq/L, although significant symptoms can develop even at higher serum [Na$^+$] levels if the rate of fall of plasma osmolality has been very rapid. The importance of duration and symptomatology relates to how well the brain has volume-adapted to the hyponatremia, and consequently its degree of risk for subsequent demyelination with rapid correction. Cases of acute hyponatremia ($\geq$48 hours in duration) are usually symptomatic if the hyponatremia is severe (i.e., $\leq$120 mEq/L). These patients are at greatest risk from neurological complications from the hyponatremia itself and should be corrected to higher plasma [Na$^+$] levels promptly. Conversely, patients with

more chronic hyponatremia >48 hours in duration) who have minimal neurological symptomatology are at little risk from complications of hyponatremia itself, but can develop demyelination following rapid correction. There is no indication to correct these patients rapidly, and they should be treated using slower-acting therapies such as fluid restriction.

Although the above extremes have clear treatment indications, most hyponatremic episodes will be of indeterminate duration and patients will have varying degrees of milder neurological symptomatology. This group presents the most challenging treatment decisions, since the hyponatremia will have been present sufficiently long to allow some degree of brain volume regulation, but not enough to prevent some brain edema and neurological symptomatology. Most recommend prompt treatment of such patients because of their symptoms, but using methods that allow a *controlled and limited* correction of their hyponatremia. Reasonable correction parameters consist of a maximal rate of correction of plasma [Na$^+$] in the range of 1 to 2 mEq $\cdot$ L^{-1} $\cdot$ h^{-1} as long as the total magnitude of correction does not exceed 25 mEq/L over the first 48 hours. Some argue that these parameters should be even more conservative with maximal correction rates of $\leq$0.5 mEq $\cdot$ L^{-1} $\cdot$ h^{-1} and magnitudes of correction that do not exceed 12 mEq/L in any 24-hour period. Treatments for individual patients should be chosen within these limits depending on their symptomatology. In patients who are only moderately symptomatic, one should proceed at the lower recommended limits of $\leq$0.5 mEq $\cdot$ L^{-1} $\cdot$ h^{-1}, while in those who manifest more severe neurological symptoms an initial correction at a rate of 1 to 2 mEq $\cdot$ L^{-1} $\cdot$ h^{-1} would be more appropriate. Controlled corrections are generally best accomplished with hypertonic (3%) NaCl solution given via continuous infusion, because patients with euvolemic hypoosmolality such as SIAD generally will not respond to isotonic NaCl. An initial infusion rate can be estimated by multiplying the patient's body weight, in kg, by the desired rate of increase in plasma [Na$^+$], in mEq $\cdot$ L^{-1} $\cdot$ h^{-1} (e.g., in a 70-kg patient an infusion of 3% NaCl at 70 mL/h will increase plasma [Na$^+$] by approximately 1 mEq $\cdot$ L^{-1} $\cdot$ h^{-1}, while infusing 35 mL/h will increase plasma [Na$^+$] by approximately 0.5 mEq $\cdot$ L^{-1} $\cdot$ h^{-1}). Furosemide (20 to 40 mg iv) should be used to treat volume overload. It should be used preemptively in patients with known cardiovascular disease. Patients with diuretic-induced hyponatremia usually respond well to isotonic NaCl and do not require 3% NaCl. Regardless of the initial rate of correction chosen, acute treatment should be interrupted once any of three endpoints is reached: (1) the patient's symptoms are abolished, (2) a safe plasma [Na$^+$] (generally $\geq$120 mEq/L) is achieved, or (3) a total magnitude of correction of 20 mEq/L is achieved. It follows from these recommendations that serum [Na$^+$] levels must be carefully monitored at frequent intervals (at least every 4 hours) during the active phases of treatment in order to adjust therapy so that the correction stays within these guidelines. Regardless of the therapy or rate initially chosen, it cannot be emphasized too strongly that it is only necessary to correct the plasma osmolality acutely to a safe range rather than completely to normonatremia. In some situations patients may spontaneously correct their hyponatremia via a water diuresis. When the hyponatremia is acute (e.g., psychogenic polydipsia with water intoxication), such patients do not appear to be at risk for subsequent demyelination; however, in cases where the hyponatremia has been chronic (e.g., hypocortisolism) intervention should be considered to limit the rate and magnitude of correction of plasma [Na$^+$] (e.g., administration of desmopressin 1 to 2 μg iv or infusion of hypotonic fluids) using the same endpoints as for active correction.

Treatment of chronic hyponatremia entails choosing among several suboptimal therapies. An important exception is patients with the reset osmostat syndrome; because the hyponatremia of such patients is not progressive but rather fluctuates around their reset level of plasma [Na$^+$], no therapy is generally required. For most other cases of mild-to-moderate SIAD, fluid restriction represents the least toxic therapy by far and is the treatment of choice. This should always be tried as the initial therapy, with pharmacologic intervention reserved for refractory cases where the degree of fluid restriction required to avoid hypoosmolality is so severe that the patient is unable, or unwilling, to maintain it. If pharmacologic treatment is necessary, the preferred drug at present is the tetracycline derivative demeclocycline, which causes nephrogenic diabetes insipidus, thereby decreasing urine concentration. The effective dose of demeclocycline ranges from 600 to 1200 mg/day; several days of therapy are necessary to achieve maximum effects, so one should wait 3 to 4 days before increasing the dose. Demeclocycline can cause reversible nephrotoxicity, especially in patients with cirrhosis; renal function should be monitored and the medication stopped if increasing azotemia occurs. Several other drugs (diphenylhydantoin, opiates, ethanol) can decrease AVP hypersecretion in selected cases, but responses are unpredictable. The current unavailability of an ideal therapeutic agent for chronic SIAD will likely change in the near future with development of specific AVP antidiuretic receptor antagonists. Such agents will likely become the treatments of choice for SIAD. However, their use to correct established hyponatremia will require judicious adherence to the same guidelines already established for other therapies to prevent complications from brain demyelination.

Bibliography

Anderson RJ, Chung H-M, Kluge R et al: Hyponatremia: A prospective analysis of its epidemiology and the pathogenetic role of vasopressin. *Ann Intern Med* 102:164–168, 1985.

Arieff AI, Llach F, Massry SG: Neurological manifestations and morbidity of hyponatremia: Correlation with brain water and electrolytes. *Medicine* 55:121–129, 1976.

Ayus JC, Wheeler JM, Arieff AI: Postoperative hyponatremic encephalopathy in menstruant women. *Ann Intern Med* 117:891–897, 1992.

Bartter FC, Schwartz WB: The syndrome of inappropriate secretion of antidiuretic hormone. *Am J Med* 42:790–806, 1967.

Berl T: Treating hyponatremia: Damned if we do and damned if we don't. *Kidney Int* 37:1006–1018, 1990.

Robertson GL, Aycinena P, Zerbe RL: Neurogenic disorders of osmoregulation. *Am J Med* 72:339–353, 1982.

Robertson GL: Posterior pituitary. In: Felig P, Baxter JD, Frohman LA (eds) *Endocrinology and Metabolism.* McGraw-Hill, New York, pp. 385–432, 1995.

Saito T, Ishikawa S, Abe K, et al: Acute aquaresis by the nonpeptide arginine vasopressin (AVP) antagonist OPC-31260 improves hyponatremia in patients with syndrome of inappropriate secretion of antidiuretic hormone (SIADH). *J Clin Endocrinol Metab* 82:1054–1057, 1997.

Schrier RW: Pathogenesis of sodium and water retention in high-output and low-output cardiac failure, nephrotic syndrome, cirrhosis and pregnancy. *N Engl J Med* 319:1065–1072; 1127–1134, 1988.

Sterns RH: Severe symptomatic hyponatremia: Treatment and outcome. A study of 64 cases. *Ann Intern Med* 107:656–664, 1987.

Sterns RH, Ocdol H, Schrier RW et al: Hyponatremia: Pathophysiology, diagnosis, and therapy. In: Narins RG (ed) *Disorders of Fluid and Electrolytes.* McGraw-Hill, New York, pp. 583–615, 1994.

Verbalis JG: Hyponatremia: Epidemiology, pathophysiology, and therapy. *Curr Opin Nephrol Hypertens* 2:636–652, 1993.

Verbalis JG: Inappropriate antidiuresis and other hypoosmolar states. In: Becker KG (ed) *Principles and Practice of Endocrinology and Metabolism.* Lippincott, Philadelphia, pp. 265–276, 1995.

Verbalis JG: The syndrome of inappropriate antidiuretic hormone secretion and other hypoosmolar disorders. In: Schrier RW, Gottschalk CW (eds) *Diseases of the Kidney.* Little, Brown & Co., Boston, pp. 2393–2427, 1996.

Zerbe R, Stropes L, Robertson G: Vasopressin function in the syndrome of inappropriate antidiuresis. *Annu Rev Med* 31:315–327, 1980.

8

HYPERNATREMIA

PAUL M. PALEVSKY

Hypernatremia is one of the two cardinal disturbances of water homeostasis. Decreases in total body water relative to total body electrolyte are characterized by an increase in the electrolyte concentration in all body fluids. In the intracellular compartment this is manifested by a decrease in cell volume and an increase in the intracellular potassium concentration. In the extracellular space, the primary manifestation is an increase in the sodium concentration, resulting in the laboratory finding of hypernatremia.

Hypernatremia does not imply an abnormality in sodium homeostasis. Rather it is a disturbance in the sodium concentration resulting from a deficit of water relative to salt. Total body sodium content is the primary determinant of extracellular volume and in the setting of intact water homeostasis does not have a primary effect on the sodium concentration. Alterations in sodium balance result in isotonic volume expansion or volume depletion unless also accompanied by a defect in water homeostasis. Hypernatremia may occur, however, with normal, increased or decreased total body sodium content, manifest by corresponding alterations in extracellular volume.

Hypernatremia is a common clinical problem, with a prevalence in hospitalized patients of 0.5 to 2%. In adults, two distinct groups of hypernatremic patients may be identified. Patients developing hypernatremia prior to hospital admission are generally elderly and debilitated and often have an intercurrent acute infection. In contrast, patients developing hypernatremia during hospitalization have an age distribution similar to that of the general hospital population. In these patients, hypernatremia is an iatrogenic complication usually associated with impaired thirst or restricted access to water combined with an inadequate prescription for water administration.

REGULATION OF WATER HOMEOSTASIS

The physiologic response to hypertonicity includes both renal water conservation and stimulation of thirst. Hypertonicity is sensed by osmoreceptors located adjacent to the anterior wall of the third ventricle in the hypothalamus. Activation of these osmoreceptors stimulates the secretion of arginine vasopressin by neurons whose cell bodies are in the supraoptic and paraventricular nuclei in the hypothalamus and whose axons terminate in the posterior pitu-

itary gland. In the kidney, arginine vasopressin modulates the hydraulic permeability of the collecting duct. In the absence of vasopressin, the collecting duct is relatively impermeant to water. Vasopressin exerts its effect on the collecting duct through the activation of V_2-vasopressin receptors located on the basolateral aspect of the tubular epithelium. The V_2-receptor is coupled to adenylate cyclase by GTP-binding proteins; receptor binding activates adenylate cyclase, which catalyzes the conversion of adenosine triphosphate (ATP) to the second messenger, cyclic-AMP (cAMP). Through incompletely elucidated mechanisms, cAMP stimulates the insertion of the aquaporin-2 water channel into the apical cell membrane. The resulting increase in the hydraulic permeability of the apical cell membrane permits the passive reabsorption of water from the collecting duct into the isotonic cortical and hypertonic medullary interstitium. The excretion of a concentrated urine is therefore dependent on the generation and maintenance of the corticomedullary osmotic gradient as well as the utilization of the gradient through the tubular response to vasopressin secretion.

The osmotic regulation of vasopressin secretion is extremely sensitive. Below a body fluid osmolality of 280 to 285 mmol/kg, vasopressin secretion is inhibited and plasma vasopressin levels are virtually undetectable. As body fluid osmolality increases above this threshold, vasopressin secretion increases linearly with increases in body fluid osmolality of as little as 1 to 2% resulting in detectable increases in plasma vasopressin levels. The renal response to changes in vasopressin secretion is also extremely sensitive. Urine is maximally dilute when vasopressin secretion is suppressed; urinary concentration increases linearly as plasma vasopressin levels rise in response to rising plasma tonicity, with maximal urinary concentration achieved at vasopressin levels that correspond to a plasma osmolality of approximately 295 mmol/kg.

While renal water conservation is important in preventing further renal water losses, it is not sufficient for the prevention of progressive hypertonicity or the restoration of plasma tonicity to normal. The ultimate defense against the development of hypertonicity and hypernatremia is the osmotic stimulation of thirst and its resultant increase in water ingestion. Thirst is also mediated by hypothalamic osmoreceptors located in the anterior wall of the third ventricle. These thirst osmoreceptors, although in proximity to the osmoreceptors modulating vasopressin secretion, are anatomically distinct. Impulses from these osmoreceptors are projected to higher levels in the cerebral cortex, where they result in the perception of thirst and water-seeking behavior. The osmotic threshold for thirst is approximately 5 mmol/kg greater than the osmotic threshold for vasopressin secretion; once this threshold is exceeded, thirst increases proportionately as body fluid osmolality rises.

PATHOPHYSIOLOGY

Hypernatremia results when there is net water loss or hypertonic sodium gain. In the normal individual, thirst is stimulated by any rise in body fluid tonicity. Water ingestion increases and the hypernatremic state is rapidly corrected. Therefore, sustained hypernatremia can occur only when the thirst mechanism is impaired and water intake does not increase in response to hypertonicity. Although increased water losses or hypertonic sodium gain usually contribute to the development of hypernatremia, abnormalities in the osmoregulation of thirst or in thirst perception or the inability to gain access to water are required for the development of sustained hypernatremia.

The importance of thirst in the pathogenesis of hypernatremia is illustrated by patients with severe diabetes insipidus. These patients are unable to concentrate their urine and excrete large volumes of dilute urine, occasionally in excess of 10 to 15 L/day. Under normal circumstances they do not develop hypernatremia—in response to their renal water losses, thirst is stimulated and they maintain body fluid tonicity at the expense of profound secondary polydipsia. If, however, they are unable to drink in response to thirst, as may occur during an intercurrent illness, hypernatremia rapidly develops.

Isolated defects in thirst (primary hypodipsia) are uncommon but may result from any process involving the hypothalamus in proximity to the anterior wall of the third ventricle (Table 1). Lesions may include a wide range of intrcranial pathology, including primary and metastatic tumors, granulomatous diseases, vascular abnormalities (most commonly involving the anterior communicating artery), trauma, and hydrocephalus. Hypodipsia has also been described in elderly patients (geriatric hypodipsia) in whom overt hypothalamic pathology is absent. Essential hypernatremia is a rare disorder in which there is an upward resetting of the thresholds for both thirst and vasopressin secretion. Patients with this condition are able to concentrate and dilute their urine, albeit around an elevated body fluid osmolality, and have an elevated set point for thirst perception. More commonly, impaired thirst results from diffuse neurologic disease which interferes with the less well-defined cerebral cortical pathways subserving thirst perception and water ingestion (secondary hypodipsia). Thus, defects in thirst are commonly associated with cerebrovascular disease, dementia, and acute illnesses that result in delirium or obtundation.

CLINICAL CLASSIFICATION

Although impaired thirst and restricted water intake underlie the development of sustained hypernatremia, the hypernatremic states are most commonly classified on the basis of the associated water loss or electrolyte gain and the corresponding changes in extracellular fluid volume (Table 2). Pure water deficits are associated with minimal change in total body sodium and relative preservation of extracellular fluid volume. When hypotonic fluid deficits are present, hypernatremia coexists with total body sodium

TABLE I
Defects in Thirst

Primary hypodipsia
    Hypothalamic lesions affecting the osmostat
    Trauma
    Craniopharyngioma or other primary suprasellar tumor
    Metastatic tumor
    Granulomatous disease
    Vascular lesions
    Essential hypernatremia
    Geriatric hypodipsia
Secondary hypodipsia
    Cerebrovascular disease
    Dementia
    Delirium
    Mental status changes

TABLE 2
Classification of Hypernatremia on the Basis of Associated Changes in Extracellular Volume

Pure water deficit (normal extracellular volume)
    Diabetes insipidus
        Hypothalamic
        Nephrogenic
    Increased insensible losses
Hypotonic fluid deficit (decreased extracellular volume)
    Renal losses
        Diuretic administration
        Osmotic diuresis
        Postobstructive diuresis
        Polyuric phase of ATN[a]
    Gastrointestinal losses
        Vomiting
        Nasogastric drainage
        Enterocutaneous fistulae
        Diarrhea
    Cutaneous losses
        Burn injuries
        Excessive perspiration
Hypertonic sodium gain (increased extracellular volume)
    Salt ingestion
    Hypertonic NaCl
    Hypertonic $NaHCO_3$
    Total parenteral nutrition

[a] ATN, acute tubular necrosis.

depletion and extracellular fluid volume contraction. Hypertonic sodium gain results in hypernatremia and extracellular fluid volume expansion. (see Fig. 1)

Pure Water Deficits

Isolated water deficits, unless of extreme magnitude, are generally not associated with clinical evidence of intravascular volume depletion. Only one-third of a pure water deficit is derived from the extracellular compartment, and only one-twelfth from the intravascular compartment. In a 70-kg individual, a 5% decrease in total body water, which would result in an increase in the plasma sodium concentration of approximately 7 mmol/L, results in a reduction in ECF volume of less than 700 mL and intravascular volume of less than 200 mL. This modest degree of volume depletion is generally not detectable on physical examination and may be manifest only by mild prerenal azotemia. With more severe water deficits, hemodynamically significant intravascular volume depletion may develop.

Pure water deficits may occur with impaired thirst unaccompanied by increased water losses. In patients with significant hypodipsia, voluntary water ingestion may not be sufficient to replace obligate gastrointestinal and insensible water losses. Despite maximal renal water conservation, progressive hypernatremia will result if supplemental water intake is not provided. More commonly, pure water deficits develop in the setting of increased insensible or renal water losses. Insensible water losses are approximately $0.6 \, \mathrm{mL} \cdot \mathrm{kg}^{-1} \cdot \mathrm{h}^{-1}$, or about 1 L/day in the average adult. These losses are not subject to osmotic regulation but may be increased by a wide variety of factors including fever, exercise, increased ambient temperature, and hyperventilation. Increased renal electrolyte-free water losses result from diabetes insipidus. Patients with increased insensible losses manifest oliguria with a maximally concentrated urine (urine osmolality >700 mmol/kg). In contrast, patients with diabetes insipidus have polyuria and a less than maximally concentrated urine.

Diabetes Insipidus

Diabetes insipidus results either from failure of the hypothalamic–pituitary axis to synthesize or release adequate amounts of vasopressin (hypothalamic diabetes insipidus) or from failure of the kidney to produce a concentrated urine despite appropriate circulating vasopressin levels (nephrogenic diabetes insipidus). In both forms of the disorder, the inability of the kidney to concentrate the

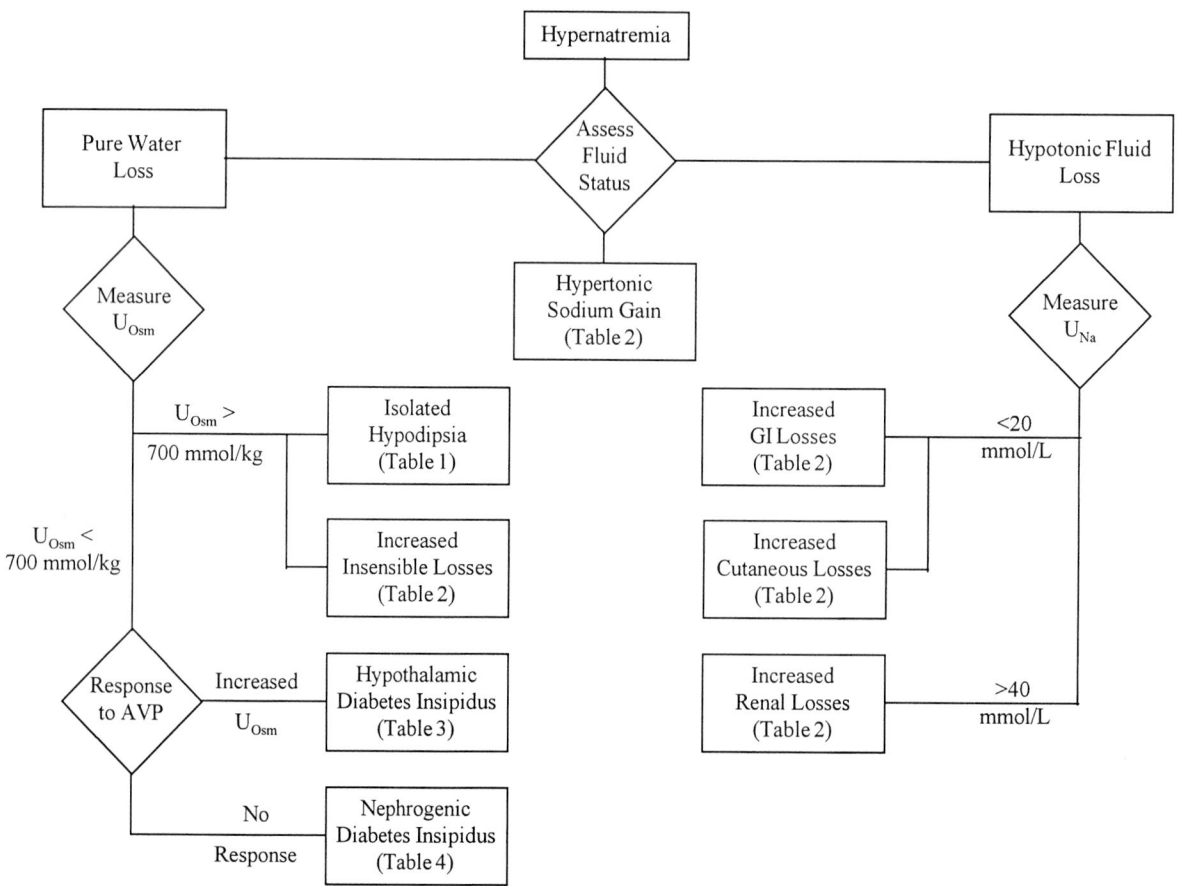

FIGURE I   Algorithm for the evaluation of hypernatremia.

urine leads to polyuria and secondary polydipsia. If water intake is adequate to replace urinary electrolyte-free water losses, hypertonicity and hypernatremia will not develop. Thus, hypernatremia is not a hallmark of diabetes insipidus.

Diabetes insipidus may occur in either complete or partial forms. In complete hypothalamic diabetes insipidus, vasopressin secretion is absent, resulting in the production of large volumes of dilute urine (urine osmolality <150 mmol/L). In partial hypothalamic diabetes insipidus, vasopressin secretion is detectable but subnormal, and a less severe defect in renal water conservation is present. Similarly, in complete nephrogenic diabetes insipidus, renal responsiveness to the hydroosmotic effect of vasopressin is absent, whereas an impaired response occurs in partial nephrogenic diabetes insipidus.

Any pathologic process involving the hypothalamic–pituitary axis may lead to vasopressin deficiency and hypothalamic diabetes insipidus (Table 3). Common etiologies include pituitary surgery, head trauma, primary and metastatic tumors, leukemia, hemorrhage, thrombosis, and granulomatous diseases. Diabetes insipidus following head trauma or surgery may be transient, may be permanent, or may follow a triphasic course. The transient form is most common, with an abrupt onset followed by resolution over a period of days to weeks. In the triphasic pattern, there is an initial period of vasopressin deficiency lasting 2 to 4 days as the result of axonal injury, a 5- to 7-day period of inappropriate vasopressin release thought to result from release of hormone by degenerating neurons, and finally permanent diabetes insipidus following neuronal death. In 30% of patients, hypothalamic diabetes insipidus is idiopathic, most probably occurring on an autoimmune

basis. A rare, hereditary form is due to mutations in the vasopressin–neurophysin gene which result in an abnormal structure and processing of the vasopressin prohormone and ultimately cell death of the vasopressin-secreting neurons.

The term nephrogenic diabetes insipidus should be restricted to those situations in which there is an intrinsic abnormality of the collecting duct that leads to vasopressin insensitivity or hyporesponsiveness. Patients with chronic tubulointerstitial renal disease may be unable to generate or maintain a normal corticomedullary osmotic gradient and are therefore unable to concentrate their urine normally. However, they rarely have significant polyuria and should not be considered to have nephrogenic diabetes insipidus.

Nephrogenic diabetes insipidus may be either acquired or congenital in origin (Table 4). The acquired form is far more common than the congenital and is most often associated with pharmacologic therapy with lithium or demeclocycline. Both agents have been demonstrated to inhibit intracellular generation of cAMP in response to vasopressin. In addition, demeclocycline also inhibits the intracellular action of cAMP. Acquired nephrogenic diabetes insipidus may also result from obstructive uropathy, hypercalcemia, or severe hypokalemia.

The congenital form of nephrogenic diabetes insipidus has been identified in multiple kindreds and is usually inherited in a sex-linked pattern with variable penetrance in hemizygous females. The genetic defect has been localized in the majority of kindreds to the vasopressin V_2-receptor gene; however, mutations in the aquaporin-2 gene have been identified in rare patients with an autosomal recessive form of nephrogenic diabetes insipidus.

The polyuria of diabetes insipidus needs to be differentiated from other forms of polyuria, including primary polydipsia, solute diuresis secondary to glycosuria, mannitol, urea, or diuretics, or resolving acute renal failure. Polyuria due to solute diuresis can usually be excluded by demonstrating that the urine osmolality is less than 150 mmol/kg. In patients with severe polyuria, formal dehydration testing is usually unnecessary and may result in severe hypernatremia and hypotension. Dehydration testing may be re-

TABLE 3
Hypothalamic Diabetes Insipidus

Pituitary surgery

Head trauma

Neoplasia
  Primary: Dysgerminoma, craniopharyngioma, suprasellar
    pituitary tumors
  Metastatic: Carcinomas of the breast and lumphoma
  Leukemia

Vascular lesions
  Aneurysms
  Cerebrovascular accidents
  Sheehan's syndrome (postpartum pituitary hemorrhage)

Infections
  Encephalitis
  Meningitis
  Tuberculosis
  Syphilis

Granulomatous disease
  Sarcoidosis
  Histiocytosis

Autoimmune

Vasopressin–neurophysin gene mutations

TABLE 4
Nephrogenic Diabetes Insipidus

Drug induced
  Lithium
  Demeclocycline
  Methoxyflurane
  Amphotericin B

Electrolyte Disorders
  Hypercalcemia
  Hypokalemia

Obstructive uropathy

Congenital
  Vasopressin V_2-receptor mutations
  Aquaporin-2 mutations

quired, however, to diagnose partial forms of diabetes insipidus.

During a dehydration test, the patient is placed on a strict fast with special care taken to ensure that the patient consumes no fluids. During the test, urine osmolality is measured hourly and plasma osmolality every 4 to 6 hours. Water deprivation is continued until body weight has declined by 3%, plasma osmolality has reached 295 mmol/kg, or urine osmolality has reached a plateau (variation of less than 5% over 3 hours). In patients with severe diabetes insipidus, urine osmolality will remain less than plasma osmolality, whereas in partial diabetes insipidus urine osmolality will be greater than plasma osmolality although submaximally concentrated (Table 5). The urinary response to exogenous vasopressin usually differentiates the hypothalamic form from the nephrogenic form. Measurement of plasma vasopressin levels at maximal dehydration (prior to exogenous vasopressin), although not routinely available, may be extremely useful in equivocal cases.

Hypotonic Fluid Deficits

Patients with inadequately replaced hypotonic fluid losses will develop both hypernatremia and extracellular volume depletion. Unlike patients with pure water losses, these individuals manifest the classic findings of intravascular volume depletion, i.e., tachycardia, hypotension, and decreased central venous pressure. Hypotonic fluid may be lost from the skin, gastrointestinal tract, or kidney. Cutaneous losses of electrolyte-containing hypotonic fluids may be significant in patients with severe burn injuries and patients with increased sensible perspiration (as opposed to insensible transpirational skin loss). The majority of gastrointestinal fluids, with the exception of pancreatic and biliary secretions, are also hypotonic. Protracted vomiting, nasogastric drainage, and diarrhea commonly contribute to the development of hypovolemic hypernatremia. Excessive renal hypotonic fluid losses are most commonly due to diuretic therapy but are also associated with osmotic diureses due to glucose, mannitol, or urea. Postobstructive diuresis, the polyuric phase of acute tubular necrosis, adrenal insufficiency, and a variety of chronic renal diseases, especially medullary cystic disease and renal tubular acidosis (types I and II), are also associated with renal-salt wasting and hypotonic urinary losses. Hypovolemic hypernatremia may

also develop in patients with "third-space" fluid losses (e.g., bowel obstruction, pancreatitis, peritonitis) if the sequestration of isotonic fluid is combined with inadequate replacement of ongoing electrolyte-free water losses.

Urinary indices are helpful in ascertaining the source of hypotonic fluid losses. When the losses have a renal origin, the urine sodium concentration is usually elevated (>20 mmol/L) and the urine is less than maximally concentrated. In contrast, nonrenal losses are associated with renal sodium avidity (urine sodium <10 mmol/L) and a maximally concentrated urine (urine osmolality >700 mmol/kg).

Hypertonic Sodium Gain

Hypertonic sodium gain produces hypernatremia and extracellular volume overload. When both thirst and renal function are intact, the volume and tonicity disturbances are transient. The increase in tonicity stimulates thirst, with a resultant increase in water intake that corrects the hypertonicity. In addition, the volume expansion stimulates a natruresis. Persistent hypernatremia implies impaired thirst or restricted water intake. Hypertonic sodium gain may result from the accidental ingestion of large quantities of sodium salts but is more commonly iatrogenic, resulting from the administration of hypertonic sodium chloride or sodium bicarbonate solutions, inappropriate electrolyte prescription for parenteral hyperalimentation solutions, or inappropriate sodium supplementation of enteral nutrition. Errors in formula preparation may result in hypernatremia in infants.

Hypertonicity Due to Nonelectrolyte Solutes

Although all hypernatremia results in body fluid hypertonicity, hypertonicity can also occur in the absence of hypernatremia. The accumulation of osmotically active nonelectrolyte solutes in the extracellular compartment may result in the development of hypertonicity accompanied by a normal, or even depressed, serum sodium concentration. The accumulation of a nonelectrolyte solute increases the osmolality of the extracellular fluids. If the solute cannot enter the intracellular compartment, water will exit the intracellular space. The net result is intracellular dehydration, cell shrinkage, expansion of the extracellular compartment, and dilution of the extracellular fluid sodium concen-

TABLE 5
Diagnosis of Diabetes Insipidus

Disorder	Urine osmolality		Plasma vasopressin level
	After dehydration	After exogenous vasopressin	
Hypothalamic DI			
Complete	<300 mmol/kg	>50% increase	<1.0 pg/mL
Partial	>300 mmol/kg	>10% increase	<1.5 pg/mL
Nephrogenic DI			
Complete	<300 mmol/kg	<50% increase	>5.0 pg/mL
Partial	>300 mmol/kg	<10% increase	>2.0 pg/mL

tration. It is important to recognize nonhypernatremic hypertonicity in order to avoid institution of inappropriate therapy for the resultant dilutional hyponatremia.

The most common nonelectrolyte solute associated causing hypertonicity is glucose. In patients with hyperglycemia, the serum sodium concentration usually declines by 1.6–2.0 mmol/L for each 100 mg/dL increase in plasma glucose above normal. Isonatremic and hyponatremic hypertonicity have also been described following administration of mannitol, maltose, sorbitol, glycerol, and radiocontrast agents. If suspected, the presence of an unmeasured solute may be confirmed by comparison of the measured plasma osmolality with an estimate of plasma osmolality derived from measurement of serum sodium, glucose, and urea nitrogen concentrations:

$$P_{Osm} = (2 \times [Na^+]) + glucose\ (mg/dL)/18 \\ + BUN\ (mg/dL)/2.8.$$

The presence of an "osmolar gap" between these two values for plasma osmolality suggests the presence of an unmeasured solute. The responsible solute can usually be ascertained by review of medications administered and may be confirmed by specific biochemical testing.

CLINICAL MANIFESTATIONS

The major clinical manifestations of hypernatremia result from alterations in brain water content. In response to hypertonicity, fluid shifts from the intracellular compartment into the extracellular compartment, maintaining osmotic equilibrium and resulting in a decrease in intracellular volume. In the central nervous system, acute hypernatremia is associated with a rapid decrease in water content and brain volume (Fig. 2). Within 24 hours, however, adaptive processes result in the uptake of electrolyte into brain cells with a partial restoration of brain volume. Subsequently, there is an increase in intracellular organic solute content, primarily through the accumulation of amino acids, polyols, and methylamines, which restores brain volume to normal. The accumulation of these intracellular solutes ("idiogenic osmoles") has important therapeutic implications. Although they minimize cerebral dehydration during hypertonicity, their accumulation increases the risk of cerebral edema during the treatment of hypernatremia.

The clinical manifestations of hypernatremia reflect its rapidity of onset, its duration, and its magnitude. In severe acute hypernatremia, brain shrinkage may be substantial, placing traction on the venous sinuses and intracerebral veins and causing their rupture. The resulting intracerebral and subarachnoid hemorrhage may produce irreversible neurologic defects or death. The manifestations of less profound hypernatremia are nonspecific and include nausea, muscle weakness, and fasciculations, and alterations in mental status ranging from lethargy to coma. Seizures, while uncommon in chronic hypernatremia, may develop after initiation of therapy in as many as 40% of patients.

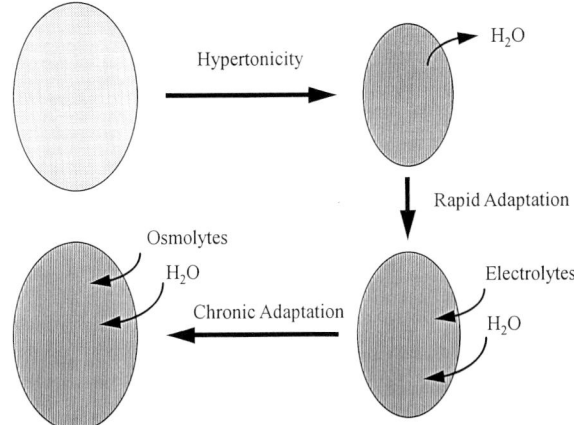

FIGURE 2 Brain adaptation to hypernatremia. Brain cell volume is indicated by the size of the oval; intracellular osmolality by the density of shading. Following the acute onset of hypernatremia, there is a rapid loss of water from the intracellular compartment resulting in a decrease in brain cell volume and an increase in brain cell osmolality. Adaptive processes are then activated which restore brain cell volume to normal. An initial phase of rapid adaptation, occurring over the first 24 hours, consists of electrolyte uptake into brain cells, partially restoring brain volume. In chronic adaptation, which is complete by Day 7, organic solutes accumulate within brain cells leading to restoration of brain volume to normal although intracellular osmolality remains elevated.

The mortality rate associated with hypernatremia has been reported to range from 40% to more than 70%, depending on the magnitude of hypernatremia and its rapidity of onset. The majority of deaths, however, are not a direct consequence of the hypernatremia but result from underlying illnesses. In a recent study, the mortality in 103 consecutive hypernatremic patients was 41%; however, in only 16% of the patients did the hypernatremia contribute to the cause of death. When mortality was analyzed on the basis of adequacy of therapy, hypernatremia contributed to mortality in 25% of patients in whom it persisted for more than 72 hours compared to only 8% of patients in whom the hypernatremia was promptly treated and resolved within 72 hours.

TREATMENT

The treatment of hypernatremia is water. The existing water deficit should be repleted and any ongoing electrolyte-free water losses replaced. The water deficit may be estimated based on the current serum sodium concentration (S_{Na}) and body weight, using the assumption that total body water is approximately 60% of body weight:

$$Water\ Deficit = 0.6 \times [Body\ Weight\ (kg)] \\ \times [(Na^+)/140) - 1].$$

Despite inaccuracies inherent in this formula, the calculation provides a useful approximation for initiating water replacement.

In acute hypernatremia, repletion of the water deficit may be rapid. The electrolytes that accumulate in the brain during acute hypernatremia are rapidly extruded into the extracellular compartment during treatment, minimizing the risk of cerebral edema. In contrast, overly rapid therapy of chronic hypernatremia may produce cerebral edema if the water replacement occurs more rapidly than the brain can dissipate the accumulated organic solutes, a process requiring approximately 24 to 48 hours. Well-controlled studies to ascertain the optimal treatment of chronic hypernatremia do not exist. However, based on knowledge of the rate of solute loss by the brain following chronic hypernatremia, prompt but gradual correction is most prudent. In symptomatic patients, rapid water replacement should be provided initially; however, the serum sodium concentration should be reduced by no more than 1 to 2 $mmol \cdot L^{-1} \cdot h^{-1}$. Once symptoms have resolved, replacement of the remainder of the water deficit should occur over 24 to 48 hours. Throughout treatment, the patient's neurologic status should be monitored carefully; deterioration after an initial improvement in neurologic symptoms suggests the development of cerebral edema and mandates temporary discontinuation of water replacement.

No individual regimen of water replacement is of documented superiority. Water may be administered enterally, either orally or by nasogastric tube, or intravenously. Intravenous repletion can consist of either hypotonic saline or 5% dextrose in water; pure water cannot be administered intravenously as the local hypotonicity at the site of administration can produce severe intravascular hemolysis. When glucose containing solutions are used, the blood glucose concentration should be monitored carefully and insulin therapy initiated, if necessary, to forestall hyperglycemia.

In addition to replacing the calculated water deficit, ongoing fluid losses must be replaced. Urinary, gastrointestinal, and other losses should be quantified and should be replaced on the basis of their volume and electrolyte content. Insensible losses must also be replaced, recognizing that they increase by approximately 20% for each 1°C increase in body temperature.

Prompt attention to reducing excessive water losses is also important. Insensible losses may be reduced by normalizing body temperature with cooling blankets and antipyretics. Hyperglycemia should be controlled and protein loading decreased in order to limit osmotic diuresis. Nasogastric drainage can be reduced by therapy with H_2-receptor antagonists or proton pump inhibitors. Diarrhea can be reduced by altering enteral feeding, treating infectious causes, discontinuing cathartic agents, or administering antidiarrheal agents. Specific therapy for diabetes insipidus should be initiated, when appropriate.

Hypothalamic diabetes insipidus is readily treated with hormone replacement. Although the native hormone, aqueous arginine vasopressin, is available, treatment is most often with desamino-8-D-arginine vasopressin (dDAVP), a synthetic analog of vasopressin with a longer half-life and less vasoconstrictive effects. Hormone replacement therapy is generally ineffective in nephrogenic diabetes insipidus. Restriction of dietary protein and sodium intake may attenuate the polyuria by reducing obligate urinary solute excretion. Thiazide diuretics may also be of benefit. Thiazides directly inhibit urinary diluting capacity and indirectly decrease distal tubular delivery by inducing mild intravascular volume contraction which increases proximal tubular sodium reabsorption. The net effect is to decrease delivery of free water to the collecting duct and to enhance vasopressin-independent water reabsorption, thereby moderating the polyuria. Nonsteroidal anti-inflammatory drugs are also useful as adjunctive therapy. Amiloride is useful in the treatment of lithium-induced nephrogenic diabetes insipidus. It is postulated that in addition to its diuretic effects amiloride blocks lithium entry into collecting duct cells, thereby reducing cellular toxicity.

Initial treatment of the patient with coexistent hypernatremia and extracellular volume depletion should be directed at restoring intravascular volume. Frank circulatory compromise should be promptly treated with isotonic saline or colloid solutions. Once adequate volume replacement has been achieved, treatment should then be directed toward replacing the water deficit. Treatment of hypernatremia in patients with volume overload generally requires both water repletion and solute removal. Because hypernatremia often develops rapidly in these patients, the compensatory mechanisms defending brain volume are ineffective and neurologic symptoms may be accentuated. In addition, the concomitant intravascular volume expansion may result in pulmonary edema and exacerbate respiratory failure. Treatment must therefore be promptly instituted in order to prevent neurologic and cardiopulmonary complications. Because water repletion will further exacerbate intravascular volume overload, a loop diuretic should be simultaneously administered to facilitate solute excretion. In patients with massive volume overload or renal failure, initiation of hemodialysis or hemofiltration may be necessary.

Bibliography

Ayus JC, Armstrong DL, Arieff AI: Effects of hypernatremia in the central nervous system and its therapy in rats and rabbits. *J Physiol* 492:243–255, 1996.

DeRubertis FR, Michelis MF, Beck N, Field JB, Davis BB: "Essential" hypernatremia due to ineffective osmotic and intact volume regulation of vasopressin secretion. *J Clin Invest* 50:97–110, 1971.

Fitzsimons JT: Physiology and pathophysiology of thirst and sodium appetite. In: *The Kidney: Physiology and Pathophysiology.* 2nd ed. Raven Press, New York, pp. 1615–1648, 1992.

Gullans SR, Verbalis JG: Control of brain volume during hyperosmolar and hypoosmolar conditions. *Annu Rev Med* 44:289–301, 1993.

Holtzman EJ, Ausiello DA: Nephrogenic diabetes insipidus: causes revealed. *Hosp Pract* 29:67–82, 1994.

Lien YH, Shapiro JI, Chan L: Effects of hypernatremia on organic brain osmoles. *J Clin Invest* 85:1427–1435, 1990.

Miller M, Dalakos T, Moses AM, et al: Recognition of partial defects in antidiuretic hormone secretion. *Ann Intern Med* 73:721–729, 1970.

Palevsky PM, Bhagrath R, Greenberg A: Hypernatremia in hospitalized patients. *Ann Intern Med* 124:197–203, 1996.

Phillips PA, Rolls BJ, Ledingham JGG, et al: Reduced thirst after water deprivation in healthy elderly men. *N Engl J Med* 311:753–759, 1984.

Robertson GL: Regulation of vasopressin secretion. In: Seldin DW, Giebisch G (eds) *The Kidney: Physiology and Pathophysiology.* 2nd ed. Raven Press, New York, pp. 1595–1613, 1992.

Ross EJ, Christie SBM: Hypernatremia. *Medicine* 48:441–478, 1969.

Seckl JR, Dunger DB: Diabetes insipidus: current treatment recommendations. *Drugs* 44:216–224, 1992.

Snyder NA, Feigal DW, Arieff AI: Hypernatremia in elderly patients. *Ann Intern Med* 107:309–319, 1987.

Zerbe RL, Robertson GL: A comparison of plasma vasopressin measurements with a standard indirect test in the differential diagnosis of polyuria. *N Engl J Med* 305:1539–1546, 1981.

9

METABOLIC ACIDOSIS

DANIEL BATLLE

Metabolic acidosis is an acid–base disorder characterized by a fall in blood bicarbonate concentration and a fall in blood pH (i.e., a rise in the hydrogen ion concentration [H+]). Respiratory compensation provides for a predictable decrease of the blood CO_2 tension (pCO_2). For each 1 mEq decrease in bicarbonate concentration the pCO_2 falls by 1.0 to 1.5 mm Hg. The importance of respiratory compensation on blood pH is illustrated with an example (Fig. 1). The presence of an inappropriate response suggests the existence of a mixed acid–base disturbance. Severe metabolic acidosis, unlike respiratory alkalosis, cannot be fully compensated despite maximal hyperventilation. Accordingly, if the blood pH is not reduced when bicarbonate is very low, a respiratory alkalosis must be present.

Metabolic acidosis occurs when bicarbonate is lost from the body (via the gastrointestinal tract or the kidney), when the kidneys fail to regenerate bicarbonate via adequate acid excretion, or when bicarbonate is consumed in the titration of excessive acid produced endogenously or from the ingestion of acid-producing compounds.

THE PLASMA ANION GAP IN THE INITIAL EVALUATION OF METABOLIC ACIDOSIS

The plasma anion gap (AG) is useful in the evaluation of the type of metabolic acidosis and the initial classification of its various causes. The AG is simply a calculation that allows the clinican to infer whether there has been a change in unmeasured anions or cations in plasma.

The use of the AG takes advantage of the principle of electroneutrality, which dictates that the number of positively charged particles in any solution must be equal to the number of negatively charged particles. The major unmeasured anions in plasma include albumin, phosphate, sulfate, and other organic anions. The major unmeasured cations in plasma include calcium, magnesium, and other less-abundant cations. That the AG actually reflects the difference between unmeasured anions (UA) and the unmeasured cations (UC) can be easily appreciated by examining the following basic equations:

Since the sum of all cations = the sum of all anions,

$$(Na^+ + K^+) + UC = (Cl^- + HCO_3^-) + UA$$
$$(Na^+ + K^+) - (Cl^- - HCO_3^-) = UA - UC.$$

Accordingly, the AG reduces to

$$AG = UA - UC$$

and

$$AG = ([Na^+] + [K^+]) - ([Cl^-] + [HCO_3^-])$$
(normally 14 ± 2 mEq/L).

Due to the small magnitude of changes in potassium concentration in the plasma, potassium is often omitted from the calculation of the AG. Thus,

$$AG = [Na^+] - ([Cl^- + [HCO_3^-])$$
(normally 10 ± 2 mEq/L).

The AG provides a convenient tool to estimate whether there has been a change in either UA or UC even before such a change can be documented by direct measurements. For instance, in metabolic acidosis due to the addition of non-chloride-containing acid (e.g., lactic acid) the added

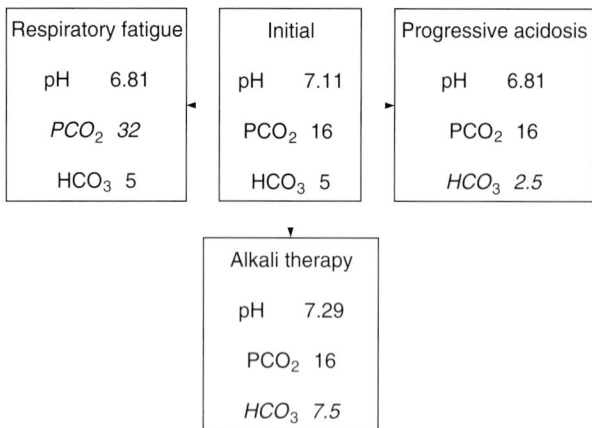

FIGURE I   The impact on pH of minimal changes in either pCO_2 or HCO_3 when plasma bicarbonate is very low is illustrated.

protons buffer the bicarbonate while the retained anion (lactate) increases the unmeasured anions. The increase in the AG from lactate will match the fall in plasma bicarbonate. In contrast, when a chloride-containing acid is added to the blood, the hydrogen ion titrates bicarbonate while exogenous chloride ion is largely retained by the kidneys. This results in a rise in the chloride concentration equivalent to the fall in bicarbonate; the AG will not change. This is described as hyperchloremic or normal AG metabolic acidosis. When the decrement in plasma bicarbonate is not matched by an equivalent increment either in plasma chloride or in the plasma AG, a mixed hyperchloremic and high AG metabolic acidosis is present. For instance, a mixed hyperchloremic/high AG metabolic acidosis can develop in a setting where the metabolic acidosis originates from two different mechanisms (e.g., diarrhea in patient with preexisting renal failure or shock).

Because the AG reflects changes in UA or UC, certain situations other than metabolic acidosis can alter the plasma AG. The level of plasma albumin influences the plasma AG and should be taken into consideration. For every fall of albumin of 10 g/L, the AG drops by about 4 mEq/L. An abnormally high concentration of unmeasured cations, as seen with the accumulation of abnormal cationic paraproteins in patients with IgG myeloma, can depress the AG. These interpretative pitfalls in the use of the plasma AG stress the need to pay careful attention to all the laboratory variables and to look for appropriate clinical correlates.

HYPERCHLOREMIC METABOLIC ACIDOSIS (OR NORMAL AG TYPE OF METABOLIC ACIDOSIS)

Hyperchloremic metabolic acidosis should be distinguished from chronic respiratory alkalosis. In either acid–base disorder plasma chloride is elevated and plasma bicarbonate is reduced. An arterial blood gas is needed to properly diagnose each acid–base disorder.

With the administration of HCl or other HCl-generating compounds a hyperchloremic metabolic acidosis develops as blood bicarbonate is titrated, while plasma chloride increases proportionally by the retention of exogenous chloride. One basic alteration underlying the generation of hyperchloremic metabolic acidosis is the loss of bicarbonate, usually in the urine or in the stools (Table 1). In individuals with metabolic acidosis associated with chronic diarrhea due to protracted laxative abuse, a chronic volume deficit ensues despite avid renal sodium retention. The virtual absence of urine sodium in some of these patients may impede a normal distal acidification response to the prevailing acidemia. This is because distal sodium delivery is necessary for optimal distal hydrogen ion secretion. When sodium excretion is increased to normal by salt replacement, urine pH falls and acid excretion increases resulting in amelioration of the metabolic acidosis.

Diversion of urine through intestinal segments can result in hyperchloremic metabolic acidosis, hypokalemia, and other electrolyte abnormalities, e.g., hypomagnesemia and hypocalcemia. Various intestinal segments have been used as conduits to substitute for the bladder. The anastomosis of a ureter into the sigmoid colon (ureterosigmoidostomy) almost always results in hyperchloremic metabolic acidosis. Consequently this technique was supplanted by the ileal conduit. Hyperchloremic metabolic acidosis, however, is still a problem in about 10% of patients with an ileal conduit, particularly those where the ileal conduit is obstructed.

RENAL CAUSES OF HYPERCHLOREMIC METABOLIC ACIDOSIS

Ingestion of an average protein-containing diet generates a net fixed acid excess of approximately 1 mEq/kg body wt daily during the course of metabolism. Addition of acid (HA) to the blood compartments results in the titration of the bicarbonate anion according to the equation

TABLE I
Causes of Hyperchloremic (or Normal AG) Metabolic Acidosis

Administration of chloride-containing acid
$\quad$ NH_4Cl, HCl
$\quad$ Hyperalimentation
$\quad$ Cholestyramine
Bicarbonate wastage
$\quad$ GI tract (diarrhea, ileus, fistula, villous adenoma)
$\quad$ Urinary tract diversions to intestine (ureterosigmoidostomy, ileal conduit)
Impaired renal H^+ secretion and reduced NH_4 excretion
$\quad$ Distal RTA (hypokalemic and some hyperkalemic types)
$\quad$ Posthypocapnia (transient)
Impaired NH_3 formation and reduced NH_4 excretion
$\quad$ Advanced renal insufficiency (GFR < 20 mL/min)
$\quad$ Hyperkalemia
$\quad$ Aldosterone deficiency

$$HA + Na\ HCO_3 \rightleftharpoons H_2O + CO_2 + Na\ A.$$

In addition to reclaiming all filtered bicarbonate, the kidney must excrete the acid anion and regenerate the bicarbonate that was consumed in the initial titration by the acid. Regeneration of bicarbonate is largely accomplished by hydrogen ion secretion in the distal nephron. Hydrogen ions secreted by the renal tubules are titrated by urinary buffers, primarily ammonia. Due to its favorable pK (6.8) and relatively high concentration in the urine, phosphate is also a major urinary buffer and contributes greatly to titratable acid excretion. Increased ammonium excretion is, by far, the major mechanism by which the kidneys can regenerate bicarbonate. Net renal acid excretion (NAE) is calculated as urinary ammonium excretion (NH_4) plus urinary titratable acid (TA) minus bicarbonate (HCO_3^-) or other potential bases (PB) that are excreted in the urine:

$$NAE \rightleftharpoons (NH_4 + TA) - (HCO_3 + PB).$$

The kidneys may fail to provide for an adequate excretion of acid because of either decreased acid excretion (NH_4, TA, or both) or increased alkali excretion (i.e., HCO_3^- wastage). The former mechanism underlies an array of syndromes collectively referred to as distal renal tubular acidosis. The latter mechanism accounts for the development of proximal renal tubular acidosis. With advanced renal failure, NH_4^+ excretion is also reduced, resulting in metabolic acidosis which is usually mixed (i.e., hyperchloremic and high AG).

PROXIMAL RENAL TUBULAR ACIDOSIS

In normal individuals, the urine bicarbonate concentration is usually very low (less than 1 mEq/24 h). In patients with proximal renal tubular acidosis (type II RTA), a large fraction of the filtered load of bicarbonate is excreted when the concentration of bicarbonate in plasma is normal or even when it is moderately reduced. In contrast, the urine of such patients is virtually bicarbonate-free when the concentration of bicarbonate in plasma falls below a critical level referred to as the renal threshold. The renal bicarbonate threshold in patients with proximal RTA varies between 15 and 20 mEq/L (normal about 24 mEq/L). When plasma bicarbonate is below the renal bicarbonate threshold, urine pH falls to levels almost as low as those seen in normal subjects (less than 5.5). This feature is helpful in distinguishing proximal RTA from some types of distal RTA where urine pH is higher than 5.5 despite severe acidemia (type I RTA and some cases of hyperkalemic RTA; see below).

In both children and adults, bicarbonate wastage may occur as a part of the Fanconi syndrome, a generalized defect in proximal tubular transport that results in inhibition of reabsorption of glucose, phosphate, uric acid, and amino acids. In this setting, glycosuria develops at normal plasma glucose concentrations, and reduced plasma phosphate and plasma uric acid levels as well as aminoaciduria may be observed.

OVERVIEW OF DEFECTS IN COLLECTING TUBULE ACIDIFICATION CAUSING THE VARIOUS DISTAL RTA SUBTYPES

The collecting tubule is the major site of urinary acidification within the distal nephron. This nephron segment displays axial heterogeneity both anatomically and functionally. In cortical collecting tubules, active sodium reabsorption generates an electrical potential (lumen-negative) that favors the secretion of H^+ and potassium. In contrast, in outer medullary collecting tubules, H^+ secretion does not appear to be under the influence of sodium transport and is not accompanied by potassium secretion. The collecting tubule contains a proton pump at its luminal surface. This pump, a proton-translocating ATPase, secretes H^+ in an electrogenic manner and can operate independently of sodium transport and despite an unfavorable transtubular electrical gradient. Alterations causing an impairment of collecting tubule acidification by primarily interfering with active H^+ secretion are referred to as secretory types of distal RTA (Table 2). Alterations in transepithelial voltage caused by either inhibition of sodium transport or enhancement of lumen to cell chloride transport can also reduce the rate of H^+ secretion, albeit indirectly, and are referred to as voltage-dependent types of distal RTA. A primary H^+ secretory defect, by definition, is limited to a defect in either the H,K-ATPase pump or the H,K-ATPase pump (Table 2).

Most patients with distal RTA appear to have a secretory defect due to H-ATPase failure. Hypokalemia can develop

TABLE 2

Classification of DRTA

Type	Example
Permeability defects	
H^+ backleak	Amphotericin B
Enhanced HCO_3^- secretion	Unknown
Secretory defects	
Diffuse collecting tubule H-ATPase defect	Chronic kidney transplant rejection
Medullary collecting tubule H-ATPase defect	Nephrocalcinosis (some cases)
Diffuse H-ATPase secretory defect	Obstructive nephropathy
Diffuse collecting H,K-ATPase defect	Endemic hypokalemic DRTA (?)
Rate-dependent defects	
Impaired Na^+ transport (Na^+ channel defect)	Amiloride, trimethoprim
Enhanced Cl transport	Pseudohypoaldosteronism type II
Aldosterone deficiency	Selective aldosterone deficiency
Aldosterone resistance	Pseudohypoaldosteronism type I
Reduced urinary buffers	Hyperkalemia
Increased intracellular pH	Cytosolic carbonic anhydrase II deficiency

in such patients as a consequence of secondary hyperaldosteronism and accelerated potassium secretion in the distal nephron. Theoretically, a defect in the H,K-ATPase pump could better explain the development of severe hypokalemia in some of these cases but evidence that such a defect causes distal RTA in humans is so far lacking. As both potassium wastage and impaired H^+ secretion are characteristic of hypokalemic distal RTA, this remains an attractive hypothesis.

In a typical patient with distal (type I or classic) RTA, urine pH during spontaneous acidosis or after acid loading cannot be lowered below 5.5 and ammonium excretion is reduced. The latter can be inferred at the bedside from the finding of a positive urine anion gap (UAG; see below). In such patients, the urine pCO_2 measured after bicarbonate loading does not increase normally (i.e., above 70 mm Hg), reflecting the reduced rate of collecting tubule H^+ secretion. The latter feature is useful in distinguishing a secretory or voltage-dependent defect from a permeability defect. Permeability defects (i.e., amphotericin B-induced RTA) do not impair the generation of a normally high urine pCO_2.

Hyperkalemic RTA

Two pathogenic subtypes of hyperkalemic distal RTA that are frequently encountered in adults with underlying renal disease have been well described (Table 3). One

TABLE 3
Causes of Hyperkalemic Metabolic Acidosis

Selective aldosterone deficiency
Low renin
  Hyporeninemic hypoaldosteronism (e.g., diabetic nephropathy)
  Prostaglandin synthesis inhibitors
Normal or high renin
  Normoreninemic hypoaldosteronism
  Hyperreninemic hypoaldosteronism in critically ill patients
  Converting enzyme inhibitors
  Corticosterone methyloxidase deficiency
  Heparin therapy
  Cyclosporine
Hyperkalemic distal renal tubular acidosis
  Obstructive uropathy
  Sickle cell hemoglobinopathies
  Renal amyloidosis
  Acute hypersensitivity interstitial nephritis
  Amiloride administration
  Trimethoprim[a]
  Cyclosporine
Aldosterone resistance
  Pseudohypoaldosteronism type I (infants)
  Pseudohypoaldosteronism type II (Gordon's syndrome)
  Adult aldosterone hyporesponsiveness and renal insufficiency
  Spironolactone administration

[a] Metabolic acidosis is usually not a feature of trimethoprim-induced hyperkalemia.

subtype, which corresponds to the animal model of selective aldosterone deficiency (SAD), is characterized by hyperkalemic hyperchloremic metabolic acidosis associated with low plasma and urinary aldosterone levels, reduced ammonium excretion, and preserved ability to lower urine pH below 5.5. This constellation of findings is also referred to as type IV distal RTA. The findings associated with SAD or type IV RTA are typified by the syndrome of hyporeninemic hypoaldosteronism. While hyperkalemia is the usual manifestation of this syndrome, the development of hyperchloremic metabolic acidosis is also very common (more than 75% of cases). In these subjects, acidosis develops because of impaired acid excretion secondary to reduced urinary buffer (ammonia) availability. Ammonia formation in these patients is suppressed as a result of both hyperkalemia and aldosterone deficiency.

In the other subtype of hyperkalemic RTA, ammonium excretion is also reduced but, characteristically, urine pH cannot be lowered below 5.5 not only during acidemia, but also after stimulation of sodium-dependent distal acidification by the administration of either sodium sulfate or loop diuretics. In this type (referred to as hyperkalemic distal RTA), plasma aldosterone levels may be normal or elevated but are more often reduced. The finding of low aldosterone levels suggests the existence of a combined defect, that is, SAD combined with a tubular defect that interferes with the ability to maximally lower urine pH despite the presence of acidosis. The mechanism underlying this subtype of hyperkalemic distal RTA, which was first described in patients with obstructive uropathy, was originally attributed to a failure to generate a favorable transtubular voltage gradient (lumen negative) in the collecting tubular that interferes with both H^+ and K^+ secretion. A recent study in patients with this subtype of hyperkalemic distal RTA suggests, however, that the defect in H^+ secretion is related to H-ATPase dysfunction and is independent of the associated defect in K^+ secretion.

RTA: CLINICAL FEATURES AND TREATMENT

A common feature of children with proximal and distal RTA is failure to thrive. Acidemia, by mechanisms not yet fully delineated, interferes with normal growth. Distal RTA may also lead to nephrolithiasis or nephrocalcinosis.

The treatment of distal RTA consists of alkali therapy. When started early in the course of the disease, alkali therapy normalizes growth. The alkali requirements of these patients are usually small compared with those of patients with proximal RTA. A dose of 1 to 2 mEq/kg body wt of sodium bicarbonate daily is sufficient in most cases. Many patients with hereditary distal RTA have a bicarbonate wastage tendency during the first years of life that gradually abates with advancing age. Hence, the dose of alkali needed to correct the acidosis decreases after 6 years of age. Alkali can be provided in the form of a sodium citrate solution, which is well tolerated because it causes less abdominal distention than bicarbonate. Each milliliter of citrate solution provides 1 mEq of bicarbonate after hepatic conversion of citrate into bicarbonate. Potassium supplements are indicated in patients with hypokalemia.

The hyperkalemic types of distal RTA usually develop in patients with an underlying tubulointerstitial renal disease and/or with moderate renal insufficiency who have aldosterone deficiency. SAD is particularly common in patients with either type I and type II diabetes, especially those who have developed nephropathy. Other common causes are listed in Table 3. Patients with hyperkalemic distal RTA should be differentiated from those with pure SAD because some patients with the latter condition are more likely to respond to treatment with mineralocorticoids. Tubular hyporesponsiveness to the action of exogenous mineralocorticoid, however, is common in some patients with SAD. High doses of mineralocorticoid may be needed to correct the hyperkalemia.

Hyperkalemia can also be treated using exchange resins such as sodium polystyrene sulfonate, which increase gastrointestinal potassium excretion. Correction of hyperkalemia has the additional salutory effect in that it improves the acidosis by increasing ammonium excretion. Loop diuretics are effective in increasing potassium excretion, and they also ameliorate the metabolic acidosis associated with SAD.

DIAGNOSTIC APPROACH TO HYPERCHLOREMIC METABOLIC ACIDOSIS

After history and physical examination, the next step in the diagnostic approach to hyperchloremic metabolic acidosis is to determine whether urinary acidification is normal (Fig. 2). Ideally, this should involve measurement of urine pH, titratable acidity, and ammonium excretion. Whether ammonium is appropriately increased or inappropriately low for the prevailing acidosis can be inferred at bedside by a simple calculation of the UAG.

$$UAG = (Na + K) - (Cl + HCO_3).$$

In a relatively acid urine (pH < 6.5), urine bicarbonate concentration is very low, and its contribution to the UAG can be considered negligible. Normally, the UAG has a negative value (0 to −50) provided that a stimulus for ammonium excretion (i.e., acidosis) is present. The UAG, by contrast, is positive in patients with various types of defects in distal urinary acidification. This reflects the inability of patients with distal RTA to excrete ammonium appropriately in the face of spontaneous acidosis.

Accordingly, the UAG is useful in the separation of those patients with reduced ammonium excretion because of impaired distal acidification from those patients with hyperchloremic metabolic acidosis from other causes, namely, gastrointestinal bicarbonate losses (Fig. 2). Normal subjects with diarrhea or given an acid load to produce metabolic acidosis display a negative UAG. The negative UAG in patients with diarrhea reflects an abundance of ammonium in the urine since the kidney's response to acidosis is appropriate (i.e., to excrete acid). In patients with diarrhea, renal acidification is greatly stimulated by acidemia, and the urine pH should be low. In some patients,

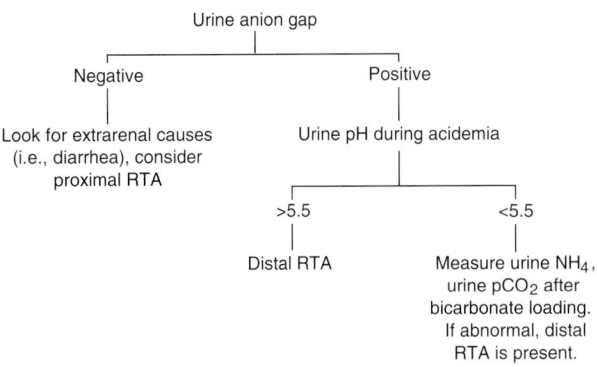

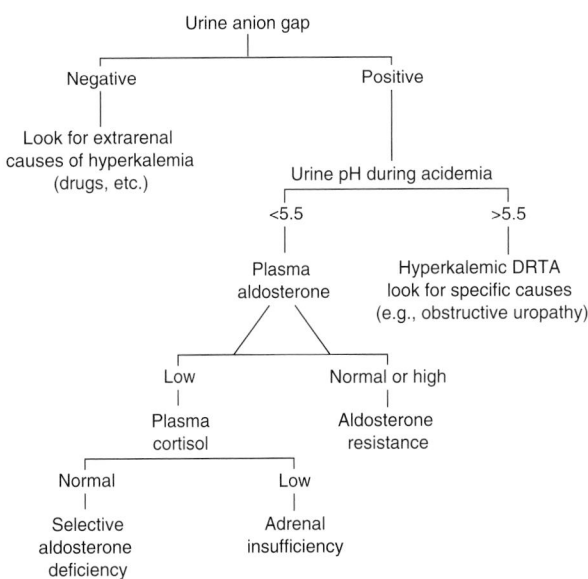

FIGURE 2   Diagnostic approach to hyperchloremic acidosis.

however, urine pH rises because of the addition of large amounts of ammonia buffer into the collecting tubule. In addition, many of these patients are volume-depleted from protracted diarrhea, so that the delivery of sodium to the collecting tubule is impaired. In this situation, urine pH may not be lowered below 5.5 despite acidemia, until distal sodium delivery is restored by the administration of salt or diuretics. The findings of hypokalemia, hyperchloremic metabolic acidosis, and a high urine pH could erroneously suggest the diagnosis of distal RTA in these patients. The key differential finding is the UAG, which is positive if the patient has distal RTA but negative if the patient has hypokalemic hyperchloremic metabolic acidosis associated with diarrhea. Patients with proximal RTA display a negative UAG insofar as they are capable of excreting substantial amounts of ammonium. Chronic respiratory alkalosis can also increase the UAG because in this condition, urinary ammonium excretion is reduced as part of a normal adaptation to hypocapnia.

Provided that respiratory alkalosis is excluded, patients with a diminished serum bicarbonate concentration who have a positive UAG should be suspected to have distal RTA, which can be separated into hyperkalemic and hypokalemic (classic) distal RTA on the basis of the plasma potassium (Fig. 2). The diagnosis of distal RTA can be confirmed by the finding of a urinary pH above 5.5 in the face of spontaneous or ammonium chloride-induced metabolic acidosis. In general, if the patient is spontaneously acidotic (pH < 7.35), there is no need to induce severe acidosis in order to evaluate urinary acidification. If the patient is suspected of having distal RTA and acidosis is mild or not present, ammonium chloride can be given (0.1 g/kg body wt daily for 3 consecutive days). Measurements of urine pH, urinary ammonium, and titratable acidity should be performed at the end of Day 3 to confirm or exclude the diagnosis of distal RTA. It should be noted that there are patients with a defect in distal acidification in whom urine pH may be less than 5.5 in the face of metabolic acidosis. This typically occurs in patients with hyperkalemic RTA associated with SAD (see Fig. 2). In some patients without hyperkalemia the ability to lower urine pH below 5.5 may also be preserved, even when distal acidification assessed by the urine pCO_2 after bicarbonate loading is defective (i.e., urine pCO_2 does not increase above 50–60 mm Hg; normal >70 mm Hg) (Table 2). This has been well documented in individuals receiving chronic lithium therapy, subjects with medullary sponge kidney, and some patients with idiopathic hypercalciuria. These patients can be considered to have incomplete distal RTA since metabolic acidosis is often absent.

HIGH AG TYPES OF METABOLIC ACIDOSIS

Renal Failure

Renal failure, both acute and chronic, is a common cause of metabolic acidosis that is usually classified as a high AG type (Table 4). It should be appreciated, however, that the fall in plasma HCO_3 associated with renal failure is mainly due to an absolute decrease in ammonium excretion as a result of reduced renal mass and that a reciprocal increase

in the AG does not need to occur. Variable degrees of anion retention (sulfate, phosphate, and organic anions) occurring as renal insufficiency progresses determine whether a high AG metabolic acidosis develops. The predominant pattern among patients with end stage renal disease on maintenance hemodialysis is a mixed one, that is, a combined high AG and hyperchloremic metabolic acidosis.

In patients with chronic renal disease an increase in ammonia production by remaining nephrons is capable of maintaining normal acid–base balance until the glomerular filtration rate has dropped below 20 to 25 mL/min. Some of the metabolic abnormalities with chronic renal insufficiency, however, may interfere with urinary acidification. In particular, chronic hyperkalemia worsens the acidosis by suppressing ammoniagenesis. An absolute decrease in overall renal ammonia production ensues when GFR is less than 20 mL/min and acidosis develops. Even with advanced renal insufficiency the urine is acid (pH < 5.5) suggesting that the collecting tubules of residual nephrons are capable of adequate H^+ secretion. In fact, when acidosis is seen in patients with moderate degrees of renal failure, a distal acidification defect should be suspected.

The acidosis is usually nonprogressive and relatively asymptomatic. The goal of alkali therapy in this group is mainly to avert the consequences of protracted acidosis on bone tissue which may be through a direct demineralization effect of acidemia or through its effects on the hormones that regulate calcium metabolism, namely, parathyroid hormone and vitamin D.

Lactic Acidosis

Lactate is formed in the cell cytosol from pyruvate. The enzyme catalyzing this reaction is lactate dehydrogenase (LDH). Under normal conditions, the rates of lactic acid regeneration and utilization are matched (about 15–20 mEq/day). The liver and, to a lesser extent, the kidneys are the major sites of lactic acid uptake and metabolism. Lactic acidosis, resulting from the accumulation of excess lactate, is usually seen in severely ill patients many of whom have tissue hypoxia due to tissue hypoperfusion from hypotension with or without hypoxemia. When the tissue oxygen supply does not meet the cellular oxygen demand, type A lactic acidosis occurs.

TABLE 4

Causes of Metabolic Acidosis with Increased Plasma Anion Gap

Etiology	Major circulating anion	Characteristic features and other comments[a]
Ketoacidosis	β-Hydroxybutyrate, acetoacetate	Diabetes, alcohol, starvation
Lactic acidosis	Lactate	Shock, tissue hypoxia, liver failure
Renal failure	Sulfate, phosphate, variety of organic acids	⇑ BUN
Methanol	Formate	Increased osmolal gap, hyperemic optic disk
Ethylene glycol	Glycolate, lactate	Increased osmolal gap; ARF, urinary oxalate crystals
Salicylates	Variety of organic acids, salicylate	Concomitant respiratory alkalosis, tinnitus, fever
Toluene	Hippurate	It also causes distal RTA and hypokalemia
Paraldehyde	Acetate?	Very rare

[a]ARF, acute renal failure; RTA, renal tubular acidosis.

Some patients with lactic acidosis, however, lack any evidence of tissue hypoxia. This condition is known as type B lactic acidosis and almost always results from impaired lactate clearance due to hepatic failure. In type A lactic acidosis, the diagnosis is usually made on the basis of the clinical setting (shock, hypoxemia, severe anemia). Type B lactic acidosis should be suspected when there is evidence of liver impairment or ingestion of substances known to produce this condition. Type B lactic acidosis can also occur with large tumors producing a large cell turnover and a marked increase in pyruvate production.

A distinctive type of lactic acidosis can occur in patients with bacterial overgrowth due, for example, to jejunoileal bypass or small-bowel resection. In this situation, intestinal bacteria can metabolize glucose into D-lactic acid, which then accumulates in the blood.

Treatment of lactic acidosis is directed toward correcting the underlying cause. Levels of plasma lactate higher than 20 mEq/L reflect very severe acidosis and are often associated with a high mortality. In monitoring the patient, one should not rely on an isolated lactate level because of the rapidly changing nature of the underlying condition. Monitoring the plasma AG provides an estimate of serum lactate changes over time and may obviate measurement of serial lactate levels.

The administration of bicarbonate is usually indicated when blood pH is very low (i.e., >7.10) despite adequate respiratory compensation. In lactic acidosis, to counteract the excessive lactic acid production, large amounts of bicarbonate are usually needed and this may lead to increased systemic CO_2 generation, a rise in cell CO_2 and thus a fall in intracellular pH. Despite this theoretical problem, the use of bicarbonate therapy in cases of severe acidemia is advisable, provided that blood pCO_2 is reduced. A more specific approach to correct lactic acidosis entails the use of dichloroacetate. This agent, now available in some hospital pharmacies, is effective in lowering lactate levels by stimulating pyruvate dehydrogenase and stimulating mitochondrial pyruvate oxidation. Despite clear-cut improvement of the acidosis, however, controlled studies have failed to demonstrate an improvement in survival in patients with lactic acidosis treated with this agent.

Diabetic Ketoacidosis

This condition is characterized by hyperglycemia of variable degree and metabolic acidosis secondary to overproduction of ketoacids. The hormonal profile of diabetic ketoacidosis comprises low insulin levels, hyperglucagonemia, high cortisol levels, high level of circulating catecholamines, and elevated growth hormone levels. These hormonal alterations trigger and maintain the ketogenesis. The accumulation of acetoacetic and β-hydroxybutyric acids results in metabolic acidosis when these acids rapidly dissociate to H^+ and the corresponding ketoanions. Some of the acetoacetic acid is nonenzymatically converted to acetone. Acetone is a volatile ketone that is excreted via the lungs producing a characteristic odor to the breath.

Although the acidosis is usually of the high AG type, a striking hyperchloremic type of acidosis may be seen when ketones are rapidly lost in the urine. If volume contraction is severe, ketoacids are retained and the AG is elevated. In this situation, the retained ketoacids provide a source of potential bicarbonate. This may contribute to a fast recovery from acidosis owing to the equimolar conversion of retained ketone salts to bicarbonate.

Metabolic acidosis in diabetic ketoacidosis is often severe. The diagnosis of ketoacidosis is established by demonstrating ketonemia or ketonuria, metabolic acidosis, and hyperglycemia (Fig. 3). Ketonuria may be undetectable if most of the offending acetoacetic acid has been converted to β-hydroxybutyric acid, which is not detected on the routine urine dipstick. Lack of a marked elevation in blood sugar may result in delayed diagnosis. Uncontrolled hyperglycemia usually has caused an osmotic diuresis with a substantial loss of sodium, chloride, and potassium. Many such patients therefore develop various degress of prerenal azotemia. A significant total body potassium deficit is usually present even in the presence of a normal serum potassium concentration. Some patients may have hyperkalemia, which is mainly due to impaired potassium transport into cells caused by the insulin deficiency. Significant phosphate depletion is usually present as a result of poor food intake and urinary phosphate wasting.

The goal of therapy is to reverse and halt the ketogenesis and to replace the electrolyte and water deficits. Insulin is needed to inhibit ketogenesis and break the cycle of lipolysis and ketogenesis. Insulin preferably should be administered as a low-dose constant intravenous infusion. Insulin should not be stopped as glucose concentrations approach the normal range. Rather, glucose should be infused and insulin continued until the ketosis has cleared. Although these patients often have more of a water than sodium deficit, isotonic saline is usually needed initially to achieve a rapid correction of the volume deficit. Correction of potassium deficit should be initiated early, even when plasma potassium concentration is normal, provided that insulin has been given and an adequate urine output is present.

The role of bicarbonate therapy in patients with diabetic ketoacidosis has been debated. In general, the use of bicarbonate is warranted when the acidosis is severe, since its potential benefits seem to outweigh the risks. Bicarbonate should be administered to patients whose arterial blood pH is less than 7.20 despite adequate hyperventilation and to those with a bicarbonate concentration below 10 mEq/L. During recovery, a high AG metabolic acidosis is sometimes replaced by hyperchloremic acidosis. The excretion of ketoanions, which represent potential bicarbonate, coupled with the administration of intravenous saline infusion and avid renal retention of chloride leads to hyperchloremia. The development of hyperchloremic acidosis is an indication for continuation of bicarbonate therapy.

Starvation Ketoacidosis

During starvation, lipolysis and gluconeogenesis provide the body with the needed calories for survival. The low

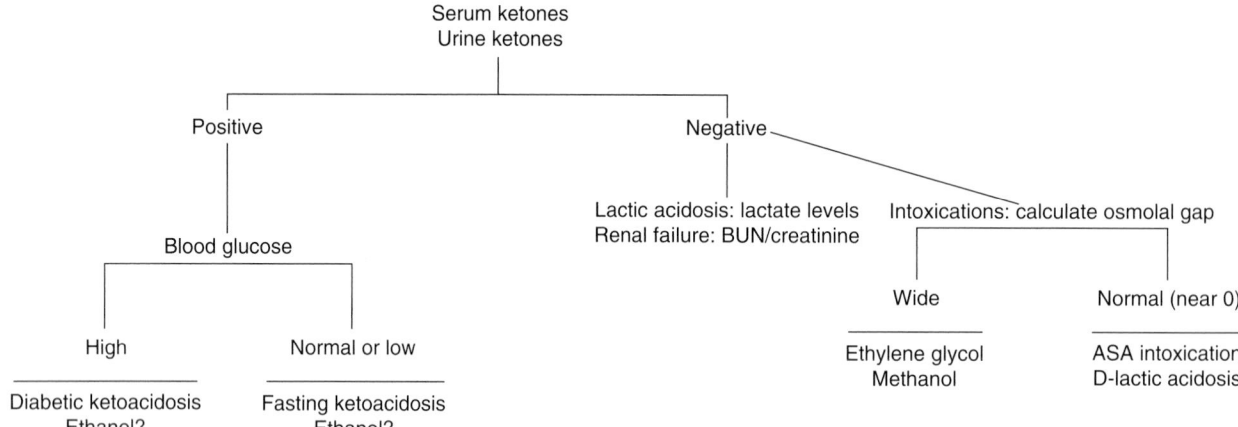

FIGURE 3 Diagnostic approach to high anion gap metabolic acidosis.

insulin levels induced by hypoglycemia and the associated increase in glucagon, epinephrine, cortisol, and growth hormone levels stimulate lipolysis with release of fatty acids. The accumulation of ketone bodies may result in metabolic acidosis which is often of mild severity. Increased net acid excretion by the kidney may correct the acidosis over the next few days, obviating the need for bicarbonate therapy. Previously malnourished individuals, however, may have inadequate ammoniagenesis and thus develop a more severe acidosis. Patients may develop metabolic alkalosis with refeeding, which may be related to the abrupt cessation of ketogenesis while urinary acidification remains stimulated.

Alcoholic Ketoacidosis

This condition is characterized by acidosis secondary to increased ketogenesis and variable blood glucose levels in the absence of clinical diabetes. Typically, the condition develops following an alcoholic binge and an episode of vomiting and starvation. Unlike starvation ketoacidosis, the acidosis in alcoholic ketoacidosis may be severe. The combination of low insulin levels (related to low food intake), high levels of epinephrine (which may be related, in part, to withdrawal of alcohol), and elevation of cortisol levels result in the stimulation of glycogenolysis, gluconeogenesis, and lipolysis. The net result is acidosis of variable severity, hyperglycemia or hypoglycemia, and a clinical picture easily confused with diabetic ketoacidosis.

There is usually a prompt improvement in response to hydration and glucose administration without need for exogenous insulin. Bicarbonate should be given if the acidosis is severe (blood pH <7.20). Therapy also includes correcting concomitant electrolyte disturbances such as hypophosphatemia, hypomagnesemia, and hypokalemia.

Salicylate Intoxication

Two distinct forms of intoxication may result from salicylate ingestion: (1) an acute form, which usually follows an acute overdose ingested accidentally or intentionally; and (2) a chronic form, which results from gradual accumulation of the drug during long-term administration. Acid–base disturbances are predominant in the acute form. Typical manifestations of acute salicylate intoxication include intense hyperventilation, fever, stupor, coma, and convulsions. Tinnitus, deafness, and vertigo are common complaints particularly in patients with chronic salicylism. Other laboratory abnormalities include hypouricemia, which is due to inhibition of renal tubule urate reabsorption by high salicylate levels.

The diagnosis of salicylate intoxication is usually obvious from the history and can be confirmed by checking the urine for salicylates using ferric chloride which produces a purple color if salicylate is present. Severe toxicity occurs when blood salicylate levels reach 100 mg/dL. In chronic salicylism, however, dose nomograms are not useful and death can occur at low blood salicylate levels.

Combined metabolic acidosis and respiratory alkalosis is a frequent finding in adult patients with acute salicylate intoxication. In children, metabolic acidosis is predominant, often overshadowing the attendant respiratory alkalosis while in adults the respiratory alkalosis usually predominates. Respiratory alkalosis is the result of direct stimulation of the respiratory center by salicylate. The amount of salicylate required to produce this effect is much less than that required to produce metabolic acidosis. The mechanism of metabolic acidosis in patients with salicylate intoxication is not totally clear. Only a small fraction of the decrement in plasma bicarbonate and the increment in unmeasured anions may be directly attributed to salicylic acid accumulation. Ketoacidosis as well as lactic acidosis may contribute to the metabolic acidosis.

Removal of the salicylate from the body starts with gastric lavage if the patient presents within 6 hours of drug administration. Repeated oral administration of oral-activated charcoal enhances whole-body drug elimination and interferes with drug absorption. Sodium bicarbonate not only corrects the acidosis but also augments the renal clearance of salicylates by producing an alkaline diuresis (urine pH > 7.0) and may limit the amount of the drug that enters the cerebrospinal fluid and brain cells. Hemodialysis is a very efficient way of removing salicylate from the body and also helps correct the acidosis and other electrolyte abnormalities.

Ethylene Glycol

Ethylene glycol is commonly found as a component of antifreeze and as a solvent in a number of industrial applications. It can cause damage to the central nervous system (CNS), the kidneys, and the cardiopulmonary system. Ethylene glycol is metabolized by alcohol dehydrogenase to glycoaldehyde, which is further metabolized to glycolic, glyoxilic, and oxalic acids—all potentially toxic compounds. Suppression of the citric acid cycle and altered intracellular redox state may lead to lactic acid overproduction. A high concentration of ethylene glycol in plasma will result in a disparity between measured and calculated plasma osmolality. This high plasma "osmolal gap" may also be seen in ethanol and methanol intoxications as well as in some cases of diabetic ketoacidosis (Fig. 2). The plasma osmolality may be estimated according to the formula

$$(Na \times 2) + \frac{glucose}{18} + \frac{BUN}{28}.$$

Calcium oxalate crystalluria is a hallmark of this type of intoxication and may cause obstructive renal failure when crystals precipitate in the renal tubules. The urine should be examined for the presence of the crystals which may be needle shaped (monohydrate) or envelope shaped (dihydrate).

Treatment includes supportive measures, diuresis, bicarbonate, ethanol administration and the provision of thiamine and pyridoxine supplements. Ethanol competes with ethylene glycol metabolism by alcohol dehydrogenase and thus slows the latter's metabolism. A serum ethanol level of 100 mg/dL can be achieved by either nasogastric or intravenous administration of ethanol. Hemodialysis may be indicated to quickly lower ethylene glycol plasma levels, to remove other potentially toxic metabolites, and to correct the acidosis.

Methanol

Methanol, or wood alcohol, is a common solvent and fuel component. It may be ingested as a substitute for ethanol, or in suicide attempts. Methanol is metabolized via alcohol dehydrogenase to formaldehyde which is rapidly converted to formate, the anion responsible for the AG and most of the toxicity. It can cause severe optic nerve as well as CNS injury. Symptoms may include blurred vision which suggests serious toxicity, respiratory depression, cya-

nosis, altered mental status, and cardiovascular collapse. There is a latent period before the onset of symptoms that averages 12 to 24 hours but that may be delayed up to 3 to 4 days if there is concomitant consumption of ethanol. Acidosis, often severe, is related to the accumulation of formate as well as lactate, ketoacids, and other organic acids. An osmolal gap is usually present. The finding of optic nerve swelling coupled with the absence of crystalluria strongly suggests the diagnosis of methanol as opposed to ethylene glycol intoxication. Therapy includes osmotic diuresis, administration of ethanol, bicarbonate infusion, and hemodialysis.

Bibliography

Adrogue HJ, Wilson H, Boyd AE, Suki WN, Eknoyan G: Plasma acid-base patterns in diabetic ketoacidosis. *N Engl J Med* 307:1603–1610, 1982.

Battle D: Hyperchloremic acidosis. In: Giebisch G and Seldin D (eds) *The Regulation of Acid-Base Balance.* Raven Press, New York, pp. 107–121, 1989.

Battle D, Flores G: Underlying defects in distal renal tubular acidosis. New understandings. *Am J Kidney Dis* 27(6):896–915, 1996.

Battle D, Arruda JAL, Kurtzman NA: Hyperkalemic distal renal tubular acidosis associated with obstructive uropathy. *N Engl J Med* 304:373–380, 1981.

Battle D, Grupp M, Gaviria M, Kurtzman NA: Distal renal tubular acidosis with intact ability to lower urine pH. *Am J Med* 72:751–758, 1982.

Battle D, vonRiotte A, Schlueter W: Urinary sodium in the evaluation of hyperchloremic metabolic acidosis. *N Engl J Med* 316:140–144, 1987.

Battle D, Hizon M, Cohen E, Gutterman C, Gupta R: The use of the urinary anion gap in the diagnosis of hyperchloremic metabolic acidosis. *N Engl J Med* 318:594–599, 1988.

Brenner RJ, Spring DB, Sebastian A, et al.: Incidence of radiographically evident bone disease, nephrocalcinosis, and nephrolithiasis in various types of renal tubular acidosis. *New Engl J Med* 307:217–221, 1982.

Emmett M, Seldin D: Overproduction acidosis. In: Giebisch G and Seldin D (eds) *The Regulation of Acid-Base Balance.* Raven Press, New York, pp. 391–429, 1989.

Fernandez PC, Cohen RM, Feldman GM: The concept of bicarbonate distribution space: The crucial role of body buffers. *Kidney Int* 36:747–752, 1989.

Gennari JR, Rimmer JM: Acid-base disorders in end stage renal disease: Part I. *Semin Dialysis* 3:81–85, 1990.

Green J, Kleeman CR: Role of bone in regulation of systemic acid-base balance. *Kidney Int* 39:9–26, 1991.

Kurtzman NA: Renal tubular acidosis: A constellation of syndromes. *Hosp Pract* 173–198, 1987.

Oh MS, Phelps KR, Traube M, Barbosa-Saldiar JL, Boxhill C, Carroll HJ: D-Lactic acidosis in a man with the short-bowel syndrome. *N Engl J Med* 301:249–252, 1979.

Peterson CD, Collins AJ, Hines JM, Bullock ML, Keane WF: Ethylene glycol poisoning: Pharmacokinetics during therapy with ethanol and hemodialysis. *N Engl J Med* 304:21–23, 1981.

Stacpoole PW, Wright EC, Baumgartner TG, et al: Dichloroacetate for lactic acidosis in adults: A controlled clinical trial of dichloroacetate for treatment of lactic acidosis in adults. *N Engl J Med* 327:1564–1569, 1992.

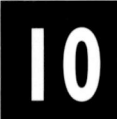

METABOLIC ALKALOSIS

EDWARD R. JONES

Metabolic alkalosis is characterized by a primary increase in the plasma bicarbonate concentration. The resultant alkalemia suppresses ventilation, yielding a secondary increase in pCO_2. An elevated bicarbonate concentration may also be observed as compensation for the hypercapnia characteristic of respiratory acidosis. Distinguishing between these disturbances, each associated with an elevated bicarbonate level and hypercapnia, requires a blood gas determination to define pH. The history and physical examination are critical in distinguishing between these two disorders and in identifying patients who have both metabolic alkalosis and respiratory acidosis. The distinctive physical characteristics of patients with chronic lung disease are helpful clues. Formulas and confidence bands to predict metabolic adaptation to hypercapnia and define the presence of simple metabolic alkalosis, respiratory alkalosis, or mixed disturbances are discussed in Chapter 12.

In a study of 13,000 arterial blood gases in 3300 hospitalized patients, metabolic alkalosis was the most frequent acid–base disturbance. Although its direct cause is poorly defined, there appears to be an increased morbidity and mortality in surgical patients with multisystem organ failure and metabolic alkalosis (blood pH > 7.55). Therefore the recognition and appropriate correction of metabolic alkalosis are important.

CLINICAL MANIFESTATIONS

Patients with metabolic alkalosis manifest symptoms related to the cause of the alkalosis, i.e., postural symptoms, weakness, and thirst are associated with volume depletion; neuromuscular symptoms and arrhythmias are associated with hypokalemia. The clinical presentation is generally a consequence of the alkalemia, which exerts significant effects on the central nervous and neuromuscular systems, cardiovascular system, and pulmonary vasculature as well as contributing to various metabolic derangements. These signs and symptoms occur in both metabolic and respiratory alkalosis. It is difficult to differentiate most of the side effects of alkalemia from the numerous other concomitant metabolic derangements in patients with metabolic alkalosis such as hypocalcemia and hypomagnesemia.

Alkalemia may contribute to the changes in mental status seen in patients with metabolic alkalosis and to a lowering of the seizure threshold. Tetany and neuromuscular irritability including carpopedal spasms and positive Chvostek or Trousseau signs may be seen.

Ventricular and supraventricular irritability as well as increased sensitivity to digoxin appears to be more frequent. Antiarrhythmics may be ineffective until the alkalemia is corrected. Decrements in cardiac output and cardiovascular instability are common.

Alkalemia decreases ionized calcium by shifting ionized calcium onto plasma proteins. Therefore, despite normocalcemia, the alkalemic patient may present with seizures or carpopedal spasms. A decrease in urinary calcium excretion may also be observed; its clinical significance is not well defined.

Alkalemia shifts potassium intracellularly, resulting in hypokalemia. In addition, metabolic alkalosis causes potassium depletion which is generally correlated with the magnitude of the alkalosis. The consequences of potassium depletion are discussed in Chapter 13.

Metabolic alkalosis causes an elevated plasma anion gap. Alkalosis stimulates glycolysis, more specifically phosphofructokinase activity, thereby increasing lactate production. The plasma lactate level may increase as much as 5 mEq/L; this can raise the anion gap by an equivalent amount. Volume contraction concentrates plasma proteins and increases the unmeasured anion. Finally, alkalemia is associated with the loss of protons from plasma proteins, uncovering negative charges and contributing to the rise in unmeasured anion.

Alkalemia also alters the oxyhemoglobin curve, shifting the curve leftward and potentially limiting oxygen availability. The clinical significance of this is unknown.

PATHOPHYSIOLOGY

Recognition and appropriate intervention to correct the many processes that result in metabolic alkalosis demand a basic understanding of the pathogenesis of metabolic alkalosis. Under normal conditions, an excess of bicarbonate from any source would be excreted by the kidney by suppressing renal acid excretion and bicarbonate reabsorption. A sustained rise in serum bicarbonate concentration can only occur if two factors are present. First there must be a source of the alkali (i.e., the generation of alkalosis), and there must be factors in place that retain the alkali or limit the ability of the kidney to excrete bicarbonate (i.e., maintenance of the alkalosis). Under normal conditions, a rise in serum bicarbonate from any source would be excreted by the kidney by suppressing renal acid excretion and bicarbonate reabsorption. In those clinical settings where metabolic alkalosis occurs, bicarbonate excretion is minimized as a result of factors which both generate and maintain the alkalosis.

Generation of Metabolic Alkalosis

The generation of bicarbonate (Table 1) results from either the renal or extrarenal loss of acid or from gain of base to the extracellular fluid. Net negative hydrogen ion balance (acid excretion exceeding production) results in a rise in extracellular fluid (ECF) bicarbonate concentration. The loss of acid translates into equimolar gain of bicarbonate.

Secretion of hydrogen ion from the gastric mucosa is associated with the addition of bicarbonate to blood. Vomiting and gastric drainage are common causes of metabolic alkalosis. Intestinal acid loss can also occur with chloride-losing diarrhea (congenital or acquired chloridorrhea).

TABLE I
Pathophysiologic Approach to Metabolic Alkalosis

Generation of Metabolic Alkalosis
Loss of acid from ECF
  Nonrenal acid loss
  Gastrointestinal fluid losses
    Gastric losses
    Chloride-losing diarrhea
  Cellular shifts: Potassium for hydrogen exchange
  Renal acid losses
    Acid secretion due to diuretics
    Nonreabsorbable anions: enhanced distal
      sodium–hydrogen exchange
    Severe potassium depletion
Gain of bicarbonate to the ECF
  Conversion of bicarbonate equivalents (citrate, acetate, lactate)
  Bicarbonate administration: parenteral or oral
  Resin exchanges plus antacids
Unchanged bicarbonate content
  Contraction of ECF bicarbonate
  Posthypercapnic state
Maintenance of Metabolic Alkalosis
Decreased GFR (decreased filtered load of bicarbonate)
Enhanced proximal bicarbonate reabsorption
  Reduced arterial blood volume—absolute or effective
  Potassium depletion (also decreased GFR)
  Hypercapnia
  Decreased parathyroid hormone
  Hypercalcemia
Increased distal tubular bicarbonate reabsorption
  Mineralocorticoid excess
  Hypokalemia
  Nonreabsorbable anion
Chloride depletion

ECF, extracellular fluid; GFR, glomerular filtration rate.

A minor rise in serum bicarbonate concentration can occur due to a translocation of protons across cells in exchange for potassium during hypokalemia. This mechanism has little or no clinical significance.

Renal loss of acid is probably the most common cause of metabolic alkalosis. Loop diuretics like furosemide as well as the thiazides stimulate acid excretion by increasing distal nephron sodium delivery and by causing secondary hyperaldosteronism. Hypokalemia enhances proton secretion and ammoniagenesis thus increasing net acid excretion.

Excessive alkali gains can be seen during the administration of bicarbonate or its equivalents during cardiopulmonary resuscitation, with massive blood transfusions (sodium citrate is used as an anticoagulant), or the administration of total parenteral nutrition formula (acetate). The addition of alkali from the gastrointestinal tract occurs during the concomitant use of exchange resins (Kayexelate) and poorly absorbable antacids.

Contraction alkalosis results from the loss of chloride-rich, bicarbonate-free fluid which increases serum bicarbonate concentration by 3 to 5 mEq/L. The metabolic alkalosis commonly seen with loop diuretics results predominately from enhanced renal acid excretion and the concomitant hypovolemia, and not contraction of ECF bicarbonate alone.

Maintenance of Metabolic Alkalosis

A sustained rise in bicarbonate concentration implies decreased renal bicarbonate excretion. Under normal circumstances, the addition of alkali to the ECF volume is associated with volume expansion and hypochloremia. The normal kidney senses the volume expansion. The alkali is excreted along with sodium, and the hypochloremia is corrected. Sustained elevations in bicarbonate concentration require one of the following: a decreased glomerular filtration rate (GFR), enhanced proximal tubular bicarbonate reabsorption (both of the latter are volume-dependent stimuli), or increased distal tubular bicarbonate reabsorption (a volume-independent mechanism).

Decrements in GFR translate into diminished filtered bicarbonate loads, limiting bicarbonate excretion. Enhanced proximal tubular bicarbonate reabsorption will sustain the ECF bicarbonate and maintain the alkalosis. Reduced effective arterial blood volume (EABV) is associated with decreased bicarbonate excretion. Hypokalemia and hypercapnia stimulate proton secretion and thus bicarbonate addition to blood. Hypokalemia may also decrease GFR, further limiting bicarbonate excretion.

Enhanced distal nephron bicarbonate reabsorption is an important factor in maintaining metabolic alkalosis. Persistent hypermineralocorticoidism, hypokalemia, and the presence of a poorly reabsorbable anion stimulate acid excretion and subsequent addition of alkali to blood.

The importance of hypochloremia in the maintenance of metabolic alkalosis is not established. Some suggest that chloride depletion itself may maintain the metabolic alkalosis and that this effect is independent of plasma volume.

Indeed, chloride depletion appears to enhance bicarbonate reabsorption while distal bicarbonate secretion decreases. Differences in location of the chloride/bicarbonate (Cl^-/HCO_3^-) exchanger within intercalated cells of the cortical collecting tubule plays a role in maintenance of metabolic alkalosis. Type A intercalated cells have the transporter on the basolateral membrane. Type B cells are thought to have these transporters on the luminal side. Hydrogen ion secretion via the H-ATPase pump and passive chloride cosecretion are enhanced on the luminal side during decreased chloride delivery. There is a concomitant enhancement of chloride entry into type A cells with subsequent HCO_3^- addition to blood. The Cl^-/HCO_3^- exchange is reversed in type B cells; thus, enhanced chloride secretion into the lumen results in decreased bicarbonate secretion. As a result, both cell types play important roles in maintaining metabolic alkalosis in chloride-depleted states.

In essence, the recognition of metabolic alkalosis and its therapeutic intervention require an understanding that subsequent metabolic alkalosis is a result of the dependent processes of generating alkali and maintaining the alkalosis. Correction of either component alone does not resolve the alkalosis. For instance, cessation of vomiting alone will not lower serum bicarbonate. Correction of the hypovolemia along with cessation of vomiting are both required to permit normalization of the ECF bicarbonate concentration.

Clinical Conditions Resulting in Metabolic Alkalosis (Fig. I; Table 2)

In keeping with the pathophysiology presented above, metabolic alkalosis is best categorized according to the volume status of the patient. Hypovolemic, chloride-deficient patients excrete less than 15 mEq/L of chloride on a random urine. These patients have been classified as having saline-responsive alkalosis. Indeed, when their plasma volume is restored with sodium chloride, a bicarbonaturia ensues.

In contrast, the ECF volume expanded (chloride-rich) patient excretes greater than 20 mEq/L of chloride. These patients, who do not respond to sodium chloride administration, have saline-resistant alkalosis.

Metabolic Alkalosis Associated with ECF Volume Contraction

An increase in bicarbonate concentration can be generated either from renal or extrarenal sources. Its maintenance results from the hypovolemia and hypokalemia that enhance proximal bicarbonate reabsorption and from the decreased GFR that limits bicarbonate excretion. In addition, the hypokalemia and excess mineralocorticoid state enhance distal acid excretion and bicarbonate addition to blood.

Renal Alkalosis

Thiazide, loop, and mercurial diuretics cause hypokalemic metabolic alkalosis, with secondary hypokalemia, hypovolemia, and hyperaldosteronism. Metabolic alkalosis occurs in 3 to 50% of patients receiving diuretics. Thiazide diuretics increase bicarbonate concentration by only 2 to 7 mEq/L. The use of loop diuretics either alone or in combination with metalazone, particularly in patients with anasarca, can increase bicarbonate concentration by 15 to 20 mEq/L.

Laboratory findings vary depending on whether the patient is still taking the diuretic. Continued diuretic consumption results in a natriuresis with a high urinary chloride, despite hypovolemia. Once the diuretic is stopped, urinary sodium and chloride fall below 15 mEq/L. This electrolyte pattern may occur with the surreptitious use of diuretics for weight loss, and may be diagnosed by a urinary diuretic screen.

The administration of poorly reabsorbable anions (e.g., ampicillin, carbenicillin, or other penicillins) results in an obligatory natriuresis with enhanced distal tubular potassium and proton losses. The resultant hypokalemia, hypovolemia, and metabolic alkalosis can be blunted or aborted with adequate potassium supplementation and volume repletion.

Bartter's syndrome is a rare disorder whose pathophysiology is still incompletely understood. The clinical presentation comprises hypokalemia, metabolic alkalosis, hypomagnesium, hyperuricemia, hyperreninism, and hyperaldosteronism but without hypertension. Prostaglandin production is increased. Patients are hyperchloruric, with potassium wasting. The majority of patients are less than 25 year olds, with common presenting symptoms of polyuria, paresthesia, and muscle weakness and cramping. Recent studies suggest that patients with Bartter's syndrome have a mutation in the sodium:potassium:2-chloride cotransporter or in a potassium secretory transporter in the thick limb of the ascending loop of Henle.

An additional syndrome which needs differentiation from Bartter's syndrome is Gitelman's syndrome. Gitelman's syndrome is a rare entity associated with hypokalemia, hypomagnesemia, and hypocalciuria. Urinary chloride levels are low and there is no juxtaglomerular apparatus hyperplasia. There is impaired transport in the cortical thick limb of the loop of Henle and reduced sodium reabsorption in the distal tubule. The former defect probably accounts for the magnesium wasting and the latter for the hypocalciuria. Indeed, data suggest that there is a defect in the gene for the thiazide-sensitive distal tubular sodium–chloride cotransporters.

Nonrenal Alkalosis

Vomiting is associated with the loss of water, electrolytes, and protons from the ECF. The loss of hydrogen ion into the gastric lumen is associated with delivery of equimolar quantities of bicarbonate into gastric venous blood increasing the filtered load. The loss of 3 or 4 L of gastric content will result in marked electrolyte and fluid losses. The hypovolemia results in hyperaldosteronism, causing a marked kaliuresis, profound potassium depletion and subsequent hypokalemia (the gastric potassium losses are trivial in this setting), hypochloremia, and severe metabolic alkalosis.

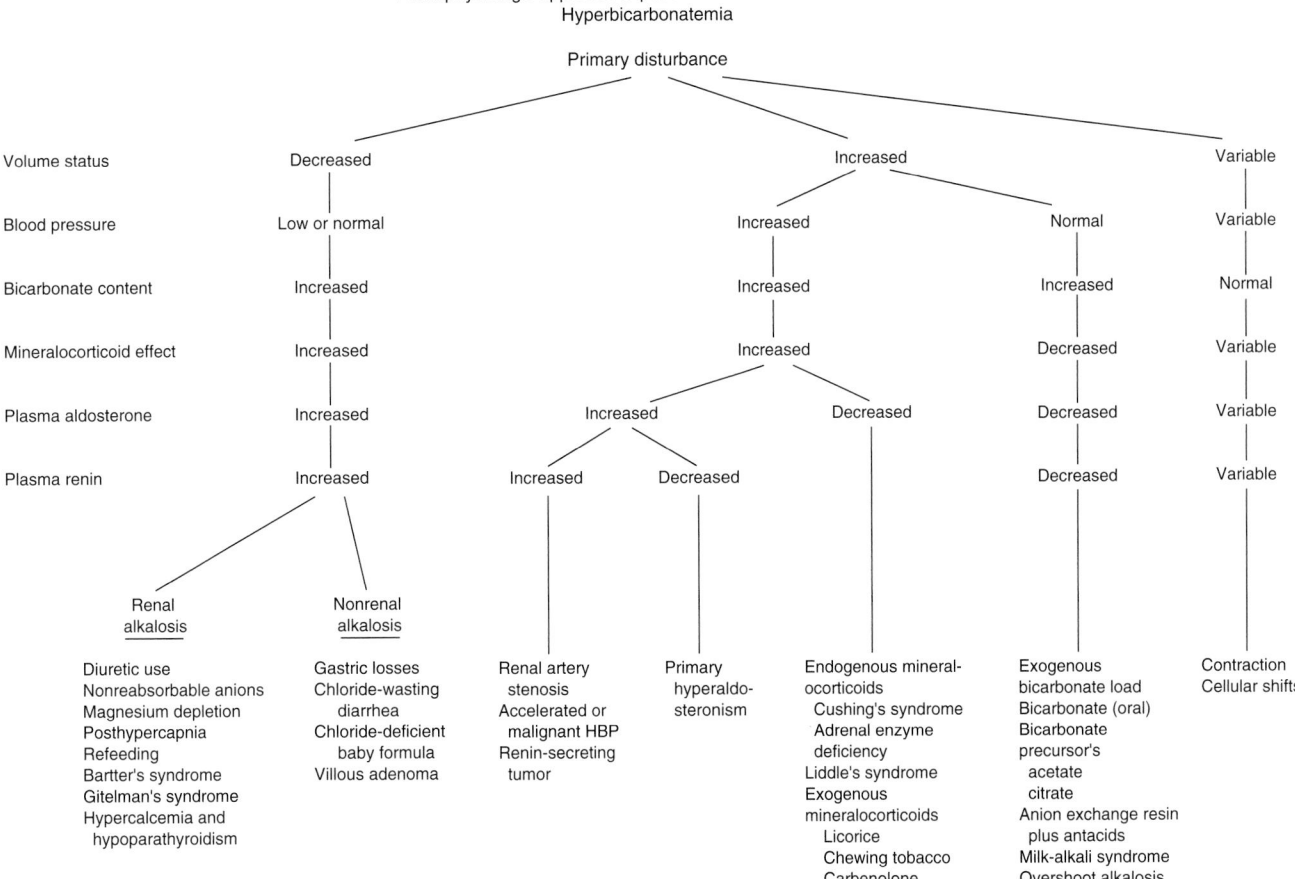

FIGURE 1   Approach to metabolic alkalosis.

TABLE 2

Differential Diagnosis of Metabolic Alkalosis

Urine chloride <15 mEq/L (chloride-responsive)
  Gastric fluid losses
  Stool losses: Chloride-losing diarrhea
  Diuretic therapy[a] (diuretic screen negative)
  Posthypercapnic state
  Refeeding
Urine chloride >20 mEq/L (chloride-resistant)
  Primary hyperaldosteronism
  Exogenous steroids
  Bartter's syndrome
  Cushing's syndrome
  Severe hypokalemia
  Alkali loading
  Hypercalcemia

---

[a] Urinary chloride will vary depending on proximity to ingestion of diuretics. Generally, a negative diuretic screen is associated with remote diuretic use and a low urine chloride.

The clinical setting of vomiting is best approached by evaluating the various phases of development of the alkalosis. The early developmental phase is associated with a rapid rise in bicarbonate, mild hypovolemia, and hypochloremia. The filtered load of bicarbonate exceeds the reabsorptive capacity of the proximal tubule. Therefore bicarbonaturia with an alkaline urine is present. Despite hypovolemia, there is a natriuresis due to an obligatory bicarbonate diuresis. Natriuresis with hypovolemia is also seen with diuretic use. Kaliuresis is marked, whereas the urine is chloride deplete. There is a positive urinary anion gap (defined as the urinary sodium plus potassium minus chloride). A positive urinary anion gap with alkaline urine implies that bicarbonate is the unmeasured anion; when the urine pH is low, nonreabsorbable anions (ketones, lactate, penicillin, etc.) account for the gap. (See Chapter 9 for a more extensive discussion of the urine anion gap.) Once gastric losses end, and the patient is profoundly hypovolemic (maintenance phase), proximal sodium reabsorption is maximized, GFR is depressed, bicarbonaturia is eliminated, and sodium is reabsorbed. The kaliuresis is lessened but persists, and approximates the low urine chloride plus an undefined quantity of anion. Urine pH falls because of the effect of aldosterone to stimulate distal proton secretion, and because the urinary anion gap is no longer significantly positive. During the correction of the alkalosis (reparative phase), as plasma volume is restored and GFR improves, bicarbonaturia resumes as do the natriuresis, alkaline urine, and positive urinary anion gap. The urine chloride remains low until volume repletion is complete. The common feature in these phases is the low urinary chloride with persistent kaliuresis.

The provision of chloride as sodium and potassium salts to avoid volume depletion can prevent significant metabolic alkalosis. The use of parenteral H_2-receptor blockers will limit gastric acid losses. Once alkalosis is present, both the generative and maintenance phase of the alkalosis must be resolved. It is critical to the gastric losses while also replenishing plasma volume in these saline-responsive patients with sodium chloride and appropriate KCl replacement.

Metabolic Alkalosis Associated with ECF Volume Expansion

The kidneys are responsible for both the generation and the maintenance of metabolic alkalosis in this setting, but the alkalosis is not responsive to saline. These patients have urinary chloride excretions greater than 20 mEq/L.

The saline unresponsive alkaloses are generally divided into those associated with or without hypertension. Further categorization according to renin/aldosterone profiles may also be helpful. The latter are generally not measured in clinical practice; this characterization is most helpful as a conceptual tool.

Hypertension with Mineralocorticoid Excess

Whether endogenous or exogenous, mineralocorticoid excess is associated with enhanced salt reabsorption with volume expansion, hypokalemia, kaliuresis, chloruresis, increased net acid excretion (enhanced ammoniagensis), and decreased GFR. The severity of the metabolic alkalosis is related to the severity of the potassium depletion.

High renin, mineralocorticoid excess states are seen most commonly with renal vascular hypertension. Approximately 20% of patients with renal artery stenosis present with severe hypokalemia and metabolic alkalosis. Malignant hypertension is generally associated with hyperreninemia due to renal ischemia and 10 to 20% of these cases are accompanied by hypokalemic metabolic alkalosis. Renin-secreting tumors of juxtaglomerular apparatus origin are associated with hypertension and metabolic alkalosis.

Low renin, mineralocorticoid excess states are most commonly seen with primary hyperaldosteronism (Conn's syndrome). Hypokalemia, metabolic alkalosis, hypernatremia, and hypertension are hallmarks of this low renin state. It accounts for less than 1 to 2% of all cases of hypertension. Marked potassium depletion (as great as 1000 mEq has been reported), together with the hyperaldosteronism, are necessary to produce the alkalosis, because aldosterone administration alone or hypokalemia alone only marginally increase serum bicarbonate concentration. The serum bi-carbonate concentration has been reported to be above 30 mEq/L in 85% of cases and above 35 mEq/L in 40% of cases.

Hypertension with Low Renin and Aldosterone

States characterized by an excess of nonaldosterone mineralocorticoids or mineralocorticoid effect will produce identical clinical findings as an excess of aldosterone, although aldosterone levels will be suppressed. The clinical syndromes include Cushing's syndrome, exogenous steroid administration, and adrenal enzyme deficiencies (11β- and 17α-hydroxylase). Use of licorice containing glycyrrhizic acid has also been associated with metabolic akalosis. Glycyrrhizic acid does not exert direct mineralocorticoid activity, rather it inhibits 11β-hydroxysteroid dehydrogenase. This enzyme is responsible for the conversion between active steroid cortisol and inactive cortisone. Liddle's syndrome is characterized by mutations that result in constitutive activation of the amiloride-sensitive collecting duct sodium channel that is ordinarily subject to stimulation by mineralocorticoids.

Volume Expanded States with Low Renin and Mineralocorticoid

Exogenous consumption of sodium bicarbonate, calcium carbonate, baking soda, Tums (10 mEq of alkali per tablet) or Rolaids (4.6 mEq per tablet) in the face of decreased renal excretion of bicarbonate can cause metabolic alkalosis.

Consumption of poorly absorbable antacids (particularly aluminum hydroxide gels used to control hyperphosphatemia or sucralfate, together with sodium polystyrene sulfonate (to treat hyperkalemia, will generate bicarbonate from the gastrointestinal tract. The resin binds cations in the gut resulting in a more soluble form of bicarbonate which is absorbed by the intestinal cell from the lumen. Renal failure perpetuates the alkalosis by impeding excretion of the excess bicarbonate added from the gastrointestinal tract.

Large volume blood transfusion can result in metabolic alkalosis. Each unit of whole blood contains 17 mEq of sodium citrate; packed red cells contain 5 mEq. The administered citrate is converted to bicarbonate, resulting in alkalosis.

Milk-alkali syndrome is a rare but frequently mentioned cause of metabolic alkalosis. The consumption of calcium-containing absorbable antacids (Oscal, oyster shell calcium, Tums, etc.) along with large quantities of milk (2–3 q/day) can produce this disorder. Hypercalcemia, hypoparathyroidism, hypercalciuria, and alkalinuria favor renal calcium-phosphorous deposition, resulting in renal failure.

DIAGNOSIS

The recognition and therapeutic intervention demand appreciation of the underlying pathophysiology. A thorough history and physical examination are necessary, centering on potential sources of alkali; particular attention should be given to the volume status of the patient. The use of the change in bicarbonate and change in anion gap or the so-called "delta-delta" gaps can uncover a metabolic alkalosis. Acid added to the extracellular fluid dissociates, yielding a proton and its related anion. The former is buffered by bicarbonate such that a rise in anion gap is reflected by an equimolar fall in bicarbonate. This results in a delta anion to delta bicarbonate (delta-delta) of one. A delta anion gap greater than the delta bicarbonate (presuming a normal starting bicarbonate) implies that excess alkali was present, and thus infers the presence of a metabolic alkalosis along with a metabolic acidosis. For example, if a patient has a bicarbonate level of 20 mEq/L (delta bicarbonate of 5 mEq/L) and an anion gap of 25 mEq/L, the delta-delta ratio is 2:1 assuming a normal anion gap of 12 mEq/L. Alternatively, to yield an anion gap of 25 mEq/L, 13 mEq/L of bicarbonate are titrated. The starting bicarbonate concentration must have been 33 mEq/L (12 + 20). Either means of assessment implies that both a metabolic alkalosis and acidosis are present.

Evaluation of urinary electrolytes to define causes of metabolic alkalosis and inferentially plasma volume presupposes normal renal and adrenal function, and the absence of diuretics. Screening for the latter may be necessary. A urinary chloride less than 15 mEq/L implies decreased effective or absolute arterial blood volume or very low salt intake. In the absence of edema, volume expansion to restore plasma volume results in bicarbonaturia and subsequent correction of the alkalosis as long as the generation of the alkalosis is also uncovered and corrected. In the presence of edema and low urinary chloride, improving EABV rather than saline infusions (which will only worsen the edema) are necessary.

Urinary chloride concentrations greater than 20 mEq/L, in the absence of polyuria, suggest that plasma volumes are normal or increased. Obviously patients with salt-wasting states in the face of volume depletion are an exception. Such patients include those with diuretic use, salt-wasting nephropathies, and nonreabsorbable anions in the urine (the early and late phases of vomiting, or penicillin use). If they are excluded on clinical grounds, mineralocorticoid excess or Bartter's syndrome are likely culprits. Hypokalemic metatabolic alkalosis from occult vomiting or diuretic consumption can be differentiated from Bartter's syndrome, but only with difficulty. Indeed some authorities have referred to these two conditions as pseudo-Bartter's syndrome. The urinary electrolytes are especially helpful in differentiating between these states.

TREATMENT

As discussed earlier, correcting the processes responsible for the generation of the alkali is necessary. Antiemetics, H_2-blockers, stopping diuretics, and preventing and correcting hypokalemia are critical. Defining and reestablishing plasma volume are mandatory. Rarely, severe alkalemia can be treated with acetazolamide (250–500 mg) with appropriate replacement of saline and potassium.

Severe metabolic alkalosis in the setting of acute or chronic renal failure, where bicarbonaturia (to correct the alkalosis) is not anticipated, may require an acidifying agent particularly in the symptomatic patient. The goal is to lower arterial pH below 7.5. Hydrochloric acid, in a concentration of 0.1 or 0.2 M (100–200 mEq/L) is infused into a central vein. The HCl distributes initially in the ECF. Therefore the amount to be infused approximates 20% of body wt times the predicted reduction in bicarbonate (in mEq/L) necessary to lower pH. The frequent determination of arterial blood gases is mandatory. Finally, in the anuric patient, an alternative is dialysis against dialysate with reduced bicarbonate content.

Bibliography

Bastani B, Purcell H, Hemken P, et al.: Expression and distribution of renal vacuolar proton-translocating adenosine triphosphatase in response to chronic acid and alkali loads in the rat. *J Clin Invest* 88:126, 1991.

Bettinelli A, Bianchetti MG, Borella P, et al: Genetic heterogeneity in tubular hypomagnesemia-hypokalemia with hypocalciuria (Gitelman's syndrome). *Kidney Int* 47:547, 1995.

Carrneiro AV, Sebastian A, Cogan MG: Reduced glomerular filtration rate can maintain a rise in plasma bicarbonate concentration in humans. *Am J Nephrol* 7:450, 1987.

Cogan MG, Liu FY, Berger BE, et al: Metabolic alkalosis. *Med Clin North Am* 67:903, 1983.

Gabow PA: Disorders associated with an altered anion gap. *Kidney Int* 27:472, 1985.

Halperin ML, Kamel KS, Narins RG: Use of urine electrolytes and osmolality: Bringing physiology to the bedside. In: Narins RG, Stein JH. *Diagnostic Techniques in Renal Diseases. Vol. 52. Contemporary Issues in Nephrology.* Churchill Livingstone, New York, p. 9, 1992.

Hodgkin JE, Soepranoff, Chan DM: Incidence of metabolic alkalemia in hospitalized patients. *Crit Care Med* 8:725, 1980.

Kassirer JP, London AM, Goldman DM, et al: On the pathogenesis of metabolic alkalosis in hyperaldosteronism. *Am J Med* 49:306, 1970.

Koch SM, Taylor RW: Chloride ion in intensive care medicine. *Crit Care Med* 20:227, 1992.

Narins RG, Jones ER, Townsend R: *Metabolic Acid Base Disorders: Pathophysiology, Classification, and Treatment. Fluid, Electrolytes and Acid Base Disorders.* Churchill Livingstone, New York, pp. 335–385, 1985.

Norris SH, Kurtzman NA: Does chloride play an independent role in the pathogenesis of metabolic alkalosis. *Semin Nephrology* 8:101, 1988.

Seldin DW, Rector FC Jr: The generation and maintenance of metabolic alkalosis. *Kidney Int* 1:305, 1972.

Stone DK, Xie XS: Proton translocating ATPases: Issues in structure and function. *Kidney Int* 33:767, 1988.

Tsukamoto T, Kobayashi T, Kawamoto K, et al: Possible Discrimination of Gitelman's Syndrome from Bartter's Syndrome by renal clearance study: Report of two cases. *Am J Kidney Dis* 25:637, 1995.

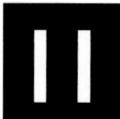

RESPIRATORY ACIDOSIS AND ALKALOSIS

NICOLAOS E. MADIAS

RESPIRATORY ACIDOSIS

Respiratory acidosis, or primary hypercapnia, is the acid–base disturbance initiated by an increase in carbon dioxide tension of body fluids. Hypercapnia acidifies body fluids and elicits an adaptive increment in plasma bicarbonate that should be viewed as an integral part of the respiratory acidosis. Arterial carbon dioxide tension (pCO_2) measured at rest and at sea level is greater than 45 mm Hg in simple respiratory acidosis. Lower values of pCO_2 might still signify the presence of primary hypercapnia in the setting of mixed acid–base disorders (e.g., eucapnia, rather than the expected hypocapnia, in the presence of metabolic acidosis).

Pathophysiology

Hypercapnia develops whenever carbon dioxide excretion by the lungs is insufficient to match carbon dioxide production, thus leading to positive carbon dioxide balance. Hypercapnia could result from increased carbon dioxide production, decreased alveolar ventilation, or both. Overproduction of carbon dioxide is usually matched by increased excretion such that generation of hypercapnia is prevented. However, patients with marked limitation in pulmonary reserve and those receiving constant mechanical ventilation might experience respiratory acidosis due to increased carbon dioxide production. Established clinical circumstances include increased physical activity, augmented work of breathing by the respiratory muscles, shivering, seizures, fever, and hyperthyroidism. Increments in carbon dioxide production might also be imposed by the administration of large carbohydrate loads (greater than 2000 kcal/day) and parenteral nutrition to semistarved, critically ill patients as well as during the decomposition of bicarbonate infused in the course of treating metabolic acidosis. By far, most cases of respiratory acidosis reflect a decrease in alveolar ventilation. Decreased alveolar ventilation can result from decreased minute ventilation, increased dead space ventilation, or a combination of both.

The major threat from carbon dioxide retention in patients breathing room air is the associated obligatory hypoxemia. Thus, in the absence of supplemental oxygen, patients suffering respiratory arrest develop critical hypoxemia within a few minutes, long before extreme hypercapnia ensues. Because of the constraints of the alveolar gas equation, it is not possible for pCO_2 to reach values much higher than 80 mm Hg while the level of pO_2 is still compatible with life. Extreme hypercapnia can only be seen during oxygen administration and, in fact, is often the result of uncontrolled oxygen therapy.

Secondary Physiological Response

An immediate increment in plasma bicarbonate concentration that is accounted for by titration of nonbicarbonate body buffers occurs in response to acute hypercapnia. This adaptation is complete within 5 to 10 minutes from the rise in pCO_2. On average, plasma bicarbonate increases by about 0.1 mEq/L for each mm Hg acute increment in pCO_2; as a result, plasma hydrogen ion concentration rises by about 0.75 nEq/L for each mm Hg acute rise in pCO_2. Therefore, the overall limit of adaptation of plasma bicarbonate in acute respiratory acidosis is quite small; even when pCO_2 rises to levels of 80 to 90 mm Hg, the increment in plasma bicarbonate does not exceed 3 to 4 mEq/L. Moderate hypoxemia does not alter the adaptive response to acute respiratory acidosis. On the other hand, preexisting hypobicarbonatemia (whether due to metabolic acidosis or chronic respiratory alkalosis) enhances the magnitude of the bicarbonate response to acute hypercapnia, whereas such a response is diminished in hyperbicarbonatemic states (whether due to metabolic alkalosis or chronic respiratory acidosis). Other electrolyte changes observed in acute respiratory acidosis include a mild rise in plasma sodium (1 to 4 mEq/L), potassium (0.1 mEq/L for each 0.1 unit fall in pH), and phosphorus, and a small decrease in plasma chloride and lactate concentrations. A small reduction in the plasma anion gap is also observed, reflecting the fall in plasma lactate and the acidic titration of plasma proteins.

The adaptive increase in plasma bicarbonate concentration observed in the acute phase of hypercapnia is amplified markedly during chronic hypercapnia as a result of generation of new bicarbonate by the kidneys. Both proximal and distal acidification mechanisms contribute to this adaptation, which requires 3 to 5 days for completion. The renal response to chronic hypercapnia includes chloruresis and generation of hypochloremia. On average, plasma bicarbonate increases by about 0.3 mEq/L for each mm Hg chronic increment in pCO_2; as a result, plasma hydrogen ion concentration rises by about 0.3 nEq/L for each mm

Hg chronic rise in pCO_2. Empirical observations indicate a limit of adaptation of plasma bicarbonate on the order of 45 mEq/L. The renal response to chronic hypercapnia is not altered appreciably by dietary sodium or chloride restriction, moderate potassium depletion, alkali loading, or moderate hypoxemia. It is currently unknown to what extent renal insufficiency of variable severity limits the renal response to chronic hypercapnia. Obviously, patients with end stage renal disease cannot mount a renal response to chronic hypercapnia and, thus, they are subject to severe acidemia. The degree of acidemia is more pronounced in patients receiving hemodialysis rather than peritoneal dialysis because the former treatment maintains, on average, a lower plasma bicarbonate concentration. Recovery from chronic hypercapnia is crippled by a chloride-deficient diet. In this circumstance, despite correction of the level of pCO_2, plasma bicarbonate concentration remains elevated as long as the state of chloride deprivation persists, thus creating the entity of "posthypercapnic metabolic alkalosis." Chronic hypercapnia is not associated with appreciable changes in the plasma concentrations of sodium, potassium, phosphorus, or anion gap.

Etiology

Respiratory acidosis can develop in patients with normal or abnormal airways and lungs. Tables 1 and 2 present causes of acute and chronic respiratory acidosis, respectively. This classification takes into consideration the usual mode of onset and duration of the various causes and emphasizes the biphasic time course that characterizes the secondary physiological response to hypercapnia. Primary hypercapnia can result from disease or malfunction within any element of the regulatory system controlling respiration, including the central and peripheral nervous system, the respiratory muscles, the thoracic cage, the pleural space, the airways, and the lung parenchyma. Not infrequently, more than one cause contributes to the development of respiratory acidosis in a given patient. Chronic lower airways obstruction resulting from bronchitis and emphysema is the most common cause of chronic hypercapnia.

Clinical Manifestations

Clinical manifestations of respiratory acidosis arising from the central nervous system are collectively known

TABLE I
Causes of Acute Respiratory Acidosis[a]

Normal airways and lungs	Abnormal airways and lungs
Central nervous system depression	Upper airways obstruction
General anesthesia	Coma-induced hypopharyngeal obstruction
Sedative overdosage	Aspiration of foreign body or vomitus
Head trauma	Laryngospasm or angioedema
Cerebrovascular accident	Obstructive sleep apnea
Central sleep apnea	Inadequate laryngeal intubation
Cerebral edema	Laryngeal obstruction postintubation
Brain tumor	Lower airways obstruction
Encephalitis	Generalized bronchospasm
Neuromuscular impairment	Severe asthma
High spinal cord injury	Bronchiolitis of infancy and adults
Guillain-Barré syndrome	Disorders involving pulmonary alveoli
Status epilepticus	Severe bilateral pneumonia
Botulism, tetanus	Infant or adult respiratory distress syndrome
Crisis in myasthenia gravis	Severe pulmonary edema
Hypokalemic myopathy	Pulmonary perfusion defect
Familial hypokalemic periodic paralysis	Cardiac arrest
Drugs or toxic agents (e.g., curare, succinylcholine, aminoglycosides, organophosphorus)	Severe circulatory failure
Ventilatory restriction	Massive pulmonary thromboembolism
Rib fractures with flail chest	Fat or air embolism
Pneumothorax	
Hemothorax	
Impaired diaphragmatic function (e.g., peritoneal dialysis, ascites)	
Iatrogenic events	
Misplacement or displacement of airway cannula during anesthesia or mechanical ventilation	
Bronchoscopy-associated hypoventilation or respiratory arrest	
Increased CO_2 production with constant mechanical ventilation (e.g., due to high carbohydrate diet or sorbent-regenerative hemodialysis)	

[a] Adapted from Madias and Adrogué (1991).

TABLE 2
Causes of Chronic Respiratory Acidosis[a]

Normal airways and lungs	Abnormal airways and lungs
Central nervous system depression	Upper airways obstruction
Sedative overdosage	Tonsillar and peritonsillar hypertrophy
Methadone/heroin addiction	Paralysis of vocal cords
Primary alveolar hypoventilation (Ondine's curse)	Tumor of the cords or larynx
Obesity–hypoventilation syndrome (Pickwickian	Airway stenosis post prolonged intubation
syndrome)	Thymoma, aortic aneurysm
Brain tumor	Lower airways obstruction
Bulbar poliomyelitis	Chronic obstructive lung disease (bronchitis, bronchiolitis, bronchiectasis,
Neuromuscular impairment	emphysema)
Poliomyelitis	Disorders involving pulmonary alveoli
Multiple sclerosis	Severe chronic pneumonitis
Muscular dystrophy	Diffuse infiltrative disease (e.g., alveolar proteinosis)
Amyotrophic lateral sclerosis	Interstitial fibrosis
Diaphragmatic paralysis	
Myxedema	
Myopathic disease	
Ventilatory restriction	
Kyphoscoliosis, spinal arthritis	
Obesity	
Fibrothorax	
Hydrothorax	
Impaired diaphragmatic function	

[a] Adapted from Madias and Adrogue (1991).

as "hypercapnic encephalopathy" and include irritability, inability to concentrate, headache, anorexia, mental cloudiness, apathy, confusion, incoherence, combativeness, hallucinations, delirium, and transient psychosis. Progressive narcosis or coma might develop in patients receiving oxygen therapy, especially those with an acute exacerbation of chronic respiratory insufficiency in whom pCO_2 levels up to 100 mm Hg or even higher can occur. In addition, frank papilledema (pseudotumor cerebri) and motor disturbances, including myoclonic jerks, flapping tremor identical to that observed in liver failure, and seizures might develop. The occurrence of neurological symptomatology in patients with respiratory acidosis depends on the magnitude of the hypercapnia, the rapidity with which it develops, the severity of the acidemia, and the degree of accompanying hypoxemia.

The hemodynamic consequences of respiratory acidosis reflect a variety of mechanisms, including a direct depressing effect on myocardial contractility. An associated sympathetic surge, sometimes intense, leads to increases in plasma catecholamines, but, during severe acidemia (generally blood pH below 7.20), receptor responsiveness to catecholamines is markedly blunted. Hypercapnia results in systemic vasodilation by a direct action on vascular smooth muscle; this effect is most obvious in the cerebral circulation where blood flow increases in direct relation to the level of pCO_2. By contrast, carbon dioxide retention can produce vasoconstriction in the pulmonary circulation as well as the kidneys; in the latter case, the hemodynamic response might be mediated via an enhanced sympathetic activity.

The composite effect of these inputs is such that mild to moderate hypercapnia is usually associated with an increased cardiac output, normal or increased blood pressure, warm skin, a bounding pulse, and diaphoresis. However, when hypercapnia is severe or considerable hypoxemia is present, decreases in both cardiac output and blood pressure might be observed. Concomitant therapy with vasoactive medications or the presence of congestive heart failure might further modify the hemodynamic response. Cardiac arrhythmias, particularly supraventricular tachyarrhythmias not associated with major hemodynamic compromise, are common. They do not result primarily from the hypercapnia, but rather reflect the associated hypoxemia and sympathetic discharge, concomitant medication, electrolyte abnormalities, and underlying cardiac disease. Salt and water retention is commonly observed in sustained hypercapnia, especially in the presence of cor pulmonale. In addition to the effects of heart failure on the kidney, multiple other factors might be involved, including the prevailing stimulation of the sympathetic nervous system and the renin-angiotensin-aldosterone axis, the increased renal vascular resistance, and the elevated levels of antidiuretic hormone and cortisol.

Diagnosis

In general, one never should rely on clinical evaluation alone to assess the adequacy of alveolar ventilation. Whenever hypoventilation is suspected, arterial blood gases should be obtained. If the patient's acid–base profile reveals hypercapnia in association with acidemia, at least an element of respiratory acidosis must be present. However, hypercapnia might be associated with a normal or an alkaline pH because of the simultaneous presence of additional acid–base disorders. Information from the patient's history, physical examination, and ancillary laboratory data should be utilized for an accurate assessment of the acid–base status.

Therapeutic Principles

Treatment of acute respiratory acidosis must be directed at prompt removal of the underlying cause whenever possible. Immediate therapeutic efforts should focus on establishing and securing a patent airway, restoring adequate oxygenation by delivering an oxygen-rich inspired mixture, and providing adequate ventilation in order to repair the abnormal gas composition. As noted, acute respiratory acidosis poses its major threat to survival not because of hypercapnia or acidemia, but because of the associated hypoxemia. Swift restoration of pCO_2 to normal levels is the therapeutic goal. Mechanical ventilation should be employed if conservative therapy fails to correct hypoxemia and hypercapnia promptly. Despite its overall merit, noninvasive oximetry should not substitute for arterial blood gas measurements in titrating F_iO_2. The presence of a component of metabolic acidosis is the primary indication for alkali therapy in patients with acute respiratory acidosis. Administration of sodium bicarbonate to patients with simple respiratory acidosis is not only of questionable efficacy, but also involves considerable risk. Concerns include pH-mediated depression of ventilation, enhanced carbon dioxide production due to bicarbonate decomposition, and volume expansion. Alkali therapy might have a special role in patients with severe bronchospasm by restoring the responsiveness of the bronchial musculature to β-adrenergic agonists. Successful management of intractable asthma in patients with blood pH below 7.00 by administering sufficient sodium bicarbonate to raise blood pH to above 7.20 has been reported.

Recent evidence indicating that lung overdistention can induce lung injury has led to a new strategy for management of disorders requiring mechanical ventilation, such as adult respiratory distress syndrome and severe airflow obstruction. The strategy entails prescription of tidal volumes of 5 to 7 mL/kg body wt (instead of the conventional level of 10 to 15 mL/kg body wt) to achieve a plateau airway pressure of ≤30 cm H_2O. Because an increase in pCO_2 might develop, this approach is termed permissive hypercapnia. If the resultant hypercapnia reduces blood pH below 7.15 to 7.20, some physicians prescribe bicarbonate; however, this strategy is controversial and others intervene only for pH values on the order of 7.00. Uncontrolled observations suggest that permissive hypercapnia affords improved clinical outcomes but controlled studies are lacking. Heavy sedation and neuromuscular blockade are frequently needed with this therapy. Following discontinuation of neuromuscular blockade, some patients develop prolonged weakness or paralysis. Contraindications to permissive hy-

percapnia include cerebral edema, increased intracranial pressure, and convulsions; depressed cardiac function and arrhythmias; and severe pulmonary hypertension.

Unfortunately, only rarely can one remove the underlying cause of chronic respiratory acidosis. Nonetheless, maximizing alveolar ventilation with relatively simple maneuvers is often rewarding. Such maneuvers include treatment with antibiotics, bronchodilators, or diuretics; avoidance of irritant inhalants, tranquilizers, or sedatives; and elimination of retained secretions. Administration of adequate quantities of chloride (usually as the potassium salt) prevents or corrects a complicating element of metabolic alkalosis (commonly diuretic induced) that can further dampen the ventilatory drive. Acetazolamide might be used as an adjunctive measure but care must be taken to avoid potassium depletion. Potassium and phosphate depletion should be corrected, because they might contribute to the development or the maintenance of respiratory failure by impairing the function of skeletal muscles. The use of pharmacologic stimulants of ventilation has been generally disappointing but a measure of benefit can be derived by some patients with central sleep apnea, obesity–hypoventilation syndrome, or chronic obstructive lung disease. In contrast to acute respiratory acidosis, administration of oxygen to patients with long-standing CO_2 retention should be carried out cautiously aiming at a pO_2 of about 60 mm Hg. Injudicious use of oxygen therapy can produce further reductions in alveolar ventilation and aggravate hypercapnia dramatically. Restoration of the chronically elevated pCO_2 to or toward normal via assisted ventilation, if indicated, should proceed gradually over many hours to a few days. Overly rapid reduction in pCO_2 in such patients risks the development of sudden, substantial alkalemia with the attendant hazards of a major reduction in cardiac output and cerebral blood flow, arrhythmias (including predisposition to digitalis intoxication), and generalized seizures. In the absence of a complicating element of metabolic acidosis and with the possible exception of the severely acidemic patient with intense generalized bronchoconstriction undergoing mechanical ventilation, there is no role for alkali administration in chronic respiratory acidosis.

RESPIRATORY ALKALOSIS

Respiratory alkalosis, or primary hypocapnia, is the acid–base disturbance initiated by a reduction in carbon dioxide tension of body fluids. Hypocapnia alkalinizes body fluids and elicits an adaptive decrement in plasma bicarbonate that should be viewed as an integral part of the respiratory alkalosis. The level of pCO_2 measured at rest and at sea level is lower than 35 mm Hg in simple respiratory alkalosis. Higher values of pCO_2 might still indicate the presence of an element of primary hypocapnia in the setting of mixed acid–base disorders (e.g., eucapnia, rather than the anticipated hypercapnia, in the presence of metabolic alkalosis).

Pathophysiology

Primary hypocapnia most commonly reflects pulmonary hyperventilation due to increased ventilatory drive. The latter results from signals arising from the lung, the peripheral chemoreceptors (carotid and aortic), the brain stem chemoreceptors, or influences originating in other centers of the brain. Additional mechanisms for the generation of primary hypocapnia include maladjusted mechanical ventilators, the extrapulmonary elimination of carbon dioxide by a dialysis device or extracorporeal circulation (e.g., heart–lung machine), and decreased carbon dioxide production (e.g., due to sedation, skeletal muscle paralysis, hypothermia) in patients receiving constant mechanical ventilation.

A condition termed pseudorespiratory alkalosis occurs in patients with profound decrements in cardiac output but relative preservation of respiratory function. In these patients, there is venous (and tissue) hypercapnia due to prolongation of transit time, resulting in a greater than normal addition of carbon dioxide per unit of blood traversing the systemic capillaries. On the other hand, arterial blood evidences hypocapnia due to increased ventilation-to-perfusion ratio causing increased removal of carbon dioxide per unit of blood traversing the pulmonary circulation. Absolute carbon dioxide excretion is decreased, however, and body carbon dioxide balance is positive. Therefore, respiratory acidosis, rather than respiratory alkalosis, is present. In addition, arterial blood might reveal normoxia or hyperoxia despite the presence of severe hypoxemia in venous blood. Thus, both arterial and mixed (or central) venous blood sampling is needed to assess the acid–base status and oxygenation of patients with critical hemodynamic compromise.

Secondary Physiological Response

Adaptation to acute hypocapnia is characterized by an immediate decrement in plasma bicarbonate that is accounted for principally by titration of nonbicarbonate body buffers. This adaptation is completed within 5 to 10 minutes after the onset of hypocapnia. Plasma bicarbonate falls, on average, by approximately 0.2 mEq/L for each mm Hg acute decrement in pCO_2; consequently, plasma hydrogen ion concentration decreases by about 0.75 nEq/L for each mm Hg acute reduction in pCO_2. The limit of this adaptation of plasma bicarbonate is on the order of 17 to 18 mEq/L. Concomitant small rises in plasma chloride, lactate, and other unmeasured anions balance the fall in plasma bicarbonate; each of these components accounts for about one third of the bicarbonate decrement. Small decreases in plasma sodium (1–3 mEq/L) and potassium (0.2 mEq/L for each 0.1 unit rise in pH) might be observed. Severe hypophosphatemia can occur in acute hypocapnia due to translocation of phosphorus into the cells.

A larger decrement in plasma bicarbonate occurs in chronic hypocapnia as a result of renal adaptation to the disorder and involves suppression of both proximal and distal acidification mechanisms. Completion of this adaptation requires 2 to 3 days. Plasma bicarbonate decreases, on average, by about 0.4 mEq/L for each mm Hg chronic decrement in pCO_2; as a consequence, plasma hydrogen ion concentration decreases by approximately 0.4 nEq/L for each mm Hg chronic reduction in pCO_2. The limit of this adaptation of plasma bicarbonate is on the order of 12 to 15 mEq/L. About two thirds of the fall in plasma bicarbonate is balanced by a rise in plasma chloride concentration, the remainder reflects an increase in plasma unmeasured anions; part of the remainder is due to the alkaline titration of plasma proteins, but most remains undefined. Plasma lactate does not rise in chronic hypocapnia, even in the presence of moderate hypoxemia. Similarly, no appreciable change in the plasma concentration of sodium occurs. In sharp contrast with acute hypocapnia, the plasma concentration of phosphorus remains essentially unchanged in chronic hypocapnia. Although plasma potassium is in the normal range in patients with chronic hypocapnia at sea level, hypokalemia and renal potassium wasting have been described in subjects in whom sustained hypocapnia was induced by exposure to high altitude. Patients with end stage renal disease are obviously at risk of developing severe alkalemia in response to chronic hypocapnia because they cannot mount a renal response. Such a risk is higher in patients receiving peritoneal dialysis rather than hemodialysis because the former treatment maintains, on average, a higher plasma bicarbonate concentration.

Etiology

Primary hypocapnia is the most frequent acid–base disturbance encountered, occurring in normal pregnancy and high-altitude residence. Table 3 lists the major causes of respiratory alkalosis. Most are associated with the abrupt appearance of hypocapnia but, in many instances, the process might be sufficiently prolonged to permit full chronic adaptation to occur. Consequently, no attempt has been made to separate these conditions into acute and chronic categories. Some of the major causes of respiratory alkalosis are benign, whereas others are life threatening. Primary hypocapnia is particularly common among the critically ill, occurring either as the simple disorder or as a component of mixed disturbances. Its presence constitutes an ominous prognostic sign, with mortality increasing in direct proportion to the severity of the hypocapnia.

Clinical Manifestations

Rapid decrements in pCO_2 to half the normal values or lower are typically accompanied by paresthesias of the extremities, chest discomfort, circumoral numbness, lightheadedness, confusion, and infrequently, tetany or generalized seizures. These manifestations are seldom present in the chronic phase. Acute hypocapnia decreases cerebral blood flow, which, in severe cases, might reach values less than 50% of normal, resulting in cerebral hypoxia. This hypoperfusion has been implicated in the pathogenesis of the neurological manifestations of acute respiratory alkalosis along with other factors, including hypocapnia per se, alkalemia, pH-induced shift of the oxyhemoglobin dissociation curve, and decrements in the level of ionized calcium

TABLE 3
Causes of Respiratory Alkalosis[a]

Hypoxemia or tissue hypoxia	Central nervous system stimulation
Decreased inspired O_2 tension	Voluntary
High altitude	Pain
Bacterial or viral pneumonia	Anxiety
Aspiration of food, foreign body, or vomitus	Psychosis
Laryngospasm	Fever
Drowning	Subarachnoid hemorrhage
Cyanotic heart disease	Cerebrovascular accident
Severe anemia	Meningoencephalitis
Left shift deviation of HbO_2 curve	Tumor
Hypotension[b]	Trauma
Severe circulatory failure[b]	**Drugs or hormones**
Pulmonary edema	Nikethamide, ethamivan
Stimulation of chest receptors	Doxapram
Pneumonia	Xanthines
Asthma	Salicylates
Pneumothorax	Catecholamines
Hemothorax	Angiotensin II
Flail chest	Vasopressor agents
Infant or adult respiratory distress syndrome	Progesterone
Cardiac failure	Medroxyprogesterone
Noncardiogenic pulmonary edema	Dinitrophenol
Pulmonary embolism	Nicotine
Interstitial lung disease	**Miscellaneous**
	Pregnancy
	Sepsis
	Hepatic failure
	Mechanical hyperventilation
	Heat exposure
	Recovery from metabolic acidosis

[a] Adapted from Madias and Adrogué (1991).
[b] Might produce pseudorespiratory alkalosis.

and potassium. Some evidence indicates that cerebral blood flow returns to normal in chronic respiratory alkalosis.

Actively hyperventilating patients manifest no appreciable changes in cardiac output or systemic blood pressure. By contrast, acute hypocapnia in the course of passive hyperventilation typically observed during mechanical ventilation in patients with depressed central nervous system or those under general anesthesia, frequently results in a major reduction in cardiac output and systemic blood pressure, increased peripheral resistance, and substantial hyperlactatemia (exceeding 2 mEq/L). Neither cardiac arrhythmias nor clinically evident signs or symptoms of coronary insufficiency develop in actively hyperventilating normal volunteers. However, patients with underlying coronary artery disease might occasionally suffer hypocapnia-induced coronary vasoconstriction resulting in angina pectoris, ischemic electrocardiographic changes, and arrhythmias. Increased cardiac excitability has been attributed to the same factors that have been held responsible for the enhanced excitability of the central nervous system associated with acute hypocapnia.

Diagnosis

Careful observation can detect abnormal patterns of breathing in some patients, yet marked hypocapnia can be present without a clinically evident increase in respiratory effort. Thus, arterial blood gases should be obtained whenever hyperventilation is suspected. In fact, the diagnosis of respiratory alkalosis, especially the chronic form, is frequently missed; physicians often misinterpret the electrolyte pattern of hyperchloremic hypobicarbonatemia as indicative of normal anion gap metabolic acidosis. If the patient's acid–base profile reveals hypocapnia in association with alkalemia, at least an element of respiratory alkalosis must be present. Primary hypocapnia, however, might be associated with a normal or an acidic pH due to the concomitant presence of other acid–base disorders. Notably, mild degrees of chronic hypocapnia commonly leave blood pH within the high-normal range. As always, proper evaluation of the patient's acid–base status requires careful assessment of the history, physical examination, and ancillary laboratory data. Once the diagnosis of respiratory alkalosis has been made, a search for its cause should be carried out. The diagnosis of respiratory alkalosis can have important clinical implications: It often provides a clue to the presence of an unrecognized, serious disorder (e.g., sepsis) or signals the severity of a known underlying disease.

Therapeutic Principles

Management of respiratory alkalosis must be directed toward correcting the underlying cause, whenever possible. Taking measures to treat the respiratory alkalosis itself is commonly not required, because the disorder, especially in its chronic form, leads to minimal or no symptoms and poses little risk to health. A notable exception is the patient with the anxiety-hyperventilation syndrome; in addition to reassurance or sedation, rebreathing into a closed system (e.g., a paper bag) might prove helpful by interrupting the vicious cycle that can result from the reinforcing effects of the symptoms of hypocapnia. Considering the risks of severe alkalemia, sedation or, in rare cases, skeletal muscle paralysis and mechanical ventilation might be required to correct temporarily marked respiratory alkalosis. Management of pseudorespiratory alkalosis must be directed at optimizing systemic hemodynamics.

Bibliography

Adrogué HJ, Rashad MN, Gorin AB, Yacoub J, Madias NE: Assessing acid-base status in circulatory failure. Differences between arterial and central venous blood. *N Engl J Med* 320:1312–1316, 1989.

Al-Awqati Q: The cellular renal response to respiratory acid-base disorders. *Kidney Int* 28:845–855, 1985.

Arbus GS, Hebert LA, Levesque PR, Etsten BE, Schwartz WB: Characterization and clinical application of the "significance band" for acute respiratory alkalosis. *N Engl J Med* 280:117–123, 1969.

Brackett NC Jr, Cohen JJ, Schwartz WB: Carbon dioxide titration curve of normal man. Effect of increasing degrees of acute hypercapnia on acid-base equilibrium. *N Engl J Med* 272:6–12, 1965.

Brackett NC Jr, Wingo CF, Muren O, Solano JT: Acid-base response to chronic hypercapnia in man. *N Engl J Med* 280:124–130, 1969.

Feihl F, Perret C: Permissive hypercapnia. How permissive should we be? *Am J Respir Crit Care Med* 150:1722–1737, 1994.

Gennari FJ, Kassirer JP: Respiratory alkalosis. In: Cohen JJ, Kassirer JP (eds) *Acid-Base.* Little, Brown, Boston, pp. 349–376, 1982.

Krapf R, Beeler I, Hertner D, Hulter HN: Chronic respiratory alkalosis. The effect of sustained hyperventilation on renal regulation of acid-base equilibrium. *N Engl J Med* 324:1394–1401, 1991.

Madias NE, Adrogué HJ. Respiratory acidosis and alkalosis. In: Adrogué JH (ed) *Contemporary Management in Critical Care: Acid-Base and Electrolyte Disorders.* Churchill Livingstone, New York, pp. 37–53, 1991.

Madias NE, Cohen JJ: Respiratory acidosis. In: Cohen JJ, Kassirer JP (eds) *Acid-Base.* Little, Brown, Boston, pp. 307–348, 1982.

Madias NE, Cohen JJ: Adaptation to respiratory acidosis and alkalosis. In: Fishman AP (ed) *Pulmonary Diseases and Disorders.* 2nd ed. McGraw-Hill Book Company, New York, Vol. 1, pp. 289–298, 1988.

Madias NE, Wolf CJ, Cohen JJ: Regulation of acid-base equilibrium in chronic hypercapnia. *Kidney Int* 27:538–543, 1985.

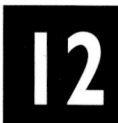

APPROACH TO ACID–BASE DISORDERS

MARTIN GOLDBERG

Acid–base disorders occur commonly in medical and surgical patients. They are particularly important in severely ill hospitalized patients. They may be present as single (simple) disorders or as a combination of simple disorders (mixed acid–base disturbances). Systematic diagnostic recognition and correction of these simple or mixed disorders is important because they may not only impact on the patient's prognosis, but also may provide clues to the nature of the underlying primary disease(s). Before discussing a systematic approach to the diagnosis of acid–base disorders, several fundamental terms require definition.

ACIDEMIA VS ALKALEMIA

These terms represent abnormal hydrogen ion concentrations of blood: either higher (acidemia) or lower (alkalemia) than the normal range of 35 to 45 nEq/L(pH = 7.35–7.45).

$$[H^+] = \text{hydrogen ion concentration}$$
$$pH = \log 1/[H^+] = -\log [H^+]$$

The Henderson–Hasselbalch equation is

$$pH = pK + \log ([HCO_3^-]/[0.03 \times pCO_2]).$$

Normally,

$$\text{Blood pH} = 6.10 + \log (24/0.03 \times 40)$$
$$= 6.10 + \log (20/1) = 7.40.$$

The Henderson equation (modified) is

$$[H^+] = 24 \times pCO_2/[HCO_3^-].$$

Normally,

$$[H^+] = 24 \times (40/24) = 40 \text{ nEq/L}.$$

ACIDOSIS VS ALKALOSIS

Alkalosis is a primary process (e.g., loss of H^+ from vomiting) which, if unopposed, would produce alkalemia. *Acidosis* is a primary process (e.g., retention of $[H^+]$ due to renal failure), which, if unopposed, would produce acidemia.

These are pathophysiological processes or abnormal states which, if unopposed by therapy or disease, would cause deviations of extracellular fluid $[H^+]$ from normal levels. They are defined independently of the $[H^+]$ or pH because two or more concomitant processes may produce either no net change in $[H^+]$ and/or may modify the body's adaptive mechanisms to a single disorder.

RESPIRATORY VS METABOLIC DISTURBANCES

Respiratory disturbances are those caused by abnormal pulmonary elimination of CO_2, producing an excess (acidosis) or deficit (alkalosis) of H_2CO_3 (in equilibrium with pCO_2) in extracellular fluid. These primarily alter the pCO_2 in the denominator of the Henderson–Haseelbalch equation. Compensatory (adaptive) adjustments involve changes in [HCO_3^-] accumulation in body fluids. Adaptation via the kidneys is slow (3–4 days); hence there are operationally four respiratory disorders: acute and chronic respiratory acidosis; acute and chronic respiratory alkalosis.

Metabolic disturbances are those caused by excessive intake, metabolic production, or losses of fixed (nonvolatile) acids or bases in the extracellular fluid. These are reflected by changes in [HCO_3^-] in blood and therefore alter primarily the numerator of the Henderson-Hasselbalch ratio. Adaptation to metabolic disorders is relatively rapid (12–36 hours); hence there are two: metabolic acidosis (a process which lowers plasma [HCO_3^-]) and metabolic alkalosis (a process which raises plasma [HCO_3^-]).

COMPENSATORY (ADAPTIVE) RESPONSES

Primary changes in the metabolic component ([HCO_3^-]) stimulate adaptive changes in ventilation, producing changes in pCO_2. Additional adaptive changes occur in extracellular and intracellular buffers and in the kidney (adjustments in H^+ secretion, HCO_3^- reabsorption and secretion, and generation of HCO_3^-).

Primary changes in the respiratory component (pCO_2) stimulate adaptive changes in [HCO_3^-] via reactions with extra- and intracellular buffers and by slower (renal) adjustments in H^+ secretion, HCO_3^- reabsorption and secretion, and HCO_3^- generation.

As a rule, compensation restores [H^+] or pH toward normal, but not to complete normality.

SIMPLE (SINGLE) VS MIXED DISORDERS

A *simple disorder* includes the primary process with the initial changes in [H^+], pCO_2 or [HCO_3^-] and all compensatory processes in reaction to these initial changes.

A *mixed disorder* is the simultaneous occurrence of two or more simple disturbances in a patient. Mixed disorders may be additive or counterbalancing regarding their net effect on [H^+] or pH; they are frequently difficult to diagnose and reflect serious illness. A mixed disorder in which there are three simultaneous primary acid–base disorders present is commonly referred to as a triple acid–base disturbance.

ACID–BASE MAPS AND FORMULAS IN DIAGNOSIS OF ACID–BASE DISORDERS

The adaptive responses for the six simple disorders (including the acute and chronic respiratory disorders) have been quantified experimentally. The 95% confidence limits can be defined, and several formulas have been developed to reflect the ranges of compensation. The acid–base map

provides the graphic representation of these ranges. (See Table 1 and Fig. 1).

In a patient with a clinical condition suggesting a simple acid–base disorder, values of pH, pCO_2, and [HCO_3^-] lying within the ranges defined by the formulas or map are compatible with the diagnosis of the specified simple disorder. This does not, however, rule out the possibility of a mixed disorder due to two or more counterbalancing processes, the net effects of which might produce values lying in the normal range, or in an area of a simple disorder. Furthermore, whereas values lying outside the range of a simple disorder suggest the diagnosis of a mixed disorder, a mixed disorder may sometimes be simulated during a transient state in which the adaptive processes to a simple disorder have not yet been completed.

ANION GAP

The anion gap (AG) is the concentration of unmeasured anions (proteinate, phosphates, sulfates, organic acid anions) which are typically associated with H^+ as it is initially generated in body fluids. It is commonly calculated as

$$AG = \text{plasma } [Na^+] - (\text{plasma } [Cl^-] + \text{plasma } [HCO_3^-]).$$

Normal values for AG are 6–13 mEq/L. An AG > 15 mEq/L generally indicates one type of metabolic acidosis (i.e., due to accumulation of organic acids as occurs in lactic acidosis, diabetic ketoacidosis, or ingested toxins). An exception to this occurs during infusions of fluids containing salts of organic anions (e.g., lactate, amino acids, high doses of penicillins).

APPROACH TO THE DIAGNOSIS OF ACID–BASE DISORDERS

Appropriate diagnosis of acid–base disorders involves analysis and synthesis of all relevant information based on the patient's history, physical examination, and laboratory data. Use of data from one of these areas alone is insufficient to define the various processes that determine the primary disorder and the body's adaptive responses. An outline of the important steps in this approach is as follows:

1. Suspect acid–base disturbances from the history.
2. Suspect acid–base disturbances from the physical examination.
3. Evaluate the venous total CO_2 (tCO_2), [Cl^-], [K^+], and AG to support suspected diagnoses and to suggest possible additional primary disorders.
4. Obtain arterial pH, pCO_2, and [HCO_3^-] to establish definitive diagnoses using formulas, acid–base map, and limits of compensation.

A careful review of the *patient's history* may reveal several commonly encountered clinical conditions which are typically associated with one or more acid–base disturbances (Table 2). The presence of these conditions should cause one to add the potential disorders to the differential diagnosis. One needs to assess the specific disease states,

TABLE I

Patterns of Arterial Blood Changes and Adaptation in Simple Acid–Base Disorders

| | Blood acid–base pattern | | | | | |
Primary disorder	pH	[H⁺]	[HCO₃⁻]	pCO₂	Adaptive response	Limits of adaptation
Metabolic acidosis	↓	↑	↓ [a]	↓ [b]	$pCO_2 = 1.5 \cdot [HCO_3^-] + 8 \pm 2$	pCO_2 not <10 mm Hg
Metabolic alkalosis	↑	↓	↑ [a]	↑ [b]	$\Delta pCO_2 = 0.5 \cdot \Delta[HCO_3^-]$	pCO_2 not >55 mm Hg
Respiratory acidosis						
Acute	↓	↑	↑ [b]	↑ [a]	$\Delta[HCO_3^-] = 0.1 \cdot \Delta pCO_2$	$[HCO_3^-]$ not >30 mEq/L
Chronic	↓	↑	↑ ↑ [b]	↑ [a]	$\Delta[HCO_3^-] = 0.4 \cdot \Delta pCO_2$	$[HCO_3^-]$ not >45 mEq/L
Respiratory alkalosis						
Acute	↑	↓	↓ [b]	↓ [a]	$\Delta[HCO_3^-] = 0.2 \cdot \Delta pCO_2$	$[HCO_3^-]$ not <17–18 mEq/L
Chronic	↑	↓	↓ ↓ [b]	↓ [a]	$\Delta[HCO_3^-] = 0.5 \cdot \Delta pCO_2$	$[HCO_3^-]$ not <12–15 mEq/L

[a] Initial event.
[b] Secondary adaptive response.
Note: Arrows indicate direction of change from normal. A double arrow indicates that the magnitude of the change is considerably greater in the chronic disorder compared to the acute disorder. Units for pCO_2 are mm Hg, and units for $[HCO_3^-]$ mEq/L. Δ = change from normal.

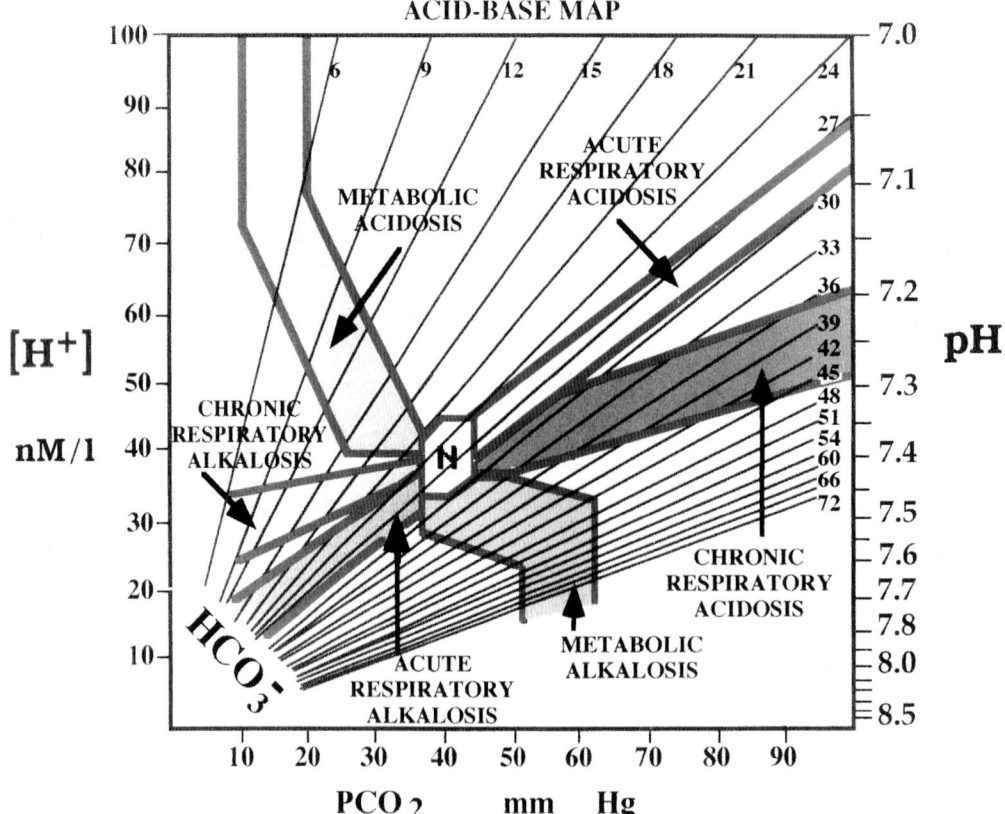

FIGURE 1   The acid–base map. Shaded areas represent the 95% confidence limits for zones of adaptation of the simple acid–base disorders. Numbered diagonal lines represent isopleths of plasma bicarbonate concentration. This map has been modified and updated from Goldberg M, Green SB, Moss ML, Marbach MS, Garfinkel D. *JAMA* 223:269–275, 1973.

TABLE 2
Common Clinical Conditions Associated With Acid–Base Disorders

Condition	Metabolic acidosis	Metabolic alkalosis	Respiratory acidosis	Respiratory alkalosis
Cardiovascular disease				
Cardiopulmonary arrest	+[a]	+[b]	+	+[b]
Pulmonary edema				+
CNS disease			+ or	+
Diabetes mellitus	+[a]			
Drugs				
Diuretics		+		
Poisonings	+[a]		+	+
Fever				+
GI disease				
Diarrhea	+			
Vomiting/gastric suction		+		
Hepatic failure	+[a]			+
Hyperkalemia	+			
Hypokalemia		+		
Pulmonary disease				
Acute asthma				+
COPD/respiratory failure			+	
Emboli				+
Pneumonia				+
Renal disease				
Renal failure	+[a]			
Renal tubular acidosis	+			
Sepsis	+[a]			+

[a] High anion gap metabolic acidosis.
[b] During treatment and recovery.

various drugs, the presence of mechanical ventilation, and nasogastric suction—all of which may be either causative of primary acid–base disorders or which may modify adaptive responses. A history of renal failure or diarrhea suggests metabolic acidosis; pneumonia, sepsis, or hepatic failure should raise the suspicion of respiratory alkalosis; therapy with the common diuretics or vomiting should alert one to the possibility of metabolic alkalosis. In particular, certain clinical catastrophes such as cardiac arrest, septic shock, various intoxications, and the heptorenal syndrome typically involve mixed acid–base disorders (see Table 2).

The *physical examination* may provide additional clues to potential acid–base disorders or may provide evidence to support those disorders suspected from the history. For example, normocalcemic tetany is compatible with severe alkalemia, and cyanosis may indicate severe hypoxia and the possibility of respiratory acidosis or lactic metabolic acidosis. Rapid and/or deep respirations in the absence of cardiac or pulmonary failure are compatible with the hyperventilation associated with severe metabolic acidosis. Metabolic alkalosis is common in patients with signs of extracellular fluid volume contraction, while high fever typically stimulates respiratory alkalosis.

Careful analysis of the routine laboratory data including the venous electrolytes may provide useful quantitative information enabling the *identification* of the possible predominant acid–base disturbance and clues to additional disorders. The presence of azotemia strengthens support for the diagnosis of renal metabolic acidosis.

Most useful is examination of the venous plasma tCO_2, $[Cl^-]$, $[K^+]$, and the AG. In the clinical laboratory, measurement of venous plasma or serum electrolytes includes an estimation of the tCO_2. This measurement reflects the sum of the numerator and the denominator of the Henderson or Henderson–Hasselbalch equations, i.e, $[HCO_3^-]$ + H_2CO_3 + dissolved CO_2 gas. Since normally and in pathophysiological states the $[HCO_3^-]$ is >90% of the tCO_2, then the venous tCO_2 is a reasonable approximation of the venous $[HCO_3^-]$. An abnormal plasma $[HCO_3^-]$ indicates an acid–base disorder (Table 1). An increased $[HCO_3^-]$ indicates either a primary metabolic alkalosis or an adaptation to respiratory acidosis. A decreased $[HCO_3^-]$ indicates either primary metabolic acidosis or an adaptation to respiratory alkalosis.

Applying knowledge of the limits of adaptation (Table 1) may help eliminate some diagnostic considerations. For example, if the plasma $[HCO_3^-] < 12$ mEq/L, which exceeds the limits of adaptation (Table 1) to respiratory alkalosis, then metabolic acidosis is definitely present. Conversely, if plasma $[HCO_3^-] > 45$ mEq/L, exceeding the adaptive limit for respiratory acidosis, then metabolic alkalosis may be diagnosed. A plasma $[HCO_3^-]$ in the normal range, on the other hand, does not exclude either a mixture of disorders which have opposing effects on $[HCO_3^-]$ (e.g., metabolic acidosis + metabolic alkalosis such as may occur in a patient with renal failure with a high AG metabolic acidosis who is also vomiting due to uremia and is losing HCl), or acute respiratory disorders in which the early adaptive changes in $[HCO_3^-]$ are small (Table 1).

Evaluating changes in plasma $[Cl^-]$ may provide additional insights into possible acid–base disorders. Remember, however, that changes in $[Cl^-]$ are important from the standpoint of acid–base disorders only when they are disproportionate to changes in plasma $[Na^+]$. When this occurs the changes in plasma $[Cl^-]$ are typically associated with reciprocal changes in plasma $[HCO_3^-]$. Thus in primary metabolic alkalosis and in the adaptation to chronic respiration acidosis, plasma $[Cl^-]$ falls as $[HCO_3^-]$ rises, whereas in primary metabolic acidosis (with normal AG) and in the adaptation to chronic respiratory alkalosis, plasma $[Cl^-]$ rises as $[HCO_3^-]$ decreases.

Abnormalities in plasma $[K^+]$ are common in patients with acid–base disorders. There is, however, no consistent quantitative relationship between changes in pH or $[HCO_3^-]$ and changes in $[K^+]$. This is because $[K^+]$ is influenced by many metabolic and physiological factors besides acid–base disturbances. Alterations in plasma $[K^+]$ are more pronounced in metabolic than in respiratory disorders. A rise in serum $[K^+]$ is more likely to be associated with an acute metabolic acidosis with normal AG and is least likely to be observed in lactic acidosis. In general a change in $[K^+]$ is useful only as a qualitative indicator in acid–base disorders; a high K^+ plus a low $[HCO_3^-]$ implies metabolic acidosis, and a low $[K^+]$ with high $[HCO_3^-]$ suggests metabolic alkalosis.

Calculation of the AG is essential in the evaluation of acid–base disorders. An elevated AG commonly signifies the presence of a metabolic acidosis regardless of the change in plasma $[HCO_3^-]$. One should be aware, however, that uncommonly the AG may be moderately increased (5–9 mEq/L) by severe volume contraction, metabolic alkalosis, and infusions of sodium salts of unmeasured anions (e.g., sulfates, lactate, carbenicillin). Nevertheless, the AG is a valuable tool in suspecting the presence of metabolic acidosis: An AG > 30 mEq/L almost always signifies a metabolic acidosis, and an AG between 20 and 30 mEq/L usually signifies metabolic acidosis.

Examination of the relationship between the change in AG (ΔAG) and the change in $[HCO_3^-]$ (ΔHCO_3^-) may be useful in diagnosing mixed acid–base disorders. In simple high AG metabolic acidosis each mEq of H^+ accumulation is associated with 1 mEq of unmeasured anion accumulation; further, each mEq of H^+ has consumed 1 mEq of HCO_3^-. Therefore increases in the AG are associated with corresponding decreases in plasma $[HCO_3^-]$, and ΔAG ap-

proximates ΔHCO_3^-. If $\Delta AG > \Delta HCO_3^-$, this suggests the presence of an additional process that generates HCO_3^- (either a metabolic alkalosis or chronic respiratory acidosis), whereas $\Delta AG < \Delta HCO_3^-$ suggests the additional presence of a hyperchloremic metabolic acidosis or a chronic respiratory alkalosis.

Arterial blood gases are used to confirm the predominant acid–base disorder and to identify and confirm mixed disturbances. From information derived from the history, physical examination, and the routine analyses of venous blood, potential acid–base disturbances can be identified, and, in many instances, a reasonable acid–base diagnosis can be established without obtaining arterial blood gases. On the other hand, it is extremely difficult to diagnose acute respiratory disturbances and most mixed acid-base disorders without knowledge of arterial pH, pCO_2, and $[HCO_3^-]$. Thus if these are distinct possibilities or if the patient is critically ill (a setting in which mixed disorders are common), arterial studies should be obtained.

The data on arterial pH, pCO_2, and $[HCO_3^-]$ should be analyzed and applied to the acid–base formulas, to the acid–base map, and to knowledge of limits of adaptation (see Table 1 and Fig. 1). The results of these analyses should be coordinated with the differential and potential diagnostic inferences derived from the history, physical examination, and routine laboratory data. Before proceeding further, however, one must ensure the internal consistency of the blood values and their compatibility with the Henderson-Hasselbalch or Henderson equations. This can readily be accomplished using the acid–base map (which also serves as a nomogram for these equations) or by converting pH values to $[H^+]$ and applying the Henderson equation. In the pH range 7.20 to 7.50, each 0.1 unit change in pH from a normal value of 7.40 corresponds to 10 nEq/L change in $[H^+]$ from a normal value of 40 nEq/L.

If the pH is abnormal then the major acid–base disturbance may be identified. Acidemia denotes a predominant acidosis, and alkalemia indicates a predominant alkalosis. Reference should then be made to the patterns for each acid–base disorder as summarized in Table 1. This will enable confirmation of the major disorder. For example, acidemia, a low $[HCO_3^-]$, and a low pCO_2 support the diagnosis of metabolic acidosis. In order to rule out an additional primary disorder as a component of a mixed disturbance, the data must be compared to the expected range of adaptation by either plotting the data on the acid-base map (Fig. 1), using one of the formulas for adaptive response in Table 1. When the pCO_2 is above or below the predicted range of compensation for a metabolic disturbance or when the $[HCO_3^-]$ is above or below the predicted levels for a respiratory disorder, a mixed disturbance is present.

Although many mixed acid–base disorders can be diagnosed using the arterial blood values in conjunction with the map or formulas, the final diagnostic conclusions require a coordinated synthesis of information derived from the clinical and laboratory data in conjunction with the arterial data. Thus, use of the map alone will not identify triple mixed acid–base disorders. Values lying within a specific zone on the map (while suggesting a simple disorder) are also compatible with a mixed disorder with counterbalancing effects on pH, $[HCO_3^-]$, or pCO_2. In order to dissect out the various components of a mixed disorder, we must apply information on changes in AG, plasma $[Cl^-]$, and the plasma $[K^+]$. In fact a normal plasma $[HCO_3^-]$ or a normal pH or a normal pCO_2 by themselves do not rule out mixed disorders; nor are normal levels of all three variables simultaneously imcompatible with mixed disorders.

Mixed disorders should be suspected in the following circumstances:

1. pH is normal and:
   a. $[HCO_3^-]$ is high (mixed metabolic alkalosis + respiratory acidosis).
   b. $[HCO_3^-]$ is low (mixed metabolic acidosis + respiratory alkalosis).
   c. $[HCO_3^-]$ is normal and AG is high (mixed metabolic acidosis + metabolic alkalosis).
2. $[HCO_3^-]$ is normal and:
   a. pH is in the acidemic range (mixed chronic respiratory acidosis and metabolic acidosis).
   b. pH is in the alkalemic range (mixed metabolic alkalosis and chronic respiratory alkalosis).
3. pCO_2 and $[HCO_3^-]$ are shifted from normal in opposite directions.
4. AG is elevated and clinical/laboratory data suggest a diagnosis other than a simple metabolic acidosis (metabolic acidosis is a component of a mixed disorder).
5. When AG is high and the $\Delta AG \neq \Delta HCO_3^-$ (see previous discussion of AG and ΔAG). Remember that a mixed disorder may include two different types or etiologies of a simple disorder (e.g., a high AG + a normal AG metabolic acidosis or an acute respiratory disorder superimposed on an underlying chronic respiratory disorder).

In conclusion, a successful approach to resolving the sometimes complex dilemmas associated with the diagnosis of acid–base disorders involves the application of a systematic, orderly, and logical series of steps. Building on a knowledge of pathophysiology, these steps involve a coordinated analysis and re-synthesis of information derived from taking a proper history, performing an adequate physical examination, and obtaining relevant laboratory data. Final success is measured not only by the intellectual satisfaction of the physician in making the correct evaluation(s), but also by the well being of the patient who has benefited from the appropriate corrective therapy.

Bibliography

Bia M, Thier SO: Mixed acid-base disturbances: A clinical approach. *Med Clin North Am* 65:347–361, 1981.

DuBose TD Jr, Cogan MG, Rector FC Jr: Acid-base disorders. In: Brenner BM, (ed) *The Kidney*. 5th ed. Saunders, Philadelphia, pp. 929–998, 1996.

Goldberg M, Green SB, Moss ML, Marbach MS, Garfinkel D: Computer-based instruction and diagnosis of acid-base disorders. *JAMA* 223:269–275, 1973.

Goodkin DA, Krishna GG, Narins RG: The role of the anion gap in detecting and managing mixed acid-based disorders. *Clin Endocrinol Metab* 13:333–350, 1984.

Hamm L: Mixed acid-based disorders. In: Kokko JP, Tannen RL (eds) *Fluids and Electrolytes*. Saunders, Philadelphia, pp. 490–495, 1990.

Kraut JA, Madias NE: Approach to diagnosis of acid-base disorders. In: Massry SG, Glassock RJ (eds) *Textbook of Nephrology*. Williams and Wilkins, Baltimore, pp. 487–493, 1995.

Laski ME, Kurtzman NA: Acid-base disorders in medicine. *Dis Mon* 42:51–125, 1996.

McCurdy DK: Mixed metabolic and respiratory acid-base disturbances: Diagnosis and treatment. *Chest* 62:35S–44S, 1972.

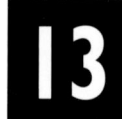

DISORDERS OF POTASSIUM METABOLISM

MICHAEL ALLON

MECHANISMS OF POTASSIUM HOMEOSTASIS

Total body potassium is about 3500 mmol. Approximately 98% of the total is intracellular, primarily in skeletal muscle, and to a lesser extent in liver. The remaining 2% (about 70 mmol) is in the extracellular fluid. Two systems help maintain potassium homeostasis. The first regulates potassium excretion (kidney and intestine). The second regulates potassium shifts between the extracellular and intracellular fluid compartments.

External Potassium Balance

The average American diet contains about 100 mmol of potassium per day but dietary potassium intake may vary widely from day to day. To maintain potassium balance, it is necessary to increase potassium excretion when dietary potassium increases, and to decrease potassium excretion when dietary potassium decreases. Normally, the kidneys excrete 90 to 95% of dietary potassium, with the remaining 5 to 10% excreted by the gut. Potassium excretion by the kidney is a relatively slow process. It takes 6 to 12 hours to excrete an acute potassium load.

Renal Handling of Potassium

To understand the physiologic factors that determine renal excretion of potassium, it is critical to review the main features of tubular potassium handling. Plasma potassium is freely filtered across the glomerular capillary into the proximal tubule. It is subsequently completely reabsorbed by the proximal tubule and loop of Henle. In the distal tubule and the collecting duct, potassium is secreted into the tubular lumen. For practical purposes, urinary excretion of potassium can be viewed as a reflection of potassium secretion into the lumen of the distal tubule and collecting duct. Thus, any factor that stimulates potassium secretion increases urinary potassium excretion; conversely, any factor that inhibits potassium secretion decreases urinary potassium excretion.

Physiologic Regulation of Renal Potassium Excretion

Five major physiologic factors stimulate distal potassium secretion, thereby increasing excretion: (1) aldosterone, (2) high distal sodium delivery, (3) high urine flow rate, (4) high $[K^+]$ in tubular cells and (5) metabolic alkalosis.

Aldosterone directly increases the activity of the Na,K-ATPase in the collecting duct cells, thereby stimulating secretion of potassium into the tubular lumen. Medical conditions that impair aldosterone production or secretion (e.g., diabetic nephropathy, chronic interstitial nephritis) or drugs that inhibit aldosterone production or action [e.g., nonsteroidal antiinflammatory drugs (NSAIDs), angiotensin converting enzyme (ACE) inhibitors, heparin, spironolactone] decrease potassium secretion by the kidney. Conversely, medical conditions associated with increased aldosterone levels (primary aldosteronism, secondary aldosteronism due to diuretics or vomiting) increase potassium excretion by the kidney. Although there is profound secondary hyperaldosteronism in congestive heart failure and cirrhosis, each of these conditions may be associated with hyperkalemia due to decreased delivery of sodium. Many diuretics increase renal potassium excretion by a number of mechanisms, including high distal sodium delivery, high urine flow rate, metabolic alkalosis, and hyperaldosteronism due to volume depletion. Poorly controlled diabetes commonly increases urinary potassium excretion, because it leads to an osmotic diuresis with a high urinary flow rate and high distal delivery of sodium.

Reabsorption of sodium in the collecting duct occurs through selective sodium channels, creating an electronegative charge within the tubular lumen relative to the tubular epithelial cell, which in turn promotes secretion of cations $(K^+$ and $H^+)$ into the lumen. Therefore, drugs that block the sodium channel in the collecting duct decrease potassium secretion. Conversely, in Liddle's syndrome, a rare genetic disorder, this sodium channel is constitutively open, resulting in avid sodium reabsorption and excessive potassium secretion.

Adaptation in Renal Failure

In patients with renal failure, the kidney compensates by increasing the efficiency of potassium excretion. Clearly, there is a limit to renal compensation, and a significant loss of kidney function impairs the ability to excrete potassium, thereby predisposing to a positive potassium balance and a tendency to hyperkalemia. In most patients with chronic renal failure, overt hyperkalemia does not occur until the creatinine clearance falls below 10 mL/min. Serum aldosterone levels are elevated in many patients with chronic renal failure. Aldosterone stimulates the activity of both Na,K-ATPase and H,K-ATPase, thereby promoting secretion of potassium in the collecting duct and defending against hyperkalemia. These adaptive mechanisms are less effective in patients with acute renal failure, as compared with chronic renal failure. Therefore, severe hyperkalemia occurs more frequently in the former group.

A subset of patients with chronic renal failure fail to increase aldosterone levels appreciably; as a result, they develop hyperkalemia at moderate levels of renal insufficiency (CrCl < 50 mL/min), typically in association with hyperchloremic, normal anion gap metabolic acidosis. This condition termed type IV renal tubular acidosis, is most commonly associated with diabetic nephropathy and chronic interstitial nephritis. Moreover, administration of drugs that inhibit aldosterone production or secretion (e.g., ACE inhibitors, angiotensin II antagonists, NSAIDs, heparin) may provoke hyperkalemia in patients with mild to moderate chronic renal failure.

Intestinal Potassium Excretion

Like the renal collecting duct, the small intestine and colon secrete potassium. Aldosterone stimulates potassium excretion by the gut. In normal individuals, intestinal potassium excretion plays a minor role in potassium homeostasis. However, in patients with significant renal failure, intestinal potassium secretion is increased three- to fourfold, thereby contributing significantly to potassium homeostasis. This adaptation is limited, and is inadequate to compensate for the loss of excretory function in patients with advanced renal failure.

Internal Potassium Balance

Overview

Extracellular fluid [K] is ~4 mEq/L, whereas the intracellular [K] is ~150 mEq/L. Because of the uneven distribution of potassium between the fluid compartments, a relatively small net shift of potassium from the intracellular to the extracellular fluid compartment produces marked increases in plasma potassium. Conversely, a relatively small net shift from the extracellular to the intracellular fluid compartment produces a marked decrease in plasma potassium. Unlike renal excretion of potassium, which requires several hours, potassium shift between the extracellular and intracellular fluid compartment (also referred to as extrarenal potassium disposal) is extremely rapid, occurring within minutes.

Clearly, in patients with advanced renal failure, whose capacity to excrete potassium is marginal, extrarenal potassium disposal plays a critical role in the prevention of life-threatening hyperkalemia following potassium-rich meals. The following example will illustrate this important principle. Suppose that a 70-kg dialysis patient with a serum potassium of 4.5 mmol/L eats one cup of pinto beans (~35 mmol potassium). Initially, the dietary potassium is absorbed into the extracellular fluid compartment ($0.2 \times 70 = 14$ L). This amount of dietary potassium will increase the serum potassium by 2.5 mmol/L (35 mmol/14 L). In the absence of extrarenal potassium disposal, the patient's serum potassium would rise acutely to 7.0 mmol/

L, a level frequently associated with serious ventricular arrhythmias. In practice, the increase in serum potassium is much smaller, due to efficient physiologic mechanisms that promote potassium shifts into the intracellular fluid compartment.

Effects of Insulin and Catecholamines on Extrarenal Potassium Disposal

The two major physiologic factors that stimulate transfer of potassium from the extracellular to the intracellular fluid compartments are insulin and epinephrine. The stimulation of extrarenal potassium disposal by insulin and β_2-adrenergic agonists are both mediated by stimulation of the Na,K-ATPase activity, primarily in skeletal muscle cells. Interference with these two physiologic mechanisms (insulin deficiency or β_2-adrenergic blockade, respectively) predisposes to hyperkalemia. On the other hand, excessive insulin or epinephrine levels predispose to hypokalemia.

The potassium-lowering effect of insulin is dose related within the physiologic range of plasma insulin and is independent of its effect on plasma glucose. Even the low physiologic levels of insulin present during fasting promote extrarenal potassium disposal. In nondiabetic individuals hyperglycemia stimulates endogenous insulin secretion, thereby decreasing the serum potassium. In insulin-dependent diabetics, endogenous insulin production is limited, and significant hyperglycemia may occur. Hyperglycemia results in plasma hypertonicity, which promotes potassium shifts out of the cells, and produces paradoxic hyperkalemia.

The potassium-lowering action of epinephrine is mediated by β_2-adrenergic stimulation and is blocked by nonselective β-blockers, but not by selective β_1-adrenergic blockers. α-Adrenergic stimulation promotes shifts of potassium out of the cells into the extracellular fluid compartment, tending to increase serum potassium. Epinephrine is a mixed α- and β-adrenergic agonist, such that its net effect on serum potassium reflects the balance between its β-adrenergic (potassium-lowering) and α-adrenergic (potassium-raising) effects. In normal individuals the β-adrenergic effect of epinephrine predominates over the α-adrenergic effect, such that the serum potassium decreases. In contrast, the α-adrenergic effect of epinephrine on potassium shifts is much more prominent in patients with severe renal failure; as a result, dialysis patients are refractory to the potassium-lowering effect of epinephrine.

Effect of Acid–Base Disorders on Extrarenal Potassium Disposal

As a general rule, metabolic alkalosis shifts potassium into the cells, whereas metabolic acidosis shifts potassium out of the cells. However, the nature of the metabolic acidosis determines its effect on serum potassium. Thus, mineral acidosis (i.e., hyperchloremic, normal anion gap metabolic acidosis) typically shifts potassium out of the cells, thereby predisposing to hyperkalemia. In contrast, organic metabolic acidosis (e.g., lactic acidosis) does not affect the serum potassium. Bicarbonate administration to individuals with normal renal function decreases serum potassium, but this effect is mainly due to enhanced urinary excretion of potassium. In contrast, bicarbonate administration to dialysis patients (in whom the capacity for urinary potassium excretion is negligible) does not lower plasma potassium acutely. Moreover, bicarbonate administration does not potentiate the potassium-lowering effects of insulin or albuterol in dialysis patients.

LABORATORY TESTS FOR DIFFERENTIAL DIAGNOSIS OF POTASSIUM DISORDERS

Differential Diagnosis of Hypokalemia and Hyperkalemia

The clinical history, review of medications, family history, and physical examination are sufficient in the rapid differential diagnosis of the etiology of most potassium disorders. In selected patients the etiology of hypokalemia or hyperkalemia is not apparent, and additional specialized laboratory tests may be useful. Measurements of the fractional excretion of potassium (FE_K) and transtubular potassium gradient (TTKG) may be useful in distinguishing between renal and nonrenal etiologies of hyperkalemia and hypokalemia. The general principle underlying these tests is that the kidney compensates for hyperkalemia by increasing potassium excretion, and compensates for hypokalemia by decreasing potassium excretion. When the serum potassium valve is abnormal and potassium excretion has not compensated appropriately, a renal etiology for the serum potassium abnormality is suggested. The optimal use of FE_K or TTKG is the differential diagnosis requires that these values be obtained before the potassium abnormality (hyperkalemia or hypokalemia) is corrected.

Fractional Excretion of Potassium

FE_K is the percentage of potassium filtered into the proximal tubule that appears in the urine. It represents potassium clearance corrected for glomerular filtration rate (GFR) or $\mathbf{Cl_K/Cl_{CR}}$. Since the clearance of any substance can be calculated from UV/P, this ratio (in bold type) can be algebraically transformed to $[(U_K V/P_K)/U_{CR} V/P_{CR})] \times 100\%$. The V in the numerator and denominator cancel out, giving the simplified formula

$$\frac{[U_K/S_K] \times 100\%}{[U_{CR}/S_{CR}]},$$

where U_K and U_{CR} are the concentrations of potassium and creatinine in the urine, and S_K and S_{CR} are the corresponding serum concentrations. For an individual with normal renal function on an average dietary potassium intake, the FE_K is approximately 10%. When hypokalemia is due to extrarenal causes (low potassium diet, GI losses, potassium shifts into cells) the kidney conserves potassium, and the FE_K is low. In contrast, hypokalemia due to renal potassium losses is associated with an increased FE_K. Similarly, in the setting of hyperkalemia, a high FE_K is consistent with appropriate renal compensation and suggests an extrarenal etiology, whereas a low FE_K suggests a renal etiology. If a urine creatinine measurement is not available, one can

often use U_K alone to differentiate between renal and extrarenal causes. Specifically, in a hypokalemic patient, $U_K > 20\,mEq/L$ suggests a renal etiology, whereas $U_K < 20\,mEq/L$ suggests an extrarenal etiology.

Transtubular Potassium Gradient

The TTKG is a formula that estimates the potassium gradient between the urine and the blood in the distal nephron. It is calculated from $[U_K/(U_{osm}/P_{osm})]/P_K$, where U_{osm} and P_{osm} are the urine and plasma osmolalities. The numerator is an estimate of the luminal potassium concentration. The U_{osm}/P_{osm} term is included to correct for the rise in U_K that is due purely to water abstraction and concentration of the urine overall. TTKG values have been derived from empiric measurements in normal individuals under a variety of physiologic conditions. In a normal individual under normal circumstances, the TTKG is about 6 to 8. Hypokalemia with a high TTKG suggests excessive renal potassium losses, whereas hypokalemia with a low TTKG suggests an extrarenal etiology. Similarly, hyperkalemia with a low TTKG suggests a renal etiology, whereas hyperkalemia with a high TTKG is consistent with an extrarenal etiology.

Several factors limit the utility of the FE_K and TTKG in the differential diagnosis of potassium disorders. The FE_K and TTKG are increased when dietary potassium is increased, and decreased when dietary potassium is decreased. Furthermore, in patients with chronic renal failure there is an adaptive increase in potassium excretion per functioning nephron, such that FE_K and TTKG increase. This means that the "normal" value for a given individual can vary substantially, making it difficult to determine the significance of a high or low FE_K or TTKG.

HYPOKALEMIA

Hypokalemia vs Potassium Deficiency

It is important to distinguish between potassium deficiency and hypokalemia. Potassium deficiency is the state resulting from a persistent negative potassium balance, i.e., potassium excretion exceeding potassium intake. Hypokalemia refers to a low plasma potassium concentration. Hypokalemia can be due either to potassium deficiency (inadequate potassium intake or excessive potassium losses) or to net potassium shifts from the extracellular to the intracellular fluid compartment. A patient may have severe potassium depletion without manifesting hypokalemia. An important example is a patient presenting with diabetic ketoacidosis. Due to hyperglycemia, such patients have typically undergone an osmotic diuresis for several days, leading to a high rate of renal potassium excretion and potassium deficiency. However, as a result of insulin deficiency, there is a concomitant shift of potassium out of the cells into the extracellular fluid compartment. At presentation to the hospital, such patients are frequently normokalemic or even hyperkalemic. Once they are treated with exogenous insulin, there is a rapid shift of potassium back into the cells, and within a few hours the patients develop significant hypokalemia. Conversely, patients hospitalized with an acute myocardial infarction commonly have hypokalemia due to stress-induced catecholamine release and enhanced extrarenal potassium disposal, even though they may have a normal external potassium balance.

Clinical Disorders Associated with Hypokalemia

Table 1 lists the most common causes of hypokalemia. The kidney can avidly conserve potassium, such that hypokalemia due to inadequate potassium intake is a rare event requiring prolonged starvation ("tea and toast diet"). Therefore, hypokalemia is usually due to excessive potassium losses from the gut or the urine or due to potassium shifts from the extracellular to the intracellular fluid compartments. Prolonged vomiting causes potassium losses, in small part due to potassium present in the gastric juice (~10 mEq/L), but mainly from renal losses due to secondary aldosteronism resulting from volume depletion. Severe diarrhea, either due to disease or laxative abuse, results in significant potassium excretion in the stool.

Excessive renal potassium losses as a cause of hypokalemia occur in a number of clinical syndromes. Conceptually, it is useful to consider separately hypokalemia associated with hypertension and hypokalemia associated with a normal blood pressure. When hypokalemia is associated with hypertension, measurements of plasma renin and aldosterone may be helpful in the differential diagnosis. Several physiologic observations are relevant:

1. Aldosterone, a mineralocorticoid, stimulates sodium reabsorption and potassium secretion in the collecting duct.
2. The physiologic stimulus for aldosterone secretion is activation of the renin-angiotensin axis. Moreover, aldosterone-induced sodium retention suppresses the renin-angiotensin axis by negative feedback.
3. Glucocorticoids at high concentrations bind to mineralocorticoid receptors and mimic their physiologic actions.
4. Glucocorticoids are stimulated by adrenocorticotropic hormone (ACTH), and suppress ACTH production by negative feedback.

Primary aldosternonism is due to autonomous (nonrenin-mediated) secretion of aldosterone by the adrenal cortex. This results in avid sodium retention and potassium secretion by the distal nephron. The patients present with volume-dependent hypertension, hypokalemia, and metabolic alkalosis. Biochemical evaluation reveals a high and nonsuppressable serum aldosterone level with a low plasma renin. Abdominal CT scan reveals either a unilateral adrenal adenoma or bilateral adrenal hyperplasia. The former is treated surgically, and the latter with spironolactone. Glucocorticoid-remediable aldosteronism (GRA) is a rare, autosomal dominant condition in which there is fusion of the 11β-hydroxylase and aldosterone synthase genes. As a result, aldosterone secretion is stimulated by ACTH, and can be suppressed by an exogenous mineralocorticoid, dexamethasone. Patients with GRA have a very similar clinical presentation to those with primary aldosteronism (volume-dependent hypertension, hypokalemia, high serum aldosterone, and low serum renin), except that they are younger and have a family history of hypertension.

Patients with renovascular hypertension, renin-secreting tumors, and severe malignant hypertension may also present with severe hypertension and hypokalemia. In contrast to patients with primary aldosteronism, these patients have secondary aldosteronism, i.e., high serum renin and aldosterone levels. Of course, patients with essential hypertension may also have hypokalemia and high plasma renin and aldosterone levels if they are treated with loop or thiazide diuretics and are volume depleted.

Patients with 11β-hydroxysteroid dehydrogenase deficiency, a rare genetic disorder, have a defect in the conversion of cortisol to cortisone in the peripheral tissues. This results in high tissue cortisol levels that activate the mineralocorticoid receptors, producing hypokalemia and hypertension. Such patients have low serum renin and aldosterone levels. Chewing tobacco, certain brands of licorice, and some French red wines contain glycyrrhizic acid, which inhibits 11β-hydroxysteroid dehydrogenase. Ingestion of these foods may produce hypokalemia, volume-dependent

TABLE I
Causes of Hypokalemia

Inadequate potassium intake (severe malnutrition)

Extrarenal potassium losses
  Vomiting
  Diarrhea

Hypokalemia due to urinary potassium losses
  Diuretics (loop, thiazides, acetazolamide)
  Osmotic diuresis (e.g., hyperglycemia)
  Hypokalemia with hypertension
    Primary aldosteronism
    Glucocorticoid remediable hypertension
    Malignant hypertension
    Renovascular hypertension
    Renin-secreting tumor
    Essential hypertension with excessive diuretics
    Liddle's syndrome
    11β-hydroxysteroid dehydrogenase deficiency
      Genetic
      Drug-induced (chewing tobacco, licorice, some French wines)
    Congenital adrenal hyperplasia
  Hypokalemia with a normal blood pressure
    Distal RTA (type I)[a]
    Proximal RTA (type II)
    Bartter's syndrome
    Gitelman's syndrome
    Hypomagnesemia (cisplatinum, alcoholism, diuretics)

Hypokalemia due to potassium shifts
  Insulin administration
  Catecholamine excess (acute stress)
  Familial periodic hypokalemic paralysis
  Thyrotoxic hypokalemic paralysis

[a] RTA, renal tubular acidosis.

hypertension, and low serum renin and aldosterone levels, similar to the clinical presentation of congenital 11β-hydroxysteroid dehydrogenase deficiency.

Patients with congenital adrenal hyperplasia have a deficiency of 11β-hydroxylasse, an enzyme required in the common pathways for mineralocorticoids and glucocorticoids. These patients have low serum renin and aldosterone levels, high levels of DOCA (a mineralocorticoid), and high levels of androgen. Males have early puberty, and females exhibit virilization, with hirsutism and clitoromegaly. This condition improves with exogenous corticosteroids to suppress ACTH.

Liddle's syndrome is a rare autosomal dominent disorder caused by a defect of the collecting duct sodium channel. It is constitutively open, resulting in an unregulated increase of sodium absorption and potassium secretion at that site. Patients present with hypokalemia, hypertension, and volume overload. Their biochemical profile reveals a low serum renin and aldosterone. The patients' blood pressure and serum potassium improves dramatically with inhibitors of the sodium channel, such as amiloride.

Hypokalemia due to excessive renal potassium excretion is also seen in a number of clinical conditions in which hypertension is infrequent. Both type I (distal) and type II (proximal) renal tubular acidosis (RTA) are associated with kaliuresis and hypokalemia; both conditions present with a normal anion gap metabolic acidosis. Type I RTA is frequently associated with hypercalciuria and calcium oxalate kidney stones. Type II RTA is rare in adults, and is often associated with a generalized defect in proximal tubular function, manifesting as glycosuria (with a normal serum glucose), hypophosphatemia with phosphaturia, and a low serum uric acid with uricosuria (see Chapter 9).

Bartter's syndrome is a rare familial disease characterized by hypokalemia, metabolic alkalosis, hypercalciuria, normal blood pressure, and high plasma renin and aldosterone levels. Recently, it has been associated with a mutation in the renal Na-K-2Cl transporter, which is responsible for active sodium reabsorption in the thick ascending limb of Henle. These patients act as if they are chronically ingesting loop diuretics; for this reason, they are difficult to distinguish clinically from patients with surreptitious diuretic ingestion. Patients with Gitelman's syndrome, a variant of Bartter's syndrome, differ in that they have hypocalciuria and hypomagnesemia. Recently, Gitelman's syndrome has been linked to a mutation in the renal thiazide-sensitive Na^+-Cl^- transporter. These patients act as if they are chronically ingesting thiazide diuretics.

Familial hypokalemic periodic paralysis is a rare, autosomal dominant disorder in which affected individuals develop periodic episodes of severe muscle weakness in association with profound hypokalemia, due to rapid shifts of potassium from the extracellular to the intracellular fluid compartment. Interestingly, even when patients have complete paralysis, the diaphragm and bulbar muscles are spared, such that the patient is able to breathe, swallow, talk, and blink. The paralysis resolves within hours of potassium ingestion. The patients are asymptomatic and have a normal serum potassium between the acute episodes.

Thyrotoxic hypokalemic paralysis is an unusual manifestation of hyperthyroidism, seen primarily in Asian patients. The clinical presentation is similar to that of hypokalemic periodic paralysis, except that the paralytic episodes cease when the hyperthyroidism is corrected.

Drug-Induced Hypokalemia

A number of drugs have the potential to cause hypokalemia—either by stimulating renal potassium excretion or by blocking extrarenal disposal. Exogenous mineralocorticoids mimic the effects of aldosterone, thereby stimulating distal potassium secretion. Glucocorticoids possess some mineralocorticoid activity; treatment with high doses of these agents has a similar effect. Most diuretics, including loop diuretics, thiazide diuretics, and acetazolamide increase renal potassium excretion. A number of drugs, including alcohol, diuretics, and cisplatinum, cause renal magnesium-wasting and hypomagnesemia. For reasons that are not well understood, hypomagnesemia impairs renal potassium conservation. Thus, these patients may have associated hypokalemia that is refractory to potassium supplementation until the magnesium deficit is corrected. (Paradoxically, cyclosporine may produce hypomagnesemia in conjunction with *hyper*kalemia.)

Drugs that promote extrarenal potassium disposal may also result in hypokalemia. This phenomenon can be seen after the administration of an acute dose of insulin. Similarly, $β_2$-agonists (either intravenous or nebulized), including albuterol and terbutaline, frequently result in acute hypokalemia.

Clinical Manifestations of Hypokalemia

Hypokalemia may produce electrocardiographic abnormalities, including a flattened T wave and a U wave (Fig. 1). Hypokalemia also increases the risk of ventricular arrhythmias in patients with ischemic heart disease or patients taking digoxin. Severe hypokalemia is associated with variable degrees of skeletal muscle weakness, even to the point of paralysis. On rare occasions, diaphragmatic paralysis from hypokalemia can lead to respiratory arrest. There may also be decreased motility of smooth muscle, manifesting itself as ileus or urinary retention. Rarely, severe hypokalemia may result in rhabdomyolysis.

Severe hypokalemia also interferes with the urinary concentrating mechanism in the distal nephron, and leads to nephrogenic diabetes insipidus. Such patients have a low urine osmolality in the face of high serum osmolality, and are refractory to vasopressin.

Treatment of Hypokalemia

The acute treatment of hypokalemia requires potassium supplementation, which can be given either intravenously or orally. The correlation between serum potassium and total potassium deficit in hypokalemia patients is quite poor. A given patient's serum potassium is a reflection of both external potassium balance and transcellular potassium shifts. The fraction of administered exogenous potas-

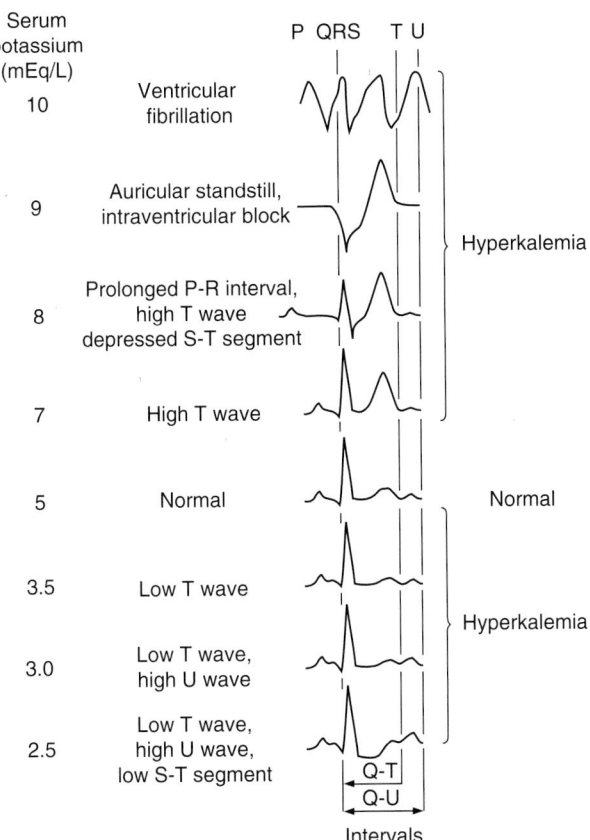

Serum
potassium
(mEq/L)

P QRS T U

10	Ventricular fibrillation	
9	Auricular standstill, intraventricular block	Hyperkalemia
8	Prolonged P-R interval, high T wave depressed S-T segment	
7	High T wave	
5	Normal	Normal
3.5	Low T wave	
3.0	Low T wave, high U wave	Hyperkalemia
2.5	Low T wave, high U wave, low S-T segment	

Q-T
Q-U
Intervals

FIGURE I   A schematic representation of EKG changes and the serum potassium levels at which such changes are typically seen. From Seldin DW, Giebisch G, eds: *The Regulation of Potassium Balance,* Raven Press, New York, 1989.

sium that remains in the extracellular fluid compartment is variable. Thus, it is difficult to predict how much potassium replacement a given hypokalemic patient will require. Without adequate monitoring, it is possible to give too much potassium, making the patient hyperkalemic. Therefore, one should give repeated small doses of potassium, with frequent checks of the serum potassium value.

Oral potassium administration is safer than the intravenous route, and is less likely to produce an overshoot in the serum potassium. Each oral dose should not exceed 20 to 40 mEq of potassium. Intravenous KCl should be reserved for severe, symptomatic hypokalemia (<3.0 mEq/ L) or for patients who cannot ingest oral potassium. Intravenous KCl should not be given any faster than 10 mmol/ h in the absence of continuous EKG monitoring. The serum potassium should be rechecked every 2 to 3 hours to confirm a clinical response and to avoid an overshoot.

Correction of the underlying medical condition may prevent recurrence of hypokalemia after its correction. If the patient has a chronic condition associated with persistent urinary potassium losses, such that hypokalemia is likely to recur, the patient should be encouraged to increase the intake of foods high in potassium (especially fresh fruits,

nuts, and legumes; see Table 2). In some patients, chronic oral potassium supplementation is necessary.

HYPERKALEMIA

Pseudohyperkalemia is a factitious elevation of the serum potassium due to in vitro release of potassium from blood cells. It may be seen with in vitro hemolysis, thrombocytosis, or severe leukocytosis. Pseudohyperkalemia due to hemolysis is readily apparent because the serum is pink. Pseudohyperkalemia due to severe thrombocytosis or leukocytosis can be confirmed by drawing simultaneous blood samples in tubes with and without anticoagulant; if the serum potassium is significantly higher than the plasma potassium, this confirms the diagnosis.

True hyperkalemia is caused by a positive potassium balance (increased potassium intake or decreased potassium excretion) or an increase in net potassium shift from the intracellular to the extracellular fluid compartment. Table 3 provides a list of the most common causes of hyperkalemia. In practice, most patients who develop severe hyperkalemia have more than one contributory factors. For example, a patient with moderate renal failure due to diabetic nephropathy may be medicated with an ACE inhibitor and have mild hyperkalemia. However, when started on indomethacin for acute gouty arthritis, the patient rapidly develops severe hyperkalemia.

Drug-Induced Hyperkalemia

Many drugs have the potential to cause hyperkalemia—either by inhibiting renal potassium excretion or by blocking extrarenal disposal (Table 4). Most individuals taking these drugs will not develop hyperkalemia. Patients at greatest risk are those with renal failure, especially if they have a high dietary potassium intake or are on an additional medication that predisposes to hyperkalemia. Most diuretics (loop diuretics, thiazide diuretics, acetazolamide) increase urinary potassium excretion and tend to cause hypokalemia. However, potassium-sparing diuretics inhibit urinary potassium excretion and predispose to hyperkalemia by one or two mechanisms. Spironolactone is a competitive inhibitor of aldosterone; it binds to the aldoster-

TABLE 2
Potassium Content of Selected Foods

Food	Potassium (mg)	Potassium (mEq)
Pinto beans (1 cup)	1370	35
Raisins (1 cup)	1106	28
Honeydew (½ melon)	939	24
Nuts (1 cup)	688	18
Blackeyed peas (1 cup)	625	16
Collard greens (1 cup)	498	13
Banana (1 medium)	440	11
Tomato (1 medium)	366	9
Orange (1 large)	333	9
Milk (1 cup)	351	9
Potato chips (10)	226	6

TABLE 3
Causes of Hyperkalemia

Pseudohyperkalemia
    Hemolysis
    Thrombocytosis
    Severe leukocytosis
    Fist clenching
Decreased renal excretion
    Acute or chronic renal failure
    Aldosterone deficiency (e.g., type IV renal tubular acidosis)
      Frequently associated with diabetic nephropathy, chronic
        interstitial nephritis, or obstructive nephropathy
    Adrenal insufficiency (Addison's disease)
    Drugs that inhibit potassium excretion (see Table 3)
    Kidney diseases that impair distal tubule function
      Sickle cell anemia
      Systemic lupus erythematosus
Abnormal potassium distribution
    Insulin deficiency
    β-blockers
    Metabolic or respiratory acidosis
    Familial hyperkalemic periodic paralysis
Abnormal potassium release from cells
    Rhabdomyolysis
    Tumor lysis syndrome

TABLE 4
Mechanisms for Drug-induced Hyperkalemia

Decrease renal potassium excretion
Block sodium channel in the distal nephron
    Potassium-sparing diuretics: amiloride, triamterene
    Antibiotics: trimethoprim, pentamidine
Block aldosterone production
    ACE inhibitors (e.g., captopril, enalapril, lisinopril,
      benazepril)
    Angiotensin II antagonists (e.g., losartan)
    NSAIDs
    Heparin
    Tacrolimus
Block aldosterone receptors
    Spironolactone
Block Na,K-ATPase activity in the distal nephron
    Cyclosporine
Inhibit extrarenal potassium disposal
    Block β_2-adrenergic mediated extrarenal potassium
      disposal—nonselective β-blockers (e.g., propranolol,
      nadolol, timolol)
    Block Na,K-ATPase activity in skeletal muscles; digoxin
      overdose (not therapeutic doses)
    Inhibit insulin release (e.g., somatostatin)
Potassium release from injured cells
    Drug-induced rhabdomyolysis (e.g., lovastatin, cocaine)
    Drug-induced tumor lysis syndrome (chemotherapy agents in
      acute leukemias, high-grade lymphomas)
Drug-induced acute renal failure

one receptors in the collecting duct, thereby inhibiting Na,K-ATPase activity, and indirectly limiting potassium secretion. Interestingly, the immunosuppressive drug cyclosporine also blocks Na,K-ATPase activity in the distal nephron. Two other potassium-sparing diuretics, amiloride and triamterene, bind to the sodium channel in the collecting duct. Blocking this channel inhibits sodium reabsorption in the distal nephron, thereby limiting the establishment of the electrochemical gradient required for potassium secretion. Two antibiotics, trimethoprim (one of the components of Bactrim) and pentamidine, have also been shown to block the sodium channel in the collecting duct and to predispose patients to hyperkalemia. In addition, trimethoprim has been shown to inhibit the collecting tubule H,K-ATPase.

Because aldosterone plays an important role in enhancing renal potassium excretion in patients with renal failure, drugs that inhibit aldosterone production (either directly or indirectly) predispose such patients to hyperkalemia. Angiotensin II is a potent stimulator of aldosterone production in the adrenal cortex. ACE inhibitors inhibit the production of angiotensin II, thereby decreasing aldosterone levels. Similarly, angiotensin II receptor blockers, such as losartan, also inhibit aldosterone production. Prostaglandin inhibitors (NSAIDs) inhibit the production of renin, thereby indirectly decreasing aldosterone production. This effect is seen even with "renal-sparing NSAIDs," such as sulindac. Heparin has been shown to inhibit the production of aldosterone in the renal cortex directly, primarily by decreasing the number and affinity of angiotensin II receptors in the zona glomerulosa. This effect occurs even with the low doses of subcutaneous heparin used for prophylaxis of venous thrombosis in hospitalized patients. The immu-

nosuppressive drug tacrolimus may also cause hyperkalemia by inhibiting aldosterone synthesis.

Given the stimulation of extrarenal potassium disposal by β-adrenergic agonists, it is not surprising that β_2-antagonists can predispose to hyperkalemia. This effect is seen primarily with nonselective β-blockers (e.g., propranolol and nadolol), rather than with selective β_1-blockers. There is significant systemic absorption of topical β-blockers, and severe hyperkalemia may rarely be provoked by timolol eyedrops. Drugs inhibiting endogenous insulin release, such as somatostatin, have rarely been implicated as a cause of hyperkalemia in patients with renal failure. Presumably, long-acting somatostatin analogs, such as octreotide, would have a similar effect on serum potassium. Digoxin overdose causes inhibition of Na,K-ATPase activity in skeletal muscle cells, and may manifest with hyperkalemia. This effect is rarely seen at therapeutic doses of the drug.

Finally, drugs can cause hyperkalemia indirectly by causing release of intracellular potassium from injured cells (e.g., rhabdomyolysis with lovastatin and cocaine, or tumor lysis syndrome occurring spontaneously or when chemotherapy is administered to patients with acute leukemia or high grade lymphoma). Moreover, drug-induced acute renal failure may be associated with secondary hyperkalemia.

Clinical Manifestations of Hyperkalemia

Hyperkalemia may produce progressive electrocardiographic abnormalities, including peaked T waves, flattening or absence of P waves, widened QRS complexes, and sine waves (see Fig. 1). The major risk of severe hyperkalemia is the development of life-threatening ventricular arrhythmias. Severe hyperkalemia with EKG changes is a medical emergency.

Severe hyperkalemia, like severe hypokalemia, can cause skeletal muscle weakness, even to the point of paralysis and respiratory failure. Hyperkalemia impairs urinary acidification by decreasing collecting tubule apical H,K-ATPase, which may result in a renal tubular acidosis (type IV RTA). Hyperkalemia stimulates endogenous aldosterone secretion.

Treatment of Hyperkalemia

Severe hyperkalemia associated with electrocardiographic changes (see Fig. 1) is a life-threatening state requiring emergent intervention. If the patient's EKG is suspicious for hyperkalemia, one should initiate therapy without waiting for the laboratory confirmation. If the patient has renal failure, urgent dialysis is required for removal of potassium from the body. Because of the inevitable delay in initiating dialysis, the following temporizing measures must be initiated promptly.

1. Stabilize the myocardium. Acute administration of intravenous calcium gluconate does not change plasma potassium, but does transiently improve the EKG. The effect is almost immediate. Give 10 mL of calcium gluconate over 1 minute. If there is no improvement in the EKG appearance within 3 to 5 minutes, the dose should be repeated.
2. Shift potassium from the extracellular to the intracellular fluid, in order to rapidly decrease the serum potassium. This involves administration of insulin and a β_2-agonist.
   a. Intravenous insulin is the fastest way to lower the serum potassium. The plasma potassium starts to decrease within 15 minutes. Intravenous glucose is given concurrently to prevent hypoglycemia. Give 10 units of regular insulin and 50 mL of 50% dextrose (1 ampule of D_{50}) as a bolus, followed by a continuous infusion of 5% dextrose at 100 mL/h to prevent late hypoglycemia. Never give dextrose without insulin for the acute treatment of hyperkalemia; in patients with inadequate endogenous insulin production, the resulting hyperglycemia can produce a paradoxical increase in serum potassium.
   b. Beta-agonists. Give 20 mg of albuterol (a β_2-agonist) by inhalation over 10 minutes. The onset of action is 30 minutes. Use the concentrated form (5 mg/mL) of the drug to minimize the volume that needs to be inhaled. The dose required to lower plasma potassium is considerably higher than that used to treat asthma, because only a small fraction of nebulized albuterol is absorbed systemically. Thus, 0.5 mg of intravenous albuterol (not available in the US) produces a comparable change in plasma potassium to that seen after 20 mg of nebulized albuterol. The potassium-lowering effect of albuterol is additive to that of insulin.
   c. Sodium bicarbonate. This is NOT useful acutely, because it takes 3 to 4 hours for an effect on serum potassium to start. Moreover, bicarbonate administration is still indicated if the patient has severe metabolic acidosis (serum bicarbonate <10 mmol/L).
3. Once the previous temporizing measures have been performed, further interventions are done to remove potassium from the body.
   a. Diuretics. These only work if the patient has adequate kidney function.
   b. Kayexalate. This resin-exchanger removes potassium from the blood via the gut, in exchange for an equal amount of sodium. It is relatively slow-acting, requiring 1 to 2 hours before plasma potassium decreases. Each gram of resin removes 0.5 to 1.0 mmol of potassium. Give 50 g in 30 mL sorbitol by mouth or 50 g in a retention enema. The rectal route is faster and more reliable.
   c. Hemodialysis. This is the definitive treatment for patients with advanced renal failure and severe hyperkalemia.

For patients with moderate hyperkalemia, not associated with electrocardiographic changes, it is frequently sufficient to provide one or two doses of exchange resin, and to discontinue the drugs predisposing to hyperkalemia.

To prevent a recurrence of hyperkalemia once the acute treatment has been provided, the following measures are useful:

1. Counsel the patient on dietary potassium restriction, 40 to 60 mEq/day (Table 2).
2. Avoid medications that interfere with renal excretion of potassium, e.g., potassium-sparing diuretics, NSAIDs, and ACE inhibitors.
3. Avoid drugs that interfere with potassium shifts from the extracellular to the intracellular compartment, e.g., β-blockers.
4. In selected patients, chronic medication with loop diuretics can be used to stimulate urinary potassium excretion.
5. Specific therapy may be indicated for the underlying etiology, when available. For example, patients with adrenal insufficiency require replacement with exogenous glucocorticoids and mineralocorticoids. In patients with hyperkalemic periodic paralysis (a rare, autosomal dominant disorder in which affected individuals develop periodic episodes of severe muscle weakness in association with profound hyperkalemia), prophylactic aerosolized albuterol can prevent both exercise-induced hyperkalemia and muscle weakness.

Bibliography

Allon M: Hyperkalemia in end-stage renal disease: mechanisms and management. *J Am Soc Nephrol* 6:1134–1142, 1995.
Allon M: Treatment and prevention of hyperkalemia in end-stage renal disease. *Kidney Int* 43:1197–1209, 1993.

DuBose TD: Hyperkalemic hyperchloremic metabolic acidosis: Pathophysiologic insights. *Kidney Int* 51:591–602, 1997.

Ethier JH, Kamel KS, Magner PO, Lemann J, Halperin ML: The transtubular potassium concentration in patients with hyperkalemia and hypokalemia. *Am J Kidney Dis* 15:309–315, 1990.

Farese RV, Biglieri EG, Shackleton CHL, Irony I, Gomez-Fontes R: Licorice-induced hypermineralocorticoidism. *N Engl J Med* 325:1223–1227, 1991.

Field MJ, Giebisch GJ: Hormonal control of renal potassium excretion. *Kidney Int* 27:379–387, 1985.

Kamel KS, Halperin ML, Faber MD, Steigerwalt SP, Heilig CW, Narins RG: Disorders of potassium balance. In: Brenner BM (ed) *The Kidney.* Saunders, Philadelphia, pp. 999–1037, 1996.

Krishna GG, Steigerwalt SP, Pikus R, et al: Hypokalemic states. In: Narins RG (ed) *Clinical Disorders of Fluid and Electrolyte Metabolism.* McGraw-Hill, New York, pp. 659–696, 1994.

Lifton RP, Dluhy RG, Powers M, et al: A chimaeric 11 beta-hydroxylase/aldosterone synthase gene causes glucocorticoid-remediable aldosteronism and human hypertension. *Nature* 355:262–265, 1992.

Salem MM, Rosa RM, Batlle DC: Extrarenal potassium tolerance in chronic renal failure: implications for the treatment of acute hyperkalemia. *Am J Kidney Dis* 18:421–440, 1991.

Shimkets RA, Warnock DG, Bositis CM, et al: Liddle's syndrome: Heritable human hypertension caused by mutations in the beta subunit of the epithelial sodium channel. *Cell* 79:407–414, 1994.

Simon DB, Nelson-Williams C, Bia MJ, et al: Gitelman's variant of Bartter's syndrome, inherited hypokalaemic alkalosis, is caused by mutations in the thiazide-sensitive Na-Cl cotransporter. *Nature Genet* 12:24–30, 1996.

Simon DB, Karet FE, Hamdan JM, et al: Bartter's syndrome, hypokalaemic alkalosis with hypercalciuria, is caused by mutations in the Na-K-2Cl cotransporter NKCC2. *Nature Genet* 13:183–188, 1996.

Tannen RL: Approach to the patient with altered potassium concentration. In: Kelley WN (ed) *Textbook of Internal Medicine.* Lippincott, Philadelphia, pp. 848–855, 1992.

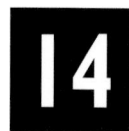

DISORDERS OF CALCIUM AND PHOSPHORUS HOMEOSTASIS

DAVID A. BUSHINSKY

CALCIUM

Calcium Homeostasis

Distribution

The vast majority (99.5%) of total body calcium is contained within the bone mineral while only about 0.1% of body calcium is in the extracellular fluid. The mineral phases of bone provide a reservoir of calcium for the smaller extra- and intracellular pools.

The concentration of calcium in the cell cytosol is approximately 100 nmol/L or approximately one-thousandth of the extracellular calcium concentration. Within the cell, the mitochondria and the sarcoplasmic and endoplasmic reticula contain the highest concentrations of calcium.

Serum Concentration

In humans the concentration of serum calcium is maintained at a constant level between 9.0 and 10.4 mg/dL or 2.25 to 2.60 mmol/L. Of the total serum calcium approximately 40% is protein bound, especially to albumin and to a lesser extent globulins and other proteins. Approximately 10% of the calcium is complexed to phosphate, citrate, carbonate, and other anions; the remaining 50% exists in the ionized form. The ionized calcium and the complexed calcium constitute what is filtered by the kidney, the ultrafiltrable calcium, which has a concentration of approximately 1.5 mmol/L.

The concentration of ionized calcium is of physiological importance and remains remarkably constant even with marked variations in the levels of total calcium. Increases in total calcium concentration lead to an increase in calcium binding to albumin, lessening the increase in ionized calcium concentration. Although a fall in serum albumin of 1 g/dL is usually associated with a fall of 0.8 mg/dL in total calcium concentration, the proportional fall in ionized calcium will be less. The fall in albumin will lessen the fraction of bound calcium and result in only a small decrease in the concentration of ionized calcium. Alterations in systemic pH will alter calcium binding by albumin. A fall in pH of 0.1 unit will cause approximately a 0.1 mEq/L rise in the concentration of ionized calcium as the increase in hydrogen ions displaces calcium from albumin. However, the concentration of ionized calcium is difficult to predict using these "rules of thumb." As most clinical laboratories have the required electrode for the direct measurement of ionized calcium, clinicians should request its measurement and become comfortable with its interpretation.

Intestinal Absorption

The average American diet contains approximately 800 mg (20 mmol) of calcium of which there is generally a net absorption of approximately 160 mg (4 mmol). Calcium absorption varies widely depending on other dietary components that may bind calcium (oxalate or phosphate) or promote absorption (lactose) and the level of serum $1,25(OH)_2D_3$. $1,25(OH)_2D_3$ is the principal hormonal regulator of intestinal calcium absorption. Calcium is absorbed in the duodenum, jejunum, and ileum. Calcium moves across the brush border down its concentration gradient by a $1,25(OH)_2D_3$-facilitated mechanism, through the cell bound to $1,25(OH)_2D_3$-induced calcium binding proteins, and then is transported across the basolateral membrane against a steep gradient utilizing a calcium ATP-ase or through a sodium for calcium exchange mechanism.

Renal Excretion

A 70-kg male with a glomerular filtration rate of 180 L/day filters approximately 270 mmol of calcium per day (180 L/day × 1.5 mmol/L). This quantity of calcium, over 10 g, is far more than the entire extracellular fluid calcium content. The kidney reabsorbs approximately 98% of the ultrafiltered calcium, leading to a urine calcium excretion of approximately 4 mmol/day. Approximately 65% of filtered calcium is reabsorbed in the proximal tubule. Proximal reabsorption is linked to sodium reabsorption and does not appear to be under hormonal control. Approximately 25% of filtered calcium is reabsorbed in the loop of Henle. In this segment, the lumen-positive voltage provides a strong driving force for calcium reabsorption. In addition, there appears to be active transport of calcium. The distal convoluted tubule is responsible for approximately 8% of calcium reabsorption, and is the major site for the regulation of urine calcium excretion. In this segment, active calcium transport occurs against both electrical and chemical gradients. Distal convoluted tubule calcium reabsorption is stimulated by parathyroid hormone (PTH) and phosphorus depletion and is inhibited by metabolic acidosis and adrenocortical excess. Thiazide diuretics increase reabsorption, whereas loop diuretics, such as furosemide, decrease reabsorption. There appears to be some, albeit quite small, calcium reabsorption in the collecting tubule.

In health, daily urine calcium excretion equals intestinal calcium absorption. However, during renal insufficiency, urine calcium excretion falls due not only to the decreased glomerular filtration rate but to enhanced calcium reabsorption secondary to the usual increase in PTH. The increase in PTH is multifactorial; it appears secondary to the decrease in renal $1,25(OH)_2D_3$ synthesis, resulting from a decrease in renal mass and from an increase in serum phosphorus due to a decrease in phosphorus excretion. The fall in $1,25(OH)_2D_3$ decreases calcium absorption, resulting in hypocalcemia and subsequent increased PTH secretion. In addition, $1,25(OH)_2D_3$ itself has a significant inhibitory effect on PTH secretion. Recent studies have shown that increased levels of serum phosphorus will increase serum levels of PTH independent of alterations in calcium or $1,25(OH)_2D_3$. Renal osteodystrophy is covered in detail in Chapter 69.

Regulation of Serum Levels

Large amounts of calcium must be transported through the extracellular fluid during periods of rapid skeletal growth and pregnancy, yet the concentration of serum calcium usually varies by less than 10%. This precise regulation of serum calcium concentration is accomplished by a complex interaction of the intestine, bone, and kidney involving the principal calcium-regulating hormones: PTH and $1,25(OH)_2D_3$. PTH stimulates renal calcium reabsorption and bone mineral turnover and increases the serum level of $1,25(OH)_2D_3$. A principal role of $1,25(OH)_2D_3$ is to stimulate intestinal calcium absorption. Numerous cellular activities are regulated by calcium or are dependent on a stable serum calcium concentration for normal function. Alterations in serum calcium concentration result in disturbances of cellular, especially neuronal, function.

DISORDERS OF CALCIUM HOMEOSTASIS

Hypocalcemia

Hypocalcemia may be defined as a reduction in the ionized component of serum calcium. Patients who have a decrease in total serum calcium concentration may, or may not, have a reduction in ionized calcium, as hypoalbuminemia is very prevalent in hospitalized patients and because albumin binds to the majority of protein-bound calcium. If there is doubt about the diagnosis, ionized calcium should be measured directly.

Clinical Presentation

The clinical presentation of patients with hypocalcemia correlates with the rapidity and magnitude of the fall in serum calcium, but symptoms are manifest in many patients with a total serum calcium of 7.0 mg/dL or less. The principal clinical findings are neurological. Perioral paresthesias are followed by carpopedal spasm. Occasionally, patients develop laryngeal stridor. Tetany may be evoked by acute respiratory alkalosis caused by hyperventilation, due to the rapid fall in ionized calcium concentration. As the pH rises (a decrease in hydrogen ion concentration), hydrogen ions dissociate from albumin, promoting increased calcium binding.

Two clinical signs may indicate hypocalcemia: Chvostek's and Trousseau's. Chvostek's sign is evoked by tapping the facial nerve and observing a grimace. Trousseau's is evoked by inflating a blood pressure cuff 3 mm Hg above the systolic pressure for at least 3 minutes and observing spasm of the outstretched hand. Trousseau's sign is more specific, as Cvostek's sign is present in approximately 10% of normocalcemic individuals.

Patients with hypocalcemia may also present with generalized seizures which represent whole body tetany. The electrocardiogram in hypocalcemic patients has a characteristic prolonged corrected QT and ST intervals. There may be peaked T waves, arrhythmias, and heart block.

Causes (Table I)

Chronic Renal Insufficiency. Decreased glomerular filtration decreases renal phosphorus excretion, resulting in hyperphosphatemia. The increased serum phosphorus not only complexes with serum calcium producing hypocalcemia but also downregulates the 1α-hydroxylase responsible for the renal conversion of $25(OH)D_3$ to $1,25(OH)_2D_3$. Chronic renal insufficiency also results in a reduction of functional renal mass and decreased $1,25(OH)_2D_3$ production. Serum levels of $1,25(OH)_2D_3$ are low, resulting in decreased intestinal calcium absorption and hypocalcemia. Levels of PTH and the osteoblastic enzyme alkaline phosphatase tend to be elevated.

Following Parathyroidectomy. Surgical reduction of parathyroid mass in patients with secondary or tertiary hyperparathyroidism usually leads to profound hypocalcemia, due to bone remineralization. This hungry bone syndrome may require prolonged and vigorous calcium replacement.

Hypoparathyroidism. Both idiopathic and postsurgical hypoparathyroidism result in a deficiency of PTH. Renal calcium excretion is increased and $1,25(OH)_2D_3$ production and bone turnover decreased. Serum levels of PTH are either low for the level of serum calcium or undetectable.

Pseudohypoparathyroidism. In this hereditary disorder, the target cell response to PTH is decreased. PTH level is elevated and, in most patients, cyclic-AMP does not rise normally in response to PTH. Patients also commonly have shortened metacarpals and metatarsals in addition to short stature, obesity, and heterotopic calcification.

Malignant Disease. The most frequent cause of a decrease in total calcium concentration in ill patients with malignant disease is a decrease in serum albumin concentration; ionized calcium may be normal. Certain malignancies, such as prostate and breast cancer, may cause enhanced osteoblastic activity and accelerated bone formation, resulting in hypocalcemia. In the tumor lysis syndrome, the rapid cell destruction in response to chemotherapy may result in an increase in serum phosphorus which then complexes serum calcium, resulting in hypocalcemia.

Rhabdomyolysis. Cellular injury, especially due to rapid crush injuries, causes a rapid release of cellular phosphorus which complexes with extracellular calcium, resulting in hypocalcemia. Associated renal failure blocks the expected PTH-induced rise in $1,25(OH)_2D_3$.

Hypomagnesemia. Hypocalcemia and hypomagnesemia frequently coexist and are often due to decreased absorption of dietary divalent cations or poor dietary intake. Hypomagnesemia may impair PTH secretion and interfere with its peripheral action.

Acute Pancreatitis. Acute pancreatitis leads to the release of pancreatic lipase which degrades retroperitoneal and omental fat which then binds calcium in the peritoneum removing it from the extracellular fluid and resulting in hypocalcemia. Hypomagnesemia and hypoalbuminemia also have been reported to contribute to the hypocalcemia of acute pancreatitis.

Septic Shock. Endotoxic shock is associated with hypocalcemia through mechanisms which are not well delineated. As myocardial function correlates directly with ionized calcium concentration, hypocalcemia in this condition may be responsible, in part, for the hypotension.

Vitamin D Deficiency. There are numerous causes of vitamin D deficiency including renal insufficiency, as noted above. Dietary deficiency is uncommon in the United States because vitamin D is added to various foods. This fat-soluble vitamin is subject to malabsorption and levels may be low in chronic liver disease and primary biliary cirrhosis. Anticonvulsant therapy with any of several agents increases the turnover of vitamin D into inactive compounds and results in a decrease in serum levels of $1,25(OH)_2D_3$.

Treatment

Acute. Patients with symptoms attributable to hypocalcemia must be treated promptly. In addition, asymptomatic patients with a serum calcium of approximately 7.0 mg/dL or less also should be treated prophylactically. Intravenous calcium is the mainstay of treatment. Calcium gluconate may be administered as 10 mL of a 10% solution (0.47 mEq calcium/mL) administered over 10 minutes. Patients on digoxin may require EKG monitoring. To avoid precipitation of the insoluble salt calcium carbonate, calcium must not be given in the same intravenous line as bicarbonate. If a patient is acidemic and hypocalcemic, in general the hypocalcemia must be treated first because the acidemia increases the proportion of ionized calcium and thus pro-

TABLE I

Principal Causes of Hypocalcemia

Chronic renal insufficiency
Following parathyroidectomy
Hypoparathyroidism
Pseudohypoparathyroidism
Malignant disease
Rhabdomyolysis
Hypomagnesemia
Acute pancreatitis
Septic shock
Vitamin D deficiency

tects the patient against symptomatic hypocalcemia. A constant infusion of calcium gluconate (50 mL of 10% calcium gluconate in 500 mL of D_5W) may be administered every 8 hours.

Chronic. In patients with normal renal function, chronic hypocalcemia is treated by administering oral calcium and $1,25(OH)_2D_3$. The former, often given as calcium carbonate, must provide at least 1 g of elemental calcium each day. $1,25(OH)_2D_3$ therapy will promote intestinal calcium absorption; however, in the case of hypoparathyroidism, it will also increase urine calcium excretion because PTH is not present to promote renal calcium reabsorption. Thus, the goal of therapy is to keep serum calcium concentration at the lower limit of normal, approximately 8.0 mg/dL, and to keep urine calcium excretion below 350 mg/day. Thiazide diuretics may be utilized to help prevent hypercalciuria and to promote normocalcemia. $1,25(OH)_2D_3$ administered without oral calcium may result in resorption of bone mineral and osteopenia.

Hypercalcemia

Hypercalcemia is defined as an increase in the concentration of serum ionized calcium.

Clinical Presentation

The clinical signs and symptoms of hypercalcemia correlate with the rapidity and magnitude of the elevation in serum calcium. As with hypocalcemia, neurologic abnormalities predominate. Often patients present with drowsiness and lethargy followed by headache and irritability. Confusion may be followed by stupor and coma. Muscle weakness, emotional problems, and depression may occur.

Polyuria is frequent in patients with hypercalcemia due to a renal concentrating defect. The excess calcium is thought to impair the renal response to antidiuretic hormone. Hypercalcemia can lead to a decline in renal function by a variety of mechanisms. Polyuria may lead to volume depletion and prerenal azotemia. Excess calcium excretion may produce nephrocalcinosis, especially in the presence of alkaline urine which decreases the solubility of calcium phosphate complexes.

Calcium directly increases cardiac contractility, and patients with hypercalcemia are thought to have an increased incidence of hypertension. Hypercalcemia shortens the corrected QT interval, may broaden the T waves, and may produce first-degree AV block. Anorexia, nausea, and severe vomiting are associated with hypercalcemia, as is constipation.

Causes (Table 2)

Primary Hyperparathyroidism. Accounting for more than 50% of patients, primary hyperparathyroidism is the leading cause of hypercalcemia. Patients are typically women 60 years of age or older. Most have a benign adenoma of a single parathyroid gland, whereas others have hyperplasia of all four glands. Parathyroid carcinoma is extremely rare. The elevated PTH levels increase both renal calcium reab-

TABLE 2
Principal Causes of Hypercalcemia

Primary hyperparathyroidism
Malignancy
Renal failure
Following renal transplant
Thiazide diuretics
Immobilization
Milk-alkali syndrome
Granulomatous disease
Familial hypocalciuric hypercalcemia
Thyrotoxicosis
Vitamin intoxication
Theophylline toxicity

sorption and phosphorus excretion. Proximal tubule bicarbonate reabsorption is impaired and, as expected, urinary cyclic-AMP is elevated. The excess PTH also increases the serum level of $1,25(OH)_2D_3$, increasing enhanced intestinal calcium absorption and bone turnover, with bone resorption predominating over bone formation.

Approximately 6% of patients with calcium-containing kidney stones have hyperparathyroidism. In this case the increased filtered load of calcium exceeds the increased renal calcium reabsorption, leading to hypercalciuria, renal stone formation, and occasionally nephrocalcinosis. Increased urinary bicarbonate alkalinizes the urine, promoting precipitation of calcium phosphorus complexes. With current automated blood chemical analysis, hypercalcemia from hyperparathyroidism is generally detected before stone formation and/or nephrocalcinosis occurs.

Malignancy. Malignancy is the second most frequent cause of hypercalcemia. Both direct bone destruction by the growing tumor and secretion of calcemic factor(s) by malignant cells may produce hypercalcemia. Patients with squamous cell lung carcinoma and metastatic carcinoma of the breast develop hypercalcemia most frequently, whereas patients with myeloma, T-cell tumors, renal cell carcinoma, and other squamous cell tumors are also prone to hypercalcemia. Many tumors produce a PTH-related peptide (PTH-rP) in which the first 13 amino acids are very similar to those in PTH and which binds to PTH receptors in the kidney and bone. Although PTHrP is not detected on standard PTH assays, commercial assays are now available. Other tumors produce factors such as transforming growth factor-α or interleukin-1, cytokines such as lymphotoxin, or hormones such as $1,25(OH)_2D_3$.

In general, the malignancy is evident when patients present with hypercalcemia. The finding of a low level of PTH and an elevated level of PTH-rP supports the diagnosis. While hypercalcemia due to an occult malignancy is rare, associated symptoms such as weight loss and fatigue should prompt a search for tumors that are frequently associated with hypercalcemia, such as those in the lung, kidney, and urogenital tract.

Renal Failure. Hypocalcemia, and not hypercalcemia, is generally found in patients with renal failure. In these patients, it is important to determine if the hypercalcemia was responsible for the renal failure. The hypercalcemia caused by diseases such as sarcoidosis, myeloma, immobilization, and milk-alkali syndrome frequently causes renal failure. Hypercalcemia may occur during the recovery phase of rhabdomyolysis-induced renal failure because calcium recently deposited in muscle and soft tissues is rapidly mobilized.

Hypercalcemia is frequently observed during excessive $1,25(OH)_2D_3$ replacement therapy of patients on dialysis, especially if they are simultaneously being given large amounts of oral calcium as a phosphorus binder. Some patients may develop severe secondary hyperparathyroidism with marked hyperplasia of the parathyroid glands and subsequent hypercalcemia. In addition, patients may have aluminum intoxication, a disorder characterized by low bone turnover, which predisposes them to hypercalcemia. These aluminum intoxicated patients often have modestly elevated PTH and alkaline phosphatase levels (see Chapter 69).

Following Renal Transplant. Frequently, patients on long-term dialysis develop parathyroid hyperplasia leading to autonomous secretion of PTH. If these patients then receive a successful renal transplant, the PTH secretion continues and hypercalcemia may develop due to enhanced, PTH-induced, renal calcium reabsorption. The hypercalcemia is generally mild and tends to decrease over the ensuing 6 to 12 months as the hypertrophied parathyroid glands involute; however, patients with prolonged marked hypercalcemia may require surgical parathyroidectomy.

Thiazide Diuretics. Thiazide diuretic therapy is often associated with mild hypercalcemia due to increased renal calcium reabsorption. If the hypercalcemia does not resolve when the thiazides are discontinued, then the patient must be investigated for other causes of hypercalcemia.

Immobilization. Immobilization leads to a rapid increase in bone resorption and may lead to hypercalcemia, especially if there is any decrement in renal calcium excretion. This disorder is most prevalent in younger patients who sustain a traumatic spinal cord injury.

Milk-Alkali Syndrome. Ingestion of large amounts of calcium-containing nonabsorbable antacids may lead to hypercalcemia, alkalemia, nephrocalcinosis, and renal insufficiency. While this disorder has become less common because ulcers are being treated with antibiotics and agents that inhibit gastric acid secretion, the use of calcium and alkali preparations is increasing in efforts to prevent and treat osteoporosis.

Granulomatous Disease. Granulomatous diseases, such as sarcoidosis, tuberculosis, and leprosy, may produce hypercalciuria and hypercalcemia due to the conversion of $25(OH)D_3$ to $1,25(OH)_2D_3$ by the granulomatous tissue. This phenomenon has been observed in anephric patients.

Familial Hypocalciuric Hypercalcemia. This autosomal dominant disorder causes mild hypercalcemia, hypophosphatemia, and reduced renal calcium excretion (often less than 100 mg/day). These patients have a mutation in the recently identified calcium receptor that causes a reduction in receptor activity. PTH levels are normal and parathyroidectomy is not indicated.

Thyrotoxicosis. Excess thyroid hormone can stimulate osteoclastic bone resorption, resulting in hypercalcemia. The hypercalcemia is generally mild and coexistent hyperparathyroidism must be excluded.

Vitamin Intoxication. Vitamin D intoxication, as noted above, is often observed in patients with end-stage renal disease treated with $1,25(OH)_2D_3$. Vitamin D intoxication can also occur in food or vitamin faddists. Vitamin A excess can also cause hypercalcemia and may be seen in the same patients.

Treatment

Treatment of hypercalcemia should be directed at the underlying disorder. However, if the patient is symptomatic and the serum calcium level is 13 mg/dL or higher acute therapy is indicated. The mainstay of treatment in patients with reasonable renal and cardiac function is intravenous saline. Rates as high as 200 to 250 mL/h of normal saline may be used to facilitate renal calcium excretion. Furosemide is calciuric and is often necessary (40 mg iv in patients with normal renal function) during volume repletion with saline to avoid pulmonary congestion. Thiazide diuretics must be avoided because they decrease renal calcium excretion. Patients with renal insufficiency may be unable to excrete the sodium load and thus hemodialysis against a low calcium bath may be necessary to lower serum calcium concentration. Patients with cardiac or renal insufficiency are at particular risk for volume overload during saline treatment and may require central monitoring and a more modest normal saline infusion.

Patients with hypercalcemia due to enhanced intestinal calcium absorption may benefit from a reduction of dietary calcium intake. Normally, Americans consume approximately 800 mg of calcium per day, reducing this by one-third is generally effective. However this should only be a short-term remedy, as the provision of a low calcium diet in a patient with normal renal function and excess $1,25(OH)_2D_3$ will promote bone demineralization. Glucocorticoids (initial dose 40 mg of prednisone) will inhibit intestinal calcium absorption but may require 1 week for maximal effect.

Patients with hypercalcemia mediated by enhanced osteoclastic bone resorption (usually patients with malignancy), will benefit from the osteoclastic inhibitor calcitonin (4–8 units/kg sc or im 6–12 hours). However, the hypocalcemic effect of calcitonin is often transient. The bisphosphonate etidronate (7.5 mg · kg body wt^{-1} · day^{-1}

infused iv for 3 days) lowers serum calcium in a few days with a maximal effect in 7 days. Pamidronate (30–90 mg/day given as a single 24-hour infusion for 3 days) is a more potent bisphosphonate than etidronate. Both bisphosphonates have been shown to cause renal insufficiency and should be avoided in patients with renal impairment. Gallium nitrate will effectively lower serum calcium; however, it is contraindicated in patients with renal insufficiency or in those receiving other nephrotoxic agents.

Oral phosphorus can be utilized to treat hypercalcemia. To prevent induction of soft-tissue and calcium degeneration, it should be employed only if the serum phosphorus is at or below the lower limit of normal. However, this form of outdated therapy is best avoided.

PHOSPHORUS

Phosphorus Homeostasis

Distribution

The majority (90%) of total body phosphorus is contained within the bone mineral while 10% is contained within the cells and 1% in the extracellular fluid.

Serum Concentration

The concentration of serum phosphorus in adults ranges from 2.5 to 4.5 mg/dL or 0.81 to 1.45 mM. Serum phosphorus levels are highest in infants and decrease in childhood reaching the normal adult levels in late adolescence. Approximately 70% of blood phosphorus is termed organic and contained within phospholipids; the remaining 30% is termed inorganic. Of the inorganic phosphorus, 85% is free and circulates as monohydrogen or dihydrogen phosphate or is complexed with sodium, magnesium or calcium. The remainder is protein bound.

Intestinal Absorption

Dietary phosphorus intake varies between 800 and 1850 mg of PO$_4$/day (26–60 mmol/day). Approximately 25 mmol/day is absorbed. Diets that are adequate in calories and protein generally contain adequate phosphorus. Phosphorus absorption is regulated by 1,25(OH)$_2$D$_3$ via a sodium-dependent active transport mechanism principally in the duodenum and by a passive phosphorus concentration dependent mechanism in the jejunum and ileum. The absorption of phosphorus is hindered by complex formation in the intestine; both aluminum and calcium can form insoluble complexes with phosphorus that hinder its absorption. During renal failure, phosphorus absorption continues. The formation of intestinal phosphorus complexes with aluminum and/or calcium is used to decrease intestinal absorption in these patients who are unable to excrete absorbed phosphorus. Use of calcium to complex intestinal phosphorus is favored over aluminum because the latter is toxic to many organs including brain and bone (see Chapters 69 and 71).

Renal Excretion

A 70-kg male with a glomerular filtration rate of 180 L/day and a mean serum phosphorus concentration of 1.25 mM filters approximately 200 mmol of phosphorus per day as approximately 85% of serum phosphorus is ultrafiltrable (180 L/day × 1.25 mmol/L × 0.85). Because urine phosphorus excretion averages about 25 mmol/day, approximately 12.5% of the glomerular filtrate is excreted in the urine. The bulk of phosphorus reabsorption (approximately 85%) occurs in the proximal tubule. Proximal phosphorus transport across the apical membrane occurs by a rate-limiting sodium–phosphorus cotransport. Phosphorus resorption occurs in the pars recta but not in the loop of Henle. A small quantity of phosphorus is reabsorbed in the distal convoluted tubule, especially in the absence of PTH. Whether there is phosphorus reabsorption more distally is not known.

Parathyroid hormone is the major hormonal regulator of phosphorus excretion. Variation in dietary phosphorus intake is the major nonhormonal regulator. PTH is phosphaturic as are 1,25(OH)$_2$D$_3$, extracellular fluid volume expansion, and a high phosphorus diet. A low phosphorus diet leads to a decrease in renal excretion. The hypophosphaturia of phosphorus depletion overrides the hyperphosphaturia induced by PTH. During renal insufficiency urine phosphorus excretion remains relatively constant until the glomerular filtration rate falls to about 25% of normal. Phosphorus excretion is maintained despite the fall in glomerular filtration rate and filtered load of phosphorus by the phosphaturic effects of elevated PTH levels. (See Renal Calcium Excretion above.)

Regulation of Serum Levels

Serum levels of phosphorus are not as tightly regulated as those of calcium. They may vary by as much as 50% over the course of a day. Although there is diurnal variation in phosphorus levels, alterations in dietary phosphorus intake are principally responsible for the swings in serum levels. In addition, serum levels are controlled by hormones such as PTH and 1,25(OH)$_2$D$_3$ and by the status of extracellular fluid volume and renal function.

DISORDERS OF PHOSPHORUS HOMEOSTASIS

Hypophosphatemia

A decrease in the level of serum phosphorus may or may not reflect total body phosphorus content because only 1% of body phosphorus is in the extracellular fluid. Moderate hypophosphatemia may be defined as a serum phosphorus between 1 mg/dL and the lower limit of normal and severe hypophosphatemia as a serum level below 1 mg/dL. While moderate hypophosphatemia is generally asymptomatic, severe hypophosphatemia is associated with a variety of clinical disturbances and, occasionally, death. Hypophosphatemia may result from a decrease in intake, and increase in excretion, or a shift of phosphorus from the extracellular environment into cells.

Clinical Presentation

Patients with severe hypophosphatemia may have neurologic dysfunction characterized by weakness, paresthesias, confusion, seizures, and coma. The weakness may be associated with muscle edema and rhabdomyolysis. Respiratory muscle paralysis may result in death.

Causes (Table 3)

Alcohol Related.   Many chronic ethanol abusers are hypophosphatemic on hospital admission or become hypophosphatemic with treatment. Although the etiology of their hypophosphatemia is multifactorial, it is due in large part to poor oral intake.

Refeeding.   When patients are fed after prolonged poor intake or starvation the calories provide a stimulus for tissue growth and utilization of phosphorus in phosphorylated intermediates such as ATP. If the diet does not contain adequate phosphorus then severe hypophosphatemia may develop after several days. Likewise, if total parenteral nutrition (TPN) solutions contain inadequate phosphorus then hypophosphatemia may become evident as the patient regains body mass.

Diabetes Mellitus.   In severe diabetic ketoacidosis, especially of prolonged duration, there is excessive urinary phosphorus loss, which is accompanied by poor oral phosphorus intake, that may lead to hypophosphatemia and also hypokalemia. The severity of the hypophosphatemia may become manifest only during treatment of the diabetic ketoacidosis.

Alkalosis.   Both respiratory and metabolic alkalosis induce hypophosphatemia; however, hypophosphatemia is far more severe in prolonged respiratory alkalosis. The extracellular alkalosis appears to cause intracellular alkalosis which results in a shift of phosphorus into the intracellular space and hypophosphatemia.

Postrenal Transplant.   Hypophosphatemia is commonly observed following renal transplantation. The etiology is multifactorial but related to a persistent elevation in serum PTH levels and an intrinsic renal tubular defect in phosphorus reabsorption that results in hyperphosphaturia. In addition, glucocorticoids used in immunosuppression inhibit renal phosphorus transport.

Urinary Loss.   Renal tubular acidosis, hypokalemia, hypomagnesemia, and other renal tubular disorders are associated with an increased urinary excretion of phosphorus.

TABLE 3
Principal Causes of Hypophosphatemia

Alcohol related
Refeeding
Diabetes mellitus
Alkalosis
Postrenal transplant
Urinary loss
Total parenteral nutrition

Treatment

The treatment of hypophosphatemia is best directed at reversing the underlying disease or nutritional process. Moderate hypophosphatemia can often be treated with oral phosphorus supplementation in the form of milk (an excellent source of phosphorus containing about 1 g of phosphorus per liter), or Neutra-Phos tablets (250 mg of phosphorus). Oral phosphorus can cause diarrhea which is usually seen at doses of over 1 g/day. Severe hypophosphatemia usually indicates a significant loss of total body phosphorus. In asymptomatic patients if oral replacement is possible, the patient should receive at least 3 g/day for 1 week. Often the patient will be symptomatic and require intravenous therapy. In this case, treatment may be initiated with 2 mg/kg body wt of phosphorus as the sodium salt infused over 6 hours. Serum phosphorus levels must be checked frequently during replacement. Intravenous phosphorus may produce hypocalcemia and metastatic calcification especially if the calcium phosphorus product exceeds 60. Concurrent hypokalemia and hypomagnesemia are often found in patients with hypophosphatemia.

Hyperphosphatemia

In adults, hyperphosphatemia is defined as an increase in the concentration of serum phosphorus to greater than 5.0 mg/dL. Because cells contain abundant phosphorus, hemolysis of the collected sample should be excluded, especially if there is associated hyperkalemia. Hypophosphatemia may be caused by decreased phosphorus excretion, an increase in phosphorus load, or a shift of phosphorus from the cells into the extracellular fluid.

Clinical Presentation

The clinical presentation of patients with hyperphosphatemia is dominated by the associated fall in serum calcium. As serum phosphorus rises there is a reciprocal fall in serum calcium. This fall is multifactorial but includes a decrease in $1,25(OH)_2D_3$ synthesis, leading to a decrease in intestinal calcium absorption and formation of calcium phosphorus complexes resulting in ectopic calcification especially of previously injured tissues. The symptoms of patients with hyperphosphatemia then are those of patients with hypocalcemia, tetany, seizures, and decreased myocardial contractility. In addition, ectopic calcification may occur in virtually any organ in the body, especially when the calcium phosphorus product exceeds 60. Calcification is especially prominent in proton-secreting organs, such as the stomach or kidney, in which basolateral bicarbonate secretion results in an increase in pH that promotes calcium hydrogen phosphate (brushite) precipitation. On a chronic basis, the hyperphosphatemia of renal failure can result in secondary hyperparathyroidism and renal osteodystrophy.

Causes (Table 4)

Renal Failure.   With a fall in the glomerular filtration rate below approximately 25 ml per minute renal excretion of phosphorus is less than intestinal absorption and hyperphosphatemia ensues. Increased levels of phosphorus have

TABLE 4

Principal Causes of Hyperphosphatemia

Renal failure
Hypoparathyroidism
Cell injury
Exogenous administration

been shown to directly increase the level of PTH. The increased levels of phosphorus also suppress renal $1,25(OH)_2D_3$ production, resulting in less calcium absorption. In addition, the excess phosphorus may bind serum calcium if the calcium phosphorus product exceeds 60. Levels of serum $1,25(OH)_2D_3$ fall due to the reduction in mass of the renal tissue that converts $25(OH)D_3$ to $1,25(OH)_2D_3$. The resulting hypocalcemia and low levels of $1,25(OH)_2D_3$ further increase PTH secretion and urine phosphorus excretion, lowering the level of serum phosphorus at the cost of hyperparathyroidism. In spite of the additional phosphorus excretion per nephron, with more profound renal insufficiency, serum phosphorus increases as the patient is unable to excrete the absorbed phosphorus. During chronic renal failure the hyperphosphatemia is less severe than during the same decrement in glomerular filtration rate in acute renal insufficiency when there has been insufficient time for adaptation (see Chapter 69).

Hypoparathyroidism. PTH promotes renal phosphorus excretion and hyperphosphatemia results when there is a lack of PTH or a resistance to its action.

Cell Injury. During effective chemotherapy, especially of rapidly lysing cells such as lymphomas, there is a marked increase in phosphorus release from cells which exceeds renal excretory capacity. The hyperphosphatemia is often associated with hyperkalemia and hyperuricemia and leads to hypocalcemia. Phosphorus can also be released from cells during acute rhabdomyolysis, crush injuries, or tissue infarction. Hyperphosphatemia is especially severe when the release of cellular phosphorus occurs in the setting of acute renal failure.

Exogenous Administration. Excess phosphorus in TPN solutions or phosphorus in laxatives may result in hyperphosphatemia. Phosphorus-containing enemas can result in hyperphosphatemia and should be avoided in patients with renal failure. Excess vitamin D not only increases calcium absorption but phosphorus absorption as well and can result in hyperphosphatemia.

Treatment

The treatment of hyperphosphatemia must be directed at the underlying cause. If renal function is intact then phosphaturia should be promoted. Extracellular fluid volume expansion with saline lowers renal phosphorus reabsorption as does increasing urine pH with sodium bicarbonate or acetazolamide. In patients with hyperphosphatemia and acute renal failure, glucose and insulin transiently increases cellular phosphorus uptake; however, phosphorus is best removed from the extracellular space with dialysis.

The successful treatment of hyperphosphatemia of chronic renal failure requires a coordinated effort among the patient, dietician, and physician. A diet devoid of phosphorus is unpalatable; however, dietary phosphorus can be reduced substantially with proper dietary supervision. Both hemodialysis and peritoneal dialysis remove phosphorus; but even with a low phosphorus diet they cannot restore phosphorus balance. Agents that bind dietary phosphorus and prevent its absorption are generally necessary to prevent and treat hyperphosphatemia. Calcium salts given with meals are effective in binding dietary phosphorus. Doses are gradually increased until the serum phosphorus is less than approximately 5 mg/dL. If hypercalcemia occurs before the serum phosphorus is controlled, then the dialysate calcium may be lowered and aluminum gels added to bind phosphorus. If patients present with severe hyperphosphatemia (serum phosphorus greater than 6.5 mg/dL), the serum phosphorus should be lowered with aluminum-binding gels prior to adding calcium salts to avoid soft tissue calcification. However, aluminum is toxic to the brain, bone, and bone marrow and should be avoided whenever possible (see Chapter 69 for details).

ACKNOWLEDGMENTS

This work was supported by grants AM-39906 and AR-33949 from the National Institutes of Health.

Bibliography

Brown EM, Pollack M, Seidman, CE, et al: Calcium-ion-sensing cell-surface receptors. *N Engl J Med* 333:234–240, 1995.

Bushinsky DA, Krieger NS: Integration of calcium metabolism in the adult. In: Coe FL, Fauus MJ (eds) *Disorders of Bone and Mineral Metabolism,* Raven Press, New York, pp. 417–432, 1992.

Bushinsky DA, Krieger NS: Role of the skeleton in calcium homeostasis. In: Seldin DW, Giebisch G (eds) *The Kidney: Physiology and Pathophysiology,* Raven Press, New York, pp. 2395–2430, 1992.

Kovach KL, Hruska KA: Phosphate balance and metabolism. In: Jacobson HR, Striker GE, Klahr S (eds) *The Principles and Practice of Nephrology,* Mosby, St. Louis, pp. 986–992, 1995.

Kumar R: Calcium metabolism. In: Jacobson HR, Striker GE, Klahr S (eds) *The Principles and Practice of Nephrology,* Mosby, St. Louis, pp. 964–971, 1995.

Levi M, Cronin RE, Knochel JP: Disorders of phosphate and magnesium metabolism. In: Coe FL, Favus MJ (eds) *Disorders of Bone and Mineral Metabolism,* Raven Press, New York, pp. 587–610, 1992.

Mundy GG: Hypercalcemia in hematologic malignancies and in solid tumors associated with extensive localized bone destruction. In: Favus MJ (ed) *Primer on the Metabolic Bone Diseases and Disorders of Mineral Metabolism,* Raven Press, New York, pp. 173–176, 1993.

Suki WN, Rouse D: Renal transport of calcium, magnesium, and phosphorus. In: Brenner BM (ed) *The Kidney,* 5th ed. Saunders, Philadelphia, pp. 472–515, 1996.

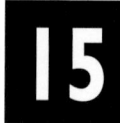

EDEMA AND THE CLINICAL USE
OF DIURETICS

DAVID H. ELLISON

Edema is usually a manifestation of expanded extracellular fluid (ECF) volume, whether it results from congestive heart failure, cirrhosis, nephrotic syndrome, or renal failure. Extracellular fluid volume expands when the kidneys retain NaCl in excess of dietary NaCl intake. Renal NaCl retention may reflect an adaptive response to inadequate effective arterial blood volume, as in patients with congestive heart failure. Renal NaCl retention may also reflect a pathological response of kidney tubules to damage, as in patients with acute renal failure. Regardless of its cause, the best treatment for edema is to restrict dietary NaCl intake and to correct the primary disorder. Despite these interventions, or when they are impossible, ECF volume frequently remains expanded unacceptably and, for this reason, diuretics are among the most commonly prescribed drugs. All of the diuretics used to treat edema increase both Na and water excretion, regardless of the underlying cause of edema. They are powerful drugs which, if used carefully, play an important role in treating symptomatic edema. The prompt and dramatic improvement of symptoms when intravenous diuretics are administered to a patient suffering from acute pulmonary edema remains one of the most gratifying responses in clinical medicine.

In addition to their use for edema, diuretic drugs are indicated for a wide variety of nonedematous disorders. Specific details of diuretic treatment of hypertension, acute renal failure, nephrolithiasis, and hyponatremia are discussed in other chapters in this volume. This chapter focuses on the renal mechanisms of diuretic action and the use of diuretics to treat edema.

THE PHYSIOLOGICAL BASIS OF DIURETIC ACTION

The amount of NaCl excreted by the kidneys is the difference between the quantity filtered by the glomeruli and the quantity reabsorbed by the renal tubules. Assuming a normal glomerular filtration rate ($\sim$150 L/day) and a normal plasma Na^+ concentration ($\sim$150 mM), $\sim$23 mol of Na^+ is filtered each day in normal humans (equivalent to about 3 lb of table salt). To maintain a normal fractional Na excretion (FE_{Na}) of <1%, more than 99% of the filtered

Na is reabsorbed. All of the diuretic drugs in clinical use act primarily on the renal tubules to inhibit Na reabsorption and increase fractional Na excretion.

A simple and clinically useful classification of diuretic drugs is based on the sites and mechanisms of their actions along the nephron (see Table 1). All active NaCl reabsorption by renal epithelial cells is driven by the Na,K-ATPase pump. This transport protein, which is present at the basolateral membrane (the blood side) of epithelial cells along the nephron, uses metabolic energy (derived from hydrolysis of ATP) to extrude Na from the cell into the bloodstream and to move K into the cell. The action of the Na,K-ATPase keeps the cellular Na concentration low and the cellular K concentration high. It also contributes to making the cell interior electrically negative with respect to the ECF. The low cellular Na concentration and the cell-negative voltage drive positively charged Na ions into the cell across the luminal membrane from tubule fluid. Although Na,K-ATPase pumps are present at the basolateral cell membranes of nearly all epithelial cells, each nephron segment possesses unique apical mechanisms that permit Na to move across the luminal membrane; these specific transport pathways at the luminal membrane form the cellular basis of diuretic action. Together, active Na extrusion from the basolateral membrane and passive Na entry across the luminal membrane permit vectorial Na transport in the absorptive direction.

Proximal Tubule Diuretics

Approximately two thirds of filtered water and NaCl are reabsorbed along the proximal tubule. Sodium moves down its electrochemical gradient from tubule lumen into proximal tubule cells coupled to the movement of other solutes against their electrochemical gradients; among these solutes are glucose, amino acids, and phosphate. Bicarbonate and chloride are indirectly coupled to Na absorption. Because the epithelium is electrically "leaky" (highly permeable to ions), large transepithelial ion gradients do not develop and solute absorption along this segment remains isoosmotic.

An important pathway by which Na crosses the luminal membrane of proximal tubule cells involves electroneutral exchange of Na^+ for H^+ (see Fig. 1). H^+ ions that are

TABLE I
Physiological Classification of Diuretic Drugs[a,b]

Proximal diuretics	Loop diuretics	DCT diuretics	CD diuretics
Carbonic anhydrase inhibitors	$Na^+–K^+–2Cl^-$ inhibitors	Na–Cl inhibitors	Na^+ channel blockers
Acetazolamide	Furosemide	Hydrochlorothiazide	Amiloride
	Bumetanide	Metolazone	Triamterene
	Torsemide	Chlorthalidone	Aldosterone antagonists
	Ethacrynic Acid	Indapamide[c]	Spironolactone
		Many others	

[a] Reproduced with permission from Ellison DH: *Ann Intern Med* 114:886–894, 1991.
[b] DCT, distal convoluted tubule; CD, collecting duct.
[c] Indapamide may have other actions as well.

extruded across the luminal membrane of proximal cells titrate bicarbonate (HCO_3^-), which has been filtered by the glomeruli, forming carbonic acid (H_2CO_3). Carbonic acid then dehydrates to CO_2 and H_2O, a reaction catalyzed by the enzyme carbonic anhydrase in the brush border of proximal tubule cells. Via these events, Na^+ and HCO_3^- are functionally reabsorbed across the luminal membrane into the cell. For transepithelial $NaHCO_3$ reabsorption to continue at steady state, Na^+ and HCO_3^- must leave the

cell across the basolateral membrane via the Na,K-ATPase pump and via a $NaHCO_3$ transport pathway. Carbonic anhydrase located within proximal tubule cells generates H^+ ions for extrusion across the apical membrane and bicarbonate ions which exit across the basolateral membrane.

Carbonic anhydrase inhibitors interfere with enzyme activity both inside the cell and within the brush border. Their action in the brush border inhibits Na^+/H^+ exchange by slowing the rate at which carbonic acid dehydrates, thereby

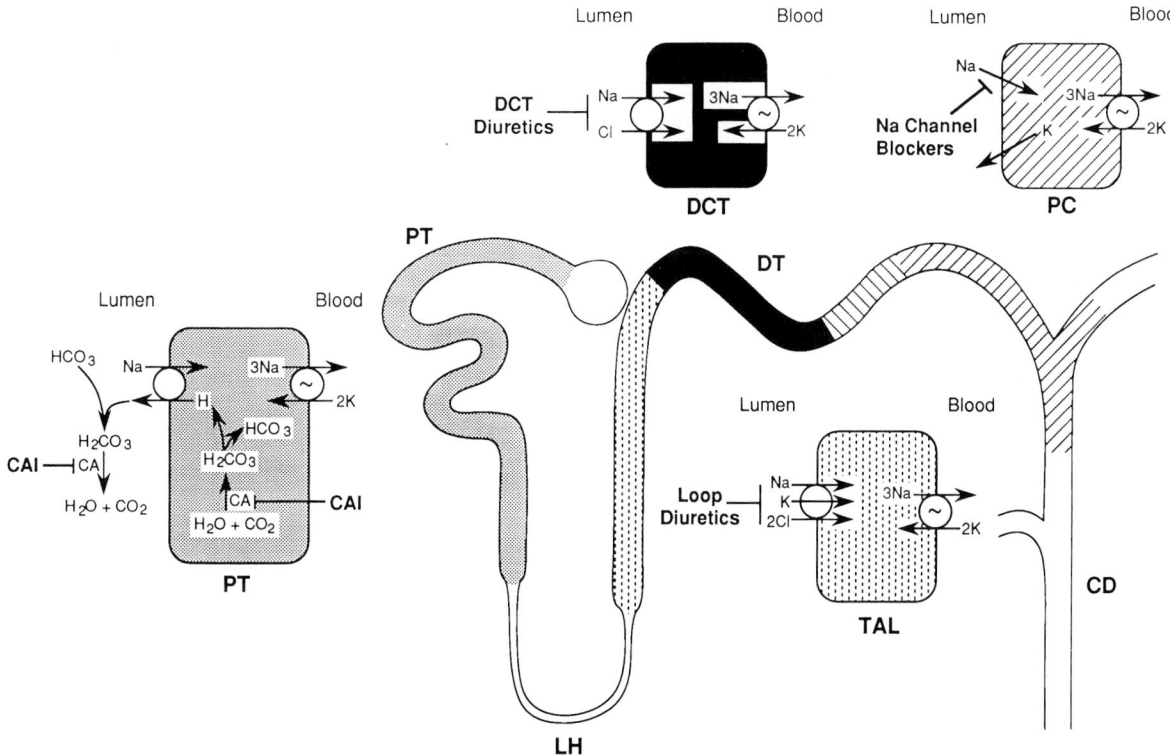

FIGURE I Predominant sites and mechanisms of action of clinically important diuretic drugs. Patterns identify sites of action along the nephron and corresponding cell types. PT, ■ proximal tubule; LH, loop of Henle; ▦ TAL, thick ascending limb cell; DT, distal tubule; ■ DCT, distal convoluted tubule cell; CD, collecting duct; ▨ PC, principal cell; CA, carbonic anhydrase inhibitors are important in their ability to reduce Na^+ reabsorption by the renal proximal tubule. Note that Na^+ channel blockers probably act along the connecting tubule ▨ as well as the collecting duct ▨. Spironolactone (not shown) is a competitive aldosterone antagonist and acts primarily in the cortical collecting tubule. Reproduced with permission from Ellison DH: *Ann Intern Med* 114:887, 1991.

acidifying tubule fluid. Their action inside the cell inhibits $NaHCO_3$ reabsorption by impairing the intracellular production of HCO_3^-, interfering with basolateral exit of HCO_3^-. The net result of carbonic anhydrase inhibition is impaired Na^+, HCO_3^- Cl^-, and water reabsorption by the proximal tubule and increased renal Na^+, Cl^-, HCO_3^- and water excretion. When administered acutely, these drugs provoke a moderate alkaline diuresis. When administered chronically, their natriuretic potency is relatively weak. Their limited potency reflects several compensatory processes that occur when carbonic anhydrase inhibitors are administered. First, when $NaHCO_3$ reabsorption along the proximal tubule is inhibited, much of the solute and fluid that escape reabsorption by the proximal tubule can be reabsorbed by more distal nephron segments. Second, inhibition of solute reabsorption along the proximal tubule leads to increased solute delivery to the macula densa. This activates the tubuloglomerular feedback mechanism, which suppresses glomerular filtration rate (GFR) and decreases the amount of Na^+, Cl^-, and HCO_3^- that is filtered. Finally, alkaline diuresis induces metabolic acidosis; when serum HCO_3^- concentrations decline, less HCO_3^- is filtered and the carbonic anhydrase-dependent component of Na^+ reabsorption falls.

Because carbonic anhydrase inhibitors are relatively weak diuretics and because they often result in metabolic acidosis, their use as diuretic drugs is limited. They are commonly employed, however, to treat open angle glaucoma, where they reduce the formation of aqueous humor by as much as 50%. Furthermore, they can be used to prevent acute mountain sickness and to treat metabolic alkalosis at times when Cl^- cannot be administered because of ECF volume expansion. This is especially useful when respiratory drive is compromised by metabolic alkalosis; careful use of carbonic anhydrase inhibitors may correct alkalosis and improve respiratory drive. Carbonic anhydrase inhibitors may also be used in conjunction with other classes of diuretics to induce diuresis in otherwise resistant patients (see "Resistance to Diuretics," below).

Loop Diuretics

Approximately 25% of the filtered NaCl is reabsorbed along the loop of Henle. Transcellular NaCl reabsorption along the medullary and cortical thick ascending limbs is driven by Na,K-ATPase at the basolateral membrane. An electroneutral pathway at the luminal membrane carries 1 Na^+, 1 K^+, and 2Cl^- from tubule fluid into the cell, driven by the electrochemical gradient for Na^+ (see Fig. 1). Much of the K^+ that is taken up via this pathway recycles across the luminal membrane through K^+ channels. The Na^+–K^+–2Cl^- pathway, therefore, generates net NaCl reabsorption and (because of the K^+ recycling) a voltage across the wall of the tubule that is oriented with the lumen positive relative to blood.

Loop diuretics such as furosemide, bumetanide, and torsemide inhibit the action of the Na^+–K^+–2Cl^- pathway directly. These diuretics are anions that circulate bound to protein so that very little diuretic reaches tubule fluid via filtration. Instead, they are secreted into the lumen of the proximal tubule by the organic anion transport pathway and travel downstream to the thick ascending limb where they bind to a Cl^- site on the transport protein. Although the mechanism by which ethacrynic acid inhibits NaCl reabsorption is not as clear, its net effect on transport along the thick ascending limb is qualitatively similar. Loop diuretics are potent ("high ceiling") drugs that promote the excretion of Na^+ and Cl^-, together with K^+. Although they inhibit K^+ reabsorption along the thick ascending limb, their effects on K^+ excretion reflect predominantly their tendency to increase K^+ secretion along the distal nephron (see "Complications of Diuretic Treatment" below). Loop diuretics increase magnesium and calcium excretion. Bumetanide, furosemide, and torsemide reduce the magnitude of the lumen positive voltage in the thick ascending limb. This tends to impair Ca^{2+} and Mg^{2+} reabsorption and appears to account for the actions of these drugs on Ca^{2+} and Mg^{2+} excretion.

Loop diuretics impair the ability of the kidney to elaborate urine that is either very concentrated or very dilute. The Na^+–K^+–2Cl^- pathway removes Na^+ and Cl^- from the lumen as fluid courses up the thick ascending limb. Because this segment of the nephron is impermeable to water, solute removal dilutes the tubule fluid. By blocking the predominant solute removal pathway, these agents inhibit free water generation. The action of the Na^+–K^+–2Cl^- pathway also provides the "single effect" that is responsible for countercurrent multiplication. Solute removal from the thick ascending limb contributes to generating a high solute concentration in the medullary interstitium which drives water reabsorption from the medullary collecting tubule. By blocking the Na^+–K^+–2Cl^- pathway, loop diuretics inhibit the kidney's ability to generate a concentrated urine; this is one reason that these diuretics can be useful for treating patients with the syndrome of inappropriate antidiuretic hormone secretion.

Loop diuretics have important hemodynamic effects—both within the kidney and systemically. They increase secretion of vasodilatory prostaglandins and often reduce cardiac preload, when administered acutely. In some situations, however, they elicit a vasoconstrictor response that may impair cardiac performance acutely; this anomalous response may be blocked by angiotensin-converting enzyme (ACE) inhibitors. Loop diuretics tend to maintain or increase the GFR, even in the face of ECF volume depletion, because they block the tubuloglomerular feedback mechanism and because diuretic-induced prostaglandin secretion dilates the afferent arteriole.

Distal Convoluted Tubule Diuretics (DCT Diuretics)

The distal tubule (the nephron segment just beyond the loop of Henle) reabsorbs 5 to 10% of the filtered NaCl. As in other nephron segments, the intracellular concentration of Na^+ is maintained low by Na,K-ATPase. Sodium and Cl^- enter the cell across the luminal membrane via a distinct Na-Cl cotransport pathway (see Fig. 1). DCT diuretics are anions that, like the loop diuretics, circulate in the bloodstream bound to protein and are secreted into the lumen of the proximal tubule by the organic anion transport pathway. They are carried downstream to the distal tubule, where they bind to the Cl⁻ site on the Na–Cl transport protein and inhibit its action. Because the distal tubule is relatively water impermeable, NaCl reabsorption along the DCT contributes to urinary dilution. DCT diuretics therefore impair urinary diluting capacity, but they have no effect on urinary concentrating ability. Most DCT diuretics, with the possible exception of metolazone, become less effective when the GFR declines below 40 mL/min.

DCT diuretics increase magnesium excretion but, in contrast to loop diuretics, they inhibit urinary calcium excretion. Two mechanisms have been invoked to explain the effects of DCT diuretics on calcium excretion. First, DCT diuretics stimulate calcium reabsorption along the proximal tubule because they contract ECF volume. Second, DCT diuretics stimulate calcium reabsorption along the distal tubule through their action on the Na–Cl cotransporter. When this pathway is blocked intracellular concentrations of Na⁺ and Cl⁻ decline. Low intracellular Cl⁻ concentrations hyperpolarize the cell membrane voltage which opens dihydropyridine-sensitive calcium channels in the luminal membrane and stimulates $Na^+–Ca^{2+}$ exchange at the basolateral cell membrane. Diuretic-induced reductions in intracellular Na⁺ concentrations may also stimulate $Na^+–Ca^{2+}$ exchange at the basolateral cell membrane. Both processes increase calcium reabsorption. The effects of DCT diuretics on calcium excretion form the basis for the use of these drugs to reduce the incidence of calcium nephrolithiasis.

Collecting Duct Diuretics

Sodium reabsorption by the collecting duct system, which amounts to only 3% of the filtered NaCl load, is primarily electrogenic (current generating), unlike transport along more proximal segments. Current moves because Na⁺ enters cells across the luminal membrane through ion channels. As in the other segments, the concentration of Na⁺ inside collecting duct (principal) cells is maintained below electrochemical equilibrium by the action of the Na,K-ATPase. As Na⁺ moves out of the lumen, it generates a voltage across the tubule wall that is oriented with the lumen negative, relative to the blood. This lumen-negative voltage helps to drive K⁺ movement in the secretory direction. Although Na⁺ and K⁺ do not traverse the same channel, their transport is coupled functionally by the transepithelial voltage.

Two major groups of diuretics act predominantly in the collecting duct. Sodium channel blockers, such as triamterene and amiloride, act from the lumen to inhibit Na⁺ movement through Na⁺ channels in principal cells. Because these drugs impair Na⁺ movement, the transepithelial voltage falls, inhibiting K⁺ secretion secondarily. This effect accounts for their K⁺ sparing action. It should be emphasized that, although amiloride inhibits renal Na⁺–H⁺ exchange in the proximal tubule, the proximal effect probably does not contribute to its diuretic action in humans because the

concentrations of amiloride achieved in the lumen of the proximal tubule during oral administration are insufficient to interfere with Na⁺–H⁺ exchange. The second class of collecting duct diuretics (CD diuretics) is represented by spironolactone, a competitive antagonist of aldosterone. Aldosterone, a mineralocorticoid hormone secreted by the adrenal gland in response to renin or high serum potassium concentrations, stimulates Na⁺ reabsorption and K⁺ secretion along the collecting duct, and increases the magnitude of the transepithelial voltage. By inhibiting the action of aldosterone, spironolactone causes mild natriuresis and potassium retention.

Because the collecting duct reabsorbs only a small percentage of the filtered Na⁺ load, collecting duct diuretics are relatively modest in potency. In the past, their use as sole agents has been limited to situations in which excessive aldosterone secretion plays a central pathogenic role; in patients with cirrhotic ascites, for example, spironolactone has been reported to be more effective than loop diuretics, as a single agent. Further, when hypertension is caused by adrenocortical hyperplasia, adequate blood pressure control can often be obtained with oral amiloride. The most common use of the collecting duct diuretics is to prevent excessive potassium wasting when combined with other, more potent, diuretics. Recently, interest in the utility of CD diuretics has been stimulated by suggestions that non renal actions of aldosterone may contribute to the pathogenesis of congestive heart failure and by suggestions that addition of these drugs to a traditional diuretic regimen may reduce the number of premature ventricular contractions in patients with congestive heart failure. A large multicenter trial is under way to examine the role of spironolactone in patients with congestive heart failure.

Osmotic Diuretics

Unlike other classes of diuretics, osmotic diuretics do not interfere directly with specific transport proteins but rather act as osmotic particles in tubule fluid. Water reabsorption throughout the nephron is driven by the osmotic gradients that are generated by solute transport. When an agent such as mannitol is administered, it is filtered but very poorly reabsorbed. Because the mannitol is retained in the tubule lumen, the osmolality of tubule fluid remains higher than normal, inhibiting fluid reabsorption. NaCl reabsorption is also inhibited, in this case because solute reabsorption dilutes tubule fluid, predisposing to NaCl backflux. Thus, these drugs tend to increase the excretion not only of fluid but of Na⁺, K⁺, Cl⁻, bicarbonate and other solutes. The urinary osmolality during osmotic diuresis tends to approach that of plasma, regardless of the state of hydration. Osmotic diuretics increase renal blood flow and wash out the medullary solute gradient, effects which contribute to the diuretic-induced impairment in urinary concentrating capacity.

Osmotic diuretics have been used to prevent acute renal failure following cardiopulmonary bypass, rhabdomyolysis, and radiocontrast exposure. Mannitol is also frequently employed to reduce cerebral edema, first by osmotic fluid removal from the brain and then by promoting diuresis. Although data in the settings of cardiopulmonary bypass and rhabdomyolysis are inconclusive, a recent, well-controlled study of patients exposed to radiocontrast agents indicated that renal failure was *more* common in the group that received mannitol than in the group that received half normal saline alone. Thus, mannitol appears to have no place in preventing contrast nephropathy.

ADAPTATION TO DIURETIC DRUGS

When a Loop diuretic is administered acutely, Na^+ and fluid excretion increase transiently. This natriuresis is followed by a period of positive NaCl balance, termed "postdiuretic NaCl retention" (see Fig. 2). The net effect of the diuretic on ECF volume during a 24-hour period is determined by the sum of NaCl losses during diuretic action (excretion > intake), and NaCl retention during periods when the drug concentration is low (intake > excretion). Factors that influence the relation between natriuresis and postdiuretic NaCl retention include the dietary NaCl intake, the dose of diuretic, its half-life, and the frequency with which it is administered. When loop diuretics are administered once daily to patients ingesting a high NaCl diet postdiuretic NaCl retention compensates entirely for NaCl losses during the period of drug action; net Na balance

remains neutral from the first day. When NaCl intake is restricted, Na avidity during the postdiuretic period cannot overcome the initial NaCl losses, Na balance is negative, and ECF volume declines. This relation between dietary NaCl intake and the net effect of diuretics accounts for the central role of dietary NaCl restriction in effective diuretic therapy.

Even when diuretic treatment does induce negative NaCl and fluid balance initially, neutral NaCl balance is achieved after several days to weeks because other adaptive mechanisms come into play, limiting the magnitude of the diuretic response (see "The Braking Phenomenon" (Fig. 2). Several mechanisms contribute to adaptation during chronic diuretic treatment. Contraction of the ECF volume, at least relative to pretreatment levels, may stimulate secretion of renin, aldosterone, and antidiuretic hormone which mediate renal NaCl and fluid retention. Contraction of the ECF volume may increase the activity of renal nerves which stimulates renal NaCl retention via direct effects on renal tubules. Contraction of the ECF volume may also reduce renal perfusion pressure and the GFR. In addition to adaptations that depend on changes in ECF volume, however, specific intrarenal effects of diuretics may also contribute to adaptation. Loop diuretics inhibit solute reabsorption by the thick ascending limb of Henle's loop, thereby increasing solute delivery to and solute reabsorp-

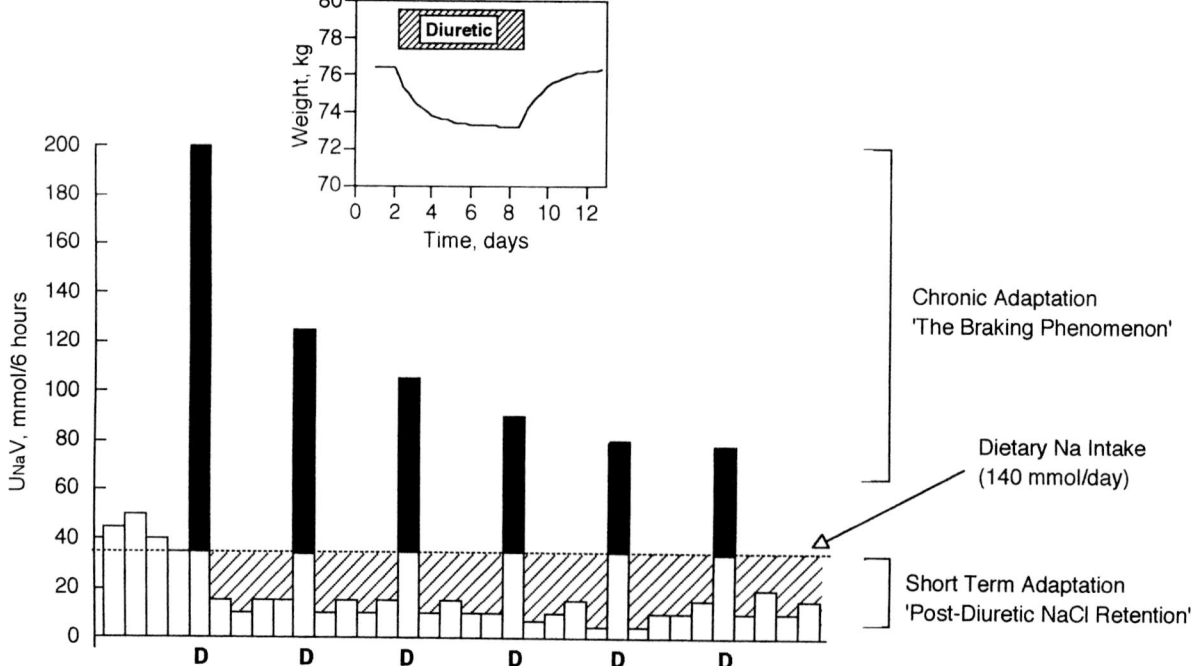

FIGURE 2 Effects of a loop diuretic on urinary Na^+ excretion. Bars represents 6 hours. Black bars indicate periods during which urinary Na^+ excretion exceeds dietary intake. Hatched areas indicate post diuretic NaCl retention, periods during which dietary Na^+ intake exceeds urinary Na^+ excretion. Changes in the magnitude of natriuretic response during several days are indicative of diuretic "braking." Dotted line indicates dietary Na^+ intake per 6-hour period. Inset is effect of diuretics on weight (and ECF volume) during several days of diuretic administration. From Ellison DH: In Sedin DW, Giebisch G (eds) *Diuretic Agents: Physiology and Pharmacology,* Academic Press, San Diego, 1997. With permission.

tion from the distal nephron. When solute delivery to the distal tubule is increased chronically (as during long-term diuretic therapy), distal tubule cells undergo substantial hypertrophy. This structural change is associated with increases in the ability of these cells to transport NaCl which participate in returning the patient to neutral NaCl balance. When these adaptive mechanisms occur prior to the achievement of acceptable levels of ECF volume, they may contribute importantly to diuretic resistance, as discussed below.

The goal of diuretic treatment of edema is not simply to increase urinary NaCl or fluid excretion. Instead, the goal is to reduce ECF volume to a clinically acceptable level and to maintain that volume chronically. To achieve this goal, urinary NaCl excretion must increase initially (Fig. 2), but excretion rates of NaCl and fluid return to pretreatment levels once steady state returns. Thus, during successful diuretic treatment of edema, when the patient's weight has stabilized, urinary NaCl excretion matches dietary intake; it is not increased above normal values.

COMPLICATIONS OF DIURETIC TREATMENT

The most common complications of diuretic treatment result directly from the effects of these drugs on renal fluid and electrolyte excretion and include ECF volume depletion, hyponatremia, and hypokalemia. Although both DCT and loop diuretics predispose to hypokalemia, disorders of K^+ homeostasis occur more frequently with DCT diuretics. Serum K^+ concentration declines by approximately 0.5 mM, when DCT diuretics are administered without KCl supplementation. Mild hypokalemia (<3.5 mM) occurs in up to 48% of patients during treatment with DCT diuretics (50 mg hydrochlorothiazide); moderate hypokalemia (<3.0 mM) occurs in up to 17%. During furosemide treatment mild hypokalemia occurs in 5% of patients, moderate hypokalemia in less than 1%. Frank hypokalemia during treatment of hypertension with a DCT diuretic should alert the clinician that increased renin or aldosterone secretion may be responsible for the hypertension (as occurs in Conn's syndrome or renovascular disease).

Several mechanisms contribute to the tendency of loop and DCT diuretics to cause hypokalemia. First, both classes of diuretics increase fluid flow through the distal nephron, the site at which K^+ secretion determines urinary K^+ excretion rates. High fluid flow rates stimulate K^+ secretion directly. Second, both loop and DCT diuretics stimulate secretion of aldosterone which also increases K^+ secretion along the distal nephron. Finally, both DCT and loop diuretics predispose to hypomagnesemia which contributes to the development of hypokalemia through unknown mechanisms. Hypokalemia has several adverse consequences. These include ventricular arrhythmias, especially during the administration of digitalis glycosides or when hypomagnesemia is present, and glucose intolerance. Hypokalemia may make control of blood pressure more difficult.

Methods to prevent or treat hypokalemia during diuretic therapy include: (1) using the lowest effective diuretic dose (especially for hypertension; see Chapter 35), (2) supplementing dietary K^+ (best administered as KCl, (3) restricting dietary Na^+, (4) preventing hypomagnesemia, and (5) using CD (K^+ sparing) diuretics together with loop or DCT diuretics. Serum concentrations of Na^+ and K^+ should be monitored in every patient who is treated with diuretics and most patients should be encouraged to consume a diet rich in K^+ and low in Na^+. Many physicians treat patients whose serum K^+ concentration falls below 3.5 mM, although some have suggested that K^+ concentrations between 3.0 and 3.5 mM do not require treatment. Certainly, if a patient is at risk for complications of hypokalemia, e.g., patients receiving digitalis glycosides or patients with hepatic cirrhosis, K concentrations should be maintained above 3.5 mM. Of note, adding a CD diuretic not only corrects hypokalemia in many patients, but may also prevent hypomagnesemia; hypomagnesemia may act synergistically with hypokalemia to predispose to ventricular arrhythmias.

Hyperkalemia is a complication of the CD diuretics. Hyperkalemia occurs most commonly in patients with renal failure or in patients taking ACE inhibitors. Triamterene metabolism is impaired in patients with cirrhosis. In addition, the drug precipitates hyperkalemia in this group of patients.

Mild metabolic alkalosis occurs frequently during treatment with loop and DCT diuretics. These drugs promote urinary losses of NaCl (leaving HCO_3^- behind). Further, they increase aldosterone secretion, which stimulates the proton secretion directly. Metabolic alkalosis can exacerbate hepatic encephalopathy and can inhibit respiratory drive. Severe metabolic alkalosis is often a manifestation of overly aggressive therapy. Loop diuretics or combination diuretic therapy (see below) may also lead to excessive ECF volume depletion and vascular collapse.

Hyponatremia may develop during treatment with loop diuretics, but this complication is more common with DCT diuretics (thiazides and their congeners). Some patients treated with thiazide diuretics develop severe and potentially life-threatening hyponatremia, often several days to weeks after initiation of diuretic therapy. The tendency for hyponatremia to recur can be assessed by measuring body weight and serum [Na] before and 6 to 8 hours after a single dose of DCT diuretic. If the serum [Na] falls below 136 mM following diuretic administration, the patient is at high risk for severe hyponatremia. In these patients, DCT diuretics appear to stimulate excessive fluid intake which contributes to weight gain and hyponatremia. Thiazide diuretics and, less commonly, loop diuretics also predispose to glucose intolerance, hyperlipidemia, and hyperuricemia, when administered chronically. Although the mechanisms by which these complications develop are not completely clear, hypokalemia and ECF volume contraction may contribute. Serum concentrations of glucose, lipids, and uric acid should be monitored in patients on chronic diuretic treatment.

Some complications of diuretic treatment are drug or group specific and reflect toxic side effects; allergic interstitial nephritis is an idiosyncratic reaction to diuretics that may precipitate skin rash and acute renal failure. Ototoxicity is a toxic effect to loop diuretics that occurs most commonly when high doses are administered rapidly (furosemide iv > 15 mg/min) to patients with renal insufficiency. Triamterene can cause renal stones and may precipitate acute renal failure when administered with indomethacin. Spironolactone causes gynecomastia, especially in patients with cirrhosis of the liver.

DIURETIC TREATMENT OF EDEMA

Edema is a manifestation of disordered NaCl homeostasis. The NaCl retention often reflects a physiological response to what the kidneys perceive as inadequate arterial blood volume, as occurs in congestive heart failure. In other situations, NaCl retention may reflect an abnormal renal response, resulting from damage to the kidney, as occurs in renal failure. In either case, therapeutic maneuvers should be aimed first at correcting the primary disorder. Often, however, such maneuvers are not available or do not contact the ECF volume adequately and more direct methods of effecting NaCl removal are needed. Before initiating treatment with diuretic drugs, it is important to begin the patient on a diet low in NaCl. Extracellular fluid volume varies directly with NaCl intake, both in normal and edematous individuals. For patients with mild ECF volume expansion, a "no added salt" diet may be appropriate (4 g Na/day); for more severe edema, a low Na diet (2 g Na/day) should be prescribed. Even when dietary restriction alone is unsuccessful and diuretic drugs are administered, the dietary Na intake must be restricted below 4 g/day for diuretics to be effective. A second important consideration before initiating diuretic therapy is to improve the general management of the patient by discontinuing, when possible, drugs that predispose to NaCl retention or interfere with diuretic efficacy. Nonsteroidal antiinflammatory drugs (NSAIDs) promote renal NaCl retention directly and interfere with the efficacy of loop and DCT diuretics. Many vasodilators promote edema; minoxidil frequently causes significant ECF volume expansion; calcium channel blockers promote edema despite intrinsic natriuretic properties, perhaps through local vasodilation. Other antihypertensive drugs may also predispose to NaCl retention by reducing renal perfusion.

Once the decision to initiate diuretic therapy has been made, the initial choice of drug and dosage depends on the underlying cause of edema and its severity. Hypertension often responds to very low doses of a DCT diuretic (e.g., 12.5 mg/day of hydrochlorothiazide), doses which tend to cause few side effects. Cirrhotic edema and ascites frequently respond to spironolactone (100–300 mg daily); spironolactone may be more effective than furosemide in these patients. Moderate edema associated with congestive heart failure may respond to a DCT diuretic such as hydrochlorothiazide, in doses of 25 to 50 mg/day; some studies suggest that a DCT diuretic may reduce ECF volume more effectively than loop diuretics in patients with very mild congestive heart failure. But when edema from congestive heart failure, cirrhosis, or nephrotic syndrome is more than mild, when renal failure is present, or in the presence of pulmonary congestion or severe symptoms, loop diuretics are the drugs of choice.

Loop diuretics have the highest natriuretic potency, are active at all levels of renal function, and act rapidly even following oral administration. The drugs have steep dose response curve; as the dose is increased, there is little response until a critical threshold is reached, above which diuretic effectiveness increases rapidly to a maximum. When a loop diuretic is administered in a dose that exceeds the threshold, most patients experience an increase in urine output that is noticeable during the several hours after diuretic ingestion. To be effective, each dose of loop diuretic must exceed this threshold. When initiating oral diuretic therapy, a target is set for weight loss and a low dose of loop diuretic (20 mg furosemide or its equivalent) is begun once daily. If urine output rises during 4 to 6 hours after diuretic ingestion, the same dose is continued on a daily basis (unless weight loss exceeds the target value). If urine output does not rise, the patient may double the dose the following day (to 40 mg once daily). If there is no response, the dose can be doubled each day until a response is obtained or until the maximum safe dose is achieved. In normal individuals, 40 mg of furosemide orally produces maximal diuresis, but in patients with edema or renal failure, larger doses are frequently necessary (even in renal failure, there is little to be gained by increasing doses beyond 240 mg furosemide or 8 mg bumetanide, iv). Often, the dose that elicits an increase in urine output can be continued indefinitely, because adaptive mechanisms such as those discussed above, bring the patient back into NaCl balance once ECF volume has been reduced. Sometimes, however, patients may be maintained with lower doses than were necessary to elicit diuresis initially, once control of the ECF volume is achieved.

DIURETIC RESISTANCE: CAUSES AND TREATMENT

Control of ECF volume expansion can be attained in most edematous patients using the approach outlined above. In some circumstances, however, moderate or high doses of loop diuretics do not reduce ECF volume to the desired level even when used appropriately, and thus the patient is deemed resistant to diuretic therapy. The determination of what ECF volume is acceptable depends on many factors including the severity of the underlying disease, patient preference, and co-morbid illness. When further reductions in ECF volume are necessary, a systematic approach (see Fig. 3) to diuretic resistance usually leads to a treatment regimen that is safe and is effective. One of the most common causes of apparent resistance to diuretic drugs is dietary indiscretion because, as discussed above, dietary NaCl excess abrogates the effect of most diuretic regimens; the influence of dietary NaCl intake is most pronounced for the loop diuretics. If the patient's weight is stable, dietary compliance can be assessed by measuring the amount of Na excreted during 24 hours. A urinary Na

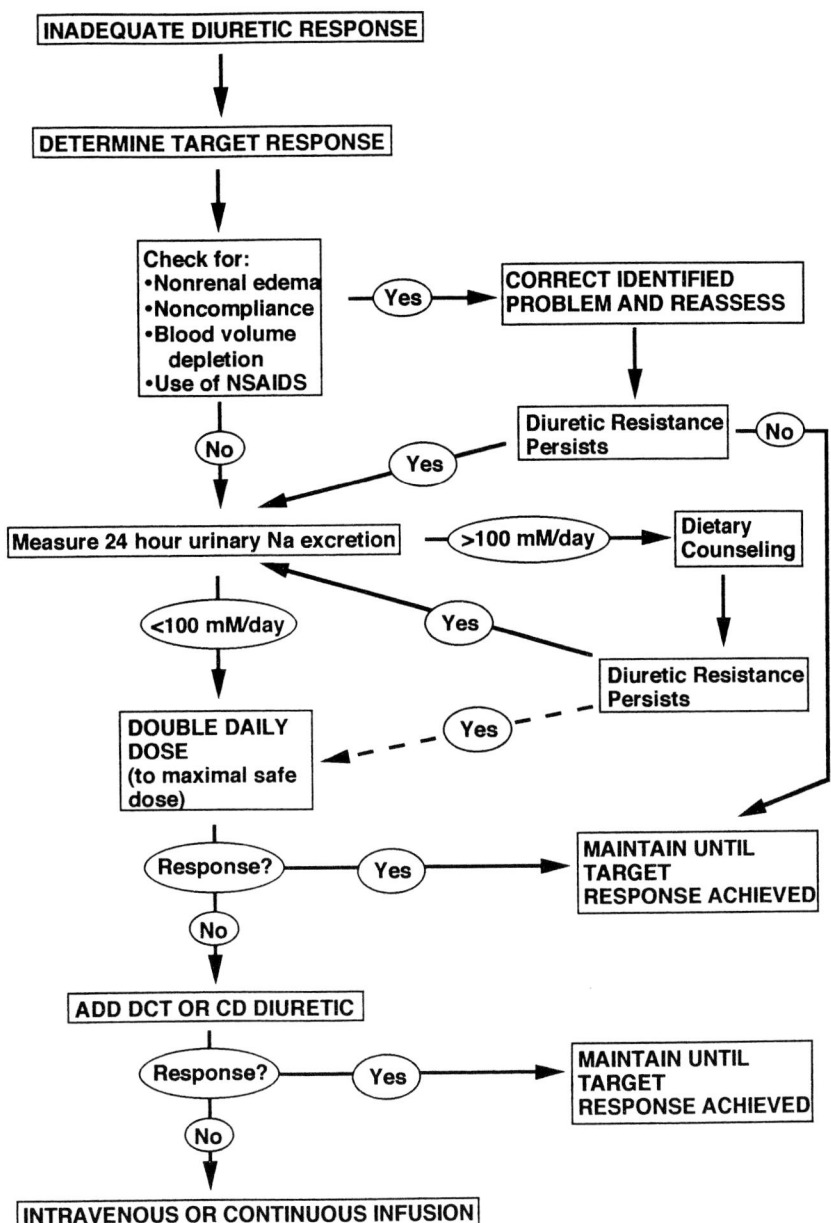

FIGURE 3 Algorithm for diuretic resistant patients. Regimens for combination therapy are given in the text. Continuous infusions can be administered according to the following schedules; furosemide: 20 to 80 mg load followed by 2 to 80 mg/h; bumetanide 1 mg load followed by 0.2 mg/h; torsemide 25 mg load followed by 1 to 50 mg/h. NSAIDs, nonsteroidal antiinflammatory drugs. From Wilcox CS: In *The Kidney,* Brenner B (ed) 5th ed. Saunders, Philadelphia, 1996.

excretion rate greater than 100 to 120 mmol (equivalent to 2–3 g Na per day) indicates both that the patient is ingesting too much NaCl and that true diuretic resistance is not present; Na excretion rates near or above 120 mmol/day should be sufficient to effect weight loss when patients ingest less than this quantity on a daily basis. Of course, dietary compliance cannot always be ensured, and more

intensive regimens (see below) may provide effective diuresis for patients who continue to ingest too much NaCl.

Absorption of many diuretics is variable. The gastrointestinal absorption of furosemide varies by as much as 60% from day to day in a single individual, averaging around 50 to 60% (this effect is true of both Lasix and other brands of furosemide). Gastrointestinal absorption may be slowed further by edema of the gut, such as occurs in some patients with congestive heart failure. When there is concern about bioavailability, it may be advantageous to use torsemide or bumetanide, rather than furosemide, because bioavailability exceeds 80% for these drugs. If a more bioavailable drug is not effective, iv therapy may be necessary until edema is controlled; at this time, diuretic absorption may improve again and oral therapy may once again become effective.

Once a loop or DCT diuretic drug has been absorbed into the bloodstream, it reaches the lumen of the kidney tubule via the organic anion secretory pathway located in the proximal tubule. This pathway also interacts with NSAIDs and probenecid, as well as with endogenous anions that accumulate in renal failure. When NSAIDs have been administered to patients with renal failure, diuretic secretion into the lumen of the proximal tubule is inhibited and less diuretic reaches its active site for any given serum concentration. To overcome the inhibition, higher serum levels are needed. This is one reason why high doses of diuretic drugs are required to elicit diuresis in patients with renal failure. Of note, although the ratio of equipotent doses of furosemide to bumetanide is 40:1 in patients with normal renal function, it falls to 20:1 in patients with renal failure because nonrenal furosemide clearance is impaired. Torsemide has both renal and nonrenal clearance. Therefore, its clearance rate is relatively stable in the face of either renal or hepatic disease. In general, when switching from intravenous to oral furosemide, twice the oral dose is given. When switching from intravenous to oral torsemide, the conversion is one to one.

Diuretic resistance is common in patients with the nephrotic syndrome. Hypoalbuminemia reduces the serum concentration of diuretics because it increases their volume of distribution (diuretics are extensively protein bound). Further, hypoalbuminemia may predispose to renal vasoconstriction. Because albumin is filtered by the abnormal glomeruli, renal clearance of diuretics is actually increased, but the diuretic in the tubule lumen may be inactive because it is bound to filtered albumin in tubule fluid and is not free to interact with the transport protein. In these situations, increasing the dose, changing from oral to intravenous therapy, or infusing diuretic mixed together with albumin may improve the therapeutic response. Experimental approaches to patients with nephrotic syndrome include administering inhibitors of diuretic–protein interactions.

Inadequate renal perfusion from any cause compromises diuretic effectiveness. For patients in whom low cardiac output contributes to Na retention, low dose dopamine $(2-4 \, \mu g \cdot kg^{-1} \cdot min^{-1})$ may increase renal plasma flow and increase urine flow (dopamine may also increase urine flow in patients with acute renal failure), but the effects of "renal dose" dopamine are controversial and poorly documented. When edema results from cirrhosis of the liver, removal of ascitic fluid by paracentesis or peritoneovenous shunting may improve renal function and Na^+ excretion. Arterial hypoxemia causes renal vasoconstriction resulting in antinatriuresis, which reverses promptly when the arterial oxygen tension increases above 60 mm Hg. Renal vasoconstric-

tors, such as NSAIDs and adrenergic agonists may also lead to diuretic resistance, in part by reducing GFR, and should be avoided in the diuretic-resistant patient. The effects of drugs used to reduce cardiac afterload on renal NaCl excretion are complex. When ACE inhibitors or nitroprusside increase cardiac output effectively, they may stimulate natriuresis and reduce edema. On the other hand, when aggressive therapy reduces blood pressure beyond a critical threshold (which may be surprisingly high in patients with severe vascular disease), it may lead to NaCl retention and even renal failure. This is especially common during concomitant administration of NSAIDs, when bilateral renal artery stenosis is present, or during very aggressive diuretic therapy.

Not uncommonly, simple approaches to diuretic resistance fail. Several strategies are available to achieve effective control of ECF volume in such patients. First loop diuretics may be administered more frequently than once a day, especially if postdiuretic Na retention is contributing importantly to NaCl retention. Recall, however, that each dose must be above the diuretic threshold to be effective. Second, a diuretic of another class may be added to a regimen that contains a loop diuretic. This strategy produces true synergism; the combination of agents is more effective than the *sum* of the responses to each agent alone. DCT diuretics are the class of drug most commonly combined with loop diuretics, although synergism occurs when loop diuretics are combined with carbonic anhydrase inhibitors and theophylline as well. These drugs act synergistically for several reasons. First, loop diuretics increase NaCl delivery to the distal tubule, a site at which NaCl transport depends on the luminal NaCl concentration. Loop diuretics, therefore, stimulate NaCl reabsorption in the DCT diuretic-sensitive segment. Adding a DCT diuretic will inhibit NaCl transport along the stimulated segment. Second, when loop diuretics are administered chronically, cells in the distal tubule enlarge, further increasing their ability to transport NaCl. DCT diuretics inhibit the increased NaCl reabsorption that accompanies hypertrophy of the distal nephron and therefore counteract the effects of hypertrophy. Third, as discussed above, the efficacy of loop diuretics reflects the balance between natriuresis during diuretic action and Na retention when diuretic concentrations decline. DCT diuretics have longer half lives than loop diuretics. The former therefore prevent or attenuate NaCl retention during the periods between doses of loop diuretics, thereby increasing the latter's net effect. Thus, at least three mechanisms contribute to the ability of DCT diuretics to act synergistically with loop acting drugs.

When two diuretics are combined, the DCT diuretic is generally administered some time before the loop diuretic (1 hour is reasonable) in order to ensure that NaCl transport in the distal nephron is blocked when it is flooded with solute. When intravenous therapy is indicated, chlorothiazide (500–1000 mg) may be employed. Metolazone is the DCT diuretic most frequently combined with loop diuretics because its half-life is relatively long (as formulated in Zaroxolyn) and because it has been reported to be effective even when renal failure is present. Other thiazide and thiazide-like diuretics, however, may be equally effective. The dramatic effectiveness of combination diuretic therapy is accompanied by complications in a significant number of patients. Massive fluid and electrolyte losses have led to circulatory collapse during combination therapy and patients must be followed carefully. The lowest effective dose of DCT diuretic should be added to the loop diuretic regimen; patients can frequently be treated with combination therapy for only a few days and then must be placed back on a single drug regimen. When continuous combination therapy is needed, low doses of DCT diuretic (2.5 mg metolazone or 25 mg hydrochlorothiazide) administered only two or three times per week may be sufficient.

For hospitalized patients who are resistant to diuretic therapy, a different approach is to infuse loop diuretics continuously (see Fig. 3). Continuous diuretic infusions have several advantages over bolus diuretic administration. First, because they avoid peaks and troughs of diuretic concentration, continuous infusions prevent periods of positive NaCl balance (postdiuretic NaCl retention) from occurring. Second, continuous infusions are more efficient than bolus therapy (the amount of NaCl excreted per mg of drug administered is greater). Third, some patients who are resistant to large doses of diuretics given by bolus have responded to continuous infusion. Fourth, diuretic response can be titrated; in the intensive care unit where obligate fluid administration must be balanced by fluid excretion, excellent control of NaCl and water excretion can be obtained. Finally, complications associated with high doses of loop diuretics, such as ototoxicity, appear to be less common when large doses are administered as continuous infusion. Total daily furosemide doses exceeding 1 g have been tolerated well when administered over 24 hours. One approach is to administer a loading dose of 20 mg furosemide followed by a continuous infusion of 4 to 60 mg/h. In patients with preserved renal function, therapy at the lower dosage range should be sufficient. When renal failure is present, higher doses may be used, but patients should be monitored carefully for side effects such as ECF volume depletion and ototoxicity.

Most patients who are deemed resistant to diuretics respond to these approaches. Rather than lack of efficacy, side effects of diuretic therapy such as increases in serum creatinine concentration often limit the ability to reduce ECF volume further. Obtaining effective control of ECF volume without provoking complications requires a thorough understanding of diuretic physiology and a commitment to use diuretics rationally and carefully. When used in this manner, diuretics remain among the most powerful drugs in clinical medicine.

Bibliography

Andreasen F, Eriksen UH, Fuul SJ, et al.: A comparison of three diuretic regimens in heart failure. *Eur J Clinical Invest* 23:234–239, 1993.

Barr CS, Lanc CC, Hanson J, Arnott M, Kennedy N, Struthers AD: Effects of adding spironolactone to an angiotensin-converting enzyme inhibitor in chronic congestive heart failure secondary to coronary artery disease. *Am J Cardiol* 76:1259–1265, 1995.

Denton MD, Chertow GM, Brady HM: "Renal-dose" dopamine for the treatment of acute renal failure: Scientific rationale, experimental studies and clinical trials. *Kidney Int* 49:4–14, 1996.

Dormans TP, Van Meyel JJ, Gerlag PG, Tan Y, Russel FG, Smits P: Diuretic efficacy of high dose furosemide in severe heart failure: Bolus injection versus continuous infusion. *J Am Coll Cardiol* 28:376–382, 1996.

Ellison DH: The physiologic basis of diuretic synergism: Its role in treating diuretic resistance. *Ann Intern Med* 114:886–894, 1991.

Ellison DH: Diuretic drugs and the treatment of edema: From clinic to bench and back again. *Am J Kidney Dis* 23:623–643, 1994.

Fliser D, Schröter M, Neubeck M, Ritz E: Coadministration of thiazides increases the efficacy of loop diuretics even in patients with advanced renal failure. *Kidney Int* 46:482–488, 1994.

Leary WP, Reyes AJ: Renal excretory actions of diuretics in man: Correction of various current errors and redefinition of basic concepts. In: Reyes AJ, Leary WP (eds) *Progress in Pharmacology.* pp. 153–166, 1988.

Martin SJ, Danziger LH: Continuous infusion of loop diuretics in the critically ill: A review of the literature. *Crit Care Med* 22:1323–1329, 1994.

Rose BD: Diuretics. *Kidney Int* 39:336–352, 1991.

Rudy DW, Voelker JR, Greene PK, Esparza FA, Brater DC: Loop diuretics for chronic renal insufficiency: A continuous infusion is more efficacious than bolus therapy. *Ann Intern Med* 115:360–366, 1991.

Solomon R, Werner C, Mann D, D'Elia J, Silva P: Effects of saline, mannitol, and furosemide on acute decreases in renal function induced by radiocontrast agents. *N Engl J Med* 331:1416–1420, 1994.

Wilcox CS: Diuretics. In: Brenner BM (ed) *The Kidney,* 5th ed. Saunders, Philadelphia, 1996, pp. 2299–2330.

Wilcox CS, Mitch WE, Kelly RA, et al: Response of the kidney to furosemide: I. Effects of salt intake and renal compensation. *J Lab Clin Med* 102:450–458, 1983.

SECTION 3

GLOMERULAR DISEASES

16

GLOMERULAR CLINICOPATHOLOGIC SYNDROMES

J. CHARLES JENNETTE AND RONALD J. FALK

Injury to glomeruli results in a variety of signs and symptoms of disease, including proteinuria caused by altered permeability of capillary walls, hematuria caused by rupture of capillary walls, azotemia caused by impaired filtration of nitrogenous wastes, oliguria or anuria caused by reduced urine production, edema caused by salt and water retention, and hypertension caused by fluid retention and disturbed renal homeostasis of blood pressure. The nature and severity of disease in a given patient is dictated by the nature and severity of glomerular injury.

Specific glomerular diseases tend to produce particular syndromes of renal dysfunction, although multiple glomerular diseases can produce the same syndrome (Tables 1 and 2). The diagnosis of a glomerular disease requires recognition of one of these syndromes, followed by collection of data to determine which specific glomerular disease is present. Alternatively if reaching a specific diagnosis is not possible or necessary, the physician should focus efforts on narrowing the differential diagnosis to a likely candidate disease.

Evaluation of pathologic features identified in a renal biopsy specimen may be required for definitive diagnosis. The pathologic features of various glomerular diseases are described in the corresponding chapters of this book. Figure 1 depicts some of the clinical and pathologic features used to resolve the differential diagnosis in patients with antibody-mediated glomerulonephritis, Figures 2–5 illustrate the distinctive ultrastructural features of some of the major categories of glomerular disease, Figure 6 illustrates some of the major patterns of immune deposition identified by immunofluorescence microscopy.

ASYMPTOMATIC HEMATURIA AND RECURRENT GROSS HEMATURIA

Hematuria is usually defined as greater than 3 red blood cells per high power field observed by microscopic examination of a centrifuged urine sediment (see Chapter 3). Asymptomatic hematuria is hematuria that a patient is unaware of and that is not accompanied by clinical manifestations of nephritis or nephrotic syndrome, that is, without azotemia, oliguria, edema, or hypertension. Asymptomatic microscopic hematuria has a prevalence of 5 to 10% in the general population. Recurrent gross hematuria may be superimposed on asymptomatic microscopic hematuria, or may occur in isolation. The patient observes urine discoloration, which often is described as tea or Cola colored.

All hematuria is not of glomerular origin. In fact, most hematuria is not of glomerular origin. Glomerular diseases cause less than 10% of hematuria in patients with no proteinuria, with almost 80% being caused by bladder, prostate, or urethral disease. Hypercalciuria and hyperuricosuria also can cause asymptomatic hematuria, especially in children.

Microscopic examination of the urine can help determine whether hematuria is of glomerular or nonglomerular origin. Chemical (e.g., osmotic) trauma to red blood cells as they pass through the nephron causes structural changes that are not present in red blood cells that have hemorrhaged directly into the urine from a gross parenchymal injury in the kidney (e.g., a neoplasm) or from a lesion in the urinary tract (e.g., renal pelvis traumatized by stones or an inflamed bladder). Dysmorphic red blood cells that have transited the urinary tract from the glomeruli usually have lost their biconcave configuration and hemoglobin, and often have multiple membrane blebs, sometimes producing acanthocytes and "Mickey Mouse cells." The presence of red blood cell casts and other sediment abnormalities typical of glomerulonephritis also supports a glomerular origin for hematuria.

Published series of renal biopsies carried out in patients with asymptomatic hematuria show differences in the frequencies of identified underlying glomerular lesions. Differences in the nature of the population analyzed (e.g., military recruits vs routine physical examination patients), and differences in pathologic analysis (e.g., failure of the earlier studies to recognize thin basement membrane nephropathy) account for the observed disparities. The data presented in Table 3 are derived from patients with hematuria who underwent diagnostic renal biopsy. The data in the first column equate with asymptomatic hematuria, and are similar to other recent series. In these patients with hematuria, less than 1 g/24 hr proteinuria and serum creatinine less than 1.5 mg/DL, the three major findings were no pathologic abnormality (30%), thin basement membrane nephropathy (26%), and IgA nephropathy (28%). Whereas

TABLE I

Clinical Manifestations of Glomerular Diseases, and Representative Diseases That Present with These Manifestations

Asymptomatic proteinuria	Acute nephritis
Focal segmental glomerulosclerosis	Acute diffuse proliferative GN
Mesangioproliferative GN	Poststreptococcal GN
	Poststaphylococcal GN
Nephrotic syndrome	Focal or diffuse proliferative GN
Minimal change glomerulopathy	IgA nephropathy
Membranous glomerulopathy	Lupus nephritis
Idiopathic (Primary)	Type I membranoproliferative GN
Secondary (e.g., lupus)	Type II membranoproliferative GN
Focal segmental glomerulosclerosis	Fibrillary GN
Mesangioproliferative GN	Rapidly progressive nephritis
Type I membranoproliferative GN	Crescentic GN
Type II membranoproliferative GN	Anti-GBM GN
Fibrillary GN	Immune complex GN
Diabetic glomerulosclerosis	ANCA GN
Amyloidosis	Pulmonary–renal vasculitic syndrome
Light-chain deposition disease	Goodpasture's (Anti-GBM) syndrome
Asymptomatic microscopic hematuria	Immune complex vasculitis
Thin basement membrane nephropathy	Lupus
IgA nephropathy	ANCA vasculitis
Mesangioproliferative GN	Microscopic polyangiitis
Alport's syndrome	Wegener's granulomatosis
Recurrent gross hematuria	Churg-Strauss syndrome
Thin basement membrane nephropathy	Chronic renal failure
IgA nephropathy	Chronic sclerosing GN
Alport's syndrome	

Note that the same manifestations can be caused by different diseases, and that the same disease can manifest in different ways. GN, glomerulonephritis; GBM, glomerular basement membrane; ANCA, antineutrophil cytoplasmic autoantibodies.

thin basement membrane nephropathy virtually always manifests as asymptomatic hematuria or recurrent gross hematuria, IgA nephropathy can manifest any of the syndromes listed in Table 1 (see Chapter 22).

Alport syndrome is an hereditary disease caused by a defect in the genes that code for basement membrane type IV collagen (see Chapter 46). In affected males, Alport syndrome initially manifests as asymptomatic microscopic hematuria, sometimes with superimposed episodes of gross hematuria. The hematuria usually begins in the first decade of life. Progressively worsening proteinuria and renal insufficiency eventually develop, although the rate of progression is quite variable. Affected females, who are almost always heterozygous, often have intermittent microscopic hematuria but may have no other manifestations of renal disease.

Renal biopsy is not usually performed to evaluate asymptomatic hematuria. Renal biopsy diagnoses rarely affect treatment in patients with asymptomatic hematuria, but occasional patients will be found to have disease that might benefit from treatment (e.g., the one patient with early crescentic glomerulonephritis identified in the cohort of patients in the first column of Table 3). Renal biopsy is also of some prognostic value. For example, thin basement membrane nephropathy has a better prognosis and a much

greater propensity for familial occurrence than IgA nephropathy. Many patients with asymptomatic hematuria are subjected to repeated invasive urologic evaluations until a definitive diagnosis can be made. In these patients, additional urologic evaluation can be prevented if renal biopsy provides a diagnosis.

In renal biopsy specimens, thin basement membrane nephropathy is diagnosed based on thinning of the glomerular basement membrane lamina densa (Fig. 3), whereas Alport's syndrome is suspected if there is marked lamination of the lamina densa. The presence of mesangial immune deposits with a dominance or codominance of immunohistologic staining for IgA is diagnostic for IgA nephropathy (Fig. 6).

ACUTE GLOMERULONEPHRITIS AND RAPIDLY PROGRESSIVE GLOMERULONEPHRITIS

Acute and rapidly progressive glomerulonephritis often present with acute onset of manifestations of nephritis, such as azotemia, oliguria, edema, hypertension, proteinuria, and hematuria with an "active" urine sediment that often contains red blood cell casts, pigmented casts, and cellular debris. Rapidly progressive glomerulonephritis leads to a 50% or greater loss of renal function within

TABLE 2

Tendencies of Glomerular Diseases to Manifest Nephrotic and Nephritic Features

	Nephrotic features	Nephritic features
Minimal change glomerulopathy	++++	−
Membranous glomerulopathy	++++	+
Diabetic glomerulosclerosis	++++	+
Amyloidosis	++++	+
Focal segmental glomerulosclerosis	+++	++
Fibrillary glomerulonephritis	+++	++
Mesangioproliferative glomerulopathy[a]	++	++
Membranoproliferative glomerulonephritis[b]	++	+++
Proliferative glomerulonephritis[a]	++	+++
Acute diffuse proliferative glomerulonephritis[c]	+	++++
Crescentic glomerulonephritis[d]	+	++++

[a] Mesangioproliferative and proliferative glomerulonephritis (focal or diffuse) are structural manifestations of a number of glomerulonephritides, including IgA nephropathy and lupus nephritis.

[b] Both type I (mesangiocapillary) and type II (dense deposit disease).

[c] Often a structural manifestation of acute poststreptococcal glomerulonephritis.

[d] Can be immune complex mediated, antiglomerular basement membrane antibody mediated, or associated with antineutrophil cytoplasmic autoantibodies.

Note that most diseases can manifest both nephrotic and nephritic features, but there usually is a tendency for one to predominate. From Jennette JC, Mandal AK (eds): *Diagnosis and Management of Renal Disease and Hypertension.* Carolina Academic Press, Durham, NC, 1994. With permission.

weeks to months. If renal failure is severe, manifestations of uremia develop, such as nausea and vomiting, hiccups, dyspnea, lethargy, pericarditis, and encephalopathy. Severe volume overload can cause congestive heart failure and pulmonary edema.

The pathologic processes that most often produce the clinical manifestations of acute or rapidly progressive nephritis are inflammatory glomerular lesions. The nature and severity of the glomerular inflammation correlate with the clinical features of the nephritis (Fig. 7). Note in Fig. 7 that the structural stages of glomerular inflammation can change over time, and this is reflected by changes in the clinical manifestations of nephritis.

The structurally least severe injury is mesangial hyperplasia alone, which usually causes asymptomatic proteinuria or hematuria rather than overt nephritis. Proliferative glomerulonephritis, which may be focal (affecting less than 50% of glomeruli), or diffuse (affecting greater than 50% of glomeruli), is characterized histologically not only by the proliferation of glomerular cells (e.g., mesangial, endothelial, and epithelial cells), but also by the influx of leukocytes, especially neutrophils and mononuclear phagocytes. Necrosis and sclerosis also may be present.

Lupus nephritis provides a paradigm of the interrelationships among pathogenic mechanisms, pathologic consequences, and clinical manifestations of glomerular disease (Fig. 4). The mildest expression of lupus nephritis (mesangioproliferative lupus glomerulonephritis, class II lupus nephritis) is induced by exclusively mesangial localization of immune complexes that usually causes only mild nephritis or asymptomatic hematuria and proteinuria. Localization

of substantial amounts of nephritogenic immune complexes in the subendothelial zones of glomerular capillaries where they are adjacent to the inflammatory mediator systems in the blood induces overt glomerular inflammation (focal or diffuse proliferative lupus glomerulonephritis, class III or IV lupus nephritis) and usually causes severe clinical manifestations of nephritis. Qualitative and quantitative characteristics of the pathogenic immune complexes that result in localization predominantly in subepithelial zones where they are not in contact with the cellular inflammatory mediator systems in the blood induces membranous lupus glomerulonephritis (class V lupus nephritis). In this form the nephrotic syndrome rather than nephritis is usually observed. As the nephritogenic immune response in a given patient changes over time and in response to treatment, transitions may occur between different lupus nephritis phenotypes (see Chapter 58).

The structurally most severe form of active glomerulonephritis is crescentic glomerulonephritis, which manifests clinically as rapidly progressive glomerulonephritis. In patients with new onset renal disease who have a nephritic sediment and a serum creatinine >3 g/24 hr, glomerulonephritis with crescents is the most common finding in renal biopsy specimens (Table 3). Crescents are proliferations of cells within Bowman's capsule that include both mononuclear phagocytes and glomerular epithelial cells. Since crescent formation is a response to glomerular rupture, it is a marker of severe glomerular injury. Crescents do not indicate the cause of glomerular injury, because many different pathogenic mechanisms can cause crescent formation. There is no consensus on how many glomeruli should

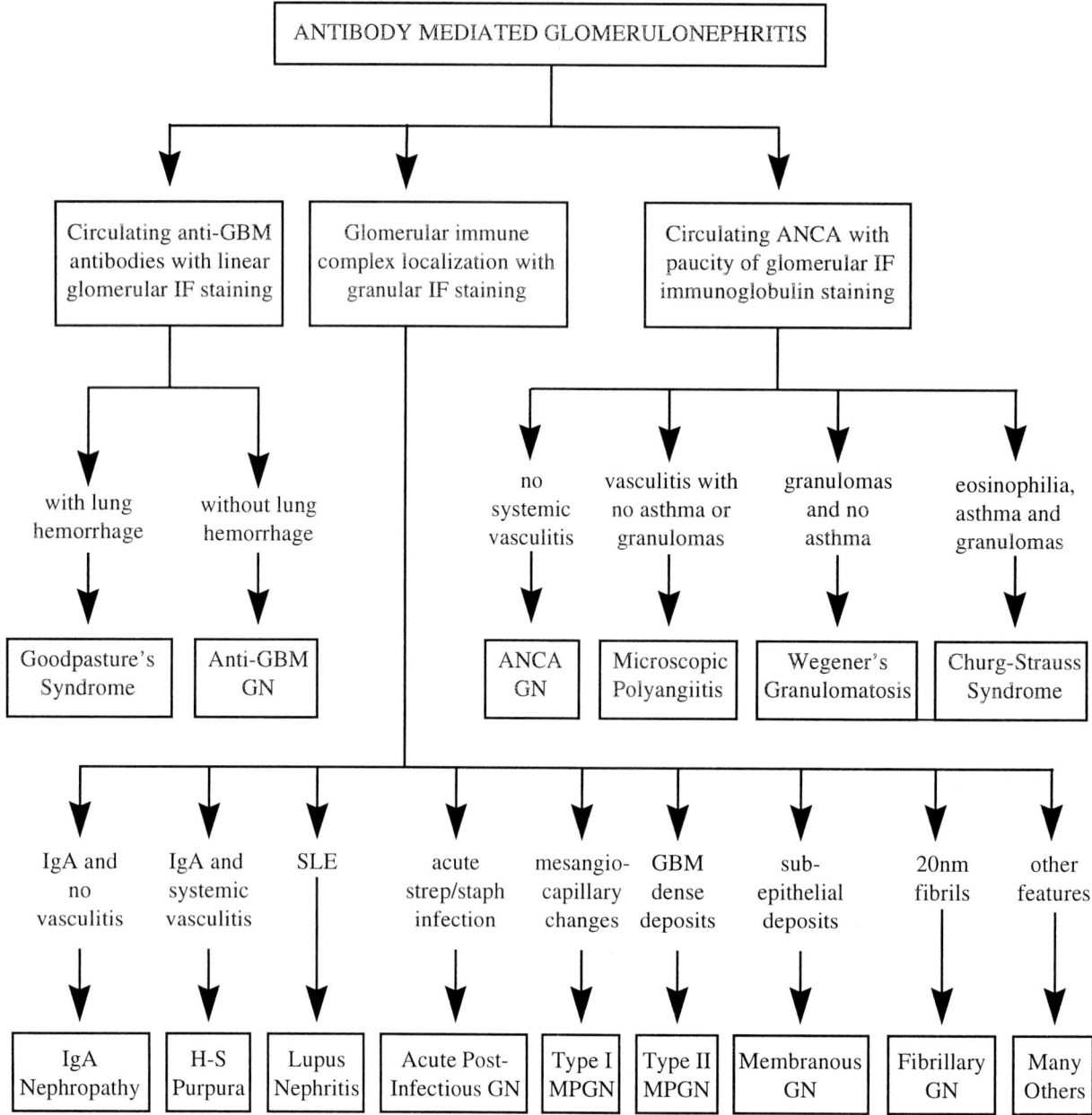

FIGURE 1 Features that distinguish different immunopathologic categories of antibody-mediated glomerulonephritis. GBM, glomerular basement membrane; IF, immunofluorescence microscopy; ANCA, anti-neutrophil cytoplasmic autoantibodies; GN, glomerulonephritis; H-S, Henoch-Schönlein; MPGN, membranoproliferative glomerulonephritis.

have crescents before the term crescentic glomerulonephritis can be applied. Most pathologists use the term when more than 50% of glomeruli have crescents, but the percenter of glomeruli with crescents should be specified in the diagnosis, even if it is less than 50% (e.g., IgA nephropathy with focal proliferative glomerulonephritis and 25% crescents). Within a specific pathogenic category of glomerulonephritis (e.g. anti-GBM disease, lupus nephritis, IgA nephropathy, poststreptococcal glomerulonephritis), the

higher the percentage of glomeruli with crescents the worse the prognosis. Among pathogenetically different glomerulonephritides, however, the pathogenic category may be more important in predicting outcome than the presence of crescents. For example, a patient with poststreptococcal glomerulonephritis with 50% crescents has a much better prognosis for renal survival, even without immunosuppressive treatment, than a patient with anti-GBM glomerulonephritis or ANCA glomerulonephritis with 25% crescents.

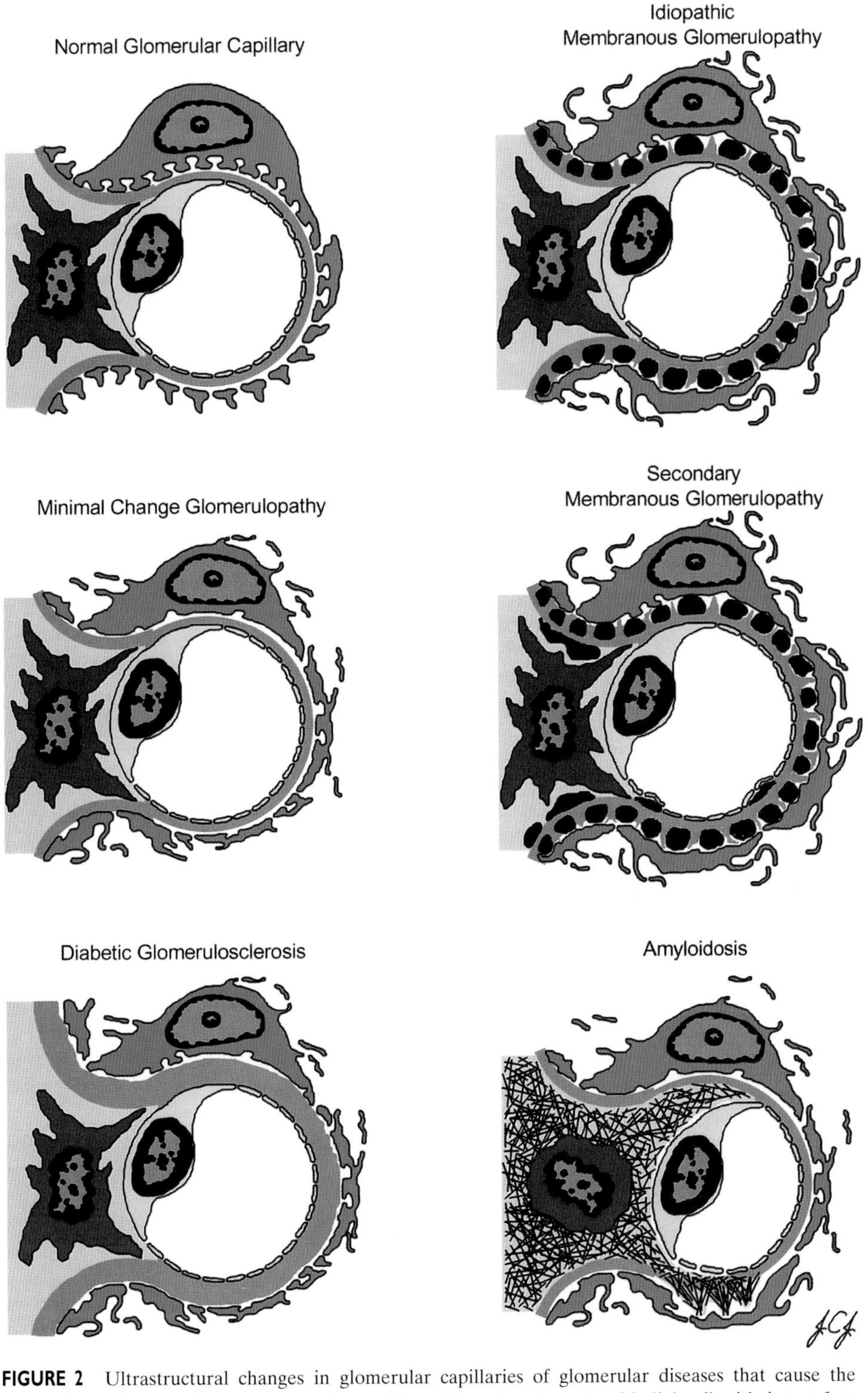

FIGURE 2 Ultrastructural changes in glomerular capillaries of glomerular diseases that cause the nephrotic syndrome. Normal glomerular capillary: Note the visceral epithelial cell with intact foot processes (green), endothelial cell with fenestrations (yellow), mesangial cell (red) with adjacent mesangial matrix (light gray), and basement membrane with lamina densa (dark gray) that does not completely surround the capillary lumen but splays out as the paramesangial basement membrane. Minimal change glomerulopathy: note the effacement of foot processes and microvillous transformation. Diabetic glomerulosclerosis: Note the thickening of the lamina densa and expansion of mesangial matrix. Idiopathic membranous glomerulopathy: Note the subepithelial dense deposits with adjacent projections of basement membrane (see also Fig. 5). Secondary membranous glomerulopathy: Note the mesangial and small subendothelial deposits in addition to the requisite subepithelial deposits. Amyloidosis: Note the fibrils within the mesangium and capillary wall. From JC Jennette, with permission.

Thin Basement Membrane
Nephropathy

Proliferative Lupus
Glomerulonephritis

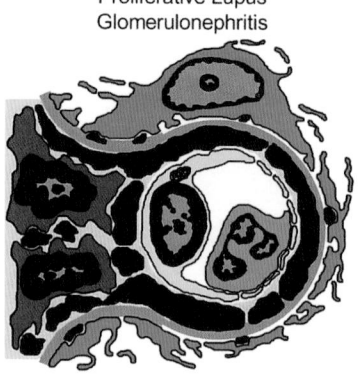

Mesangioproliferative
Glomerulonephritis

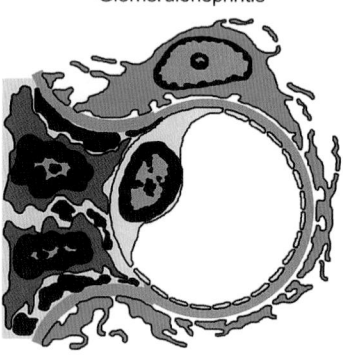

Type I Membranoproliferative
Glomerulonephritis

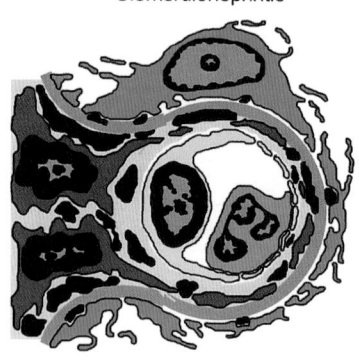

Acute Postinfectious
Glomerulonephritis

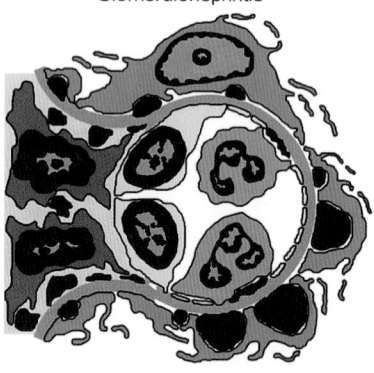

Type II Membranoproliferative
Glomerulonephritis

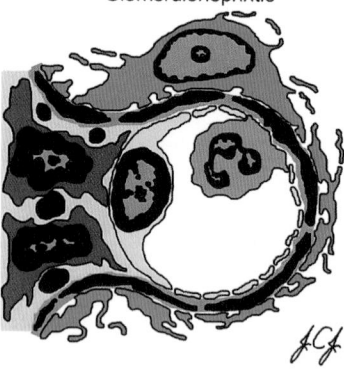

FIGURE 3 Ultrastructural changes in glomerular capillaries of glomerular diseases that cause hematuria and the nephritic syndrome. Thin basement membrane nephropathy: Note the thin lamina densa of the basement membrane. Mesangioproliferative glomerulonephritis (e.g., mild lupus nephritis or IgA nephropathy): Note the mesangial dense deposits and mesangial hypercellularity. Acute diffuse proliferative glomerulonephritis (e.g., poststreptococcal glomerulonephritis): Note the endocapillary hypercellularity contributed to by leukocytes, endothelial cells, and mesangial cells and the dense deposits, including not only conspicuous subepithelial "humps" but also inconspicuous subendothelial and mesangial deposits. Proliferative lupus glomerulonephritis (see also Fig. 4): Note the extensive subendothelial and mesangial dense deposits. Type I membranoproliferative glomerulonephritis (mesangiocapillary glomerulonephritis): Note the subendothelial deposits with associated subendothelial interposition of mesangial cytoplasm and deposition of new matrix material resulting in basement membrane replication. Type II membranoproliferative glomerulonephritis (dense deposit disease): Note the intramembranous and mesangial dense deposits. From JC Jennette, with permission.

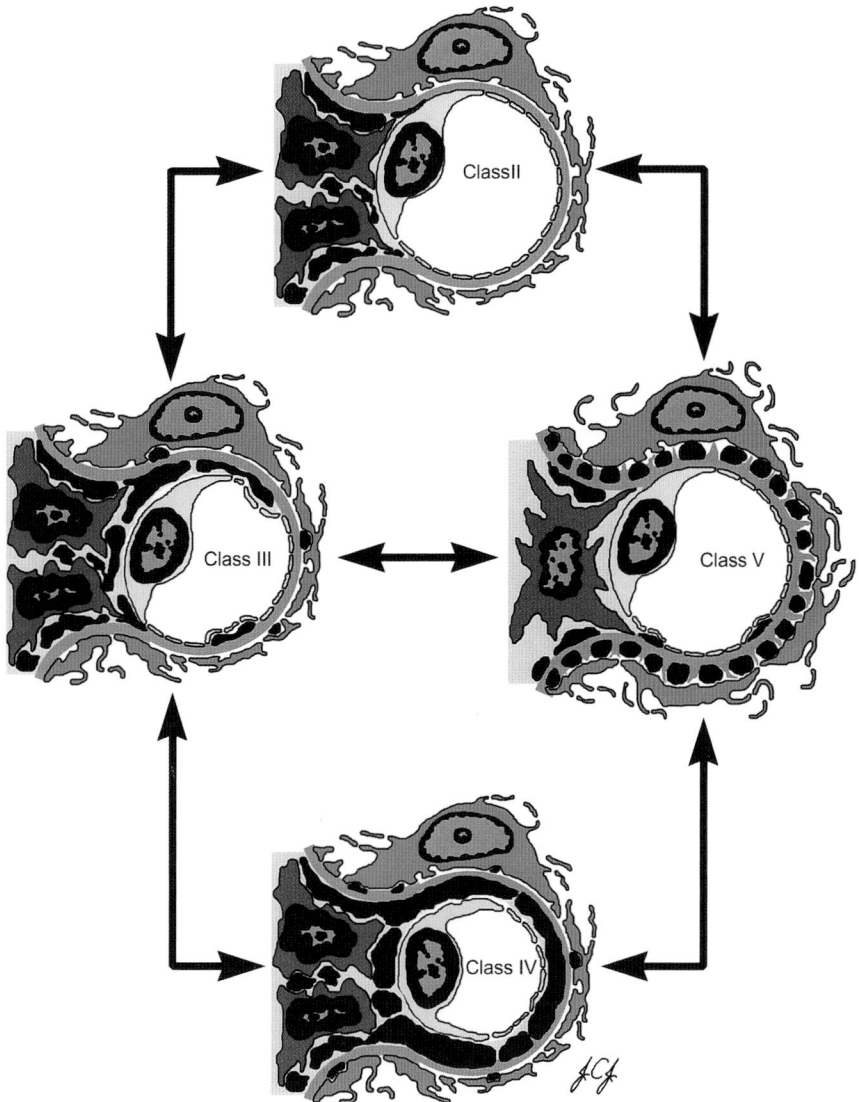

FIGURE 4 Ultrastructural features of the major classes of lupus nephritis. The sequestration of immune deposits within the mesangium in class II (mesangioproliferative) lupus glomerulonephritis causes only mesangial hyperplasia and mild renal dysfunction. Substantial amounts of subendothelial immune deposits, which are adjacent to the inflammatory mediator systems of the blood, cause focal (class III) or diffuse (class IV) proliferative lupus glomerulonephritis with overt nephritic signs and symptoms. Localization of immune deposits predominantly in the subepithelial zone causes membranous (class V) lupus glomerulonephritis, which usually manifests predominantly as the nephrotic syndrome. From JC Jennette, with permission.

This importance of pathogenic category in predicting the natural history of glomerulonephritis indicates that the pathologic separation of glomerulonephritis into the light microscopic morphologic categories in Fig. 7 is not sufficient for patient management. In addition to establishing the type of glomerular terms present, the pathogenic or immunopathologic category of disease must be determined as well. If a renal biopsy is performed, this determination is usually based on immunohistology and electron microscopy (Figs. 1–6). Immunohistology reveals the presence or absence of immunoglobulins and complement components.

The distribution (e.g., capillary wall, mesangium), pattern (e.g., granular, linear), and composition (e.g., IgA-dominant, IgG-dominant, IgM-dominant) of immunoglobulin is useful for determining specific types of glomerulonephritis (as will be discussed in detail in later chapters in this primer).

Table 4 gives the frequencies of the major immunopathologic categories of glomerulonephritis in patients with crescents who have undergone renal biopsy. The immune complex category contains a variety of diseases, including lupus nephritis, IgA nephropathy, and poststreptococcal glomer-

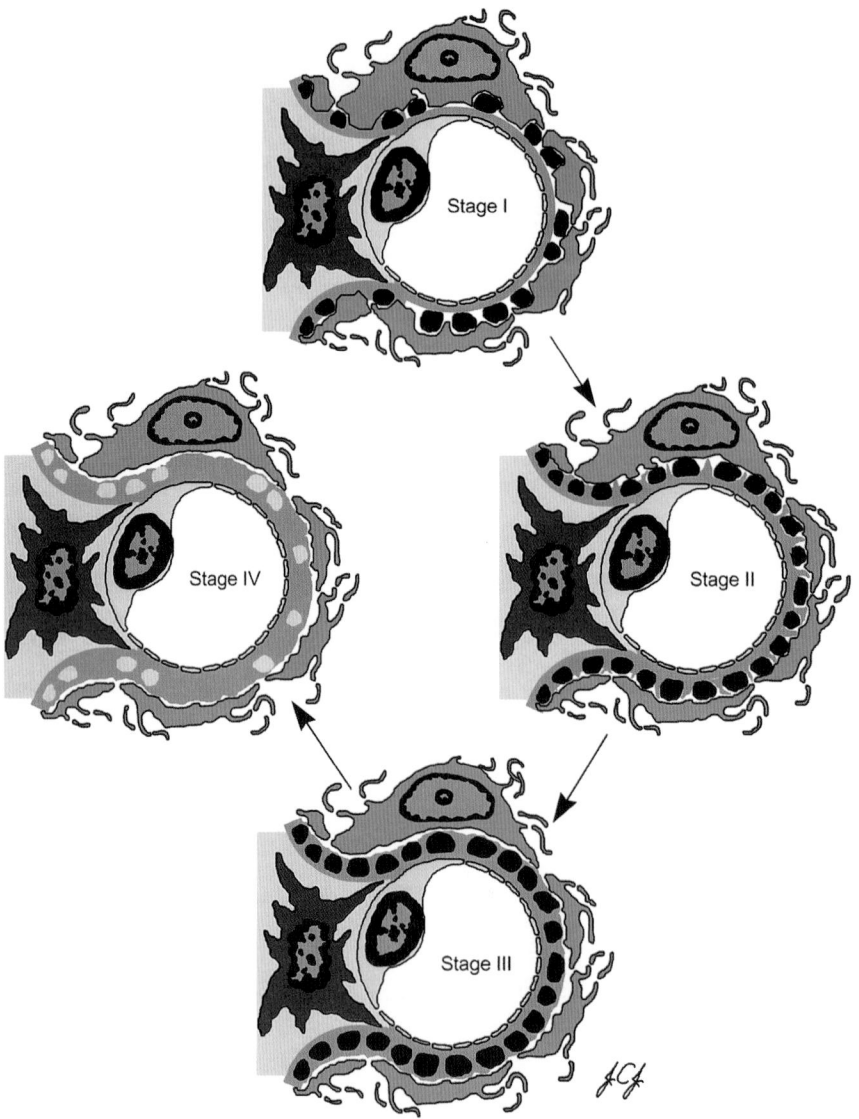

FIGURE 5 Ultrastructural stages in the progression of membranous glomerulopathy. Stage I has subepithelial electron-dense immune complex deposits without adjacent projections of basement membrane material. Stage II has adjacent GBM projections that eventually surround the electron-dense immune deposits in stage III. Stage IV has a markedly thickened GBM with electron lucent zones replacing the electron-dense deposits. From JC Jennette, with permission.

ulonephritis. Note that the majority of patients with >50% crescents have little or no immunohistologic evidence for immune complex or anti-GBM antibody localization within glomeruli (i.e., the term is pauciimmune). More than 80% of these patients with pauciimmune crescentic glomerulonephritis have circulating antineutrophil cytoplasmic auto-antibodies (ANCA).

Because both the structural severity (e.g., morphologic stages in Fig. 7) and immunopathologic category of disease (e.g., the categories given in Figs. 1–6, such as IgA nephropathy, lupus nephritis, anti-GBM disease) are important in predicting the course of disease in a patient with glomerulonephritis, the most useful diagnostic term should include

information about both (e.g., focal proliferative IgA nephropathy, diffuse proliferative lupus glomerulonephritis, crescentic anti-GBM glomerulonephritis).

Because they often are immune-mediated inflammatory diseases, many types of glomerulonephritis are treated with corticosteroids, cytotoxic drugs or other antiinflammatory and immunosuppressive agents. The aggressiveness of the treatment, of course, should match the aggressiveness of the disease. For example, active class IV lupus nephritis warrants immunosuppressive treatment, whereas class II lupus nephritis dose not.

The two most aggressive forms of glomerulonephritis are anti-GBM crescentic glomerulonephritis and ANCA

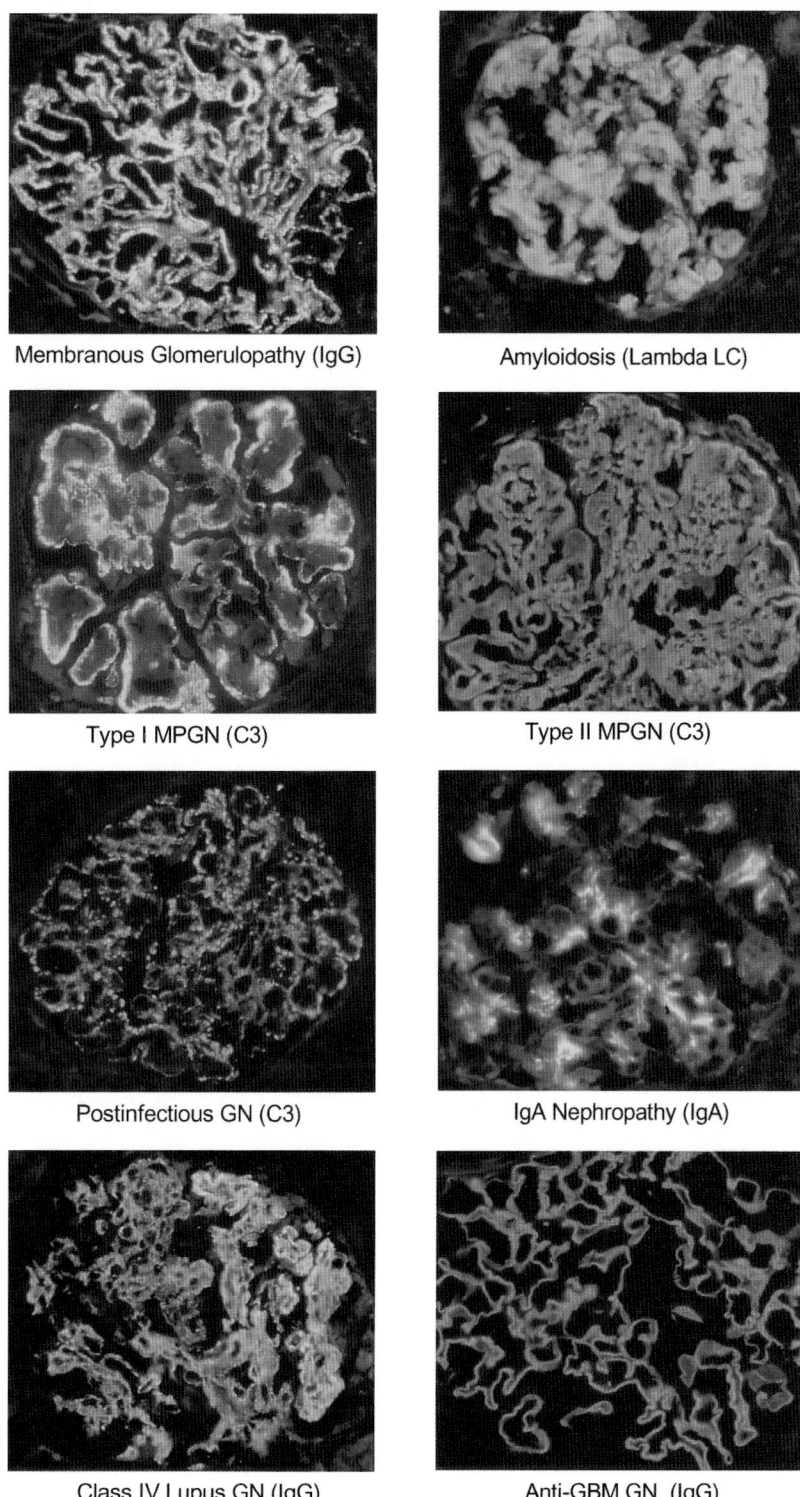

Membranous Glomerulopathy (IgG)

Amyloidosis (Lambda LC)

Type I MPGN (C3)

Type II MPGN (C3)

Postinfectious GN (C3)

IgA Nephropathy (IgA)

Class IV Lupus GN (IgG)

Anti-GBM GN (IgG)

FIGURE 6 Immunofluorescence microscopy staining patterns for membranous glomerulopathy: Note the global granular capillary wall staining for IgG. AL amyloidosis: Note the
irregular fluffy staining for light chains. Type I membranoproliferative glomerulonephritis
(MPGN): Note the peripheral granular to band-like staining for C3. Type II MPGN:
Note the band-like capillary wall and coarsely granular mesangial staining for C3. Acute
postinfectious glomerulonephritis: Note the coarsely granular capillary wall staining for
C3. IgA nephropathy: Note the mesangial staining for IgA. Class IV lupus nephritis:
Note the segmentally variable capillary wall and mesangial staining for IgG. Anti-GBM
glomerulonephritis: Note the linear GBM staining for IgG.

TABLE 3
Renal Disease in Patients with Hematuria Undergoing Renal Biopsy

	Prot <1 Cr <1.5	Prot 1–3	Cr 1.5–3.0	Cr >3
No abnormality	30%	2%	1%	0%
Thin BM nephropathy	26%	4%	3%	0%
IgA nephropathy	28%	24%	14%	8%
GN without crescents[a]	9%	26%	37%	23%
GN with crescents[a]	2%	24%	21%	44%
Other renal disease[b]	5%	20%	24%	25%
Total	100%	100%	100%	100%
	n = 43	n = 123	n = 179	n = 255

[a] Proliferative or necrotizing GN other than IgA nephropathy or lupus nephritis.

[b] Includes causes for the nephrotic syndrome, such as membranous glomerulopathy and focal segmental glomerulosclerosis.

Note: This is an analysis of renal biopsy specimens evaluated at by the University of North Carolina Nephropathology Laboratory. Patients with systemic lupus erythematosus have been excluded from the analysis. GN, glomerulonephritis; BM, basement membrane; P, proteinuria (g/24hr); Cr, serum creatinine (mg/dL). Derived from Caldas MLR, Jennette JC, Falk RJ, Wilkman AS: NC Glomerular Disease Collaborative Network: What is found by renal biopsy in patients with hematuria? *Lab Invest* 62:15A, 1990.

crescentic glomerulonephritis. The most important factor in renal outcome is early diagnosis and treatment. Both diseases are treated with immunosuppressive regimens (e.g., pulse methylprednisolone and intravenous or oral cyclophosphamide). Plasmapheresis is usually added to the regimen for anti-GBM disease. Immunosuppressive treatment generally can be terminated after 4 to 5 months in patients with anti-GBM glomerulonephritis with very little risk of recurrence (see Chapter 23). The initial induction of remission for ANCA-glomerulonephritis often is carried

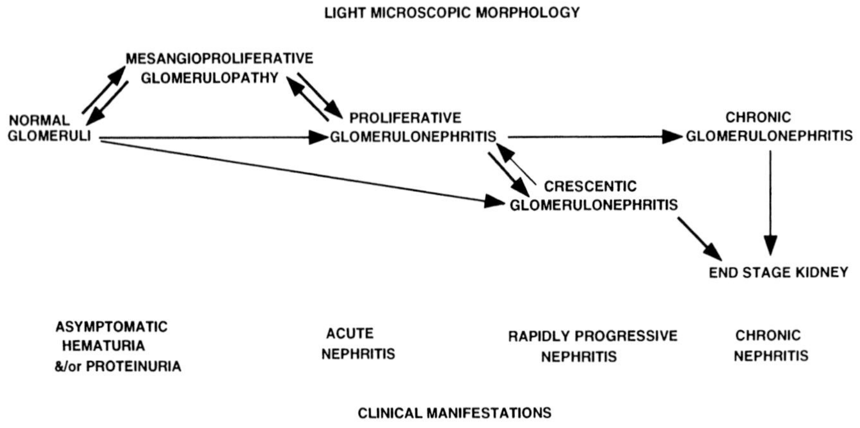

FIGURE 7 Morphologic stages of glomerulonephritis (top of diagram) aligned with the usual clinical manifestations (bottom of diagram). Certain glomerular diseases, such as anti-GBM and ANCA glomerulonephritis, usually have crescentic glomerulonephritis with rapid progression of renal failure if not promptly treated. Others, such as lupus nephritis, have a predilection for causing focal or diffuse proliferative glomerulonephritis with variable rates of progression dependent on the activity of the glomerular lesions. Some, such as IgA nephropathy, tend to begin as mild mesangioproliferative lesions but may progress into more severe proliferative lesions. Poststreptococcal glomerulonephritis and similar diseases typically initially develop a very active acute proliferative glomerulonephritis but then resolve through a mesangioproliferative phase to normal: Still others, such as IgM mesangial nephropathy, rarely progress past the mesangioproliferative phase. Reprinted with permission from Jennette JC, Mandal AK: Syndrome of glomerulonephritis. In: Mandal AK, Jennette JC (eds), *Diagnosis and Management of Renal Disease and Hypertension* (2nd Ed.). Carolina Academic Press, Durham, NC, 1994.

TABLE 4

Frequency of Immunopathologic Categories of Crescentic Glomerulonephritis in More Than
3000 Consecutive Nontransplant Renal Biopsies Evaluated by Immunofluorescence Microscopy
in the University of North Carolina Nephropathology Laboratory

	Any crescents ($n = 540$)	>50% crescents ($n = 195$)	Arteritis in biopsy ($n = 37$)
Immunohistology			
Pauciimmune (<2 + Ig)	51% (277/540)	61% (118/195)[a]	84% (31/37)
Immune complex (≥2 + Ig)	44% (238/540)	29% (56/195)	14% (5/37)[c]
Anti-GBM	5% (25/540)[b]	11% (21/195)	3% (1/37)[d]

[a] 70 of 77 patients tested for ANCA were positive (91%). (44 P-ANCA and 26 C-ANCA)
[b] 3 of 19 patients tested for ANCA were positive (16%). (2 P-ANCA and 1 C-ANCA)
[c] Four patients had lupus and one had poststreptococcal glomerulonephritis.
[d] This patient also had a P-ANCA (MPO-ANCA).
From Jennette JC, Falk RJ: The pathology of vasculitis involving the kidney. *Am J Kidney Dis* 24: 1994.

out for 6 to 12 months, and even then there is an approximately 25% risk for recurrence that will require additional immunosuppression.

GLOMERULONEPHRITIS ASSOCIATED WITH SYSTEMIC DISEASES

Some patients with acute or rapidly progressive glomerulonephritis have a pathogenetically related systemic disease. Immune complex-mediated glomerulonephritides that are induced by infections may have an antecedent or concurrent infection, such as streptococcal pharyngitis or pyoderma preceding acute poststreptococcal glomerulonephritis or hepatitis C infection concurrent with type I membranoproliferative glomerulonephritis. As noted earlier, glomerulonephritis with any of morphologic expressions shown in Fig. 7, as well as membranous glomerulopathy, can be caused by systemic lupus erythematosus (Fig. 4).

Because glomeruli are vessels, glomerulonephritis is a frequent manifestation of systemic small vessel vasculitides, such as Henoch-Schönlein purpura, cryoglobulinemic vasculitis, microscopic polyangiitis (microscopic polyarteritis), Wegener's granulomatosis, or Churg-Strauss syndrome. Henoch-Schönlein purpura is caused by vascular localization of IgA-dominant immune complexes, which manifests as IgA nephropathy in the glomeruli. Cryoglobulinemic vasculitis is caused by cryoglobulin deposition in vessels, and often is associated with hepatitis C infection. In glomeruli, cryoglobulinemia usually causes type I membranoproliferative glomerulonephritis. Microscopic polyangiitis, Wegener's granulomatosis, or Churg-Strauss syndrome have a paucity of immune deposits in vessel walls and are associated with circulating ANCA. ANCA glomerulonephritis is characterized pathologically by fibrinoid necrosis and crescent formation, and often manifests as rapidly progressive renal failure. Patients with vasculitis-associated glomerulonephritis typically have clinical manifestations of vascular inflammation in multiple organs, such as skin purpura caused by dermal angiitis, hemoptysis caused by alveolar capillary hemorrhage, abdominal pain caused by gut infarcts, and mononeuritis multiplex caused by vasculitis in the epineural and perineural vessels of peripheral nerves.

A distinctive and severe clinical presentation for glomerulonephritis is pulmonary–renal vasculitic syndrome, which usually has rapidly progressive glomerulonephritis combined with pulmonary hemorrhage. Table 1 lists the most common causes for pulmonary–renal vasculitic syndrome. Histologic and immunohistologic examination of involved vessels, including glomeruli in renal biopsy specimens, is useful in making a definitive diagnosis (Fig. 1) Serologic analysis for anti-GBM antibodies, ANCA, and markers for immune complex disease (e.g., antinuclear antibodies, cryoglobulins, antihepatitis C and B antibodies, complement levels) also may indicate the appropriate diagnosis (Fig. 1).

ASYMPTOMATIC PROTEINURIA AND NEPHROTIC SYNDROME

When proteinuria is severe, it causes the nephrotic syndrome. Less severe proteinuria, or severe proteinuria of short duration, may be asymptomatic. The nephrotic syndrome is characterized by massive proteinuria (>3 g $\cdot$ 24hr^1 $\cdot$ 1.73 m^{-2}), hypoproteinemia (especially hypoalbuminemia), edema, hyperlipidemia, and lipiduria. The most specific microscopic urinalysis finding is the presence of oval fat bodies. These are sloughed tubular epithelial cells that have resorbed some of the excess lipids and lipoproteins in the urine (see Chapter 3, Fig. 3).

Severe nephrotic syndrome predisposes to thrombosis secondary to loss of hemostasis control proteins (e.g., antithrombin III, protein S, and protein C), infection secondary to loss of immunoglobulins and, possibly, accelerated atherosclerosis because of the hyperlipidemia. Dehydration and inactivity may increase the risk for venous thrombosis in nephrotic patients. In nephrotic patients with frequent bacterial infections, administration of intravenous gamma globulin may be required.

Any type of glomerular disease can cause proteinuria. In fact, proteinuria is a very sensitive indicator of glomerular damage. All proteinuria, however, is not of glomerular origin. For example, tubular damage can cause proteinuria, but rarely more than 2 g/24 hr.

As noted in Table 2, some glomerular diseases are more likely to manifest the nephrotic syndrome than others, although virtually any form may cause the nephrotic syndrome. The two primary renal diseases that most often manifest as nephrotic syndrome are minimal change glomerulopathy and membranous glomerulopathy, and the two secondary forms of renal disease that most often manifest as nephrotic syndrome are diabetic glomerulosclerosis and amyloidosis (specifically, AL and AA amyloidosis).

Age is a major influence on the frequency of causes for the nephrotic syndrome. In children under 10 years old, about 80% of the nephrotic syndrome is caused by minimal change glomerulopathy. Throughout adulthood, minimal change glomerulopathy accounts for only 10 to 15% of primary nephrotic syndrome.

Membranous glomerulopathy is the most common cause of primary nephrotic syndrome in adults, but it accounts for less than 50% of cases. As shown in Fig. 8, a variety of glomerular diseases account for the remaining cases of nephrotic syndrome that are identified at the time of renal biopsy. The data in Fig. 8 are derived from patients with nephrotic range proteinuria who have undergone renal biopsy. The frequency of causes for the nephrotic syndrome that are not always examined by renal biopsy, especially diabetic glomerulosclerosis, are not accurately represented in Fig. 8.

Membranous glomerulopathy is most frequent in the fifth and sixth decades of life. It is characterized pathologically by numerous subepithelial immune complex deposits (Figs. 2, 5, and 6). The glomerular lesion evolves over time, with progressive accumulation of basement membrane material around the capillary wall immune complexes (Fig. 5) and eventual development of chronic tubulointerstitial injury in those patients with progressive disease (see Chapter 21). If the Heymann nephritis animal model is analogous to human disease, idiopathic (primary) membranous glomerulopathy may be caused by autoantibodies specific for antigens on visceral epithelial cells, which would allow immune complex formation in the subepithelial zone but not in the subendothelial zone or mesangium of glomeruli. In addition to the numerous subepithelial immune deposits, membranous glomerulopathy secondary to immune complexes composed of antigens and antibodies in the systemic circulation often has immune complex deposits in the mesangium, and may have small subendothelial deposits (Fig. 2). Thus, the ultrastructural identification of mesangial or subendothelial deposits should raise the level of suspicion for secondary membranous glomerulopathy, such as membranous glomerulopathy caused by a systemic autoimmune disease (e.g., lupus, mixed connective tissue disease, autoimmune thyroiditis), infection (e.g., hepatitis B or C, syphi-

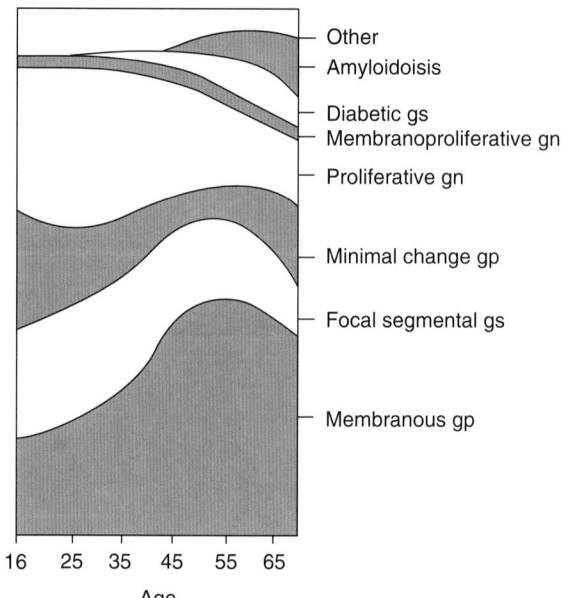

FIGURE 8 Diagram demonstrating the approximate frequency of different renal diseases in patients with the nephrotic range proteinuria *who had renal biopsies* that were evaluated in the University of North Carolina Nephropathology Laboratory. Note the variation in frequency with age. The proliferative glomerulonephritis category includes all forms of proliferative glomerulonephritis, including lupus nephritis, IgA nephropathy, IgM mesangial nephropathy and others. gn, glomerulonephritis; gp, glomerulopathy; gs, glomerulosclerosis. Reprinted with permission from Jennette JC, Mandal AK: The nephrotic syndrome. In: Mandal AK, Jennette JC (eds), *Diagnosis and Management of Renal Disease and Hypertension* (2nd ed.). Carolina Academic Press, Durham, NC, 1994.

lis), or neoplasm (e.g., lung or gut carcinoma). In very young and very old patients, the likelihood of secondary membranous glomerulopathy is greater, although still uncommon. Membranous glomerulopathy occurring in young patients raises the possibility of systemic lupus erythematosus or hepatitis B infection, and in very old patients raises the possibility of occult carcinoma.

Both type I and II membranoproliferative glomerulonephritis (MPGN) typically manifest mixed nephrotic and nephritic features, sometimes accompanied by hypocomplementemia and C3 nephritic factor, which is an autoantibody against the C3 convertase of the alternative complement activation pathway (see Chapter 19). Both types often have glomerular capillary wall thickening and hypercellularity by light microscopy. Type I MPGN (mesangiocapillary glomerulonephritis) is characterized ultrastructurally by subendothelial immune complex deposits that stimulate subendothelial mesangial interposition and replication of basement membrane material, whereas type II MPGN (dense deposit disease) has pathognomonic intramembranous dense deposits (Fig. 3). Both types have extensive glomerular staining for C3 (Fig. 6), with type I having more immunoglobulin staining than type II. Type I MPGN may be secondary to cryoglobulinemia, neoplasms, or chronic infections (e.g., hepatitis C and B, and infected prostheses, such as a ventriculoatrial shunt).

When taken as a group, focal and diffuse proliferative glomerulonephritides account for a substantial proportion of patients who have nephrotic range proteinuria. Patients with proliferative glomerulonephritis and marked proteinuria usually also have features of nephritis, especially hematuria. Included in this group would be patients with lupus nephritis and IgA nephropathy who have nephrotic range proteinuria.

Amyloidosis as a cause for the nephrotic syndrome is most frequent in older adults (Fig. 8). Currently in the United States, amyloid causing the nephrotic syndrome is approximately 75% AL amyloid rather than AA, and AL amyloid is approximately 75% lambda rather than kappa light-chain composition. Patients with kappa light-chain paraproteins and the nephrotic syndrome are more likely to have light-chain deposition disease (i.e., nodular sclerosis without amyloid fibrils) rather than amyloidosis (see Chapter 30). Amyloid composition can be determined by immunofluorescence microscopy (Fig. 6).

CHRONIC GLOMERULONEPHRITIS AND END STAGE RENAL DISEASE

Most glomerular disease, with possible exceptions being uncomplicated minimal change glomerulopathy and thin basement membrane nephropathy, can progress to chronic glomerular sclerosis with progressive renal failure and eventually to end stage renal disease (ESRD). Chronic glomerular disease is the third leading cause of ESRD in the United States, following hypertensive and diabetic renal disease in frequency. Clinicopathologic studies of different glomerular diseases have revealed marked differences in their natural histories. Diseases such as anti-GBM and ANCA crescentic glomerulonephritis have high risk for rapid progression to ESRD unless treated. Other diseases such as IgA nephropathy and focal segmental glomerulosclerosis, have more indolent but persistent courses. A few glomerulonephritides, for example poststreptococcal glomerulonephritis, may initially manifest a rather severe nephritis, but usually resolve completely with little risk for progression to ESRD. And some diseases are very unpredictable. For example, membranous glomerulopathy may remit spontaneously, have persistent nephrosis for decades without renal failure, or progress over several years to ESRD.

Chronic glomerulonephritis is characterized pathologically by varying degrees of glomerular scarring, which is always accompanied by cortical tubular atrophy, interstitial fibrosis, interstitial infiltration by chronic inflammatory cells, and arteriosclerosis. As the glomerular, interstitial, and vascular sclerosis worsen, they eventually reach a point at which histologic evaluation of the renal tissue cannot reveal the initial cause for the renal injury, and a pathologic diagnosis of ESRD is all that can be concluded.

Clinically, chronic glomerulonephritis that is progressing to ESRD eventually results in uremia that must be managed by dialysis or renal transplantation. As the term implies, patients with uremia have accumulation of nitrogenous wastes (urea, uric acid, creatinine) in the blood. Other clinical manifestations of uremia include nausea and vomiting, hiccups, anorexia, pruritis, lethargy, pericarditis, myopathies, neuropathies and encephalopathy (see Chapter 62).

RENAL BIOPSY: INDICATIONS AND METHODS

In a patient with renal disease, a renal biopsy provides tissue that can be used to determine the diagnosis, indicate the cause, predict the prognosis, direct treatment, and collect data for research, although not all potential applications are accomplished by every renal biopsy.

Renal biopsy is indicated in a patient with renal disease when all three of the following conditions are met: (1) the cause cannot be determined or adequately predicted by less invasive diagnostic procedures; (2) the signs and symptoms suggest parenchymal disease that can be diagnosed by pathologic evaluation; and (3) the differential diagnosis includes diseases that have different treatments, different prognoses, or both. Situations in which a renal biopsy serves an important diagnostic function include nephrotic syndrome in adults, steroid-resistant nephrotic syndrome in children, glomerulonephritis in adults other than clear-cut acute poststreptococcal glomerulonephritis or lupus nephritis, and acute renal failure of unknown cause. In some renal diseases for which the diagnosis is relatively certain from clinical data, a renal biopsy may be of value not only for confirming the diagnosis but also for assessing the activity, chronicity, and severity of injury; for example, in patients with suspected lupus nephritis. Although the diagnosis is strongly supported by positive serologic results in patients with anti-GBM and ANCA-glomerulonephritis, the extremely toxic treatment that is used for these diseases warrants the additional level of confirmation that a renal biopsy provides. A renal biopsy also provides information about the severity and potential reversibility of the glomerular damage. Table 5 demonstrates the types of native renal disease that have prompted renal biopsy among the nephrologists who refer specimens to the University of North Carolina Nephropathology Laboratory. Approximately 80% of these biopsies were performed by nephrologists in community practice. Diseases that typically cause nephrotic syndrome were the most frequent impetus for biopsy, followed by diseases that cause nephritis.

Contraindications to percutaneous renal biopsy include an uncooperative patient, solitary kidney, hemorrhagic diathesis, uncontrolled severe hypertension, severe anemia or dehydration, cystic kidney, hydronephrosis, multiple renal arterial aneurysms, acute pyelonephritis or perinephric abscess, renal neoplasm, and ESRD.

Clinically significant complications of renal biopsy are relatively infrequent but must be kept in mind when determining the risk–benefit ratio of the procedure. Small perirenal hematomas that can be seen by imaging studies (e.g., ultrasound) are relatively common if looked for carefully. Gross hematuria occurs in <10% of patients, arteriovenous

TABLE 5

Frequency of Various Diagnoses Among 7257 Renal Biopsies Evaluated in the University of North Carolina
Nephropathology Laboratory

Diseases that often cause nephrotic syndrome (42%)	3067	Diseases that often cause hematuria and nephritis (29%)	2109
Idiopathic membranous glomerulopathy	847	Lupus nephritis (all classes)	636
Focal segmental glomerulosclerosis (FSGS)	768	IgA nephropathy	538
Minimal change glomerulopathy	398	Other immune complex proliferative GN	375
Diabetic glomerulosclerosis	246	Pauciimmune/ANCA GN	301
Type I membranoproliferative GN	190	Acute diffuse proliferative (postinfectious) GN	86
Mesangioproliferative GN	145	Thin basement membrane nephropathy	82
Amyloidosis	108	Anti-GBM GN	56
Clq nephropathy	99	Alport's syndrome	35
Collapsing variant of FSGS	87	Diseases that often cause chronic renal failure (8%)	583
Glomerular tip lesion variant of FSGS	65	Arterionephrosclerosis	229
Fibrillary GN	59	Chronic sclerosing GN	166
Light-chain deposition disease	26	End stage renal disease	114
Type II membranoproliferative GN	14	Chronic tubulointerstitial nephritis	74
Preeclampsia/eclampsia	6	Miscellaneous other diseases (3%)	199
Immunotactoid glomerulopathy	6	No pathologic lesion identified[b] (2%)	141
Collagenofibrotic glomerulopathy	3	Adequate tissue with nonspecific abnormalities[b] (5%)	370
Diseases that often cause acute renal failure[a] (5%)	371	Inadequate tissue for definitive diagnosis[b] (6%)	417
Thrombotic microangiopathy (all types)	126		
Acute tubulointerstitial nephritis	101		
Acute tubular necrosis	69		
Atheroembolization	34		
Light-chain cast nephropathy	31		
Coritcal necrosis	10		

[a] Other than glomerulonephritis.

[b] Specimens with nonspecific abnormalities (e.g., interstitial fibrosis, tubular atrophy, glomerular scarring, arteriosclerosis), specimens with no identifiable pathologic abnormality (e.g., in a patient with asymptomatic hematuria), and some specimens with inadequate tissue for definitive diagnosis (e.g., a very small specimen with only a few glomeruli but with negative immunofluorescence microscopy) may provide useful clinical information, especially with respect to ruling out diseases that were in the differential diagnosis.

GN, glomerulonephritis.

fistula in <1%, hemorrhage that requires surgery in <1%, and mortality in <0.1%.

Current percutaneous needle biopsy procedures usually employ localization of the kidney by real-time ultrasound guidance, determination of kidney location and depth by ultrasound immediately prior to biopsy, or CT guided localization of the kidney. Many varieties of biopsy needles have been used over the years—most of which are effective in experienced hands. Recently, there has been a major shift toward utilization of spring-loaded disposable gun devices.

Light microscopy alone is not adequate for the diagnosis of most native kidney diseases, although it may be adequate for assessing the basis for renal allograft dysfunction during the first few weeks after transplantation. All native kidney biopsies should be processed for at least light microscopy and immunofluorescence microscopy. Most renal pathologists advocate performing electron microscopy on all native kidney biopsies, but some believe that tissue for electron microscopy should be fixed as a contingency and electron microscopy performed only if the other microscopic findings suggest that it will be useful.

The needle biopsy core should be examined with a magnifying glass (e.g., 15X) or a dissecting microscope to con-

firm that renal tissue is present and to determine whether it is cortex or medulla. When gently prodded and pulled with forceps, adipose tissue is mushy and strings out, skeletal muscle tissue falls apart into little clumps, and renal tissue maintains a cylindrical shape. At 15X magnification, adipose tissue looks like clusters of tiny fat droplets (cells), skeletal muscle is red-brown with irregular fiber bundles, and renal tissue is pale pink-tan. Glomeruli in the renal cortex appear as reddish blushes or hemispheres projecting from the surface of the core. Straight red striations produced by the vasa recta are markers for the medulla. When there is extensive glomerular hematuria, the convoluted tubules in the cortex appear as red corkscrews. Once the tissue landmarks are identified, portions of tissue should be separated for processing for light, immunofluorescence, and electron microscopy.

In our experience with renal biopsy specimens sent to us from more than 100 different nephrologists per year, most of whom are in private practice, approximately 6% of renal biopsy specimens are inadequate for a definitive diagnosis (Table 5). The most common inadequacy is renal tissue with too little or no cortex. This can be remedied by beginning the sampling procedure with the biopsy needle just barely into the outer cortex. Obviously, if the biopsy needle is inserted too deeply into or through the cortex, the sampling procedure will obtain only medulla. Even specimens that are considered inadequate for a definitive diagnosis may provide useful information. For example, in a patient with the nephrotic syndrome, a renal biopsy specimen that has no glomeruli for light or electron microscopy, but has one glomerulus that stains negative for immunoglobulins and complement by immunofluorescence microscopy, rules out any form of immune complex glomerulonephritis, such as membranous glomerulopathy, and focuses the differential diagnosis on minimal change glomerulopathy vs. focal segmental glomerulosclerosis.

Bibliography

Appel GB: Renal biopsy: The clinician's viewpoint. In: Silva FG, D'Agati VD, Nadasdy T (eds) *Renal Biopsy Interpretation.* Churchill Livingstone, New York, pp. 21–29, 1996.

Bolton WK: Goodpasture's syndrome. *Kidney Int* 50:1753–1766, 1996.

Cameron JS: The nephrotic syndrome and its complications. *Am J Kidney Dis* 10:157–171, 1987.

Cohen AH, Nast CC, Adler SG, Kopple JD: Clinical utility of kidney biopsies in the diagnosis and management of renal disease. *Am J Nephrol* 9:309–315, 1989.

Couser WG: Rapidly progressive glomerulonephritis: Classification, pathogenetic mechanisms, and therapy. *Am J Kidney Dis* 11:449–464, 1988.

Dische F, Parsons V, Taube D: Thin-basement-membrane nephropathy. *N Engl J Med* 320:1752–1753, 1989.

Galla JH: IgA nephropathy. *Kidney Int* 47:377–387, 1995.

Glassock RJ, Cohen AH: The primary glomerulopathies. *Disease A Month* 42:329–383, 1996.

Jennette JC, Falk RJ: Diagnosis and management of glomerulonephritis and vasculitis presenting as acute renal failure. In: Mandal AK, Hebert LA (eds), *Medical Clinics of North America: Renal Failure and Transplantation.* Saunders, Philadelphia, pp. 893–908, 1990.

Mariani AJ, Mariani MC, Macchioni C, Stams UK, Hariharan A, Moriera A: The significance of adult hematuria: 1,000 hematuria evaluations including a risk-benefit and cost-effectiveness analysis. *J Urol* 141:350–355, 1989.

Tiebosch ATMG, Frederik PM, van Breda Vriesman PJC, et al.: Thin-basement-membrane nephropathy in adults with persistent hematuria. *N Engl J Med* 320:14–28, 1989.

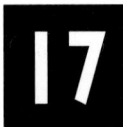

IMMUNOPATHOGENESIS OF RENAL DISEASE

DIANE M. CIBRIK AND JOHN R. SEDOR

The mechanisms of renal injury that lead to progressive disease are becoming better understood. Both humoral and cell-mediated immunity are implicated in the primary processes (i.e., the mechanisms that induce kidney injury) and the secondary events (i.e., the cascade of tissue responses activated by the initial renal damage) that mediate renal inflammation and fibrosis. Experimental models of kidney disease can be initiated by intrarenal antibody deposition or by immune effector cells. The extent and character of subsequent tissue immunologic injury is influenced by the ongoing accessibility and distribution of the kidney antigens, the biochemical characteristics of the antibody deposited and the specific, secondary inflammatory mediators induced by the primary injury process. Nonimmunologic mechanisms, although not the subject of this chapter, also can propagate ongoing injury. These processes include adaptive hemodynamic and physical forces that can cause intraglomerular hypertension and abnormal intravascular stress and strain (see Chapter 66). Although not well studied in renal model systems, information obtained with other experimental systems shows that these stimuli can alter the proteins synthesized by the target cells in a manner that contributes to persisting inflammatory tissue injury.

This chapter presents an overview of basic immunology, including the pertinent differences between humoral and cellular immunity and the concepts of self-tolerance and autoimmunity. With these fundamental mechanisms of immune injury in mind, the immunopathogenesis of kidney disease will be explored as it relates to in situ immune complex disease, circulating immune complex disease, and cell-mediated injury of the kidney. Finally, the role of complement activation in the context of renal disease will be discussed. Although these pathways of immune-mediated renal injury are dealt with individually within this chapter, many of these effector pathogenetic mechanisms often act in concert in vivo to cause renal damage (Fig. 1).

IMMUNE RESPONSE

A specific immune response can be generated by both the cellular and humoral immune systems (Fig. 2). T cells, for the most part, direct the cellular immune response, whereas antibodies derived from B cells direct the humoral immune response. Antigen-presenting cells (APC) in conjunction with T cells are essential in the initiation of the immune response. Examples of APCs include monocytes, macrophages, dendritic cells, and B cells. These cells express multi-subunit, major histocompatibility complex (MHC) proteins on their cell surfaces. These MHC molecules consist of class I and class II molecules which differ in their function, chemical structure, cell distribution, and length of peptide fragment that they will bind. Class I MHC molecules are present on all nucleated cells, whereas constitutive class II MHC molecule expression is restricted to specific cells such as macrophages, B cells, certain endothelial cells, and some activated T cells. The expression of class I MHC molecules on most cell types can be increased by proinflammatory mediators such as interferons as an amplification mechanism for certain T cell responses.

Cytokine-inducible increases in class II molecules on mononuclear phagocytes are also an important means of increasing expression on these cells from constitutively low levels. Both in vitro and in vivo studies suggest that cytokines can stimulate nonimmune cells to express class II molecules, but the functional consequences of these observations remain unclear. Self or nonself peptide fragments which interact with MHC molecules can be generated by one of two intracellular pathways: (1) the degradation of cytosolic proteins (e.g., viral proteins) within proteasomes with subsequent processing to permit interaction with class I MHC molecules and transport to the cell surface (i.e., presentation), or (2) the endocytosis of exogenous proteins (self or nonself) from the external milieu for association with, and presentation by, class II MHC proteins. The subunits of both classes of MHC molecules associate to form a "groove" or pocket where the peptide fragments bind to specific amino acid residues and are subsequently monitored by surveying T cells. Class I and class II are recognized by counter-receptors on CD8+ or CD4+ (helper) T cells, respectively. Although the MHC is extremely polymorphic within a given species, an individual's complement of MHC proteins can bind only a distinct subset of peptide fragments. This restriction influences the character of an individual immune response against a specific antigen.

Surveying T cells interact with the peptide:MHC complex through the highly variable regions of the T cell receptor (TCR). The binding of the MHC with the TCR confers specificity on the immune response, but this association alone is not sufficient to induce T cell activation. In order to activate T cells, a second interaction is necessary between

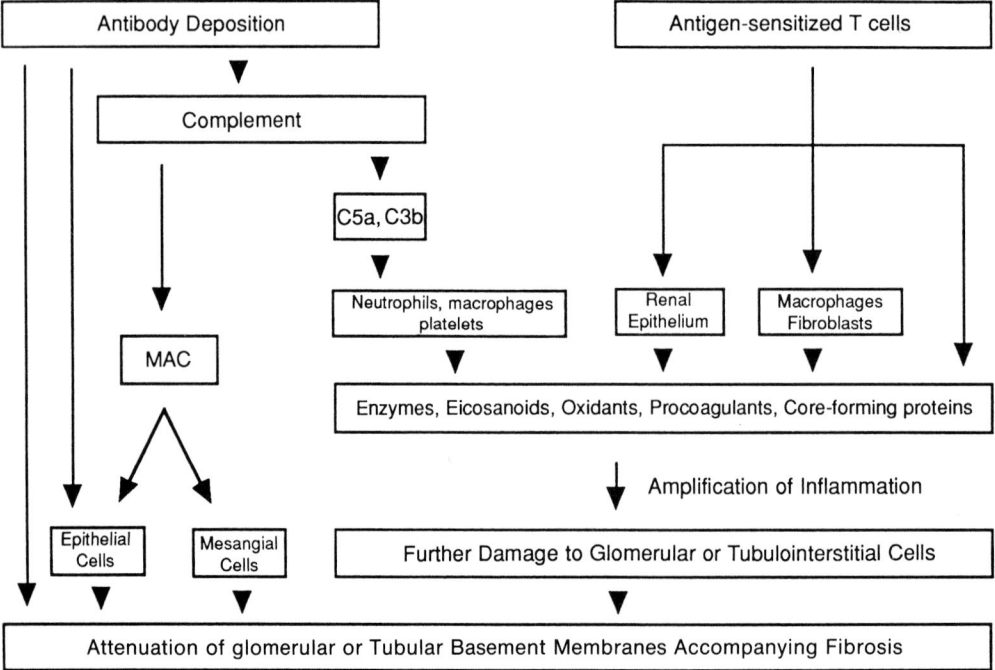

FIGURE 1 Effector pathways of the immune response which mediate renal injury in animal models. From Couser WG: *J Am Soc Nephrol* 1:13–29, 1990.

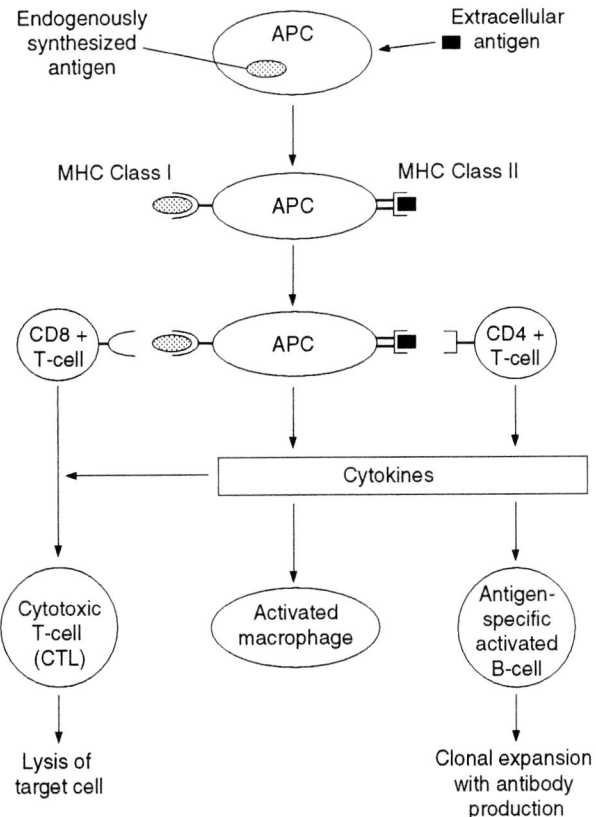

FIGURE 2 Activation of the immune response. Antigen-presenting cells (APC) present endogenous or exogenous antigen via MHC class I or class II molecules, respectively, to the T-cell receptor (TCR). The interaction between the TCR and MHC: antigen complex, in conjunction with costimulator activities (see text), induces T-cell activation and proliferation and APC activation. Activated APCs and T cells release cytokines that promote cytotoxic T lymphocyte (CTL) formation and antigen-specific, clonal B-cell expansion.

cell surface molecules present on the APC (i.e., B7 or ICAM-1) and their counter-receptors expressed on the T cell. This interaction, known as costimulation, aids in T cell–APC adhesion and stimulates the intracellular signal transduction events necessary for T cell activation. By requiring two signals for activation, the T cell can monitor self from nonself (foreign) peptides and control its subsequent responses. Recognition of the first signal (MHC: peptide complex binding to the TCR) without the second, costimulatory signal may lead to anergy, or may lead to deletion of self-reactive T cells from the repertoire in some instances. The production and release of soluble mediators (i.e., cytokines from APCs and T cells) also requires both T cell activation signals. These mediators, in turn, can amplify the immune response by enhancing APC activation, T cell proliferation, and monoclonal B cell expansion. Thus, many interactive signals are required to generate an effective immune response.

Humoral immunity is also important in generating an extracellular immune response. B cells can be activated to secrete antibodies by one of two mechanisms. In the first, B cells can bind specific antigen directly via crosslinking immunoglobulin (Ig) molecules present on the cell surface, resulting in stimulation of biochemical signals within the cell. Together with the help of cytokines, these intracellular signals stimulate B cell proliferation and differentiation into antibody-forming cells. In the second mechanism, B cells act as APCs by internalizing antigen bound weakly to surface Ig. Processed antigen is loaded onto class II MHC molecules and brought to the cell surface where it can be recognized by CD4+ T cells. In conjunction with the secretion of cytokines by T cells and other costimulatory activities, this B cell–T cell interaction stimulates antigen-specific, B cell proliferation and differentiation, and clonal expansion with subsequent antibody production (Fig. 2).

Autoimmunity, either directly or indirectly, has been implicated in the immunopathogenesis of many renal diseases. Knowledge of the mechanisms that control self-tolerance is important to understanding the immunopathogenesis of kidney disease. Humoral and cellular immune responses against self antigens can result in autoimmune diseases. However, many normal individuals produce auto-antibodies or autoreactive T cells when challenged by a foreign protein but fail to mount an autoimmune response. Why don't these individuals develop an autoimmune disease? Immunologic tolerance is a physiological state in which a potentially destructive immune response does not develop against self-antigens. Several specific immune mechanisms protect against potentially, self-destructive processes. Clonal deletion, clonal anergy, and T cell peripheral suppression are three ways in which immunologic tolerance is achieved within the immune system. In clonal deletion, self-reactive T and B cells in the thymus and bone marrow, respectively, bind to autologous antigen during maturation and are lost via negative selection. Functional inactivation of T cells (clonal anergy) occurs when APCs, presenting self-antigen, lack secondary costimulatory signals, such as B7. In peripheral suppression, cellular (suppressor T cells) and humoral molecules (antiinflammatory cytokines) can suppress autoreactive lymphocytes. Because of these three mechanisms, immunologic tolerance is maintained and autoimmune disease states are only rare and aberrant events.

Autoimmunity and disease occur when all mechanisms of self-tolerance are overcome and an immune response against self-antigens is generated. Several important concepts about autoimmunity which are applicable to renal disease have evolved from the experimental and clinical literature. First, the response to a specific self-antigen occurs on a spectrum ranging from immunologic tolerance to immune self-destruction. In the aggregate, environmental factors such as microbial infection, genetic background, and specific immunologic abnormalities influence the response. Aberrant function of a single control component alone is insufficient to generate an autoimmune response. Second, autoimmune diseases can be systemic or organ-specific. Finally, multiple effectors mediate tissue injury in autoimmune diseases.

A number of mechanisms have been postulated to cause loss of self-tolerance. First, peripheral tolerance may be overcome. T and B-cell anergy is induced by antigen recognition in the absence of APC costimulatory activities or T-cell help, respectively. If local infection or inflammation stimulates the expression of costimulator molecules on APCs or activates helper T cells that can interact with potentially autoreactive B cells, anergy may be lost. Second, antigen-independent stimuli may activate self-reactive lymphocytes not depleted during development. For example, previously anergic B-cell clones can be stimulated nonspecifically by endotoxin from microorganisms or by viral infection to cause polyclonal B-cell activation that includes self-reactive B cells. Third, antibodies or activated T cells produced in the normal immune response to a pathogen may recognize (i.e., crossreact with) native or modified self proteins. One hypothesized mechanism of poststreptococcal glomerulonephritis suggests that antibodies against streptococci crossreact with normal basement protein or glomerular cell surface protein epitopes, a phenomenon termed antigenic or molecular mimicry. Antigenic crossreactivity between foreign and self proteins can also occur if the self protein is modified by complexing with haptens, such as drugs, or by partial degradation to expose neoantigenic determinants. Fourth, loss of self-tolerance may also occur when a neoantigen sequestered during development is exposed by tissue damage and viewed as foreign. This mechanism has been implicated in human Goodpasture's disease (see below). Finally, loss of suppressor T-cell function or excessive T-cell help may create an imbalance between suppressor and helper influences to result in loss of immunologic tolerance. Excessive cytokine production may "break" T-cell tolerance or stimulate previously silent B-cell clones to produce high levels of antibody. Through specific and nonspecific immune mechanisms, autoimmunization plays a critical role in the loss of self-tolerance and has been implicated in the pathogenesis of both experimental and human kidney disease.

IMMUNE MECHANISMS OF GLOMERULAR INJURY

Immune mechanisms are central to the pathogenesis of most types of glomerulonephritis. These mechanisms can be divided into two categories; humoral and cell-mediated. Most of the focus in the past has been on antibody-mediated injury. Two forms have been established: in situ immune complex disease and circulating immune complex disease (Fig. 3). Although these mechanisms of immune injury are not mutually exclusive, each produces a distinct immunofluorescence pattern within the glomerulus. The requisite antibodies may be generated through the autoimmunization mechanisms described above. However, antibody deposition by itself is not sufficient to cause renal injury. Cell-mediated tissue injury can occur through the release of cytokine growth factors or other mediators of inflammation. In addition, in vitro results suggest that inflammatory cells may directly injure the glomerulus, as in pauci-immune glomerulonephritis. Activation of the complement cascade, either by the classical or alternative pathway, also plays a significant role in glomerular damage.

Humoral Immunity

In Situ Immune Complex Disease

The binding of antibody to antigen (i.e., formation of an immune complex) localized to within a specific tissue is known as in situ immune complex formation. In situ immune complex disease can occur in one of two ways: either by antibodies binding to "native" antigen or to "planted" antigen. Native antigens are intrinsic glomerular protein constituents. Two well-established experimental models of "native" antigen immune complex disease exist: antiglomerular basement membrane (GBM) nephritis which models human Goodpasture's disease and Heymann's nephritis, an experimental model of human membranous nephropathy (Fig. 3). In anti-GBM nephritis, antibodies are directed against intrinsic fixed antigens within the glomerular base-

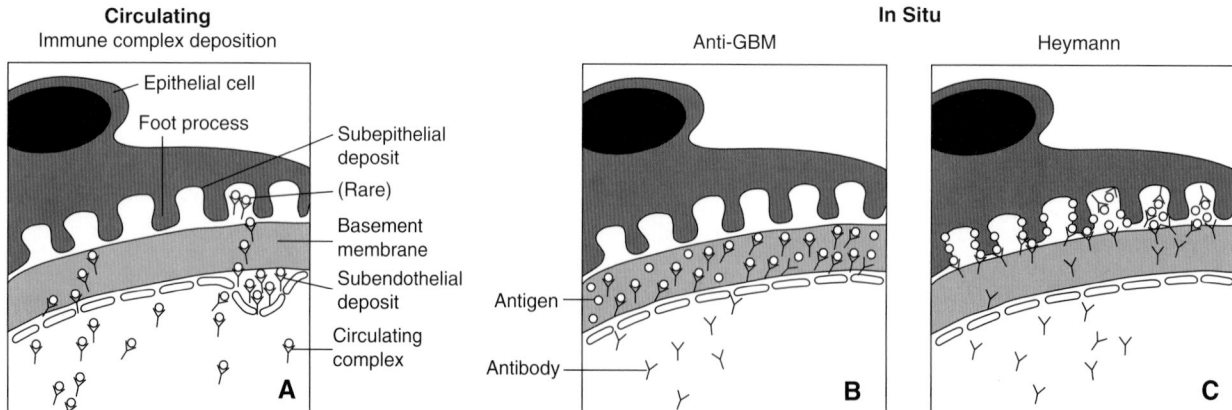

FIGURE 3 Antibody-mediated glomerular disease. Circulating Immune complexes (A) deposit in the subendothelial space and subsequently can be modified and rearranged to facilitate movement within the glomerulus. In situ immune complex formation is illustrated by the deposition of anti-GBM antibodies in anti-GBM disease (B) or anti-megalin antibodies in Heymann nephritis (C). From Cotran RS, Kumar V, Robbins SL: *Pathologic Basis of Disease.* WB Saunders Co., Philadelphia 1994.

ment membrane. In the experimental model, antibodies generated in rabbits immunized with rat kidney tissue are injected into normal rats with the subsequent development of anti-GBM nephritis. These antibodies can also crossreact with basement membrane present in lung alveoli, yielding simultaneous lung and kidney lesions, or Goodpasture's syndrome. In this syndrome, the human basement membrane antigen recently has been identified as two discontinuous epitopes within the noncollagenous domain of the α3 chain of collagen type IV. The current model of the pathogenesis of Goodpasture's syndrome proposes that these antigenic epitopes are concealed during the normal assembly of type IV collagen into basement membrane. Subsequent exposure of these privileged epitopes, possibly caused by modification of the GBM in response to smoke, hydrocarbons, infections, or other precipitating factors results in the formation of an antigenic structure, antibody production, and inflammation.

In the Heymann's nephritis model, rats are immunized with preparations of proximal tubular brush border. The animals subsequently develop renal lesions that resemble human membranous nephropathy. The rat Heymann antigen has been identified as gp330 or megalin, a 330-kD glycoprotein member of the LDL receptor superfamily which is localized in the clathrin-coated pits of visceral epithelial cells and on the proximal tubule brush border. Antibody binding to gp330 results in alternative pathway complement activation with subsequent shedding of the immune complexes from the cell surface into the subepithelial space. In membranous nephropathy, no cellular infiltrates are seen on light microscopy, most likely because the immune deposits form within the subepithelial surface of the glomerular capillary wall and are not in direct contact with circulating immune cells. However, these immune deposits can interact with soluble mediators to initiate an inflammatory response.

Complement is the best studied of these mediator systems. Experimental evidence demonstrates that complement pathways are activated by the immune complexes deposited within kidney (see below). The complement membrane-attack complex (MAC, C5b-9) can initiate glomerular capillary wall damage that results in proteinuria, although the specific mechanisms by which MAC causes proteinuria are unknown. In vitro studies have demonstrated that MAC is a potent stimulus for glomerular cells to produce oxidants, proteases, prostaglandins, and cytokines. Through these processes, MAC may be responsible for the alteration in the GBM permeability seen in membranous nephropathy. Megalin, like other members of the LDL receptor superfamily, may bind and clear proteases that escape through the glomerular filtration barrier. When antibody binding interferes with normal, receptor-mediated endocytosis to fix megalin and any associated proteins in immune deposits, megalin-associated enzymes may degrade the matrix constituents of the glomerular basement membrane or activate other soluble mediator systems.

In contrast to these native antigens, "planted" antigens are not intrinsic to the glomerulus. They may become trapped within the glomerulus because of charge and size characteristics, molecular configuration, or carbohydrate content. For example, segments of the glomerular filtration barrier can interact with positively charged proteins which act as "planted" antigens to form in situ immune complexes. Occasionally, immunoglobulins themselves are "planted" antigens and attract antiidiotypic antibodies, such as rheumatoid factors, to augment in situ immune complex formation. "Planted" antigens fall into two groups: endogenous and exogenous. Examples of endogenous antigens are DNA, IgA, and other immunoglobulins. DNA has an affinity for the moieties present on the GBM, whereas immunoglobulin aggregates can get trapped within the mesangium. In one rat model for anti-GBM nephritis, rabbit anti-rat GBM antibodies, in amounts insufficient to directly cause glomerular injury, can serve as foreign antigen and initiate an antiidiotypic response. The possibilities for exogenous antigens are endless. Drugs, lectins, and infectious agents can have an affinity for glomerular constituents. Thus "planted" antigens can either be trapped nonspecifically within the glomerulus or specifically bind to glomerular constituents.

Circulating Immune Complex Disease

In this form of immune complex disease, soluble circulating antigen-antibody complexes become passively trapped within the glomerulus, subsequently resulting in renal injury through complement activation, leukocyte infiltration, and often glomerular cell proliferation. Unlike the antibodies that form in situ immune complexes, the antibodies that make up these complexes have no specificity for glomerular components. Although usually cleared by the reticuloendothelial phagocytes, circulating immune complexes can deposit within the glomerulus and other vessel walls if they have appropriate physical and chemical characteristics. Due to their charge and size characteristics, circulating immune complexes initially lodge in the subendothelial space, rarely progressing further into the basement membrane. As a result subendothelial deposits or paramesangial deposits are commonly identified in renal biopsies. Once formed, however, deposited immune complexes can be modified and rearranged in situ as a result of changing antigen:antibody ratios. Free antibody will bind to other antigenic epitopes, increasing the size of the immune complex deposits. Excess antigen may actually dissolve already formed deposits. Several studies have suggested that this ongoing in situ modification can facilitate movement from one glomerular site, such as the subendothelial space, to another, such as the subepithelial glomerular basement membrane.

The noncovalent nature of the antigen and IgG interaction may allow the circulating immune complex to separate within the kidney circulation into component antibody and antigen. Intrarenal immune complex formation can result from the free antigen planting within the GBM followed by subsequent binding of antibody. These models suggest that circulating immune complexes do not directly deposit in the kidney. However, several studies in which covalently (and therefore irreversibly)-linked antigen and antibody complexes were injected into rodents clearly have demonstrated glomerular immune complex deposition, suggesting that circulating complexes can directly deposit in the kidney. The net charge of the injected complexes determined the site of their intraglomerular localization.

The classic experimental models for glomerular injury induced by circulating immune complexes are acute and chronic serum sickness. In these models, rabbits are immunized with a heterologous protein, bovine serum albumin (BSA). Glomerulonephritis, which is characterized by subendothelial and mesangial immune deposits, develops after the animals develop anti-BSA antibodies. Circulating immune complexes also have been implicated in the pathogenesis of human renal diseases such as the autoimmune nephritides associated with cryoglobulinemia and lupus erythematosus, poststreptococcal glomerulonephritis, and tumor-antigen associated membranous nephropathy. Human serum sickness, also associated with circulating immune complex-mediated renal disease, has become rare but can be seen with antivenom therapy for poisonous snake, fish, and spider bites and with experimental therapies using mouse monoclonal antibodies. As already indicated in the discussion of in situ complex disease (above), circulating immune complexes can contain either endogenous or exogenous antigens. Examples of endogenous antigens identified in circulating immune complexes and implicated in human glomerulonephritis include DNA, thyroglobulin, thyroid antigens, immunoglobulins, red cell stroma, and tumor neoantigens. Exogenous antigens implicated in glomerulonephritis are primarily derived from microbes, such as bacteria (streptococci) and viruses (hepatitis B and C). Fungi and parasites also can serve as exogenous antigen. Soluble foreign serum proteins (cow, goat etc.), food antigens, and chemicals, such as gold and mercury, act as exogenous antigens to generate circulating immune complexes that can result in serum sickness or renal disease.

Cell-Mediated Immunity

Many types of glomerulonephritis exhibit hypercellularity upon light microscopic examination, reflecting infiltration of the kidney by inflammatory cells such as neutrophils, monocytes, T cells, or platelets, or proliferation of resident glomerular cells. The location of the glomerular immune complex deposits controls, in part, whether inflammatory cells will be involved in mediating glomerular injury. As previously discussed, immune complexes at the subepithelial site are separated from the circulation by the GBM, limiting leukocyte access. Therefore, as exemplified by membranous nephropathy, a nonproliferative lesion results because complement-derived chemoattractants and antibody cannot interact directly with circulating immune cells. In contrast, immune deposits within subendothelial or mesangial sites are more readily accessible to circulating inflammatory cells and can lead to cell adhesion, activation, and transmigration across the capillary wall. Many human renal inflammatory diseases, such as diffuse proliferative lupus nephritis, IgA nephropathy, type I membranoproliferative glomerulonephritis, Henoch-Schönlein purpura,

and some types of acute postinfectious nephritis result from deposition of immune complexes at mesangial and subendothelial sites. Once localized, inflammatory cells mediate immune injury by releasing soluble mediators such as cytokines, proteolytic enzymes, or reactive oxygen metabolites (Table 1). These mediators can amplify the existing immune response, directly injure nearby glomerular cells, or degrade or denature the matrix protein constituents of the glomerular filtration barrier.

Mediators of immune glomerular injury can be divided into two groups: primary and secondary. Antibody (discussed previously) and T cells are primary mediators, whereas complement, other inflammatory cells, and their secretagogues are secondary mediators of the immune response. Recently, a number of studies using animal models of glomerulonephritis have strongly implicated T-cell mediated, immune mechanisms of kidney injury, which are independent of antibody deposition. For example, transfer of sensitized T cells from donors with progressive glomerulonephritis to normal recipients can initiate glomerular injury in the absence of immune complex deposition. In a rat

TABLE I
Immune Mediators Implicated in Renal Injury

Complement
  Membrane attack complex (C5b-9)
  C3b
  C5a

Reactive oxygen metabolites
  Hydroxy radicals
  Hydrogen peroxides
  Superoxides
  Hypochlorous acids

Enzymes
  PMN myeloperoxidase
  Neutral serine proteases (elastase, cathepsin G)
  Cysteine proteases (cathepsin B & H)
  Metalloproteinases (gelatinase)

Cell adhesion molecules

Cytokines and growth factors (secretory mediators)
  IL-1β
  TNFα
  TGFβ
  Basic FGF
  Prostaglandins
  PDGF
  Plasminogen activator
  Eicosanoids (thromboxanes, leukotrienes)
  Polypeptide growth factors

Coagulation cascade
  Thrombin
  Plasmin
  Plasminogen activators
  Plasminogen activator inhibitors

Note: A wide variety of proinflammatory and immunomodulatory mediators have been associated with renal immune/inflammatory injury. The above list is not intended to be exhaustive.

model of granulomatous nephritis with proteinuria induced by a chemically reactive form of a well-studied hapten, adoptive transfer of T cells from hapten-immunized animals, but not administration of antihapten antibody, induced disease in naive recipients. These studies suggest that intrinsic kidney cells can present antigen in vivo and that cell-mediated immune mechanisms can cause renal injury. In a rat model of nephrotoxic serum nephritis, depletion of CD8+ T cells prior to the administration of nephrotoxic serum completely prevented proteinuria, although the amount of antibody present in the glomeruli of CD8+ T-cell-depleted animals was similar to control animals. In another experimental model employing chickens, in which B cell development was arrested by neonatal bursectomy, immunization with GBM induces a severe proliferative glomerulonephritis characterized by T cells within the glomeruli without evidence of anti-GBM antibodies.

Besides T cells, other inflammatory leukocytes, such as neutrophils, macrophages, and platelets, can migrate into and localize within the glomerulus to promote immune injury. Release of cytokines, proteases, and/or oxidants from these cells (Tables 1 and 2) can damage the GBM resulting in detachment of the epithelial cells foot processes from the filtration barrier with subsequent protein leakage. Effacement of epithelial foot processes is an electron micrographic hallmark of proteinuric renal disease. Neutrophils can infiltrate the glomerulus via Fc receptor-mediated adherence, interactions with adhesion molecules expressed on endothelial cell surfaces, and by the actions of chemoattractants such as C5a from complement activation. The major soluble mediators released by neutrophils are reactive oxygen metabolites such as peroxide, hydroxyl radicals, oxygen free radicals, and superoxides. Myeloperoxidase, a positively charged enzyme found within polymorphonuclear neutrophils, binds to anionic sites within the glomerulus and catalyzes the reaction between peroxide and halide anion to generate hypohalous acids. These acids are thought to directly damage the GBM, leading to proteinuria. In addition to these reactive oxygen metabolites, activated neutrophils release neutral serine proteases such as elastase and cathepsin G that have been shown to degrade the GBM in vitro. Macrophages localize within the glomerulus in response to chemoattractant cytokines (chemokines) derived from cell-mediated immune reactions or in response to antibody deposition via their Fc receptor. Activated macrophages secrete numerous proinflammatory and immunomodulatory molecules, including IL-1β and TNF-α, TGF-β, prostaglandins, and lipid mediators such as platelet-activating factor and lipoxygenase products (see Tables 1 and 2).

Many of these molecules enhance the immune response or alter the character and functions of resident glomerular cells. For example, platelet-derived growth factor stimulates mesangial cell proliferation, which in turn, leads to the increased production of mesangial cell proteases, resulting in glomerular injury. TGF-β activates mesangial cells to increase extracellular matrix deposition, which leads to scarring and glomerulosclerosis. Antibodies, complement, and immune complexes as well can activate mesangial cells to produce various cytokines that can amplify the immune response or promote glomerular injury and sclerosis. Platelets localize within the glomerulus in a complement-dependent manner during immune-mediated injury and release growth factors and eicosanoids which may influence glomerular permeability. In models of experimental glomerulonephritis, depletion of platelets by antiplatelet antibody reduces proteinuria significantly, supporting a role for platelets in glomerular injury. Although each of the inflammatory cells has been discussed individually, each, along with its many soluble mediators, can act in concert with the others to produce immune injury (Fig. 1).

Complement pathway activation may produce immune-mediated renal injury in one of two ways: by recruitment of inflammatory cells to the site of immune injury or by generation of the C5b-9 membrane attack complex (MAC). C5a, a product of the complement cascade activation attracts neutrophils to the site of immune complex deposition and leads to their adherence via their C3b receptors. In Heymann nephritis, complement depletion abolishes proteinuria. In contrast, leukocyte depletion has little effect on indices of renal injury. These results suggest that proteinuria in Heymann nephritis is a complement dependent process mediated by MAC and that complement-induced renal injury can occur without involvement of inflammatory cells. The mechanisms by which MAC causes proteinuria have yet to be determined. In vitro complement compo-

TABLE 2
Cellular Sources of Immune Mediators

Circulating cells	
PMNs	Reactive oxygen metabolites
	Proteases
	Myeloperoxidase
Macrophages	Reactive oxygen metabolites
	Cytokines
	Prostaglandins
	Platelet-derived growth factor
	Eicosanoids
	Coagulation factors
Platelets	Platelet-activating factor
	Eicosanoids
	Platelet-derived growth factor
Renal cells	
Mesangial cells	Reactive oxygen metabolites
	Neutral proteases
	Cytokines
	Prostaglandins
	Plasminogen activator
	Platelet-derived growth factor
	Basic fibroblast growth factor
Endothelial cells	Adhesion molecules
	Cytokines
	Growth factors
Glomerular epithelial cells	Proteolytic enzymes
	Megalin
	Oxygen radicals
Tubular epithelial cells	Class II MHC proteins
	Cytokines

nents activate glomerular epithelial cells (GEC) to produce proinflammatory mediators such as oxidants, proteases, and cytokines which may alter the permeability of the GBM. MAC may also stimulate the GEC to produce excess extracellular matrix components that lead to an altered GBM architecture and increased permeability. Lastly, MAC may alter the binding of extracellular matrix proteins to their receptors (integrins) on GEC, leading to detachment of the GEC and proteinuria.

The alternative pathway of complement activation has been specifically implicated in the pathogenesis of membranoproliferative glomerulonephritis (MPGN) and IgA nephropathy. Seventy percent of patients with a particular type of MPGN (type II) have C3 nephritic factor present in their sera. This factor, instead of properdin, binds and stabilizes alternative C3 convertase. The C3 nephritic factor is an autoantibody to the alternative C3 convertase, suggesting that MPGN is an autoimmune disease. In IgA nephropathy, IgA codeposits along with C3 and properdin in the mesangium. In both diseases, early complement components are usually absent in glomeruli, suggesting a role for the alternative pathway in the immunopathogenesis of both these glomerulonephritides.

In contrast to the glomerulonephritides discussed above, which are associated with antibody-mediated immune injury, necrotizing and crescentic glomerulonephritis, also known as pauci-immune glomerulonephritis, lacks any evidence of glomerular antibody deposition. The immunopathogenesis of this disease remains unclear, but approximately 90% of patients with pauci-immune vasculitis or glomerulonephritis have circulating antineutrophil cytoplasmic antibodies (ANCA) (see Chapter 27). Examples of ANCA-associated diseases are polyarteritis nodosa, leukocytoclastic angiitis, and Wegener's granulomatosis. ANCAs have been implicated in the pathogenesis of these diseases and can be classified into two groups based on their characteristic immunohistochemical staining patterns of neutrophils. C-ANCA yields a cytoplasmic staining pattern, whereas P-ANCA gives a perinuclear staining pattern. The antibodies are specific for enzymes present within the primary granules of neutrophils. For C-ANCA, the enzyme is serine protease 3 and for P-ANCA it is myeloperoxidase. The mechanisms by which ANCA cause glomerulonephritis remain to be elucidated. In vitro evidence suggests that these antibodies stimulate neutrophils to release toxic oxygen radicals and proteolytic enzymes, which subsequently cause fibrinoid necrosis. Antimyeloperoxidase ANCA antibodies along with TNF and endotoxin can stimulate neutrophils to damage human endothelial cells in a dose-dependent manner in vitro.

TUBULOINTERSTITIAL NEPHRITIS

Humoral and cell-mediated immune mechanisms similar to those characterized in the immunopathogenesis of experimental glomerular disease also have been implicated in primary tubulointerstitial immune injury. In situ immune complexes can form and circulating immune complexes can deposit within the tubulointerstitium. Possible mechanisms of tubulointerstial immune complex deposition include "overflow" of glomerular immune complex "binding" sites resulting in tubulointerstitial immune complex formation, cross-reactivity between glomerular and tubulointerstitial antigenic epitopes and simultaneous production of autoreactive antibodies against multiple self-antigens.

Cell-mediated pathways of immune injury appear to be the primary mechanisms of tubulointerstitial nephritis and have been best characterized in a model of tubulointerstitial nephritis produced by antitubular basement membrane antibodies. Although initiated by heterologous antibodies in susceptible rodents, antibody-mediated injury is minimal. Rather, sensitized T cells are required for disease in both an acquired model as well as in an inbred mouse strain (*kdkd*) that spontaneously develops tubulointerstitial nephritis. The target antigen, 3M-L, is synthesized by proximal tubular epithelial cells. Antibody binding to its antigenic epitope activates the mechanisms of immune injury described in detail in the preceding sections.

Tubulointerstitial inflammation almost always accompanies proteinuric renal disease, and some of the most intriguing recent work in renal immunopathogenesis has attempted to elucidate the molecular signals that underlie this link between glomerular and interstitial pathology. Proximal tubular cells actively reabsorb proteins via clathrin-coated pits via a receptor or constitutive pathway. Reabsorbed proteins are degraded by lysosomes into amino acids. The increase in proteinuria that accompanies many renal diseases may overwhelm the capacity of the tubular epithelial cell to perform this function. Accumulation of abnormally high amounts of protein in the endolysosomes leads to organelle rupture and leak of lysosomal enzymes into the cytoplasm. In addition, protein congestion may increase intracellular oxidant stress, a process known to activate a number of signaling enzymes and transcription factors. For example, the activity of the transcription factor NF-κB regulates expression of many proinflammatory cytokines and is increased by oxygen radicals. Thus, tubular protein overload, a nonimmunologic stimulus of renal injury, can activate interstitial immune mechanisms to cause tubulointerstitial inflammation.

Bibliography

Abbas A, Lichtman AH, Pober JS: *Cellular and Molecular Immunology*. WB Saunders Company, Philadelphia, 1994.

Bolton WK, Tucker FL, Sturgill BC: New avian model of experimental glomerulonephritis consistent with mediation by cellular immunity. *J Clin Invest* 73:1263—276, 1984.

Brady HR, Papuyianni A, Serhan CN: Leukocyte adhesion promotes biosynthesis of lipoxygenase products by transcellular routes. *Kidney Int* 45:S-90–S97, 1994.

Cotran RS, Kumar V, Robbins SL: *Pathologic Basis of Disease*. WB Saunders Company, Philadelphia, pp. 171-240 and 927-990, 1994.

Couser WG: Mediators of immune glomerular injury. *Clin Investig* 71:808–811, 1993.

Couser WG: Pathogenesis of glomerulonephritis. *Kidney Int* 44:S519-S526, 1993

Emancipator SN, Sedor JR. Cytokines and Renal Function. In: Remick DG, Kunkel SL (eds) *Cytokines in Health and Disease;*

Physiology and Pathophysiology. Dekker, New York, pp. 467–488, 1992.

Ewert BH, Jennette JC, Falk RJ: Anti-myeloperoxidase antibodies stimulate neutrophils to damage human endothelial cells. *Kidney Int* 41:375–383, 1992.

Farquhar MG: Molecular analysis of the pathological autoimmune antigens of Heymann nephritis. *Am J Pathol* 148:1331–1337, 1996.

Glassock RJ: The glomerulopathies. In: Schrier RW (ed) *Renal and Electrolyte Disorders.* Little, Brown, Co., Boston, pp. 727–806, 1992.

Kawasaki K, Yaoita E, Yamamoto T, et al.: Depletion of CD8 positive cells in nephrotoxic serum nephritis of Wky rats. *Kidney Int* 41:1517–1526, 1992.

Kelly CJ. Tomaszewski J, Neilson EG: Immunopathogenic mechanisms of tubulointerstitial injury. In: Brenner BM, Tisher CC (eds) *Renal Pathology.* 2nd ed., Lippincott, Philadelphia, 2. pp. 699–722, 1996

Makker SP: Mediators of immune glomerular injury. *Am J Nephrol* 13:324–336, 1993.

Neilson EG: Pathogenesis and therapy of interstitial nephritis. *Kidney Int* 35:1257–1270, 1989

Paul WE: The immune system: An introduction. In: Paul WE (ed) *Fundamental Immunology.* Raven Press, New York, pp. 1–20, 1993

Remuzzi G, Ruggenenti P, Benigni A: Understanding the nature of renal disease progression. *Kidney Int* 51:2–15, 1997.

Rennke HG, Klein PS, Sandstrom DJ et al.: Cell mediated injury in the kidney: Acute nephritis induced in the rat by azobenzene-arsonate. *Kidney Int* 45:1044–1056, 1994.

Roy S, Scherer MT, Briner TJ et al.: Murine MHC polymorphism and T-cell specificities. *Science* 244:572–574, 1989

Sedor JR: Cytokines, growth factors and glomerulonephritis immune-mediated renal disease. *Semin Nephrol* 12:428–440, 1992.

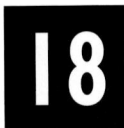

MINIMAL CHANGE NEPHROPATHY

NORMAN J. SIEGEL

OVERVIEW AND TERMINOLOGY

Minimal change nephropathy or minimal change disease (MCD) is a histopathologic lesion which is almost always associated with the nephrotic syndrome at the onset of disease. Other terms such as lipoid nephrosis, nil disease, and idiopathic nephrotic syndrome have been used, interchangeably, with minimal change nephropathy. Because of the finding of lipids in renal tubule cells and the urine of patients with nephrotic syndrome, the term *lipoid nephrosis* has been used to describe patients with steroid-responsive nephrotic syndrome. However, this term is not synonymous with MCD because other histologic lesions may also show a response to steroid therapy. The term *nil disease* is an oversimplification of the histopathology seen in patients with minimal change disease because it refers predominantly to the findings by light microscopy alone. *Idiopathic nephrotic syndrome* actually refers to a wide variety of histopathologic lesions which are associated with primary nephrotic syndrome. Thus, while each of these terms is prevalent in the literature, contemporary understanding of the natural history and therapeutic options requires more precise terminology.

HISTOPATHOLOGY

Minimal change nephropathy is defined on light microscopy by a lack of definitive alteration in glomerular structure. While the degree of alterations which may remove a biopsy from this category has been debated, it is generally agreed that the cellularity of the glomerulus must be *minimal* and that the tubular and interstitial structures must also be normal. There may be some doubly refractile appearance or lipid droplets in the tubule cells but there is no evidence of tubular atrophy or interstitial fibrosis. Immunofluorescent staining also shows no change from normal and an absence of immunoglobulin or complement protein deposition. The most obvious and consistent finding in patients with MCD is a characteristic fusion of epithelial foot processes seen on electron microscopy (Fig. 1). There is normal fenestration of the endothelial cells lining the capillary loop; the glomerular basement membrane is uniform in thickness and structure, but the epithelial cells show swelling and continuous contact with the glomerular basement membrane. Because a biopsy is susceptible to sampling error, it must be remembered that lesions which affect only some glomeruli, such as focal and segmental

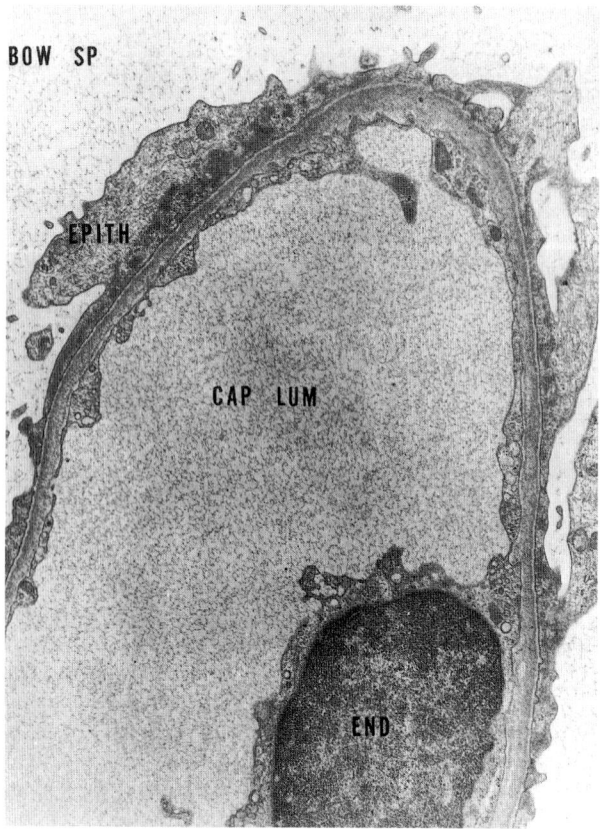

FIGURE I   Electron micrograph of glomerular capillary loop in patient with MCD. The endothelial cell (End) and basement membrane are normal in content and structure. The epithelial cell (Epith) demonstrates diffuse swelling of the pseudopods, footprocess fusion. There are no electron dense deposits.

glomerulosclerosis, may be inadvertently misdiagnosed as MCD.

The role of a renal biopsy in the initial management of patients who present with nephrotic syndrome is controversial. In most cases, children are treated with a course of steroids and biopsies are reserved for those who are steroid resistant. Because of the lower prevalence of steroid-responsive lesions, adolescents and adults are usually biopsied prior to treatment. For those patients of any age with a complicated clinical presentation or course of disease, an assessment of histopathologic changes is essential.

CLINICAL PRESENTATION

Although generally thought to be a childhood disease, MCD presents in both children and adults. The insidious onset of nephrotic syndrome, usually manifested by edema formation, is the most common presentation. In children, the onset of disease is after the first year of life, with a peak incidence between 24 and 36 months of age and a strong male predominance. In preadolescent children, 85 to 95% with idiopathic or primary nephrotic syndrome will have MCD. In adolescents and young adults, the prevalence

of MCD declines to approximately 50% and the male predominance begins to disappear. In patients over the age of 40 years with primary nephrotic syndrome, the incidence of MCD is 20 to 25% and there is a nearly equal distribution between males and females.

In patients presenting with the typical features of MCD, a relatively "pure" nephrotic syndrome is usually observed. Nephritic features such as hypertension, hematuria, and reduced renal function are relatively uncommon. Any one of these nephritic features may occur in 15 to 20% of patients with MCD but the combination of two or more of these factors is decidedly unusual and should make one consider a different diagnosis. The finding of gross hematuria or red cell casts would generally not be considered compatible with the diagnosis of MCD. Thus, the predominant clinical features are those of nephrotic syndrome with heavy proteinuria, low serum albumin, edema formation, and elevated serum cholesterol. Other than the findings of oval fat bodies which appear as maltese crosses on examination of the urine under a polarized lens (see Chapter 3, Fig. 3) the urinalysis is normal. Serum complement levels are normal and antinuclear antibodies and cryoglobulins absent. Serum immunoglobulins may be abnormal with a reduction of serum IgG levels to 20% or less of normal values, a less severe reduction in IgA, and a mild increase in IgM and IgE levels.

Although MCD is usually associated with a primary or idiopathic nephrotic syndrome, secondary MCD also occurs (Table 1). In 80 to 90% of children, MCD is idiopathic although cases associated with the ingestion of heavy metals such as mercury or lead as well as acquired immunodeficiency syndrome have been reported. In adult patients, especially the elderly, the association of this MCD with nonsteroidal anti-inflammatory drugs is particularly important because of their very frequent use. Hodgkin's disease and lymphoproliferative disorders must be kept in

TABLE I
Secondary Causes of Minimal
Change Nephropathy

Drugs
    Nonsteroidal antiinflammatory agents
    Ampicillin/penicillin
    Trimethadione
Toxins
    Mercury
    Lead
    Bee stings
Infection
    Mononucleosis
    HIV
    Immunizations
Tumors
    Hodgkin's lymphoma
    Other lymphoproliferative diseases
    Carcinoma
Obesity

mind when older patients present with MCD. Although most patients with obesity and nephrotic syndrome have focal segmental glomerulosclerosis, some of these patients have responded to steroids or been documented to have MCD.

RESPONSE TO THERAPY

The benchmark for therapy in MCD is the use of corticosteroids. No other cause of nephrotic syndrome is as exquisitely sensitive to treatment with steroid therapy as MCD. Because of the high prevalence of this lesion in children, disappearance of proteinuria in response to the oral administration of prednisone is considered diagnostic for MCD. Characteristically, these young children respond to treatment with a diuresis and clearing of proteinuria within about two weeks of initiation of prednisone therapy, usually at a dose of 2 mg · kg^{-1} · day^{-1} not to exceed 60 mg/day. Some children may have a slower response to initial therapy and not clear their proteinuria for 6 to 8 weeks. A response to therapy in 80 to 90% of adolescents and adults with MCD has also been documented. However, in these age groups, the response is slower and a prolonged period of therapy, in some cases up to 16 weeks, may be required before complete remission of proteinuria is achieved. Unfortunately, this distinct effect of steroids on MCD has been used to presume that remission of proteinuria while on prednisone implies underlying MCD.

The clinical course of MCD is frequently described in terms of the patient's response to steroids (Table 2). Complete remission is defined as complete resolution of proteinuria for at least 3 to 5 consecutive days; a partial remission is a reduction in the degree of proteinuria without complete clearing; and a relapse is a reoccurrence of proteinuria for at least 3 to 5 consecutive days. Children and adolescents tend to have complete remissions whereas partial remissions are more frequent in adult patients. The clinical outcome for children with MCD, as related to steroid therapy, is outlined in Fig. 2. A similar, although not identical, pattern can be expected in adults. About 10% of patients initially treated with steroid therapy will not respond to treatment and will have early steroid resistance. Alternative methods of administration of steroids have been at-

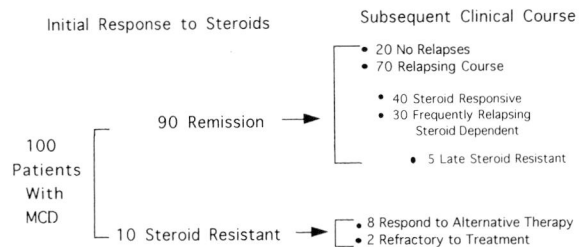

FIGURE 2 Clinical outcome for children with MCD.

tempted in this group of patients, but have not been particularly successful. These patients frequently respond to cytotoxic or immunosuppressive therapies.

Of the patients who achieve a remission on initial steroid therapy, 75 to 85% experience one or more relapses (Fig. 2). In those patients who are destined to follow a relapsing course, the first relapse usually occurs within 6 to 12 months of the onset of their disease, although in some patients the first relapse may be delayed as long as 24 to 30 months. In patients with a relapsing course, 50 to 65% can be expected to have a steroid-responsive clinical profile with frequent relapses occurring over 3 to 5 years. However, for 25 to 30% of patients with MCD, a more protracted clinical course occurs and their disease is described as being frequently relapsing or steroid dependent. A small proportion of these patients may develop late steroid resistance at which point a repeat renal biopsy may show evolution to other histopathologic patterns such as focal segmental glomerular sclerosis. Thus, the majority of patients with MCD have a good response to initial steroid therapy, and a disease course characterized by relapses of their nephrotic syndrome but, overall, an excellent long-term prognosis.

Patients with frequently relapsing/steroid-dependent MCD present the greatest therapeutic challenge. In the long run, the relapsing nature of their disease is likely to disappear; however, over the short term, deleterious side effects of continued steroid therapy may occur—particularly in adults and geriatric patients. Most often, when a patient has a frequently relapsing/steroid-dependent clinical pattern, an attempt is made to decrease the frequency of relapses by maintaining the patient on chronic low dose corticosteroid therapy. Many patients will tolerate low doses of prednisone on a daily or alternate day basis without significant side effects. For those patients who require large doses of medication to remain in remission or who develop significant side effects, alternative therapy must be considered.

Cyclophosphamide and chlorambucil have proved to be the most effective alternative therapies for patients with MCD. These drugs have been shown to be effective in both children and adults with frequently relapsing/steroid-dependent nephrotic syndrome. Typically, prednisone will be used to induce remission, then an 8- to 12-week course of cyclophosphamide in a dose of 2 mg · kg^{-1} · day^{-1} or chlorambucil in a dose of 0.1 to 0.2 mg · kg^{-1} · day^{-1} will be added. The most pronounced and dramatic effect is the prolonged period of remission of the nephrotic syndrome

---

TABLE 2

Clinical Course of Minimal Change Disease as Related to Steroid Therapy

Steroid responsive
  Complete remission of proteinuria within 8–12 weeks with
    infrequent relapses

Frequently relapsing steroid dependent
  Relapses occur during the taper of steroids
  Relapses occur at rate of twice every 6 months or six times
    every 18 months
  Relapses occur within 2 weeks of cessation of therapy

Steroid resistant
  Failure to obtain a remission within 12 weeks

---

152 — Norman J. Siegel

which is achieved in patients treated with these agents. After cessation of the cytotoxic agent, 30 to 40% of patients will have no subsequent relapses. Among relapsers, the average period of remission is 18 to 24 months. Subsequent relapses are usually more steroid responsive than prior to cytotoxic therapy. Thus, steroid-related side effects such as a cushingoid appearance or growth retardation can be markedly diminished and reversed. In patients unable to tolerate steroids, it is also possible to induce a remission of the nephrotic syndrome with either of these agents alone; in the elderly, alkylating agents have been used as initial therapy. These agents have a number of serious side effects, including cystitis, alopecia, leukopenia, gonadal toxicity, potential for malignancy formation, and seizures; their use requires caution and careful judgment.

Other medications have also been used to treat patients with either steroid refractory or frequently relapsing/steroid-dependent disease. Cyclosporine has been reported to be effective in some adult and pediatric patients with an initial steroid-resistant course. Its primary utility is to achieve a steroid-sparing effect because the relapse rate is high after cyclosporine is discontinued. The prolonged period of remission produced by treatment with cyclophosphamide or chlorambucil is not observed. In addition, long-term therapy with cyclosporine may be complicated by nephrotoxicity. Despite multiple clinical trials, cyclosporine remains a late therapeutic option for patients with MCD. Levamisole has also been used to achieve a steroid-sparing effect.

For patients unresponsive to these therapeutic interventions, symptomatic control of edema formation with salt restriction and diuretics are the mainstays of therapy. If complications of anasarca occur, such as pleural or pericardial effusions, severe hyponatremia, or fascitis, the infusion of albumin can be beneficial to mobilize the extracellular fluid and prevent pulmonary or cardiac decompensation. This therapy, however, should be undertaken with caution because the shifts in intravascular volume associated with albumin infusion can result in severe hypertension or congestive heart failure and because the beneficial effect is short term since the albumin is rapidly excreted in a patient with heavy proteinuria. Proteinuria can be reduced with nonsteroidal antiinflammatory drugs (NSAIDS) and angiotensin converting enzyme (ACE) inhibitors. These therapies may be of benefit in patients who are refractory to treatment of their nephrotic syndrome, have severe proteinuria, and who are developing malnutrition because of the quantity of protein lost in the urine. However, the reduction in proteinuria in patients treated with either of these medications is, in large part, related to alterations in renal blood flow and glomerular filtration rate rather than a direct effect on the mechanisms of the proteinuria. Consequently, patients with MCD who are treated with either NSAIDS or ACE inhibitors are particularly susceptible to alterations in intravascular volume and renal perfusion and are prone to the development of acute renal failure or hyperkalemia. While these drugs are generally well tolerated and may be beneficial in a selected subset of patients, careful monitoring of patients receiving them is essential.

COMPLICATIONS AND LONG-TERM OUTCOME

The primary complications of MCD are related to persistent nephrotic syndrome or to side effects of therapy. The most common complications of steroid therapy include cushingoid facies, stria, and acne, as well as cataracts. In general, these medications are much better tolerated in children than in adults. The induction of a prolonged remission by a cytotoxic agent permits regression of the majority of the steroid-related side effects. Stria and cataracts usually persist; however, catch-up growth frequently occurs and the cushingoid appearance disappears. Complications of cytotoxic agents are substantial but can be avoided with the careful dosing of these drugs, limitations of their use to short courses, and appropriate precautions such as adequate hydration. Indeed, in the majority of studies in children and adults, minimal side effects of either chlorambucil or cyclophosphamide have been reported and the drugs have been well tolerated. One of the most disturbing side effects of cyclophosphamide therapy, gonadal toxicity, appears to be dose related and reversible in the majority of young patients treated with this medication.

Peritonitis is an important complication of the nephrotic syndrome for those patients particularly children, who are unable to achieve a remission of their proteinuria. Peritonitis occurs during periods of severe edema formation particularly when ascites is present. The most common infecting agent is *Streptococcus* pneumonia. However, infections with *Escherichia coli* and *Hemophilus influenzae* have also been reported. Prior to antibiotic therapy, peritonitis was the major cause of death in children and adults with MCD.

Reversible acute renal failure has also been reported in patients with MCD. This complication appears to occur much more frequently in adult patients than in children. It is usually associated with a state of severe edema formation. A period of rapid weight accumulation immediately precedes the onset of the renal failure. The pathophysiology of acute renal failure in patients with MCD is poorly understood and cannot be clearly related to intravascular volume depletion, acute tubular necrosis, or vascular obstruction such as renal vein thrombosis.

The development of chronic renal failure in patients with MCD is rare in children and adults with a steroid-responsive clinical course. Patients at highest risk are those who either do not have an initial response to steroid therapy or those who become late nonsteroid responders (Fig. 2). In both of these situations the possibility that the histopathologic lesion may be different or have evolved into a pattern different than MCD must be considered and may be the dominant factor in overall prognosis. For the majority of children the relapsing nature of their disease will begin to dissipate about 10 years after onset and the majority will be free of proteinuria after puberty. However, late relapses after long-term remissions of the nephrotic syndrome in patients who have had their initial episode at a very young age have been well documented. Similarly, adult patients with MCD have a very good prognosis with 85 to 90% survival rate 10 years or more after the onset of disease. The major morbidity is related to complications of therapy.

Bibliography

Berns JS, Gaudio KM, Krassner LS, et al.: Steroid-responsive nephrotic syndrome of childhood: A long-term study of clinical course, histopathology, efficacy of cyclophosphamide therapy, and effects on growth. *Am J Kidney Dis* 9:108–114, 1987.

Habib R, Kleinknecht C: The primary nephrotic syndrome of childhood: Classification and clinicopathologic study of 406 cases. In: Sommers SC (ed) *Pathology Annual.* Appleton-Century-Crofts, New York, pp. 417–474, 1971.

International Study of Kidney Disease in Children: Nephrotic syndrome in children: Prediction of histopathology from clinical and laboratory characteristics at time of diagnosis. *Kidney Int* 13:159–165, 1996.

Nolasco F, Cameron JS, Heywood EF, et al.: Adult-onset minimal change nephrotic syndrome: A long-term follow-up. *Kidney Int* 29:1215–1223, 1986.

Siegel NJ, Goldberg B, Krassner LS, Hayslett JP: Long-term follow-up of children with steroid-responsive nephrotic syndrome. *J Pediatr* 81:251–258, 1972.

Smith JD, Hayslett JP: Reversible renal failure in the nephrotic syndrome. *Am J Kidney Dis* 21:201–213, 1992.

White RHR, Glasgow EF, Mills RJ: Clinicopathologic study of nephrotic syndrome in childhood. *Lancet* 1:1353–1359, 1970.

Korbet SM: Management of idiopathic nephrosis in adults, including steroid-resistant nephrosis. *Curr Opin Nephrol Hypertens* 4(2): 169–16, 1995.

19

MEMBRANOPROLIFERATIVE GLOMERULONEPHRITIS

VIVETTE D'AGATI

Membranoproliferative glomerulonephritis (MPGN) is a morphologic entity which is primarily defined at the light microscopic level. The membranoproliferative pattern of glomerular injury is characterized by mesangial proliferation and thickening of the glomerular capillary walls due to peripheral capillary wall immune deposits, mesangial interposition, and double contours ("tram-tracks") of the glomerular basement membrane, each of which may be present to varying degrees. Because MPGN manifests mesangial proliferation and extension of cells into the peripheral capillaries, thereby causing accentuation of the glomerular lobularity, the terms "mesangiocapillary glomerulonephritis" and "lobular glomerulonephritis" have been used synonymously. An important concept in approaching this entity is that MPGN is a nonspecific pattern of glomerular response to injury and as such includes primary (or idiopathic) forms which are subdivided into types I, II, and III, as well as a large number of secondary forms listed in Table 1. These secondary conditions are actually more common than the idiopathic forms and include various systemic autoimmune, infectious, and neoplastic disorders. Secondary causes of MPGN must be excluded by careful integration of the renal histologic, immunofluorescence, and electron microscopic findings

with the clinical and laboratory features, before a diagnosis of primary MPGN can be made. Whereas most cases of MPGN occurring in children are idiopathic, secondary forms tend to predominate in the adult population.

PATHOLOGY

Idiopathic MPGN

Idiopathic MPGN occurs in several morphologically distinct forms, each of which may correspond to a different clinicopathologic disease entity. Type I is the most common. It consists of mesangial expansion owing to increased mesangial cell number and matrix containing mesangial immune deposits, sometimes imparting a nodular quality to the mesangium Fig. 1. The peripheral capillary walls are thickened by extensive circumferential mesangial interposition, subendothelial deposits, and double contours of the glomerular basement membrane best delineated with the Jones methenamine silver stain. The degree of glomerular hypercellularity varies from mild to marked, and the severe forms generally have highly exaggerated lobularity. Infiltrating neutrophils and monocytes may contribute to the glomerular hypercellularity. Glomeruli tend to be affected

TABLE I

Membranoproliferative Glomerulonephritis

Primary or idiopathic
    Type I   Mesangiocapillary glomerulonephritis
    Type II   Dense deposit disease
    Type III   With mixed features of type I MPGN and membranous GN (Burkholder et al., 1970)
                    With complex intramembranous deposits (Strife et al., 1984; Anders et al., 1977)

Secondary (associated with other diseases)
  With immune deposits
    Infections   Cryoglobulinemia (predominantly type II, also type III)
                 Hepatitis B, Hepatitis C, Endocarditis, Visceral abscesses, Infected ventriculoatrial shunts, Malaria,
                    Schistosomiasis, Mycoplasma, EBV, HIV
    Autoimmune diseases
                 SLE, Rheumatoid arthritis, Sjogren's syndrome
    Dysproteinemias
                 Light chain deposition disease, Cryoglobulinemia type I or II
                 Waldenstrom's macroglobulinemia, Immunotactoid and Fibrillary glomerulopathy
  Without immune deposits
    Chronic liver disease
                 Cirrhosis, α_1-antitrypsin deficiency
    Thrombotic microangiopathies (subacute phase)
                 HUS/TTP, Anti-phospholipid antibody syndrome, Radiation nephritis, Sickle cell anemia, Transplant
                 glomerulopathy

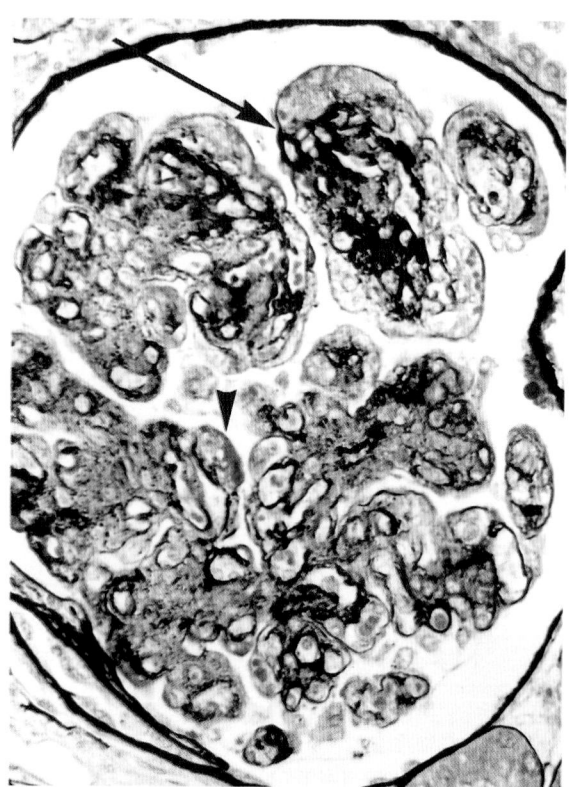

FIGURE I MPGN type I showing lobular accentuation of the tuft with global mesangial hypercellularity and sclerosis, with nodular enlargement of the mesangium (arrow). There are frequent double contours in association with subendothelial deposits (arrowhead) (Jones methenamine silver, X300).

uniformly, in a global and diffuse manner, although mild cases may have more focal and segmental lesions. By immunofluorescence, the immune deposits usually consist of immunoglobulins and complement components distributed in a combined granular mesangial pattern and granular to semilinear subendothelial pattern which outlines the lobular contours. Although IgG and C3 usually predominate, weaker and more variable staining for IgM, IgA, and C1q may also be found. A minority of cases will exhibit staining for C3 only without codeposits of immunoglobulin. By electron microscopy, the mesangial areas are expanded by mesangial proliferation and mesangial immune deposits, with increasing mesangial sclerosis and nodularity as the disease progresses. Mesangial cells migrate into the peripheral capillaries by interposing their cell processes between the original glomerular basement membrane (GBM) and the endothelium ("mesangial interposition" or "peripheral mesangial extension"), often in association with subendothelial electron dense deposits Fig. 2. There is debate whether monocytes or endothelial cells are also capable of cellular interposition. In this peripheral location, irregular neomembrane is produced internal to the original GBM, producing a double contour or tram-track, which may be partial or circumferential.

Type II MPGN is the least common form of idiopathic MPGN, also known as "dense deposit disease." The degree of mesangial hypercellularity is highly variable and less uniform than in type I, and double contours of the GBM tend to be less well developed Fig. 3. The defining feature is a band-like thickening of the lamina densa of the GBM, some tubular basement membranes, and the basal lamina of Bowman's capsule by intramembranous deposits of PAS-positive, silver-positive material. By electron microscopy, these consist of distinctive highly electron dense deposits

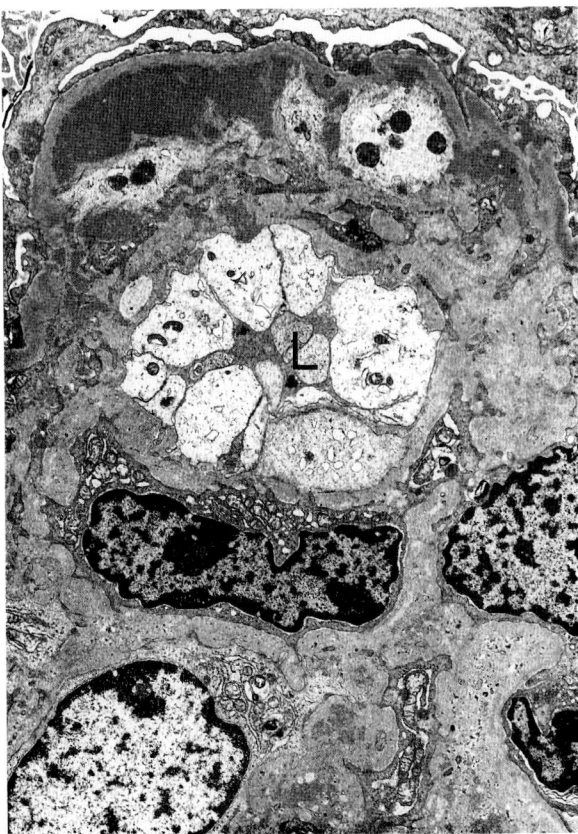

FIGURE 2 MPGN type I. Electron micrograph showing narrowing of the capillary lumen (L) by subendothelial deposits, circumferential extension of mesangial cells and subendothelial neomembrane, producing a double contour (X3000).

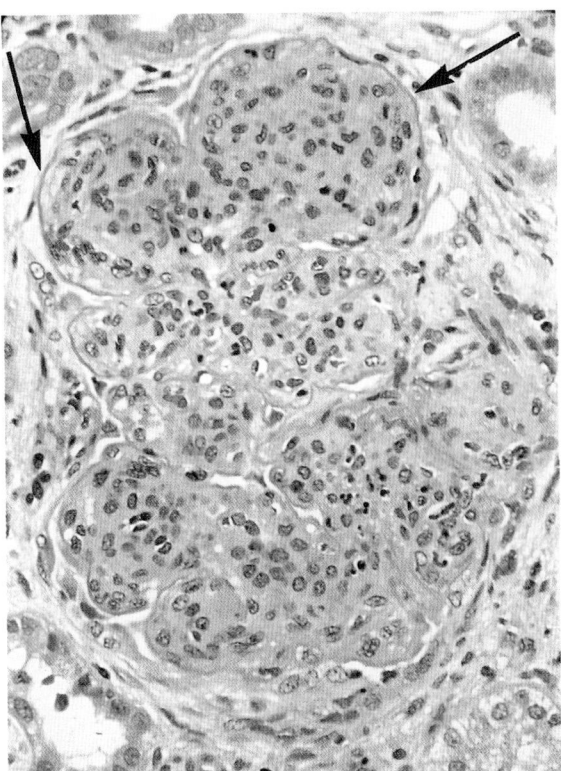

FIGURE 3 MPGN type II. A severe example with exuberant lobular accentuation of the tuft by mesangial proliferation. There is band-like thickening of the glomerular basement membranes (arrows) (hematoxylin-eosin, X300).

which replace and transform the lamina densa, producing smooth, ribbon-like thickenings Fig. 4. More nodular mesangial electron dense deposits are also usually found. By immunofluorescence there is typically positivity for C3 only in a linear or double-contoured distribution along the glomerular basement membranes and as nodular "ring forms" in the mesangium. More focal and often discontinuous linear C3 deposits are also found in Bowman's capsule and some tubular basement membranes.

Type III MPGN is a relatively uncommon and controversial variant. Two subtypes have been defined. The first displays combined features of MPGN type I and membranous glomerulonephritis with variable deposits in mesangial, subendothelial, and subepithelial locations. These usually consist of immunoglobulins (particularly IgG) and complement (C3 and C1), although up to half of cases may have staining for C3 only. By electron microscopy the glomerular capillary walls exhibit a complex thickening due to electron dense deposits in mixed subendothelial and subepithelial locations, often with associated tramtracks on the inner aspect, and basement membrane spikes separating the subepithelial deposits on the outer aspect. Correspondingly, at the light microscopic level, silver stain highlights the combined GBM double contours and spikes,

giving a complex, woven, and multilayered appearance to the glomerular capillary wall. The second variant is less well accepted. It resembles a hybrid between type I and type II MPGN, with combined subendothelial and extensive intramembranous deposits which cause highly irregular thickenings of the glomerular capillary wall, often extending from the subendothelial to the subepithelial aspect. These intramembranous deposits lack the smooth, ribbon-like appearance of the dense deposits in type II disease. The intramembranous deposits are silver negative and cause severe disruption and fraying of the lamina densa. Correspondingly, by light microscopy, the glomerular basement membranes appear markedly thickened and usually fail to take the silver stain. Tubular basement membrane deposits occur with less regularity than in MPGN type II.

Secondary MPGN

Although the many entities listed in Table 1 share membranoproliferative features at the light microscopic level, they can usually be distinguished from the primary form by integrating clinical and serologic data with the immunofluorescence and electron microscopic features. Some secondary forms of MPGN have immune complex deposits similar to the primary forms, whereas others have mesangiocapillary proliferative features without immune deposits

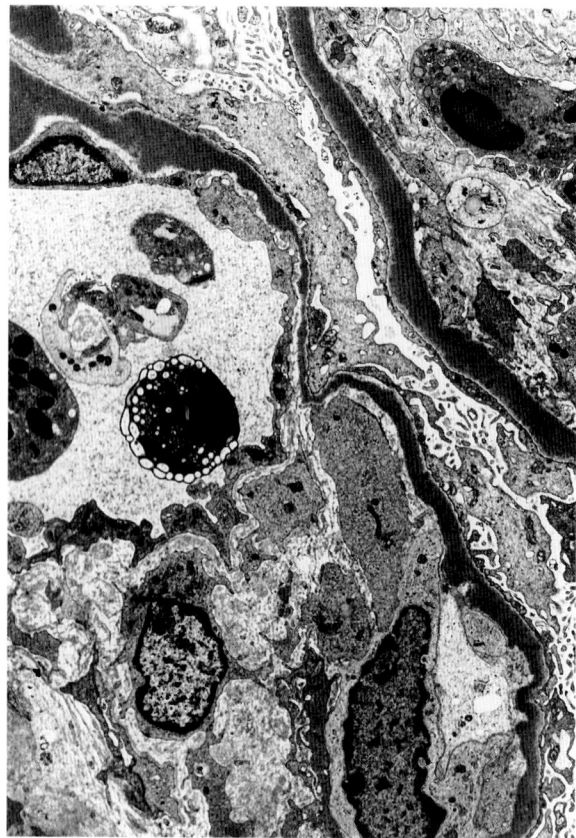

FIGURE 4 MPGN type II. Electron micrograph showing smooth ribbon-like dense deposits within the lamina densa of two adjacent glomerular capillaries (X2000).

(as in chronic thrombotic microangiopathy). For example, in light chain deposition disease, the deposits consist of light chain only (usually kappa), without associated Ig heavy chain or complement. In thrombotic microangiopathies, the subendothelial material found between the double contours of GBM consists of organizing products of coagulation rather than immune deposits and thus stains predominantly for fibrinogen. In fibrillary glomerulopathy, the deposits consist of polyclonal IgG and complement and have a characteristic ultrastructural appearance of randomly oriented fibrils 16 to 24 nm in diameter.

In cryoglobulinemia, the glomerular deposits reflect the composition of the cryoprecipitate detected in the serum. In type I cryoglobulinemia, these consist of a single monoclonal immunoglobulin component, (such as IgG kappa). In the more common type II cryoglobulinemia, the deposits usually stain for both IgG and IgM but with IgM dominance since the cryoglobulins typically consist of a monoclonal IgM kappa component complexed to polyclonal IgG. C3 is usually more intense than C1q. Type II cryoglobulinemia is the form most frequently identified in "mixed essential" cryoglobulinemia, of which most cases have now been linked to chronic hepatitis C infection. Type III cryoglobulins consisting of two polyclonal immunoglobulins are common in autoimmune and infectious diseases but are less

frequently implicated in MPGN. In MPGN secondary to cryoglobulinemia, large intracapillary glomerular deposits ("protein thrombi") are common. By electron microscopy, glomerular electron dense deposits may be of the usual granular type or exhibit an organized annular-tubular (25 to 35 nm) or fibrillar substructure (Fig. 5). In some patients with cryoglobulinemic glomerulonephritis, the deposits may be relatively scanty at both the immunofluorescence and ultrastructural level. Vasculitis with arterial cryoglobulin deposits can also sometimes be demonstrated on renal biopsy.

PATHOGENESIS

Although the nature of the antigenic stimulus in most forms of MPGN is unknown, the demonstration of circulating immune complexes (ICs) in over half of patients and hypocomplementemia in nearly three quarters strongly supports an IC pathogenesis. A process of IC deposition in the mesangium and glomerular capillary wall followed by complement activation, leukocyte chemotaxis, platelet activation, and release of cytokines mitogenic for mesangial cells is likely central to its mediation. Experimental models of chronic serum sickness produced by repeated injection of foreign antigen closely mimic MPGN, although the relative contribution of passive deposition of preformed ICs and in situ IC formation following local Ag planting are in dispute. In models of passive administration of preformed ICs, complexes of intermediate size and variable charge (cationic, neutral, or anionic) tend to deposit in the mesangium and subendothelial zones and could be augmented by complement activation and binding of antiidiotypic antibodies or rheumatoid factors. Experimentally, cationic antigens have a particular affinity for the negatively charged lamina rara interna and could act as a source of subendothelial Ag planting. Hepatitis B viral antigens (surface, core, and e antigen), hepatitis C nucleocapsid/core protein C22-3, and DNA-histones are examples of antigens which have been identified in the circulating ICs or glomerular deposits of patients with secondary forms of MPGN due to infections and SLE. Whereas many cases of MPGN type I follow an upper respiratory tract infection or other infectious process, the inciting antigen in the idiopathic forms remains unknown.

The pathogenesis of MPGN type II is likely to be quite different from the schema of IC deposition outlined above. In dense deposit disease, no circulating ICs have been identified and glomerular deposits consist of C3 only, without Ig. These patients have evidence of systemic dense deposits affecting splenic sinusoids and Bruch's membrane of the retina, and some have associated partial lipodystrophy. Lipid extraction techniques applied to the ultrathin sections for electron microscopy cause the dense deposits to lose their electron dense appearance, suggesting that they may consist of lipids rich in unsaturated fatty acids, although their chemical composition and origin are unknown. It has been postulated that factor D of the complement system, a serine protease "adipsin" synthesized by adipocytes which converts factor B of the preconvertase C3bB to its activated

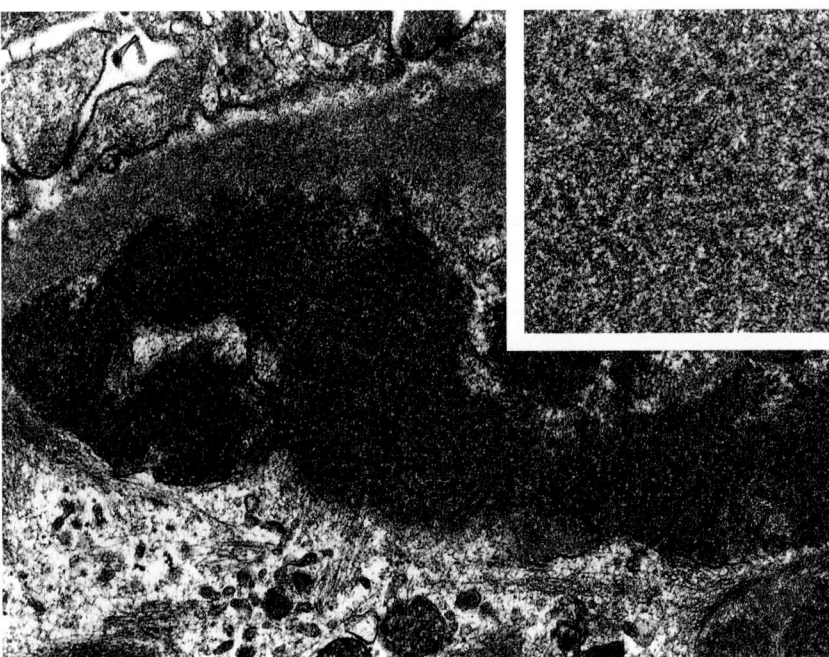

FIGURE 5 Cryoglobulinemic glomerulonephritis. Electron micrograph showing subendothe-lial electron dense deposits with organized substructure (X10,000). The inset shows a higher magnification of the subendothelial deposits with hollow annular-tubular structures approximately 30 nm in diameter (X24,000).

form C3bBb, may provide a pathogenetic link between partial lipodystrophy and MPGN type II.

CLINICAL FEATURES AND OUTCOME

Idiopathic MPGN

Complement activation and hypocomplementemia are integral features of all three types of MPGN, and thus the term "hypocomplementemic glomerulonephritis" was used in the past. Although there is considerable overlap, the patterns of complement activation tend to differ between the three forms. In type I, serum C3 and CH50 levels are reduced in up to one half of patients. Concentrations of C1q, C4, properdin, and factor B are borderline or reduced in less than half of cases. These findings are consistent with the hypothesis of both classic complement pathway activation by ICs as well as alternative pathway complement activation. Inherited complement deficiencies (C2, C3, C6, C7, and C8) and reduced hepatic synthesis of complement likely contribute to the hypocomplementemia in some patients with MPGN, particularly types I and III. In type II, there is persistent and often profound depression of C3, with normal levels of early complement components C1q and C4. This persistent marked C3 reduction is likely mediated by C3 nephritic factor (Nfa), an autoantibody to C3bBb, the C3 convertase of the alternative pathway, which is demonstrable in more than 70% of patients with MPGN type II. By binding to the C3 convertase, C3 nephritic factor stabilizes the convertase and prevents the action of C3b inactivator, thereby maintaining the convert-

ase in a continually activated state. C3 nephritic factor is not unique to MPGN type II but can be identified in about a quarter of patients with type I disease and some autoimmune conditions such as SLE, cryoglobulinemia, and shunt nephritis. In type III MPGN, C3 levels are reduced in up to 50% of patients, C4 levels are usually normal, and C3 nephritic factor is absent. The presence of reduced C5, C6, C7, and C9 in some patients with type III MPGN has been linked to a separate terminal pathway nephritic factor (NFt) which activates complement more distally in the complement cascade.

In its primary form, MPGN is most common in older children and young adults, (ages 7 to 30). It is equally prevalent in both sexes, with white racial predominance. The renal manifestations include nephrotic and nephritic features, often present in combination. In two thirds of patients with MPGN type I, features of nephrotic syndrome dominate the clinical presentation. Other presenting features include asymptomatic hematuria with erythrocyte casts, acute nephritic syndrome, subnephrotic proteinuria with stable or slowly progressive renal insufficiency, and recurrent episodes of gross hematuria. An upper respiratory tract infection including streptococcal pharyngitis commonly precedes first clinical recognition of renal disease. The failure of the nephritis to resolve, with persistence of proteinuria, hematuria, and hypocomplementemia beyond 6 weeks, are ominous clues that the disease is other than acute poststreptococcal glomerulonephritis, which must then be confirmed by renal biopsy.

MPGN type I tends to be a slowly progressive disease and there are few spontaneous remissions. The reported

10-year renal survival is 50%. Median renal survival for both children and adults ranges from 9 to 12 years. Treatment may lead to partial or complete clinical remission in a subgroup of patients. Repeat renal biopsies performed after a prolonged course of therapy have documented regression of the mesangiocapillary lesions but with frequent persistence of mesangial hypercellularity.

Type II MPGN is much rarer than MPGN type I, constituting less than 5% of all cases of idiopathic MPGN seen at Columbia Presbyterian Medical Center. Mean age of onset is slightly younger than in type I and common presentations include acute nephritic syndrome or recurrent macroscopic hematuria. Median renal survival ranges from 5 to 12 years. The course of MPGN type II is generally more aggressive than type I, although up to 20% of patients may exhibit a relatively stable, more indolent course.

In all types of MPGN, features which portend a poor outcome include greater percentage of sclerotic glomeruli, numerous crescents and more severe tubular atrophy, and interstitial fibrosis at biopsy. Negative clinical prognostic features include elevated serum creatinine and hypertension at biopsy as well as a course of severe, unremitting nephrotic syndrome. Outcome appears to be better in patients with asymptomatic hematuria and subnephrotic proteinuria who have more focal and milder membranoproliferative features on renal biopsy.

Secondary MPGN

A major cause of secondary MPGN is cryoglobulinemia. Cryoglobulins are immunoglobulins which share the physical property of precipitation in the cold. Three main types have been identified. Type I cryoglobulins consist of a single monoclonal immunoglobulin. This type occurs in dysproteinemias such as B cell lymphoma, Waldenstrom's macroglobulinemia, and myeloma. Type II and III cryoglobulins are mixed cryoglobulins containing two immunoglobulins, often with rheumatoid factor activity. Type II cryoglobulins consist of one monoclonal immunoglobulin (usually IgM) complexed to a polyclonal IgG. Type III cryoglobulins consist of two polyclonal immunoglobulins (usually IgG and IgM). These mixed forms are often found in autoimmune diseases, chronic infections, chronic liver disease and, in the case of type II, some dysproteinemias. Recently, the majority of cases of mixed essential cryoglobulinemia have been linked to hepatitis C virus (HCV) infection. In fact, IgG directed to HCV core (C22-3) protein has been found to be enriched in the circulating cryoglobulins.

Clinical manifestations of cryoglobulinemia resemble those of multisystem vasculitis. These include palpable purpura due to leukocytoclastic vasculitis, arthralgias and arthritis, distal necroses and skin ulcerations, Raynaud's phenomenon, peripheral neuropathy, abdominal pain, and glomerulonephritis of the MPGN type, sometimes with associated vasculitis of renal arterioles, small arteries and veins.

A significant fraction of cases of apparently "idiopathic" MPGN in adults may actually be related to HCV infection.

However, the incidence of HCV infection in patients with MPGN has not been studied in any systematic way. The increasing recognition of hepatitis C-associated MPGN in adults has only become possible with the availability of highly sensitive serum assays for antibody to HCV [including second generation enzyme-linked immunoassay (EIA II) and recombinant immunoblot assay (RIBA) which test for antibody to four HCV antigens] as well as polymerase chain reaction (PCR) for viral genome in patient serum. Acute hepatitis due to HCV is often subclinical and anicteric but leads to chronic active hepatitis in a significant percentage of cases. The development of glomerulonephritis and cryoglobulinemia are late complications of hepatitis C infection. Among patients with HCV-associated MPGN, only one fifth have signs of liver disease but two thirds have mild elevations of their liver transaminases. Primary risk factors for HCV infection in this group include IVDA in over half and blood transfusions in about one fifth. Other cases may be caused by perinatal transmission from mother to fetus. Cryoglobulinemia can be detected in about two thirds of patients but less than half have extrarenal manifestations (such as purpura, arthralgias, neuropathy, and cardiomyopathy). Decreased CH50 is detectable in 90%, with reduced C4 in 70%, reduced C3 in 50%, and positive rheumatoid factor in more them 70%. In some cases, diagnosis of HCV-associated MPGN may precede by months or years the clinical demonstration of cryoglobulinemia. About one third of cases of HCV-associated MPGN never develop evidence of cryoglobulinemia. The most common renal presentation is proteinuria (which is nephrotic in about 70%) and mild azotemia. Hematuria and nephritic features are present in about 25%. The most common pattern of glomerulonephritis is MPGN type I (>80%), with fewer cases of MPGN type III or acute exudative glomerulonephritis.

TREATMENT

Idiopathic MPGN

In neither children nor adults is the optimal therapy for idiopathic MPGN clearly defined. Only limited data are available for types II and III MPGN, and most of the randomized clinical trials are flawed by short-term follow-up periods of only 1 to 4 years. Interpretation of the findings is made difficult by the failure of earlier studies to identify HCV as an associated risk factor.

The major treatment modalities employed in children and adults with idiopathic MPGN include corticosteroids and antiplatelet agents. In the pediatric population, early studies showed stabilization of renal function in most children treated with alternate day steroids (2 mg/kg every other day for 1 year, tapered gradually to 20 mg every other day for up to 5 to 10 years). In a subsequent controlled trial by the International Study of Kidney Disease in Children, alternate day prednisone administered for 3 to 4 years led to stabilized or improved renal function in 61% of patients, compared to 12% of controls. However, treatment failures occurred in 40% of the prednisone-treated group compared to 55% of those receiving placebo. Problems related to steroid toxicity, such as hypertension and seizures, in children treated with this regimen have led to trials of shorter courses of steroids coupled with aggressive antihypertensive therapy. In one uncontrolled pediatric study of 19 patients, prednisone 2 mg/kg daily was administered for a maximum of 8 weeks, followed by taper to 20 mg every other day for 2 to 3 years, in conjunction with one or more antihypertensive medications. At 2 years following onset of treatment, there was significant improvement in GFR and proteinuria in most patients, with reversion to inactive urinary sediment.

A role for corticosteroid therapy in adults with idiopathic MPGN is less clear. Convincing evidence of benefit has been difficult to demonstrate in several retrospective studies. On the other hand, one study has demonstrated that antiplatelet agents (aspirin 975 mg/day and dipyridamole 225 mg/day) administered for 1 year reduced the incidence of renal failure at 3 to 5 years, but without a difference in outcome at 10 years. These findings suggest that more prolonged therapy may be required. A small controlled trial of aspirin (500 mg/day) and dipyridamole (75 mg/day) versus placebo, together with antihypertensives and protein restriction for 3 years, showed greater reduction in proteinuria in those treated with aspirin and dipyridamole. Larger, long-term studies are required to better define the role of these agents in children and adults.

In sum, conformity of opinion on how to treat idiopathic MPGN is lacking. Based on the available data, it seems judicious to treat children with idiopathic MPGN who have significant active disease and nephrotic syndrome with a prolonged course of low-dose corticosteroids. A similar regimen may be considered in adults with type I MPGN in whom secondary forms (in particular, HCV infection) have been excluded. Treatment has not been shown to be efficacious for type II or type III MPGN in adults. The role of antiplatelet agents as first-line therapy remains to be defined in long-term studies. Nonetheless, antiplatelet therapy appears a reasonable alternative to steroids in selected cases.

Compared to earlier 10-year renal survivals of approximately 50%, more recent studies of patients receiving various therapies for MPGN have reported improved survivals of 60 to 85% for both children and adults. This apparently improved outcome is likely due in part to bias in the study design, since survival for the treated group was calculated from onset of therapy whereas survivals in historical controls were calculated from time of clinical onset of disease.

Secondary MPGN

Choice of therapy in secondary forms of MPGN depends on the underlying condition. For example, membranoproliferative variants of lupus nephritis will usually respond to immunosuppressive regimens used to treat other examples of class IV lupus with comparable activity. Partial or complete remission can be attained in MPGN secondary to bacterial endocarditis or infected atrioventricular shunts with use of appropriate antimicrobial therapy. In hepatitis

B-associated MPGN, the glomerulonephritis often resolves spontaneously and immunosuppressive therapy may be contraindicated because of the increased risk of activation of the hepatitis.

In hepatitis C-associated MPGN with or without cryoglobulinemia, therapeutic strategies have included prednisone, pulse methylprednisolone, cyclophosphamide, plasmapheresis, and interferon-α. When 19 patients with HCV-associated MPGN were treated for 6 months or more with interferon-α, there was a significant reduction in proteinuria (5.8 to 2.0 g/day), but no significant change in renal function at the end of the study period. In a controlled Italian study of 53 patients with HCV-associated cryoglobulinemia, of whom two thirds had clinical evidence of renal disease, patients randomized to receive interferon for 6 months had significant improvement in cutaneous vasculitis, circulating cryoglobulin levels, and renal function compared to those receiving conventional therapy. Unfortunately, in this and a number of other studies, relapses of renal disease and cryoglobulinemia are common after discontinuation of interferon therapy, suggesting that long-term interferon use may be more beneficial. Interferon-α's efficacy correlates with its ability to reduce viral burden; however, significant side effects including fever, flu-like symptoms, and myalgias may limit its use in some patients. A course of aggressive immunosuppressive therapy (pulse methylprednisolone followed by oral steroids and cyclophosphamide) is usually reserved for patients with severe acute vasculitic multisystem manifestations but runs the risk of promoting HCV viral replication or lymphoma in the long term. In patients with severe acute disease, plasmapheresis (two or three times weekly) for up to 4 weeks has been used successfully to remove the circulating cryoglobulin, and can be administered in conjunction with immunosuppressive therapy. Cryofiltration, which precipitates out the cryoglobulins by cooling of the patient's plasma and then reinfuses the patient's own rewarmed plasma, can obviate the need for replacement fluid. Most centers now advocate plasmapheresis combined with an immunosuppressive regimen that includes steroids and cyclophosphamide to control the severe acute systemic vasculitis, whereas long-term therapy with interferon alone remains the mainstay for the chronic phase of the disease.

TRANSPLANTATION

For those patients with idiopathic MPGN who progress to end stage renal disease and receive a renal transplant, recurrence of MPGN in the allograft is a frequent occurrence, particularly within the first 6 months to 1 year posttransplant. Approximately 30% of transplanted children with MPGN type I develop recurrence, some in several successive allografts. Up to 40% of these recurrences lead to graft failure. In type II MPGN, recurrence is even more common and may be as high as 80 to 100%, depending on how carefully it is sought. However, recurrences tend to be clinically mild and fewer than 10 to 20% of recurrences are responsible for graft loss. The recurrence rate of MPGN type III is not known. Recurrences must be differentiated from transplant glomerulopathy, which also has membra-noproliferative features but lacks immune deposits. Rare cases of de novo MPGN related to hepatitis C infection have also been reported in allografts.

Bibliography

Anders D, Agricola B, Sippel M, et al.: Basement membrane changes in membranoproliferative glomerulonephritis. II. Characterization of a third type by silver impregnation of ultra thin sections. *Virchows Arch [Pathol Anat]* 376: 1–19, 1977.

Burkholder PM, Marchand A, Krueger RP: Mixed membranous and proliferative glomerulonephritis. *Lab Invest* 23: 459–479, 1970.

Cameron JS, Turner DR, Heaton J, et al.: Idiopathic mesangio-capillary glomerulonephritis. comparison of types I and II in children and adults and long-term prognosis. *Am J Med* 74: 175–192, 1983.

D'Amico G, Fornasieri A: Cryoglobulinemic glomerulonephritis: A membranoproliferative glomerulonephritis induced by hepatitis C virus. *Am J Kidney Dis* 25: 361–369, 1995.

Donadio JV, Anderson CF, Mitchell JC, et al.: Membranoproliferative glomerulonephritis. A prospective clinical trial of antiplatelet therapy. *N Engl J Med* 310: 1421–1426, 1984.

Donadio JV, Offord KP: Reassessment of treatment results in membranoproliferative glomerulonephritis. *Am J Kidney Dis* 14: 445–451, 1989.

Ford DM, Briscoe DM, Shanley PF, Lum GM: Childhood membranoproliferative glomerulonephritis type I: Limited steroid therapy. *Kidney Int* 41: 1606–1612, 1992.

Habib R. Gubler MC, Loirat C, et al.: Dense deposit disease: A variant of membranoproliferative glomerulonephritis. *Kidney Int* 7: 204–215, 1975.

Habib R, Kleinknecht C, Gubler MC, et al.: Idiopathic membrano-proliferative glomerulonephritis in children. Report of 105 cases. *Clin Nephrol* 1: 194–214, 1973.

Holley KE, Donadio JV, Jr: Membranoproliferative glomerulonephritis. In: Tisher CC, Brenner BM (eds) *Renal Pathology, with Clinical and Functional Correlations.* 2nd ed., Lippincott, Philadelphia, pp. 294–329, 1994.

Johnson RJ, Gretch DR, Couser WG, et al.: Hepatitis C virus-associated glomerulonephritis. Effect of alpha-interferon therapy. *Kidney Int* 46: 1700–1704, 1994.

Johnson RJ, Gretch DR, Yamabe H, et al.: Membranoproliferative glomerulonephritis associated with hepatitis C virus infection. *N Engl J Med* 328: 465–470, 1993.

Johnson RJ, Willson R, Yamabe H, et al.: Renal manifestations of hepatitis C virus infection. *Kidney Int* 46: 1255–1263, 1994.

McEnery PT, McAdams AJ, West CD: The effect of prednisone in a high-dose, alternate-day regimen on the natural history of idiopathic membranoproliferative glomerulonephritis. *Medicine* 64: 401–424, 1985.

Misiani R. Bellavita P, Fenili D, et al.: Interferon alfa - 2a therapy in cryoglobulinemia associated with hepatitis C virus. *N Engl J Med* 330: 751–756, 1994.

Strife CF, Jackson EC, McAdams AJ: Type III membranoproliferative glomerulonephritis: Long-term clinical and morphologic evaluation. *Clin Nephrol* 21: 323–334, 1984.

Tarshish P, Bernstein J, Tobin JN, Edelmann CM: Treatment of mesangiocapillary glomerulonephritis with alternate-day prednisone—A report of the International Study of Kidney Disease in Children. *Pediatr Nephrol* 6: 123–130, 1992.

Varade WS, Forristal J, West CD: Patterns of complement activation in idiopathic membranoproliferative glomerulonephritis types I, II and II. *Am J Kidney Dis* 16: 196–206, 1990.

West CD: Childhood membranoproliferative glomerulonephritis: An approach to management. *Kidney Int* 29: 1077–1093, 1986.

20

FOCAL SEGMENTAL GLOMERULOSCLEROSIS

GERALD B. APPEL

Focal segmental glomerulosclerosis (FSGS) is a clinical and histopathologic entity with a pattern of glomerular injury which may occur in an idiopathic or secondary form (see Table 1). The most common manifestation is proteinuria, which can range from minor amounts to nephrotic levels. FSGS accounts for less than 15% of cases of idiopathic nephrotic syndrome in children, but is more frequent in adults. Recent studies performed at several institutions have documented an increased incidence of FSGS in biopsies of adult patients that is especially noteworthy among nephrotic patients. FSGS appears to be the most common pattern of idiopathic nephrotic syndrome among African-Americans and may now be the most common pattern in all races. Idiopathic FSGS frequently progresses to end stage renal failure (ESRD). While potentially treatable, the appropriate type of therapy, duration of treat-

TABLE I

Etiologies of Focal Sclerosis

Primary idiopathic

Focal segmental glomerulosclerosis

Variants of minimal change disease
  IgM nephropathy
  Diffuse mesangial hypercellularity

Variants of FSGS
  Glomerular tip lesion
  Collapsing FSGS

Secondary

Unilateral renal agenesis

Renal ablation—remnant kidney

Sickle cell disease

Morbid obesity (with or without sleep apnea)

Congenital cyanotic heart disease

Heroin nephropathy

HIV nephropathy

Aging kidney

Healed focal proliferative or necrotizing GN

Vesicoureteral reflux

FSGS, focal segmental glomerulosclerosis; GN, glomerulonephritis.

ment, and response rate to treatment are all subjects of controversy.

PATHOLOGY

There are no uniformly agreed on diagnostic criteria for FSGS. The pathologic diagnosis of FSGS usually depends on identifying in some glomeruli (focal lesions) areas of glomerulosclerosis in parts of the glomerular tufts (segmental lesions) (Fig. 1). In addition, fusion or effacement of foot processes is found to some extent in all of the glomeruli,

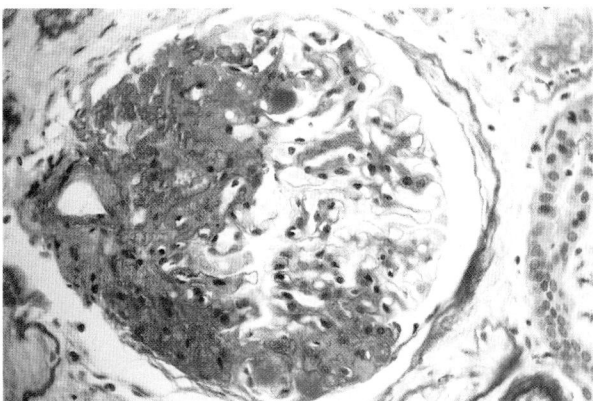

FIGURE I Glomerulus from a patient with focal segmental glomerulosclerosis showing perihilar sclerosis with adhesion to Bowman's capsule (periodic acid–Schiff stain). Courtesy of Dr. J. C. Jennette.

including those unaffected by areas of segmental sclerosis. The term "idiopathic" FSGS may be used only if the lesions of other types of focal glomerulonephritis that could heal as focal sclerosing lesions are absent and if there is no evidence of immune complex deposition by electron microscopy (EM). Focal areas of IgM and C3 deposition isolated to the areas of segmental sclerosis are thought to result from entrapment of immunoglobulin and complement components rather than from true immune complex deposition. The remainder of the glomerular tuft and the glomeruli unaffected by glomerulosclerosis typically have some degree of foot process effacement noted by EM, but they do not have evidence of immune complex deposition by IF. Although large amounts of proteinuria and uniform foot process fusion may be present, biopsies taken early in the course of FSGS, when renal function is still normal, show few glomeruli with segmental sclerosing lesions and almost no global sclerosis. At a later stage, as renal function deteriorates, many glomeruli will show segmental or global sclerosis. Some investigators believe the segmental sclerosing lesions are initially present in the juxtamedullary glomeruli and then spread outward in time to involve the remaining renal cortex. Interstitial fibrosis is also a common finding in biopsies with significant glomerulosclerosis. The mechanism responsible for this damage is unclear but may relate to changes in the postglomerular circulation, absorption of filtered proteins and lipoproteins across tubular epithelia, or incitement of cytokine and growth factors by abnormally filtered substances. The presence of increased tubulointerstitial damage correlates with a poor renal prognosis.

Several variants of FSGS deserve comment. The glomerular tip lesion is characterized by swelling, vacuolation, and proliferation of epithelial cells and, later, sclerosis and hyalinosis in the segment of the glomerulus adjacent to the origin of the proximal tubule. The remainder of the glomerulus has changes similar by light microscopy (LM) and EM to those seen in minimal change nephrotic syndrome. Another variant of FSGS is associated with focal or global glomerular capillary collapse and sclerosis with visceral epithelial cell swelling similar to that seen in HIV glomerulopathy (see Fig. 1, Chapter 33). This so-called "collapsing" or "malignant" variant of glomerulosclerosis is more common in African-Americans, and has a distinctive and more ominous clinical course than other forms of idiopathic FSGS. In addition, a number of lesions that are often considered variants of minimal change nephrotic syndrome may evolve into FSGS, including IgM nephropathy (a presentation of minimal change by LM but with IF positivity for IgM and, in some patients, mesangial dense deposits on EM), and diffuse mesangial hypercellularity (mild proliferation of cells limited to the glomerular mesangium).

PATHOGENESIS

By definition, the pathogenesis of idiopathic FSGS is unknown. Some patients who appear on initial biopsy to have minimal change disease evolve into FSGS, which can be demonstrated on a subsequent biopsy. While the sample of glomeruli observed on initial biopsy in some of these patients may have missed segmental lesions present in only a few juxtamedullary glomeruli, other patients with repeated relapses of the nephrotic syndrome after discontinuation of steroid therapy seem more convincingly to have experienced evolution of the lesion. Moreover, all the glomeruli in classic FSGS have fusion of foot processes and are responsible for the proteinuria. As in minimal change nephrotic syndrome, the loss of the charge barrier of the glomerular capillary wall may allow negatively charged albumin to pass through the altered capillary wall into Bowman's space. These alterations may be in response to lymphokine production or other circulating humoral mechanisms. Evidence for the latter includes studies describing a circulating permeability factor that promotes the in vitro permeability of glomeruli to albumin. The presence of this permeability factor, a 50 kDa protein that is not an immunoglobulin, has been used to predict the rapid development of proteinuria in the allograft of some FSGS patients who reach ESRD and undergo transplantation. Moreover, some patients with recurrent FSGS in the allograft respond to plasmapheresis or to use of a protein absorption column with a reduction in proteinuria.

Proteinuria in FSGS is often less selective than in minimal change disease (vide infra), implying leakage of larger macromolecules through "larger pores" in the glomerular basement membrane. Drug-induced (e.g., puromycin nephrosis, adriamycin nephrosis) minimal change lesions in some animals can develop a picture of FSGS with nonselective proteinuria. In one such model, the lifting off of the visceral epithelial cells from the glomerular basement membrane has been correlated with the nonselective proteinuria.

The pathogenesis of the sclerosing lesions and their progressive nature is also debated. Humans with idiopathic FSGS or remnant kidney FSGS initially have a high glomerular filtration rate (GFR) and evidence of hyperfiltration, suggesting that hyperfiltration and increased intracapillary glomerular pressure may be mediators of FSGS. Likewise, patients with glomerulomegaly, as seen in remnant kidneys or due to obesity or hypoxemia in sleep apnea, also have a high incidence of the nephrotic syndrome and FSGS. FSGS without increased glomerular capillary pressure or glomerulomegaly may relate to hyperlipidemia or intra-glomerular coagulation.

It is possible and even likely that the pattern of FSGS seen on biopsy represents a common pathway for a number of distinct entities with different pathogenetic mechanisms and clinical courses.

CLINICAL FEATURES

Most patients with idiopathic FSGS present with either asymptomatic proteinuria or the full nephrotic syndrome. The 10 to 30% of cases with asymptomatic proteinuria are typically children whose proteinuria is detected during routine pediatric checkups or camp or sports physicals; in adults, detection of asymptomatic cases occurs most often at military induction examinations, routine gynecologic or obstetric check-ups, and insurance or employment physicals. Patients with the nephrotic syndrome present with edema.

Hypertension is found in 30 to 50% of children and adults with FSGS. Microscopic hematuria is found in 25 to 75% of these patients: likewise, a decreased GFR is noted at presentation in 20 to 30% of these patients. Daily urinary protein excretion ranges from less than 1 g to 20 to 30 g/day. Proteinuria is typically nonselective, i.e., it contains higher molecular weight proteins as well as albumin. Nevertheless, albumin still comprises the largest component of the urine protein. Complement levels and other serologic tests are normal. Occasional patients will have glycosuria, aminoaciduria, phosphaturia, or a concentrating defect indicating tubular damage as well as glomerular injury.

DIAGNOSIS

The diagnosis of FSGS requires a renal biopsy. Early on, only a minority of the glomeruli show the segmental sclerosing lesion. Even these lesions may have a predilection for the juxtamedullary region of the kidney, so the renal biopsy may look identical to that of minimal change nephrotic syndrome. This is especially likely when a very superficial biopsy contains only a small number of glomeruli. Likewise, a small sample of glomeruli in a biopsy in an older adult may show some glomeruli identical to minimal change disease and one or two globally sclerotic glomeruli. They may be the result of FSGS or merely the obsolescent glomeruli that are found in the kidneys of older individuals without renal disease. The finding of tubulointerstitial damage in such biopsies should suggest the possibility of unobserved scarred glomeruli and FSGS, but in neither situation can the diagnosis of FSGS be firmly established. Clinically, patients who are thought to have a minimal change pattern nephrotic syndrome with a poor response to corticosteroids or other immunosuppressive agents are likely to have FSGS. The biopsy may also provide clues to a secondary form of FSGS. In heroin nephropathy there is often more severe tubulointerstitial disease than in idiopathic FSGS. In HIV nephropathy there is often a collapsing variant of glomerulosclerosis with global rather than segmental involvement, and tubuloreticular inclusions are commonly found on EM. In patients with remnant kidneys and hyperfiltration-induced FSGS there is often less effacement of the foot processes than in idiopathic FSGS.

THERAPY AND OUTCOME

Although variable in the individual patient, the course of untreated FSGS is usually one of progressive proteinuria and declining GFR. Patients with asymptomatic proteinuria typically develop the nephrotic syndrome over time. Only a small minority of patients experience a spontaneous remission of proteinuria or the nephrotic syndrome. Both children and adults usually develop ESRD 5 to 20 years from presentation. Some patients with the collapsing variant (or so-called malignant FSGS) will have a more rapid course to ESRD in 2 to 3 years. The features which have been associated with a more rapid progression to renal failure in idiopathic FSGS include higher grade proteinuria (> 10–15 g day), a higher serum creatinine at time of biopsy, a greater degree of glomerulosclerosis on biopsy, and more tubulointerstitial damage on renal biopsy.

Idiopathic FSGS may recur in the transplanted kidney with severe proteinuria and the nephrotic syndrome. Patients who present with more severe degrees of proteinuria and a more rapid course to renal failure are at greater risk for recurrence in the allograft.

The therapy of FSGS is controversial. There are few randomized, controlled trials upon which to base decisions. In general, those patients with a sustained remission of their nephrotic syndrome are unlikely to progress to ESRD, whereas those with unremitting nephrotic syndrome are likely to have progression. In most studies before 1985, only 10 to 30% of patients appeared to respond to a course of corticosteroids with a remission of proteinuria. Moreover, only a low response rate to other immunosuppressive agents such as azathioprine, cyclophosphamide, and chlorambucil was recorded, and the relapse rate after treatment was also high. As a result most American nephrologists considered FSGS to be unresponsive to therapy and did not advocate immunosuppressive treatment.

A seminal Canadian study in 1987 noted that 44% of children with FSGS responded with a remission of proteinuria. While the response rate for treated adults was similar (39%), most adults did not receive any specific therapy. Recent studies of the use of immunosuppressives in FSGS have confirmed initial response rates of 25 to 60%. A collaborative Italian study using much longer courses of prednisone, cyclophosphamide, and/or azathioprine found 60% of FSGS patients to have a complete remission of the nephrotic syndrome. Those patients with a complete remission had an excellent long-term renal survival, without the occurrence of ESRD. An uncontrolled trial in children using combined pulse steroids and long-term immunosuppression with corticosteroids and cytotoxics has also found a 60% complete remission rate and a 16% partial remission rate of the nephrotic syndrome and a low rate of progression to renal failure. A recent American study of more than 50 nephrotic adults with nephrotic syndrome due to FSGS also showed a better than 50% response rate as well as long-term improvement in renal survival in the treated group. Finally a number of trials have used low dose cyclosporine (4–6 mg · kg^{-1} · day^{-1}, for 2–6 months) to treat steroid-resistant FSGS patients. Three controlled trials have had complete and partial remission rates of 60 to > 90% with use of cyclosporine vs 17 to 33% in the placebo group. The largest of these studies, The North American Collaborative Study of Cylosporine in Nephrotic Syndrome, found 12% complete remission and > 70 % complete or partial remission with use of cyclosporine in steroid-resistant FSGS. Even some FSGS patients who have been unresponsive to cytotoxic agents may respond to this therapy. Unfortunately, some patients will experience renal damage from the cyclosporine.

At present the ideal regimen to treat idiopathic FSGS is unknown. Many clinicians would not treat patients with subnephrotic levels of proteinuria and little damage on their renal biopsies. Others would treat these patients with angiotensin converting enzyme (ACE) inhibitors to reduce proteinuria and its side effects but would not use immunosuppressives to treat the specific glomerular lesion. Patients at increased risk of renal failure such as those with nephrotic range proteinuria, elevated serum creatinines, and interstitial scarring on biopsy may be treated with a prolonged course (6–9 months) of daily or every other day corticosteroids (starting with 60 mg of prednisone daily or 120 mg every other day and tapering to lower doses after several months), or other immunosuppressive medication in the hope of inducing a remission of the nephrotic syndrome and preventing eventual ESRD.

For patients with secondary forms of FSGS, treatment of the primary etiology, although rarely possible, is the first step in management. Patients with FSGS secondary to obesity and heroin nephropathy have had remissions of proteinuria after weight reduction or cessation of drug use, respectively. Use of ACE inhibitors and other nonspecific methods to reduce proteinuria and the manifestations of the nephrotic syndrome may also be beneficial. Immunosuppressive medications have not proved effective in any form of secondary FSGS. In those patients with either primary idiopathic or secondary forms of the FSGS who remain nephrotic, control of fluid retention and edema can be managed with salt restriction and diuretics. In addition, attention should be given to hypertension control with antihypertensive medication, hyperlipidemia control with diet and antihyperlipidemic medications, and perhaps to prevent hyperfiltration with low protein diets.

Bibliography

Arturo M, Biava C, Amend W, Tomlanovich S, Vincenti F: Recurrent focal glomerulosclerosis: Natural history and response to treatment. *Am J Med* 92:375, 1992.

Banfi G, Moriggi M, Sabadini E, Fellin G, D'Amico G, Ponticelli C: The impact of prolonged immunosuppression on the outcome of idiopathic focal-segmental glomerulosclerosis with nephrotic syndrome in adults. *Clin Nephrol* 36: 53–59, 1991.

Barisoni L, Valeri A, Radhakrishnan J, Nash M, Appel GB, D'Agati V: FSGS: A 20 years epidemiologic study. *J Am Soc Nephrol.* 5:347, 1994.

Cattran D, Greenwood C, Bernstein K, et al.: Results of a 6 month randomized trial of cyclosporine vs. placebo in adults with FSGS. *J Am Soc Nephrol* 6:413, 1995.

D'Agati V: Nephrology forum. The many masks of FSGS. *Kidney Int* 46:1223–1241, 1994.

Dantal J, Bigot E, Bogers W, et al.: Effect of plasma protein absorption on protein excretion in kidney transplant recipients with recurrent nephrotic syndrome. *N Engl, J Med* 330: 7–14, 1994.

Detwiler RK, Falk RJ, Hogan SL, Jennette JC: Collapsing glomerulopathy: A clinically and pathologically distinct variant of FSGS. *Kidney Int* 45: 1416–1424, 1994.

Fogo A: Internephron heterogeneity of growth factors and sclerosis. *Kidney Int* 45:S24–s26, 1994.

Haas M, Spargo BH, Coventry S: Increasing incidence of FSGS among adult nephropathies: A 20-year renal biopsy study. *Am J Kidney Dis* 26: 740–750, 1995.

Jennette JC, Marquis A, Falk RJ, Bodick N: Glomerulomegaly in focal segmental glomerulosclerosis but not in minimal change glomerulopathy. *Lab Invest* 62: 48A, 1990.

Korbet SM, Schwartz M, Lewis EJ: Primary FSGS: Clinical course, and response to therapy. *Am J Kidney Dis* 23:773–783, 1994.

Lieberman KV, Tejani A, for the NY-NJ Pediatric Nephrology Study Group: A randomized double-blind placebo-controlled trial of cyclosporine in steroid resistant FSGS in children. *J Am Soc Nephrol* 7: 56–63, 1996.

Pei Y, Cattran D, Delmore T, Katz A, Lang A, Rance P: Evidence suggesting under-treatment of adults with idiopathic focal segmental glomerulosclerosis. *Am J Med* 82: 938–944, 1987.

Ponticelli C, Rizzoni G, Edefonti A, Alt et al.: A randomized trial of cyclosporine in steroid-resistant idiopathic nephrotic syndrome. *Kidney Int* 43:1377–1384, 1993.

Rennke H, Klein PS: Pathogenesis and significance of non-primary focal and segmental glomerulosclerosis. *Am J Kidney Dis* 13: 443–455, 1989.

Rydell JJ, Korbet SM, Borok RZ, Schwartz MM: FSGS in adults: Presentation, course, and response to treatment. *Am J Kidney Dis* 25:534–542, 1995.

Savin VJ, Artero M, Sharma R, et al.: Circulating factor associated with increased glomerular permeability to albumin in recurrent focal segmental sclerosis. *N Engl J Med* 334:878–882, 1996.

Tune BM, Kirpekar R, Sibley RK, Reznik VM, Griswold WR, Mendoza SA: Intravenous methylprednisolone and alkylating agent therapy of prednisone-resistant pediatric FSGS: A long-term follow-up. *Clin Nephrol* 43: 84–88, 1995.

Valeri A, Barisoni L, Appel GB, Seigle R, D'Agati V:Idiopathic collapsing FSGS: A clinicopathologic study. *Kidney Int* 50:1734–1746, 1996.

21

MEMBRANOUS NEPHROPATHY

SHARON G. ADLER AND CYNTHIA C. NAST

Membranous nephropathy is a histologic diagnosis based on the presence of subepithelial deposits along an often thickened glomerular basement membrane. In the nephropathology literature, the terms epi-, peri-, or extramembranous have occasionally been substituted for membranous, and the term glomerulonephritis has been used interchangeably with glomerulopathy and nephropathy. Membranous nephropathy is the histological diagnosis in 15 to 25% of adult patients with no associated systemic illness who undergo renal biopsies for heavy proteinuria. In this setting, membranous nephropathy is referred to as "idiopathic." However, in up to 30% of patients with renal biopsy-proven membranous nephropathy, medications or associated systemic illnesses appear to play a pathogenetic role in the initiation of the glomerular disorder. Table 1 summarizes those entities reported to be associated with so-called "secondary" membranous nephropathy. Idiopathic and secondary membranous nephropathy are often distinguishable by clinical, laboratory, or histological features, and therapeutic strategies for treatment tend to differ. However, it should be noted that in routine clinical practice, it often proves difficult or impossible to rigorously exclude underlying causes. In fact, on occasion membranous nephropathy may precede by many months or even years the clinical presentation of an associated systemic illness. While a relatively common cause of nephrotic syndrome in adults, membranous glomerulopathy in children occurs less frequently than minimal change disease.

CLINICAL FEATURES

The clinical presentation is characterized by heavy proteinuria in more than 80% of patients, most often in association with the full expression of the nephrotic syndrome. The remaining patients have asymptomatic proteinuria. A minority have accompanying microscopic hematuria. The onset of symptomatology tends to be insidious. Hypertension and azotemia are usually not features at initial presentation, although hypertension may be present in a minority of patients at presentation, and certainly develops as progressive renal insufficiency ensues. Males tend to be affected more often and more severely than females. Although idiopathic membranous nephropathy can occur at any age, 80 to 90% of patients are older than 30 years at diagnosis. The older the patient, the greater the likelihood that there is associated malignancy. This may be present in up to 20% of patients over the age of 60.

Manifestations of the nephrotic syndrome may be quite severe in patients with membranous nephropathy, includ-

Immunologic Disorders—Systemic lupus erythematosus, mixed connective tissue disease, rheumatoid arthritis, Sjögren's syndrome, dermatomyositis, sarcoidosis, Hashimoto's thyroiditis, dermatitis herpetiformis, myasthenia gravis, Gullain-Barré syndrome, Weber-Christian panniculitis, bullous pemphigoid, anticardiolipin antibody syndrome.

Neoplasms—Carcinoma (lung, colon, breast, stomach, kidney, esophagus, carotid body), melanoma, leukemia, lymphoma (especially non-Hodgkin's).

Infections—Hepatitis B, secondary or congenital syphilis, quartan malaria, leprosy, schistosomiasis, filariasis, scabies.

Medications—Penicillamine, organic gold, mercury-containing compounds, captopril, probenicid, trimethadione, nonsteroidal anti-inflammatory drugs.

Miscellaneous—Sickle cell anemia, Fanconi's syndrome, sclerosing cholangitis, systemic mastocytosis, volatile hydrocarbon exposure, Kimura's disease, Gardner-Diamond syndrome, diabetes, de novo in renal allografts.

ing anorexia, malaise, edema, and occasionally anasarca. Ascites, pericardial, and pleural effusions are less common in adults, even with severe nephrotic syndrome, than in children. Hyperlipidemia is common. It is characterized by increases in total and LDL cholesterol, Apo B, C-II, C-III, triglycerides, VLDL, and sometimes Lp(a), and by abnormalities in the distribution of HDL cholesterol, particularly an increase in HDL fraction 3 and a decrease in HDL fraction 2. In the general population these changes are associated with an increase in atherogenesis and cardiovascular disease. By inference, it is presumed that these same risks are also conferred on patients with nephrotic syndrome with these changes, but this has not been studied longitudinally in this population. Growth retardation in children with severe nephrotic syndrome is a difficult clinical problem. Predisposition to arterial and venous thromboses have been noted. The incidence of renal vein thrombosis is high. The precise frequency is difficult to ascertain since its determination would require venography, an invasive measure that is rarely undertaken unless symptomatically indicated. Similarly, pulmonary embolus has been reported, rarely as the presenting manifestation of the nephrotic syndrome.

PATHOLOGY

Primary (Idiopathic) Membranous Nephropathy

On light microscopy, glomeruli have mesangial regions of normal width which do not display hypercellularity. In very early membranous nephropathy, the glomeruli may appear completely normal. With more well-developed lesions, capillary walls are thickened with patent capillary lumina, occasionally with a rounded configuration. Subepithelial fuchsinophilic deposits are observed with Masson's trichrome staining. Methenamine silver stain discloses sub-

epithelial projections ("spikes") along the capillary walls, corresponding to the deposition of new basement membrane material adjacent to the deposits (Fig. 1). When capillary walls are tangentially sectioned, the deposits and "spikes" may appear as holes within the basement membranes. In advanced membranous glomerulopathy the deposits are often within the capillary basement membrane, having been completely covered by the new basement membrane material, and capillary walls may display "double contours." Crescent formation is uncommon in membranous nephropathy. When present, crescents may be associated with late stages of the disease or, rarely, the formation of antiglomerular basement membrane antibodies.

Immunofluorescence microscopy always demonstrates strong granular capillary wall staining for IgG, with C3 and both light chains usually present in the same pattern. Weaker IgA and IgM staining are infrequently observed.

The ultrastructural features of membranous nephropathy have been used to classify the disease into four stages. Stage I is associated with normal light microscopy; by electron microscopy there are few to many small or medium-size electron-dense deposits along the capillary walls in a subepithelial position, with effacement of the overlying visceral epithelial foot processes. Stage II is characterized by more numerous and larger deposits with the formation of subepithelial projections of basement membrane material lateral to the deposits ("spikes"). In stage III the new extracellular material surrounds the deposits which become incorporated into the capillary basement membrane. Stage IV has markedly thickened capillary walls with rarefaction and lucent areas in the intramembranous deposits and layering of the basement membrane. In all stages, resolution of the disease is associated with fading of the deposits as they undergo resorption, and fresh homogeneous deposits are observed when the disease is active. Mesangial deposits are very rarely encountered in primary membranous nephropathy.

Secondary Membranous Nephropathy

The capillary wall changes are similar to those of the primary disease, although there may be fewer deposits. Mesangial regions are frequently expanded and hypercellular, most strikingly in lupus nephritis; mesangial deposits are common in secondary forms, particularly those related to infections. Subendothelial deposits may occur infrequently. In membranous lupus nephritis, glomerular staining for all immunoglobulins and C1q is common, as are subendothelial and extraglomerular deposits and tubuloreticular structures in endothelial cell cytoplasm. Recurrent and de novo membranous nephropathy occurring in renal transplants in the absence of other glomerular abnormalities usually appears histologically similar to primary membranous glomerulopathy.

PATHOGENESIS

Membranous nephropathy is an immune-mediated disease in which immune complexes localize in the subepithe-

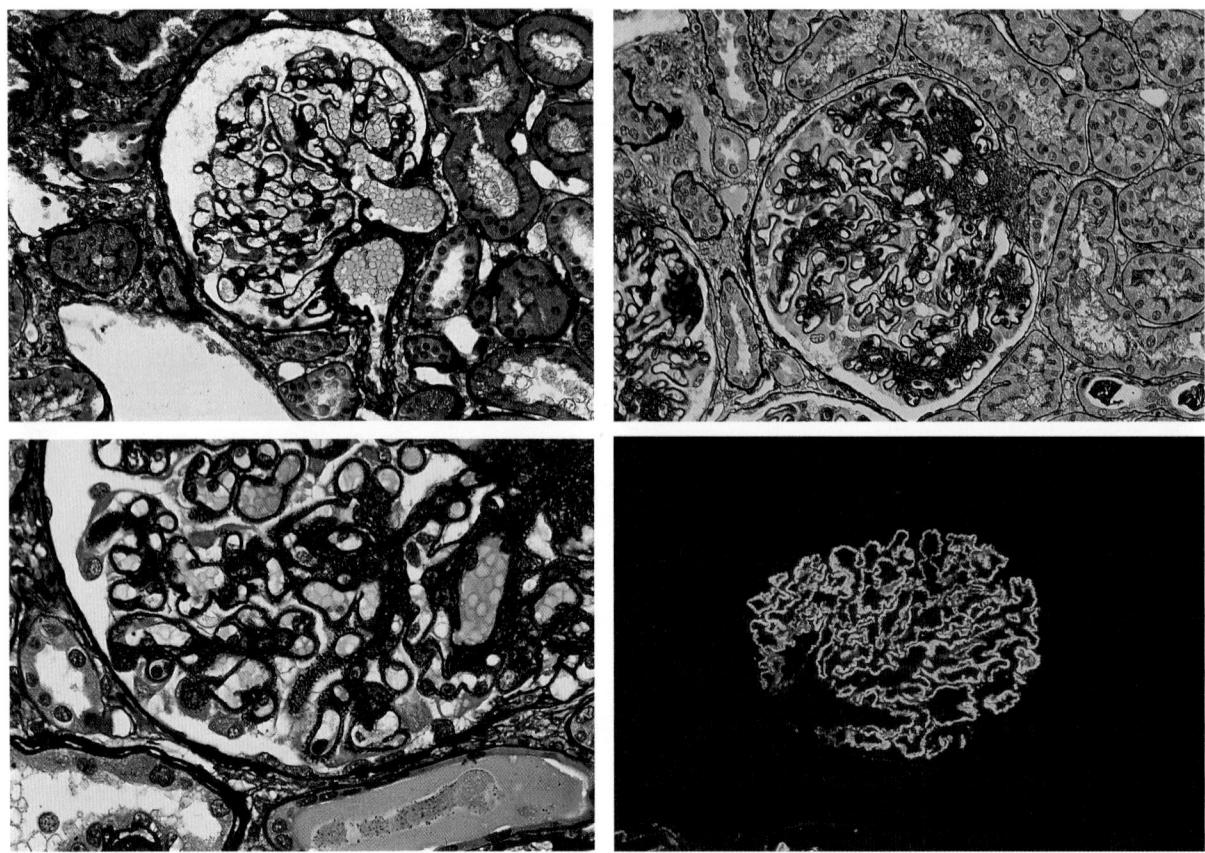

FIGURE I (A) Glomerulus from a patient with primary membranous nephropathy. Capillary walls are slightly thickened without mesangial abnormalities [silver stain (Jones), ×230]. (B) Glomerulus from a patient with membranous lupus glomerulonephritis. Note the mesangial hypercellularity in addition to the thickened capillary walls [silver stain (Jones), ×230]. (C) Glomerular capillary walls showing subepithelial projections (spikes) of silver-positive basement membrane material (arrows) [silver stain (Jones), ×700]. (D) Glomerulus showing granular capillary wall staining by immunofluorescence using anti-IgG antibody in primary membranous nephropathy (×480).

lial aspect of glomerular capillary walls. Antigen-antibody complexes could develop at this location by the production of immune complexes in situ (the most likely mechanism) or by the deposition of circulating immune complexes. Immune complexes forming in situ at the subepithelial capillary wall site can involve the binding of a circulating antibody to an intrinsic glomerular antigen. In one experimental form of membranous nephropathy (Heymann's nephritis), the intrinsic antigen is a glycoprotein synthesized by glomerular visceral epithelial cells. In situ complex formation can also be initiated by the deposition of an extrinsic "planted" antigen. Size and charge are critical factors in the localization of "planted antigens" to the subepithelial aspects of capillary walls with subsequent immunoglobulin deposition. Cationic proteins have been "planted" by intravenous injection to induce membranous nephropathy experimentally. Antigens may also become trapped in the capillary wall by direct binding, binding related to biochemical factors, or autoimmune mechanisms. Low-avidity antibody predisposes to subepithelial deposit formation. Finally, circulating immune complexes with a suitable cationic charge and of the appropriate size may traverse the capillary basement membrane, lodging in the subepithelial

space and binding to anionic sites in the capillary wall. However circulating complexes are not uniformly found in patients with membranous nephropathy and currently are not thought to account for the majority of cases of this disorder.

The antigen(s) involved in primary human membranous nephropathy are not known. In secondary membranous nephropathy, many of the antigens have not been discerned; however, hepatitis B surface and e antigens have been identified in immune deposits, as have thyroid antigens in occasional patients with thyroiditis. In both primary and secondary forms, complement is activated at the capillary wall site and appears to be related to the development of proteinuria, but it is not required for the development of the morphologic lesion. The finding of urinary complement membrane attack complex (C5b-C9) has been suggested as a diagnostic test for following disease activity. It may be more useful when the glomerular antigen is intrinsic than when it is "planted."

DIAGNOSIS

Idiopathic membranous nephropathy is a diagnosis based on histological findings in a patient whose history, physical examination, and appropriate laboratory testing exclude the likelihood of a secondary cause. Approximately 80% of patients have poorly selective proteinuria. The majority of patients have proteinuria exceeding 3.5 g per day. A full-blown nephrotic syndrome is common, including hypoalbuminemia, hyperlipidemia, and lipiduria. The urinary sediment is usually inactive and characterized by heavy proteinuria. Lipiduria and oval fat bodies may be present when the nephrotic syndrome occurs. Microhematuria occurs in less than a quarter of patients. Serum complement levels are usually normal. Low serum complement levels suggest a secondary form of membranous nephropathy or an alternative diagnosis. Serum protein electrophoresis commonly shows broad band increments in β and γ globulins as a nonspecific feature of the nephrotic syndrome. The following laboratory tests are usually negative or normal in patients with idiopathic membranous glomerulopathy, and abnormalities should suggest a secondary form of the disorder: antinuclear antibodies, anti-DNA antibodies, rheumatoid factor, glycosylated hemoglobin, hepatitis antigen or antibody, thyroid antibodies, carcinoembryonic antigen, and cryoglobulins. Circulating immune complexes, when sought, have been found in idiopathic membranous nephropathy by some but not all investigators and is not diagnostically helpful. Increased risk for the development of idiopathic membranous glomerulopathy appears to be associated with the presence of the histocompatibility antigens DR3 in Caucasians and Chinese and DR2 in Japanese.

COURSE

The course of untreated idiopathic membranous nephropathy is highly variable. Among patients initially presenting with the nephrotic syndrome and a normal serum creatinine level, the probability of a spontaneous complete remission and a stable glomerular filtration rate (GFR) for up to 20 years is approximately 30%. The probability of a spontaneous partial remission with stable GFR is approximately 25%. An additional 20-25% of patients experience persistent nephrotic syndrome with stable or very slowly progressive loss of GFR. Twenty to twenty-five percent of patients progress to end-stage renal disease over a 20- to 30-year period of follow-up. On initial presentation, it is difficult to predict the likely outcome of an individual patient. However, the following factors have been suggested as portending risk for a poor outcome: significant tubulointerstitial fibrosis and elevated serum creatinine at the time of initial renal biopsy, male sex, older age at onset, heavy proteinuria (e.g., >10 g/day), hypertension, and stage IV lesions. The outcome in patients with secondary membranous nephropathy is affected by the associated underlying disorders. Complete remissions are reported in patients with treated infections, occasionally with treated neoplasms, and often in association with discontinuation of offending drugs. Complete or partial remissions may also be achieved with immunosuppressive therapy for patients with membranous nephropathy secondary to immunologic disorders.

THERAPY

Controversy and uncertainty continue to envelop the decision-making process with regard to the treatment of idiopathic membranous nephropathy. These difficulties emerge largely as a result of the clinical heterogeneity of these patients. Given the overall good prognosis for most, the lack of uniform benefit from treatment regimens involving steroids and/or cytotoxics, and the inherent risks involved with the employment of these agents, many have advocated palliative therapy for the patient with normal renal function and few adverse symptoms. This might begin with sodium restriction and diuretics, taking care not to induce a state of marked prerenal azotemia.

A number of strategies have been advocated to diminish heavy proteinuria. Nonsteroidal anti-inflammatory drugs (NSAIDS) have been reported to decrease proteinuria in some patients with the nephrotic syndrome. An accompanying decrement in GFR is almost always seen, though the decrease in proteinuria is often greater. Indomethacin and meclofenamate have been the drugs most often used for this purpose. Despite their utility in occasional patients with heavy proteinuria, for the majority of patients with nephrotic syndrome, the overall impact of NSAIDS in substantially diminishing proteinuria appears disappointing. Dietary protein restriction in the range of 0.6-0.8 g · kg^{-1} day^{-1} has been suggested as a further means of diminishing proteinuria, although longterm studies regarding nutritional safety are still necessary in patients with heavy proteinuria.

Small, prospective clinical trials performed in patients with membranous nephropathy have demonstrated reductions in proteinuria averaging approximately 50% in patients treated with ACE inhibitors. Furthermore, a randomized prospective trial involving 583 patients with chronic renal insufficiency of varying etiologies (192 of whom had glomerular disease), demonstrated that the use of an ACE inhibitor (in this case, benazepril) slowed the progression of chronic renal insufficiency. Over the 3-year follow-up period, the risk reduction for a doubling of serum creatinine was 53%. ACE inhibitors offer the obvious collateral benefit of blood pressure control in these patients, and a recent analysis of data from the Modification of Renal Disease Study suggests that in patients with >1 g of proteinuria, a mean arterial pressure of <92 mm Hg slows the rate of renal functional decline. Thus, ACE inhibitors offer benefits for those patients with membranous nephropathy for whom immunosuppressive therapy is not indicated.

The hyperlipidemia of nephrotic syndrome may contribute to accelerated atherogenesis. Although dietary fat restriction is reasonable, it rarely normalizes the hyperlipidemia of nephrosis. Use of the newer HMG-CoA reductase inhibitors (3-hydroxy-3-methylglutamyl-coenzyme A) or agents such as gemifibrizol often lower serum LDL cholesterol and triglyceride levels substantially in nephrotics. However, currently it is unclear whether this will have long-term benefit on atherogenesis. For the patient experiencing hypercoagulability with venous, or less commonly arterial, thrombosis or pulmonary emboli, long-term anticoagulation for the duration of the nephrotic syndrome is recommended.

Patients at higher risk for progressive disease, patients who actually have progressive disease, and those with particularly severe nephrotic complications are candidates for immunosuppressive therapy. Historically, corticosteroid therapy used alone without the addition of cytotoxic drugs had long been advocated as the mainstay of treatment for idiopathic membranous nephropathy. Three large prospective randomized clinical trials examined the usefulness of steroids in achieving remissions in proteinuria and preventing progressive loss of kidney function. The earliest of these three studies suggested that remissions of proteinuria were more common and progressive loss of renal function was less frequent in steroid-treated than in control patients. However, later studies failed to confirm these findings. Thus, currently, most available data do not suggest benefit from the use of corticosteroids alone in the therapy of most patients with idiopathic membranous nephropathy.

Additional data suggest that treatment for idiopathic membranous glomerulopathy may be improved by combining corticosteroids with cytotoxic agents. In the largest series of such patients with the longest follow-up, control patients received no specific therapy. During a 6-month course, treated patients were given intravenous methylprednisolone followed by daily oral prednisone during months 1, 3, and 5 and oral chlorambucil during months 2, 4, and 6. After a median follow-up of 5 years, the treated group experienced more partial and complete remissions of nephrotic syndrome and had lower serum creatinines than did the untreated controls. However, no patient with a serum creatinine >1.7 mg/dL at entry participated in this trial. Additional analyses showed that while the treatment regimen increased the probability of remission compared to controls, this probability was somewhat reduced by the presence of a serum creatinine >1 mg/dL and proteinuria >5 g/day. Thus, it has been argued that the data cannot be applied to many of the patients most needy of an aggressive therapeutic approach. To determine whether the chlorambucil contributed significantly to the beneficial effects of the regimen, an additional study was performed comparing combination treatment with steroids alone. While more patients given the steroids plus chlorambucil were in remission in the first 3 years of follow-up than those given steroids alone, by Year 4 the differences were no longer statistically significant. Thus, the apparent dilemma in the use of combined prednisone and chlorambucil is twofold. First, in order to maximize response rate, patients need to be treated early, thereby exposing to risk patients who might otherwise undergo spontaneous remissions. Second, given the relapses that may occur in the treated group and the late spontaneous remissions that may occur in the untreated group, the added benefit of cytotoxics over the long term are still not yet clearly defined.

In studies attempting to address the first dilemma, steroids have been used either with chlorambucil or with longer-term cyclophosphamide in small numbers of patients with idiopathic membranous nephropathy and more

advanced renal insufficiency. Limited success has been reported in diminishing proteinuria and/or improving renal function using chlorambucil or oral cyclophosphamide. However, patients with renal insufficiency who are treated with alkylating agents tend to experience more severe side effects, including leukopenia and clinically significant, sometimes life-threatening infections. To further complicate matters, in a recently reported prospective, randomized controlled trial using intravenous cyclophosphamide with steroids in patients with membranous nephropathy and renal insufficiency, alkylator therapy was not shown to be a better treatment than steroids alone. Furthermore in a randomized controlled trial involving 18 patients with membranous nephropathy and progressive renal insufficiency, steroids and low-dose chlorambucil, but not steroids and intravenous cyclophosphamide were effective in improving renal function. The efficacy of cyclosporine in treating patients with membranous nephropathy who have a poor prognosis was examined by Cattran et al. Seventeen patients who had been followed for 1 year with dietary therapy alone and who continued to have proteinuria and a decline in creatinine clearance of at least 8 mL/min were randomized to receive either cyclosporine or no additional treatment for 12 months. The patients treated with cyclosporine had improved proteinuria and creatinine clearance compared to the untreated group, and 6 of 8 maintained their decrement in proteinuria up to 9 months after cyclosporine discontinuation. However, the treated group had a higher incidence of hypertension and a larger number of transient rises in serum creatinine. Although only a small number of patients have been studied to date, and follow-up is short, these data nevertheless suggest that cyclosporine therapy may be useful in selected patients with membranous nephropathy. Confirmatory data in larger groups of patients with longer term follow-up are needed to better evaluate the usefulness of this therapy. Intravenous immunoglobulin has been used in a small number of patients, but more experience will be required to assess its potential.

To summarize, the treatment of idiopathic membranous nephropathy remains highly controversial and should be individualized. To a great extent, the choices regarding therapy have more to do with the patient's perception of the benefits and risks of the therapies and the illness than they do about the physician's sense of them. It is therefore incumbent on physicians to provide patients with a balanced view of the available information regarding treatment options, along with their specific recommendation for treatment, in the hope that the patient will be able to make an informed consent regarding therapy. In low-risk patients, (e.g., those with normal renal function, relatively low proteinuria, and manageable nephrotic syndrome), nonspecific therapies are indicated. These might include salt restriction and diuretics for the management of edema, angiotensin converting enzyme (ACE) inhibitors and perhaps nonsteroidal anti-inflammatory drugs to decrease proteinuria and HMG-CoA reductase inhibitors to improve hyperlipidemia. Anticoagulation may be used to treat a thrombotic event, and perhaps also as prophylaxis against thrombotic events, particularly in patients with serum albumin <1.5 mg/dL. In high-risk patients, particularly those with azotemia, histological evidence of tubulointerstitial fibrosis, very heavy proteinuria, hypertension, or morbid events from the nephrotic syndrome, the use of steroids in combination with chlorambucil or oral cyclophosphamide, or perhaps, in selected patients, cyclosporine or intravenous immunoglobulin may be beneficial. However, the prescription of these agents should be tempered by the knowledge that they may be least effective when used under the circumstances of highest risk and that their side-effect potential in this setting may be heightened.

Therapies for the secondary forms of membranous nephropathy are guided by the nature of the underlying cause. Lupus membranous nephritis is discussed in Chapter 28. Discontinuation of offending drugs and treatment of infections frequently induce complete remission. The use of interferon for the treatment of chronic active hepatitis B has been reported to achieve complete remission in some patients with associated membranous nephropathy. Remission appears more likely in patients who were infected during adulthood, compared to patients who were infected perinatally or in early childhood. Of note, the liver disease of patients with hepatitis B and membranous nephropathy may be exacerbated by the use of high-dose long-term steroids. Thus, steroids are currently discouraged as a sole treatment for patients with membranous nephropathy and hepatitis. Since malignancy is uncommon as an underlying cause of membranous nephropathy in patients under the age of 50, an exhaustive search for malignancy seems unwarranted unless a neoplastic process is suggested by a thorough history, physical examination, chest X-ray, and routine clinical chemistries. In older patients, the addition of mammography in women, stool guaiac examinations, and endoscopic examination of the colon may be considered. It should be noted that even this would not detect all potential underlying neoplasms, as the origin of an underlying tumor may include numerous organs, and the neoplasm may be occult at the time of initial presentation with nephropathy. Medical or surgical treatments of neoplasms have occasionally been associated with remission. In these patients, recurrence may be heralded by a relapse of the nephrotic syndrome.

Bibliography

Austin HA III, Antonyvich TT, MacKay K, Boumpas DT, Balow JE: NIH conference. Membranous nephropathy. *Ann Intern Med* 110:672–82, 1992.

Bruns FJ, Adler S. Fraley DS, Segel DP: Sustained remission of membranous glomrulonephritis after cyclophosphamide and prednisone. Ann Int Med 114:725–730. 1991

Burstein DM, Korbet SM, Schwartz MM: Membranous glomerulopathy and malignancy. Am J Kidney Dis 22:5–10, 1993

Cattran DC, Greenwood C, Ritchie S, et al.: A controlled trial of cyclosporine in patients with progressive membranous nephropathy. Canadian Glomerulonephritis Study Group. *Kidney Int* 47:1130–1135, 1995.

Falk RJ, Hogan SL, Muller KE, Jennette JC, and the Glomerular Disease Collaborative Network: Treatment of progressive membranous glomerulopathy: A randomized trial comparing cyclophosphamide and corticosteroids with corticosteroids alone. Ann Int Med 116:438–445, 1992

Gabbai FB, Goshwa LC, Wilson CB, Blantz RC: An evaluation of the development of experimental membranous nephropathy. Kidney Int 31:1267–1278, 1987

Maschio G, Alberti D, Janin G, et al.: Effect of the angiotensin-converting-enzyme inhibitor benazepril on the progression of chronic renal insufficiency. N Engl J Med 334:939–945, 1996.

Noel LH, Zonetti M, Droz D. Long-term prognosis of idiopathic membranous glomerulonephritis. Am J Med 66:82–90, 1979

Peterson JC, Adler S, Burkart JM, et al.: Blood pressure control, proteinuria, and the progression of renal disease. The Modification of Diet in Renal Disease Study. *Ann Intern Med* 123:754–762, 1995.

Ponticelli C, Zucchelli P, Imbasciati E, Cagnole L, Pozzi C, Passerini P, Grassi C, Limido D, Pasquali S, Volpini T, Sasdelli M, Locatelli F: Controlled trial of methylprednisolone and chlorambucil in idiopathic membranous nephropathy. N Engl J Med 310:946–950, 1984

Ponticelli C, Zucchelli P, Passerini P, Cesana B, and the Italian Idiopathic Membranous Nephropathy Treatment Study Group: Methylprednisolone plus chlorambucil as compared with methylprednisolone alone for the treatment of idiopathic membranous nephropathy. N Engl J Med 327:599–603, 1992

Reichert LJM, Huysmans FTM, Assmann K, Koene RAP, Wetzels JFM: Preserving renal function in patients with membranous nephropathy: Daily oral chlorambucil compared with intermittent monthly pulses of cyclophosphamide. *Ann Intern Med* 121:328–333, 1994.

Ronco P, Allegri L, Brianti E, Chatelet F, VanLeer EHG, Verroust P: Antigenic targets in epimembranous glomerulonephritis. Appl Pathol 7:85–98, 1989

Rostoker G, Ben Maadi A, Remy P, Lang P, Lagrue G, Weil B: Low-dose angiotensin-converting enzyme inhibitor captopril to reduce proteinuria in adult idiopathic membranous nephropathy: a prospective study of long-term treatment. *Nephrol Dial Transplant* 10:25–21, 1995.

Schiepatti A, Mosconi L, Peina L, et al.: Progression of untreated patients with idiopathic membranous nephropathy. *N Engl J Med* 329:85–89, 1993.

Wheeler DB, Bernard DB: Lipid abnormalities in the nephrotic syndrome: causes, consequences and treatment. *Am J Kidney Dis* 23:331–346, 1994.

22

IgA NEPHROPATHY AND
RELATED DISORDERS

BRUCE A. JULIAN

In 1968 Berger and Hinglais in France described the unique renal immunohistologic features of IgA nephropathy. In the subsequent 29 years, it has been recognized as the most common form of primary glomerulonephritis in the world and accounts for about 10% of patients reaching endstage renal failure in many countries. Because of the enthusiasm of its champion and evolving controversies about the pathogenesis, the eponym Berger's disease has gained increasing favor. The same renal immunohistologic features may be found in patients with nephritis due to Henoch-Schönlein purpura, perhaps the systemic form of the disease process causing IgA nephropathy. These two entities have been grouped as *primary* IgA nephropathy, in distinction to *secondary* IgA nephropathy in patients with other disorders in which the IgA deposits in the renal mesangium due to increased production or decreased extrarenal clearance: alcoholic cirrhosis, dermatitis herpetiformis, psoriasis, ankylosing spondylitis, celiac disease, inflammatory bowel disease, carcinoma at various sites, and mycosis fungoides.

PATHOLOGY

Immunohistology

The diagnosis of IgA nephropathy requires immunofluorescence examination of kidney tissue. IgA is the predominant or sole immunoglobulin and is in the mesangium of all glomeruli, even those with a normal histologic appearance (Fig. 1). In occasional patients the IgA deposits extend to the peripheral capillary loops. The IgA is predominantly of the IgA1 subclass. The intensity of staining for lambda light chains often exceeds that for the kappa isotype. In about three fourths of patients a second immunoglobulin, IgG or IgM (sometimes both), is detected with staining intensity equal to or less than that for IgA. Staining for C3 (the third component of complement) is usually observed in areas with IgA, although the deposits do not always coincide. Other components of the alternative complement pathway, including properdin and factor H (β1H), as well as the membrane attack complex (C5b-9) are often detected. C4 binding protein is detected in about one third of patients, sometimes accompanied by a second complement

protein of the classical pathway. In renal biopsy specimens with IgG, the minimal or no staining for C1q is a useful criterion to distinguish IgA nephropathy from lupus nephritis.

IgA deposits in the capillaries of skin biopsy specimens have been reported in some patients with IgA nephropathy without cutaneous manifestations of a vasculitis. This finding is often cited as support for the hypothesis that IgA nephropathy and Henoch-Schönlein purpura constitute the spectrum of one disease. However, the frequency of this finding is variable and a skin biopsy does not replace a renal biopsy for the diagnosis.

Light Microscopy

The characteristic light microscopic finding is mesangial enlargement due to proliferation of mesangial cells, increased mesangial matrix, or both (Fig. 2). The abnormalities may be focal (not all glomeruli affected) and segmental (only a portion of a glomerulus affected). Most patients exhibit mesangial changes in all glomeruli, whereas a few patients show no significant glomerular abnormality. Segmental sclerosing lesions are found in many patients. Proliferation of the glomerular epithelial cells causing crescents is observed occasionally and is more common when the IgA deposits extend to the glomerular basement membranes, or in patients with acute renal insufficiency or macroscopic hematuria. Circumferential crescents are rare. Focal necrosis of a glomerular capillary suggesting a vasculitis may be found in patients with Henoch-Schönlein purpura and occasionally in the biopsy samples from patients with primary IgA nephropathy

The severity of the findings in the interstitium (fibrosis, tubular damage, infiltration of lymphocytes) and vascular sclerosis generally correlates with the extent of the glomerular pathology. A few patients undergoing renal biopsy at the time of macroscopic hematuria with acute renal insufficiency have sloughing of the tubular epithelial cells ("acute tubular necrosis") with red blood cell casts.

Electron Microscopy

The mesangium is enlarged by proliferation of mesangial cells with abundant cytoplasm, often with increased mesan-

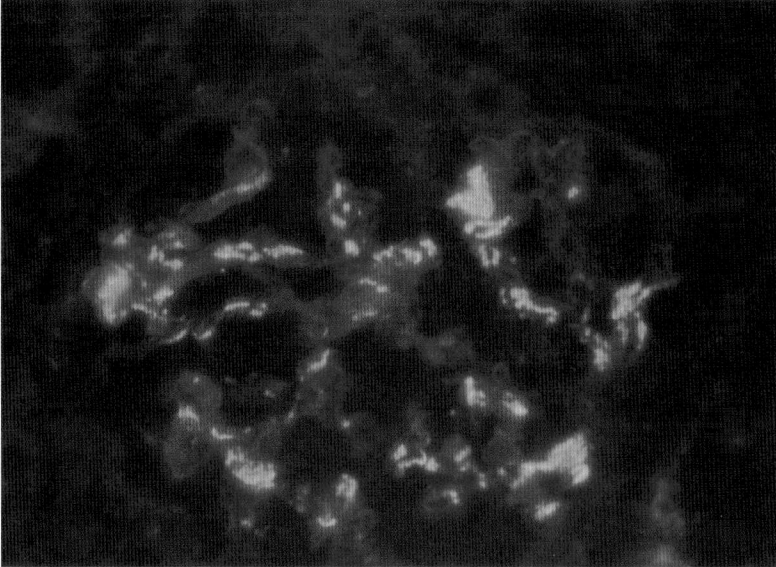

FIGURE 1 Direct immunofluorescence microscopy of a glomerulus with normal architecture by light microscopy using FTIC-conjugated anti-human IgA. Staining is limited to the mesangial areas (x350).

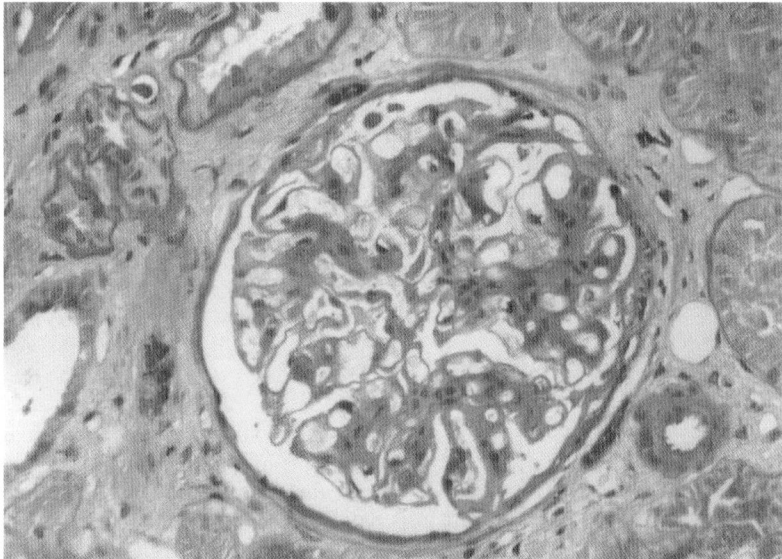

FIGURE 2 Light microscopic histology of glomerulus with increased mesangial cells and matrix (periodic acid–Schiff, x350).

gial matrix. Electron-dense deposits in the mesangial and paramesangial areas correspond to the immune deposits. Some deposits may extend into the subendothelial area of the glomerular basement membrane. Deposits in the subepithelial and intramembranous areas are uncommon. One third of patients exhibit abnormalities of the glomerular basement membranes: focal thinning, splitting, and lamination. The focal distribution of these changes distinguishes IgA nephropathy from the more diffuse patterns in Alport's syndrome and thin basement membrane syndrome.

CLINICAL FEATURES

Epidemiology

Primary IgA nephropathy may be diagnosed in individuals of all ages, but is most common in children and young adults. Males are affected two to three times more often than females. The frequency of the disease varies substantially between countries. In southern Europe, Asia, and Australia IgA nephropathy accounts for 20 to 40% of patients with primary glomerular disease. Japan has the highest frequency, probably due to widespread screening of school children for urinary abnormalities. The United States and Canada have the lowest frequencies, and IgA nephropathy is rare in central Africa.

The wide range in disease prevalence may reflect differences in criteria for performing the requisite renal biopsy, as well as genetically determined differences in the development of renal disease. In the United States the prevalence of IgA nephropathy is high among some Native American groups, but very low in African Americans. Several large families with multiple members with IgA nephropathy have been described. The clinical features may vary widely among these relatives; some have Henoch-Schönlein purpura. Familial IgA nephropathy has not yet been linked to an HLA antigen, restriction fragment length polymorphism, or other genetic marker. The mode of inheritance of familial IgA nephropathy remains uncertain.

Clinical Presentation

Patients with primary IgA nephropathy usually present with one of three syndromes (Table 1). The most distinctive is an episode of macroscopic hematuria concurrent with an infection of the upper respiratory tract. In contrast to a 10-14 day delay for the onset of macroscopic hematuria in patients with poststreptococcal glomerulonephritis, the urine becomes red or tea-colored 1 to 2 days after the onset of symptoms; this feature has been labeled "synpharyngitic" hematuria. The patient is usually asymptomatic, but sometimes reports malaise, fatigue, or myalgia. Hypertension and peripheral edema of the nephritic syndrome, common in poststreptococcal glomerulonephritis, are rare. Some patients, especially children, experience loin pain. Bleeding may last hours to many days; episodes may recur months or years later with pharyngitis, a febrile illness of another cause, or extreme exercise. Macroscopic hematuria is more common in children than adults, and the interval between episodes lengthens with increasing age. A few patients with macroscopic hematuria develop acute renal dysfunction that generally improves with supportive therapy; dialysis is occasionally necessary.

TABLE I
Clinical Presentation of IgA Nephropathy

Common
    Synpharyngitic macroscopic hematuria
    Asymptomatic microscopic hematuria
    Henoch-Schönlein purpura
Uncommon
    Nephrotic syndrome
    Chronic renal insufficiency with hypertension

A second presentation is asymptomatic microscopic hematuria with variable degrees of proteinuria. Such patients are often adults undergoing routine urinalysis as part of an insurance or employment physical. Proteinuria is usually less than 1 g/day. These patients rarely experience macroscopic hematuria after ascertainment.

Henoch-Schönlein purpura is a third common mode of presentation and develops much more frequently in children than in adults. Patients also manifest skin, joint, and intestinal involvement. The skin lesions are characteristically more numerous on the legs and lower trunk. The rash is frequently morbiliform early in the course and rapidly becomes purpuric. Arthralgias are not usually accompanied by features of inflamed joints. Gastrointestinal symptoms may be striking, including severe abdominal pain, ileus, or bloody diarrhea. Nephritis often develops after the initial symptoms subside; therefore, a urinalysis should be checked at a 1-month follow-up visit. Some patients, especially young children, never exhibit nephritis.

A less common presentation is the nephrotic syndrome. These patients may have advanced glomerular disease with hypertension and renal insufficiency. Alternatively, the nephrotic syndrome may be the initial clinical feature of patients with normal renal function and normal blood pressure. Proteinuria in the latter setting is often selective, comprised primarily of smaller proteins such as albumin. Renal biopsy shows histologic features similar to minimal-change glomerulonephritis, but with diffuse staining for IgA in all mesangia. Whether these few patients comprise a subset of IgA nephropathy patients or have two separate diseases is controversial. Chronic renal insufficiency and hypertension (occasionally malignant) are the initial manifestations for a minority of patients.

Laboratory Findings

Because the glomerular IgA is apparently derived from the circulation, much attention has focused on the serum levels of IgA or IgA-containing immune complexes. Serum IgA concentrations are increased in about 50% of patients. However, this finding is neither unique to patients with IgA nephropathy nor consistent when multiple assays are performed for an individual patient over several months. Serum concentrations of complement components are usually normal. Levels of circulating IgA-containing immune complexes are frequently increased. The complexes may contain C3, IgG, or both, but an antigen such as a viral or dietary protein has not been identified. Discovery of circulating IgA-fibronectin complexes in some patients sparked interest as a possible screening tool, but the specificity and sensitivity are too poor. Renal biopsy remains the standard for the diagnosis.

Natural History

IgA nephropathy is a chronic disease. Although clinical remission (resolution of microscopic hematuria and proteinuria with a normal serum creatinine concentration) may develop in as many as one third of patients several years after renal biopsy, disappearance of the IgA from glomeruli has been only rarely documented. Renal function progressively worsens in about 40% of patients, about half of whom reach endstage renal failure after 20 years of clinically apparent disease. For patients with modest proteinuria at biopsy, an increase in magnitude of proteinuria often portends a rise in serum creatinine concentration. About 10% of patients with renal insufficiency develop the nephrotic syndrome. Nearly one third of patients exhibit a benign course with chronic microscopic hematuria and normal serum creatinine concentration; proteinuria generally remains less than 1 g/day.

Hypertension in patients with primary IgA nephropathy is at least as common as in patients with membranous or membranoproliferative glomerulonephritis, but probably less frequent than in patients with idiopathic focal segmental glomerulosclerosis. Hypertension is more common in patients whose biopsy specimens show vascular sclerosis. Malignant hypertension develops in about 5% of patients. Among patients whose urinalysis becomes normal with prolonged observation, half remain hypertensive.

Prognostic Markers

Clinicopathological parameters shown by multivariate analysis in studies at separate centers to predict a poor long-term clinical outcome are shown in Table 2. These features are more useful for a group of patients than for an individual. Patients with a history of macroscopic hematuria also have a better long-term outlook. This clinical feature is more common in pediatric patients who may have had a shorter duration of disease than adults. Nonetheless, it remains a marker for a good prognosis even after taking patient age into account. Variations in the gene encoding angiotensin converting enzyme may predict the clinical course. In some, but not all, studies, patients homozygous for the D (deletion) allele had a worse prognosis than those homozygous the I (insertion) allele. The prognostic value of other clinical variables, including older age at diagnosis (with an unknown duration of disease) and male gender, are less well defined. In contrast, several laboratory or histologic parameters have not been helpful in predicting outcome, including serum IgA concentration, intensity of immunofluorescence staining for IgA in the biopsy specimen, and the isotype of any additional immu-

noglobulin in the mesangium. The long-term prognosis differs between some ethnic groups, perhaps reflecting varied methods of ascertainment and differences in criteria for performing renal biopsies.

PATHOGENESIS

The pathogenesis of IgA nephropathy is not yet understood. There is no evidence, however, that the process is different in patients with macroscopic hematuria or familial disease as compared with those without these clinical features. Multiple mechanisms likely play a role in the primary and secondary forms of the disease. Research has focused on the characteristics of the IgA molecules in the mesangium, the source of these molecules, the mechanism of deposition in the mesangium, and the inflammatory response that culminates in glomerular damage.

Primary IgA Nephropathy

Immunofluorescence and electron microscopic findings of granular mesangial deposits of IgA and C3 resemble the pattern in experimental immune complex glomerulonephritis. However, it is uncertain whether the IgA and C3 are deposited as an immune complex from the circulation or whether they combine locally through an in situ mechanism. IgA1 is the predominant IgA subclass in the renal deposits, whereas the other IgA subclass, IgA2, is rarely detected. For technical reasons, the relative contribution of the molecular forms, monomers and polymers, is difficult to establish. The question of polymeric vs monomeric form in the mesangium is relevant for the induction of inflammation damaging glomeruli. Polymeric IgA is much more active phlogistically than monomeric IgA.

Several observations support the hypothesis that the mesangial IgA is derived from the circulation: recurrence of mesangial IgA in a transplanted allograft, clearance of renal IgA deposits in an allograft inadvertently transplanted from a donor with subclinical IgA nephropathy, restriction of the mesangial IgA to the IgA1 subclass, and increased plasma levels of IgA1 (with normal levels of IgA2) and IgA1-containing immune complexes.

Increased levels of these complexes could be caused by increased synthesis or decreased hepatic catabolism. Increased production of IgA1 has been shown, but alone is is not usually sufficient to cause IgA nephropathy. For example, patients with IgA1 myeloma or infection with HIV have high plasma levels of IgA1 but rarely exhibit glomerular deposits. Thus, a qualitative abnormality of circulating IgA appears necessary for mesangial deposition. Recent studies have shown that IgA molecules in the blood of patients with IgA nephropathy contain decreased numbers of galactose residues in the O-linked glycans in the hinge region. This abnormality may decrease uptake by hepatic receptors, thereby bypassing metabolism in the liver and increasing the amount circulating through the kidneys. Moreover, the decreased content of galactose may enhance binding of IgA molecules to renal mesangial cells, leading to greater glomerular sclerosis and damage. Some

TABLE 2
Markers of Poor Outcome in IgA Nephropathy

Hypertension

Proteinuria greater than 2 g/24 hr

Renal insufficiency at biopsy

Biopsy changes
    Severe proliferative and sclerotic changes in glomeruli
    Interstitial fibrosis
    Vascular sclerosis
    Extension of IgA deposits to peripheral capillary walls

of the circulating IgA complexes also contain fibronectin that facilitates attachment of IgA to collagen in the mesangial matrix, but this binding is not specific for patients with IgA nephropathy. In addition, IgA molecules may also attach to type V collagen in the matrix by a mechanism independent of fibronectin.

The process by which mesangial deposits of IgA damage glomeruli has not been elucidated. Activation of complement appears important, as in other types of glomerulonephritis. Immunohistologic findings suggest involvement predominantly of the alternative pathway, although the classical complement pathway may participate in some patients. Cells infiltrating glomeruli from the circulation may accentuate the inflammatory response by secreting cytokines. Furthermore, mesangial cells synthesize an array of inflammatory mediators and express receptors for some of them. On activation, the mesangial cells proliferate and secrete extra matrix.

Secondary IgA Nephropathy

The pathogenetic mechanisms of secondary IgA nephropathy are uncertain. Decreased hepatic clearance of IgA-containing immune complexes has been postulated for patients with alcoholic cirrhosis. Increased systemic exposure to dietary antigen leading to increased production of IgA has been proposed for patients with celiac disease, inflammatory bowel disease, and dermatitis herpetiformis. However, the basis for glomerular deposition of IgA in patients with various other diseases, such as carcinoma of the respiratory or gastrointestinal tract, is unknown.

TREATMENT

Treatment of secondary IgA nephropathy is generally directed toward the associated medical condition. Clearance of mesangial IgA deposits has been described in patients whose principal disorder resolved. Alternatively, no consensus has emerged about a disease-specific approach for patients with primary IgA nephropathy. Unfortunately, only a few controlled treatment trials have been conducted. One approach to treatment is to separate patients into two clinical categories: acute and chronic.

Acute Disease

Acute renal dysfunction affects a small minority of patients. The renal biopsy specimen may show glomerular epithelial crescents. No consensus has been reached about the approach to these patients, but treatment has included glucocorticoids, cytotoxic agents, anticoagulants, or plasmapheresis, alone or in combination. Many centers favor glucocorticoid therapy, often given as three 0.5 to 1.0 g intravenous doses of methylprednisolone followed by an oral prednisone regimen for several months. Assessment of the apparent benefit is complicated by spontaneous resolution of renal dysfunction in some patients. Early treatment-associated improvement in renal function is frequently shortlived.

For patients with macroscopic hematuria and tubular necrosis without glomerular crescents, renal function often returns to baseline with supportive therapy with control of blood pressure and dialysis as necessary.

A few patients with normal renal function develop the nephrotic syndrome with light microscopic histologic features of minimal-change glomerulonephritis. Treatment with glucocorticoids clears the nephrotic syndrome, but the IgA deposits usually persist.

Chronic Disease

Most patients with chronic IgA nephropathy are hypertensive and control of their blood pressure is the cornerstone of therapy. An angiotensin converting enzyme (ACE) inhibitor appears to be the agent of choice. Not only is blood pressure usually well controlled, but the rate of decline of creatinine clearance is frequently slowed or stabilized, possibly due to better control of intraglomerular capillary hypertension or decreased cytokine-induced glomerular sclerosis. Proteinuria often improves, but a decrement does not always predict a favorable effect on creatinine clearance. Enthusiasm for this class of agents recently increased because patients homozygous for the D allele of the gene encoding angiotensin converting enzyme had the highest circulating levels of the enzyme, and the largest decrement in proteinuria after treatment.

Use of an ACE inhibitor in normotensive patients is more controversial. These patients often have a normal serum creatinine and may become hypotensive with treatment. In one study of adults, therapy for 4 months significantly decreased proteinuria; however, no study has evaluated the long-term preservation of renal function in this setting.

Because macroscopic hematuria frequently coincides with an upper respiratory tract infection, infection may accentuate glomerular damage, perhaps by increasing synthesis of IgA or various cytokines that augment the inflammatory process. Although chronic antibiotic prophylaxis has no proven benefit, tonsillectomy in some studies decreased the magnitude of hematuria; however, its effects on renal function have not been adequately evaluated. Phenytoin decreases serum IgA concentrations and treatment may decrease the frequency of macroscopic hematuria, but histologic features do not improve.

In the absence of a disease-specific therapy, investigators have tried various other approaches. In a nonrandomized study, children with histologic features associated with progressive disease treated with alternate-day prednisone preserved renal function with resolution of proteinuria and hematuria. In a separate study, daily prednisone therapy of adults preserved renal function when the initial creatinine clearance was greater than 70 ml/min. Fish oil rich in omega-3 fatty acids given for 2 years was found to preserve creatinine clearance in patients with proteinuria at least 1 g/day in a multicenter, placebo-controlled, randomized study. Proteinuria was not altered. Therapy was well tolerated: No bleeding complication or increase in plasma cholesterol or triglyceride concentrations was observed. Prior results with fish oil had been more controversial; only two of four trials showed a beneficial effect. Treatment for 9 months with pooled intravenous followed by intramuscular immunoglobulins slowed the decline in renal function and lessened proteinuria in one study, but the effect was frequently shortlived after stopping therapy. Several immunosuppressive or antiinflammatory agents, alone or in combination, have not consistently shown benefit: azathioprine, cyclosporine, aspirin, dipyridamole, dapsone, and danazol. Unfortunately, there is little agreement about these therapeutic options.

Two general treatment options may be helpful. Moderate salt restriction usually enhances an antihypertensive regimen. Also, restriction of dietary protein intake to 0.6 g/kg body weight per day may slow loss of renal function in patients with various chronic renal diseases such as IgA nephropathy, but patients should be monitored for protein malnutrition.

For patients reaching endstage renal failure, transplantation affords an excellent option. Recurrent disease (the appearance of the immunohistologic features) has been documented in about 50% of patients 2 years posttransplant, but loss of the allograft from recurrent disease is uncommon. Kidneys from living-related donors are not at greater risk than cadaveric allografts for recurrent disease.

BIBLIOGRAPHY

Berger J: Recurrence of IgA nephropathy in renal allografts. *Am J Kidney Dis* 12:371–372, 1988.

Cameron JS: Henoch-Schönlein purpura: clinical presentation. *Contrib Nephrol* 40:246–249,1984.

Cattran DC, Greenwood C, Ritchie S: Long-term benefit of angiotensin-converting enzyme inhibitor therapy in patients with severe immunoglobulin A nephropathy: A comparison to patients receiving treatment with other antihypertensive agents and to patients receiving no therapy. *Am J Kidney Dis* 23:247–254,1994.

Donadio JV Jr, Bergstralh EJ, Offord KP, et al.: A controlled trial of fish oil in IgA nephropathy. *N Engl J Med* 331:1194–1199,1994.

Galla JH: IgA nephropathy. *Kidney Int* 47:377–387,1995.

Isbels LS, Gyory AZ: IgA nephropathy: Analysis of the natural history, important factors in the progression of renal disease, and a review of the literature. *Medicine* 73:79–102, 1994.

Julian BA: Treatment options in IgA nephropathy. *Nephrology* 3:103–108, 1997.

Mestecky J, Tomana M, Crowley-Nowick PA, et al.: Defective galactosylation and clearance of IgA1 molecules as a possible etiopathogenetic factor in IgA nephropathy. *Contrib Nephrol* 104:172–182,1993.

Mustonen J, Pasternack A: Associated diseases in IgA nephropathy. In: Clarkson AR (ed) IgA Nephropathy. Martinus Nijhoff Publishing, Boston, pp. 47–65, 1987.

van Es LA: Pathogenesis of IgA nephropathy. *Kidney Int* 41:1720–1729,1992.

Wyatt RJ, Kritchevsky SB, Woodford SY, et al.: IgA nephropathy: Long-term prognosis for pediatric patients. *J Pediatr* 127:913–919, 1995.

Yoshida H, Kon V, Ichikawa I: Polymorphisms of the renin-angiotensin system genes in progressive renal diseases. *Kidney Int* 50:732–744,1996.

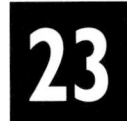

GOODPASTURE'S SYNDROME AND ANTI-GBM DISEASE

CAROLINE O.S. SAVAGE

INTRODUCTION

Goodpasture's syndrome is defined as the concurrence of pulmonary hemorrhage and focal necrotizing glomerulonephritis. This pulmonary–renal syndrome is seen most commonly in the context of systemic vasculitis and thenmost frequently in the presence of antineutrophil cytoplasm antibodies (ANCA). Confusingly, Goodpasture's name is also associated with the occurrence of antiglomerular basement membrane (GBM) antibodies. Today, many prefer to use the term Goodpasture's *disease* to specifically describe those patients with focal necrotizing glomerulonephritis, often accompanied by pulmonary hemorrhage, who demonstrate autoimmunity to the GBM.

Causes of Goodpasture's syndrome, specifically pulmonary–renal vasculitic syndromes, are given in Table 1. Goodpasture's syndrome needs to be distinguished from the presence of lung and renal disease occurring together either with (e.g., sarcoidosis) or without (e.g., presence of pulmonary emboli, infection, or cancer occurring in patients with diverse types of nephritis) immediate pathogenic relationship. This chapter deals specifically with Goodpasture's disease or anti-GBM disease.

GOODPASTURE'S DISEASE

Clinical and Pathological Features

Goodpasture's disease has a peak incidence in the third to sixth decades but all ages may be affected and there is a secondary peak in incidence in the sixth and seventh decades. The full syndrome with pulmonary hemorrhage and nephritis is more common in young males, perhaps reflecting smoking habits, wherever elderly females tend to present with nephritis alone. Whites are more commonly affected than individuals of African ancestry. Patients with overt pulmonary hemorrhage tend to present at an earlier stage and before oliguria develops, while in the absence of overt pulmonary hemorrhage patients often present in renal failure. Smoking predisposes to development of pulmonary hemorrhage. Pulmonary hemorrhage occurs in about two thirds of patients in most series.

Features of pulmonary hemorrhage include symptoms of continuous or episodic dyspnea, and of hemoptysis. Hemoptysis may be minimal or massive and absence of this feature does not exclude presence of pulmonary hemorrhage. Symptoms can develop rapidly over hours. Signs may include tachypnea, cyanosis in severe cases, and inspiratory crackles or bronchial breathing over the basal lung fields. The chest radiograph usually shows patchy or diffuse infiltrates involving the central lung fields; the changes are usually but not always symmetrical (Fig. 1). Blood gas

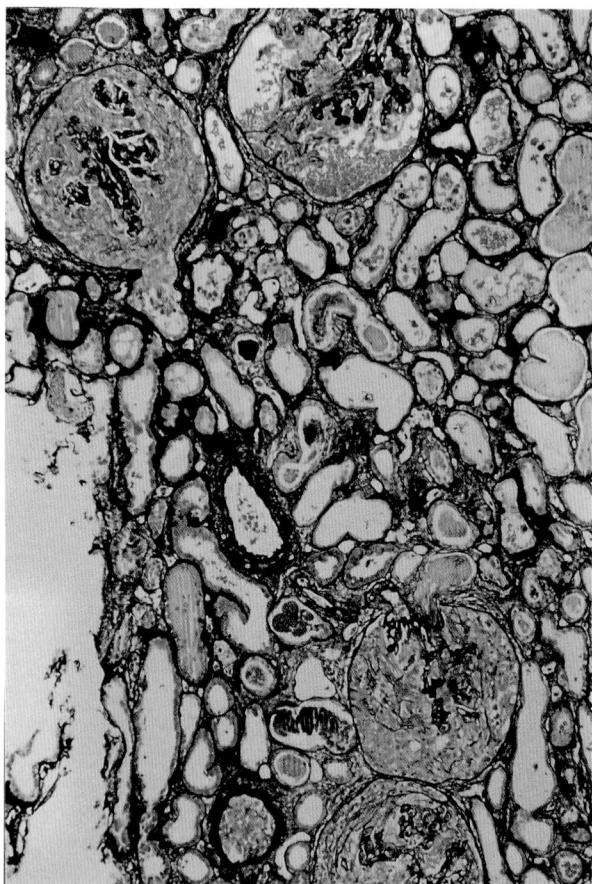

FIGURE 2 Acute crescentic glomerulonephritis associated with Goodpasture's syndrome.

analysis reveals a reduced pO_2. A rise in transfer factor, the rate of transfer of a small concentration of CO in the inspired air onto hemoglobin, is indicative of bleeding within alveoli; correction should be made for hemoglobin concentration because transfer factor varies directly with this. Significant blood loss into the lungs may cause a fall in circulating hemoglobin concentration, while actual bleeding may be visualized at bronchoscopy. Occasionally subclinical hemorrhage leads to iron deficiency anemia. Lung biopsy and histology may document intra-alveolar red blood cells or hemosiderin-laden macrophages. Immunofluorescence and immunoperoxidase staining is difficult in the lung, but when possible, studies have demonstrated linear fixation of IgG along the pulmonary basement membrane.

Nephritis is associated with hematuria on urinanalysis; the urinary sediment reveals red blood cell casts and distorted red blood cells, due to bleeding directly from glomeruli into renal tubules. Proteinuria may be present but is usually less than 5 g /24 hr. If renal function is not already impaired on measurement of BUN and Serum creatinine levels, it may rapidly and inexorably deteriorate if treatment is not instituted as an emergency. Kidney size is usually normal on renal ultrasound and percutaneous renal

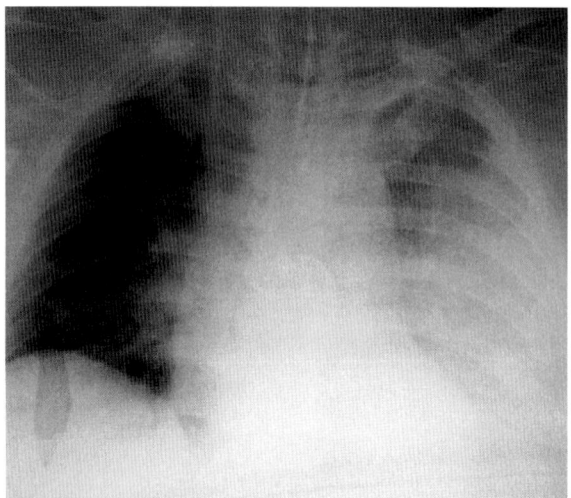

FIGURE I Chest radiograph of a patient with Goodpasture's disease who had pulmonary hemorrhage.

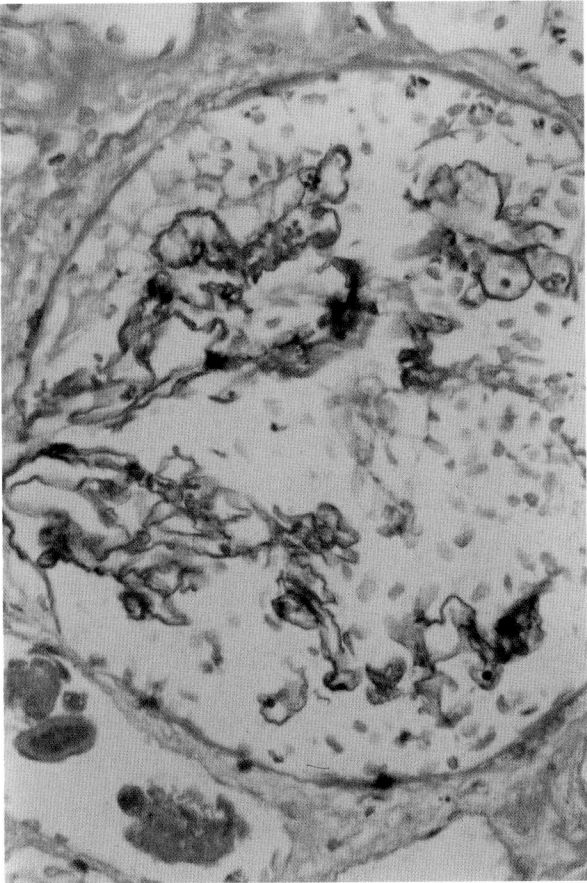

FIGURE 3 Immunoperoxidase staining showing linear fixation of IgG along the GBM in Goodpasture's syndrome.

biopsy permits a histological renal diagnosis. Typically, there is a diffuse nephritis with focal or total necrosis of glomerular tufts and segmental or circumferential cellular crescents around some or all glomeruli (Fig. 2). By immunofluorescence or immunoperoxidase staining, linear IgG fixation is present along the GBM (Fig. 3) and may be accompanied by other immunoglobulins. Linear or granu-

TABLE I

Pulmonary–Renal Vasculitic Syndrome

Disease	Diagnostic test assay
Microscopic polyangiitis	ANCA[a]
Wegener's granulomatosis	ANCA
Goodpasture's disease	Anti-GBM antibodies
Systemic lupus erythematosus	Anti-DNA antibodies
Churg-Strauss syndrome	ANCA present in about half of cases
Henoch-Schönlein purpura	IgA deposition in skin and kidney
Behçet's disease	Clinical only
Rheumatoid vasculitis	Rheumatoid factor
Penicillamine	Drug history

[a] ANCA, antineutrophil cytoplasm antibodies.

lar C3 is present in about two thirds of biopsies. It is worth remembering that other conditions can cause linear staining on direct immunostaining including systemic lupus erythematosus, diabetes mellitus, normal autopsy kidney, cadaveric kidney after perfusion, and renal transplants in patients with Alport's syndrome.

Diagnosis

The diagnosis of Goodpasture's disease is confirmed by presence of linear IgG. (detected by direct immunofluorescence), along the GBM in renal biopsy tissue and by detection of circulating anti-GBM antibodies. These latter may be detected within serum samples by using specific ELISA or, as used in some reference laboratories, by radioimmunoassay. In both, the principle is to coat purified GBM components that have been digested by collagenase (or, as is increasingly used, $NC1\alpha3IV$ peptides) onto a solid-phase support such as plastic microtiter plates. Diluted serum is applied and anti-GBM antibodies bind to the GBM components. Binding is subsequently detected using anti-human IgG reagents labeled a marker agent.

Concurrence with Other Diseases

A number of well-documented cases of membranous glomerulonephritis have evolved into Goodpasture's disease with presence of circulating and fixed anti-GBM antibodies. Patients with Goodpasture's disease and anti-GBM antibodies may sometimes have clinical evidence of vasculitis with circulating ANCA. Finally, Goodpasture's disease can arise within the transplanted kidneys of patients with Alport's syndrome. The native kidneys of these individuals lack the Goodpasture antigen (the underlying inherited defect of $\alpha5(IV)$-chains causes a secondary loss of $\alpha3(IV)$-chains) predisposing them to develop an immune response to the previously unseen antigen that is present within the allograft.

Autoantigens and Autoantibodies

The pathogenesis of Goodpasture's disease is believed to be directly linked to development of autoimmunity to the noncollagenous 1 domain of the $\alpha3$ chain of type IV collagen ($NC1\alpha3IV$). The type IV collagen molecule is composed of three $a(IV)$-chains which are folded into a globular NC1 domain at the C-terminal region. There are five chains for type IV collagen and a sixth gene has been identified. The $\alpha1(IV)$ and $\alpha2(IV)$ chains are ubiquitous while the $\alpha3(IV)$, $\alpha4(IV)$ and $\alpha5(IV)$-chains colocalize and are only present in specialized basement membranes, including those within the kidney, lung, eye, cochlea, and choroid plexus.

Development of autoantibodies to $NC1\alpha3IV$ is closely linked to clinical evidence of disease, and passively injected anti-GBM antibodies can cause disease in subhuman primates and in sheep. Binding of autoantibodies to glomerular or pulmonary basement membranes initiates an inflammatory response with complement deposition, leukocyte recruitment, and eventual tissue injury.

Genetics

Many autoimmune diseases demonstrate association with antigens of the major histocompatibility (MHC) complex. Goodpasture's disease shows a strong association with HLA-DR2. HLA-DR2 has been divided into two specificities—DRw15 and DRw16—each of which consists of a number of alleles. More recent studies using molecular analysis of HLA class II genes in Goodpasture's disease has shown that the association is with the DRw15 (DRB1*1501 and *1502) alleles. These alleles are in strong linkage disequilibrium with DQw6 (DQA1*01 and DQB1*06) and so there is also an association with this entire haplotype.

Environmental Influences

There are a number of reports suggesting geographical case clustering on occasion, possibly indicative of environmental factors that might initiate or reveal disease. Smoking or infections may act to aggravate tissue injury and so reveal disease. There are also reports of association with exposure to organic solvents or hydrocarbons.

Therapy

Therapies are directed toward removing the pathogenic anti-GBM antibodies as quickly as possible, preventing further synthesis and reinstituting tolerance to NC1α3IV. This was the reasoning behind the introduction of plasma exchange, used in conjunction with powerful immunosuppressive therapy, in the 1970s. Most therapeutic protocols now use a combination of prednisolone, cyclophosphamide, and plasma exchange (Table 2). Response to treatment can be monitored by serum creatinine, chest radiograph changes, improvement in lung transfer factor, and by monitoring anti-GBM antibody titers. Blood count measurements are important not only to exclude further falls in hemoglobin due to lung hemorrhage but also to ensure that cyclophosphamide therapy does not induce life-threatening bone marrow suppression. It is important to avoid infection as far as is possible not only because the patient is immunosuppressed but also because infection may precipitate worsening of disease and tissue injury during the early stages of treatment.

TABLE 2
Treatment Protocol for Goodpasture's Syndrome

Prednisolone	$1 \text{ mg} \cdot \text{kg}^{-1} \cdot 24 \text{ hr}^{-1}$ orally (maximum 80 mg). Weekly dose reduction to 20 mg and then more slowly to 1–2 years
Cyclophosphamide	$2.5 \text{ mg} \cdot \text{kg}^{-1} \cdot \text{d}^{-1}$ orally (maximum 150 mg/d). Continue for 4 months, white blood cell count permitting, then change to azathioprine for 1–2 year
Plasma exchange	Daily 4 L exchanges for 4.5% albumin for 14 days or until anti-GBM antibodies are undetectable

The observation that patients presenting with end stage renal failure who are dialysis dependent and who have a severe crescentic renal biopsy rarely recover renal function has led to the recommendation that such patients should be spared immunosuppressive therapy. Predictors of a poor renal prognosis include a serum creatinine greater than 7 mg/dL and crescent formation in more than 50% of the glomeruli on renal biopsy. The exception would be those individuals who have concurrent pulmonary hemorrhage who should receive full immunosuppressive therapy. The use of methylprednisolone has been advocated instead of plasma exchange in this setting and while there are no controlled clinical trials that directly compare use of plasma exchange with methylprednisolone, methylprednisolone may be associated with a greater risk of opportunistic infections, which may considerably worsen the prognosis. In those patients in whom immunosuppressive therapy is withheld, anti-GBM antibody titers fall spontaneously with a mean time to baseline values of about 11 months. Once anti-GBM antibodies are undetectable, these patients may be safely transplanted.

Plasma Exchange

Plasma exchange involves the extracorporeal separation of plasma from cellular elements of blood, with return of cells to the individual together with a substitute fluid for the removed plasma. Automated methods are based on either centrifugation principles, with continuous or discontinuous flow techniques, or filtration principles. In both methods, blood is processed in an extracorporeal circuit and exchange of 2 to 4 L may be achieved in 2 hours. The procedure requires vascular access that is capable of withstanding flow rates of 60 to 150 mL/min (e.g., via antecubital veins or indwelling catheters inserted into the internal jugular or subclavian veins), adequate anticoagulation (e.g., heparin, acid citrate dextrose B form), and suitable replacement fluids or combinations of fluids (e.g., albumin solutions, fresh frozen plasma, synthetic plasma expanders, crystalloids). Fresh frozen plasma (300–400 ml) may be given at the end of the exchange when there is fresh pulmonary hemorrhage or within 24 hours of an invasive procedure.

Complications include the following; anaphylactoid reactions, most common with use of fresh frozen plasma; metabolic alkalosis in patients with renal failure due to infusion of solutions containing high citrate and low chloride levels; citrate toxicity especially if liver disease is present; hemorrhage particularly in patients with thrombocytopenia or defective clotting; thrombosis related to access procedures; posttransfusion hepatitis; cardiovascular complications associated with administration of sodium citrate, ionic alterations, and use of central vascular access; pulmonary edema caused by alveolar lesions induced by presence of leukocyte alloantibodies in replacement plasma; nausea, vomiting, and rigors due to endotoxin contamination of replacement fluids.

Course of the Disease

Effective immunosuppressive therapy usually leads to abolition of the circulating anti-GBM antibodies, although linear antibody may remain fixed within the kidney for a year or more. It is possible but highly unusual for patients with Goodpasture's disease to relapse, unlike patients with systemic vasculitis who relapse frequently. In Goodpasture's disease, even severe lung lesions have the capacity to resolve completely, and it is unusual for patients who have survived serious lung hemorrhage to be left with significant pulmonary impairment or with radiological evidence of fibrosis. The same is not true of the nephritis; patients presenting with a creatinine above 6–7 mg/dL, with oligoanuria, or with extensive crescent formation within the renal biopsy, do not recover renal function.

Bibliography

Burns AP, Fisher M, Li P, et al.: Molecular analysis of HLA class II genes in Goodpasture's disease. *Q J Med* 88:93–100, 1995.

Fleming SJ, Savage COS, McWilliam LJ, et al.: Anti-GBM antibody mediated nephritis complicating transplantation in a patient with Alport's syndrome. *Clin Nephrol* 46:857–859, 1988.

Flores JC, Taube D, Savage COS, et al.: Clinical and immunological evolution of oliguric anti-GBM nephritis treated by haemodialysis. *Lancet* 1:5–8, 1986.

Haworth SJ, Savage COS, Carr D, et al.: Pulmonary hemorrhage complicating Wegener's granulomatosis and microscopic polyarteritis. *Br Med J* 290:1775–1778, 1985.

Lerner RA, Glassock RJ, Dixon FJ: The role of anti-glomerular basement membrane antibody in the pathogenesis of human glomerulonephritis. *J Exp Med* 126:989–1004, 1967.

Merkel F, Pullig O, Marx M, et al.: Course and prognosis of anti-basement membrane antibody (anti-BM-Ab)-mediated disease: Report of 35 cases. *Nephrol Dial Transplant* 9:372–376, 1994

Niles JL, Bottinger EP, Saurina GR, et al.: The syndrome of lung hemorrhage and nephritis is usually an ANCA-associated condition. *Arch Intern Med* 156:440–445, 1996.

Phelps RG, Turner AN: Goodpasture's syndrome; New insights into pathogenesis and clinical picture. *J Nephrol* 9:111–117, 1996.

Saus J, Wieslander J, Langeveld JPM, et al.: Identification of the Goodpasture antigen as the alpha3(IV) chain of collagen IV. *J Biol Chem* 263:13374–13380, 1988.

Savage COS, Pusey CD, Bowman C, et al.: Antiglomerular basement membrane antibody mediated disease in the British Isles 1980-1984. *Br Med J* 292:301–304, 1986.

Short AK, Esnault VLM, Lockwood CM: Antineutrophil cytoplasm antibodies and antiglomerular basement-membrane antibodies - 2 coexisting distinct autoreactivities detectable in patients with rapidly progressive glomerulonephritis. *Am J Kidney Dis* 26:439–445, 1995.

Turner AN, Rees AJ: Goodpasture's disease and Alports syndromes. *Annu Rev Med* 47:377–386, 1996.

SECTION 4

THE KIDNEY IN SYSTEMIC DISEASE

24

RENAL FUNCTION IN CONGESTIVE HEART FAILURE

WILLIAM T. ABRAHAM AND ROBERT W. SCHRIER

Chronic congestive heart failure (CHF) affects more than 4 million Americans, or approximately 1 to 1.5% of the U.S. population. For those age 65 to 74 years, the prevalence of CHF is about 5%, while for those older than 75 years, the prevalence of CHF exceeds 10%. Currently, there are 700,000 new cases of CHF diagnosed each year in the United States. Moreover, CHF is now the most common hospital discharge diagnosis for those over the age of 65 years and the fourth leading cause of hospitalization in US adults. In 1992, the estimated total direct costs of heart failure in the US exceeded 10 billion dollars, while hospitalization costs for heart failure surpassed those for myocardial infarction and cancer combined.

A major cause of morbidity and mortality in patients with symptomatic CHF relates to alterations in renal function which cause avid sodium and water retention. Sodium and water retention in patients with CHF results in expansion of intravascular fluid volume, which leads to increased cardiac preload and subsequently to an enlargement of extravascular and interstitial fluid volumes manifested clinically as pulmonary and peripheral edema. This increase in cardiac preload contributes to the two most common symptoms of heart failure—dyspnea and fatigue—and may contribute to the progressive decline in cardiac performance that comprises the natural history of CHF. Knowledge of the pathogenesis of this renal sodium and water retention permits the rational use of conventional and investigational medical therapy in CHF.

AFFERENT MECHANISMS INVOLVED IN THE SODIUM AND WATER RETENTION OF CHF

In normal humans, an expansion of the extracellular fluid (ECF) volume due to an increase in sodium and water intake is associated with an increase in renal sodium and water excretion followed by restoration of the normal ECF volume. However, in certain edematous states, including cardiac failure, cirrhosis, and pregnancy, avid renal sodium and water retention persists despite expansion of the ECF volume. In fact, this clinical paradox of continued renal sodium and water retention despite total body sodium and water excess defines these edematous disorders. In these clinical circumstances, it is clear that the integrity of the

kidney as the ultimate effector organ of body fluid regulation is intact. Thus, in such edematous states, the kidney must be responding to extrarenal signals from the afferent (i.e., "sensor") limb of a volume regulatory system by decreasing renal sodium and water excretion. The exact nature of these afferent mechanisms has been a major focus of research.

A proposed body fluid volume regulation hypothesis indicates that the relative integrity or "fullness" of the arterial circulation constitutes the primary afferent signal through which the kidneys either increase or decrease their excretion of sodium and water (Fig. 1). This hypothesis explains how an increase in the volume of blood on the venous side of the circulation may cause a rise in total blood volume while a decrease in the *relative* volume of blood in the arterial circulation may promote continued renal sodium and water retention. A decrease in cardiac output is the most obvious means whereby a decrease in arterial circulatory integrity may occur. However this cannot be the only afferent signal for underfilling of the arterial circulation because several edematous disorders, such as cirrhosis, high-output cardiac failure, pregnancy, and large arteriovenous fistulae, are associated with increased cardiac output. Thus, peripheral arterial vascular resistance and the compliance of the arterial vasculature has been proposed as the second determinant of the fullness of the arterial circulation. Peripheral arterial vasodilation therefore provides another afferent signal for arterial underfilling which causes renal sodium and water retention. Thus, a diminished cardiac output could initiate sodium and water retention in low-output heart failure, whereas arterial vasodilation is the proposed mechanism in high-output CHF and other edematous states (Fig. 1).

Arterial blood pressure is not a sensitive index of the presence of arterial underfilling in cardiac failure or other edematous states, because of the rapidity of the compensatory efferent (i.e., "effector") responses. Rather, it is only with advanced disease states that the compensatory responses to arterial underfilling are insufficient to maintain mean arterial pressure. Even if sensitive methods for accurately measuring the volume of blood in the arterial circulation (which is generally less than 2% of total body fluid) were available, the absolute measured arterial blood vol-

BODY FLUID VOLUME REGULATION
HYPOTHESIS

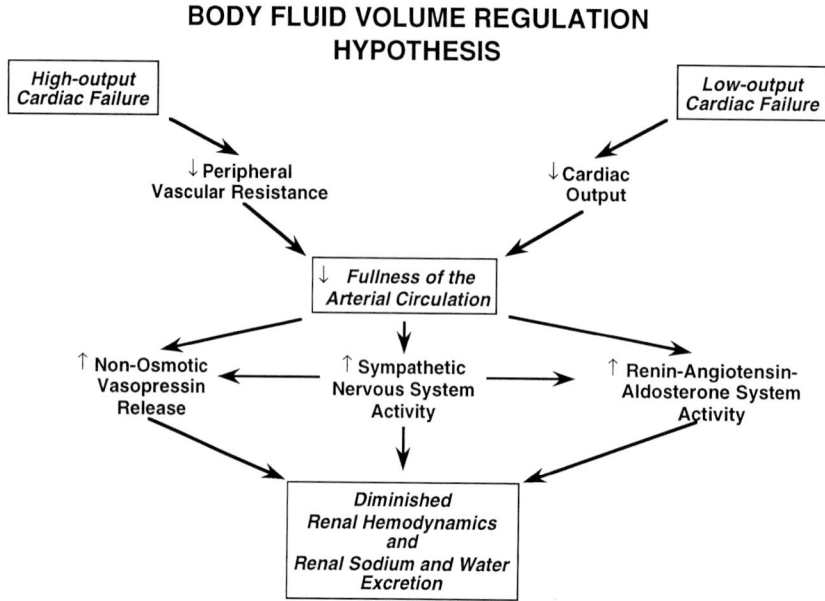

FIGURE 1 Proposed mechanism of renal sodium and water retention in high-output and low-output cardiac failure. A decrease in cardiac output initiates sodium and water retention in low-output heart failure. In high-output CHF, arterial vasodilation starts the sequence of events leading to diminished renal hemodynamics and reduced renal sodium and water excretion. From Schrier RW: *N Engl J Med* 319:1065–1072, 1988. (With permission from the Massachusetts Medical Society.)

ume could be increased as compared to that of normal subjects despite relative arterial underfilling caused by peripheral arterial vasodilation.

Afferent Volume Receptors

The afferent volume receptors must reside in the arterial vascular compartment and predominate over low-pressure receptors. While stimulation of the low-pressure volume receptors of the thorax, including the atria, right ventricle, and pulmonary vessels, results in enhanced release of atrial natriuretic peptide (ANP) and suppression of arginine vasopressin (AVP), patients with advanced CHF exhibit avid sodium and water retention despite the presence of elevated atrial pressures and increased circulating concentrations of ANP. Thus, the high-pressure baroreceptors in the left ventricle, carotid sinus, aortic arch, and juxtaglomerular apparatus have been implicated as the primary afferent receptors involved in this volume regulatory system. Unloading of these ventricular and arterial receptors results in diminution of the tonic inhibitory effect of afferent vagal and glossopharyngeal neural traffic to the central nervous system and initiates the nonosmotic release of vasopressin, activation of the renin-angiotensin-aldosterone system, and stimulation of the adrenergic nervous system. The activation of these three neurohumoral vasoconstrictor systems, by altering renal hemodynamics and tubular function, mediates the avid renal sodium and water retention characteristic of patients with advanced CHF.

EFFERENT MECHANISMS INVOLVED IN THE SODIUM AND WATER RETENTION OF CHF

As noted, the changes in renal hemodynamics and tubular sodium and water handling that occur in CHF are primarily mediated by activation of neurohormonal systems. In this regard, the previously mentioned major neurohormonal vasoconstrictor systems predominate in advanced or decompensated CHF. However, vasodilating hormones such as the natriuretic peptides and renal prostaglandins may play important counterregulatory roles. The renal effects of activation of these neurohormonal systems in CHF are reviewed below and are summarized in Tables 1 and 2.

Changes in Renal Hemodynamics in CHF

The glomerular filtration rate (GFR) is usually normal in mild heart failure and is reduced only as cardiac performance becomes more severely impaired. Renal vascular resistance is increased with a concomitant decrease in renal blood flow (RBF). Generally, RBF decreases in proportion to the decrease in cardiac performance. Therefore the filtration fraction, the ratio of GFR to RBF, is usually increased in patients with cardiac failure. This increased filtration fraction is a consequence of predominant constriction of the efferent arterioles within the kidney. This efferent arteriolar vasoconstriction is mediated by increased renal adrenergic nerve activity and angiotensin II. These changes in renal hemodynamics alter the hydrostatic and oncotic forces in the peritubular capillaries to favor

TABLE 1

Renal Effects of Neurohormonal Vasoconstrictors in
Congestive Heart Failure

Renal nerves
  Promote efferent greater than afferent arteriolar constriction
  Enhance sodium reabsorption in the proximal tubule
  Stimulate renal renin release
Angiotensin II
  Promotes efferent greater than afferent arteriolar constriction
  Enhances sodium reabsorption in the proximal tubule
  Stimulates adrenal aldosterone synthesis and release
Aldosterone
  Enhances sodium reabsorption and potassium and hydrogen
    ion secretion in the collecting duct
Arginine vasopressin
  Increases water reabsorption in the cortical and medullary
    collecting duct
  Increases sodium chloride reabsorption in the medullary
    ascending limb of Henle's loop

From Hosenpud JD, Greenberg BH (eds): *Congestive Heart
Failure: Pathophysiology, Diagnosis, and Comprehensive Approach to Management.* Springer-Verlag, New York, pp. 161–173,
1994. With permission.

TABLE 2

Renal Effects of Hormonal Vasodilators in Congestive
Heart Failure

Natriuretic peptides
  Increases glomerular filtration rate
  Promotes diminished sodium reabsorption in the collecting
    duct
  Suppresses renin activity
  Inhibits aldosterone synthesis and release
  Possibly inhibits vasopressin release
Renal prostaglandins
  Promote renal vasodilation
  Decrease tubular sodium reabsorption in the ascending limb
    of Henle's loop
  Inhibit vasopressin hydroosmotic action in the collecting duct

From Hosenpud JD, Greenberg BH (eds): *Congestive Heart
Failure: Pathophysiology, Diagnosis, and Comprehensive Approach to Management.* Springer-Verlag, New York, pp. 161–173,
1994. With permission.

increased proximal tubular reabsorption of sodium and
water.

Renal Effects of Neurohormonal Vasoconstrictor Activation in CHF

As mentioned, increased renal adrenergic nerve activity
and angiotensin II cause efferent arteriolar vasoconstriction which increases the filtration fraction and moves the
balance of hemodynamic forces in the peritubular capillaries in favor of enhanced proximal tubular sodium reabsorption. In addition to this indirect effect to increase sodium
reabsorption in the proximal tubule, both renal adrenergic
nerves and angiotensin II exhibit a direct effect in the
proximal tubule to enhance sodium reabsorption. Renal
nerves also stimulate renal renin release which contributes
to the increase in circulating angiotensin II concentration
seen in CHF, and angiotensin II stimulates adrenal aldosterone synthesis and release. The latter enhances sodium
reabsorption in the collecting duct. In support of a role for
increased renal adrenergic nerve activity in the sodium and
water retention of CHF is the observation that intrarenal
adrenergic blockade results in a natriuresis in experimental
animals and humans with CHF. For example, in rats with
CHF, the intravenous administration of the central $alpha_2$
receptor agonist, clonidine, results in a marked decrease
in renal adrenergic nerve activity and a concomitant increase in urinary volume excretion.

A role for the renin-angiotensin-aldosterone system in
the sodium retention of CHF is suggested by the observation that urinary sodium excretion inversely correlates with
plasma renin activity and urinary aldosterone excretion
in patients with CHF. However, the administration of an
angiotensin converting enzyme (ACE) inhibitor to patients

with CHF does not consistently increase urinary sodium
excretion despite a consistent decrease in plasma aldosterone concentration. The simultaneous fall in blood pressure
due to decreased circulating concentrations of angiotensin
II or an excessive fall in glomerular capillary pressure due
to decreased angiotensin II and increased bradykinin may
obscure the natriuretic response to ACE inhibition. The
observation that furosemide-induced natriuresis is augmented by very low doses but not by standard doses of
an ACE inhibitor is compatible with this hypothesis. In
addition, an important role for aldosterone in the sodium
retention of CHF has been demonstrated using the specific
aldosterone antagonist, spironolactone.

Arginine vasopressin increases water reabsorption in the
cortical and medullary collecting duct and increases sodium
chloride reabsorption in the medullary ascending limb of
Henle's loop. Two lines of evidence implicate the nonosmotic release of AVP in the abnormal water retention of
CHF. In experimental CHF, the absence of a pituitary
source of AVP is associated with normal or near normal
water excretion. In addition, the use of investigational antagonists to the renal, or V_2, receptor of AVP may reverse
the abnormal water retention in experimental and human CHF.

Renal Effects of Hormonal Vasodilator Activation in CHF

The natriuretic peptides, ANP and brain natriuretic peptide (BNP), increase GFR, promote diminished sodium
reabsorption in the collecting duct, and suppress renin activity and aldosterone synthesis and release. The tubular
sites of action for these neurohormonal agents are shown
in Fig. 2. Experimental observations suggest that the natriuretic peptides play an important role in attenuating the
renal sodium and water retention associated with CHF.
Circulating concentrations of ANP and BNP are elevated
in CHF; however, the natriuretic effect of both endogenous
and exogenous natriuretic peptides is often blunted in CHF

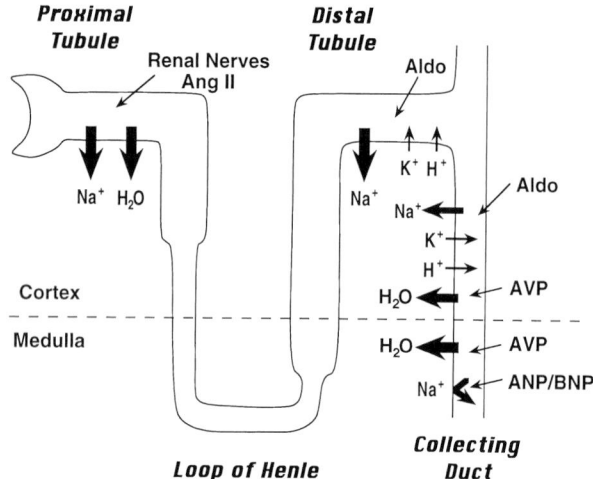

Proximal Tubule

Distal Tubule

Renal Nerves Ang II

Aldo

Na^+ H_2O

K^+ H^+

Na^+

Aldo

Na^+

K^+

H^+

Cortex

H_2O AVP

Medulla

H_2O AVP

Na^+ ANP/BNP

Loop of Henle

Collecting Duct

FIGURE 2 Sites of action of some important neurohormonal systems which alter the tubular handling of sodium and water in CHF. Renal nerves and angiotensin II (Ang II) enhance sodium reabsorption in the proximal tubule. Aldosterone (Aldo) increases sodium reabsorption and promotes potassium and hydrogen ion secretion in the distal nephron. Arginine vasopressin (AVP) acts to increase water reabsorption in the cortical and medullary collecting duct. Atrial (ANP) and brain (BNP) natriuretic peptides inhibit sodium reabsorption in the collecting duct. From Hosenpud JD, Greenberg BH (eds): *Congestive Heart Failure: Pathophysiology, Diagnosis, and Comprehensive Approach to Management.* Springer-Verlag, New York, pp. 161–173, 1994. With permission.

patients. Based on the observation of a positive correlation among endogenous ANP levels, urinary cyclic guanosine monophosphate (cGMP, the second messenger for the natriuretic effect of ANP and BNP in vivo), and cardiac filling pressures, it has been suggested that the natriuretic peptide resistance seen in CHF patients may be due to decreased sodium delivery to the distal tubular site of natriuretic peptide action rather than a direct impairment of the receptor-signal transduction system involving cGMP. This possibility may be analogous to the impairment in aldosterone escape seen in patients with CHF and other chronic sodium-retaining states. This diminished distal tubular sodium delivery hypothesis of natriuretic peptide resistance is also supported by the observation that maneuvers which increase distal tubular sodium delivery (e.g., low-dose mannitol, renal denervation, and angiotensin II blockade) restore renal responsiveness to ANP in CHF and in other edematous disorders. In patients with advanced CHF the natriuretic response to BNP correlates most strongly with the change in distal tubular sodium delivery during BNP infusion. Other mechanisms, such as intracellular factors acting beyond cGMP, may also contribute to natriuretic peptide resistance in CHF.

Renal prostaglandins promote renal vasodilation, decrease sodium reabsorption in the ascending limb of Henle's loop, and inhibit AVP hydroosmotic action in the collecting duct. The administration of acetylsalicylic acid to patients with moderate CHF and a normal sodium intake in doses that decrease the synthesis of renal prostaglandin

E_2 results in a significant reduction in urinary sodium excretion and suggests a possible counterregulatory role for vasodilating prostaglandins in CHF. Moreover, it has been well documented that the administration of a cyclooxygenase inhibitor to patients with CHF may result in acute reversible renal failure, an effect that is thought to be due to inhibition of renal prostaglandins.

IMPLICATIONS FOR MEDICAL THERAPY OF CHF

Medical therapy of CHF with diuretics and direct-acting vasodilators may further activate neurohormonal vasoconstrictor systems and diminish circulating concentrations of ANP. The emergence of diuretic resistance or vasodilator tolerance in patients with chronic heart failure may be due, in part, to further activation of vasoconstrictor mechanisms induced by these therapeutic agents. For example, the administration of the loop diuretic, furosemide, increases plasma norepinephrine, renin activity, and aldosterone and decreases plasma ANP in patients with acute or chronic heart failure. These neurohormonal effects of diuretic therapy may contribute to the development of diuretic resistance, because increased renal nerve activity and angiotensin II enhance proximal tubular sodium reabsorption thereby obscuring the beneficial effect of a diuretic that acts in the loop of Henle or in a more distal segment of the nephron. Continuous vasodilator therapy with nitroglycerin results in the rapid development of drug tolerance and in fluid retention, occurring simultaneously with activation of the renin-angiotensin-aldosterone system. That this nitrate tolerance is prevented by the concomitant administration of an ACE inhibitor further implicates drug-induced activation of neurohormonal vasoconstrictor mechanisms in the fluid retention associated with these agents.

This further activation of neurohormonal vasoconstrictor systems in response to diuretic or nitrate administration is compatible with the aforementioned arterial underfilling hypothesis in CHF. Diuretic- or vasodilator-induced reductions in cardiac preload, although effective in decreasing the congestive signs and symptoms of CHF, move the myocardial length-tension relationship in a direction that further diminishes ventricular performance. In contrast, the administration of a positive inotrope to patients with CHF results in an upward and leftward shift of the Starling curve and an increase in ventricular performance which may restore the integrity of the arterial circulation and improve the neurohormonal milieu.

These observations suggest that inhibition of vasoconstrictor mechanisms by neurohormonal antagonists or positive inotropes may be more beneficial than or additive to nonspecific diuretic or vasodilator therapy in CHF. The proven beneficial effects of ACE inhibition on symptoms, hemodynamics, and survival in heart failure patients support the routine use of these agents in CHF. However, as mentioned above, the administration of an ACE inhibitor during heart failure does not consistently increase urinary sodium excretion. Adrenergic-blocking agents, renin antagonists, angiotensin II antagonists, AVP antagonists, natriuretic peptides, vasodilating prostaglandins, and a variety of positive inotropes are all under active investigation in heart failure patients. A recent study in human heart failure suggests that angiotensin II receptor antagonism may exert a more favorable effect on the kidney when compared to ACE inhibition. However, this observation awaits confirmation by large clinical trials. V_2 receptor AVP antagonists, now in phase I–II clinical development in the United States, are promising agents for reversing the dilutional hyponatremia of CHF.

Low or "renal" doses of dopamine ($1-2 \mu g \cdot kg^{-1} \cdot min^{-1}$) may improve renal blood flow and GFR, promote natriuresis via a direct effect on the proximal tubule, and facilitate diuresis in some patients with advanced decompensated CHF. However, the indiscriminate use of dopamine in patients with heart failure should be avoided, because large-scale randomized clinical efficacy trials have not been performed. In a careful study of six diuretic-sensitive CHF patients, dopamine did not improve the responsiveness to furosemide. Thus, the empiric use of dopamine should probably be reserved for patients with decompensated CHF and some degree of diuretic resistance. In this setting, urine output should be followed prior to and during dopamine infusion to assess its clinical efficacy and indication for continued administration.

Finally, the pharmacologic management of CHF is frequently complicated by the coexistence of chronic renal failure. The use of ACE inhibitors in such patients may be complicated by altered pharmacokinetics and worsening renal dysfunction. The former concern applies to all but one of the ACE inhibitors and may be overcome by modest dose reduction. The latter complication is seen most frequently in the setting of advanced heart failure, where preservation of glomerular capillary pressure may be particularly dependent on angiotensin II-induced efferent arteriolar constriction and maintenance of systemic blood pressure. However, with careful drug titration, many patients with heart failure and chronic renal insufficiency will tolerate ACE inhibition. As the GFR falls below 30 mL/min, the efficacy of distal tubular diuretics (thiazides and potassium-conserving agents) is lost. Thus, loop diuretics and metolazone are preferred in such patients. Finally, digoxin intoxication is common in patients with coexistent cardiac and renal disease. Because digoxin is eliminated primarily via the kidneys, dose adjustment is necessary as the GFR falls.

Bibliography

Abraham WT: New neurohormonal antagonists and natriuretic peptides in the treatment of congestive heart failure. *Coronary Artery Dis.* 5:127–136, 1994.

Abraham WT: Physiology and therapeutic implications of natriuretic peptides in chronic heart failue. *Heart Failure* 12:55–72, 1996.

Abraham WT, Schrier RW: Renal salt and water handling in congestive heart failure. In: Hosenpud JD, Greenberg JH (eds) *Congestive Heart Failure: Pathophysiology, Differential Diagnosis, and Comprehensive Approach to Therapy.* Springer-Verlag, New York, pp. 161–173, 1993.

Abraham WT, Schrier RW: Use of furosemide in the treatment of congestive heart failure. In: *Aspects of Diuretic Therapy with Furosemide: An Update.* International Clinical Practice Series. Wells Medical Ltd., Kent, pp. 23–33, 1993.

Abraham WT, Schrier RW: Cardiac failure, liver disease, and nephrotic syndrome. In: Schrier RW, Gottschalk CW. (eds) *Diseases of the Kidney.* 6th ed. Little, Brown Co., Boston, pp. 2353–2392, 1996.

Schrier RW. Pathogenesis of sodium and water retention in high-output and low-output cardiac failure, nephrotic syndrome, cirrhosis, and pregnancy. *N Engl J Med* 319:1065–1072 (Part 1); 1127–1134 (Part 2), 1988.

Schrier RW: Body fluid volume regulation in health and disease: A unifying hypothesis. *Ann Intern Med* 113:155–159, 1990.

Schrier RW. A unifying hypothesis of body fluid volume regulation: The Lilly Lecture 1992. *J Royal Coll Physicians London* 1992; 26:295-306.

Schrier RW: An odyssey into the milieu interieur: Pondering the enigmas. *J Am Soc Nephrol* 2:1549–1559, 1992.

25

RENAL FUNCTION IN LIVER DISEASE

MURRAY EPSTEIN

A variety of alterations in renal function and electrolyte metabolism frequently accompany liver disease. These diverse complications vary from those that have little clinical significance to others that constitute serious derangements requiring therapeutic intervention. This chapter emphasizes abnormalities of renal sodium and water handling, and on the hepatorenal syndrome.

RENAL SODIUM HANDLING

Clinical Features

Patients with Läennec's cirrhosis manifest a remarkable capacity for sodium chloride retention; indeed, they frequently excrete urine that is virtually free of sodium. Extracellular fluid accumulates excessively and eventually becomes manifest as clinically detectable ascites and edema. It should be emphasized that cirrhotic patients who are unable to excrete sodium will continue to gain weight and accumulate ascites and edema as long as dietary sodium content exceeds maximal urinary sodium excretion. If access to sodium is not curtailed, the relentless retention of this ion may lead to the accumulation of vast amounts of ascites (on occasion up to 20 L). Weight gain and ascites formation promptly cease when sodium intake is limited.

The abnormality of renal sodium handling in cirrhosis is not a static and unalterable condition. Rather, patients with cirrhosis may undergo a spontaneous diuresis followed by a return to avid salt retention. While a significant number of patients who are maintained on a sodium-restricted dietary program may undergo a spontaneous diuresis, there is inadequate information concerning the incidence of this phenomenon and the predictability of its occurrence in any particular patient. The primary renal excretory abnormality causing fluid retention is a disturbance of sodium rather than water excretion. Many sodium-retaining patients with ascites and edema can excrete large volumes of dilute urine when given excessive amounts of water without sodium.

Pathogenesis

The pathogenetic events leading to the deranged sodium homeostasis of cirrhosis are exceedingly complex and remain the subject of continuing controversy. At least two hypotheses have been advanced. Traditionally, it has been proposed that ascites formation in cirrhotic patients begins when a critical imbalance of Starling forces in the hepatic sinusoids and splanchnic capillaries causes an excessive amount of lymph formation, which exceeds the capacity of the thoracic duct to return it to the circulation. Consequently, excess lymph accumulates in the peritoneal space as ascites. Simultaneously, vasodilatation and opening of arteriovenous shunts expands the space in which the plasma volume is contained; renal sodium retention is activated and the relative disparity between plasma volume and the circulatory space is perceived as "effective" plasma volume contraction. The renal retention of sodium may be successful in restoring absolute total plasma volume to a normal or even supranormal value; however, because of the enlargement of the circulatory space in which this volume is contained, a state of relative or "effective" plasma volume contraction persists. This may explain the apparent paradox of unremitting renal sodium retention even with an apparently expanded absolute plasma volume. The term "effective" plasma volume refers to the part of the total circulating volume that is effective in stimulating volume receptors. The concept is elusive because the actual volume receptors remain incompletely defined. The diminished effective volume is thought to constitute an afferent signal that triggers events leading to augmentation of salt and water reabsorption by the renal tubule. Thus, the traditional formulation implies that the renal retention of sodium is a secondary rather than primary event.

In contrast, the "overflow" hypothesis for ascites formation suggests that the primary event is the inappropriate retention of excessive sodium by the kidney with a resultant expansion of plasma volume. In the setting of abnormal Starling forces (both portal venous hypertension and a reduction in plasma colloid osmotic pressure) in the portal venous bed and hepatic sinusoids, the expanded plasma volume is sequestered preferentially in the peritoneal space with ascites formation. Thus, according to this formulation, renal sodium retention and plasma volume expansion precede rather than follow the formation of ascites.

A third hypothesis to account for renal sodium and water retention in cirrhosis has been proposed. This theory, termed the "peripheral arterial vasodilation hypothesis," postulates that peripheral vasodilation is the initial determinant of intravascular underfilling, i.e., that an imbalance between an expanded capacitance and the available volume constitutes a diminished effective volume. This "peripheral vasodilatation" theory is not a separate hypothesis, but rather represents a revision of the "underfill" theory.

Efferent Factors

Initial attempts to explain the renal abnormalities responsible for sodium retention focused on the decrement in glomerular filtration rate (GFR) that frequently occurs in patients with advanced liver disease. A number of observations indicated, however, that a decrease in GFR cannot constitute the major determinant of the abnormalities in renal sodium handling, because sodium retention occurred despite normal or supranormal GFR. Thus, renal sodium retention accompanying cirrhosis is due primarily to enhanced tubular reabsorption rather than to alterations in the filtered load of sodium.

The mediators for the enhanced tubular reabsorption of sodium in cirrhosis and their relative role in this process have not been elucidated completely. Several mechanisms have been suggested, including (1) hyperaldosteronism, (2) alterations in intrarenal blood flow distribution, (3) an increase in renal sympathetic nervous system activity, (4) alterations in eicosanoids including a relative diminution of renal vasodilatory prostaglandins, (5) a relative impairment of renal kallikrein generation, (6) alterations in atrial natriuretic peptide, and (7) modulation of a possible humoral natriuretic factor.

MANAGEMENT OF ASCITES AND EDEMA

The approach to the cirrhotic patient with ascites should be grounded on the realization that ascites, unless massive, may not require treatment per se. The initial goal of any treatment program should be an attempt to obtain spontaneous diuresis by consistent and scrupulous adherence to rigid dietary sodium restriction (500 mg per day). While the frequency with which such dietary management successfully relieves ascites is unsettled, if feasible such a diet should be prescribed to all patients since it is impossible to predict which patients will respond. When the response to dietary management is inadequate or when the imposition of rigid dietary sodium restriction is not feasible because of cost or unpalatability of the diet, diuretic agents should be prescribed.

If there is no compelling reason for rapidly mobilizing excessive fluid, treatment should begin with one of the distal potassium-sparing diuretics. It is reasonable to start with spironolactone, 100 mg/day twice daily. If this dosage of spironolactone does not induce a natriuresis, the dosage may be increased in stepwise fashion every 3 to 5 days to a maximum of 400 mg/day. Spironolactone's onset of action is slow, requiring 3 to 5 days for the peak effect to become manifest, and thus natriuresis will not occur during the initial 2 to 3 days of therapy. If no natriuresis occurs with the maximum dosage of spironolactone, one can add a loop diuretic such as furosemide to the regimen.

Loop diuretics most be delivered into the lumen of the renal tubule to produce a pharmacologic effect. Studies in patients with cirrhosis disclose wide variability in response,

but some patients clearly have diminished ability to attain sufficient drug in the urine to cause a response. Such patients may require 2 to $2\frac{1}{2}$ times greater doses of loop diuretics to attain "normal" amounts at the site of action. Hence, a reasonable therapeutic strategy is first to administer conventional doses of a loop diuretic (e.g., 40 mg of IV furosemide = 80 mg of oral furosemide = 1 mg of iv or oral bumetamide). If no response or an inadequate response ensues, the dose may be increased by at most $2\frac{1}{2}$ fold. There appears to be no justification for higher doses. Such a strategy should compensate for any changes in the disposition of loop diuretics in patients with liver disease and still be safe. Because of recent trends emphasizing reduction of hospital length of stay, many clinicians short-circuit this approach by utilizing large-volume paracentesis.

Large-Volume Paracentesis

Because large-volume paracentesis may induce hypovolemia, hyponatremia, renal failure, and encephalopathy, until recently its use in the treatment of refractory ascites has been limited. Previous studies have demonstrated a varied decrease in plasma volume following paracentesis. Furthermore, it has been suggested that ascites per se may have a negative influence on cardiac function. Recently, several groups of investigators have reevaluated the effects of large-volume (4 to 25 L per day until disappearance of ascites) or total paracentesis (complete mobilization of ascites in only one paracentesis session) and concluded that it constitutes effective and relatively safe therapy for mobilizing ascites. Extensive studies by the Barcelona group have clearly established a role for large-volume paracentesis in the therapeutic armamentarium of refractory ascites. Their experience and that of others would dictate that there are relatively few side effects associated with this procedure. The intravenous administration of albumin or other plasma expanders is initiated at the end of the procedure to obviate the adverse effects on renal function. In cases of massive ascites treated by total paracentesis (>8 L), half of the dose of plasma expanders should be administered at the end of the procedure and half 6 hours later to prevent excessively rapid plasma volume expansion, which may lead to variceal bleeding. In most patients, peripheral edema rapidly reabsorbs following mobilization of ascites and usually disappears within the first 2 days after treatment.

RENAL WATER HANDLING IN CIRRHOSIS

Clinical Features

Impairment of renal diluting capacity occurs frequently in cirrhosis. Hyponatremia, the expression of this impaired capacity to excrete water, is a commonly encountered clinical problem in cirrhotic patients. Although this abnormality may reflect the severity of the hepatic disease, the available data suggest difficulty in correlating the impairment of maximal water diuresis with specific clinical features, such as the degree of ascites or the level of jaundice.

The majority of patients with compensated liver disease excrete water normally wherever those with decompensated hepatic illness manifest widely varying responses to oral loading. Prospective studies have indicated that the transition from compensation to decompensation, or vice versa, is not necessarily accompanied by concomitant changes in renal water handling.

Pathogenesis

The mechanism responsible for the impairment of water diuresis in cirrhosis is not fully established. Four factors have been proposed: (1) enhanced antidiuretic hormone (ADH) activity; (2) a decreased delivery of filtrate to the diluting segments of the nephron; (3) a decrease in the release of prostaglandins; and (4) an increase in renal sympathetic nervous system activity.

Treatment of Hyponatremia

An impaired diluting ability has important management implications for many patients with advanced liver disease. Because hyponatremia connotes a dilutional state secondary to an impaired capacity to excrete water, fluid restriction constitutes the basis for treatment. Appropriate fluid restriction will eventually repair this abnormality, regardless of the degree of dilutional impairment.

Unfortunately, this seemingly simple goal is often elusive. In many hospitals, adherence to the physician's orders for fluid restriction is erratic. Because paramedical and nursing personnel may not consider the fluids administered with medication as part of fluid intake, patients who are supposedly on rigid fluid restriction regimens may be receiving as much as 1500 and even 2000 mL fluid per day. Because of this problem, it is sometimes necessary to resort to absolute fluid restriction (0 to 200 mL/day) for the first few days in order to initiate normalization of serum sodium.

Of interest, several vasopressin antagonists under development promise to become important adjuncts normal type not hold in the management of refractory hyponatremia.

SYNDROMES OF ACUTE AZOTEMIA

Acute renal failure occurs with increased frequency in patients with hepatic and biliary disease. While acute azotemia may often be due to classic acute renal failure, cirrhotic patients can also develop a unique form of renal failure called the hepatorenal syndrome.

Hepatorenal Syndrome

Progressive oliguric renal failure commonly complicates the course of patients with advanced hepatic disease. While this condition has been designated by many names including "functional renal failure" and "the renal failure of cirrhosis," the more appealing, albeit less specific, term "hepatorenal syndrome" (HRS) is widely applied. Hepatorenal syndrome may be defined as unexplained renal failure occurring in patients with liver disease in the ab-

sence of clinical, laboratory, or anatomical evidence of other known causes of renal failure.

Clinical Features

The clinical presentation and course of HRS are characterized by marked variability. HRS develops usually in patients who have advanced chronic hepatic failure and portal hypertension. Although this form of renal failure can complicate the course of virtually all forms of severe liver disease, most studies performed in the United States have identified alcoholic cirrhosis as the underlying disorder.

Renal failure may develop with great rapidity, occasionally occurring in patients in whom normal GFR and concentrating ability were documented a few days before the onset of HRS. Although HRS may follow events that reduce effective blood volume, including abdominal paracentesis, vigorous diuretic therapy, and gastrointestinal bleeding, it can occur in the absence of an apparent precipitating factor. Patients with cirrhosis often develop HRS following admission to the hospital, raising the question as to whether events in the hospital might precipitate HRS. Generally, HRS develops in patients who have ascites, which is often tense, as well as other clinical stigmata of portal hypertension and chronic liver disease. Rarely, HRS can occur with little evidence of severe hepatic dysfunction.

A substantial body of evidence lends strong support to the concept that the renal failure in HRS is functional in nature. Direct evidence is derived (1) from the demonstration that kidneys transplanted from patients with HRS are capable of resuming normal function in the recipient and (2) by the return of renal function when the patient with HRS successfully receives a liver transplant. Laboratory studies confirm the severity of hepatic disease. Prothrombin time is prolonged, serum albumin concentration is reduced, and bilirubin concentration is increased although the degree of jaundice is extremely variable. Most patients have a modest decrease in systemic blood pressure. Urine volume is reduced (<800 mL/day), oliguria is common (<400 mL/day), but anuria is rare. The serum creatinine and blood urea nitrogen (BUN) are elevated but seldom approach the high values seen in patients with endstage renal failure due to primary renal disease. The degree of renal impairment is underestimated by our reliance on the BUN and serum creatinine concentrations as indices of renal function. These parameters are misleading because BUN levels tend to be depressed in cirrhotics owing to reduced protein intake from anorexia and limited hepatic synthesis of urea. Similarly, endogenous creatinine production declines as muscle wasting develops in protein-malnourished cirrhotics, thereby lowering serum creatinine concentration at any level of creatinine clearance. The urine is usually acid; mild proteinuria, granular casts, and microscopic hematuria are not infrequent. The urine is virtually free of sodium chloride (<10 mEq/L) and modestly concentrated (500 to 700 mOsm/kg H_2O). Occasionally, urine sodium concentrations of 20 to 30 mEq/L may be seen. This may be due to superimposed acute tubular necrosis (ATN) or acute metabolic alkalosis due to vomiting; in the former, urinary chloride would be commensurate with that of sodium, while in the latter, urinary chloride would be low. Toward the end of the clinical course, urinary sodium excretion may increase and urine osmolality decrease toward isotonicity, probably due to superimposed ATN. Urinary lysozyme, a marker of tubule cell injury, is also low in contrast to the levels in typical ATN.

The prognosis of HRS is grave. The majority of patients die within a few weeks of onset of azotemia, although 5 to 10% of the patients may survive several months of mild azotemia. Complete recovery in those with advanced renal failure is rare.

Differential Diagnosis

As has been discussed earlier, the abrupt onset of oliguria in a cirrhotic patient may have other etiologies than HRS. Prerenal causes are important to differentiate, particularly because they constitute reversible conditions if recognized and treated in the incipient phase. Volume contraction or cardiac pump failure may present as a "pseudohepatorenal" syndrome. As already mentioned, it is common for patients with alcoholic cirrhosis to develop classic ATN. In many instances, the differentiation from HRS can be made readily by recognition of the precipitating event and characteristic laboratory findings. Table 1 lists laboratory features helpful in differentiating the three principal causes of acute azotemia in patients with liver disease. The most common finding in the urine of HRS patients is a strikingly low sodium concentration, usually less than 10 mEq/L, and occasionally as low as 2 to 5 mEq/L. Similarly, prerenal azotemia is associated with low urinary sodium concentrations. In contrast, patients with oliguric ATN frequently have urinary sodium concentrations exceeding 30 mEq/L, sometimes higher. Both HRS and prerenal azotemia manifest well-maintained urinary concentrating ability characterized by a urine to plasma osmolality ratio (U/Posm) >1.0, whereas ATN patients excrete an isoosmotic urine. Urine to plasma creatinine ratio (U/P creatinine) is >30 in both prerenal failure and HRS, whereas U/P

creatinine is <20:1 in ATN. Proteinuria is absent or minimal in HRS.

In summary, the finding of a low urinary sodium concentration in the presence of oliguric ATN precludes the diagnosis of ATN. Only when prerenal failure and ATN are excluded can one establish the diagnosis of HRS.

Because HRS and prerenal azotemia have similar urinary diagnostic indices, one must often use a functional maneuver, i.e., the administration of volume expanders, to differentiate between the two entities. In this regard, it should be underscored that our frame of reference for the cirrhotic patient may be quite different from that pertaining to other disease states. The degree of volume expansion necessary to replete the cirrhotic patient may at times be marked, occasionally requiring the infusion of massive amounts of colloid.

Treatment

The management of HRS is discouraging in view of the absence of any reproducibly effective treatment modality. Because knowledge today about the pathogenesis of HRS remains inferential and incomplete, therapy must be primarily supportive. The initial step in management is not to equate decreased renal function with HRS, but rather to search diligently for and treat correctable causes of azotemia such as volume contraction, cardiac decompensation, and urinary tract obstruction. The diagnosis of ATN should be considered, since the cirrhotic patients with ATN may recover, if supported with dialytic therapy.

Once the correctable causes of renal functional impairment are excluded, the mainstay of therapy is careful restriction of sodium and fluid intake. A number of specific therapeutic measures have been attempted, but few have proved to be of practical value. Attempts at volume expansion with different exogenous expanders result in only transient improvement in renal hemodynamics and function without significant improvement in the outcome. Similarly, attempts at reinfusion of ascites utilizing peritoneal fluid which has been concentrated have not provided any lasting improvement.

TABLE I

Differential Diagnosis of Acute Azotemia in Patients with Liver Disease

Biochemical characteristics	Important differential urinary findings		
	Prerenal azotemia	Hepatorenal syndrome	Acute renal failure (Acute tubular necrosis)
Urine sodium concentration (mEq/L)	<10	<10	<30[a]
Urine to plasma creatinine ratio	<30:1	>30:1	<20:1
Urine osmolality	At least 100 mOsm > plasma osmolality	At least 100 mOsm > plasma osmolality	Equal to plasma osmolality
Urine sediment	Normal	Unremarkable	Casts, cellular debris

[a] It has recently been appreciated that radiocontrast agents and sepsis may lower urinary sodium concentration in patients with acute tubular necrosis.

In view of the prominent role assigned to renal cortical ischemia in the pathogenesis of HRS, it is not altogether surprising that numerous attempts to treat HRS with vasodilators have their made. Intrarenal infusion of nonspecific vasodilators such as acetylcholine improve renal blood flow but do not augment GFR. Similarly, blockade of vasoconstrictor α-adrenergic nerves by intrarenal infusion of phentolamine or phenoxybenzamine has no significant effect on GFR. Infusions of vasodilator prostaglandins to correct a possible renal prostaglandin deficiency have been unrewarding.

Dialysis has been reported to be ineffective in the management of HRS. Increasing experience, however, suggests that such a sweeping condemnation should be qualified. Although most of the early published literature indeed suggests a dismal prognosis for patients who are dialyzed, such reports have dealt with patients with chronic end-stage liver disease. In a few instances, dialysis has been undertaken with an ultimately favorable outcome in HRS patients with *acute* hepatic disease. These observations indicate that in selected patients, i.e., patients with acute hepatic dysfunction in whom there is reason to believe that renal failure may reverse with resolution of the acute hepatic insult, dialytic therapy is indicated. Recently, the role of dialysis has been expanding as a supportive measure for patients awaiting hepatic transplantation.

Because many patients undergoing liver transplantation with or without acute renal failure exhibit hemodynamic instability, treatment with continuous hemofiltration may be better tolerated. Fluid removal may facilitate overall management and allow liberal replacement of clotting factors and other fluids during the perioperative period. In addition, continuous renal replacement therapy may help control hepatic encephalopathy and the associated increases in intracranial pressure.

There has been a flurry of enthusiasm for the use of the peritoneal jugular shunt (LeVeen shunt) in the management of HRS. Because the underlying abnormality is thought to be maldistribution of extracellular fluid with a resultant diminished effective blood volume, attention has focused on developing procedures that can redistribute body fluids between compartments, so that the central compartment is replenished at a time when ascites is decreasing.

Only two prospective randomized studies of the role of the PVS in the treatment of HRS have been performed. The first prospectively compared the effects of the PVS shunt ($n = 10$) or medical therapy ($n = 10$) on renal function and mortality in 20 patients with the HRS associated with alcoholic liver disease. After 48 to 72 hours, body weight and serum creatinine were increased with medical therapy and decreased in patients with the shunt. Despite improvement of renal function only one patient with the PVS had a prolonged survival (210 days). In the second, there were seven long-term survivals in a group of 14 patients treated with PVS, but the results were not statistically significant when compared to those of a group of 19 patients undergoing medical therapy. The mean half-life of patients treated with the shunt did not differ significantly from that of controls. Based on the available data, it is apparent that a beneficial role for the PVS in the treatment of the HRS has not been established.

Transjugular Intrahepatic Porto-systemic Shunt

Recently, a few anecdotal reports have appeared describing improvement in renal function in HRS patients following insertion of a transjugular intrahepatic porto-systemic shunt (TIPS). The rationale for this procedure is similar to that for the establishment of a side-to-side portacaval shunt, thereby creating a portal to systemic vascular pathway that serves to decompress portacaval system. Although TIPS obviates the need for performing major vascular surgery, it is not as simple and innocuous a procedure as some of its adherents propose. It is operator-dependent, requiring skilled and experienced interventional radiologists for its successful insertion. The available data supporting its use consist mainly of a few preliminary and anecdotal reports.

Orthotopic Liver Transplantation

Orthotopic liver transplantation (OLTX) has recently become the accepted treatment for end-stage liver disease. Of interest, many of these patients present with varying degrees of concomitant renal dysfunction, including HRS. OLTX has been reported to reverse HRS acutely. A large, recent study reported a good, long-term survival with return of acceptable renal function for prolonged periods after OLTX. Of More than 800 patients undergoing transplantation in Dallas, 59 had HRS. Of the patients surviving liver transplant, four required subsequent renal transplant for nonreturn of function. Of the remaining patients without hepatorenal syndrome (more than 650), two required subsequent kidney transplant. These results and others clearly indicate that patients with HRS have good survival rates following liver transplant action, although the rates are statistically inferior compared with patients without HRS. With aggressive pre- and posttransplant management, one can anticipate excellent results following OLTX in patients with HRS.

Acknowledgments

Portions of this chapter have been adapted from two earlier reviews by the author: Epstein M: "Renal sodium handling in liver disease" and "The hepatorenal syndrome". Both are in Epstein M (ed) *The Kidney in Liver Disease,* 4th ed., Hanley & Belfus, Philadelphia, 1996.

Bibliography

Epstein M: The LeVeen shunt for ascites and hepatorenal syndrome. *N Engl J Med* 302:628–630, 1980.

Epstein M: Derangements of renal water handling in liver disease. *Gastroenterology* 89:1415–1425, 1989.

Epstein M: Atrial natriuretic factor in patients with liver disease. *Am J Nephrol* 9:89–100, 1989.

Epstein M: Renal effects of head-out water immersion in humans: A 15-year update. *Physiol Rev* 72:563–621, 1992.

Epstein M, Berk DP, Hollenberg NK, et al.: Renal failure in the patient with cirrhosis: the role of active vasoconstriction. *Am J Med* 49:175–185, 1970.

Epstein M: Hepatorenal syndrome. In: Epstein M (ed.) *The Kidney in Liver Disease.* 4th ed. Hanley & Belfus, pp. 75–108, 1996.

Epstein M. Renal sodium handling in liver disease. In: Epstein M (ed.) *The Kidney in Liver Disease.* 4th ed. Hanley & Belfus, pp. 3–31, 1996.

Ginés P, Arroyo V, Vargas V, et al.: Paracentesis with intravenous infusion of albumin as compared with peritoneovenous shunting in cirrhosis with refractory ascites. *N Engl J Med* 325:829–835, 1991.

Gonwa TA, Wilkinson AH: Liver transplantation and renal function: Results in patients with and without hepatorenal syndrome. In: Epstein M (ed.) *The Kidney in Liver Disease.* 4th ed. Philadelphia, Hanley & Belfus, pp. 529–542, 1996.

Levy M: Pathophysiology of ascites formation. In: Epstein M (ed.) *The Kidney in Liver Disease.* 4th ed. Philadelphia, Hanley & Belfus, pp. 179–220, 1996.

Linas SL, Schaffer JW, Moore EE, Good JT Jr, Giansiracusa R: Peritoneovenous shunt in the management of the hepatorenal syndrome. *Kidney Int* 30:736–740, 1986.

Perez GO, Epstein M, Oster JR: Dialysis, hemofiltration, and other extracorporeal techniques in the treatment of the renal complications of liver disease. In: Epstein M (ed.) *The Kidney in Liver Disease.* 4th ed. Philadelphia, Hanley & Belfus, pp. 517–528, 1996.

Stanley MM, Ochi S, Lee KK, et al.: Peritoneovenous shunting as compared with medical treatment in patients with alcoholic cirrhosis and massive ascites. *N Engl J Med* 321:1632–1638, 1989.

Vaamonde CA. Renal water handling in liver disease. In: Epstein M (ed.) *The Kidney in Liver Disease.* 4th ed. Philadelphia, Hanley & Belfus, pp. 33–74, 1996.

Somberg KA. Transjugular intrahepatic portosystemic shunt in the treatment of refractory ascites and hepatorenal syndrome. In: Epstein M (ed.) *The Kidney in Liver Disease.* 4th ed. Philadelphia, Hanley & Belfus, pp. 507–516, 1996.

26

POSTSTREPTOCOCCAL AND OTHER INFECTION-RELATED GLOMERULONEPHRITIDES

ASHA MOUDGIL, ARVIND BAGGA, RAGINI FREDRICH, AND STANLEY C. JORDAN

Glomerulonephritis (GN) is characterized by proliferation and inflammation of the glomeruli secondary to immune complex deposition within the glomerular capillary walls and the mesangium. GN may occur as a consequence of infections or autoimmune diseases or may be idiopathic. This chapter focuses on GN resulting from infections. Nephritogenic antigens derived from infectious agents may either bind directly to glomerular sites forming in situ immune complexes with cognate antibody, or circulating immune complexes may become trapped in the glomeruli. Either mechanism initiates inflammation of the glomeruli through complement activation and chemotaxis of polymorphonuclear leukocytes. Immunochemical analysis of immune complexes isolated from affected glomeruli has demonstrated antigenic structures specific for infectious agents.

The onset of clinical symptoms may be acute, with hypertension, edema, gross hematuria, variable degrees of proteinuria, oliguria, and azotemia. Some patients may have an insidious onset of edema, hematuria, proteinuria, and renal insufficiency. Patients presenting with features of acute GN (AGN) often have evidence of a recent infection of the pharynx or skin with group A β-hemolytic streptococci. However, other bacterial, viral, and parasitic agents have also been implicated in the pathogenesis of GN (Table 1). In patients with GN associated with infections other than group A β-hemolytic streptococci, the onset is often insidious and the course protracted. Some of these patients

TABLE I

Infectious Agents Associated with Immune
Complex Glomerulonephritis

Bacterial	Parasitic
Group A β-hemolytic streptococci	*Plasmodium malariae*
Staphylococcus aureus	Toxoplasma
Staphylococcus epidermidis	Filaria
Gram-negative bacilli	Schistosomia
Streptococcus pneumoniae	Trichinella
Treponema pallidum	Trypanosome
Salmonella typhi	Rickettsial
Meningococcus	Scrub typhus
Leptospirosis	Fungal
Viral	*Coccidioides immitis*
Hepatitis B and C	
Cytomegalovirus	
Enteroviruses	
Measles	
Parvovirus	
Oncornavirus	
Mumps virus	
Rubella	
Varicella	

may develop chronic renal failure. In developed countries, GN associated with nonstreptococcal infections is assuming greater importance. This is thought to be secondary to a decline in the incidence of group A streptococcal infections and a relative increase in the incidence of other infection-related glomerulonephritides in alcoholics and intravenous drug abusers.

POSTSTREPTOCOCCAL GLOMERULONEPHRITIS

Poststreptococcal glomerulonephritis (PSGN) is the most common form of GN in children. If follows either pharyngeal or skin infection with group A β-hemolytic streptococci. Streptococcal pharyngitis occurs more commonly during the winter and early spring, whereas impetigo is more common in summer. Only certain serologic types of streptococci, known as "nephritogenic strains," are associated with PSGN. The nephritogenic strains associated with pharyngeal infections include protein M types 1, 3, 4, 6, 12, 25, and 49 and those with skin infections types 2, 49, 55, 57, and 60. Serotype 49 is the most common strain associated with PSGN.

The occurrence of PSGN following infection with a nephritogenic strain is variable and dependent on environmental, host, and genetic factors. The risk of developing AGN is 10 to 15% during epidemics of infection with these strains. Subclinical episodes occur 4 to 10 times more frequently than overt clinical disease. Asymptomatic contacts of patients with PSGN may have abnormal urinary findings, most commonly hematuria.

Clinical Features

Poststreptococcal glomerulonephritis is primarily a disease of children, mostly occurring between 5 and 15 years

of age; it is rare under 2 years and over 40 years. A male preponderance (2:1) is reported. The onset of GN is usually abrupt and preceded by streptococcal pharyngitis or pyoderma by 1 to 4 weeks. This latent period is 7 to 14 days for the postpharyngitic and 14 to 28 days for the postpyoderma forms of GN.

Hematuria and edema are the most common complaints (Table 2). Gross hematuria, classically described as cola-colored, smoky, reddish brown urine, is seen in 70% and microscopic hematuria in virtually all patients. Typically the edema is periorbital and worse in the morning. Weight gain may occur without evidence of edema. The etiology of fluid accumulation is multifactorial; contributing factors include reduction in glomerular filtration rate, sodium and water retention, and, to a lesser degree, proteinuria. Most patients with PSGN have oliguria. Anuria is infrequent and if persistent suggests rapidly progressive GN.

Hypertension is usually mild to moderate and most likely secondary to increased sodium and water retention. The hypertension may be severe enough to cause hypertensive encephalopathy with headache, visual disturbances, altered sensorium, coma, or convulsions. Serious neurologic manifestations have been described even in the absence of severe hypertension. Circulatory congestion secondary to expansion of the extracellular fluid volume is present in the majority of patients and may result in dyspnea, orthopnea, cough, cardiomegaly, gallop rhythm, pleural effusions, and pulmonary edema. In such cases, an incorrect diagnosis of primary cardiovascular disease may be made if examination of the urinary sediment is omitted. Pallor frequently develops in patients with PSGN, secondary to dilutional anemia and edema. Systemic symptoms such as mild fever, nausea, vomiting, and abdominal pain may be present, especially in children.

Patients with PSGN may not have all the clinical features mentioned above. Therefore, the diagnosis of PSGN should be considered in patients with sudden unexplained onset of edema, oliguria, hypertension, or encephalopathy. Subclinical cases may be discovered on examination of the urine sediment during investigation of family contacts of patients with overt disease.

Because there is a latent period between streptococcal pharyngeal infection and the onset of hematuria, PSGN is

TABLE 2

Clinical Manifestations of Acute
Poststreptococcal Glomerulonephritis

Common	Variable
Hematuria	Circulatory congestion
Edema	Encephalopathy
Hypertension	Headache
Oliguria	Somnolence
Uncommon	Convulsions
Anuria and renal failure	Systemic symptoms
	Mild fever
	Nausea
	Abdominal pain
	Pallor

often referred to as "postpharyngitic nephritis." Viral and bacterial upper respiratory infections may trigger inflammation in an already damaged glomerulus resulting in concomitant, or "synpharyngitic hematuria." This is commonly observed with IgA nephropathy, Henoch-Schönlein purpura, familial nephritis, and membranoproliferative GN. Synpharyngitic nephritis can also occasionally be seen with streptococcal infections and represents an exacerbation of an underlying chronic renal disease. In these patients, hematuria abates rapidly, in contrast to PSGN where it may last for more than 1 year.

Laboratory Findings

Urinalysis

Hematuria is present in virtually all patients and may be gross or microscopic. The majority of red blood cells in the urinary sediment are dysmorphic. Red cell casts are present in fresh urine in 60 to 85% of hospitalized patients. Leukocyte casts, tubular epithelial cell casts, and granular casts are common. Proteinuria is often present, usually less than $2 \text{ g} \cdot \text{m}^{-2} \cdot \text{day}^{-1}$; its severity often parallels that of hematuria. In 30% of the patients, proteinuria may be in the nephrotic range. Proteinuria is nonselective and often contains fibrin degradation products.

Blood Chemistry

Serum creatinine levels are usually normal, although blood urea nitrogen may be increased disproportionately. Renal tubular function including the urine concentrating ability is usually preserved. The fractional excretion of sodium is less than 0.5% during the acute phase of the illness. Dilutional hyponatremia and hyperchloremic metabolic acidosis with mild hyperkalemia, consistent with the diagnosis of type IV renal tubular acidosis, may occur. Renal tubular acidosis is considered to occur from suppression of plasma renin activity and aldosterone secretion by an expanded extracellular volume. Serum albumin is often reduced because of dilution and urinary losses of protein.

Cultures for Streptococci

Despite a latent period between the streptococcal infection and PSGN, throat or skin cultures may show group A streptococci. Family contacts of patients may have positive cultures even in the absence of nephritis. Because about 20% of children are asymptomatic carriers of streptococci in the nasopharynx, a positive throat culture cannot be used as the sole criterion to diagnose PSGN.

Serologic Findings

Antibodies against extracellular products of streptococci constitute indirect evidence of recent infection. These antibodies include antistreptolysin O (ASO), antistreptokinase, antihyaluronidase (AH), antideoxyribonuclease B (ADNase B) and antinicotyladenine dinucleotidase (NADase). The ASO titers begin to rise 10 to 14 days after streptococcal pharyngitis, peak at 3 to 4 weeks, and then decrease. Early antibiotic treatment can blunt the rise in titers of these antibodies. The magnitude of ASO titers bears no relation to the development of nephritis or its severity. In streptococcal skin infections, binding of the streptolysin to skin lipids may blunt the immunologic response to this antigen, resulting in a low ASO titer. In these situations, ADNase B and AH are more specific and positive in 90% of the cases. Antibodies against endostreptosin (an antigen derived from nephritogenic streptococci) are usually increased for a prolonged duration in PSGN. The Streptozyme test, a slide agglutination test, detects antibodies against erythrocytes coated with a mixture of streptococcal extracellular antigens (streptolysin O, hyaluronidase, DNase B, streptokinase, and NADase). It has not proved to be a reliable substitute for ASO and ADNase B because of a high rate of false positives and negatives. In 1986, the World Health Organization advised against its use.

Depression of hemolytic complement activity (CH 50) and C3 levels is seen in 90 to 100% of cases of active PSGN. Similar depression of C3 is seen in siblings of patients with PSGN despite absence of hematuria. The early complement components (C1q, C2, C4) may also be mildly reduced, initially. Serum properdin and C5 levels are decreased in 60% of patients, usually in association with reduced C3 levels, suggesting activation of the alternative complement pathway. C3 nephritic factor activity may be detected initially but becomes undetectable with normalization of C3 levels. There is no correlation between the depression of C3 level and severity of nephritis. C3 levels return to normal within 6 to 8 weeks after the onset of disease in more than 90% of patients. Persistently low C3 levels suggest underlying membranoproliferative GN, lupus nephritis, or GN related to endocarditis or occult visceral abscess.

Circulating cryoglobulins and immune complexes may be found in most patients in the first few weeks of the illness. High-molecular-weight fibrinogen complexes are present in severe cases. Circulating antibodies to basement membrane constituents (type IV collagen and laminin) may also be found.

Hematology

The normocytic normochromic anemia is usually dilutional rather than secondary to hematuria or hemolysis. Shortened erythrocyte survival, secondary to rapid elimination of red cells coated with immune complexes, has also been described. Thrombocytopenia is rarely reported. Fibrinogen, factor VIII, and plasmin are elevated acutely and are thought to correlate with disease activity.

Indications for Renal Biopsy

Renal biopsy is rarely indicated in PSGN, but should be considered in patients with: (1) atypical presentation such as prolonged oliguria, anuria, severe proteinuria, marked azotemia, and no serologic evidence of preceding streptococcal infection; (2) significant hypertension and macroscopic hematuria for 2 to 3 weeks or persistent proteinuria with or without hematuria lasting more than 6 months; and (3) persistently low C3 levels. Renal biopsy is done to assess prognosis or detect the presence of other underlying glomerular diseases such as systemic lupus erythematosus, antineutrophil cytoplasmic autoantibody associated vasculitis, or membranoproliferative GN.

Pathology

As indicated above, renal biopsy is generally not required for the diagnosis of PSGN. Information on pathology has been derived from patients with severe nephritis or from autopsy material. Primary acute abnormalities include a generalized and diffuse endocapillary and mesangial cell proliferation accompanied by infiltration with polymorphonuclear leukocytes, monocytes, and eosinophils within the capillary lumina and mesangium. The glomeruli may enlarge and show lobular accentuation of the tufts (Fig. 1). Epithelial cells are rarely involved in the proliferative process; significant crescent formation is limited to patients with severe disease. Crescents in 50% or more glomeruli suggests a guarded prognosis for complete recovery. In cases biopsied after clinical resolution, the hypercellularity subsides beginning with disappearance of the neutrophils, and the capillary lumina become patent. However, glomeruli may retain some abnormal morphological features and diffuse or segmental mesangial proliferation may persist for prolonged periods.

On electron microscopy, the presence of discrete electron-dense, dome-shaped subepithelial deposits is characteristic (Fig. 2). These "humps" are present early in the clinical course and diminish after 4 to 6 weeks. Small mesangial and subendothelial deposits also are usually present. Incomplete clinical resolution may occur when they are present in large numbers and in contiguous areas. Immunofluorescence examination shows deposition of IgG and C3 in a granular pattern along the glomerular basement membrane and in the mesangium. Most deposits disappear after a few weeks, but mesangial deposits may persist for prolonged periods.

Pathogenesis

Poststreptococcal glomerulonephritis is an immune complex disease. However, the precise nature of the antigens involved in the formation of nephritogenic immune complexes is unknown. Soluble streptococcal antigenic products in the glomeruli have been detected inconsistently.

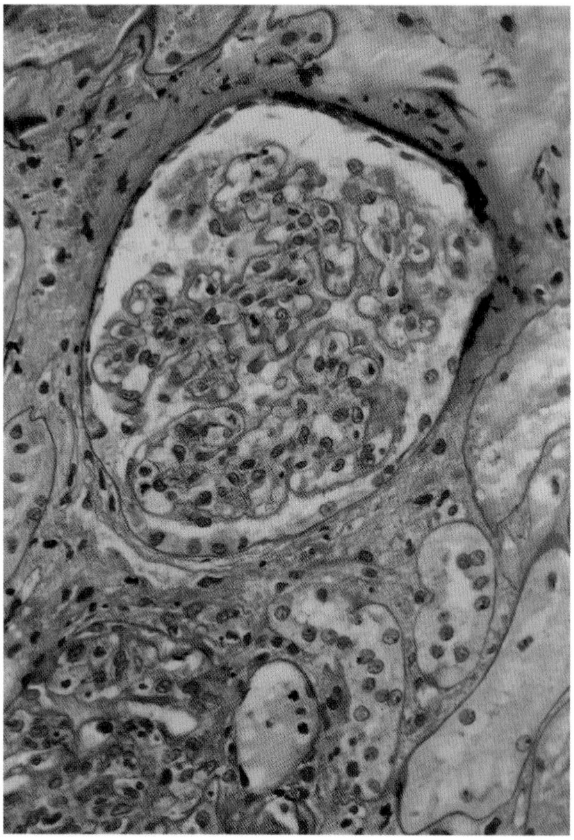

FIGURE 1 Light microscopy of acute poststreptococcal glomerulonephritis showing a hypercellular glomerulus with polymorphonuclear leukocytes within the capillary lumen. Part of the second glomerulus in the figure shows increased endocapillary proliferation with narrowing of the lumen (hematoxylin–eosin). Courtesy of Dr. A. H. Cohen.

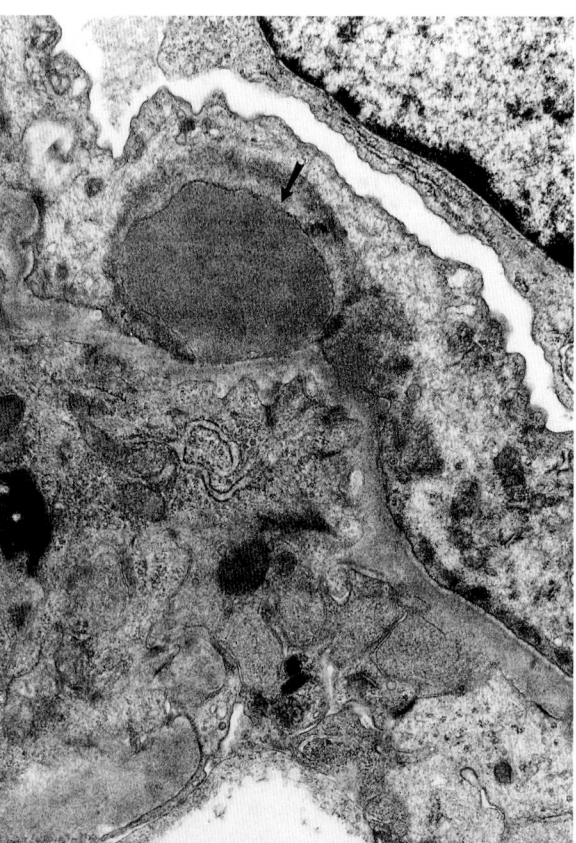

FIGURE 2 Electron micrograph of a glomerular capillary from a patient with acute poststreptococcal glomerulonephritis showing a large dome-shaped subepithelial electron-dense deposit (arrow). Effacement of foot processes is present. Courtesy of Dr. A. H. Cohen.

The reasons for this inconsistency include possible denaturization of antigenic material in the glomeruli and saturation of antigen with specific antibody, therefore blocking recognition by immunochemical probes. Endostreptosin has been identified in the mesangium, but not in the "humps" that are characteristic of the disease.

IgG, C3, and streptococcal extracellular antigens have been detected in circulating immune complexes of patients with PSGN. However, similar complexes are also found in patients with impetigo without nephritis. Since streptococcal antigens are not always nephritogenic, other mechanisms may be involved. It has been suggested that these antigens may induce alterations of autologous IgG or glomerular components rendering them immunogenic or cross-reactive with normal glomerular constituents. Another possible mechanism is that endostreptosin, or other cationic cytoplasmic antigens, may bind to glomerular structures and serve as "fixed" or "planted" antigen for development of in situ immune complexes. Glomerular immune complex deposition may then result in complement activation, activation of kinin or coagulation cascades, release of polymorphonuclear chemotactic factors, and acute glomerular injury.

Prevention and Treatment

A long-term protective immunity against nephritogenic streptococci cannot be achieved with active immunization and complete eradication of the organism in the population is also not feasible. Early antimicrobial therapy of affected persons and immediate family members may prevent the spread of streptococcal infections but does not prevent the development of PSGN. It may, however, attenuate the severity of clinical disease. Widespread use of antimicrobials and better hygiene has greatly reduced the incidence of PSGN in developed countries.

Treatment of patients with acute PSGN is symptomatic. Fluid and sodium restriction and judicious use of loop diuretics are useful in patients with circulatory congestion, hypertension, and edema. Severe hypertension with or without encephalopathy is an emergency and usually responds to treatment with nifedipine and furosemide. Calcium channel blockers and loop diuretics may also be used for treatment of moderate hypertension. Because plasma renin activity is reduced in these patients, angiotensin-converting enzyme inhibitors and β-blockers could be predicted to be less useful. Despite this, captopril has been shown to lower blood pressure and increase creatinine clearance in these patients.

Bed rest has no beneficial effect but has been traditionally recommended for treatment of severe hypertension, hematuria, and marked edema. Restriction of protein may be necessary in the presence of marked azotemia. Hyperkalemia may be treated with ion exchange resins. Occasionally dialysis may be necessary. Antibiotic therapy has no influence on the course of the disease; however, appropriate therapy should be instituted for patients with positive cultures for group A β-hemolytic streptococci. Since subsequent encounters with nephritogenic strains of group A β-hemolytic streptococci are unlikely, penicillin prophylaxis is not recommended.

Course and Prognosis

The acute clinical episode of PSGN is usually self-limited and most patients will undergo diuresis within 7 to 10 days of onset of the illness. Hypertension and azotemia subside within 1 to 2 weeks. Hematuria and proteinuria disappear by 6 months in more than 90% of children. Microscopic hematuria may persist for 1 to 2 years. In adults, proteinuria may be present in 60% for more than 1 year and in 30% for 2 or more years.

Follow-up of pediatric patients with PSGN has revealed a paucity of chronic sequelae. In the majority of patients, with no evidence of preexisting renal disease, heavy proteinuria or extensive crescentic glomerular lesions at the onset, the prognosis is excellent. However, in children with disease severe enough to require hospitalization, the outcome may not always be benign. Most investigators believe that the severity of disease at the onset correlates with the development of chronicity and chronic glomerulonephritis does not evolve from mild or unrecognized PSGN.

In contrast to children, the prognosis in adults is less favorable. Long-term studies of patients with PSGN have reported progression to endstage renal failure in some instances. Data from Trinidad and South Australia, however, have indicated that recovery is the rule even though complete histological and clinical healing may take as long as 9 years. The long-term prognosis of PSGN occurring in association with epidemics appear to be more favorable than those occurring sporadically. This may represent selection bias.

Since immunity to streptococcal M-protein is type specific and long lasting and nephritogenic serotypes are limited in number, recurrent episodes of PSGN are rare.

GLOMERULONEPHRITIS ASSOCIATED WITH INFECTIONS OTHER THAN GROUP A β-HEMOLYTIC STREPTOCOCCI

GN Associated with Sepsis, Bacterial Endocarditis, and Visceral Abscesses

GN may be seen in association with a variety of infections other than group A β-hemolytic streptococci (Table 1). It may also occasionally occur with group D streptococci, gonococci, and gram-negative rods. The incidence of GN due to staphylococcal and gram-negative infections has increased in the past two or three decades, particularly in immunocompromised adults, alcoholics, intravenous drug abusers, and the elderly. Some of these patients develop bacterial endocarditis and visceral abscesses. The clinical features in these patients may be indistinguishable from PSGN; occasionally, however, the onset may be insidious and the course protracted. GN is of varying severity and may show focal or diffuse endocapillary proliferation with or without crescents. The total complement and C3 levels are usually decreased. Cryoglobulins and circulating immune complexes are frequently detected. It is important to distinguish these patients from PSGN patients because appropriate antibiotic therapy leads to resolution of symptoms. Valve replacement surgery may be indicated in patients with bacterial endocarditis and persistent infection despite proper antimicrobial treatment. Surgery may also be required to drain a valve ring abscess. Delay in institution of proper treatment may lead to increased patient mortality and or incomplete renal recovery leading to chronic renal failure.

Shunt Nephritis

GN associated with a chronically infected shunts used for relieving hydrocephalus and infected vascular grafts or venous catheters is known as shunt nephritis. *Stapylococcus epidermidis,* an organism found on normal skin, is the most common infecting organism and may be cultured either from the blood or from the shunt. Other organisms implicated include *Staphylococcus aureus* and gram-negative bacteria. Clinical features are usually indolent and include fever, arthralgias, lethargy, weight loss, pallor, purpuric rash, lymphadenopathy, and hepatosplenomegaly. Patients may have microscopic hematuria, proteinuria, and impaired renal function. Gross hematuria, hypertension, and nephrotic syndrome are uncommon. Serum complement levels are usually low. Serum concentrations of factor B and properdin are only occasionally decreased, indicating predominant activation of the classical complement pathway. Rheumatoid factor, circulating immune complexes, and cryoglobulins are frequently present in the serum. Renal histology generally shows features of membranoproliferative GN and sometimes of focal proliferative GN. Renal biopsy is not usually indicated. Most patients recover with removal of shunts and antibiotic therapy. Some patients may be left with residual renal impairment.

Glomerulonephritis Associated with Syphilis

Renal involvement is known to occur in congenital and, rarely, acquired syphilis. Patients generally present with nephrotic syndrome, but may occasionally show features of AGN. The renal disease is usually associated with other manifestations of congenital syphilis, including hepatosplenomegaly, skin rash, and mucosal involvement. The diagnosis is confirmed by positive serologic test results for syphilis. Complement levels of C1q, C4, C3, and C5 are decreased in congenital syphilis and return to normal following treatment with penicillin. The serum levels of complement are usually normal in acquired syphilis. Membranous nephropathy or diffuse proliferative GN may be seen on renal biopsy. Renal disease is thought to be secondary to an immunologically mediated reaction to treponemal antigens. Treatment of both congenital and acquired syphilis results in rapid improvement of renal manifestations.

Glomerulonephritis Associated with Hepatitis B and C

Hepatitis B infection is associated with glomerular disease, (usually a membranous nephropathy), membrano-

proliferative GN, mesangial proliferative GN, and vasculitic involvement of the kidney may also occur. The patients generally present with nephrotic syndrome, but may also present with AGN. These patients have circulating HBsAg, and a high proportion also show HBe antigenemia. Serum C3 and C4 levels are usually decreased, and cryoglobulins and circulating immune complexes are often detected. HBV particles may be seen in the glomerular capillary wall on electron microscopy, and HBsAg and HBeAg have been detected in the glomerular capillaries by immunofluorescence.

Hepatitis C virus infection is also associated with the development of GN. The spectrum of glomerular lesions found in association with hepatitis C infection is similar to that seen in hepatitis B. Hepatitis C infection is more commonly associated with proliferative GN, whereas hepatitis B infection is more common in membranous nephropathy. Figure 3 shows light microscopy of a patient with hepatitis C related GN illustrating mesangial proliferation in some capillary loops whereas others are unaffected. It also shows thickening of glomerular basement membrane in some capillaries. Patients may develop hematuria, proteinuria, or nephrotic syndrome. The pathogenesis of GN is thought to be similiar to that associated with hepatitis B.

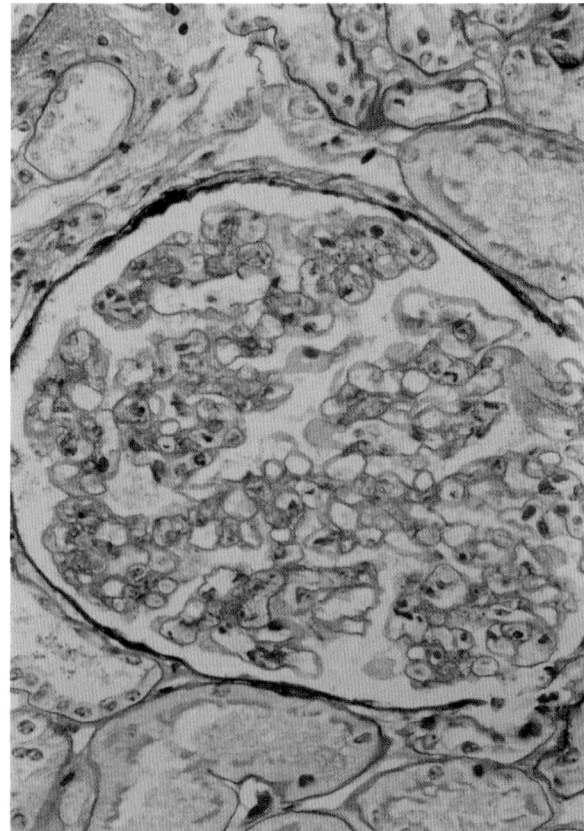

FIGURE 3 Light microscopic histology of hepatitis C related glomerulonephritis showing focal mesangial proliferation and thickening of the capillary wall (periodic acid–Schiff). Courtesy of Dr. A. H. Cohen.

Hepatitis C particles have, however, not been conclusively demonstrated in the glomerular capillaries, but have been identified in cryoglobulins and immune complexes.

Immunosupressive therapy is not indicated in the treatment of hepatitis B or hepatitis C associated GN since it impairs the host's ability to clear these viruses from the circulation and may actually stimulate viral replication. Some patients, particularly those with hepatitis B associated GN, may go into spontaneous remission. Antiviral therapy with interferon-α may be useful, but relapses are common (see Chapter 19)

Other Infections Reported in Association with GN

GN secondary to typhoid fever, brucellosis, leptospirosis, cytomegalovirus, measles, mumps, and infectious mononucleosis has also been described. The nephritis seen with these organisms is usually mild and often presents with hematuria and proteinuria. The absence of bacteriological and serological evidence of a prior streptococcal illness and the temporal association with these infections suggest the diagnosis of infectious GN of nonstreptococcal origin.

GN Associated with Parvovirus B19 and Hantavirus

Infection with parvovirus B19, in patients with sickle cell disease, has been recently reported to cause focal segmental GN. These patients presented with nephrotic syndrome approximately 1 week after the onset of aplastic crisis. Most of these patients showed progression to chronic renal failure. Focal segmental glomerulosclerosis was seen in one patient who was biopsied late in the course of disease.

Hantavirus infection, originally discovered in Korea, is known to cause hemorrhagic fever with renal involvement. A few cases have been described in the United States and other developed countries. It primarily causes tubulointerstitial nephritis and acute renal failure. Slight glomerular mesangial changes may be seen on renal biopsy in some patients.

With the availabilty of newer and powerful diagnostic tools such as polymerase chain reaction/insitu hybridization to detect infectious agents, the list of viruses and other infectious agents associated with GN will probably continue to grow. These advances will help us to understand more about the pathogenesis of so called "idiopathic GN" and even focal segmental glomerulosclerosis.

Bibliography

Arze RS, Rashid H, Morley R, et al.: Shunt nephritis: report of 2 cases and review of the literature. *Clin Nephrol* 19 (1):48–53, 1983

Baldwin DS, Gluck MC, Schacht RG, et al.: The long term course of poststreptococcal glomerulonephritis. *Ann Intern Med* 80 (3):342–358, 1974.

Beaufils M, Liliane MM, Sraer JD, et al.: Acute renal failure of glomerular origin during visceral abscesses. *N Engl J Med* 295 (4):185–189, 1976.

Centers for disease control and prevention. Update:Hantavirus disase in United States. *MMWR* 42:612–614, 1993.

Conjeevaram HS, Hoofnagle JH, Austin HA, et al.: Long term outcome of hepatitis B virus related glomerulonephritis after therapy with interferon alfa. *Gastroenterology* 109 (2):540–546, 1995.

Dodge WF, Spargo BH, Travis LB, et al.: Poststreptococcal glomerulonephritis: A prospective study in children. *N Engl J Med* 286 (6):273–278, 1972.

Gumber SC, Chopra S: Hepatitis C: A multifaceted disease. Review of extrahepatic manifestations. *Ann Intern Med* 123 (8): 615–620, 1995.

Hruby Z, Kuzniar J, Rabczynski J, et al.: The variety of clinical and histopathologic presentations of glomerulonephritis associated with latent syphilis. *Int Urol Nephrol* 24(5):541–547, 1992.

Montseny JJ, Meyrier A, Kleinknecht D, et al.: The current spectrum of infectious glomerulonephritis. Experience with 76 patients and review of the literature. *Medicine* 74 (2): 63–73, 1995.

Neugarten J, Gallo GR, Baldwin DS: Glomerulonephritis in bacterial endocarditis. *Am J Kidney Dis* 3(5): 371–379, 1984.

Potter EV, Lipschultz SA, Abidh S, et al.: Twelve to seventeen year follow-up of patients with poststreptococcal acute glomerulonephritis in Trinidad. *N Engl J Med* 307 (12):725–729, 1982.

Ronco P, Verroust P, Morel-Maroger L: Viruses and glomerulonephritis. *Nephron* 31 (2):97–102, 1982.

Simckes AM, Spitzer A: Poststreptococcal acute glomerulonephritis. *Pediatr Review* 16 (7): 278–279, 1995.

Seligson G, Lange K, Majeed MA, et al.: Significance of endostreptosin antibody titres in poststreptoccal glomerulonephritis. *Clin Nephrol* 24 (2):69–75, 1985.

Vogl W, Renke M, Mayer-Eichberger D, et al.: Long-term prognosis for endocapillary glomerulonephritis of poststreptococcal type in children and adults. *Nephron* 44 (1):58–65, 1986.

Wierenga KJ, Pattison JR, Brink N, et al.: Glomerulonephritis after human parvovirus infection in homozygous sickle-cell disease. *Lancet* 346 (8973):475–476, 1995.

27

RENAL INVOLVEMENT IN SYSTEMIC VASCULITIS

J. CHARLES JENNETTE AND RONALD J. FALK

The kidneys are affected by many systemic vasculitides (Fig. 1). Large vessel vasculitides, such as giant cell (temporal) arteritis and Takayasu arteritis, can narrow the abdominal aorta or renal arteries, resulting in renal ischemia and renovascular hypertension. Medium-sized vessel vasculitides, such as polyarteritis nodosa and Kawasaki disease, also can reduce flow through the renal artery and may affect intrarenal arteries, resulting in infarction and hemorrhage. Small vessel vasculitides, such as microscopic polyangiitis (microscopic polyarteritis), Wegener's granulomatosis, Henoch-Schönlein purpura, and cryoglobulinemic vasculitis, frequently involve the kidneys, especially glomerular capillaries.

PATHOLOGY

As depicted in Fig. 1 and described in Table 1, different types of systemic vasculitis have a predilection for affecting different vessels within the kidney. In addition, different types of vasculitis have different histologic and immunohistologic features.

Giant cell (temporal) arteritis and Takayasu arteritis have a predilection for the aorta and its major branches, and only rarely cause clinically significant renal disease, although asymptomatic pathologic involvement is more common. Giant cell (temporal) arteritis often involves the extracranial branches of the carotid arteries, including the temporal artery. Some patients, however, do not have temporal artery involvement, and patients with other types of vasculitis (e.g., microscopic polyangiitis and Wegener's granulomatosis) may have temporal artery involvement. Therefore, temporal artery disease is neither a required nor a sufficient pathologic feature of giant cell (temporal) arteritis.

Histologically, both giant cell (temporal) arteritis and Takayasu arteritis are characterized by focal granulomatous inflammation, often with multinucleated giant cells. With chronicity, the inflammatory injury evolves into fibrosis and frequently results in vascular narrowing.

Polyarteritis nodosa and Kawasaki disease have a predilection for medium-sized arteries (i.e., main visceral arteries), such as the mesenteric arteries, hepatic arteries, coronary arteries, and main renal arteries. Polyarteritis nodosa often involves the renal arteries, whereas Kawasaki disease only rarely affects the renal arteries. These diseases also may involve small arteries, such as arteries within the parenchyma of skeletal muscle, liver, heart, pancreas, spleen, and kidney. By the definitions in Table 1, these vasculitides do not affect vessels smaller than arteries (i.e., arterioles, capillaries, venules), and thus do not cause glomerulonephritis. The presence of arteritis and glomerulonephritis indicates some form of small vessel vasculitis, such as microscopic polyangiitis.

Histologically, the acute arterial injury of Kawasaki disease and polyarteritis nodosa is characterized by focal vessel wall fibrinoid necrosis and infiltration of inflammatory cells. Fibrinoid necrosis results from plasma coagulation factors spilling into the necrotic areas, where they are activated to form fibrin. Early in the inflammatory process, neutrophils predominate, but later mononuclear leukocytes are most numerous. Thrombosis may occur at the site of inflammation, resulting in infarction. Focal necrotizing injury to vessels erodes into the vessel wall and adjacent tissue producing an inflammatory aneurysm, which may rupture and cause hemorrhage.

Although small vessel vasculitides may affect medium-sized arteries, they have a predilection for small vessels such as arterioles, postcapillary venules (e.g., in the dermis), and capillaries (e.g., in glomeruli and pulmonary alveoli) (Fig. 1). As described in Table 1, a variety of clinically and pathogenetically distinct forms of small vessel vasculitis have in common focal necrotizing inflammation of small vessels. In the acute phase, this injury is characterized histologically by segmental fibrinoid necrosis and neutrophil infiltration (Fig. 2), sometimes with secondary thrombosis. The neutrophils often undergo karyorrhexis (leukocytoclasia). With chronicity, mononuclear leukocytes become predominant and fibrosis develops.

The distinctive features of each form of vasculitis are described in Table 1 and Fig. 1. For example, Wegener's granulomatosis has necrotizing granulomatous inflammation, Churg-Strauss syndrome has eosinophilia and asthma, Henoch-Schönlein purpura has IgA-dominant vascular immune deposits, cryoglobulinemic vasculitis has cryoglobulins, and microscopic polyangiitis has none of these features.

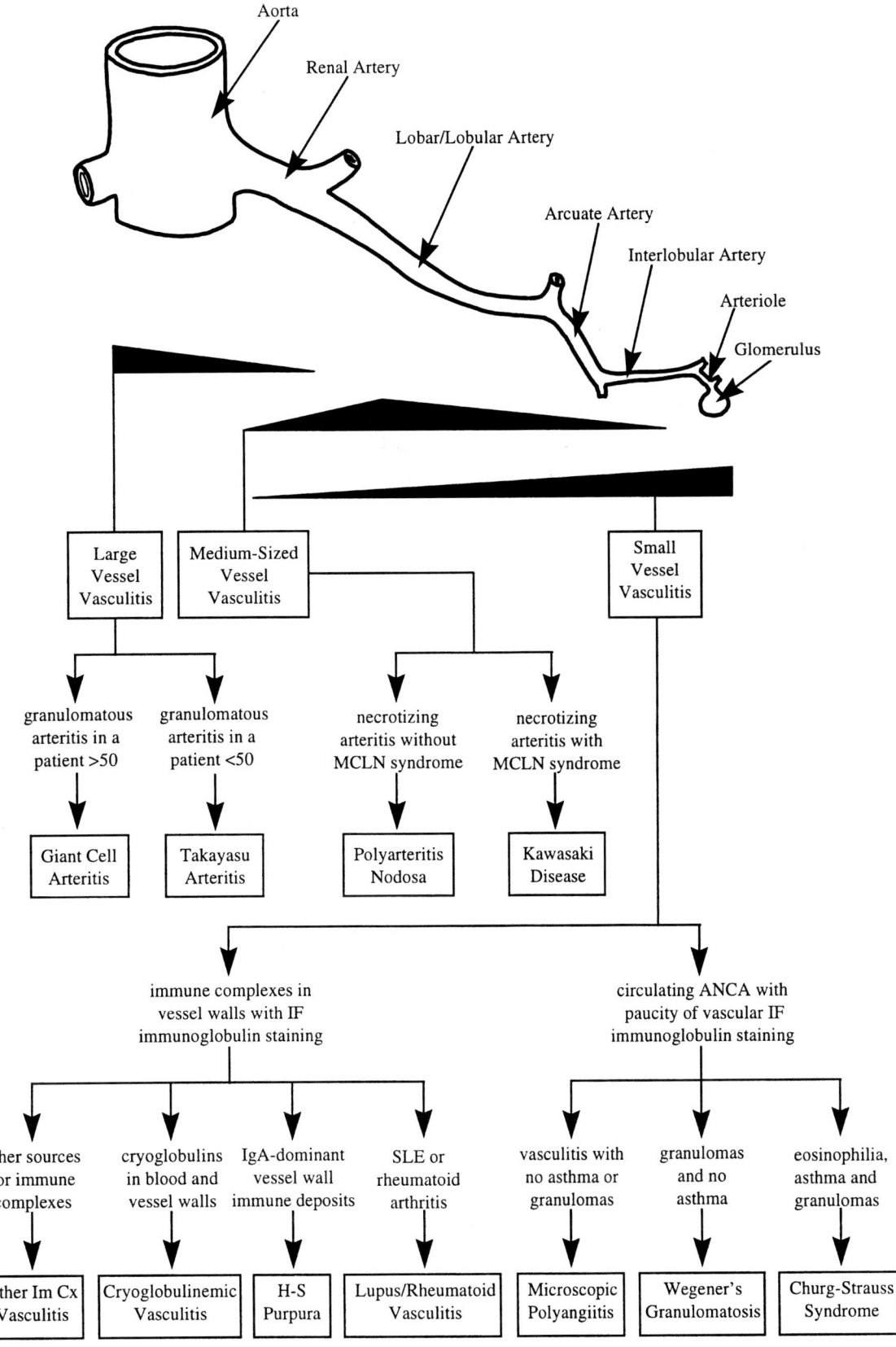

FIGURE I Predominant distribution of renal vascular involvement by systemic vasculitides and diagnostic clinical and pathologic features that distinguish among them. The width of the black triangles indicates the predilection of small, medium, and large vessel vasculitides for various portions of the renal vasculature. Note that medium-sized renal arteries can be affected by large, medium, and small vessel vasculitides, but arterioles and glomeruli are affected by small vessel vasculitides alone based on the definitions in Table 1. MCLN; mucocutaneous lymph node syndrome.

TABLE I

Names and Definitions of Vasculitis Adopted by the Chapel Hill Consensus Conference on the Nomenclature of
Systemic Vasculitis

Large vessels vasculitis[a]	
Giant cell (temporal) arteritis	Granulomatous arteritis of the aorta and its major branches, with a predilection for the extracranial branches of the carotid artery. Often involves the temporal artery. Usually occurs in patients older than 50 and often is associated with polymyalgia rheumatica.
Takayasu arteritis	Granulomatous inflammation of the aorta and its major branches. Usually occurs in patients younger than 50.
Medium-sized vessel vasculitis[a]	
Polyarteritis nodosa (classic polyarteritis nodosa)	Necrotizing inflammation of medium-sized or small arteries without glomerulonephritis or vasculitis in arterioles, capillaries, or venules.
Kawasaki disease	Arteritis involving large, medium-sized, and small arteries, and associated with mucocutaneous lymph node syndrome. Coronary arteries are often involved. Aorta and veins may be involved. Usually occurs in children.
Small vessel vasculitis[a]	
Wegener's granulomatosis[b,c]	Granulomatous inflammation involving the respiratory tract, and necrotizing vasculitis affecting small to medium-sized vessels, e.g., capillaries, venules, arterioles, and arteries. Necrotizing glomerulonephritis is common.
Churg-Strauss syndrome[b,c]	Eosinophil-rich and granulomatous inflammation involving the respiratory tract and necrotizing vasculitis affecting small to medium-sized vessels, and is associated with asthma and blood eosinophilia
Microscopic polyangiitis (microscopic polyarteritis)[b,c]	Necrotizing vasculitis with few or no immune deposits affecting small vessels, i.e., capillaries, venules, or arterioles. Necrotizing arteritis involving small and medium-sized arteries may be present. Necrotizing glomerulonephritis is very common. Pulmonary capillaritis often occurs.
Henoch-Schonlein purpura[c]	Vasculitis with IgA-dominant immune deposits affecting small vessls, i.e., capillaries, venules, or arterioles. Typically involves skin, gut, and glomeruli, and is associated with arthralgias or arthritis.
Essential cryoglobulinemic vasculitis[c]	Vasculitis with cryoglobulin immune deposits affecting small vessels, i.e., capillaries, venules, or arterioles, and associated with cryoglobulins in serum. Skin and glomeruli are often involved.
Cutaneous leukocytoclastic angiitis	Isolated cutaneous leukocytoclastic angiitis without systemic vasculitis or glomerulonephritis.

Note. Modified from Jennette JC, Falk RJ, Andrassy K, et al.: Nomenclature of systemic vasculitides: the proposal of an international consensus conference. *Arthritis Rheum,* 1994;37:187–192.

[a] Large artery refers to the aorta and the largest branches directed toward major body regions (e.g., to the extremities and the head and neck); medium-sized artery refers to the main visceral arteries (e.g. renal, hepatic, coronary and mesenteric arteries), and small vessel refers to the distal arterial radicals that connect with arterioles (e.g., renal arcuate and interlobular arteries), as well as arterioles, capillaries, and venules. Note that some small and large vessel vasculitides may involve medium-sized arteries; but large and medium-sized vessel vasculitides do not involve vessels smaller than (other than) arteries.

[b] Strongly associated with antineutrophil cytoplasmic autoantibodies (ANCA).

[c] May be accompanied by glomerulonephritis and can manifest as nephritis or pulmonary-renal vasculitic syndrome.

The glomerular lesions of microscopic polyangiitis, Wegener's granulomatosis, and Churg-Strauss syndrome (i.e., the ANCA vasculitides) are identical pathologically and are characterized by segmental fibrinoid necrosis and crescent formation (Fig. 3). The glomerulonephritis of Henoch-Schonlein purpura is identical to IgA nephropathy. The glomerulonephritis of cryoglobulinemic vasculitis is a secondary form of type I membranoproliferative glomerulonephritis (mesangiocapillary glomerulonephritis).

Leukocytoclastic angiitis of medullary vasa recta (Fig. 4) also occurs in the ANCA-vasculitides, and rarely may be severe enough to cause papillary necrosis.

PATHOGENESIS

Vasculitides are caused by the activation of inflammatory mediator systems in vessel walls. The initiating event (i.e., the etiology), however, is unknown for most vasculitides. An immune response to heterologus antigens (e.g., hepatitis B or C antigens in some forms of immune complex vasculitis) or autoantigens (e.g., endothelial antigens in Kawasaki disease) is presumed to be the etiologic event in many vasculitides, but this can be documented in only a few patients. Table 2 categorizes vasculitides based on putative immunologic mechanisms.

Except for cellular vascular rejection in transplanted organs, there is no well-documented example of T-cell-

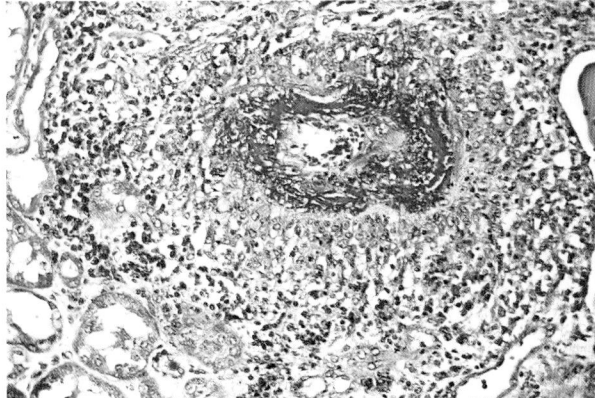

FIGURE 2   Renal interlobular artery with fibrinoid necrosis from a patient with microscopic polyangiitis (Masson trichrome stain).

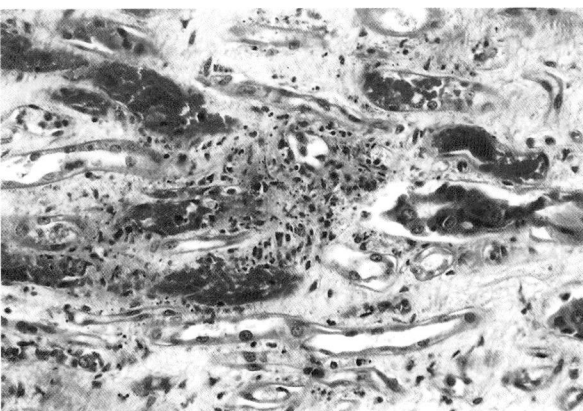

FIGURE 4   Medullary vasa recta with leukocytoclastic angiitis from a patient with Wegener's granulomatosis (hematoxylin and eosin).

mediated vasculitis. Primarily because of the pattern of inflammation, cell-mediated inflammation has been incriminated in the pathogenesis of giant cell (temporal) arteritis and Takayasu arteritis, but there is no strong experimental support for this.

The vasculitides listed in the immune complex mediated category in Table 2 all immunohistologic evidence for vessel wall immune complex localization, i.e., granular staining for immunoglobulins and complement. In these vasculitides, the presence of antibodies bound to antigens in vessel walls activates humoral inflammatory mediator systems (e.g., complement, coagulation, fibrinolytic and kinin systems), which attract and activate neutrophils and monocytes. These activated leukocytes releaser generate toxic oxygen metabolites and release enzymes that cause matrix lysis and cellular apoptosis, resulting in necrotizing inflammatory injury to vessel walls.

This same final pathway of inflammatory injury also can be reached by antibodies binding to antigens that are inte-

gral components of vessel walls. The best documented example of this is anti-GBM antibody mediated glomerulonephritis and Goodpasture's syndrome. A less well-documented example of direct antibody attack is Kawasaki disease. There is evidence that patients with Kawasaki disease have antiendothelial antibodies that react with antigens that are expressed on the surface of stimulated endothelial cells.

A very important group of necrotizing systemic small vessel vasculitides, which frequently involve the kidneys, has no immunohistologic evidence for vascular immune

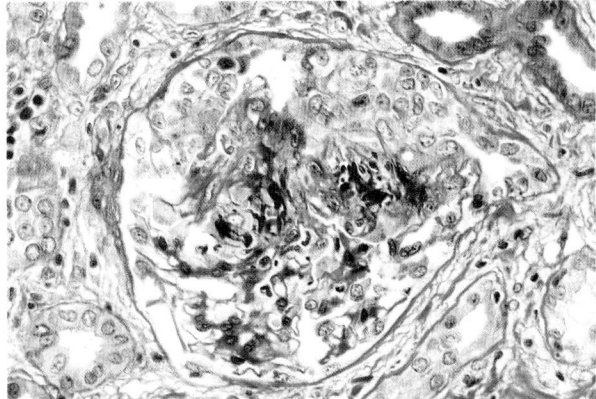

FIGURE 3   Glomerulus with segmental fibrinoid necrosis with red (fuchsinophilic) fibrinous material and an adjacent cellular crescent from a patient with ANCA-small vessel vasculitis (Masson trichrome stain).

TABLE 2

Putative Immunologic Causes of Vasculitis

Immune complex mediated
   Henoch-Schonlein purpura[a]
   Cryoglobulinemic vasculitis[a]
   Lupus vasculitis[a]
   Serum sickness vasculitis[a]
   Rheumatoid vasculitis
   Polyarteritis nodosa
   Infection-induced immune complex vasculitis[a]
      Viral (e.g., hepatitis B and C virus)
      Bacterial (e.g., streptococcal)

Direct antibody attack mediated
   Goodpasture's syndrome (antibasement membrane antibodies)[a]
   Kawasaki disease (antiendothelial antibodies)

ANCA-associated and possibly ANCA-mediated
   Wegener's granulomatosis[a]
   Microscopic polyangiitis[a]
   Churg-Strauss syndrome[a]

Cell mediated
   Allograft cellular vascular rejection
   Giant cell (temporal) arteritis
   Takayasu arteritis

[a] May be accompanied by glomerulonephritis and can manifest as nephritis or pulmonary-renal vasculitic syndrome.

complex localization or direct antibody binding. This paucity of immune deposits has fostered the designation pauci-immune for this group of vasculitides, which includes microscopic polyangiitis (microscopic polyarteritis), Wegener's granulomatosis, and Churg-Strauss syndrome. The pathogenesis of these vasculitides is unknown, but their close association with antineutrophil cytoplasmic autoantibodies (ANCA) has lead to speculation that they result from ANCA-induced leukocyte activation and vascular injury.

ANCA are autoantibodies specific for proteins within the granules of neutrophils and lysosomes of monocytes. They often are detected in patient serum by indirect immunofluorescence microscopy using alcohol-fixed normal human neutrophils as substrate. Using this assay, two patterns of neutrophil staining discriminate between the two major subtypes of ANCA: cytoplasmic staining (C-ANCA) and perinuclear staining (P-ANCA). Using specific immunochemical assays, such as enzyme-linked immunosorbent assays or radioimmunoassays, most C-ANCA are specific for a neutrophil and monocyte proteinase called proteinase 3 (PR3) and most P-ANCA are specific for myeloperoxidase (MPO).

One hypothesis about the pathogenesis of ANCA-associated vasculitides proposes that ANCA react with cytoplasmic antigens (e.g., PR3 and MPO) that are released at the surface of cytokine-stimulated leukocytes, causing the leukocytes to adhere to vessel walls, degranulate, and generate toxic oxygen metabolites. ANCA antigens also may become planted in vessel walls or even produced by endothelial cells, thus providing a nidus for in situ immune complex formation in vessel walls. If such in situ formation is present, it must be at a level that cannot be detected by immunofluorescence microscopy, because of the pauciimmune character of ANCA vasculitis.

CLINICAL FEATURES

The clinical features of systemic vasculitides are extremely varied and are dictated by the category of vasculitis, the type of vessel involved, and the organ system distribution of vascular injury. Irrespective of the type of vasculitis, most patients will have accompanying constitutional features of inflammatory disease, such as fever, arthralgias, myalgias, and weight loss. These are probably caused by increased circulating levels of proinflammatory cytokines.

Giant cell (temporal) arteritis and Takayasu arteritis typically present with evidence for ischemia in tissues supplied by involved arteries. Patients with Takayasu arteritis often develop claudication (especially in the upper extremities), absent pulses, and bruits. Approximately 40% of patients with Takayasu arteritis develop renovascular hypertension, but this is rare with giant cell arteritis.

Giant cell (temporal) arteritis can affect virtually any organ in the body, but signs and symptoms of involvement of arteries in the head and neck are the most common clinical manifestations. Superficial arteries (e.g., the tempo-

ral artery) may be swollen and tender. Arterial narrowing causes ischemic manifestations in affected tissues, such as headache, jaw claudication, and loss of vision. About half of the patients with giant cell (temporal) arteritis have polymyalgia rheumatica, which is characterized by aching and stiffness in the neck, shoulder girdle, or pelvic girdle.

Medium-sized vessel vasculitides (i.e., polyarteritis nodosa and Kawasaki disease) often present with clinical evidence for infarction in multiple organs, such as abdominal pain with occult blood in the stool and skeletal muscle pain and cardiac pain with elevated serum muscle enzymes. Laboratory evaluation often demonstrates clinically silent organ damage, such as liver injury with elevated liver function tests and pancreatic injury with elevated serum amylase.

Polyarteritis nodosa frequently causes multiple renal infarcts and aneurysms. Unlike microscopic polyangiitis, polyarteritis nodosa usually does not cause severe renal failure. Rupture of arterial aneurysms with massive retroperitoneal or intraperitoneal hemorrhage is a life-threatening complication of polyarteritis nodosa.

Kawasaki disease almost always occurs in young children and has a predilection for coronary, axillary, and iliac arteries. Kawasaki disease is accompanied by the mucocutaneous lymph node syndrome, which includes fever, nonpurulent lymphadenopathy, and mucosal and cutaneous inflammation. Although the renal arteries frequently are involved histologically, clinically significant renal disease is very rare in patients with Kawasaki disease.

The small vessel vasculitides often present with evidence for inflammation in vessels in multiple organs, but may initially manifest with involvement of only one organ, followed by development of disease in other organs. Hematuria, proteinuria, and renal insufficiency caused by glomerulonephritis are frequent clinical features of all of the small vessel vasculitides listed in Table 1. Other manifestations include purpura caused by leukocytoclastic angiitis in dermal venules and arterioles, abdominal pain and occult blood in the stool from mucosal and bowel wall infarcts, mononeuritis multiplex from arteriolitis and arteritis in peripheral nerves, necrotizing sinusitis from upper respiratory tract mucosal angiitis, and pulmonary hemorrhage from necrotizing alveolar capillaritis.

In addition to the features just described, which are common to patients with all types of small vessel vasculitis, patients with Wegener's granulomatosis and Churg-Strauss syndrome have distinctive clinical features that set them apart. Patients with Wegener's granulomatosis have necrotizing granulomatous inflammation in the upper or lower respiratory tract, and rarely in other tissues (e.g., skin, orbit). In the lungs, this inflammation produces irregular nodular lesions that can be observed by radiography. These lesions may cavitate and hemorrhage, but massive pulmonary hemorrhage in patients with Wegener's granulomatosis is usually caused by capillaritis rather than granulomatous inflammation. By definition, patients with Churg-Strauss syndrome have blood eosinophilia and a history of asthma. They also develop eosinophil-rich tissue inflammation, especially in the lungs and gut.

DIAGNOSIS

Multisystem disease in a patient with constitutional signs and symptoms of inflammation, such as fever, arthralgias, myalgias, and weight loss, should raise suspicion of systemic vasculitis. Data that will resolving the differential diagnosis include the patient's age, organ distribution of injury, concurrent syndromes (e.g., mucocutaneous lymph node syndrome, polymyalgia rheumatica, asthma), type of vessel involved (e.g., artery, arteriole, venules capillary), lesion histology (e.g., granulomatous, necrotizing), lesion immunohistology (e.g., immune deposits, pauciimune), and laboratory data (e.g., cryoglobulins, ANCA) (Fig. 1).

Signs and symptoms of tissue ischemia along with angiography demonstrating irregularity, stenosis, occlusion, or, less commonly, aneurysms of large and medium-sized arteries should suggest giant cell (temporal) arteritis or Takayasu arteritis. A useful discriminator between giant cell arteritis and Takayasu arteritis is age, with the former rarely occurring before 50 years of age and the latter rarely occurring after 50. The presence of polymyalgia rheumatica is a clinical marker for giant cell arteritis.

Polyarteritis nodosa and Kawasaki disease cause organ ischemia and have a preference for internal viscera, such as the heart, kidneys, liver, spleen, and gut. Arteritis in skeletal muscle and subcutaneous tissues causes tender nodules that can be identified on physical examination. Medium-sized artery aneurysms observed angiographically (e.g., in renal arteries) indicate some type of vasculitis, but this is not very disease-specific because giant cell (temporal) arteritis, Takayasu arteritis, polyarteritis nodosa, Kawasaki disease, Wegener's granulomatosis, microscopic polyarteritis, and Churg-Strauss syndrome can all produce them. Kawasaki disease occurs almost always in children under 5 years old and is accompanied by the mucocutaneous lymph node syndrome.

A small vessel vasculitis should be suspected when there is evidence for inflammation of vessels smaller than arteries, such as glomerular capillaries (hematuria and proteinuria), dermal postcapillary venules (purpura), and alveolar capillaries (hemoptysis). To discriminate among the small vessel vasculitides, evaluation of serology data, vessel immunohistology, or concurrent nonvasculitic disease (e.g., asthma, eosinophilia) is required (Fig. 1).

Evaluation of vessels in biopsy specimens, such as glomerular capillaries in renal biopsies or alveolar capillaries in a lung biopsies, can be helpful, especially if immunohistology is performed. The pauciimmune vasculitides (i.e., microscopic polyangiitis, Wegener's granulomatosis, Churg-Strauss syndrome) will lack immune deposits, anti-GBM disease will have linear immunoglobulin deposits, and the immune complex vasculitides will have granular immune deposits.

Serology, especially, ANCA analysis is useful in differentiating among the small vessel vasculitides. Wegener's granulomatosis, microscopic polyangiitis (microscopic polyarteritis), and Churg-Strauss syndrome are strongly associated with ANCA. As depicted in Fig. 5, most patients with active untreated Wegener's granulomatosis have C-ANCA (PR3-ANCA). A minority of patients will have P-ANCA (MPO-ANCA). Therefore, C-ANCA are a very sensitive serologic marker for active Wegener's granulomatosis; however, C-ANCA are not completely specific for Wegener's granulomatosis because some patients with C-ANCA will have systemic small vessel vasculitis without granulomatous inflammation (i.e., microscopic polyangiitis) and others will have pauciimune necrotizing and crescentic glomerulonephritis alone. Approximately 80% of patients with microscopic polyangiitis have either C-ANCA or P-ANCA, with most having P-ANCA (MPO-ANCA). Patients with Churg-Strauss syndrome usually have either P-ANCA or C-ANCA. A minority of patients with immune-complex-mediated vasculitis or anti-GBM disease will have concurrent ANCA-associated disease.

Diagnostic serologic tests for immune-complex-mediated vasculitides include assays for circulating immune complexes (e.g., cryoglobulins in cryoglobulinemic vasculitis), assays for antibodies known to participate in immune complex formation or to mark the presence of a disease that generates immune complexes (e.g., antibodies to hepatitis B or C, streptococci, DNA), and assays for consumption or activation of humoral inflammatory mediator system components (e.g., assays for reduced complement components or for activated membrane attack complex).

THERAPY AND OUTCOME

All of the vasculitides discussed in this chapter respond to anti-inflammatory or immunosuppressive therapy. The aggressiveness of treatment should match the aggressiveness of the disease.

Takayasu arteritis and giant cell (temporal) arteritis usually respond well to high-dose corticosteroid treatment (e.g., 1 mg/kg body wt per day prednisone) during the acute phase of the disease, followed by tapering and low-dose maintenance for several months to a year depending on disease activity. Occasional patients with severe disease or steroid toxicity benefit from cytotoxic agents (e.g., cyclophosphamide). If present, renovascular hypertension should be controlled. After the inflammatory phase is past and the sclerotic phase has developed, reconstructive vascular surgery may be required to improve flow to ischemic tissues, especially in patients with Takayasu arteritis.

Corticosteroid treatment is not recommended for Kawasaki disease because it appears to worsen coronary artery disease, which is the most life-threatening aspect of Kawasaki disease. The preferred treatment is a combination of aspirin and high-dose intravenous gamma globulins. This controls the inflammatory manifestations of the disease (e.g., the mucocutaneous lymph node syndrome), prevents

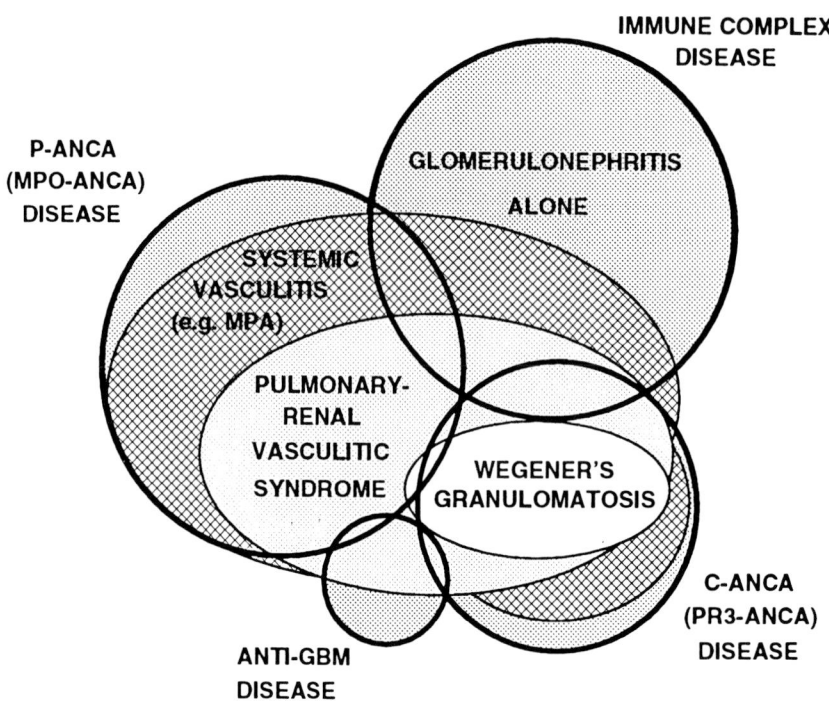

FIGURE 5 Relationship of vasculitic clinicopathologic syndromes to immunopathologic categories of vascular injury in patients with crescentic glomerulonephritis. The circles represent the major immunopathologic categories of vascular inflammation that affect the kidneys, and the shaded ovals the clinicopathologic expressions of the vascular inflammation. Note that clinical syndromes can be caused by multiple immunopathologic processes, e.g., pulmonary-renal vasculitic syndrome can be caused by anti-GBM antibodies (i.e., Goodpasture's syndrome), immune complex localization (e.g., systemic lupus erythematosus), or ANCA-associated disease (e.g., microscopic polyangiitis and Wegener's granulomatosis). Reproduced with permission from Jennette JC: Anti-neutrophil cytoplasmic autoantibody-associated disease: A pathologist's perspective. *Am J Kidney Dis* 1991;18:164–170.

thrombosis of injured arteries, and limits of coronary artery involvement. With appropriate treatment, more than 90% of patients with Kawasaki disease have complete resolution of the disease.

Most patients with Henoch-Schönlein purpura have mild self-limited disease that requires only supportive care. Arthralgias are relieved by nonsteroidal antiinflammatory drugs. Corticosteroid treatment is beneficial in patients who have severe abdominal pain caused by intestinal vasculitis. The treatment of severe glomerulonephritis in patients with Henoch-Schönlein purpura is controversial. There is anecdotal evidence that aggressive crescent glomerulonephritis should be treated with high-dose corticosteroids, cytotoxic agents, and/or plasmapheresis, but this has not been documented in controlled trials (see Chapter 28).

The course and treatment of cryoglobulinemic vasculitis depend in part on the presence of associated diseases. In patients with multiple myeloma or other lymphoproliferative diseases, treatment should be directed at the primary disease. Up to 25% of patients with cryoglobulinemic vasculitis caused by hepatitis C may respond to interferon-α treatment. In patients with severe vascular inflammation,

treatment with corticosteroids, cytotoxic drugs, and plasmapheresis may be required (see Chapter 19).

High-dose corticosteroids (e.g., pulse methylprednisolone) and cytotoxic agents (e.g., cyclophosphamide) are recommended for controlling severe major organ damage caused by microscopic polyangiitis, Wegener's granulomatosis, and Churg-Strauss syndrome. In patients with mild disease, or disease of limited extent (e.g., polyarteritis nodosa confined to the skin or Wegener's granulomatosis limited to the upper respiratory tract), corticosteroids alone may be adequate. Trimethoprim-sulfamethoxazole may be adequate treatment for mild Wegener's granulomatosis of the upper respiratory tract, and perhaps for preventing nasal relapse in patients with Wegener's granulomatosis that is in remission.

Important indicators for aggressive treatment in patients with microscopic polyangiitis and Wegener's granulomatosis are the development of rapidly progressive glomerulonephritis or massive pulmonary hemorrhage. Patients with these complications should be treated with high-dose corticosteroids (e.g., pulse methylprednisolone 7 mg·kg^{-1}·day^{-1} for 3 days followed by daily oral prednisone) and oral or intravenous cyclophosphamide. Oral cyclophosphamide can be initiated at a dose of 2 mg · kg^{-1} · day^{-1}, or intravenous cyclophosphamide can be begun at 0.5 g · m^{-2} · month^{-1} adjusted upward to 1 g/m^2 based on the leukocyte count. The optimum duration of cyclophosphamide treatment is controversial. One approach is to stop treatment when there is disease remission, or after 6 months. Plasmapheresis and high-dose intravenous gamma globulin also may be beneficial, but this is not well documented.

As many as 80% of ANCA vasculitis patients will enter remission with aggressive immunosuppression, but approximately a third will have a relapse within 2 years. There is controversy over how best to treat relapses. A frequent approach is to re-treat overt vasculitic relapses with a repeat course of corticosteroids and cyclophosphamide.

Bibliography

Agnello V, Chung RT, Kaplan LM: A role for hepatitis C virus infection in type II cryoglobulinemia *N Engl J Med* 327:1490–1495, 1992.

Churg J, Churg A. Idiopathic and secondary vasculitis: A review. *Mod Pathol* 2:144–60, 1989.

DeRemee RA, McDonald TJ, Harrison EG, et al.: Wegener's granulomatosis. Anatomic correlates, a proposed classification. *Mayo Clin Proc* 51:777–781, 1976.

Falk RJ, Hogan S, Carey TS, Jennette JC: Clinical course of antineutrophil cytoplasmic autoantibody-associated glomerulonephritis and systemic vasculitis: the Glomerular Disease Collaborative Network. *Ann Intern Med* 113:656–663, 1990.

Hagen EC, Ballieux BE, van Es LA, Daha MR, van der Woude FJ: Antineutrophil cytoplasmic autoantibodies: A review of the antigens involved, the assays, and the clinical and possible pathogenetic consequences. *Blood* 81:1996–2002, 1993.

Hoffman GS, Kerr GS, Leavitt RY, et al.: Wegener's granulomatosis: An analysis of 158 patients. *Ann Intern Med* 116:488–498, 1992.

Hunder GG, Arend WP, Bloch DA, C et al.: The American College of Rheumatology 1990 criteria for the classification of vasculitis. *Arthritis Rheum* 3:1065–1067, 1990.

Jennette JC, Falk RJ: The pathology of vasculitis involving the kidney. *Am J Kidney Dis* 24:130–141, 1994.

Jennette JC, Falk RJ, Andrassy K, et al.: Nomenclature of systemic vasculitides: proposal of an international consensus conference. *Arthritis Rheum* 37:187–192, 1994.

Leung DYM, Collins T, Lapierre LA, et al.: Immunoglobulin M antibodies present in the acute phase of Kawasaki syndrome lyse cultured vascular endothelial cells stimulated by gamma interferon. *J Clin Invest* 77:1428–1435, 1986.

Lie JT: Systemic and isolated vasculitis: A rational approach to classification and pathologic diagnosis. *Pathol Annu* 24(Pt 1):25–114, 1989.

Niles JL, Pan GL, Collins AB, et al.: Antigen-specific radioimmunoassays for anti-neutrophil cytoplasmic antibodies in the diagnosis of rapidly progressive glomerulonephritis. *J Am Soc Nephrol* 2:27–36, 1991.

Nachman PH, Hogan SL, Jennette JC, Falk RJ: Treatment response and relapse in ANCA-associated microscopic polyangiitis and glomerulonephritis. *J Am Soc Nephrol* 7:23–32, 1996.

Ronco P, Verroust P, Mignon F, et al.: Immunopathological studies of polyarteritis nodosa and Wegener's Granulomatosis: A report of 43 patients with 51 renal biopsies. *Q J Med* 206:212–223, 1983.

Serra A, Cameron JS, Turner DR, et al.: Vasculitis affecting the kidney: Presentation, histopathology and long-term outcome. *Q J Med* 53:181–207, 1984.

Smith DL. Spontaneous rupture of a renal artery aneurysm in polyarteritis nodosa: Critical review of the literature and report of a case. *Am J Med* 87:464–467, 1989.

RENAL MANIFESTATIONS OF SYSTEMIC LUPUS ERYTHEMATOSUS AND OTHER RHEUMATIC DISORDERS

JAMES E. BALOW

The kidney is affected in many rheumatic diseases as well as by some of the drugs used to treat them. Some of these topics are covered elsewhere: systemic vasculitis (Chapter 27), membranoproliferative glomerulonephritis and cryoglobulinemia (Chapter 19), dysproteinemias and amyloidosis (Chapter 30), and nonsteroidal anti-inflammatory drugs and the kidney (Chapter 42). This chapter focuses primarily on systemic lupus erythematosus, Henoch-Schönlein purpura, and systemic sclerosis, which regularly and often dramatically affect the kidney.

SYSTEMIC LUPUS ERYTHEMATOSUS

Systemic lupus erythematosus (SLE) is the classic autoimmune disease, with deposition of immune complexes and infiltration of inflammatory cells in diverse tissue sites. The spectrum of systemic involvement is reflected in part by the multiplicity of standard criteria for diagnosis and classification of SLE listed in Table 1. For research purposes, four or more of these criteria are conventionally used to classify patients with a diagnosis of SLE. For clinical purposes, diagnosis of SLE may be appropriate with less than four of the formal criteria, especially in the presence of other signs, such as alopecia and Raynaud's phenomenon. Autoantibodies are prominent in the diagnosis of SLE. A synopsis of the autoantibodies found in SLE and the other rheumatic diseases with renal components discussed in this chapter is shown in Table 2.

Chronic fatigue, arthralgias, and skin rashes are among the most intrusive symptoms and signs of SLE. Paradoxically, major visceral disease, while representing a greater threat to long-term survival, often produces fewer and less imposing subjective manifestations and can easily go undetected until substantial damage has accrued. Such is the case with renal involvement where asymptomatic hematuria or proteinuria are common initial manifestations and are often overlooked or misinterpreted as signs of minor genitourinary tract disorders. It is critically important for the clinician, at a minimum, to ask laboratory personnel to examine the urine in light of suspicion of glomerular disease, or preferably to examine the urine sediment personally. Lupus nephritis is all too frequently unrecognized until full-blown nephritic and/or nephrotic syndromes emerge. Renal insufficiency is not a common early manifestation because compensatory hypertrophy and hyperfiltration in less affected nephrons often mask significant injury in others. Nonetheless, the diligent physician should be able to recognize renal involvement early in the course of lupus nephritis when intervention will be the most effective.

A renal biopsy is often used in defining the prognosis and formulating plans for treatment of lupus nephritis. Clinicopathologic correlations in the various forms of lupus nephritis are shown in Table 3. Mesangial nephropathy can be considered the lowest common denominator of lupus nephritis. In some cases, mesangial abnormalities are the expression of intrinsically mild lupus nephritis which does not warrant specific treatment. More commonly, mesangial nephropathy represents the early stage of glomerular disease in transition to proliferative or membranous forms of lupus nephritis, but criteria for preemptive treatment have not been defined. Focal and diffuse proliferative lupus nephritis exhibit pathologic renal lesions which are qualitatively similar and, in essence, represent mild and severe forms of proliferative disease. Thus, focal and diffuse proliferative lupus nephritis are separated arbitrarily by the presence of pathologic lesions which obliterate glomerular capillaries in less than or more than 50% of nephrons, respectively. Typical lesions of proliferative lupus nephritis include endocapillary hypercellularity and "wire loop" lesions which represent large but irregular subendothelial immune complex deposits affecting certain glomerular capillaries (Fig. 1).

In general, the functional consequences of proliferative lupus nephritis are related to the extent of obliterative lesions along the filtration surface of glomerular capillaries. However, many active proliferative lesions are reversible with effective therapy (e.g., hypercellularity, inflammatory infiltrates) and renal prognosis depends on the extent of lesions that heal mostly by scarring (e.g., cellular crescents, fibrinoid necrosis) or are already irreversible prior to therapy (e.g., glomerular sclerosis, fibrous crescents, tubular atrophy, interstitial fibrosis). Analysis of renal biopsies is

208

TABLE I
Diagnosis of Systemic Lupus Erythematosus

Criterion	Description
1. Malar rash	Erythema (flat or raised) of malar eminences
2. Discoid rash	Erythematous, scaling plaques with variable skin atrophy
3. Photosensitivity	Sunlight-induced or exacerbated rashes
4. Oral ulcers	Mucous membrane ulcerations
5. Arthritis	Nonerosive, nondeforming arthritis of small joints
6. Serositis	Pleuritis, or pericarditis
7. Renal disease	Persistent proteinuria (>0.5 g/d or 3+ dipstick), or cellular (red, white, tubular, or mixed cell) casts
8. Neurologic disease	Seizures (in the absence of other causes) or psychosis (in the absence of other causes)
9. Hematologic disease	Hemolytic anemia or leukopenia ($<4000/\mu L$ on two or more occasions), or lymphopenia ($<1500/\mu L$ on two or more occasions, or thrombocytopenia ($<100,000/\mu L$)
10. Immunologic disease	LE cell prep, or anti-DNA antibody, or anti-Sm antibody, or false positive serologic test for syphilis (STS)
11. Antinuclear antibody	Abnormal titer (in absence of predisposing drugs)

From Tan EM, Cohen AS, Fries JF: *Arthritis Rheum* 25:1271–1277, 1982.

facilitated by systematic scoring of pathologic lesions and creation of an activity index (glomerular cellularity, leukocyte exudation, hyaline deposits, necrosis, cellular crescents, and interstitial inflammation) and a chronicity (damage) index (glomerulosclerosis, fibrous crescents, tubular atrophy, and interstitial fibrosis).

Transitions occur among the various major classes of lupus nephritis. Mesangial nephropathy may represent an inherently mild form of disease which may remain as such; alternatively, mesangial nephropathy may represent an early stage of disease in evolution to proliferative or membranous forms of lupus nephritis. Proliferative nephropathies may "heal" by regression of hypercellularity and resorption of subendothelial deposits leaving the appearance of membranous nephropathy (thickened capillary loops and subepithelial deposits) (Fig. 2). True mixed membranous and proliferative forms of lupus nephritis may coexist; such cases have a particularly ominous prognosis and treatment should be focused on the proliferative element. Extraglomerular renal vasculopathy occurs in lupus nephritis but

it is rarely due to frank vasculitis. SLE-associated antiphospholipid antibodies seem to increase risk of vasculopathy.

The prognosis of the various forms of lupus nephritis is estimated from a composite of clinical and pathologic features. Nephritic urinary sediment and/or worsening nephrotic syndrome, particularly when combined with progressive deterioration of renal function, is ominous and constitutes a major indication for therapy. The levels of activity and chronicity indexes in the renal biopsy help to define prognosis and supplement the clinical indications for therapy. On renal biopsy, high-grade proliferation, fibrinoid necrosis, cellular crescents, and/or extensive subendothelial immune complex deposits portend a poor prognosis and hence are also considered strong indications for intensive therapy (Table 3). While isolated laboratory tests are rarely dependable predictors of an adverse course, falling serum complement levels or rising anti-DNA antibody titers should prompt an intensified search for other direct evidence of incipient renal flares. Conversely, fixed nonnephrotic proteinuria, fixed azotemia, or high chronicity index

TABLE 2
Characteristic Autoantibodies in the Renal-Rheumatic Diseases

Disorder	Autoantibodies
Systemic lupus erythematosus	Anti-nuclear antibodies (ANA) diffuse pattern, anti-DNA, anti-Sm, anti-phospholipid (cardiolipin)
Henoch-Schönlein purpura	None
Systemic sclerosis	ANA (speckled), anti-Scl-70 (topoisomerase 1), anticentromere
Mixed connective tissue disease	ANA, anti-RNP (ribonucleoprotein)
Sjögren's syndrome	ANA, anti-Ro (anti-SS-A), anti-La (anti-SS-B)
Rheumatoid arthritis	Rheumatoid factor (mostly IgM antibody to IgG)
Behçet's syndrome	None
Relapsing polychondritis	None (occasional antibodies to type 2 collagen)
Familial Mediterranean fever	None

TABLE 3
Typical Clinicopathological Features and Correlations in Lupus Nephritis

Morphologic class	Clinical renal manifestations	Characteristic renal pathology
I. Normal or minimal abnormality	Usually asymptomatic	Minimal glomerular abnormalities by light microscopy No glomerular immune deposits
II. Mesangial nephropathy	Low-grade hematuria and/or proteinuria Normal renal function	Mesangial expansion but mostly patent capillaries Mesangial immune deposits
III. Focal proliferative lupus nephritis	Nephritic urinary sediment Variable but usually nonnephrotic proteinuria	Predominantly segmental proliferation, necrosis, crescents in <50% of glomeruli Predominantly mesangial and subendothelial immune deposits
IV. Diffuse proliferative lupus nephritis	Nephritic and nephrotic syndromes Hypertension Variable renal insufficiency	Predominantly global proliferation, necrosis, crescents in >50% of glomeruli Variable sclerosis, atrophy, fibrosis Predominantly mesangial and subendothelial immune deposits
V. Membranous nephropathy	Nephrotic syndrome	Uniform capillary loop thickening Subepithelial (and mesangial) immune deposits
VI. Sclerosing nephropathy	Inactive urinary sediment: broad, waxy (chronic renal failure) casts	Glomerular obsolescence, tubular atrophy, and interstitial fibrosis Few if any immune deposits

on renal biopsy when present in isolation indicate a poor prognosis and are relative contraindications to treatment.

Corticosteroids are the backbone of treatment of SLE. However, the threat of pernicious long-term complications (e.g., osteoporosis, avascular necrosis of bone, cataracts, and atherosclerosis) mandates that corticosteroid therapy be used with restraint; this means limited duration of high doses, frequent attempts at tapering, and alternate day prednisone therapy whenever possible. Some mild cases of proliferative lupus nephritis may respond to corticosteroids alone. When remission of renal disease is prompt and nearly complete, simply tapering to alternate-day prednisone over the subsequent month and establishment of a low maintenance dose may be acceptable. However, in most forms of proliferative lupus nephritis, the renal response is delayed and incomplete and most consultants would institute pulse cyclophosphamide as an adjunct to prednisone within 4 to 8 weeks of starting treatment. Indeed, there is broad agreement that cyclophosphamide treatment is warranted for severe focal (crescents or necrosis in >25% of glomeruli) and almost all cases of diffuse proliferative lupus nephritis from the outset. Intermittent pulse cyclophosphamide is favored because of reduced long-term toxicity (e.g., bone marrow, gonads, and bladder) compared to conventional daily oral cyclophosphamide. Pulse cyclophosphamide is commonly administered monthly for 6 months as induction therapy; this is followed by quarterly pulse cyclophosphamide maintenance treatments until remission of nephritis has been sustained for 1 year or longer (see below). Azathioprine has been proposed as an acceptable alternative to the extended courses of pulse cyclophosphamide during the maintenance period. The practical roles of cyclosporine or mycophenolate for either induction or maintenance therapy are uncertain and undefined. Several controlled studies have failed to show that plasma exchange therapy is useful in proliferative lupus nephritis.

Stabilization and gradual improvement in clinical and laboratory features occur in the majority of cases of proliferative lupus nephritis within several weeks of the initiation of corticosteroid and pulse cyclophosphamide therapy. However, complete remission of lupus nephritis (i.e., inactive urinary sediment, proteinuria <1 g/day, inactive lupus serologies) is typically not seen for many months. Exacerbations of lupus nephritis continue to be problematic following all current forms of therapy. Indeed, each major relapse produces cumulative damage and progressive compromise of renal function no matter how effective is each induction therapy program. Recent studies have shown that major exacerbations of severe lupus nephritis are significantly more common after short (6-month) induction courses of pulse cyclophosphamide than they are after an extended course of low-intensity maintenance therapy. Thus, there is a growing consensus that low-intensity maintenance therapy is preferable to repeated episodes of high-intensity corticosteroid and cyclophosphamide treatment for proliferative lupus nephritis.

The renal prognosis of proliferative lupus nephritis has markedly improved during the last half of the 20th century. The likelihood of end-stage renal failure or death within 10 years of diagnosis has fallen from more than 80% to less than 20% in racially diverse populations. The improved prognosis is due to a composite of medical advances, including more effective antibiotics and antihypertensives, as well as safer immunosuppressive regimens, particularly pulse cyclophosphamide therapy. The prognosis of lupus nephri-

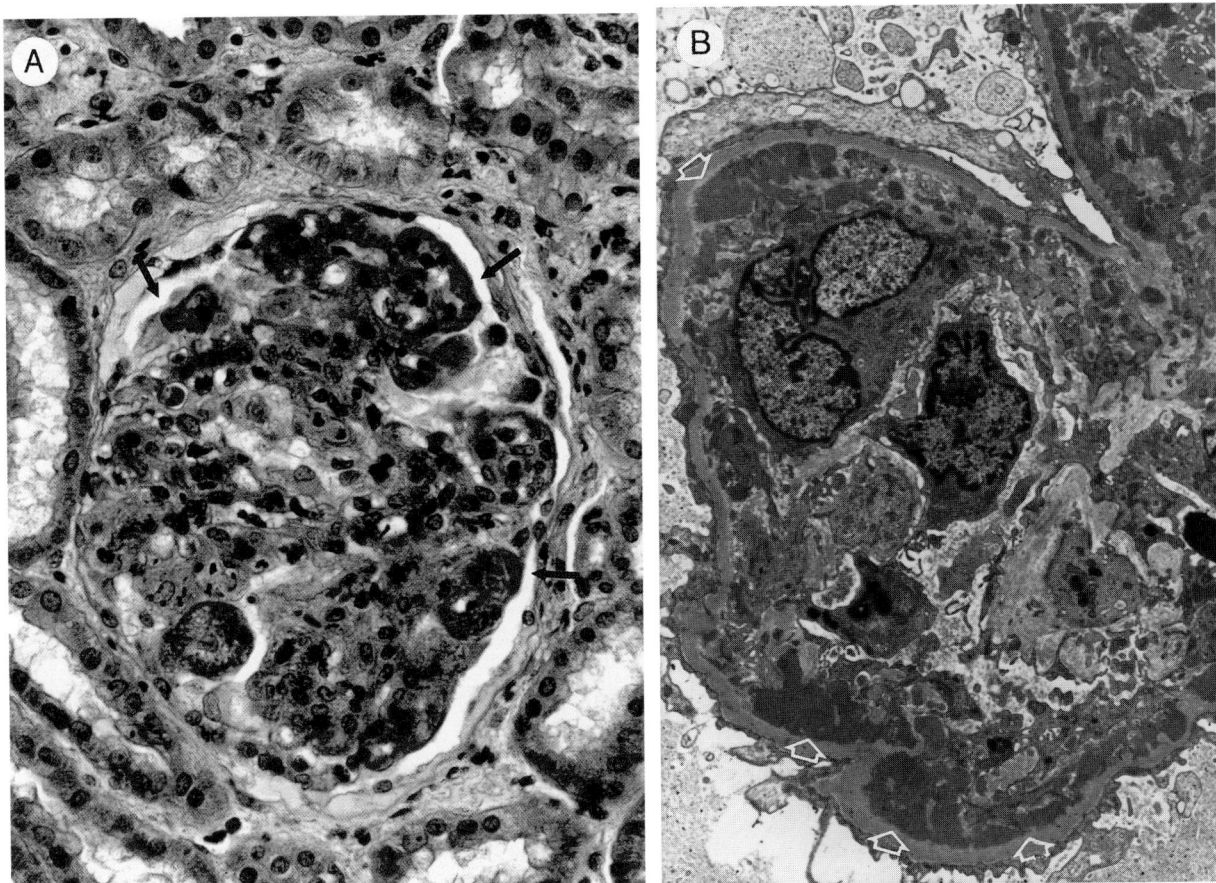

FIGURE 1 Diffuse proliferative (Class IV) glomerulonephritis. (A) Light microscopy shows global hypercellularity and increased mesangial matrix which compromise the filtration surface of the glomerular capillaries. So called "wire loop" lesions (arrows) formed by massive but irregular immune complex deposits cause irregular thickening of the capillary loops (hematoxylin and eosin stain). (B) Electron microscopy shows extensive dark-staining subendothelial immune complex deposits (arrows) disrupting the integrity of the endothelial cells and compromising the capillary lumen. Epithelial foot process fusion is seen along the outer surface of the glomerular basement membrane. Courtesy of Dr. Sharda Sabnis, Nephropathology Section, Armed Forces Institute of Pathology, Washington, DC.

tis is worse in African-American patients than in comparably treated whites. The basis for this observation is unknown, but differences in racial mix in various clinical reports may contribute to the discrepancies in apparent treatment effects in proliferative lupus nephritis.

The indications for treatment of membranous lupus nephropathy are controversial. The prognosis measured by risk of renal failure is relatively low (approximately 25% at 15 years). Male gender and massive proteinuria (>10 g/day) may define subsets of patients with higher risk of renal progression. Recent reports indicate that the atherogenic cardiovascular disease and thromboembolic events brought on by persistent nephrotic syndrome may be additional reasons for attempting to treat membranous nephropathy. Angiotensin-converting enzyme inhibitors are commonly used to reduce proteinuria and HMG-CoA reductase inhibitors are used to reduce hypercholesterolemia, but responses are usually partial until remission of nephrotic syndrome occurs either spontaneously or with immunosuppressive drug therapy. High-dose alternate-day prednisone

tapered after approximately 2 months is the most commonly used approach. Clinical trials are in progress to evaluate the benefits of adjunctive pulse cyclophosphamide or low-dose cyclosporine in membranous lupus nephropathy.

HENOCH-SCHÖNLEIN PURPURA

Henoch-Schönlein purpura (HSP) is a systemic disease, is found mainly in children and adolescents, and has characteristic features of purpuric rash, arthritis, gastrointestinal hemorrhage, and glomerulonephritis. The skin lesions are those of a cutaneous vasculitis, specifically a leukocytoclastic vasculitis with secondary hemorrhage. There are no recognized autoantibodies, but Henoch-Schönlein disease is characterized by IgA deposits in the skin and kidneys, suggesting a relationship to IgA nephropathy. Transient, asymptomatic hematuria and proteinuria occur in more than half of the cases, but they do not warrant treatment. Hypertension, early appearance of nephrotic syndrome, persistent nephritic urinary sediment, or progressive azote-

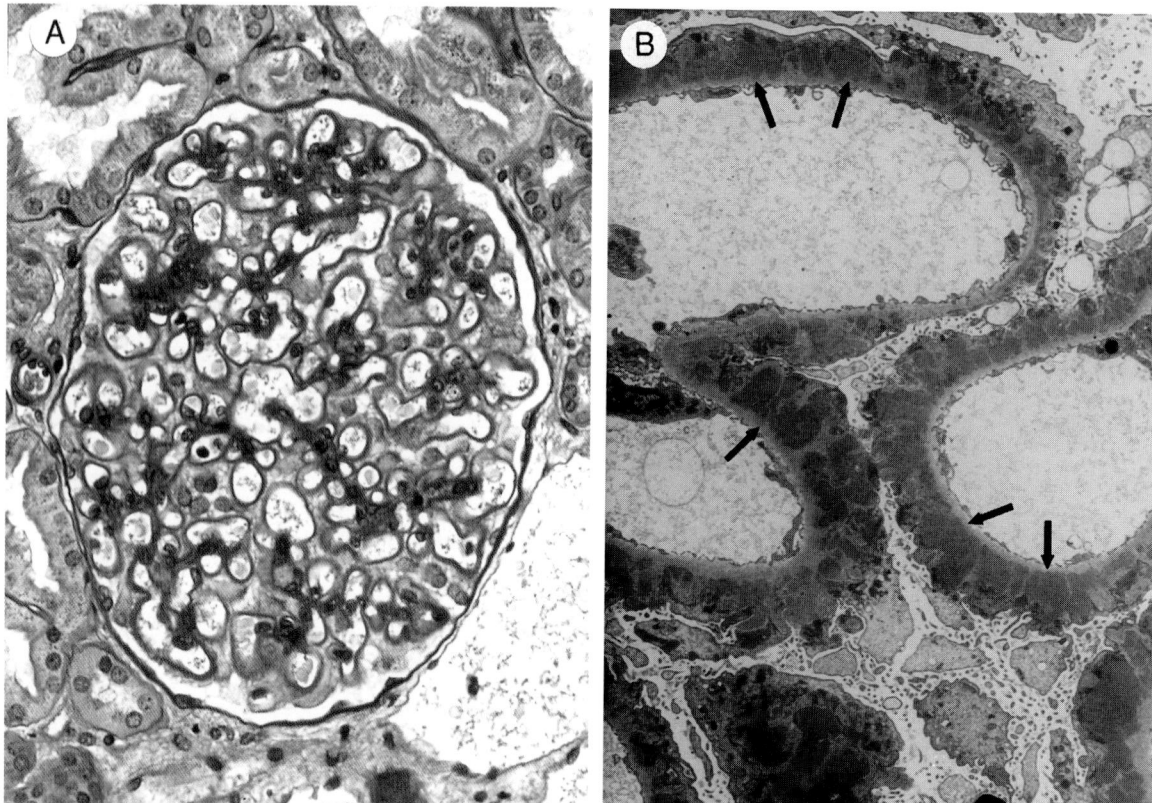

FIGURE 2 Membranous (Class V) lupus nephropathy. (A) Light microscopy shows uniformly thickened but widely patent glomerular capillary loops. Hypercellularity is limited to mild mesangial expansion (periodic acid–Schiff stain). (B) Electron microscopy shows well-preserved but uniformly thickened capillary loops. Extensive dark staining deposits are seen on the external (subepithelial) side of the glomerular basement membranes. Some examples are marked with arrows. Courtesy of Dr. Sharda Sabnis, Nephropathology Section, Armed Forces Institute of Pathology, Washington, DC.

mia reflects proliferative glomerulonephritis. More than 50% glomerular cellular crescents forebode an unfavorable prognosis and are important indications for treatment. Relapsing or chronic courses of Henoch-Schönlein purpura are unusual, but they increase the likelihood of progressive nephritis.

Immunosuppressive therapy is warranted in a minority of patients with Henoch-Schönlein nephritis. In patients with severe and/or rapidly progressive Henoch-Schönlein nephritis, high-dose corticosteroids, especially pulse methylprednisolone, are indicated. Cytotoxic drugs, such as cyclophosphamide and azathioprine, and plasma exchange are often used in refractory cases, but their supplemental benefits over corticosteroids alone are unproven.

SYSTEMIC SCLEROSIS

Systemic sclerosis or scleroderma is characterized by hardening of skin and dysfunction of certain internal organs due to massive connective tissue (notably collagen) accumulation and vasculopathy. Raynaud's syndrome, skin thickening, digital pulp atrophy (sclerodactyly), and tel-

angectasia are the primary clinical manifestations of systemic sclerosis. Musculoskeletal involvement includes periarticular tendon and nerve entrapment, flexion contractures, acral osteolysis, and myopathy. Alimentary tract dysfunction includes esophageal dysmotility and malabsorption, which are major causes of morbidity. Pulmonary hypertension and interstitial fibrosis, cardiomyopathy, and scleroderma renal crisis are the major causes of mortality. While antibodies to nuclear (ANA) and to specific Scl-70 (topoisomerase 1) antigen (Table 2) are present in at least two-thirds and one-fifth of patients, respectively, very little is known of the pathogenesis of systemic sclerosis. Current theories focus on primary disturbances in the vascular endothelium, in the immune and cytokine systems, and in collagen biosynthesis.

The kidney is affected in about one third of patients with systemic sclerosis. The clinical spectrum includes renin-mediated hypertension, microangiopathic hemolytic anemia (Fig. 3), low-grade proteinuria, and azotemia. In aggressive cases, malignant hypertension and rapidly progressive renal failure ensue (scleroderma renal crisis). The kidney pathology includes an occlusive vasculopathy due

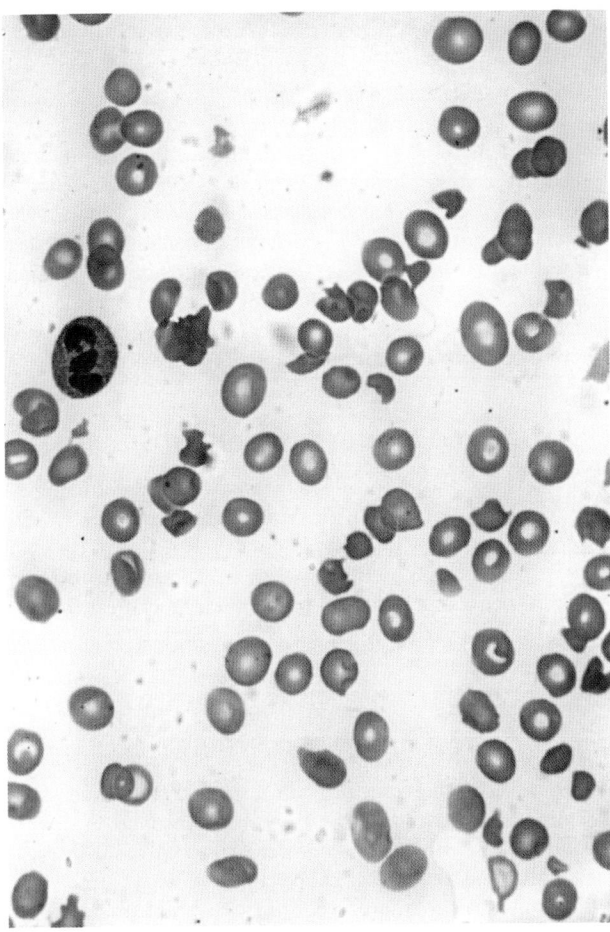

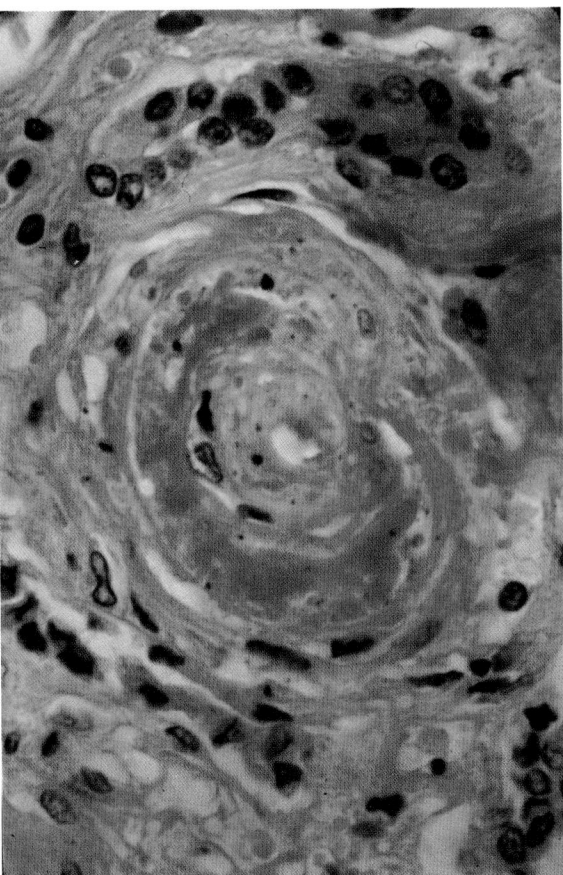

FIGURE 3 Microangiopathic hemolytic anemia. Peripheral blood smear showing fragmented red blood cells of various shapes and sizes, but few platelets (Wright stain). In addition to scleroderma renal crisis, thrombotic microangiopathy is seen in various forms of malignant hypertension, disseminated intravascular coagulation, thrombotic thrombocytopenic purpura, hemolytic uremic syndrome, and necrotizing vasculitis.

FIGURE 4 Vasculopathy of scleroderma renal crisis. Interlobular artery shows severe mucoid intimal thickening with fibrin exudation (red, amorphous deposits). Compromise of the vessel lumen produces a viscous cycle of malignant hypertension and worsening thrombotic microangiopathy (hematoxylin and eosin stain).

to intimal swelling, fibrinoid necrosis and fragmentation, and duplication of the elastic lamina (Fig. 4). Thrombotic microangiopathy and rapidly progressive renal failure sometimes occur in the absence of hypertension and rarely even before characteristic clinical features indicate a diagnosis of systemic sclerosis.

Although considered an immunologic disorder, systemic sclerosis does not appear to benefit substantively from currently available immunosuppressive drugs. Corticosteroids may in fact be deleterious in systemic sclerosis. Overall, 5-year survival for diffuse scleroderma is approximately 60%; in an uncontrolled study of diffuse scleroderma, penicillamine treatment improved survival to 80%. Cardiac, pulmonary, and especially renal involvement worsens prognosis significantly. At present, medical therapy in the face of renal involvement is focused on interrupting the vicious cycle of vasculopathy, hypertension, and azotemia. The prognosis of scleroderma renal crisis has historically been extremely poor. However, in recent years, survival has dramatically improved as the result of therapy with angiotensin-converting enzyme inhibitors early in the course (with the onset of hypertension but before creatinine levels exceed 3 mg/dL). The prognosis of patients with scleroderma renal crisis treated with angiotensin-converting enzyme inhibitors has improved from <10% to >50% patient and renal survival. Nearly half of patients needing dialysis have return of renal function if blood pressure is effectively controlled.

MIXED CONNECTIVE TISSUE DISEASE

Overlap syndromes occur among the rheumatic diseases, most often with features of systemic lupus, rheumatoid arthritis, Sjögren syndrome, systemic sclerosis, and polymyositis. Some authors favor assigning diagnosis to the nearest discrete connective tissue disease category depending on the dominant symptoms and signs; others favor using a separate diagnosis of mixed connective tissue disease

(MCTD). The latter approach is supported by autoantibodies to extractable nuclear antigens (ENA), particularly to ribonuclear protein (RNP), which is characteristic of patients with MCTD (Table 2). Renal involvement is variable; when present in MCTD, the glomerular disease is most akin to that of mesangial and membranous forms of lupus nephritis. In dermatomyositis or polymyositis (whether idiopathic or as the predominant component of MCTD), renal involvement is distinctly uncommon.

SJÖGREN'S SYNDROME

Sjögren's syndrome may be primary or may be a secondary feature of rheumatoid arthritis, systemic lupus, MCTD, systemic sclerosis, or polymyositis. It is characterized by parotid and other exocrine gland swelling and dysfunction due to lymphoid infiltration; the resulting mucus secretory defect produces dry mucous membranes (sicca complex). Characteristically, Sjögren's is accompanied by profound hyperglobulinemia and a high frequency of type 1 (distal) renal tubular acidosis. The long-term positive hydrogen ion balance must be countered by base (sodium bicarbonate or sodium citrate) supplementation in order to avert osteoporosis, hypercalciuria, nephrocalcinosis, and nephrolithiasis. Rare cases of glomerulonephritis have been seen in patients with primary Sjögren's syndrome. The clinical and pathologic features, as well as indications for treatment, are akin to those of membranous or proliferative forms of lupus nephritis.

RHEUMATOID ARTHRITIS

Rheumatoid arthritis is a chronic symmetrical polyarthritis accompanied by periarticular osteoporosis and bone erosions. Rheumatoid factor (IgM antibody against IgG) is characteristic and rheumatoid nodules often develop in patients with high titers of these autoantibodies. Progressive glomerular disease is uncommon in the natural history of rheumatoid arthritis. On the other hand, isolated hematuria due to mild mesangial nephropathy is recognized with increasing frequency, but treatment is usually unnecessary. Side effects of treatments for rheumatoid arthritis are quite often the causes of renal disease. Rare cases of nephrotic syndrome are mostly due to membranous nephropathy; predilection to membranous nephropathy seems to be increased by gold and penicillamine therapy. Proteinuria and abnormal urine sediment are considered reasons to discontinue these treatments for rheumatoid arthritis. Secondary (AA) amyloidosis is an uncommon cause of nephrotic syndrome in severe, debilitated patients with rheumatoid arthritis. Treatment of AA amyloidosis of the kidney is usually ineffective and most cases inexorably progress to end-stage renal failure. Proliferative glomerulonephritis caused by cryoglobulinemia or rheumatoid (necrotizing) vasculitis is an additional rare cause of renal disease in rheumatoid arthritis; institution or intensification of cytotoxic drug therapy may be effective in reducing cryoglobulinemia and in controlling renal vasculitis.

BEHÇET'S SYNDROME

Behçet's syndrome is a male-predominant vasculitic disease characterized by painful oral and genital ulcers, arthritis, rash, iritis, uveitis, retinitis, and focal central nervous system deficits. A thrombotic diathesis leads to vascular occlusive events which overlap with those of vasculitic lesions. There are no laboratory criteria for this clinical syndrome. Major systemic involvement, including renal disease due to a vasculitic-like process, may occur in a small minority of patients. Rapidly progressive, crescentic glomerulonephritis has been described as a very rare component of Behçet's syndrome.

RELAPSING POLYCHONDRITIS

Relapsing polychondritis is characterized by inflammation of the cartilage of the ears, joints, nose, eyes, and respiratory tract. Clinically, many of the features are akin to Wegener's granulomatosis. As in Behçet's syndrome, on rare occasions relapsing polychondritis can escalate to a severe vasculitis associated with a rapidly progressive glomerulonephritis.

FAMILIAL MEDITERRANEAN FEVER

Familial Mediterranean fever is an autosomal recessive disorder characterized by relapsing episodes of fever, polyserositis, arthritis, and erythematous skin rash. Secondary (AA) amyloidosis is a cause of nephrotic syndrome and subsequent renal failure in certain susceptible populations, particularly those of Turkish, Armenian, and Sephardic Jewish descent. Colchicine is effective in treating the acute episodes of familial Mediterranean fever and in preventing secondary amyloidosis.

Bibliography

Austin HA, Balow JE: Henoch-Schönlein nephritis: Prognostic features and the challenge of therapy. *Am J Kidney Dis* 2:512–520, 1983.

Balow JE, Boumpas DT, Austin HA: Renal Disease. In: Schur P (ed) *The Clinical Management of Systemic Lupus Erythematosus*. 2nd ed. Lippincott-Raven, Philadelphia, pp. 109–126, 1996.

Boumpas DT, Austin HA, Vaughan EM, et al.: Severe lupus nephritis: Controlled trial of pulse methylprednisolone versus two different regimens of pulse cyclophosphamide. *Lancet* 340:741–745, 1992.

Chang-Miller A, Okamura M, Torres VE, et al.: Renal involvement in relapsing polychondritis. *Medicine (Baltimore)* 66:202–217, 1987.

Churg J, Bernstein J, Glassock RJ: *Renal Disease: Classification and Atlas of Glomerular Diseases*. Igaku-Shoin, New York, 1995.

Donnelly S, Jothy S, Barre P: Crescentic glomerulonephritis in Behçet's syndrome—Results of therapy and review of the literature. *Clin Nephrol* 31:213–218, 1989.

Donohoe JF: Scleroderma and the kidney. *Kidney Int* 41:462–477, 1992.

El-Mallakh RS, Bryan RK, Masi AT, Kelly CE, Rakowski KJ: Long-term low-dose glucocorticoid therapy associated with remission of overt renal tubular acidosis in Sjögren's syndrome. *Am J Med* 79:509–514, 1985.

Goldstein AR, White RH, Akuse R, Chantler C: Long-term follow-up of childhood Henoch-Schönlein nephritis. *Lancet* 339: 280–282, 1992.

Grishman E, Churg J, Needle MA, Venkataseshan VS (eds): *The Kidney in Collagen-Vascular Diseases.* Raven Press, New York, 1993.

Helin HJ, Korpela MM, Mustonen JT, Pasternak AI: Renal biopsy findings and clinicopathologic correlations in rheumatoid arthritis. *Arthritis Rheum* 38:242–247, 1995.

Kitridou RC, Akmal M, Turkel SB, Ehresmann GR, Quismorio FP, Massry SG: Renal involvement in mixed connective tissue

disease: A longitudinal clinicopathologic study. *Semin Arthritis Rheum* 16:135–145, 1986.

Klippel JH, Dieppe PA (eds). *Practical Rheumatology.* Mosby, London, 1995.

Said R, Hamzeh Y, Said S, Tarawneh M, al-Khateeb M: Spectrum of renal involvement in familial Mediterranean fever. *Kidney Int* 41:414–419, 1992.

Steen VD. Renal involvement in systemic sclerosis. *Clin Dermatol* 12:253–258, 1994.

Steen VD, Costantino JP, Shapiro AP, Medsger TA: Outcome of renal crisis in systemic sclerosis: relation to availability of angiotensin converting enzyme (ACE) inhibitors. *Ann Intern Med* 113:352–357, 1990.

29

DIABETIC NEPHROPATHY

JULIA BREYER

Diabetic nephropathy is the leading cause of end-stage renal disease (ESRD) in the United States. Patients with diabetes currently account for 35% of all the patients enrolled in the Medicare ESRD program. Sixty-three percent of the patients with diabetic nephropathy have type II diabetes mellitus. The cost to Medicare for ESRD patients with diabetes mellitus exceeded $2 billion per year in 1990. In addition to its significant impact on health care costs, the development of diabetic kidney disease has a dramatic impact on the morbidity and mortality of patients with diabetes. It has been estimated that patients with type I diabetes mellitus and nephropathy as manifested by proteinuria have a 100-fold greater risk of dying relative to a nondiabetic population. Diabetic patients without proteinuria have only a 2-fold increase in relative mortality.

EPIDEMIOLOGY

Diabetic nephropathy with proteinuria rarely develops before ten years duration of diabetes. The cumulative incidence of proteinuria in patients with type I diabetes after 40 years duration of diabetes is 40%. However, the annual incidence of diabetic nephropathy in type I patients peaks just before 20 years duration of diabetes and thereafter declines. This suggests that the risk of developing diabetic nephropathy is not constant over the duration of diabetes

and that a pool of susceptible patients becomes exhausted. Thus, if a patient survives 35 years of diabetes without developing nephropathy, the patient is at extremely low risk of doing so in the future. Studies of type II diabetes mellitus in Pima Indians and in western Europe show results similar to those of studies of patients with type I diabetes mellitus; approximately 40% of these patients will also develop diabetic nephropathy.

Diabetic African Americans, Mexican Americans, American Indians, Maori, and Polynesians are among the minority populations who have a greater risk of developing diabetic nephropathy and a more rapid progression to ESRD. It is not known whether these racial differences are due to genetic, environmental, or other factors.

PATHOGENESIS

Many factors have been postulated to be important in the pathogenesis of diabetic nephropathy. Normal kidneys transplanted into patients with diabetes develop diabetic lesions, where kidneys from patients with diabetes that were inadvertently transplanted into nondiabetic ESRD patients resolved their diabetic lesions. These observations strongly support the notion that exposure to the diabetic milieu rather than an intrinsic defect in the kidneys predisposes patients to the development of diabetic nephropathy.

Not only hyperglycemia but also insulin deficiency, augmented glucagon and growth hormone levels, and increased ketone bodies have been implicated in the pathogenesis of diabetic nephropathy. Recently, it has been demonstrated that hyperglycemia leads to the accumulation of advanced glycosylation endproducts in tissues in patients with diabetes. It has been postulated that this, at least in part, may be responsible for the endorgan complications of diabetes. Glucose forms chemically reversible early glycosylation products with proteins at a rate proportional to the glucose concentration. Some of these early glycosylation endproducts on long-lived proteins undergo a complex series of chemical rearrangements, forming covalent crosslinks that do not reverse with correction of hyperglycemia. The presence of these irreversibly cross-linked advanced glycosylation endproducts (AGE) results in a series of interactions that produce the endorgan damage seen in diabetes, at least in animal models. AGEs accumulate faster than normal in patients with diabetes and their accumulation parallels the severity of renal disease.

In studies in diabetic rats and in humans with diabetes, unilateral renal artery stenosis has been reported to protect the kidney distal to the blocked renal artery from developing the morphologic changes of diabetes. This suggests that exposure to the systemic blood pressure is an important factor in the development of diabetic kidney disease. Additionally, abnormal intraglomerular pressures have been demonstrated to contribute to the development of glomerulosclerosis in the diabetic rat. It has been demonstrated in diabetic rats that decreasing intraglomerular pressures by decreasing angiotensin II-mediated efferent arteriolar vasoconstriction preserves the structure and function of the glomerulus. Thus, both systemic blood pressure and intraglomerular pressure appear to have an important role in the development of diabetic kidney disease.

Finally, other factors have been implicated in the pathogenesis of diabetic nephropathy including dietary protein excess, alterations in the renin angiotensin axis, altered prostaglandin production, elevated kinin production, and elevated atrial naturetic factor levels.

NATURAL HISTORY

At the onset of type I diabetes, functional changes are present in virtually all patients (Fig. 1). Within a few years, morphologic changes occur in the kidneys of most patients. Early nephropathy is manifested by the development of microalbuminuria. Hyperfiltration, elevations in the mean arterial blood pressure, and poor blood sugar control can all be features of this early period. Approximately 17 ± 6 years after the onset of type I diabetes, frank proteinuria is manifested. Once proteinuria is established, renal function inexorably declines with 50% of patients reaching ESRD 7 to 10 years after the onset of proteinuria.

Patients with type II diabetes in whom the true time of onset of diabetes (e.g., the Pima Indians) is known appear to have a very similar natural history. However, for most patients with type II diabetes, the time of onset of diabetes is unknown and they have likely had diabetes for many years by the time the diagnosis is made. Thus, they may have proteinuria and declining renal function even at the time their diabetes is diagnosed.

Functional Changes

At the time of diagnosis of diabetes, functional changes present in the kidney include increased kidney size, albuminuria that reverses with blood sugar control, and glomerular hyperfiltration. Increased glomerular filtration rate (GFR) at the time of diagnosis of type I diabetes has been shown to be predictive of the development of clinically overt diabetic nephropathy on average 20 years later. Glomerular hyperfiltration in animal models of diabetes is associated with increments in renal plasma flow, due to renal vasodilatation, and increases in the glomerular transcapillary hydraulic pressure gradient, which lead to glomerulosclerosis.

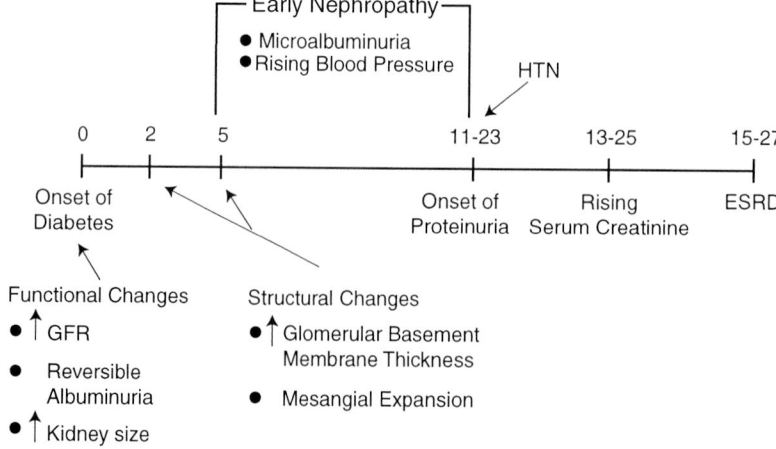

FIGURE 1 The natural history of diabetic nephropathy. HTN, hypertension; ESRD, end stage renal disease.

Pathology

At the onset of type I diabetes, renal biopsies are normal. Within 1 1/2 to 2 1/2 years glomerular basement membrane (GBM) thickening, a sensitive indicator for the presence of diabetes, appears. In addition to GBM thickening, other distinctive lesions include nodular (Kimmelstiel-Wilson) and diffuse forms of intracapillary glomerulosclerosis, the capsular drop lesion, the fibrin cap, and mesangial matrix expansion (Fig. 2). These changes, along with afferent and efferent arteriolar hyalinosis and increased renal extracellular membrane albumin and IgG localization in the glomeruli as demonstrated by immunofluorescence microscopy are diagnostic of diabetic nephropathy. Mesangial expansion correlates with creatinine clearance although no correlation exists between the GBM thickening and clinical renal function. Diabetes is primarily a vascular (including glomerular) disease; however, altered structure and function of the renal tubules and interstitium are also present (i.e. interstitial fibrous and tubular atrophy). The degree of interstitial fibrosis correlates with the reduction in GFR. However, no one has yet demonstrated that renal biopsies done before the onset of proteinuria will distinguish those patients who will later develop proteinuria and declining renal function from those who will not. Biopsies from patients with type II diabetes are indistinguishable from biopsies in type I patients.

Microalbuminuria and Early Nephropathy

A sensitive assay for urinary albumin excretion has shown that subclinical elevations of urinary albumin excretion in diabetic patients without overt proteinuria predict the later development of proteinuria and ESRD. Normal urinary albumin excretion is less than 30 mg/24. Patients with overt proteinuria have elevated urinary albumin excretion in excess of 300 mg/24 h. With this sensitive assay, patients with urinary albumin excretion between 30 and 300 mg/24 h can be identified, and this is the range that defines microalbuminuria. The presence of microalbuminuria in type I diabetes patients is highly predictive of progres-

sion to proteinuria and renal insufficiency during the next 10 to 15 years. Patients with type II diabetes also develop microalbuminuria which predicts progression to proteinuria and declining renal function. Excessive cardiovascular mortality has been reported in patients with type II diabetes and microalbuminuria. Due to premature cardiovascular deaths, there is a discrepancy between the number of patients with early nephropathy and those who develop ESRD.

Elevated blood pressure has also been demonstrated to precede and perhaps predict the development of diabetic nephropathy. Patients with microalbuminia or overt nephropathy are predisposed to hypertension, as indicated by elevated sodium–lithium countertransport activity in erythrocytes and a strong parental history of hypertension, compared to patients with diabetes but without nephropathy. Poor glycemic control also synergistically increases the risk of nephropathy in patients who are genetically predisposed to hypertension.

Proteinuria and Declining Renal Function

The presence of persistent proteinuria heralds the overt phase of diabetic nephropathy. Once proteinuria is established, renal function inevitably declines. The proteinuria can be as little as 500 mg/24 h or greater than 20 g/24 h.

In the vast majority of patients, GFR begins to decline with the onset of proteinuria, with the average time of ESRD being 10 years after the onset of proteinuria (Fig. 1). Renal function can also be adversely affected by other complications of diabetes, such as neurogenic bladder, urinary tract infection, and papillary necrosis. As renal function declines, uremia ensues. Insulin requirements decrease in uremia in part because the kidney is responsible for 30 to 40% of the catabolism of insulin and also because patients lose their appetite as renal function declines. Diabetes is also the most common cause of type IV renal tubular acidosis, which results in hyperkalemia and a hyperchloremic metabolic acidosis. Thus, patients with this tubular defect can have hyperkalemia and acidosis despite relatively well-preserved GFR.

SCREENING

Based on current recommendations, all patients with type I diabetes of greater than 5 years duration should have annual screens for microalbuminuria to identify this high-risk population. It is important to specifically order testing for urinary albumin excretion or microalbuminuria since routine urine protein determinations are not sensitive enough to detect microalbuminuria. A complete 24-hour urine collection, an overnight urine collection, which can be extrapolated to 24 hours, or a spot morning urine with measurement of the albumin : creatinine ratio may be employed. As shown in Table 1, hyperglycemia, uncontrolled hypertension or congestive heart failure, urinary tract infections, and excessive physical exercise must be considered as potential causes of transient microalbuminuria. Thus, if the urinary albumin excretion rate is elevated in a single

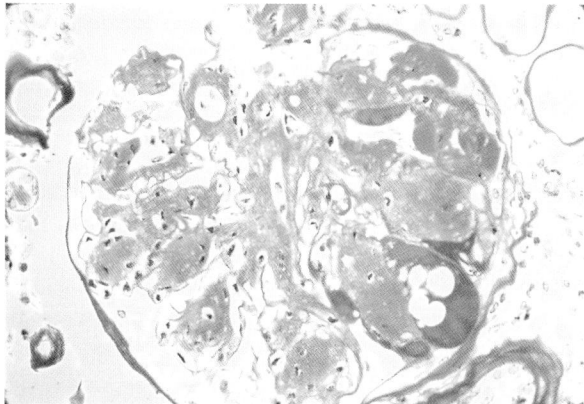

FIGURE 2 Diffuse and early nodular diabetic glomerulosclerosis. The peripheral structures at the right that consist of hyalinized eosinophilic material are fibrin caps. (periodic acid–Schiff stain).

TABLE I
Measurement of Microalbuminuria

Test IDDM patients of greater than 5 years duration every year. Test NIDDM patients at the time of diagnosis and every year.

Rule out causes of transient microalbuminuria: hyperglycemia, UTI, PE, essential HTN, CHF, water loading.

If the albumin excretion rate is elevated, repeat three times over 3–6 months to define persistent microalbuminuria.

Normal albumin excretion: <30 mg/24 h; microalbuminuria: 30–300 mg/24 h; proteinuria: >300 mg/24 h

IDDM, insulin-dependent diabetes mellitus; NIDDM, non-insulin-dependent diabetes mellitus; UTI, urinary tract infection; PE, physical exercise; HTN, hypertension; CHF, congestive heart failure.

collection, persistent microalbuminuria should be confirmed with three additional collections over 3 to 6 months. Patients with type II diabetes should be screened at the time of diagnosis and yearly thereafter.

When the patient with diabetes develops proteinuria, an evaluation for the cause of proteinuria should be undertaken. Ninety to 95% of type I patients with diabetic nephropathy will have diabetic retinopathy. The absence of retinopathy should make one suspect a cause of proteinuria other than diabetic nephropathy. In patients with type I diabetes, proteinuria from diabetic nephropathy occurs in a particular time frame: 17 ± 6 years after the onset of diabetes. If a patient with type I diabetes first manifests proteinuria after 5 years of diabetes or after 30 years of diabetes they are unlikely to have diabetic nephropathy as the cause. Patients should be evaluated carefully for the presence of other systemic diseases that can cause proteinuria such as hepatitis B, systemic lupus erythematosus, or amyloidosis. Renal ultrasounds should be performed to rule out anatomic abnormalities. If any evidence of another disease process is present, a renal biopsy should be considered. The presence of significant hematuria or red blood cell casts should also prompt consideration of a renal biopsy. However, for the vast majority of patients with diabetes and proteinuria who present with retinopathy, a benign urinalysis, no evidence of another systemic disease, and proteinuria in the appropriate time frame, a renal biopsy is not necessary for diagnosis.

TREATMENT OF PROGRESSIVE DISEASE

The major therapeutic interventions that have been evaluated include: improved glycemic control, antihypertensive therapy, treatment with angiotensin converting enzyme (ACE) inhibitors, and restriction of dietary protein intake.

Tight control of blood glucose prevents the development of and ameliorates established diabetic nephropathy in animal studies. Multiple epidemiologic studies have implicated hyperglycemia in the pathogenesis of the long-term complications of diabetes in humans. Recently, the Stockholm Diabetes Intervention Study demonstrated a beneficial effect of intensive blood sugar control in patients with type I diabetes and established complications.

The Diabetes Control and Complications Trial (DCCT) randomly assigned 1441 patients with type I diabetes to either intensive therapy, achieving a mean hemoglobin A_1C of 7%, or conventional therapy, achieving a mean hemoglobin A_1C of 9%. At baseline, the patients were in two cohorts: 726 with no evidence of end organ complications (the primary cohort), and 715 patients with early complications primarily of mild retinopathy (the secondary cohort). In both cohorts, microalbuminuria developed in fewer patients in the intensive therapy group than in the conventional therapy group, with a risk reduction of 34% within the primary cohort and 43% in the secondary cohort. The risk of developing proteinuria was reduced by 56% in the secondary cohort. The chief adverse effect associated with intensive blood sugar control was a two-to three fold increase in severe hypoglycemic episodes requiring assistance. In the secondary analysis, the beneficial effects of intensive blood sugar control were a continuous function, so that any decrease in hemoglobin A_1C values was associated with decreased risk of developing diabetic nephropathy. Thus, intensive blood sugar control prevents the development and progression of early diabetic nephropathy. In patients with type II diabetes, far fewer studies have been completed, although several are ongoing to examine the impact of intensive blood sugar control in preventing the development of diabetic nephropathy.

Multiple studies have demonstrated that in type I diabetes patients with proteinuria and declining renal function, lowering the systemic blood pressure slows the rate of decline in renal function and improves patient survival. Similar results have been found in patients with type II diabetes. Also, in patients with early diabetic nephropathy manifested by microalbuminuria, lowering the systemic blood pressure has been demonstrated to lower urinary albumin excretion rates. Thus, even in early diabetic kidney disease, the lowering of systemic blood pressure appears to be of benefit. The definition of adequate blood pressure control in patients with diabetic nephropathy is unclear. The current target recommendation is a blood pressure at or below 135/85 mm Hg. It has also been suggested that the goal of blood pressure therapy should be a documented decrease in urinary albumin excretion rate or proteinuria.

Studies in animals with diabetic kidney disease demonstrated that ACE inhibitors preserved renal structure and function independent of their effect on systemic blood pressure. In these diabetic animals, the mechanism of protection was interruption of the vasoconstrictor effect of angiotensin II on the efferent arteriole, leading to lower glomerular intracapillary pressures while preserving renal plasma flow. Treatment with ACE inhibitors in patients with microalbuminuria has been reported to decrease the urinary albumin excretion rate and decrease the progression to overt proteinuria.

In a clinical trial, patients with type I diabetes and diabetic nephropathy (manifested by ≥ 500 mg proteinuria per 24 hours and serum creatinine $=2.5$ mg/dL) were randomized to receive either captopril 25 mg three times a day or placebo. The primary outcome was time to doubling of serum creatinine to at least 2 mg/dL, which approximated halving the patient's GFR. Patients receiving captopril had a 48% risk reduction for doubling of serum creatinine and a 50% risk reduction for the secondary outcome of time to death, dialysis, or transplantation compared to the placebo group. The renoprotective effect of ACE inhibition was independent of its effect on systemic blood pressure. ACE inhibitors were equally efficacious in normotensive and hypertensive patients. Thus, the use of ACE inhibition is of clear benefit in patients with type I diabetes and established nephropathy. A beneficial effect of ACE inhibitors in patients with type II diabetes is less well established.

A beneficial effect of calcium channel blockers in diabetic nephropathy has not been established. Far fewer studies have been performed and the available studies were done with small numbers of patients, most of whom had type II diabetes. Recently it has been suggested that a combination of ACE inhibitors and calcium channel blockers may be of benefit. But again, few data support this recommendation.

In many experimental animal models of renal disease, including diabetes, high dietary protein intake accelerates the deterioration of renal function. Several studies done in small numbers of patients with diabetes and diabetic nephropathy have suggested a beneficial effect of low protein diets in slowing the rate of decline of renal function.

A variety of other interventions have been attempted in small studies in either diabetic rats or humans, including the use of aldose reductase inhibitors, treatment with inhibitors of the formation of AGES, treatment of dyslipidemia, treatment with octreotide, treatment with antiplatelet drugs, treatment with thromboxane synthetase inhibitors, and treatment with the protease inhibitor camostate mesilate. None of those interventions have as yet been proven efficacious.

The 40% of patients with diabetes who develop diabetic nephropathy must be identified as early in their course as possible. Interventions noted above can be implemented to slow and halt the progression of their renal disease even at very early stages such as when the patient has only microalbuminuria. Once persistent elevation of the urinary albumin excretion is found, the patient should be referred to a nephrologist for further evaluation and for consideration of implementation of specific therapeutic interventions. The nephrologist can also evaluate the patient to ensure that no other cause of the proteinuria besides diabetic nephropathy is present. In addition to implementing specific therapeutic interventions it is important to help preserve the patients remaining renal function by avoiding other insults such as excessive use of nonsteroidal antiinflammatory agents, the unnecessary use of aminoglycoside antibiotics, and by properly managing urinary tract infections or distinctive uropathy due to diabetic neurogenic bladder. Patients with established diabetic nephropathy are at particularly high risk for developing acute renal failure secondary to exposure to IV contrast agents. Because of their high incidence of vascular complications, patients with diabetes are often candidates for radiocontrast administra-

tion for cardiac catherizations or other diagnostic procedures. Minimizing exposure to radiocontrast agents plays an important role in preserving residual renal function. If exposure to a radiocontrast agent is necessary, ensuring adequate intravascular volume at the time of the study is critical. (see Chapters 6 and 36).

Lastly, patients with diabetes develop uremia and require renal replacement therapy earlier than patients with other forms of renal disease. Patients with diabetes will often have a lower GFR for any given serum creatinine than a nondiabetic patient with renal insufficiency. Thus, it is not uncommon for a patient with diabetes to be near ESRD, even with a serum creatinine as low as 2 to 3 mg/dL. Diabetic patients also develop symptoms of uremia at higher GFR levels (10–15 mL/min) than patients with nondiabetic kidney disease. Establishing a vascular access for hemodialysis may be difficult because of coexistent vascular disease. Because diabetic patients have a high prevalence of cardiovascular disease, their transplantation evaluations may require extensive cardiac testing. For all of these reasons, dialysis teaching and planning as well as transplant evaluations should begin early.

TREATMENT OF ESRD

Once patients with diabetic nephropathy reach ESRD, their options are hemodialysis, peritoneal dialysis, or transplantation. Figure 4 in Chapter 65 shows the first year mortality rates for dialysis patients by year of first ESRD therapy and primary cause of ESRD. Patients with diabetes have the highest first year mortality throughout the years shown. Encouraging, however, is the overall decline in adjusted one year death rates for patients with diabetes from 1983 through 1993. Patients with diabetes who receive a cadaveric renal transplant also have a higher morbidity and mortality than the nondiabetic transplant patient. However, 2-year renal graft and patient survival rates in the type I patient with a living related donor transplant are comparable to nondiabetic ESRD patients. Survival is longer for the patient with diabetes who receives a living related donor transplant compared to a patient who remains on dialysis. Combined renal pancreas transplants have a higher morbidity rate than renal transplant alone but have improved glycemic control and motor and sensory nerve function, as well as less extensive morphologic changes of diabetic nephropathy in the allograft. No benefits are accrued in pancreatic polypeptide secretion, preservation of kidney function, or retinopathy, however.

The increased morbidity and mortality rates in ESRD patients with diabetes are primarily secondary to complications of atherosclerotic disease. Multiple investigators have demonstrated that the risk of cardiovascular disease in type I patients with renal disease far exceeds that in duration matched type I patients without nephropathy (Fig. 3). There are not only increased rates of cardiovascular events, but also excessive cerebral and peripheral vascular complications in patients with diabetes on dialysis or posttransplant. Malnutrition, as evidenced by low serum albumin values and infections, also complicate the renal replace-

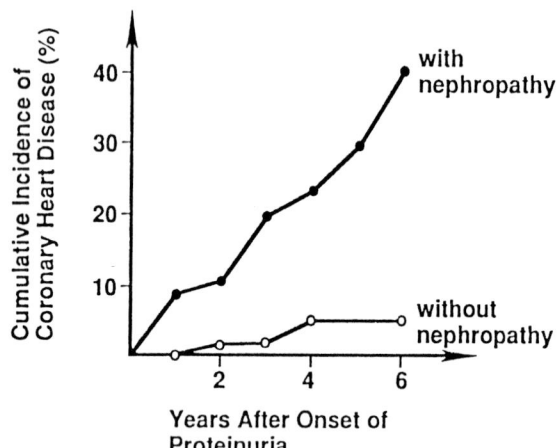

FIGURE 3 Cumulative incidence of coronary heart disease in patients with (●) and without (○) nephropathy. (Reprinted from Breyer, 1992, with permission.)

ment therapy of patients with diabetes. Thus, despite advances in renal replacement therapies, malnutrition, infection, and atherosclerotic disease shorten the life of the patient with diabetes and ESRD.

Bibliography

Bennett PH, Haffner S, Kasiske BL, et al.: Screening and management of microalbuminura in patients with diabetes mellitus: Recommendations to the scientific Advisory Board of the National Kidney Foundation from an ad hoc committee of the Council on Diabetes Mellitus of the National Kidney Foundation. *Am J Kidney* Dis 25:107–112, 1995.

Breyer JA: Diabetic nephropathy in insulin-dependent patients. *Am J Kidney Dis* 6:533–547, 1992.

Breyer JA: Medical management of nephropathy in type I diabetes mellitus: Current recommendations. *J Am Soc Nephrol* 6:1523–1529, 1995

DeFronzo RA: Diabetic nephropathy: Etiologic and therapeutic considerations. *Diabetes Rev* 3:510–564, 1995.

The Diabetes Control and Complications Trial Research Group. The effect of intensive treatment of diabetes on the development and progression of long-term complications in insulin-dependent diabetes mellitus. *N Engl J Med* 329:977–986, 1993.

The Diabetes Control and Complications Research Group: Effect of intensive therapy on the development and progression of diabetic nephropathy in the Diabetes control and Complications Trial. *Kidney Int* 7:1703–1720, 1995.

Humphrey LL, Ballard DJ, Frohnert PP, et al.: Chronic renal failure in non-insulin-dependent diabetes mellitus. *Ann Intern Med* 111:788–796, 1989.

Lewis EJ, Hunsicker LG, Bain RP, et al.: The effect of angiotensin-converting enzyme inhibition on diabetic nephropathy. *N Engl J Med* 329:1456–1462, 1993.

Mattock MB, Morrish NJ, Viberti G, et al.: Prospective study of microalbuminuria as predictor of mortality in NIDDM. *Diabetes* 41:736–741, 1992.

Mogensen CE: Microalbuminuria as a predictor of clinical diabetic nephropathy. *Kidney Int* 3:673–689, 1987.

Ritz E Stefanski A: Diabetic nephropathy in type II diabetes *Am J Kindey Dis* 27:167–194, 1996.

Tuck ML, Corry, DB: Pathophysiology and management of hypertension in diabetes. *Annu Rev Med* 42:533–58, 1991.

DYSPROTEINEMIAS AND AMYLOIDOSIS

PAUL W. SANDERS

LIGHT-CHAIN-RELATED RENAL DISEASES

Overview

Following the description of an abnormal urinary protein initially identified by Dr. William Macintyre and subsequently characterized by Dr. Henry Bence Jones in 1847, Bence Jones proteins have been found to represent immunoglobulin light chains, and the multiple renal lesions associated with deposition of these proteins have been studied extensively. Plasma cells synthesize light chains that become part of the immunoglobulin molecule. Each light chain possesses two independent globular regions, termed constant and variable domains. The variable domain forms part of the antigen-binding site and derives from rearrangement of more than 20 gene segments. Thus, despite similar biochemical properties, no two light chains are identical. Disulfide bonding among two light chains with higher molecular weight proteins (heavy chains) occurs during or shortly after heavy-chain synthesis, forming the classical immunoglobulin G molecule that is then secreted. A slight excess production of light, compared to heavy, chains appears to be required for efficient immunoglobulin synthesis, but may result in release of free light chains. Light chains can also form homodimers through disulfide bonding to another light chain before secretion.

Once in the circulation, light chains are handled similarly to other low-molecular-weight proteins, which are cleared by the kidney. Unlike albumin, monomers (~22 kDa) and dimers (~44 kDa) are readily filtered at the glomerulus and reabsorbed by the proximal tubule. In the proximal tubule, endocytosis of light chains occurs through a single class of receptors with relative selectivity for these proteins. The isoelectric point of light chains does not influence reabsorption rate. After endocytosis, lysosomal enzymes hydrolyze the proteins, and the amino acid components are returned to the circulation. Reabsorption is saturable and allows the delivery of light chains to the distal nephron and their ultimate appearance in the urine as Bence Jones proteins.

Urinary Bence Jones proteins possess unusual heat solubility properties. When heated to 60°C, the proteins precipitate, but upon further heating to 100°C, the proteins resolubilize. Although this unusual thermal property was the standard screening test for the presence of Bence Jones proteins, it is very insensitive and positive only when significant quantities are excreted in the urine. The qualitative urine dipstick test for protein also has low sensitivity for light chains. In healthy adults, the approximate urinary concentration of light chain proteins, which are polyclonal because of escape into the circulation of small amounts of free light chain produced during normal immunoglobulin assembly, is 2.5 μg/mL. Urinary light chain concentration is generally between 20 and 500 μg/mL in patients with monoclonal gammopathies of undetermined significance, and is usually much higher (range 0.02–11.8 mg/mL) in patients with multiple myeloma or Waldenström's macroglobulinemia. The amount of light chain excreted is often insufficient for detection using turbidimetric and heat tests. In addition, because of the insensitivity of routine serum protein electrophoresis (SPEP) and urinary protein electrophoresis (UPEP), these tests are no longer recommended. Identification therefore rests with antibody detection assays (immunofixation electrophoresis or immunoelectrophoresis) using serum and urine. Immunofixation electrophoresis is very sensitive and detects monoclonal light chains and immunoglobulins even in very low concentrations. The causes of monoclonal light-chain proteinuria, a hallmark of plasma cell dyscrasias, are listed (Table 1). The most common cause of light chain proteinuria is multiple myeloma.

Virtually every compartment of the kidney can be damaged from monoclonal light-chain deposition (Table 2). Histologic examination of necropsy specimens from 57 pa-

TABLE 1
Causes of Bence Jones Proteinuria

Multiple myeloma
AL-amyloidosis
Light-chain deposition disease
Waldenstrom's macroglobulinemia
Monoclonal gammopathy of undetermined significance
Heavy-chain disease (μ) (rare)
Lymphoproliferative disease (rare)
Rifampin therapy (rare)

tients demonstrated renal lesions in 48 to 49%. Sixty-five percent of those patients with renal lesions had cast nephropathy, or "myeloma kidney," while 21% had AL-amyloidosis and 11% had monoclonal light chain deposition disease (LCDD). The light chain takes the center stage in the pathogenesis of these renal lesions. The type of renal lesion induced depends on the physicochemical properties of the light claim, and the simultaneous occurrence of two or more of these lesions in the same patient is unusual.

Cast Nephropathy

Pathology

Cast nephropathy is a noninflammatory tubulointerstitial renal lesion. Characteristically, multiple intraluminal proteinaceous casts are identified mainly in the distal portion of the nephrons (Fig. 1). Casts may also be seen in the proximal tubule, or even in glomeruli when they are abundant. The casts are usually acellular, homogeneous, and eosinophilic with multiple fracture lines. Immunofluorescence and immunoelectron microscopy confirm that the casts contain light chains and Tamm-Horsfall glycoprotein. Persistence of the casts produces giant cell inflammation and tubular atrophy that typify myeloma kidney. Glomeruli are usually normal.

TABLE 2
Light-Chain-Related Renal Lesions

Glomerulopathies
Light-chain deposition disease
AL-amyloidosis
Cryoglobulinemia
Fibrillary glomerulonephritis (rare)
Immunotactoid glomerulopathy (rare)
Tubulointerstitial lesions
Cast nephropathy ("myeloma kidney")
Fanconi syndrome
Proximal tubule injury (acute tubular necrosis)
Tubulointerstitial nephritis (rare)
Vascular lesions
Asymptomatic Bence Jones proteinuria
Hyperviscosity syndrome
Neoplastic cell infiltration (rare)

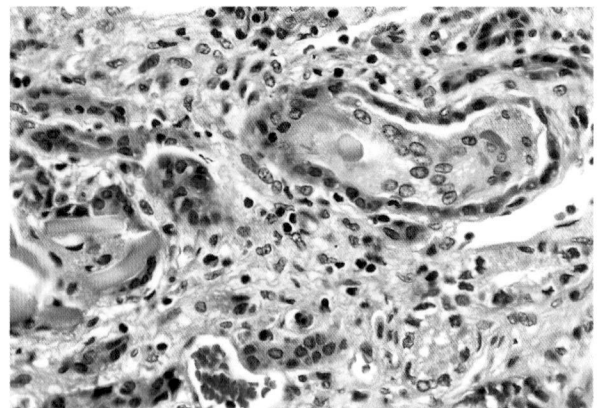

FIGURE 1 Renal biopsy tissue from a patient with myeloma cast nephropathy showing tubules with multinucleated giant cells that contain cast material. Some of the cast material has angular or rhomboid contours. Note that there is also tubular epithelial atrophy as well as interstitial edema, fibrosis, and infiltration by mononuclear leukocytes (hematoxylin–eosin stain).

Clinical Features

Renal failure from this lesion may present acutely or as a chronic progressive disease and may develop at any stage of the disease. The diagnosis is usually evident when chronic bone pain, pathologic fractures, and hypercalcemia are complicated by proteinuria and renal failure. Recently, more patients present with symptoms of renal failure or undefined proteinuria; further evaluation then confirms a malignant process. Cast nephropathy should therefore be considered when proteinuria (often more than 3 g/day), particularly without concomitant hypoalbuminemia or albuminuria, is found in a patient who is in the fourth decade of life or older. Hypertension is not common in cast nephropathy. The diagnosis may be confirmed by finding monoclonal immunoglobulins or light chains in the serum and urine and typical intraluminal cast formation on kidney biopsy. Virtually all patients with cast nephropathy have detectable monoclonal light chains in the urine or blood.

Pathogenesis

Myeloma casts contain Tamm-Horsfall glycoprotein and occur initially in the distal nephron, which provides an optimum environment for precipitation of light chains (Table 3). Casts occur in part because light chains coaggre-

gate with Tamm-Horsfall glycoprotein. Tamm-Horsfall glycoprotein, which is synthesized exclusively by cells of the thick ascending limb of the loop of Henle, is the major fraction of urinary protein and the predominant constituent of urinary casts in normal individuals. Cast-forming Bence Jones proteins bind to a common portion of the peptide backbone of Tamm-Horsfall glycoprotein; binding results in coaggregation of these proteins and subsequent occlusion of the tubule lumen by precipitated protein complexes. Intranephronal obstruction and renal failure ensue. Light chains with high affinities for Tamm-Horsfall glycoprotein are potentially nephrotoxic. Intravenous infusion of nephrotoxic human light chains in rats elevates proximal tubule pressure and decreases single nephron glomerular filtration rate; intraluminal protein casts can be identified in these kidneys.

Coaggregation of Tamm-Horsfall glycoprotein with light chains also depends upon the ionic environment and the physicochemical properties of the light chain, because not all patients with myeloma develop cast nephropathy, even when the urinary excretion of light chains is significant. Increasing concentrations of sodium chloride or calcium, but not magnesium, facilitate coaggregation. The loop diuretic furosemide augments coaggregation and accelerates intraluminal obstruction in vivo in the rat. Finally, the lower tubule fluid flow rates of the distal nephron allow more time for light chains to interact with Tamm-Horsfall glycoprotein and subsequently to obstruct the lumen. Situations where flow rates are reduced, such as volume depletion, can accelerate tubule obstruction or convert nontoxic light chains into cast-forming proteins.

Treatment and Prognosis

The principles used to treat cast nephropathy include decreasing circulating light chain and preventing coaggregation of light chain with Tamm-Horsfall glycoprotein (Table 4). Prompt and effective chemotherapy should start on diagnosis of multiple myeloma. Standard treatment employs alkylating agents and steroids. Intermittent treatment with melphalan and prednisone decreases circulating levels of light chains and stabilizes or improves renal function in two thirds of patients who present with renal failure. Fanconi syndrome may also resolve with this therapy. An alternative chemotherapeutic regimen that includes vincristine, adriamycin, and either methylprednisolone (VAMP) or dexamethasone (VAD) has been used successfully. VAD can induce a remission more rapidly than melphalan and prednisone and allow faster reduction in the amount of

---

TABLE 3

Factors Affecting Cast Formation

Concentration and type of light chain
Concentration and carbohydrate content of Tamm-Horsfall
  glycoprotein
Distal nephron [NaCl]
Distal nephron [Ca^{2+}]
Tubule fluid flow rate
Presence of furosemide or radiocontrast agents
Acidic urine

TABLE 4

Standard Therapies for Cast Nephropathy

Chemotherapy to decrease light-chain production
Increase free water intake to 2–3 L per day as tolerated
Treat hypercalcemia aggressively
Avoid exposure to furosemide, radiocontrast agents, and
  nonsteroidal anti-inflammatory agents
Alkalinize urine

circulating light chains. Dosing of VAD may be easier since the elimination of melphalan, which is mainly excreted in the urine, is problematic in patients with renal failure. Thus, VAD may be particularly beneficial in the setting of renal failure related to deposition of light chains, and the physician can rapidly determine the efficacy of such an approach. Myeloablative therapy followed by allogeneic bone marrow transplantation may also prove effective in controlling renal failure in myeloma, but it has a significant mortality and its use is currently limited to the small population who are suitable and have an HLA-compatible relative. The role of autologous bone marrow transplantation is uncertain. Plasmapheresis removes light chains from bloodstream effectively over a short period and is useful primarily in the setting of acute renal failure or hyperviscosity syndrome.

Prevention of aggregation of light chains with Tamm-Horsfall glycoprotein is the second cornerstone of therapy. Volume repletion, normalization of electrolytes, and avoidance of complicating factors such as furosemide, radiocontrast material, and nonsteroidal anti-inflammatory agents are helpful in preserving and improving renal function. Daily fluid intake, up to 3 L in the form of electrolyte-free fluids, should be encourated as long as defects in osmoregulation do not manifest. Alkalinization of the urine with oral sodium bicarbonate (or citrate) to keep the urine pH >7 may also be therapeutic and should be attempted.

Hypercalcemia occurs in more than 25% of patients with multiple myeloma. In addition to being directly nephrotoxic, hypercalcemia enhances the nephrotoxicity of light chains. In most cases, treatment of volume contraction with the infusion of saline will correct the hypercalcemia. Loop diuretics also increase calcium excretion, but furosemide, because it may facilitate nephrotoxicity from light chains, should not be administered until the patient is clinically euvolemic. Glucocorticoid therapy (prednisone, 60 mg/day) is helpful for acute management of the multiple myeloma as well as hypercalcemia. However, the response to the latter is not dramatic. Rarely, more aggressive management is necessary. The bisphosphonates, pamidronate and etidronate, are used to treat moderate hypercalcemia (serum calcium >3.25 mmol/L, or 13 mg/dL) unresponsive to other measures. Though the exact mechanism of action is debated, bisphosphonates lower serum calcium by interfering with osteoclastic bone resorption. While hypercalcemia of myeloma responds to bisphosphonates, these agents are nephrotoxic and should be administered only to euvolemic patients. Therapy with pamidronate allows out-patient management of mild hypercalcemia. Although their efficacy is transient, use of the bisphosphonates may allow time for chemotherapy and hydration to prevent recurrence of hypercalcemia.

Dialysis should be used as indicated. Perhaps 5 to 10% of patients who are dialysis dependent because of cast nephropathy will regain sufficient renal function to stop dialysis. Renal transplantation has also been successfully performed in selected patients with multiple myeloma in remission.

Renal failure decreases survival in multiple myeloma. Median survival for patients with renal failure is 20 months, compared with a median survival of 20 to 40 months for the general population of patients with myeloma. Major predictors of survival include the stage of the disease, decline in serum creatinine concentration at 1 month into treatment to 3.4 mg/dL, and response to chemotherapy. Response to chemotherapy is important: Median survival time is 36 months for responders, but only 10 months for nonresponders.

Other Tubulointerstitial Renal Lesions

Proximal tubule injury, including Fanconi syndrome, and tubulointerstitial nephritis can also rarely occur. Fanconi syndrome may precede overt multiple myeloma. Plasma cell dyscrasia should therefore be considered in the differential diagnosis when this syndrome occurs in adults. More severe damage to proximal tubule epithelium can produce clinical manifestations of acute renal failure. The mechanism of damage to the proximal epithelium is related to accumulation of toxic light chains in the endolysosomal system. An inflammatory tubulointerstitial nephritis with cellular infiltrates including eosinophils and active tubular damage has also been described. A careful search usually detects subtle light chain deposits along the tubular basement membranes almost exclusively in the areas of interstitial inflammation. This interstitial inflammatory pattern is sometimes associated with glomerular involvement, and cast formation is rare. Without detection of the deposits of light chains along the basement membrane, this lesion may be mistakenly considered to be a hypersensitivity reaction to drugs, most notably nonsteroidal antiinflammatory agents.

Light-Chain Deposition Disease

Light-chain deposition disease (LCDD) is a systemic disease but typically manifests renal failure related to a glomerular lesion associated with nonamyloid electron-dense granular deposits of monoclonal light chains with or without heavy chains. LCDD may be accompanied by other clinical features of multiple myeloma or another lymphoproliferative disorder, or may be the sole manifestation of a plasma cell dyscrasia.

Pathology

Nodular glomerulopathy with distortion of the glomerular architecture by deposition of amorphous, eosinophilic material is the most common pathologic finding observed with light microscopy (Fig. 2). These nodules, which are composed of light chains and extracellular matrix proteins, begin in the mesangium, and their appearance is reminiscent of diabetic nephropathy. Less commonly, other glomerular morphologic lesions besides nodular glomerulopathy can be seen in LCDD. Immunofluorescence microscopy demonstrates the presence of monotypical light chains in the glomeruli. Under electron microscopy, linear deposits of light-chain proteins are present in a subendothelial position along the glomerular capillary wall, along the outer aspect of tubular basement membranes, and in the mesan-

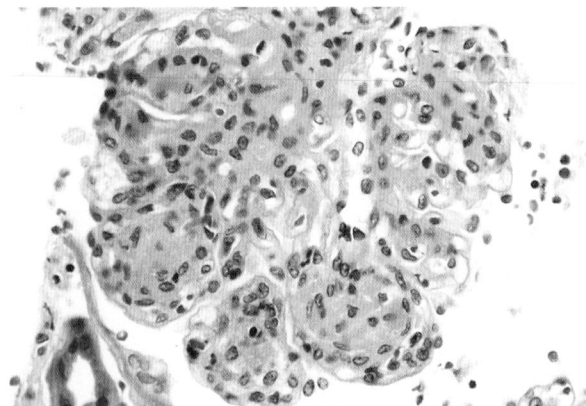

FIGURE 2 Glomerulus from a patient with κ light-chain deposition disease showing marked nodular mesangial matrix expansion with slight hypercellularity (hematoxylin–eosin stain).

gium. Tubular cell damage is also notable and obvious in some patients, even in the early stage of the disease.

Clinical Features

The clinical presentation is typical of a progressive glomerulonephritis. The major symptoms of LCDD are proteinuria, sometimes in the nephrotic range, microscopic hematuria, and renal failure. Albumin and monoclonal light chains are dominant proteins in the urine, and the presence of albuminuria and other findings of nephrotic syndrome are important clues to the presence of a glomerular lesion. The amount of excreted light chain is usually less than that found in cast nephropathy. Although extrarenal manifestations of overt multiple myeloma can manifest at presentation or over time, a majority (74%) of patients with LCDD will not develop myeloma or other malignant lymphoproliferative disease. Other organ dysfunction, especially liver and heart, can develop and is related to deposition of light chains in those organs. Development of renal failure in untreated patients is common. Because renal manifestations generally predominate and are often the sole presenting features, the diagnosis of their plasma cell dyscrasia is not infrequently first made during the evaluation of unexplained renal abnormalities. Renal biopsy, which is necessary to establish the diagnosis, is recommended early in the course.

Pathogenesis

LCDD has a pathogenesis different from that of cast nephropathy. The response to light-chain deposition includes expansion of the mesangium by extracellular matrix proteins to form nodules and eventually glomerular sclerosis. Recent experimental studies have shown that mesangial cells exposed to light chains obtained from patients with biopsy-proven LCDD produce transforming growth factor-β, which serves as an autacoid to stimulate these same cells to produce matrix proteins, including type IV collagen, laminin, and fibronectin. Thus, transforming growth factor-β plays a central role in glomerular sclerosis from LCDD.

While light chains play an important pathogenetic role in these glomerular lesions, heavy chains, along with light chains, can be identified in the deposits, prompting some authors to suggest the term monoclonal light-chain and heavy-chain deposition disease. In those specimens, the punctate electron-dense deposits appear larger and more extensive than those deposits that contain only light chains, but it is unclear whether the clinical course of these patients differs from the course of isolated light-chain deposition without heavy-chain components.

Treatment and Prognosis

The treatment of LCDD is difficult. Randomized controlled trials for treatment of this light chain-related renal disease are unavailable, but these patients appear to benefit from the same chemotherapy as that given for multiple myeloma, particularly if renal failure is mild at presentation. Five of eight patients with serum creatinine concentrations less than 4.0 mg/dL at the time of diagnosis did not progress with chemotherapy, while 9 of 11 patients with higher creatinine concentrations progressed to end-stage renal failure despite therapy. The 5-year survival is approximately 70%, and is reduced by coexistent myeloma.

AL-Amyloidosis

Amyloid represents a family of proteins. Fifteen different types of amyloid have been identified and are named according to the precursor protein that is involved in production of the amyloid. AL-amyloidosis, which is also known as "primary amyloidosis," represents a plasma cell dyscrasia that is usually characterized by systemic deposition of amyloid and a mild increase in monoclonal plasma cells in the bone marrow. However, about 20% of patients with AL-amyloidosis have overt multiple myeloma or other lymphoproliferative disorder. In AL-amyloidosis, the amyloid deposits are composed of immunoglobulin light chains.

AL-amyloidosis is a systemic disease characterized by extracellular deposition of AL-amyloid in a variety of organs (Table 5). Cardiac infiltration frequently produces congestive heart failure and is a common presenting manifestation of primary amyloidosis. Infiltration of the lungs and gastrointestinal tract is also common, but often produces few clinical manifestations. Dysesthesias, orthostatic hypotension, diarrhea, and bladder dysfunction from peripheral and autonomic neuropathies can also occur. Amyloid deposition can also produce an arthropathy that resembles rheumatoid arthritis, a bleeding diathesis, and a variety of skin manifestations that include purpura. Kidney involvement is common in primary amyloidosis.

Pathology

Glomerular lesions are the dominant renal features of AL-amyloidosis, and are characterized by the presence of mesangial nodules and glomerular sclerosis (Fig. 3). In the early stage, amyloid deposits are usually found in the mesangium and are not associated with an increase in mesangial cellularity. Deposits may also be seen along the subepithelial space of capillary loops in more advanced

TABLE 5

Relative Frequency of Organ Infiltration by Light Chains in LCDD and AL-Amyloidosis

		Organ involvement					
	Isotype	Renal	Cardiac	Liver	Neurologic	GI	Pulmonary
LCDD	$\kappa > \lambda$	++++	+++	+++	+	rare	rare
AL-amyloid	$\lambda > \kappa$	+++	++	+	+	+++	++++

Note: +, uncommon but occurs during the course of the disease; ++++, extremely common during the course of the disease.

stages. Immunohistochemistry demonstrates that the deposits consist of light chains. On electron microscopy, the deposits are characteristic randomly oriented, nonbranching fibrils 7 to 10 nm in diameter. In some cases of early amyloidosis, glomeruli may appear normal on light microscopy. Careful examination, however, will identify scattered monotypic light chains on immunofluorescence microscopy. Ultrastructural examination with immunoelectron microscopy to reveal the fibrils of AL-amyloid may be required to establish the diagnosis. As the disease advances, mesangial deposits progressively enlarge to form nodules that compress the filtering surfaces of the glomeruli and cause renal failure. Epithelial proliferation and crescent formation are rare in AL-amyloidosis.

There are significant differences between amyloidosis and LCDD. For amyloid deposition to occur, amyloid P glycoprotein must also be present. The amyloid P component is not part of the amyloid fibrils, but binds them. This glycoprotein is a constituent of normal human glomerular basement membrane and elastic fibrils. In contrast to AL-amyloid, in LCDD the light-chain deposits are punctate, granular, and electron-dense and are identified in the mesangium and/or subendothelial space. Amyloid P component is absent. Amyloid has characteristic tinctorial properties and stains with Congo red, which produces an apple-green birefringence when the tissue section is examined under polarized light, and with thioflavin T and S. These special stains are not taken up by the granular light-

chain deposits of LCDD. Another difference between these lesions is the tendency for κ light chains to compose the granular deposits of LCDD, while usually λ light chains constitute AL-amyloid. Both diseases can involve organs other than the kidney (Table 5). Amyloidosis more commonly involves the gastrointestinal tract and lungs, whereas deposits of LCDD infiltrate the liver more frequently than amyloidosis.

Clinical Features

Proteinuria and renal insufficiency are the two main renal manifestations of AL-amyloidosis. Proteinuria ranges from asymptomatic nonnephrotic proteinuria to nephrotic syndrome. More than 90% of patient have monoclonal light chains in the urine or blood, and renal insufficiency is present in 58 to 70% at the time of diagnosis. Isolated microscopic hematuria is not common in AL-amyloidosis. Biopsies of the kidney or other affected organ with ultrastructural studies and immunohistochemistry are important tools to establish the diagnosis. Scintigraphy using ^{123}I-labeled P component, which binds to amyloid, can often diagnose the degree of organ involvement from amyloid infiltration.

Pathogenesis

The pathogenesis of AL-amyloidosis is not completely understood. Recently, internalization and processing of light chains by mesangial cells has been shown to cause amyloid formation. The finding that N-terminal sequences of light-chain fragments in amyloid are identical to the sequence of soluble light chains suggests that proteolytic cleavage of light chains may play a role in causing amyloid. Presumably, intracellular oxidation or proteolysis of light chains allows formation of amyloid, which is then extruded into the extracellular space. With continued production of amyloid, the mesangium expands, compressing the filtering surface of the glomeruli and producing progressive renal failure.

Treatment and Prognosis

A recent randomized trial compared colchicine therapy alone (0.6 mg twice daily) to colchicine plus melphalan and prednisone in doses used for multiple myeloma. A 1-year course of intermittent melphalan and prednisone along with colchicine increased survival from 6.7 to 12.2 months, thus supporting the use of chemotherapy in AL-amyloidosis not associated with multiple myeloma. Colchicine should probably be continued indefinitely but

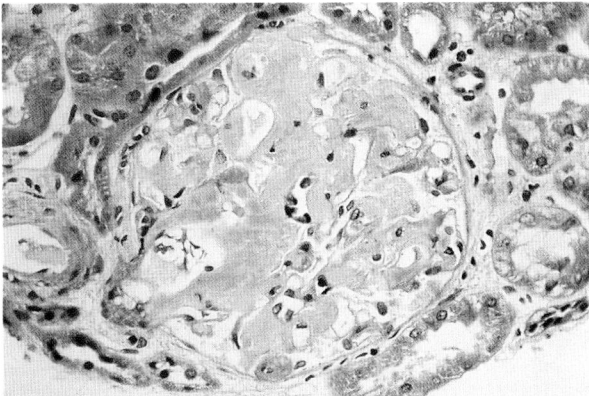

FIGURE 3 Glomerulus from a patient with AL amyloidosis showing segmentally variable accumulation of amorphous acidophilic material that is effacing portions of the glomerular architecture (hematoxylin–eosin stain).

the total dose of melphalan should be limited 600 mg because melphalan promotes development of myelodysplasia or leukemia. In another retrospective study, patients with nephrotic syndrome, a normal serum creatinine concentration, and no echocardiographic evidence of cardiac amyloidosis had the best response rate (39%) to melphalan and prednisone. Response in this subset required 11.7 months of treatment, but the median survival was 89.4 months, with 78% surviving 5 years. Eleven of seventeen patients who responded to treatment had complete resolution of nephrotic syndrome and 6 others had a 50% reduction in urinary protein excretion; only 3 of the 17 had persistent nephrotic-range proteinuria. Toxicity was significant in this series; acute leukemia or myelodysplasia developed in 7 of the responders. Survival for patients with AL-amyloidosis averages 12.2 months with chemotherapy. At present, there are no controlled trials showing that patients who do not respond to melphalan and prednisone will respond to more aggressive chemotherapeutic regimens.

Fibrillary Glomerulonephritis and Immunotactoid Glomerulopathy

Fibrillary glomerulonephritis is a rare disorder characterized ultrastructurally by the presence of amyloid-like, randomly arranged, fibrillary deposits in the capillary wall. Unlike amyloid, these fibrils are thicker (18 to 22 nm) and Congo red and thioflavin T stains are negative (Fig. 4). Most patients with fibrillary glomerulonephritis do not have a plasma cell dyscrasia; however, occasionally a plasma cell dyscrasia is present, so screening is advisable. Patients typically manifest nephrotic syndrome and varying degrees of renal failure; progression to end stage renal failure is the rule. No standard treatment for the idiopathic variety is currently available. Immunotactoid, or microtubular, glomerulopathy is usually associated with a plasma

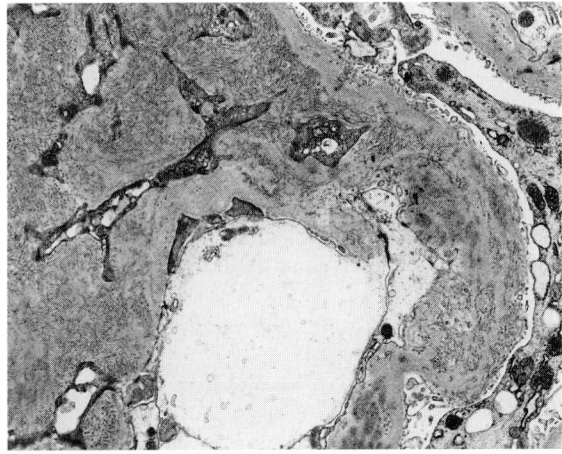

FIGURE 4 Electron micrograph of a glomerulus from a patient with fibrillary glomerulonephritis. Note the randomly arranged relatively straight fibrils with a diameter of approximately 20 nm. The overall ultrastructural appearance resembles amyloid except that the fibrils are approximately twice as thick.

cell dyscrasia. The deposits in this lesion contain thick (>30 nm), organized, microtubular structures that are located in the mesangium and along capillary walls. Cryoglobulinemia, (see Chapter 19), should be considered in the differential diagnosis and ruled out clinically. Treatment of the underlying plasma cell dyscrasia is indicated for this rare disorder.

WALDENSTRÖM'S MACROGLOBULINEMIA

This disorder constitutes about 5% of monoclonal gammopathies and is characterized by the presence of a monoclonal population of lymphocytoid plasma cells. This condition clinically behaves more like lymphoma, although the malignant cell secretes IgM (macroglobulin). IgM is not excreted and accumulates in the plasma to produce hyperviscosity syndrome. Lytic bone lesions are uncommon, but hepatosplenomegaly and lymphadenopathy are frequently identified. Hyperviscosity syndrome produces neurologic symptoms, visual impairment, bleeding diathesis, renal failure, and symptoms of hypervolemia. Renal failure is usually mild but occurs in about 30% of patients. Hyperviscosity syndrome and precipitation of IgM in the glomerular capillaries are the most common causes of renal failure. About 10 to 15% of patients develop AL-amyloidosis, but cast nephropathy is rare.

Because of the typically advanced age at presentation (sixth to seventh decade) and slowly progressive course, the major therapeutic goal is relief of symptoms. Treatment is generally plasmapheresis for hyperviscosity syndrome, followed by alkylating agents alone. All patients with monoclonal IgM levels >3 g/dL should have a serum viscosity check. Plasmapheresis is indicated in symptomatic patients and should be continued until symptoms resolve and serum viscosity normalizes. Initial chemotherapy is usually chlorambucil, which is adjusted to control serum IgM concentration and organomegaly, without inducing cytopenias. Severe renal failure requiring renal replacement therapy is uncommon. Median survival is about 3 years and is related to the advanced age at onset of this disorder.

Bibliography

Alexanian R, Dimopoulos, m: The treatment of multiple myeloma. *N Engl J Med* 330:484–489, 1994.

Buxbaum JN, J Chuba JV, Hellman GC, et al.: Monoclonal immunoglobulin deposition disease: Light chain and light and heavy chain deposition diseases and their relation to light chain amyloidosis. *Ann Intern Med* 112:455–464, 1990.

Ganeval D, Noël L-H, Preud'Homme J-L, et al.: Light-chain deposition disease: Its relation with AL-type amyloidosis. *Kidney Int* 26:1–9, 1984.

Ganeval D, Rabian C, Guérin V, et al.: Treatment of multiple myeloma with renal involvement. *Adv Nephrol* 21:347–370, 1992.

Gertz MA, Kyle RA, Greipp PR: Response rates and survival in primary systemic amyloidosis. *Blood* 77:257–262, 1991.

Heilman RL, Velosa JA, Holley KE, et al.: Long-term follow-up and response to chemotherapy in patients with light-chain deposition disease. *Am J Kidney Dis* 20:34–41, 1992.

Iványi B: Frequency of light chain deposition nephropathy relative to renal amyloidosis and Bence Jones cast nephropathy in a necropsy study of patients with myeloma. *Arch Pathol Lab Med* 114:986–987, 1990.

Jones HB: Papers on chemical pathology: Prefaced by the Gulstonian Lectures, read at the Royal College of Physicians, 1846. *Lancet* 2:88–92, 1847.

Preud'homme J-L, Aucouturier P, Touchard G, et al: Monoclonal immunoglobulin deposition disease (Randall type). Relationship with structural abnormalities of immunoglobulin chains. *Kidney Int* 46:965–972, 1994.

Sanders PW, Herrera GA, Kirk KA, et al.: Spectrum of glomerular and tubulointerstitial renal lesions associated with monotypical immunoglobulin light chain deposition. *Lab Invest* 64:527–537, 1991.

Sanders PW, Herrera GA: Monoclonal immunoglobulin light chain-related renal diseases. *Semin Nephrol* 13:324–341, 1993.

Skinner M, Anderson JJ, Simms R, et al.: Treatment of 100 patients with primary amyloidosis: A randomized trial of melphalan, prednisone, and colchicine versus colchicine only. *Am J Med* 100:290–298, 1996.

Solomon A, Weiss DT, Kattine AA:. Nephrotoxic potential of Bence Jones proteins. *N Engl J Med* 324:1845–1851, 1991.

Tagouri YM, Sanders PW, Pickens MM, et al.: In vitro AL-amyloid formation by rat and human mesangial cells. *Lab Invest* 74:290–302, 1996.

Zhu L, Herrera GA, Murphy-Ullrich JE, et al.: Pathogenesis of glomerulosclerosis in light chain deposition disease: Role for transforming growth factor-β. *Am J Pathol* 147:375–385, 1995.

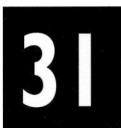

RENAL AND UROLOGIC COMPLICATIONS OF CANCER AND ITS TREATMENT

MARC B. GARNICK

Nephrourologic complications of cancer constitute a major source of morbidity and oftentimes mortality in patients with neoplastic disorders. These complications may take many forms. Cancer may be associated with glomerulonephritis, often of the immune complex variety. Urinary tract obstruction may cause significant functional and structural changes within the kidney, pelvis, and ureter, leading to acute or chronic renal failure as well as predisposing to urinary tract infection. Malignant cells may arise in or invade the renal parenchyma, leading to renal dysfunction. Cancer therapy itself may also cause renal and urothelial damage. Finally, abnormalities of urinary tract function can occur secondary to spontaneous or chemotherapy-induced tumor cell lysis in which the kidney is overwhelmed by breakdown products of rapid cellular dissolution.

GLOMERULAR DISEASE

Secondary nephrotic syndrome has been reported with adenocarcinomas of the gastrointestinal tract, including colon, rectum, stomach, and pancreas, as well as with lung, breast, ovary, skin, prostate, renal cell, and other tumors. Secondary membranous nephropathy is the histologic lesion in two thirds of patients with nephrotic syndrome and carcinomas. The nephropathy is immune-complex-mediated; carcinoembryonic and other antigens have been eluted from renal tissue of some patients. Less frequently, proliferative lesions with a nephritic picture are found.

Hodgkin's disease is associated with nephrotic syndrome, which is usually due to minimal change nephropathy. Other histologic patterns, including amyloidosis, have been observed. The activity of the minimal change nephropathy often parallels activity of the underlying lymphoma. The nephrotic syndrome responds to therapy of the lymphoma and a relapse of proteinuria may herald relapse of the tumor. Non-Hodgkin's lymphomas are associated with membranous nephropathy. Minimal change nephropathy or proliferative glomerulopathies are less frequently found.

With the use of interferons (both α and γ), rare cases of reversible, immune-mediated glomerulonephritis have been reported.

COMPLICATIONS RESULTING FROM ANATOMIC ABNORMALITIES RELATED TO THE PRIMARY DISEASE PROCESS

Urinary Tract Obstruction

Retroperitoneal tumors causing ureteral obstruction can occur with any solid neoplasm. Urologic and gynecologic cancers, together with lymphomas, are the most common causes of ureteral obstruction. Anatomically, the retroperitoneal lymph nodes which are often the drainage site for urologic or gynecological cancers or the sites of lymphomatous infiltration are along paraaortic, paracaval, and periureteral locations in the retroperitoneal space. Lymphadenopathy of mild to moderate degree which is strategically placed along the course of the ureter can result in unilateral hydronephrosis in a relatively short time. Likewise, retroperitoneal lymph node metastases or primary retroperitoneal tumors can attain a large size without ever causing ureteral obstruction because of their location with respect to the course of the ureter. Prostate cancer causes distal urinary tract obstruction due to obstruction at the bladder neck. This is also the case for advanced cervical cancer which, in addition to causing obstruction of the bladder neck, may infiltrate the retroperitoneal surfaces and obstruct the ureters. Testicular cancer, especially seminoma, can invade the retroperitoneal space and result in large bulky tumors capable of obstructing both ureters simultaneously. In addition, metastatic neoplasms of many sources can invade the retroperitoneal areolar tissues forming a plaque-like sheet of tumor, sometimes thin, that can involve and obstruct the ureters. Adenopathy may not be evident on imaging studies, making diagnosis difficult. Metastatic breast cancer, for example, may result in a desmoplastic reaction which may mimic primary retroperitoneal fibrosis. Regardless of what the cause of urinary obstruction is, prompt diagnosis and treatment are imperative, since the ability to deliver potentially nephrotoxic drugs that are curative, such as cisplatin, will be compromised early on if there is irreparable renal damage resulting from obstruction.

The management of obstructive uropathy due to cancer requires consideration of the underlying malignancy and its location, prognosis, and expected response to therapy. Obstructive uropathy is discussed in detail in Chapter 54.

Renal Parenchymal Infiltration

Renal failure resulting from bilateral replacement of the kidneys by tumor has been reported in leukemia and lymphoma. While 30 to 50% of autopsied patients with leukemia may show infiltration of the kidneys by leukemic cells, actual compromise of renal function is rare. The leukemic infiltrate is usually diffuse, but may be nodular or focal and may result in as much as a ten-fold increase in kidney size. Radiographically, renal enlargement and elongation of the calyces are common. Among the leukemias, the form most commonly associated with acute renal failure is acute lymphocytic leukemia. Radiation to the kidneys in doses of 600 to 1000 rads accompanied by cytotoxic chemotherapy is the treatment of choice for this condition.

Renal parenchymal infiltration by Hodgkin's and non-Hodgkin's lymphomas has been reported in one third of autopsied cases. Clinically, the diagnosis is suggested by flank masses or enlarged renal outlines on radiograms, but uremia from lymphomatous renal infiltration can also occur in normal-sized kidneys. Other clues incude mild, nonnephrotic proteinuria or hypertension, the latter presumably due to distention of intrarenal arteries. Pathologically, multiple discrete kidney nodules appear more frequently than diffuse enlargement. Despite the high prevalence of lymphomatous renal infiltration, however, death directly attributable to acute renal failure secondary to such tumor invasion is uncommon. In the absence of a known diagnosis of lymphoma, acute renal failure of unknown etiology merits an extensive evaluation which often includes a kidney biopsy. In the setting of widespread lymphoma and enlarged kidneys, however, an invasive diagnostic procedure is usually not indicated. When lymphoma has been shown to be the cause of acute renal failure, radiotherapy and chemotherapy in conjunction with dialysis have transiently improved renal function.

Myloma and other plasma cell dyscrasias may also cause renal dysfunction related to structural abnormalities of the kidney. These findings are discussed in Chapter 30.

COMPLICATIONS SECONDARY TO CANCER THERAPY

Genitourinary Hemorrhage

One of the most dramatic clinical events in cancer management is the development of uncontrollable urinary tract hemorrhage. Although in the past this was often due to bleeding from the bladder secondary to radiation therapy and/or cyclophosphamide or ifosfamide treatment, it is fortunately an uncommon event. Now, the use of Mesna with ifosfamide has greatly reduced the urothelial damage from this alkylating agent. Mesna is able to inactivate the toxic metabolites of ifosfamide on uroepithelial surfaces. Bleeding diathesis superimposed upon urothelial damage from toxic drugs or their metabolites in the urine is most often the etiology of urinary tract hemorrhage. Additional agents implicated in urinary tract hemorrhage, however, include L-asparaginase, actinocyceri-D, mitomycin-C, mithramycin, and 6-mercaptopurine. Patients with cancer often receivie anticoagulants and may receive antibiotics with anticoagulant effects. Together these may place the urinary tract at increased risk for bleeding.

The management of hemorrhagic cystitis requires the combined efforts of urologist and oncologist alike. Catheter drainage and continuous irrigation, intravesical cautery, and intravesical therapy with formalin have all been used with reported success. For refractory bleeding, surgical approaches including cystotomy with installation of phenol and ligation of the bladder vessels have been required. Urinary diversion and removal of the organ to stop life-threatening bleeding have on occasion been necessary.

Drug-Specific Effects

Table 1 lists potentially nephrotoxic agents.

Cisplatin

With its wide spectrum of activities, cisplatin is one of the most commonly used anticancer agents. It is primarily excreted by the kidney and accumulates in renal tubular cells selectively. Platinum resorption in the tubules leads to enzyme inhibition, alkylation of specific molecules, and generalized cellular injury that is worse in the distal nephron. Pathologic changes in the kidney include interstitial edema and tubular dilatation with relative glomerular sparing. Cisplatin damage may lead to acute renal failure, but, more commonly, a gradual and irreversible decline in renal function occurs with cumulative dosing. The presence of chloride favors the persistence of cisplatin rather than the formation of the active chemotherapeutic species, aquated dihydroxydiamino platinum. Therefore, vigorous hydration with saline should be employed when cisplatin is administered, with the goal of maintaining a urine output in excess of 200 mL/h before and for at least 18 hours after the dose. Diuretics may be employed. Most nephrotoxicity is traceable to underhydration and inattentive supervision of urinary volumes.

Cyclophosphamide

Cyclophosphamide has a wide spectrum of urological effects, including hemorrhagic cystitis (see above). The most commonly described defect of renal function is impaired water excretion, most commonly seen with the high doses (usually greater than 50 mg/kg) used for bone marrow transplantation. Laboratory manifestations of cyclophosphamide-induced impaired water excretion include hyponatremia, decreased serum osmolality, and elevated urinary sodium, but normal serum vasopressin levels. These abnormalities probably result from a direct toxic effect of cyclophosphamide metabolites on distal tubules and collecting ducts. Hypotonic solutions and solutions that induce hyponatremia should be avoided when effecting the diuresis needed to prevent hemorrhagic cystitis.

Streptozotocin

Renal damage is common following streptozotocin therapy and may present as tubular dysfunction with phosphate wasting or a complete Fanconi syndrome with aminoaciduria, proteinuria, or renal insufficiency. Careful and diligent monitoring of renal function must occur following administration.

TABLE I

Potentially Nephrotoxic Chemotherapeutic Agents

Drug	Risk High	Risk Int	Risk Low	Type Acute	Type Chronic	Specific tubular damage	Time Course Immed	Time Course Delayed
Alkylating agents								
Cisplatin	X			X	X	X	X	X
Cyclophosphamide			X			X		X
Streptozotocin[a]	X			X	X	X		X
Semustine (methyl CCNU)		X			X			X
Carmustine (BCNU)			X		X			X
Lomustine (CCNU)			X		X			X
Antimetabolites								
Methotrexate[b]	X			X			X	
Cytocine arabinoside (Ara-C)			X	X			X	
5-Fluorouracil (5-FU)[c]			X	X	X		X	
5-Azacytidine			X	X			X	
6-Thioguanine			X	X			X	
Antitumor antibiotics								
Mitomycin[d]			X		X		X	X
Mithramycin[e]	X			X			X	
Adriamycin			X	X		X		
Biologic agents								
Interferon-α			X	X			X	
Interferon-γ		X		X			X	
Corynebacterium parvum			X	X			X	
Interleukin-2		X		X			X	

From Weber B, Garnick MB, Rieselbach RE: Nephropathies due to antineoplastic agents. In: Massry SG, Glassock RJ (eds) *Textbook of Nephrology.* 2nd ed., Vol 1. Williams & Wilkins, Baltimore, pp. 818–822, 1989. With permission.

[a] Fanconi's syndrome as the most severe manifestation.
[b] Only seen with intermediate to high dose regimens.
[c] Only seen where given in combination with mitomycin C.
[d] Hemolytic-uremic syndrome as the most severe manifestation.
[e] Frequent with antineoplastic doses, rare in doses used for hypercalcemia.

Semustine (CCNU)

Nitrosoureas are excreted primarily in the urine. Dose-related renal dysfunction occurs with cumulative semustine doses, usually after 1500 mg/m^2 has been administered. The onset of renal dysfunction may also be delayed for years following completion of therapy. Pathologic examination demonstrates glomerular and interstitial fibrosis.

Methotrexate

Methotrexate competitively binds to dihydrofolate reductase, the enzyme responsible for converting folic acid to reduced folate cofactors. Drug-induced nephrotoxicity can be a prominent feature of higher dose methotrexate therapy. Although the exact mechanism of damage is unclear, three explanatory hypotheses have been suggested. The first relates to methotrexate or methotrexate metabolites precipitating in the renal tubules causing an obstructive nephropathy. Methotrexate also may have a direct effect on renal tubular cells altering regeneration of epithelial cells and ion secretory channels and other metabolic processes with a secondary feedback decrease in GFR. A third possibility relates to a direct effect on glomular perfusion causing a direct decrease in glomular filtration rate.

Toxicity is dose-related. The urinary solubility of methotrexate and its metabolites is increased at higher urine pH. Thus hydration and urinary alkalinization have been shown to be useful in minimizing toxicity. Rescue agents such as leucovorin, thymidine, carboxypeptidase, and dihydrofolate reductase that correct or bypass the effect of methotrexate have also been employed.

Mitomycin C

Mitomycin C, an antitumor antibiotic isolated from *Streptomyces caespitosis*, is primarily used in the treatment of gastrointestinal and breast cancers. Nephrotoxicity is dose-related and cumulative. Clinically, a rising blood urea nitrogen and creatinine and proteinuria are the most common features.

The hemolytic uremic syndrome may be a severe consequence of mitomycin C therapy, usually after 60 mg of the drug has been administered. Characterized by endothelial damage leading to micro-angiopathic hemolytic anemia (fragmented red blood cells on smear), irreversible uremia, and thrombocytopenia, this syndrome may also be associated with hypertension, neuropathies, and pulmonary edema. Although most commonly associated with mitomycin C, other chemotherapies have been implicated in the development of this syndrome. Once recognized, blood products should be avoided, as this may exacerbate symptoms.

Mithramycin

Mithramycin is rarely used as an antineoplastic agent; it is more frequently employed to treat cancer-related hypercalcemia. The doses required for hypercalcemia, 25 μg/kg, are much lower than the antitumor dose and rarely result in renal dysfunction. However, mithramycin may be nephrotoxic in up to 40% of patients receiving antitumor doses of 125 to 250 μg/kg. Usually mithramycin nephrotoxicity is characterized by proteinuria and a diminution in creatinine clearance, but hemolytic uremic syndrome may also occur.

Biological Response Modifiers

Biological response modifiers are receiving widespread use in the treatment of many disorders including neoplasia, chemotherapy-induced cytopenias, and viral hepatitis. Interferon-α interferon γ, corynebacterium parvum, interleukin-2, and the newly introduced colony stimulating factors, G-CSF and GM-CSF, have all occasionally been associated with nephrotoxicity. The most prominent of these is interleukin-2, administered with or without associated LAK cell therapy. Early studies with IL-2 reported a nearly 50% incidence of oliguria and azotemia. In one study of adoptive immunotherapy with IL-2, 10 of 20 patients developed creatinine elevations between 2.1 and 10 mg/dL during the course of therapy, although these elevations were usually rapidly reversible on cessation of therapy. Renal physiology studies with IL-2 administration have demonstrated universal diminution in GFR and reduction in FENa, similar to what is seen in endotoxic shock. With more recent alterations in dosing schedules, IL-2 nephrotoxicity has been diminished, although not eliminated. In one study of weekly "low-dose" IL-2, reversible nephrotoxicity occurred in 2 of 33 patients.

Renal Complications of Bone Marrow Transplantation, High-Dose Chemotherapy, and Total Body Irradiation

Over the past decade, the use of high-dose chemotherapy (HDC; with or without total body irradiation), accompanied by bone marrow transplantation and peripheral blood stem cell progenitor support, has assumed an important role in oncologic practice. Although commonly used in selected patients with lymphoma, breast cancer, and certain leukemias, this treatment modality continues to be investigated in other hematologic neoplasms, such as myeloma and solid tumors such as melanoma and testis cancer. Many of the chemotherapeutic agents listed in Table 1 have intrinsic nephrotoxicity when used in conventional doses. When super high doses are administered, a broadened range of renal derangements may occur, especially when concomitant total body irradiation (TBI) is administered as part of the preparative regimen prior to transplantation. The additional need for potentially nephrotoxic antibiotics, antifungals, and immunosuppressants may increase the incidence of nephrotoxicity.

In one study of 84 patients treated with HDC and TBI for hematologic neoplasms, the presence of significant renal dysfunction was correlated with the dose of TBI given and the presence of graft vs host disease (GVHD). Ninety-three percent (93%) of patients receiving lower doses of TBI without GVHD were free of renal dysfunction at 18 months posttransplantation compared to 52% of patients who received higher radiation doses and GVHD. Renal shielding should be recommended and renal doses carefully monitored in these patients. Another study with longer follow-up reported frequent renal dysfunction in recipients of transplantation with accompanying TBI.

The concomitant use of nonchemotherapeutic nephrotoxins, such as cyclosporine, amphotericin, and aminoglycoside antibiotics, must be scrupulously monitored to avoid synergistic adverse effects. The incidence of renal toxicity may be diminished by monitoring blood levels of these agents, as well as performing detailed pharmacokinetic profiling of the individual chemotherapeutic agents. In one study, the development (and subsequent avoidance) of potentially fatal nephrotoxicity was predicted early in the course of therapy by using real-time pharmacokinetic guided dosing.

Metabolic Complications of Tumor Lysis

Acute uric acid nephropathy may occur in a cancer patient when there is a rapid turnover of cellular contents, usually secondary to lysis of tumors sensitive to chemotherapy or radiation. Plasma levels of urate become elevated due to nucleic acid breakdown. In response to hyperuricemia, the kidney increases the tubular secretion of urate. Uric acid solubility decreases at low pH. Because of the acidification mechanisms within the distal tubule, uric acid precipitation and tubular obstruction may occur.

Uric acid nephropathy most often occurs in association with chemotherapy responsive tumors such as leukemias and lymphomas, especially Burkitt's lymphoma. It is important to anticipate the development of this complication prior to the initiation of therapy. Vigorous hydration, prophylactic use of allopurinol both before and during antineoplastic therapy, and meticulous attention to serum electrolytes, especially potassium, calcium, and phosphate, are crucial in the overall management of patients undergoing cytoreductive therapy. Urate nephropathy and the tumor lysis syndrome are discussed in detail in Chapter 25.

Radiation Nephropathy

Although uncommon today, radiation damage to the kidney had been a major complication of curative therapy of large abdominal and retroperitoneal neoplasms in which both kidneys were included in the radiation therapy port. Physiologically, alterations in glomerular filtration rate, renal plasma flow, and tubular excretory capacity occur following as little as 400 cGy delivered to the bulk of both kidneys. Urinalysis findings with radiation nephropathy include microscopic hematuria, albuminuria, and hyaline and granular casts. Pathologically the kidneys are scarred and shrunken with evidence of arteriolar fibrinoid necrosis, tubular atrophy and glomerulosclerosis. These changes usually occur over 6 to 12 months following the delivery of greater than 2300 cGy to both kidneys during a 4- to 5-week period. Acute radiation nephropathy presents with renal dysfunction and signs and symptoms referable to cardiovascular compromise secondary to hypertension, which may be accelerated or malignant. Chronic radiation nephropathy may be insidious occurring as late as 10 years following the radiation therapy treatment. Patients may present with asymptomatic renal failure and *a* clinical syndrome suggestive of chronic glomerulonephritis or tubulointerstitial disease. Today, the most effective treatment for radiation nephropathy is prevention through careful localization of the kidneys during treatment field planning and limitation of dosage and volume. It appears that the delivery of 200 cGy in 10 fractions in a 10-week period is a reasonably safe treatment plan for large abdominal tumors that are going to encompass both kidneys. There is also some potential for synergistic radiation nephropathy to occur in association with nephrotoxic agents such as dactinomycin.

Bibliography

Abelson HT. Garnick MB: Renal failure induced by cancer chemotherapy. In: Rieselbach RE, Garnick MB (eds) *Cancer and the Kidney*. Lea & Febiger, Philadelphia, pp 769–813, 1982.

Alpers CE, Cotran RS: Neoplasia and glomerular injury. *Kidney Int* 30:465–473, 1986

Averbuch SD, Austin H, Sherwin S, et al.: Acute interstitial nephritis with the nephrotic syndrome following recombinant leukocyte A interferon therapy for mycosis fungoides. *N Engl J Med* 310:32–35, 1984

Cadman E, Lundberg W, Bertino J: Hyperphosphatemia and hypocalcemia accompanying rapid cell lysis in a patient with Burkitt's lymphoma and Burkitt cell leukemia. *Am J Med* 62:283, 1977.

DeFronzo RA, Colvin OM, Braine H, et al.: Cyclophosphamide and the kidney. Cancer 33:483–491, 1973

Garnick MB: Urologic complications of cancer and its treatment. In: Holland JF, Frei III E (eds) *Cancer Medicine*, 3rd ed. Lea & Febiger, Philadelphia. pp. 2323–2331, 1993.

Garnick MG, Mayer RJ: Acute renal failure associated with neoplastic disease and its treatment. *Semin Oncol* 5:155–165, 1978.

Garnick MB, Mayer RJ, Abelson HT: Acute renal failure associated with cancer treatment. In: Brenner BM, Lazarus JM (eds) *Acute Renal Failure*, 2nd ed. Churchill-Livingstone, New York, pp. 621–657, 1988.

Harmon WE, Cohen HT, Schneeberger E, et al.: Chronic renal failure in children treated with methyl CCNU. *N Engl J Med* 300:1200–1203, 1979

Leblond V, Sutton L, Jacquiaud C, et al.: Evaluation of renal function in 60 long-term survivors of bone marrow transplantation. *J Am Soc Nephrol* 6:1661–1665, 1995.

Miralbell R, Bieri S, Mermillod B, et al.: Renal toxicity after allogeneic bone marrow transplantation: The combined effects of total-body irradiation and graft-versus-host disease. *J Clin Oncol* 14:579–585, 1996.

Morel-Maroger Striker L, Striker GE: Glomerular lesions in malignancies. *Contrib Nephrol* 48:111–124, 1985

Price TM, Murgo AJ, Keveney JJ, et al.: Renal failure and hemolytic anemia associated with mitomycin C. *Cancer* 55:51–56, 1989.

Rieselbach RE, Garnick MB: Renal diseases induced by antineoplastic agents. In: Schrier RW, Gottschalk CW (eds) *Diseases of the Kidney*, 5th ed., Vol 2. Little Brown. Boston, pp. 1165–1186, 1993.

Wright JE, Elias A, Tretyakov O, et al.: High-dose ifosfamide, caraboplatin and etoposide pharmacokinetics: Correlation of plasma drug levels with renal toxicity. *Cancer Chemother Pharmacol* 36:345–351, 1995.

32

HEMOLYTIC UREMIC SYNDROME/THROMBOTIC THROMBOCYTOPENIC PURPURA

RICHARD L. SIEGLER

Hemolytic uremic syndrome (HUS) and thrombotic thrombocytopenic purpura (TTP) are both characterized by a thrombotic microangiopathy (TMA) in target organs (Fig. 1). However, the epidemiology, clinical expression, response to therapy, and natural history of classic postdiarrheal (D⁺) HUS and TTP are sufficiently distinct to warrant viewing them as different, but similar, disorders. It must be acknowledged, however, that some cases of nondiarrheal (atypical) HUS, especially those cases seen in adults, are indistinguishable from TTP. This has led to the concept that HUS and TTP should be viewed as variable expressions of a single disorder. TTP was first described by Moschowitz in 1925 when he reported a 16-year-old female who succumbed to anemia and multiorgan TMA. Although Gasser is credited with first describing childhood HUS 30 years later, we owe much of our understanding of the clinical features and natural history of postdiarrheal (D⁺) HUS to the observations of Gianantonio in the 1960s and 1970s. A major contribution was also made by Karmali in 1983 when he recognized the syndrome's association with cytotoxin producing enterohemorrhagic *Escherichia coli* (e.g., *E. coli* O157:H7).

HEMOLYTIC UREMIC SYNDROME

Epidemiology

Ninety percent of childhood HUS, but less than 50% of adult cases, are preceded by diarrhea (D⁺) that is usually bloody (Table 1). There is persuasive evidence that the diarrhea is caused by enterohemorrhagic *E. coli* (EHEC) that produce potent cytotoxins known as Shiga-like toxins (SLT) or verotoxins. About 90% of EHEC cases in the United States are of the O157:H7 serotype, but dozens of other toxin-producing EHEC serotypes exist.

Vectors for EHEC include meat, especially beef hamburger and fermented salami. Other vectors include contaminated water, fruits, and vegetables, as well as unpasteurized apple juice, apple cider, and dairy products. Person-to-person spread has been responsible for numerous outbreaks. Cattle intestines are natural reservoirs for the bacteria. Therefore, contamination of beef with cattle feces during the slaughtering process sets the stage for HUS. Hamburger is the single most commonly recognized vector because surface contamination of sides of beef used to make hamburger results in the mixing of pathogens throughout the beef patty. Thereafter, only thorough cooking kills the toxin-producing organisms. Classic postdiarrheal (D⁺) HUS occurs predominately during the warmer months of the year; there is no clear-cut gender predilection. The median age for children is 2 years (mean age 4 years), but it also occurs in adolescents and adults. The incidence varies between different regions of the United States, but the overall annual incidence is probably about 1 to 1.5 cases for every 100,000 children less than 18 years of age. The incidence rises dramatically in infants aged 1 to 2 years (e.g., 7 cases/100,000). There are few incidence data available for D⁺ HUS in adults. A study of *E. coli* O157:H7 associated HUS in Washington State, however, demonstrated an annual incidence of approximately 1 case/100,000 population for those ages 20 to 49 years, 0.5 case/100,000 population for those 50 to 59 years of age, and close to 2 cases/100,000 population for those 60 years of age and older. Washington experiences more cases than most regions of the country, so the overall national incidence in adults is probably much lower.

Ten percent of childhood HUS and more than one-half of adult cases are not preceded by diarrhea. Nondiarrheal (D⁻) HUS, also known as atypical HUS, can be secondary or idiopathic. As with TTP, it can occur in association with nonenteric infections, during pregnancy and the postpartum period, or with primary glomerulonephritis, malignant hypertension, drugs, bone marrow transplant, cancer, and collagen vascular disorders such as systemic lupus erythematosus (SLE) and scleroderma. The most common nonenteric infection associated with HUS is pneumococcal pneumonia or meningitis, but HIV is also emerging as a causative agent. Preeclampsia can progress to HUS, which can also occur as late as 3 months following a normal delivery. Examples of drug-related causes in-

232

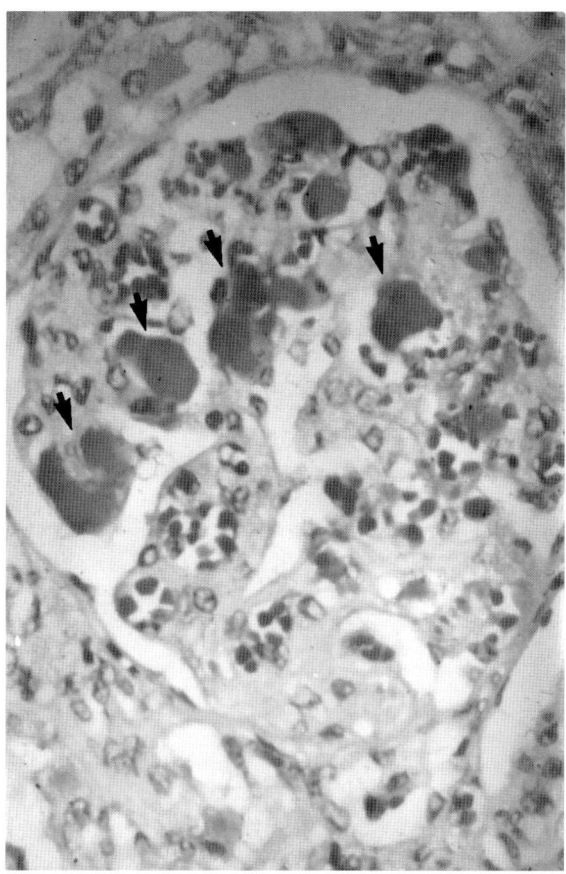

FIGURE 1 A glomerulus from a child with postdiarrheal HUS, showing microthrombi of glomerular capillaries.

clude oral contraceptives, mitomycin, and cyclosporine. Approximately 10% of patients with systemic sclerosis (scleroderma) experience rapid onset of acute renal failure with clinical and histological features of HUS. Most also have malignant hypertension. Very severe hypertension, without associated scleroderma can, on occasion, also progress to secondary HUS. Although secondary HUS accounts for the majority of D⁻ cases in adulthood, it is rare in children. The bulk of the D⁻ cases in children, and a minority in adults, are idiopathic. Some of these cases are familial.

TABLE I
Epidemiology

	D^+ HUS	TTP
Age (mean)	4 yr	35 years
Gender	Equal	70% women
Seasonality	Warm months	All year
Incidence	1–1.5/100,000	0.37/100,000
	(<18 years age)	(all ages)
Antecedents	Diarrhea	Varied

Pathogenic Cascades

The pathogenic cascade for classic postdiarrheal HUS is becoming better understood. Ingested EHEC colonize the distal ileum and large intestines via bacterial fimbrial attachment and cause a severe (hemorrhagic) colitis. This severe inflammatory response facilitates the entry of Shiga-like toxins, and probably lipopolysaccharide, into the circulation. Shiga-like toxins are 71-kDa protein subunit toxins comproised of five B subunits and one A subunit; they exist in several forms (i.e., SLT-1, SLT-2, SLT-2 variants). Following absorption into the circulation, the SLT B subunits rapidly attach to glycolipid (GB₃) receptors in the gut, kidneys, and, occasionally, other organs (e.g., brain, pancreas). The single A subunit is then internalized and inhibits protein synthesis, thereby causing cell injury or death. Even though microvascular endothelial cell injury is central to the TMA that characterizes HUS/TTP, it is not clear that the endothelial cell is the initial renal target for the toxin. There is some evidence that the renal tubular epithelial cell is initially injured in D⁺ HUS.

Shiga-like-toxins-mediated endothelial cell injury results in thickened glomerular capillary walls due to endothelial cell swelling, detachment of endothelial cells from the underlying basement membrane, and accumulation of fluffy material between the endothelial cells and basement membrane. The endothelial cell injury also results in the release of von Willebrand factor (vWF) multimers and platelet activating factor and activation of platelets, and, to a lesser extent, the coagulation cascade. Concomitantly, there are perturbations of multiple additional pathogenic cascades, including production of cytokines (e.g., tumor necrosis factor, interleukin-6, interleukin-8), as well as increased synthesis of thromboxane and endothelin coupled with decreased production of prostacyclin (PGI₂), which together impair the renal microcirculation by facilitating both microthrombotic obstruction and renal vasoconstriction.

The pathogenesis for D⁻ HUS is less well understood. Secondary HUS is presumably caused by drugs (e.g., oral contraceptives, mitomycin, cyclosporine) or condition (e.g., malignant hypertension, cancer, SLE, scleroderma) that either damage endothelial cells or favor microthrombus formation (e.g., anticardiolipin antibodies, reduced PGI₂ production). Idiopathic D⁻ HUS is sometimes familial (autosomal dominant or recessive). Low serum complement concentrations are common, and, in some families, there is deficient production of the antithrombotic prostaglandin PGI₂.

Prodrome

Classic postdiarrheal HUS is preceded by colitis that becomes bloody in about 75% of patients. Most children also experience vomiting. Abdominal pain can be severe and is sometimes initially misdiagnosed as acute appendicitis or ulcerative colitis. Rectal prolapse, intussusception, and bowel necrosis with perforation can occur. Children with nondiarrheal (D⁻) HUS usually have vomiting without diarrhea. Low-grade fever occurs in almost half, and upper respiratory infection in about one-fourth.

Clinical Features

After about 1 week of diarrhea (range 1–14 days) (Table 2), the onset of HUS is heralded by pallor, diminished urine output, lethargy, and irritability and, in close to 10% of cases, seizures. Jaundice, petechia, or purpura occur occasionally. Mild cases, with little or no renal failure, and examples of incomplete syndrome (i.e., lacking the triad of hemolytic anemia, thrombocytopenia, and acute renal failure) have been reported. Most children experience oliguric renal failure that lasts on average about 1 week. Close to one-half have a period of anuria with a duration of 3 days. Prolonged oliguria occurs occasionally.

Hypertension is present in the majority of cases of D⁺ HUS. Usually it is mild to moderate and labile, and resolves by the time of discharge from the hospital.

Seizures and other forms of severe central nervous system involvement used to be seen in close to 50% of cases. Now, however, as a result of more timely diagnoses, greater attention to fluid and electrolyte management, and earlier initiation of dialysis, metabolic encephalopathy (e.g., seizures, coma, semicoma) occurs in only about 20% of cases. A 3 to 5% incidence of stroke or generalized cerebral edema is still observed.

Pancreatic involvement is seen in approximately 20% of cases. It is usually expressed as elevated serum amylase and lipase enzyme concentrations, with or without pain, tenderness, or vomiting; pseudocysts or necrosis have not been reported. Of greater concern is insulin-dependent diabetes mellitus that has been reported to occur in close to 10% of cases; on occasion it can be permanent. On rare occasions the TMA can involve the heart, lungs, eyes, parotid gland, skin, or muscle.

Although the clinical features of nondiarrheal HUS in children can be very similar to those of classic D⁺ disease, there is a subset of D⁻ patients who present with the insidious onset of nonoliguric renal failure and malignant hypertension that often leads to congestive heart failure. The clinical expression of D⁻ HUS in adults is generally severe. Cases associated with preeclampsia are usually accompanied by fetal distress, liver involvement, and, in about one-third of cases, disseminated intravascular coagulation. Postpartum HUS typically includes severe renal failure and hypertension. Fever and neurological involvement are frequent. Cancer (especially gastric and metastatic carcinoma) and mitomycin-associated HUS are associated with a very malignant and rapidly progressive clinical course.

Laboratory features include microangiopathic hemolytic anemia, thrombocytopenia, and azotemia. The anemia is largely due to mechanical fragmentation of red blood cells (RBC) as they pass through partially occluded renal vessels. It is characterized by fragmented RBCs (e.g., burr cells, shistocytes) on blood smear and elevated serum lactic dehydrogenase concentrations. A low platelet count can be documented in about 95% of cases, but severe thrombocytopenia occurs infrequently. Prothrombin times and partial thromboplastin times are usually normal. Increased serum concentrations of hepatic enzymes, uric acid, triglycerides, and bilirubin are commonly seen.

Management

Supportive therapy continues to be the cornerstone in managing children with classic postdiarrheal HUS. Numerous therapies, including heparin, antiplatelet agents, fibrinolytic agents, vitamin E, prostacyclin, intravenous IgG, and infusion of fresh frozen plasma, have been tried, but have been found to be either too risky or of no, or only marginal, benefit. High doses of intravenous furosemide may decrease the need for dialysis in some patients.

In contrast to TTP (vide infra), the value of plasma exchange in D⁺ HUS is unclear. Although there are anecdotal reports suggesting benefit, there was only one prospective controlled clinical trial in children; it included both D⁺ and D⁻ patients. The results of this study suggest that it may be helpful in certain high-risk patients. The response, if any, to plasma exchange is certainly not dramatic, however, and in no way approaches the response seen in most cases of TTP. Moreover, the difficulty in obtaining vascular access in small infants, the high volume of blood required for operation of some systems, the expense, and the risk of infection in infusing fresh frozen plasma, coupled with the usually favorable outcome for those treated conservatively, argue against its routine use. There is a temptation to initiate plasma exchange for those doing poorly, especially for those with severe central nervous system dysfunction. Even so, if used, plasma exchange should be done with the understanding that it is of unproven value in improving the outcome in these unfortunate patients.

There is greater enthusiasm for using plasma exchange in children with atypical (nondiarrheal) HUS, and some

TABLE 2
Features

	D⁺ HUS	TTP
Severe colitis	Usually	Rarely
Fever	Mild	Prominent
Encephalopathy	20%	>90%
Thrombocytopenia	Moderate	Severe
Hemorrhage, multiorgan	Rarely	Usually
Hematuria/proteinuria	100%	75%
Oligoanuria	Usually	Occasionally
Renal failure	Usually	Occasionally
Multiorgan involvement	Occasionally	Usually
Death[a]	5%	15%
Recurrences	1%	20%

[a] With optimal therapy.

reports suggest benefit compared to historical controls who did not receive plasma exchange. There are no published prospective controlled studies to support its recommended use, however. Plasma manipulation (infusion or exchange) is commonly used to treat D⁻ HUS in adults, especially if there is neurological involvement or a relapsing course. Anecdotal reports suggest benefit, but its efficacy has not been tested in large prospective trials.

HUS occurring during pregnancy usually resolves following delivery; cases secondary to scleroderma and associated malignant hypertension benefit from treatment with angiotensin-converting enzyme (ACE) inhibitors.

Therefore, meticulous attention to fluid and electrolyte balance, control of any seizures or hypertension, blood transfusions for severe anemia, the appropriate use of dialysis, and aggressive nutritional support constitute appropriate management. Packed red blood cells should be administered for severe anemia. Since some survivors will eventually require a renal transplant, consideration should be given to using leukocyte-poor blood in order to avoid presensitization. Patients with D⁻ pneumococcal-related HUS should receive blood products that are free of anti-T antibody. Maintaining the hematocrit between 33 and 35% may improve CNS oxygen delivery in those with severe encephalopathy. Platelet transfusions should be used sparingly and limited to those with severe bleeding or those about to undergo potentially dangerous invasive vascular procedures (e.g., placement of subclavian dialysis lines), since administering platelets may provide substrate for additional platelet microthrombi deposition. Total parenteral nutrition will be necessary for those with severe colitis. Because most children have severe hypertriglyceridemia, it may not be possible to administer lipids. Because pancreatic TMA with subsequent insulin-dependent diabetes mellitus can occur, frequent blood sugar measurements are necessary, especially in those receiving high concentrations of dextrose.

Outcome

Approximately 5% of children die during the acute phase of D⁺ HUS, usually from extrarenal disease. Brain involvement (e.g., infarction, generalized edema) accounts for the majority of fatal complications, but bowel infarction, as well as heart or lung TMA, can be fatal. An additional 5% are left with chronic brain damage or end-stage renal disease (ESRD). The remaining 90% experience functional recovery, though about 5% are left with chronic hypertension and approximately half have either proteinuria or diminished glomerular filtration rate (GFR). Sometimes chronic abnormalities appear after a period of apparent recovery. Approximately 10% are left with both chronic proteinuria and low GFR and are therefore at high risk for eventually developing ESRD. Those who experience prolonged oliguria (e.g., >10 days) are at very high risk for chronic renal damage. Additional sequelae include rectal stricture (3%), diabetes mellitus (8%) that can be perma-

nent, and neurological deficits (e.g., hemiparesis) from stroke (3%). Sequelae secondary to involvement of the retina, heart, or lungs are rare (<1%). Although a recurrence occurs in only about 1% of D⁺ cases, it happens in approximately 10% of those with ESRD who receive a kidney transplant. Children with D⁻ HUS, however, experience about a 20% recurrence rate. Moreover, in most parts of the world, those with D⁻ HUS experience greater mortality and more ESRD than those with D⁺ disease. The outcome is worse in adults. Overall mortality is approximately 15 to 30%, chronic renal failure occurs in 20 to 30% of survivors, and recurrence is seen in about 25% of cases. This difference in outcome appears to be largely, but not entirely, due to the much higher incidence of D⁻ cases in the adult population. Adults who have familial HUS experience a high incidence of ESRD, and postpartum, cancer, and mitomycin-associated HUS patients experience a 50% or greater mortality rate.

THROMBOTIC THROMBOCYTOPENIC PURPURA

Epidemiology

Although there are a few reports of TTP following EHEC (e.g., *E. coli* O157:H7), enteric infections, postdiarrheal TTP is uncommon. It usually occurs during or after pregnancy, in association with certain drugs (e.g., birth control medications, mitomycin, and cyclosporine), systemic disorders (e.g., systemic lupus erythematous and scleroderma) and malignant hypertension. More reports of AIDS-associated TTP are appearing in the literature.

In contrast to D⁺ HUS, there is no seasonal variation for TTP. There is a higher incidence of disease in women, who account for about 70% of all cases. Even though the disease occurs at all ages, it is rare during infancy and in the very elderly (>80 years of age). In most series the peak incidence is during the third and fourth decades, with an average age of about 35 years. The incidence of TTP appears to be increasing, but it cannot be entirely attributed to the AIDS epidemic. The current estimate is 0.37 case per 100,000 persons per year. African Americans are afflicted more often than whites, with a relative risk ratio of 3.4.

Pathogenic Cascades

The pathogenic cascade of TTP has not been studied to the same extent as that of D⁺ HUS, but it is probably similar. Even though it is assumed that damage to endothelial cells of involved organs is also pivotal in TTP, the cause of the damage is usually obscure. Moreover, patients with TTP, but usually not those with HUS, have very large vWF multimers in their circulation during the acute phase of their disease; multimers tend to persist in those with chronic relapsing TTP. The very large multimeric forms of vWF strongly react with platelets and promote their aggregation.

Prodrome

TTP is only rarely preceded by diarrhea, but may follow a viral-flu-like syndrome characterized by fatigue, fever, abdominal pain, nausea, and vomiting.

Clinical Features

In contrast to classic D^+ HUS, patients with TTP generally present with fever (Table 2), bleeding and, in about half of the cases, CNS dysfunction. Brain involvement eventually occurs in approximately 90% of cases and is usually the dominant feature of the syndrome. Headache, somnolence, confusion, aphasia, hemiparesis, and minor motor irritability (e.g., tremor, jerkiness) are very common. Seizures occur in about one-third of patients, and coma in approximately 10%. The neurological findings often fluctuate and can be fleeting. Hemorrhage, in the form of gastrointestinal (GI) bleeding, is seen in the majority of cases, and purpura is very common. Retinal lesions occur in close to 20% of cases. Although the majority of patients show signs of renal involvement (i.e., hematuria, proteinuria, and azotemia), in contrast to HUS, oliguric renal failure with severe azotemia is uncommon. However, life-threatening involvement of other vital organs (e.g., heart, lungs) is seen much more frequently than in HUS. Laboratory findings are similar to those described for HUS, except that the thrombocytopenia tends to be more severe. This may explain the higher incidence of epistaxis, menorrhagia, purpura, and GI bleeding.

Management

The supportive therapy guidelines for HUS mentioned above also apply to treatment of TTP, but in contrast to D^+ HUS, there are also specific therapies of value. It is difficult to determine the relative efficacy of the various specific therapies, however, since in most reported series two or more therapies were administered concurrently.

Even so, there is a consensus that plasma therapies offer the greatest benefit, and they should be initiated as soon as the diagnosis is established. Plasma exchange is probably the most effective modality and with good response in 70 to 90% of cases. Its efficacy is assumed to result from removal of harmful mediators of TMA, coupled with the replacement of factors needed to inhibit the disease process. The initial replacement solution should be fresh frozen plasma; those who fail to respond can sometimes be salvaged by changing the replacement solution to cyrosupernatant, which lacks the very largest VWF multimers. There is no consensus as to frequency and duration of therapy, but seven consecutive daily treatments followed by alternate day exchanges in those showing improvement, using a total exchange volume per treatment of 1 to 1.5 times the patients predicted plasma volume, is reasonable. Treatment should be continued until remission is achieved. It is not certain that plasma exchange is superior to the infusion of fresh frozen plasma alone. The better results reported with plasma exchange may be because plasma exchange allows the infusion of much larger volumes of fresh frozen plasma, especially in those with oligoanuria. Periodic infusions of fresh frozen plasma (without plasma exchange) are often effective in preventing relapses in those with recurrent TTP.

Vincristine is probably of value in those who fail to respond to plasma exchange. Corticosteroids, iv immunoglobulins (gamma globulin), and antiplatelet agents (e.g., dipyridamole, dextran 70, ticlodipine) have all been used, usually in combination with other modalities, making if difficult to evaluate their efficacy. Splenectomy may be helpful for those who fail to respond to plasma manipulation and vincristine, or who continue to experience recurrences in spite of prophylactic infusions of fresh frozen plasma. However, this procedure carries a very high risk.

In summary, plasma exchange is the treatment of choice and should be instituted promptly. Those who fail to respond can be treated with vincristine. Splenectomy should be reserved for those who fail to benefit from less extreme therapies.

Outcome

Both mortality and recurrence are higher in TTP than in D^+ HUS. Without treatment, the death rate approaches 90%; even with modern plasma therapy there is approximately a 15% mortality rate. Uncontrollable multisystem involvement (e.g., brain, heart, lungs) accounts for most deaths. Recurrences occur in approximately 20% of cases. The relative infrequency of TTP, compared to D^+ HUS, has hampered the acquisition of long-term outcome information.

Bibliography

Bell WR, Braine HG, Ness PM, Kickler TS: Improved survival in thrombotic thrombocytopenic purpura—hemolytic uremic syndomre. Clinical experience in 108 patients. *N Engl J Med* 325:398–403, 1991.

Hayward CPM, Sutton DMC, Carter Jr WH, et al.: Treatment outcomes in patients with adult thrombotic thrombocytopenic purpura—hemolytic uremic syndrome. *Arch Intern Med* 154:982–987, 1994.

Melnyk AMS, Solez K, Kjellstrand CM: Adult hemolytic-uremic syndrome. A review of 27 cases. *Arch Intern Med* 155:2077–2084, 1995.

Remuzzi G: HUS and TTP: Variable expression of a single entity. *Kidney Int* 32:292–308, 1987.

Remuzzi G, Ruggenenti P: The hemolytic uremic syndrome. *Kidney Int* 47:2–19, 1995.

Rock GA, Shumak KH, Buskar NA, et al.: Comparison of plasma exchange with plasma infusion in the treatment of thrombotic thrombocytopenic purpura. *N Engl J Med* 325:393–397, 1991.

Ruggenenti P: Thrombotic thrombocytopenic purpura and related disorders. *Hematol/Oncol Clin North Am* 4:219–241, 1990.

Ruggenenti P, Remuzzi G: The pathophysiology and management of thrombotic thrombocytopenic purpura. *Eur J Haematol* 56:191–207, 1996.

Schieppati A, Ruggenenti P, Cornejo RP, et al.: Renal function at hospital admission as a prognostic factor in adult hemolytic uremic syndrome. *J Am Soc Nephrol* 2:1640–1644, 1992.

Siegler RL: Management of hemolytic-uremic syndrome. *J Pediatr* 112:1014–1020, 1988.

Siegler RL: Spectrum of extrarenal involvement in postdiarrheal hemolytic-uremic syndrome. *J Pediatr* 125:511–518, 1994.

Siegler RL: The hemolytic uremic sydnrome. *Pediatr Clin North Am* 42:1505–1529, 1995.

Siegler RL: Atypical hemolytic-uremic syndrome: A comparison with postdiarrheal disease. *J Pediatr* 128:505–511, 1996.

Siegler RL, Milligan MK, Burningham TH, Christofferson RD, Chang S-Y, Jorde LB: Long-term outcome and prognostic indicators in the hemolytic-uremic syndrome. *J Pediatr* 118:195–200, 1991.

Siegler RL, Pavia AT, Christofferson RD, Milligan MK: A 20 year population-based study of postdiarrheal hemolytic uremic syndrome in Utah. *Pediatrics* 94:35–40, 1994.

RENAL MANIFESTATIONS OF HIV

PATRICIA Y. SCHOENFELD

Human immunodeficiency virus (HIV) infection causes structural as well as functional abnormalities of the kidney that can occur at all stages of the illness. However, most of the acute complications are more common during later stages of disease, when clinical acquired immunodeficiency syndrome (AIDS) is present. Most clinical interest has focused on the occurrence of specific patterns of glomerular disease, such as HIV-associated nephropathy (HIVAN), but immune complex glomerulonephritis occurs in 35% of biopsied patients with HIV infection and other forms of renal disease that may be related to HIV co-infections such as hepatitis C (HCV) and hepatitis B (HBV) infection are also being recognized with greater frequency. It is well recognized that fluid, electrolyte, and acid–base disturbances and associated endocrine abnormalities occur with regularity in HIV-infected patients. Acute renal failure due to drug-induced nephrotoxicity or acute tubular necrosis associated with hypovolemia and septic shock is common in sick, hospitalized patients. Finally, end-stage renal failure (ESRD) requiring dialysis is growing in frequency and patients are surviving longer with more successful AIDS therapy and appropriate dialysis treatment.

FLUID AND ELECTROLYTE ABNORMALITIES

Hyponatremia

Of the commonly encountered fluid and electrolyte disturbances summarized in Table 1, the most frequent abnormality is hyponatremia. This disorder has been found in 30 to 60% of patients hospitalized with HIV infection. More than half of those patients develop hyponatremia from volume depletion, usually due to extrarenal losses such as diarrhea and vomiting. Inadequate volume replacement or restoration of losses with dilute fluids results in dilutional hyponatremia superimposed on absolute sodium depletion. Clinical management includes replacement of salt and water deficits, as well as measures to treat the underlying cause of volume depletion.

Hyponatremia can also occur as a result of inappropriate secretion of antidiuretic hormone (SIADH) associated with common pulmonary and intracranial diseases such as *Pneumocystis carinii* pneumonia, toxoplasmosis, and tuberculosis. Treatment of SIADH consists of fluid restriction, resulting in negative water balance and a rise in serum sodium. Persistent release of ADH due to infections that are slowly responsive to treatment may also be managed with the use of demeclocycline 600 to 1200 mg/day to block the action of ADH on the renal tubule (see Chapter 7).

HYPOKALEMIA

Abnormalities of serum potassium concentration are summarized in Table 1. Severe diarrhea due to gastrointestinal infection can often present with volume depletion, hypokalemia, and metabolic acidosis. Treatment of the underlying cause of diarrhea is of principal benefit, but most patients require large quantities of volume with bicarbonate and potassium replacement to correct the electrolyte abnormalities. A number of drugs frequently used in pa-

TABLE I
Fluid and Electrolyte Abnormalities in HIV Infection

Disorders of serum sodium concentration
  Hyponatremia
    Extrarenal salt and water loss with dilute fluid replacement
    Syndrome of inappropriate antidiuretic hormone secretion
     (SIADH)
    Adrenal dysfunction
    ? Renal salt wasting
  Hypernatremia
    Drug-induced nephrogenic diabetes insipidus
Disorders of serum potassium concentration
  Hypokalemia
    Severe diarrhea
    Drug-induced tubular dysfunction
  Hyperkalemia
    Adrenal insufficiency or isolated mineralocorticoid
     deficiency
    Renal failure
     Primary renal disease
     Drug induced renal disease
    Hyporeninemic hypoaldosteronism
    Drug related
     Trimethoprim
     Pentamidine
Acid-base disorders
  Respiratory alkalosis and acidosis
  Metabolic acidosis
    Bicarbonate loss from diarrhea
    Renal acidosis from renal failure
    Lactic acidosis
Other disorders
  Hypocalcemia
    Foscarnet
    Pentamidine
  Hypercalcemia
    CMV infection
    MAC complex
    Lymphoma
  Hyperphosphatemia
    Foscarnet induction therapy (2nd week)
  Nephrogenic diabetes insipidus
    Foscarnet
    Amphotericin B
  Increased serum uric acid concentration
    Rifampin
    Ethambutol
    Pyrazinamide
    Didanosine (ddl)

tients with AIDS can also result in hypokalemia, due to tubular dysfunction, such as that seen with amphotericin B (see Chapter 3).

HYPERKALEMIA

Hyperkalemia is most often seen in the setting of renal insufficiency associated with acute or chronic renal parenchymal disease. It may also be a manifestation of mineralo-corticoid deficiency due to either Addison's disease or more selective defects in aldosterone biosynthesis. Renal tubular abnormalities caused by interstitial nephritis, as well as adrenal dysfunction, have been reported to result in deficient production of renin and aldosterone [hyporeninemic hypoaldosteronism (HRHA)], which is clinically manifested by metabolic acidosis, hyperkalemia, and mild hyponatremia. Clinical HRHA has been reported to occur in 50% of patients with unexplained persistant hyperkalemia. This disorder, termed type IV renal tubular acidosis, will often respond clinically to treatment of the underlying disorder and the use of loop diuretics or fludrocortisone to correct the distal tubular defects in potassium and acid secretion (see Chapters 9 and 13).

Pentamidine has been shown to inhibit distal nephron reabsorption of sodium by blocking apical sodium channels in a fashion similar to the potassium-sparing diuretic amiloride. This results in a decrease in the electrochemical gradient that drives distal potassium secretion and thus can result in hyperkalemia. High-dose trimethoprim-sulfamethoxazole (20 and 100 mg · kg^{-1} · day^{-1}, respectively) and trimethoprim dapsone has also been reported to cause an increase in serum potassium in 20 to 53% of patients, due to the action of trimethoprim, which also mimicks that of amiloride. This side effect usually occurs 7 to 10 days after the start of treatment and can increase further with continuing therapy. Patients require close monitoring of serum potassium to prevent life-threatening hyperkalemia.

ACID–BASE DISORDERS

The most common acid–base disturbances in AIDS patients are respiratory alkalosis and respiratory acidosis due to pulmonary and central nervous system opportunistic infection. Respiratory alkalosis is often the initial disturbance, but as lung disease worsens and gas exchange deteriorates, hypercapnia and respiratory acidosis will occur. Metabolic acidosis occurs as a result of several different causes listed in Table 1.

1. Hyperchloremic metabolic acidosis occurs in patients with large diarrheal losses of alkali in the stool secondary to intestinal infection. This type of acidosis can also present as renal tubular acidosis due to distal tubular dysfunction associated with drug toxicity or in patients with isolated hypoaldosteronism or, more rarely, adrenal insufficiency.
2. Patients with acute or progressive chronic renal insufficiency develop metabolic acidosis, which may be accompanied by an increase in anion gap.
3. Lactic acidosis manifested by markedly elevated blood lactate levels, has been reported in a small number of patients, but without associated hypoxemia, tissue hypoperfusion, malignancy, or sepsis. Some patients were taking Zidovudine, which suggests a possible relationship between the drug and mitochondrial dysfunction. While this is a rare complication, its serious nature requires

prompt diagnosis and treatment with conventional measures as well as thiamine.

Other Electrolyte Disturbances

Abnormalities in serum calcium, phosphorus, magnesium, and uric acid concentrations have been reported, although the causes of these disturbances are not well understood. The use of Foscarnet has been found to produce a dose-related drop in ionized calcium with normal total serum calcium. It is also frequently associated with transient hyperphosphatemia during the second week of induction therapy. Granulomatous infections, disseminated cytomegalovirus infection, human T cell leukemia, and lymphoma can cause hypercalcemia, with the latter being due to the production of 25-hydroxylase by tumor cells resulting in increased hydoxylation of 25-hydroxyvitamin D to dihydroxyvitamin D3. Other drugs listed in Tables 1 and 2 can cause various disturbances in these electrolytes. Infection with *P. carinii* pneumonia is associated with macrophage dysfunction, which has been reported to result in abnormal vitamin D metabolism and elevated 1,25-dihydroxyvitamin D levels, which corrects with treatment of the pneumonia. Hypercalcemia may be missed due to the frequent occurrence of hypoalbuminemia in HIV-infected patients. However, measurement of the ionized calcium level will reveal the presence of this complication.

TABLE 2
Cause of Acute Renal Failure in HIV-Infected Patients

Drug toxicity	ATN	TIN	Other
TMP-SMX		+++	Hyperkalemia
Foscarnet	+++	+/−	Crystalluria
Amphotericin B	+++		Hypokalemia
Pentamidine	++		Hyperkalemia
Rifampin	+++		
Acyclovir	++	+	Crystalluria/ obstruction
Dapsone (rare)	+		Papillary necrosis
Sulfadiazine		++	
Interferon-α			MPGN

Acute tubular necrosis

Rhabdomyolysis

Hemolytic uremic syndrome/thrombotic thrombocytopenic purpura

Postinfectious GN

Plasmacytic interstitial nephritis

Obstructive uropathy
    Crystalluria (acyclovir, sulfadiazine, uric acid)
    Tumor lysis syndrome (increased PO_4, uric acid)
    Retroperitoneal fibrosis
    Ureteral compression (tumor, lymph nodes)

ATN, Acute tubular necrosis; TIN, tubulointerstitial nephritis; GN, glomerulonephritis; MPGN, membranoproliferative glomerulonephritis

ACUTE RENAL FAILURE

Acute renal failure (ARF) has been reported to occur in 3 to 4 % of HIV-infected patients in New York and Miami; another center in New York reported an incidence of 20% in a retrospective analysis of AIDS patients in the mid-1980s. These figures compare to an incidence rate of 4 to 5% in hospitalized non–HIV-infected patients. The cause of ARF in 88 patients from the latter study was volume depletion in 30%, drug toxicity in 42%, and shock or hemodynamic instability in 17%. Others have reported drug toxicity (59%) or sepsis, either directly or indirectly (75%), to be the major cause of ARF. Table 2 summarizes the major factors causing ARF, including some of the more common drugs responsible for nephrotoxicity. Both oliguric and nonoliguric forms of renal failure can be encountered, and the natural course of the renal disease is similar to that associated with other acute illness. Survival and recovery from ARF are usually dependent on the nature and severity of the underlying illness, and the mortality rate in AIDS patients is about 50 to 60%—a figure that is not different from the general population. Dialytic and conventional support measures are often successful in reversing renal insufficiency, particularly in patients whose HIV infection is not as advanced.

STRUCTURAL RENAL DISEASE

HIV-Associated Nephropathy (HIVAN)

This unique clinical and histopathological renal disease is thought to be the direct result of HIV in the kidney. It occurs in about 5 to 10% of HIV-infected patients, but the prevalence and geographical distribution are not uniform and depend on specific risk factors for HIV which are race, gender, and social behavior dependent. There is a striking predilection of HIVAN for African-American individuals, as is also true for focal segmental glomerulosclerosis (FSGS) associated with intravenous drug use (IDU). This is in contrast to IgA nephropathy, which has been reported primarily in whites, and other forms of immune complex disease, which occur in all racial groups. HIVAN is 7 to 10 times more common in men than women, and 30 to 60% have a history of IDU. Thus, in the United States, the typical patient with HIVAN is a young black male with a history of IDU who presents with the typical clinical presentation shown in Table 3. HIVAN has been reported

TABLE 3
Clinical Manifestations of HIVAN

Heavy proteinura
Azotemia
Enlarged kidneys
Normal blood pressure
Rapid progression to ESRD without treatment
Improved renal function and delayed progression with combination antiviral treatment

ESRD, end-stage renal disease.

to occur in about 8% of children with AIDS from the University of Miami.

The pathology of HIVAN has been well characterized and is summarized in Table 4 and Figs. 1 and 2. There are characteristic glomerular, tubulointerstitial, and ultrastructural lesions. The glomeruli show diffuse epithelial cell changes with prominent collapse of the glomerular tuft. Most biopsies show FSGS and obsolescent glomeruli; earlier stages have visceral epithelial cell swelling and hypertrophy with periodic acid–Schiff positive inclusion droplets which stain with immunoglobulin sera on immunofluorescence. There are typically large dilated tubules containing hyaline occlusive casts and prominent lymphocytic infiltration of the interstitium. Ultrastructural changes consist of numerous tubuloreticular structures in the endoplasmic reticulum of glomerular and endothelial cells and in interstitial leukocytes. Nuclear bodies are noted in greater frequency. The ultrastructural changes are not unique to HIVAN, as they are also seen in idiopathic FSGS and heroin nephropathy. They may represent a common viral marker for different forms of renal disease. Collectively,

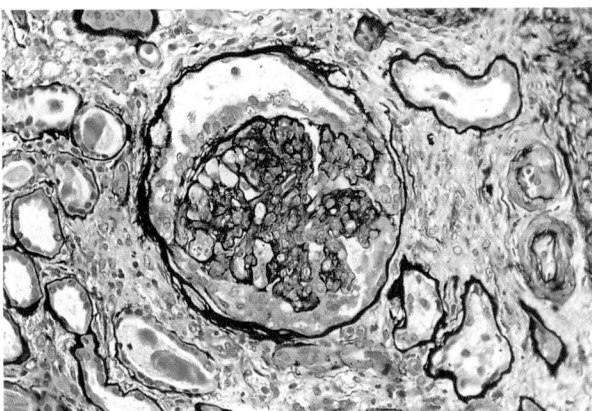

FIGURE 1   Glomerulus from a patient with HIV-associated nephropathy showing extensive global collapse of capillaries and hypertrophy and slight hyperplasia of visceral epithelial cells. Also note interstitial fibrosis and tubular atrophy (henatoxylin–eosin–methionine stain). Courtesy of Dr. J.C. Jennette.

TABLE 4

Pathology of the Kidney in HIV Infection

Interstitial renal disease
  Infections
    CMV
    Cryptococcosis
    Histoplasmosis
    Mycobacteria
    Fungal agents (candida, aspergillosis)
  Malignancy
    Kaposi's sarcoma
    Lymphoma
  Acute tubular necrosis

HIV-associated nephropathy (HIVAN)
  FSGS
    Widespread visceral epithelial changes
    Global collapse of the glomerular tuft
  Interstitial fibrosis
  Tubular dilatation with proteinaceous casts
  Ultrastructural changes
    Tubuloreticular inclusions
    Nuclear bodies
    Granulofibrillary transformation

Other glomerular disease
  Immune complex glomerulonephritis
    Membranoproliferative GN (HCV and cryoglobulinemia,
      HBV related)
    IgA nephropathy
    Membraneous nephropathy
    Postinfectious GN
    Diffuse proliferative GN
  Mesangial hyperplasia
  Minimal change disease
  AA Amyloidosis

Note: CMV, cytomegalovirus; FSGS, focal segmental glomerulosclerosis; GN, glomerulonephritis; HBV, hepatitis B virus; HCV, hepatitis C virus

the histological findings above are the basis for defining HIVAN as a distinct renal disease, different from the other causes of FSGS.

The pathogenesis of HIVAN has been intensely studied over the past 10 years, and the accumulated data provide substantial evidence that HIVAN is caused by localization of the virus in the kidney. However, the mechanism by which HIV leads to glomerulosclerosis remains unknown. Mesangial cells of the normal kidney express CD4 antigen, which is the receptor for the gp120 envelope protein of HIV. HIV core p24 antigen has been localized by immunochemistry in tubular epithelial cell cytoplasm. The HIV genome has been found in tubular and glomerular epithelial cells using in situ hybridization and a cDNA nucleic probe in patients with HIVAN, but not in patients with immune-mediated glomerulonephritis or HIV seronegative patients. Several investigators have succeeded in infecting glomerular cells by exposing them to HIV in vitro. With more sensitive PCR techniques, HIV DNA has been detected in HIV-infected patients with proteinuria, and the genome was present in all renal cell types except interstitial cells. All these studies suggest that the HIV genome is ubiquitous in renal tissue of HIV-infected patients, regardless of type of renal disease. However, the genome itself is probably not enough for the development of sclerosis, and other mechanisms are necessary for the induction of the disease. Other possible factors in the pathogenesis of renal disease, especially the interstitial pathology, include the presence of many different infectious agents that have been found in kidneys of patients dying with AIDS. Cytokines and growth factors are important in the progression of idiopathic FSGS and may contribute to the rapid progression in HIV patients.

Until recently the clinical course of HIVAN has been one of inexorable progression to ESRD in 6 to 12 months. As summarized in Table 5, different types of treatment have been attempted with some modest success to date. These include the use of antiviral agents such as the nucleo-

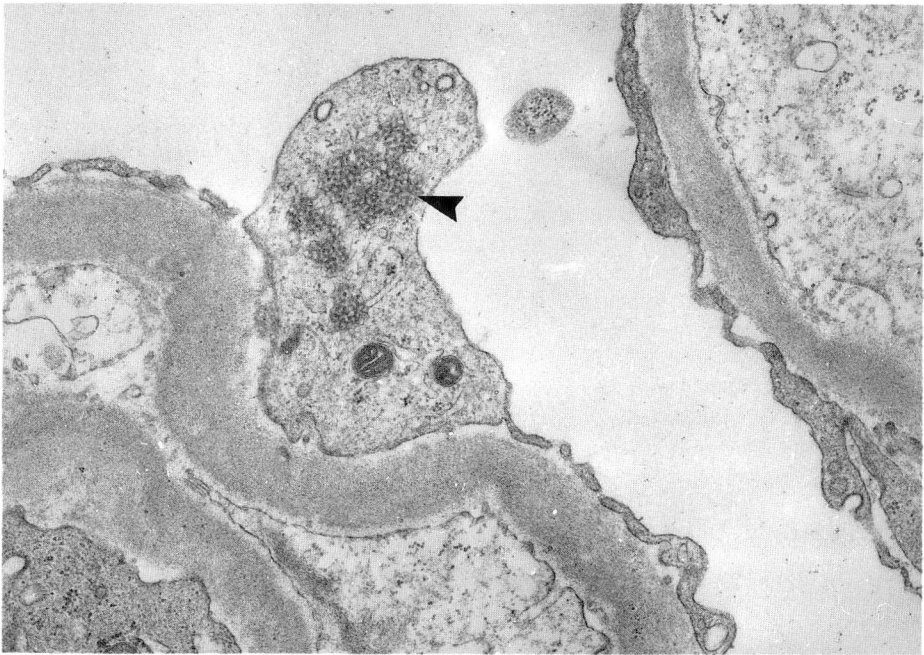

FIGURE 2   Electron micrograph of glomerular capillary from a patient with HIV-associated nephropathy, demonstrating endothelial tubuloreticular inclusions (arrow).

side analogues Zidovudine (AZT) and /or didanosine (ddI), which have been used by several groups who reported temporary remission or delay of progression of renal disease for as long as 33 months. The most benefit with these agents appears to be in patients who are treated early and before azotemia develops. The use of immunomodulator therapy has been reported to improve renal function and to delay progression in small number of patients. However, steroid-induced complications were significant and patients relapsed when the drug was stopped. Recently, even greater hope for HIV-infected patients with renal disease has emerged with the institution of combination antiviral therapy which includes nucleoside analogues and a protease inhibitor, such as AZT, 3TC, and Indinavir. Several reports have demonstrated striking falls in viral

load with the use of protease inhibitors, and preliminary experience with this type of drug regimen in predialysis patients and one dialyzed patient in our clinics has shown improvement in renal function associated with large decreases in viral load measurements to undetectable levels (less than 500 copies). When to start such treatment remains controversial, but all agree that it should be used in advanced HIV disease and many would use it in patients with CD4 counts below 300 to 400 or with viral loads greater than 5000 copies. Use in patients with renal disease is not well defined, but it would seem logical to start treatment when HIV-related kidney disease is diagnosed, especially HIVAN. Experience with this regimen in the treatment of immune-mediated renal disease in HIV-infected patients (see below) is not available. It is recommended that viral load measurements be used for following the course of disease and obtained twice at 1-month intervals to establish a baseline, then quarterly, and 4 weeks after establishing new therapy.

TABLE 5

Treatment of HIVAN

Nucleoside analogues
  AZT (zidovudine)
  ddI (Didanosine)
  3TC (Lamivudine)

Immunomodulators
  Steroids
  Cyclosporine

Angiotensin-converting enzyme inhibitors

Combination nucleoside analogue and protease inhibitor antiretroviral therapy
  AZT, 3TC, Indinavir

Immune-Mediated Renal Disease

As mentioned earlier, 25 to 50% of patients with HIV infection have been found to have renal histopathological abnormalities on renal biopsy consistent with a diagnosis of immune-mediated renal disease, which may be associated with some features of HIVAN. Membranoproliferative and diffuse proliferative glomerulonephritis, membranous, and IgA nephropathy have been found on renal biopsy in patients with HIV infection. The significance of such disparate types of renal disease is unclear, but the possible pathogenetic mechanisms include the deposition of HIV antigen–antibody immune complexes in response to infectious agents or as a specific immune complex directly causing renal disease. In some cases, the renal disease may be indirectly related or even unrelated to the HIV, but influenced by the patient's genetic makeup, infectious complications of AIDS, HIV therapy, or differences in systemic host responses.

The diagnoses most commonly reported include IgA nephropathy, focal proliferative, and membranoproliferative glomerulonephritis. IgA nephropathy occurs mostly in whites and tends to be mild or slowly progressive compared to the more rapid course of HIVAN. The relationship of IgA nephropathy to HIV is unclear, but increased circulating levels of IgA and the presence of circulating immune complexes containing IgA are common findings in HIV-infected patients and may result from abnormal IgA regulation, which leads to deposition in the kidney and renal disease.

HCV and HIV co-infection are common, especially in patients with a history of IDU as the primary risk factor for these infections. Such patients presenting with hematuria and cryoglobulinemia frequently have membranoproliferative glomerulonephritis on renal biopsy, a finding in about 50% of HIV-infected patients presenting with hematuria to our renal clinic. It is unclear whether the cryoprecipitate is related to anti-HCV associated antibodies or whether immune complexes containing HIV antigens are involved as well.

Other forms of renal disease including minimal change disease, AA amyloidosis, hemolytic uremic syndrome/thrombotic thrombocytopenic purpura, and tumor invasion of the kidneys have been reported with less frequency.

END-STAGE RENAL DISEASE

While renal transplantation is not currently an option for most patients with ESRD and HIV, many patients are treated successfully with chronic dialysis therapy. The incidence of centers providing dialysis for Patients with HIV has increased from 11% in 1985 to 37% in 1994. During 1994, 1.5% or 3144 dialyzed patients had HIV; however since only 28% of centers tested for the AIDS virus at entry to dialysis, this probably represents an underestimate of the prevalence of dialyzed patients with HIV. Incidence figures are not available. However, in the dialysis program at San Francisco General Hospital, 15% of new dialysis patients each year are positive for HIV.

The choice of dialysis modality has implications not present in the non–HIV-infected patient, including risk of disease transmission, care of patients with communicable diseases, ethical issues related to the care of the terminally ill, and shortened survival. For many of these considerations, peritoneal dialysis (PD) has had distinct medical advantages, including fewer invasive procedures, less exposure to potential infections, and possibly less stimulation of the immune system by blood membrane interactions. Staff who care for HIV-infected patients on PD have fewer risks

of needle stick, less equipment involved, and less overall contact with patients with communicable diseases. Potential disadvantages to PD therapy include increased frequency of peritonitis in some patients, peritonitis due to fungal or other opportunistic organisms, and technique failure as advanced AIDS-related complications may limit the ability to do self-care.

Survival of dialyzed patients with HIV has been recently reviewed for a 10-year period from 1985 to 1995 in a group of 62 patients treated at the University of California Renal Center at San Francisco Hospital. The median survival for all patients was 10 months compared to 17 months for AIDS patients without ESRD followed by the Department of Public Health in San Francisco. In patients with CD4 counts above 200 cells/mL, survival was substantially better, 33 months compared to 7 months in patients with CD4 counts below 200. Patients able to do PD had a significantly longer survival than patients treated with hemodialysis, but some of this advantage may be due to earlier stage of disease in those patients. Survival was positively correlated with CD4 count, as well as serum albumin concentration, which fell progressively with disease progression. HIV-related cognitive motor complex was more common in dialyzed patients than reported for the general AIDS population, and also correlated significantly with overall survival.

The diagnosis and clinical care of HIV-infected patients with renal disease are challenging and require a concerted effort from nephrology and AIDS care professionals. Appropriate antiviral agents, prophylactic care to prevent complications, and adequate dialysis therapy are all required to prolong survival. New regimens of combination antiviral therapy, including protease inhibitors, assessment of the stage of illness with viral load measurements, and earlier treatment of infection and renal disease offer new hope for the delay of progression to ESRD and for optimizing survival in those treated with chronic dialysis.

Bibliography

Carpenter CCJ, Fischl MA, Hammer SM, et al.: Antiretroviral therapy for HIV infection in 1996. Recommendations of an International Panel. *JAMA* 276: 146–154, 1996.

Cohen AH: Renal pathology of HIV-associated nephropathy. In: Kinmel PL, Berns JS (eds) *Renal and Urologic Aspects of HIV Infection*. Churchill Liningstone, New York, pp. 155–180, 1995.

D'Agati V, Appel GB: HIV infection and the Kidney. *J Am Soc Nephrol* 8:138–152, 1997.

Humphreys MH: Human immunodeficiency virus-associated renal disease. *Kidney Int* 48: 311–320, 1995.

Humphreys MH, Schoenfeld P: Electrolyte, acid-base, and endocrine disturbances in patients with HIV infection. In: Kinmel PL, Berns JS (eds). *Renal and Urologic Aspects of HIV Infection*. Churchill Livingstone, New York, pp. 27–40, 1995.

Mellors JW, Rinaldo CR, Gupta P, et al.: Prognosis in HIV-1 infection predicted by the quantity of virus in the plasma. *Science* 272: 1167–11170, 1996.

Pardo V, Strauss J, Abitbol C, Zilleruelo G: Renal disease in children with HIV infection: In: Kimmel PL, Berns JS (eds)

Renal and Urologic Aspects of HIV Infection. Churchill Livingstone, New York, pp. 135–153, 1995.

Rao TK, Friedman EA, Nicastri AD: The types of renal disease in the aquired immunodeficiency syndrome. *N Engl J Med* 316: 1062–1068, 1987.

Rao TK, Friedman EA: Outcome of severe renal failure in patients with acquired immunodeficiency syndrome. *Am J Kidney Dis* 25: 309–398, 1995.

Rao TKS: Renal complications in HIV disease. Management of the HIV-Infected patient, Part I. In *Medical Clinics of North America* 80 (6), 1996.

Schoenfeld P, Mendelson M, Rodriquez R: Survival of ESRD patients with HIV infection. *J Am Soc Nephrol* 6:561, 1995.

Schoenfeld P, Rodriquez R: Renal aspects of HIV disease. In: Cohen PT, Sande MA, Volberding PA (eds) *The AIDS Knowledge Base.* 3rd ed. Little, Brown & Co., Boston, 1997, in press.

SECTION 5

ACUTE RENAL FAILURE

34

PATHOPHYSIOLOGY OF ACUTE RENAL FAILURE

ROBERT SAFIRSTEIN

The syndrome of acute renal failure (ARF) is defined as a reduction of glomerular filtration rate (GFR) that is often reversible. The syndrome may occur in three clinical settings: (1) as an adaptive response to severe volume depletion and hypotension with structurally and functionally intact nephrons; (2) in response to cytotoxic insults to the kidney when both renal structure and function are abnormal; and (3) when the passage of urine is blocked. Thus ARF may be classified as prerenal, intrinsic, and postrenal. While this classification is useful in establishing a differential diagnosis, it is now evident that many pathophysiologic features are shared among the different categories. The intrinsic form of the syndrome may be accompanied by a well-defined sequence of events: an initiation phase characterized by daily increases in serum creatinine and reduced urinary volume; a maintenance phase, where GFR is relatively stable and urine volume may be increased; and a recovery phase in which serum creatinine falls and tubule function is restored. This sequence of events is not always apparent and oliguria may not be present at all. The reason for this lack of uniform clinical presentation is most probably a reflection of the variable nature of the injury. It is also useful to classify ARF as oliguric or nonoliguric based on the daily urine excretion. Oliguria is defined as a daily urine volume of less than 350 to 400 mL/day. Stratification of the renal failure along these lines helps in decision making, such as the timing of dialysis, and seems to be an important criterion for response to therapy (see below). This chapter considers the pathophysiology of the syndrome, focusing especially on the intrinsic form of the disease, and introducing newer concepts of what causes the syndrome, based on recent observations in human and animal forms of the disease. This better understanding of ARF has lead to newer approaches to treatment that is hoped will improve outcome in this group of patients.

MORPHOLOGY OF ARF

The changes in renal epithelial morphology that accompany ARF are subtle. At least four cellular fates can be identified in ARF: cells may die either by frank necrosis or in apoptosis; they may replicate and divide; or they may appear indifferent to the stress (Fig. 1). Frank necrosis, as is often seen experimentally, is not prominent in the vast majority of human cases. Necrosis is usually patchy, involving individual cells or small clusters of cells, sometimes resulting in small areas of denuded basement membrane. Less obvious injury is more often noted, including loss of brush borders, flattening of the epithelium, detachment of cells, intratubular cast formation, and dilatation of the lumen. While proximal tubules show many of these changes, injury to the distal nephron can also be demonstrated when human biopsy material is closely examined. The distal nephron is also the site of obstruction by desquamated cells and cellular debris.

Apoptosis has been noted in ischemic and nephrotoxic forms of ARF. This form of cell death differs from frank necrosis in that it requires the activation of a regulated program that leads to DNA fragmentation, cytoplasmic condensation, and cell loss without precipitating an inflammatory response (Table 1). In contradistinction to necrosis, the principal site of apoptotic cell death is the distal nephron.

Disruption of the cell cytoskeleton seems to be an important determinant of many of the early morphologic changes, especially in ischemic injury. Loss of the integrity of the actin cytoskeleton leads to flattening of the epithelium, with loss of the brush border, loss of focal cell contacts and subsequent disengagement of the cell from the underlying substratum. Membrane proteins, including the integrins and the Na, K-ATPase, redistribute in the plasma membrane as cells lose their polarity. The functional impact of these changes is great as cells lose their capacity to achieve vectorial transport, and the redistribution of the adhesion molecules from the basolateral membrane sites provokes intratubular obstruction. These sublethal changes contribute considerably to the severe impairment of function (see section later on treatment of ARF), and may help explain the often disproportionate decline in renal function when compared to the minor morphologic changes observed.

Molecular Responses to Renal Injury: Implications for Cell Fate

In sections of the kidney taken from patients with ARF, regeneration and necrosis coexist, indicating how early the

247

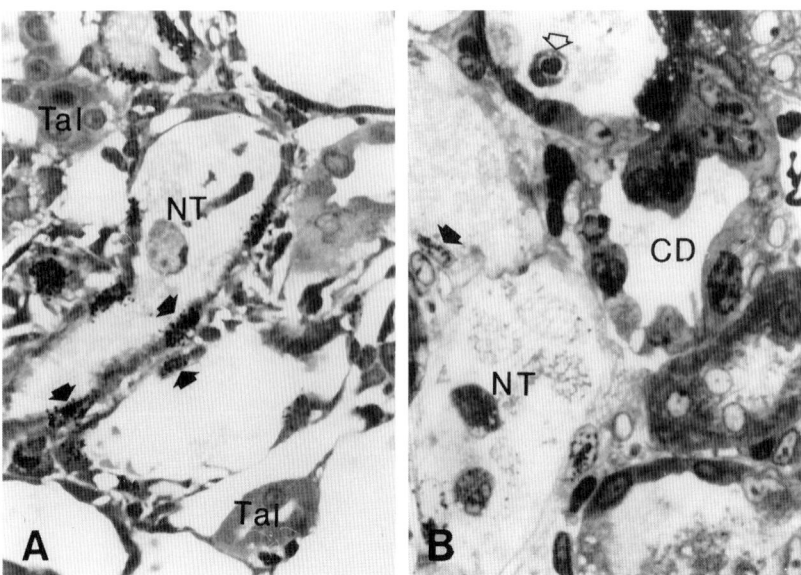

FIGURE I   Representative photomicrographs of outer stripe of outer medulla of rat kidney 5 days after cisplatin injection (5 mg/kg body wt) demonstrating cell fate during acute renal failure. (A) Necrosis of the S3 segment of the proximal convoluted tubule is apparent (NT). The solid arrows show regenerating tubules, indicated by the uptake of ^{3}H-thymidine. (B) The open arrow shows an apoptotic body. Thick ascending limbs (Tal) and collecting ducts (CD) are without apparent morphological damage.

attempt to repair the kidney is initiated in the course of renal failure. Even in its most severe form, few patients who survive initial dialysis require long-term dialysis, indicating how effective this repair process is. The regeneration process is accompanied by increased renal DNA synthesis and is proceeded by prominent changes in gene expression. The changes in renal gene expression can be grouped in at least three major categories (Table 2).

Many of the genes that are expressed after renal injury are involved in cell cycle regulation and are similar to those expressed when growth factors are added to cells to stimulate them to enter the growth cycle. Although the endogenous growth factors that serve this response have not been identified, administration of growth factors exogenously has been shown to ameliorate and hasten recovery from ARF (see Section later on treatment of ARF).

Another group of genes are proinflammatory and chemotactic and may be responsible for the apparent inflammatory aspects of ARF. Depletion of neutrophils, and blockade of neutrophil adhesion each reduce renal injury following ischemia indicating that the inflammatory response is in part responsible for some features of ARF. This mechanism may be especially prominent in posttransplant ARF. This proinflammatory state may also be important in the prescription of dialysis, especially in sepsis where consideration should be given to whether the procedure will enhance or reduce cytokine production (see below).

These two aspects of the renal molecular response to injury—the increases in protooncogene and chemokine expression—resemble what is observed in cells exposed to adverse environmental conditions such as ionizing radiation, oxidants, and hypertonicity, and have been termed

TABLE I

Comparison between Apoptotic and Necrotic Cell Death

	Apoptosis	**Necrosis**
Stimuli	Physiologic	Pathologic
Occurrence	Single cells	Groups of cells
Adhesion between cells	Lost (early)	Lost (late)
Nucleus	Convolution of nuclear outline and breakdown (karyorrhexis)	Disappearance (Karyolysis)
Nuclear chromatin	Compaction in uniformly dense masses	Clumping not sharply defined
DNA cleavage	Internucleosomal, "laddering" appearance of distinct fragments on agarose gels	Random; "smear" pattern on agarose gels
Phagocytosis by other cells	Present	Absent
Inflammation	Absent	Present

TABLE 2
Molecular Responses to Renal Ischemia

Increased gene expression
    Genes involved in cell fate determinations: regeneration, apoptosis
        Transcription factors: c-*jun*, c-*fos*
        Cyclin dependent kinase inhibitors: p21
    Genes involved in inflammation
        Chemokines: MCP-1, IL-8
        Adhesion molecules: ICAM-1, integrins
Decreased gene expression—loss of mature phenotype
    Prepro epidermal growth factor
    Tamm-Horsfall protein
    Aquaporin-2
    Sodium proton exchanger 3 (*NHE3*)

the stress response (Fig. 2). This response is thought to be a major determinant of whether cells survive the insult or not, and might be necessary for the repair of injured cells. In some circumstances, the stress response leads to apoptosis rather than survival, and is probably a function of the duration of the stress response, its degree, and the specific cell in which the response takes place. In the ischemia/reperfusion model of renal injury, which may also involve DNA damage, these genes are expressed for the most part in the distal nephron, a site of both cell survival and apoptosis (see above).

A summary of these important features of the renal stress pathway and its possible consequences is given in Fig. 2. It can be seen that initiation of the stress response may ultimately determine much of the proinflammatory, reparative, cytoreductive, and functional aspects of renal failure. Particular limbs of the response can be targeted for up-or

downregulation to limit injury or improve function. The recent data using growth factors (presumably to tip the balance between cell gain and cell loss), as well as the data on antiadhesion molecules to reduce inflammation, support the notion that the renal stress response is an appropriate target for therapy (see discussion on treatment of ARF).

The last group of changes involves what appears to be a loss of the mature phenotype of the kidney, because many of the changes in gene expression involve the loss of proteins that are only expressed maximally during the maturation of the kidney. These include the prepro epidermal growth factor and Tamm-Horsfall protein genes, whose functions are unknown in the kidney, but also include the downregulation of important membrane transporter genes, such as *Aquaporin-2,* and *NHE3*. The loss of these latter proteins may be responsible, in part, for the tubular reabsorptive defects typical of ARF (see below).

Pathophysiology of the Cell Injury

The mechanism of the changes in cell viability during renal injury are complex and incompletely understood. Most of the experimental data have been derived from the ischemia-reperfusion model of acute renal failure and have focused on necrotic cell death. Because as many as 50% of patients have ischemia-induced ARF, the observations should be relevant to a large portion of the patients at risk. As mentioned above, different stresses initiate common biochemical events, so that understanding the relevant pathways of one stress will most likely be applicable to others. Such studies have focused on three biochemical pathways: intracellular calcium homeostasis, reactive oxygen species, and phospholipases.

Depletion of intracellular ATP that accompanies ischemia increases the cytosolic concentration of calcium. Such

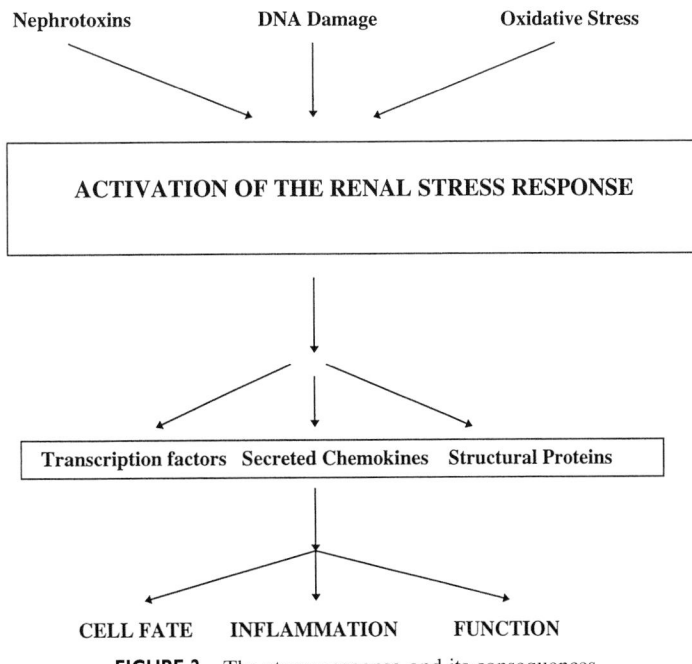

FIGURE 2 The stress response and its consequences.

increases in intracellular calcium can damage epithelial cells by activating proteases and phospholipases, and can disrupt cellular integrity. Controversy remains, however, about the importance of this change even in the generation of ischemic injury.

Restoration of renal blood flow after ischemia produces a burst of reduced oxygen species from a variety of processes. Resultant lipid, protein, and DNA damage could lead to necrosis. Direct tests of their role in human ARF by the use of oxygen scavengers have been disappointing so far, however.

Members of the phospholipase family, which hydrolyze membrane lipids, could contribute to ischemic renal injury as they appear to do in other organs injured by ischemia. Several products of phospholipid breakdown are vasoconstrictive and chemotactic and could participate in the functional and cytotoxic events of renal failure. Adequate assessment of their role in the cytotoxicity of ischemia awaits the availability of useful inhibitors of the various members of the family.

PATHOPHYSIOLOGY OF ABNORMAL FUNCTION

Reduced GFR

From a consideration of the forces and flows at the glomerular capillary vascular bed it is possible to form a conceptual framework in which to analyze the causes of reduced GFR in ARF (Table 3).

Intrarenal vasoconstriction is the dominant mechanism for the reduced GFR in acute renal failure, especially in its initial phases. Reduction in renal blood flow reduces net ultrafiltration pressure because it increases the rate of rise of π_{GC} along the length of the glomerular capillary, thus reducing net ultrafiltration pressure. If accompanied by a reduction in arterial pressure or selective afferent arteriolar vasoconstriction, P_{GC} would also fall. The mediators of this vasoconstriction are unknown but tubule injury seems to be an important concomitant finding. There is some evidence experimentally that a low ultrafiltration coefficient may also play a role in reducing GFR during acute renal failure, presumably due to mesangial cell contraction

and consequent reduction in the area available for filtration. While obstruction to the outflow of urine into the collecting system is an obvious cause of reduced net ultrafiltration, less obvious is the intratubular obstruction that results from sloughed cells and cellular debris that evolves in the course of renal failure. The importance of this mechanism is highlighted by the improvement in renal function that follows relief of such intratubular obstruction. Also, when obstruction is prolonged (longer than a few hours), intrarenal vasoconstriction is prominent. Damaged renal epithelium are also abnormally permeable to inulin, and thus backleak of glomerular filtrate may be an additional mechanism of renal failure. Each of these mechanisms— vasoconstriction, mesangial cell contraction, tubular obstruction, and backleak—contribute individually or in combination during the course of ARF.

Apart from the increase in basal renal vascular tone observed during ARF, it is also true that the stressed renal microvasculature is more sensitive to otherwise tolerated manipulations of the renal vascular bed. For example, the use of nonsteroidal antiinflammatory drugs in patients with severe liver disease may precipitate ARF. As a result, a prerenal state may progress to an intrinsic form of renal failure and thus reduce GFR further. Prolonged vasoconstriction may evolve into intrinsic ARF especially when there is concomitant large vessel arterial disease. This latter form of renal failure is often induced by the use of angiotensinconvertingenzyme inhibitors and/or diuretics. The vasculature of the injured kidney has an impaired vasodilatory response and loses its autoregulatory behavior. This latter phenomenon has important clinical relevance as the frequent reduction in systemic pressure during intermittent hemodialysis may provoke additional damage that could delay recovery of ARF.

PATHOPHYSIOLOGY OF THE CONCENTRATING DEFECT

Another physiologic hallmark of intrinsic ARF is the failure to concentrate urine maximally. The defect is not responsive to pharmacologic doses of vasopressin and is postreceptor in nature. The injured kidney fails to generate and maintain a high medullary solute gradient. Because the accumulation of solute in the medulla depends on normal distal nephron function, this is yet another example of the role of the distal nephron in the pathophysiology of ARF. The mechanism of this defect is not simply a function of lethally injured proximal tubules, because necrosis is not prominent in the distal nephron, but rather may involve more subtle affects on function, such as the observed loss of Aquaporin 2 expression following renal ischemia. The failure to excrete a concentrated urine even in the face of oliguria is a helpful diagnostic tool to distinguish prerenal from intrinsic renal disease.

DIAGNOSTIC INDICES OF GLOMERULAR AND TUBULAR FUNCTION USED IN THE DIFFERENTIAL DIAGNOSIS OF ARF

A rapid rise in serum creatinine, which is sometimes associated with a reduced urine volume, declares the pres-

---

TABLE 3

Determinants of Glomerular Filtration Rate

$$\text{GFR} = L_p A \times P_{net}$$

L_pA is the ultrafiltration coefficient, consisting of the hydraulic permeability and area of the glomerular membrane

$P_{net} = \Delta P - \Delta \pi$ is the net ultrafiltration pressure across the entire glomerular capillary, where

$\Delta P = P_{GC} - P_{PT}$ is the hydrostatic pressure difference between the glomerular capillary and Bowman's space, P_{GC} is the glomerular capillary hydrostatic pressure, and P_{PT} is the intratubular hydrostatic pressure

$\Delta \pi$ is the net glomerular oncotic pressure, the difference between glomerular oncotic pressure (π_{GC}) and tubule oncotic pressure (π_{PT})

ence of ARF. Given the conceptual framework discussed above, determination of whether the cause of the renal failure is prerenal, intrinsic, or postrenal usually requires only a few noninvasive tests, in addition to history and physical.

If a prerenal cause of ARF is suggested by history, confirmation of the adaptive nature of the response can be obtained by examining the urine and searching for evidence of enhanced renal water and solute reabsorption. The findings of a highly concentrated urine with a low pH in the absence of cellular elements is suggestive adaptive responses to volume depletion. These findings, combined with a disproportionate rise of blood urea nitrogen as compared to creatinine and an elevated serum concentration of uric acid, all point to prerenal causes.

A widely used aid to discriminate between prerenal and intrinsic ARF is the determination of the fractional excretion of sodium,

$$FE_{Na} = (U_{Na}/P_{Na})/(U_{Cr}/ \times 100.$$

Low (<1%) fractional excretion indicates salt and water avidity and is consistent with prerenal causes of renal failure. Lethal and sublethal renal cell injury, on the other hand, would lead to diminished salt reclamation and failure to reach maximum urine concentration, and, as a result, FE_{Na} rises and exceeds 1%. This index is helpful when the patient is oliguric.

A reliance on any of these determinations alone is hazardous because the regulation of salt and water metabolism is complex and other factors besides the fullness of the intravascular space may be present. For example, the fractional excretion of sodium may be low in intrinsic ARF when there are other comorbid events that enhance salt reabsorption. Coexistent heart and liver disease enhance renal sodium retention even in the diseased kidney. Also, the common use of diuretics may also confound interpretation of high fractional sodium excretion even when prerenal causes predominate. Accurate history and physical are a great help in this regard.

Postrenal causes are detected by renal sonography. Renal perfusion scans do not usually help distinguish among the various causes of reduced renal perfusion except when there is asymmetric perfusion suggestive of renal vascular lesions. In this case, the presence of such lesions should be confirmed by MRI and/or renal angiography.

TREATMENT OF ARF RE: IMPLICATIONS DERIVED FROM NEWER UNDERSTANDING OF ITS PATHOPHYSIOLOGY

The mortality of ARF is still high, especially in those patients who require dialysis. This high mortality is in part due to a sicker and older population of patients receiving potentially nephrotoxic medical and surgical therapies. Recent insights into the pathophysiology of ARF have provided newer targets for therapy with the hope of improving outcome in these patients. Such approaches are summarized in Table 4.

TABLE 4
Therapeutic Targets of Treatment

Offsetting vasoconstriction	Calcium channel blockage
	Atrial natriuretic factor
	Endothelin blockade
	Nitric oxide regulation
Limiting inflammation	Antiadhesion strategies, anti-ICAM antiintegrins
	Biocompatible membranes
	Cytokine absorbing biomembranes
Altering cell outcome	Growth factors and "survival" factors
Dialysis dose adjustments	Hi flux membranes
	Continuous arteriovenous hemodialysis (CAVHD)
	Continuous venovenous hemodialysis (CVVHD)
	Continuous venovenous hemofiltration (CVVH)

Therapeutic Interventions Directed at Renal Vasodilation

Although the effector pathway for the intense vasoconstriction during ARF is as yet unknown, a variety of therapeutic approaches have been used to limit the decline in GFR with inconsistent results. Calciumchannel blockade to relax the renal vasculature and ameliorate renal failure may be useful in ARF seen after renal transplantation, cyclosporine, and radiocontrast dyes. It has not been effective in most other forms of renal failure. Dopamine, which vasodilates the normal renal vasculature and increases sodium excretion, has not been effective clinically and is associated with significant side effects, especially in the critically ill patient. Atrial natriuretic peptide may improve renal function in oliguric ARF patients, but not in those who are nonoliguric. Isotonic saline infusion at relatively modest rates, (which would increase renal blood flow and provoke a diuresis), has been shown to ameliorate radiocontrast-induced ARF in patients with modest reduction of renal function before exposure. Antagonism of the potent renal vasoconstictive effects of endothelin shows promise experimentally in ischemic renal failure, but there is no clinical experience at present. Finally, modifying nitric oxide production has also been shown to protect kidneys experimentally. Identification of the effector pathways responsible for the renal vasoconstriction offers the hope of more successful therapy.

Approaches Based on Modifying the Inflammatory Aspects of ARF

Several aspects of the renal stress response are proinflammatory in nature, including the increased expression of the potent monocyte and neutrophil chemotactic chemokines monocyte chemotoctic protein 1 (MCP-1) and interleukin-8 (IL-8). Overproduction of cytokines may be

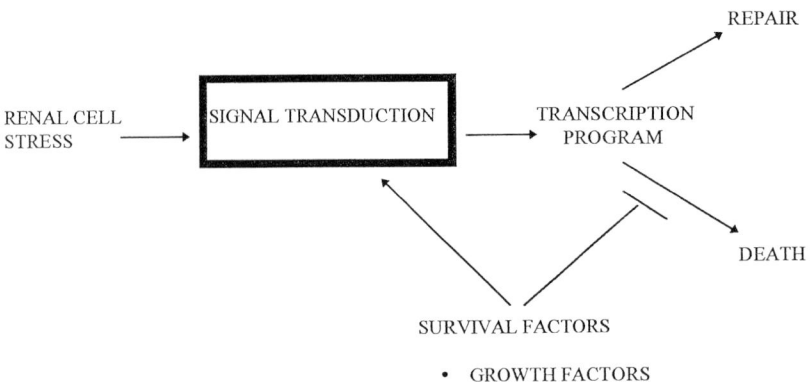

FIGURE 3 Survival factors and cell fate during renal cell stress.

a factor in many aspects of renal failure, including vasocon-striction and leukocyte invasion. Blockade of intracellular adhesion molecule I and integrin-mediated adhesion is a promising new approach, which is mediated perhaps by interfering with inflammation. Strategies directed against the integrins may also operate by reducing intratubular obstruction, as stated above. Additional insight into how these chemokines work in the kidney will most likely yield additional approaches.

Survival Factors

As dicussed above renal stress initiates a transcriptional program that is intimately involved in cell fate. Some cells participating in this response will survive and repair, whereas others will die by apoptosis. What determines whether a cell will recover from such injury or undergo cell death by necrosis or apoptosis is probably a function of the severity of the stress, the specific changes in gene regulation that the cell is capable of mounting, and the availability of survival factors in the cell's external milieu. An example of these internal and external influences on cell survival after toxic exposure is given by the sensitivity of cells derived from patients with Xeroderma pigmentosa. Such cells lack a critical DNA repair pathway and do not survive otherwise tolerated doses of radiation. Also, the survival of bone marrow cells damaged by cancer chemo-therapeutic agents may be prevented by addition of IL-3. Figure 3 provides the conceptual framework for this approach. The provision of survival factors, such as trophic cytokines and growth factors, in addition to accelerating entry of cells into replicative phases of the cell cycle and hence increase the rate at which cells reline injured tubules, may also alter an apoptotic or even necrotic outcome to one of survival and repair. Early success with exogenously administered growth factors such as EGF and IGF (among others) show promise in this regard. Survival factors identi-fied during early morphogenesis of the kidney are also likely to be used in treatment of the injured kidney in this way, or be used prior to exposure to mitigate the injury.

Renal Replacement Therapy

The decision to offer renal replacement therapy should be made cautiously, given the instability of the renal vascu-lature, the hypotension acute intermittent hemodialysis provokes, and the proinflammatory state of the injured kidney. For these reasons, hemodialysis via high flux bio-compatible membranes that limit the frequency of hypoten-sive episodes and diminish cytokine production show great promise in the treatment of ARF.

SUMMARY

(Great strides) have been made in the understanding of the pathophysiology of ARF. Morphologic and molecular information have broadened our notions of how the kidney loses function and recovers from cytotoxic insults. The study of the stress response and its consequences, the cell cycle and its regulation, as well as continued advances in the understanding of the embryology of the kidney, will likely yield specific targets for therapy and newer survival factors that could limit injury and hasten repair.

Bibliography

Chan L, Chittinandana A, Shapiro JI, Stanley P F Schrier RW: Effect of an endothelin-receptor antagonist on ischemic acute renal failure. *Am J Physiol* 266:F135–F138, 1994.

Chertow GM, Christiansen CL, Cleary PD, Munro C, Lazarus JM: Prognostic stratification in critically ill patients with acute renal failure requiring dialysis. *Arch Intern Med* 155:1505–1511, 1995.

Conger J, Robinette JB, Hammond WS: Differences in vascular reactivity in models of ischemic acute renal failure. *Kidney Int* 39:1087–1097, 1991.

Di Mari JF, Saggi S, Aronson P, Safirstein R: Renal ischemia reperfusion injury reduces Aquaporin-2 and NHE3 Expression. *J Am Sec Nephrol* 7:1823, 1996.

Donohoe JF, Venkatachalam MA, Bernard DB, Levinsky N: Tu-bular leakage and obstruction after renal ischemia: structural-functional correlations. *Kidney Int* 13:208–222, 1978.

Goligorsky MS, Lieberthal W, Racusen LC, Simon EE: Integrin receptors in renal tubular epithelium: new insights into patho-physiology of acute renal failure. *Am J Physiol* 264:F1, 1993.

Hakim RM: Clinical implications of hemodialysis membrane bio-compatibility. *Kidney Int* 44:484–494, 1993.

Holbrook NJ, Fornace AJ, Jr: Response to adversity: molecular control of gene activation following genotoxic stress. *New Biol* 3:825–833, 1991.

Kelly KJ, Williams LWW, Colvin RB, Bonventre JN: Antibody to intracellular adhesion molecule-I protects the kidney against ischemic injury. *Proc Natl Acad Sci USA* 91:812, 1994.

Noiri E, Peresleni T, Miller F, Goligorsky MS: In vivo targeting of inducible NO synthase with oligodeoxynucleotides protects rat kidney against ischemia. *J Clin Invest* 97:2377–2383, 1996.

Nouwen E, Verstrepen W, Buyssens N, Zhu M, De Broe M: Hyperplasia, hypertrophy, and phenotypic alterations in the distal nephron after acute proximal tubular injury in the rat. *Lab Invest* 70:479–493, 1994.

Paller MS: Effect of neutrophil depletion on ischemic renal injury in the rat. *J Lab Clin Med* 113:379–386, 1989.

Safirstein R, Miller P, Dikman S, Lyman N, Shapiro C: Cisplatin nephrotoxicity in rats: defect in papillary hypertonicity. *Am J Physiol* 241:F175–F185, 1981.

Safirstein R, Bonventre JV: Molecular response to ischemic and nephrotoxic acute renal failure. In: Schlondorff D, Bonventre

JV (eds) Molecular nephrology: Kidney function in health and disease. D. Marcel Dekker, New York, 1995, pp. 839–854.

Schumer M, Colombel MC, Sawczuk IS: Morphologic, biochemical, and molecular evidence of apoptosis during the reperfusion phase after brief periods of renal ischemia. *Am J Pathol* 140:831–838, 1992.

Solez K, Finckh ES: Is there a correlation between morphologic and functional changes in human acute renal failure? Data of Finckh, Jeremy, and Whyte re-examined twenty years later. In: Solez K, Whelton A (eds) Acute Renal Failure: Correlations between Morphology and Function. Dekker New York, 1984.

Solomon R, Werner C, Mann D, D'Elia J, Silva P: Effects of saline, mannitol, and furosemide to prevent acute decreases in renal function induced by radiocontrast agents. *N Engl J Med* 331:1416–1420, 1994.

Thadhani R, Pascual M, Bonventre JV: Acute renal failure. *N Engl J Med* 334:1448–1460, 1996.

van Bommel E, Bowry N, So K et al: Acute dialytic support for the critically ill: Intermittent hemodialysis versus continuous arteriovenous hemodiafiltration. *Am J Nephrol* 15:192–200, 1995.

APPROACH TO THE PATIENT WITH ACUTE RENAL FAILURE

ROBERT D. TOTO

INTRODUCTION

Acute renal failure (ARF) is defined as an abrupt reduction in renal function sufficient to result in azotemia. Establishing the correct diagnosis and correctly assessing the cardiovascular and volume status of the patient are the key elements in patient management. As such, the approach to the patient with ARF requires a careful history and physical examination in combination with routine laboratory tests including complete blood count, blood biochemistries urinalysis, and urine electrolytes. Renal imaging is often useful, and in some cases, a renal biopsy is necessary.

Fortunately, in most instances the primary cause of ARF can be identified from the history, physical examination, urinalysis, and renal sonogram.

ACUTE VS CHRONIC RENAL FAILURE

Distinguishing acute from chronic renal failure can be difficult. A history of chronic symptoms of fatigue, anorexia, nocturia, pruritus, or restless legs may point to chronic renal failure. The renal sonographic finding of small contracted kidneys signals chronic renal failure; normal-size kidneys can be observed with either acute or chronic renal failure. Although rare, radiographic findings of renal osteodystrophy are also helpful when present since hyperparathyroid changes occur only in chronic renal failure.

CAUSES OF ARF

ARF is often multifactorial, particularly in an ICU patient. For example, septic shock causing ischemia in combination with a nephrotoxic antibiotics or myoglobinuria is not an uncommon combination in this setting. ARF is usually classified according to whether the renal circulation (prerenal), the renal parenchyma (intrinsic renal) or the urinary flow tract (postrenal) are altered as shown in Table 1.

TABLE I
Causes of ARF

Prerenal (decreased renal blood flow)
  Hypotension from any cause
  Congestive heart failure
  Volume depletion
    Renal loss: Addisonian crisis, vomiting, DKA
    Extrarenal loss: Vomiting, diarrhea, burns, excessive
      sweating
  Hypercalcemia
  Prostaglandin inhibition (NSAIDs), cyclosporine, ACE
    inhibitors, other
Intrarenal
Ischemia
  Hypoperfusion from systemic hypotension of any cause
  Sepsis syndrome
  Atheroembolism
  Thromboembolism: Renal artery thrombosis, aortic
    thrombosis
  Thrombotic microangiopathy from TTP, HUS/verotoxins,
    drugs
  Systemic necrotizing vasculitides (e.g., polyarteritis nodosa)
Toxins
  Endogenous
    Myoglobin, hemoglobin, uric acid, calcium-phosphate
      complexes
  Exogenous
    Drugs including aminoglycosides, cephalosporins, acyclovir,
      amphotericin
    Chemotherapeutic agents, e.g., cisplatinum, methotrexate,
      mitomycin C
Inflammation
  Acute glomerulonephritis, acute tubulointerstitial nephritis
Tumor
  Tumor infiltration, myeloma kidney
Postrenal (Obstruction)
  Prostate hypertrophy
  Intratubular obstruction: Uric acid, calcium oxalate, acyclovir,
    others
  Intra- and extraluminal: Stone, tumor, fibrosis, clot, abscess

NSAIDS, nonsteroidal anti-inflammatory drugs; TTP, thrombotic thrombocytopenic purpura; ACE inhibitors, angiotensin-converting enzyme inhibitors

Prerenal Azotemia

In prerenal azotemia, renal blood flow is markedly decreased, usually because of intense, compensatory renal afferent arteriolar vasoconstriction. Because renal plasma flow rate is the main determinant of glomerular filtration rate (GFR), filtration rate decreases markedly. Common clinical situations in which this is the major or only mechanism of ARF include hypotension from any cause, severe extracellular fluid volume depletion, hemorrhage, gastrointestinal losses, and third-space losses from burns, peritonitis, pancreatitis, or liver disease, as well as renal salt losses, severe congestive heart failure, and hepatorenal syndrome. Various drugs including nonsteroidal antiinflammatory drugs, cyclosporine, osmotic diuretic agents (including glucose and mannitol), and angiotensin-converting enzyme inhibitors can precipitate ARF when mild degrees of volume depletion or CHF are present. Vascular diseases may also cause prerenal ARF by reducing glomerular blood flow. Among the responsible disorders are renal artery emboli, thrombotic occlusion of the aortorenal bifurcation, and atheroembolic renal disease. Despite the fall in GFR, renal tubular structure and function remain normal. Vasculitides and thrombotic thrombocytopenic purpura/hemolytic uremic syndrome may also lead to ARF in this fashion, but more commonly they also cause significant glomerular injury including endothelial damage, increased permeability to proteins, and inflammatory infiltration. In prerenal azotemia, increased reabsorption of sodium and water with elaboration of a concentrated urine with a low sodium concentration is typical. As urea reabsorption is also increased, a disproportionate increase in BUN relative to creatinine occur; hence the BUN/S_{cr} ratio is often $> 20:1$.

Intrarenal ARF

The most common cause of intrinsic renal failure is acute tubular necrosis (ATN). This lesion is typically found after ischemic or toxic insults. Tubular necrosis leads to sloughing of tubular cells into the lumina with partial or total obstruction of nephron flow, thereby contributing to the reduction in GFR. The urinalysis typically reveals granular casts and renal tubular cells indicative of injured tubules. Damaged tubules do not transport solutes normally, leading to elaboration of a dilute urine with a high sodium concentration. Acute glomerulonephritis leads to ARF because of impaired ultrafiltration across the glomerular basement membrane. Damage to glomerlar capillaries leads to proteinuria and hematuria; red blood cell casts may be observed. Another common cause of intrinsic renal failure is acute interstitial nephritis caused by drugs or other toxins (see Chapter 40). In this situation interstitial inflammation leads to tubular injury and necrosis. Pyuria, hematuria, proteinuria with granular casts, and renal tubular epithelial cells in the urine reflect the inflammation and tubular damage in the kidney. Also, elaboration of a dilute urine with a high sodium concentration is typical.

Postrenal ARF

Obstruction of the collecting system generally must involve both kidneys or a solitary kidney to cause significant renal failure. Obstruction of the urinary tract at any level may cause acute renal failure (see Chapter 54). Thus bladder outlet obstruction from prostate enlargement, tumor, or urethral stricture; ureteral obstruction from tumor, stone, papillae or fibrosis; or even massive crystal (uric acid, acyclovir, calcium oxalate) deposition in the tubules can cause acute obstruction leading to renal failure. Distension of the bladder may cause pain and a palpable mass. Obstruction should be considered in patients with acute anuria, particularly in those with a recent history of polyuria alternating with oliguria.

HISTORY

Obtaining a careful history is essential to determining the etiology of ARF. The history should focus initially in two key areas: (1) factors known to lower renal perfusion and (2) known and potential nephrotoxins. Attention should be directed to recent events that could lead to alterations in cardiovascular and volume status and use of drugs/toxins should be sought. For example, patients with volume depleted states may present with orthostatic dizziness, presyncope, or syncope as their main problem. In this instance, a careful history of factors that cause volume depletion such as vomiting, diarrhea, excessive sweating, burns, and renal salt wasting (e.g., diabetic ketoacidosis) should be sought. In contrast, headaches caused by hypertension, dyspnea caused by pulmonary congestion, and peripheral edema caused by extracellular fluid volume expansion are common complaints in patients with congestive heart failure or renal salt retention due to glomerulonephritis or other glomerular/vascular disorders (e.g., hemolytic-uremic syndrome or atheroembolic renal disease) causing ARF. A history of recent trauma with blood loss or muscle trauma should raise the possibility of renal failure due to ischemia and/or myoglobin-induced tubular necrosis. Fever, skin rash, and joint pains should raise the possibility of a rheumatic disease such as SLE, a vasculitis, endocarditis, or a drug allergy causing intrinsic renal failure. A history or dyspnea or pulmonary hemorrhage should raise the possibilities of Goodpasture's syndrome, Wegener's granulomatosis, Churg-Strauss vasculitis and pulmonary edema due to volume overload from glomerulonephritis. Constitutional and non-specific symptoms including low grade fever, malaise, myalgias, arthralgias, weakness and fatigue are common in patients presenting with acute renal failure due to rapidly progressive glomerulonephritis.

Both endogenous and exogenous toxins can give rise to renal failure (Table 1). Therefore, a history of nephrotoxin exposure is an extremely important component of the evaluation of a patient with ARF. A careful and thorough review of the patient's history (and chart) for nephrotoxin exposure is an extremely important component of the evaluation of a patient with ARF. Over-the-counter drugs, including acetaminophen, antibiotics, antihypertensives, and poisons, should be considered in all patients in which the cause of ARF is inapparent. For example, occult ingestion of ethylene glycol can lead to renal failure with prominent metabolic acidosis (see Chapter 9). A patient may survive the initial metabolic acidosis and present later with renal failure, sometimes in association with cranial nerve (especially VI) palsies or other neurologic effects.

Endogenous toxins include myoglobin, hemoglobin, and calcium-phosphorus complexes. ARF may be the presenting finding in patients with nontraumatic rhabdomyolysis from cocaine use or infections, and hemoglobinuric renal failure may be the initial presentation in a patient with an acute intravascular hemolytic event. Occupational exposure history is also important because various heavy metals can cause acute tubular necrosis. For example, exposure to mercury vapor or liquid, lead, cadmium, or other heavy metals can be encountered by welders and miners.

A history of recent infections is important. A wide variety of infections can cause renal failure either by direct invasion of the kidney or indirectly by activation of the immune system in which the kidney is an innocent bystander. It is important to review the patient's urine color, volume, and pattern of output. Abrupt anuria suggests an acute obstruction, severe acute glomerulonephritis, or a sudden vascular catastrophe such as renal artery emboli or atherosclerotic occlusion of the aortorenal bifurcation. A gradually diminishing urine output may indicate a urethral stricture or, in an older male, bladder outlet obstruction due to prostate enlargement. Painless, gross hematuria in the setting of ARF suggests acute glomerulonephritis, whereas painful gross hematuria suggests obstruction of the ureter by tumor, blood clots, or necrotic renal papillae.

PHYSICAL EXAMINATION

The physical examination may provide many clues to the underlying cause and potential therapy for ARF.

Skin

Examination of the skin for petechiae, purpura, and ecchymoses provides clues to inflammatory and vascular causes of renal failure, including infectious diseases, thrombocytopenic purpura, and disseminated intravascular coagulation. Also, skin infarction from embolic phenomena and cutaneous vasculitis presenting as palpable purpura occur frequently in patients with septic shock, atheroembolic disease, systemic vasculitis, and infective endocarditis and should be looked for carefully (Fig. 1).

Ocular Findings

Examination of the eye may reveal evidence of uveitis (interstitial nephritis and necrotizing vasculitis), ocular muscle paralysis (ethylene glycol poisoning and necrotizing vasculitis), signs of severe hypertension, atheroembolic lesions (Hollenhorst crystals), and Roth spots (endocarditis) Cytoid bodies (cotton wool exudates) may be seen in systemic lupus erythematosus (SLE). In addition, ophthal-

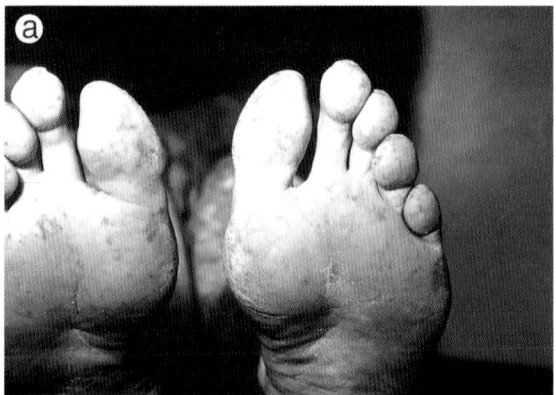

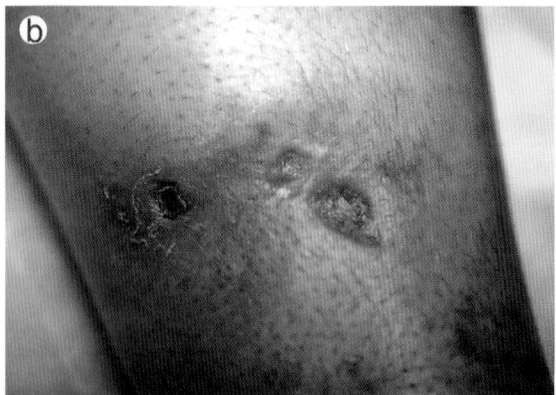

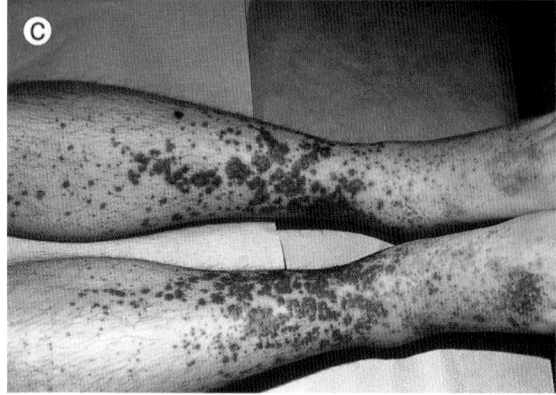

FIGURE 1 Cutaneous lesions in patients with (a) atheroembolic disease (b) systemic necrotizing vasculitis; (c) cryoglobulinemia.

moplegia may be present in patients with systemic necrotizing vasculitis with renal failure.

Cardiovascular and Volume Status

A careful determination of the cardiovascular and volume status is the most important aspect in the diagnosis and initial management of ARF. Evaluating daily intake and output and body weight are extremely useful in estimating volume status. A table illustrating the trends in fluid balance and weights is helpful in establishing an accurate estimate of volume status. Pulse rate and blood pressure should be measured in the supine and standing (or seated with legs dangling) positions. Close inspection of the neck for jugular venous pulse level, careful examination of the heart and lungs, and an assessment of peripheral edema are essential.

The volume status of patients with prerenal azotemia may vary substantially. Characteristic hypotension, low urine output, and low urine sodium are observed both with severe extracellular volume depletion and with severe congestive heart failure. The decrease in arterial blood volume in the former leads to findings similar to those found with the decrease in effective arterial volume (despite extracellular fluid volume expansion) in the latter.

Importantly, the management of these two presentations is completely opposite; patients with heart failure require vasodilators, inotropes, and diuretics, whereas the volume-depleted patient requires saline, blood products, etc. Evidence for volume depletion, including orthostatic hypotension, dry mucous membranes, decreased skin turgor as well as signs of sepsis, congestive heart failure, or cardiac tamponade, should be sought in patients with low blood pressure or overt hypotension. Often it is difficult to assess the volume status from the examination alone, particularly in elderly, obese, or severely edematous patients. In such cases, placement of a central venous catheter or a pulmonary artery catheter to measure right heart pressures, cardiac output, and systemic vascular resistance may be necessary.

Severe hypertension should raise the possibility of renal failure due to malignant nephrosclerosis, glomerulonephritis, vasculitis, or atheroembolic disease. Cardiac murmurs may be a sign of endocarditis, which can produce fulminant glomerulonephritis with ARF. A pericardial friction rub in a patient with ARF not only is an indication for emergency hemodialysis but also may be a premonitory sign of impending cardiac tamponade. Hypotension due to tamponade can be temporarily stabilized by increasing cardiac preload with a rapid intravenous fluid bolus.

Abdominal Examination

Abdominal examination may reveal signs of urinary obstruction (palpable bladder), tenderness in the upper quadrants (associated with ureteral obstruction or renal infarction), or ascites which may be associated with hepatic failure, severe nephrotic syndrome, or Budd-Chiari syndrome. An abdominal bruit should raise the possibility of severe atherosclerotic disease, which can engender renal failure from a number of related disorders, including renal artery stenosis, thrombosis of the real artery origin, or atheroembolic renal disease. Obstruction may be accompanied by a flank mass due to tumor or retroperitoneal fibrosis.

Extremities

Examination of the extremities for signs of edema, tissue ischemia, muscle tenderness from rhabdomyolysis, and arthritis (e.g., SLE, rheumatoid arthritis, relapsing polychondritis, infections) may provide clues to the diagnosis of renal failure. Nail findings of hypoalbuminemia (paired bands of pallor in the nailbed—Muehrcke's lines) may be a clue to underlying nephrotic syndrome which may rarely predispose a patient to ATN.

Neuropsychiatric Abnormalities

Neuropsychiatric abnormalities are common in renal failure and range from signs of uremic encephalopathy (confusion, somnolence, stupor, coma, seizures) to neurologic abnormalities associated with specific diseases. As mentioned above, cranial nerve palsies can be seen in patients with ethylene glycol poisoning and vasculitides, including Wegener's granulomatosis and polyarteritis nodosa. Altered and changing mental status is common in both thrombotic microangiopathy and systemic atheroembolism.

DIAGNOSTIC TESTS

Serum Biochemistry Tests

Increases in BUN and creatinine are hallmarks of renal failure. Typically, the serum creatinine increases 1 to 2 $mg \cdot dL^{-1} \cdot day^{-1}$; however, increases of $> 5mg \cdot dL^{-1} \cdot day^{-1}$ can occur in patients with rhabdomyolysis since muscle is a major source of creatine, the precursor of creatinine. In cases of prerenal azotemia and in some patients with obstructive uropathy, the BUN/S_{cr} ratio is elevated above 20 : 1 because of enhanced reabsorption of urea. Also, in cases where significant upper gastrointestinal bleeding occurs, the BUN/S_{cr} ratio may increase further as digested protein from blood is absorbed and metabolized by the liver.

Urinalysis

The urinalysis is the most important test in the initial evaluation of ARF (see Chapter 3). An abnormal urinalysis strongly suggests intrinsic renal failure. Gross color changes in the urine may be seen with various intrinsic renal diseases. The urine in acute tubular necrosis from ischemia and toxins frequently appears "dirty" brown and opaque owing to the presence of tubular casts. Reddish brown urine or "cola-colored" urine is present in patients with acute glomerulonephritis and is some times observed in patients with pigment-associated tubular necrosis including myoglobinuria and hemoglobinuria. Dipstick tests positive for proteinuria and blood are particularly useful for diagnosing intrinsic renal diseases, including glomerulonephritides, acute interstitial nephritis, toxic and infectious causes of tubular necrosis, and vascular diseases. Examination of the spun urine sediment is extremely helpful for differentiating prerenal from intrarenal causes of renal failure. As shown in Table 2, the urine sediment typically reveals granular "muddy" casts and renal tubular cells in ATN. Interstitial nephritis is often accompanied by pyuria, WBC casts, and microhematuria. In allergic interstitial nephritis, eosinophiluria may be present on Wright and Hansel's stains

but eosinophiluria is nonspecific and can be seen in urinary tract infections, glomerulonephritis, and atheroembolic renal disease as well. Glomerulonephritis is heralded by hematuria and RBC casts. In addition, granular casts, fat globules, and oval fat bodies may be seen in glomerulopathies associated with heavy proteinuria. Uric acid crystals may be present in ATN associated with acute uric acid nephropathy, calcium oxalate crystals may be present in ethylene glycol poisoning with acute renal failure due to nephrocalcinosis, and acetaminophen crystals may be observed in ATN from acute poisoning with this drug. Some of the ordinary findings in ATN are shown in Chapter 3, Figs. 1D, 2B, and 2D.

Urine Electrolytes

In a patient with ARF, urine electrolytes can serve as an indicator of the functional integrity of the renal tubules. The determination is most helpful when performed in the setting of hypotension and oliguric renal failure. The single most informative test is the fractional excretion of sodium (FE_{Na}). FE_{Na} is defined as:

$$((\text{Urine [Na]/Plasma [Na]})/(\text{Urine [Cr] / Plasma [Cr]})) \times 100.$$

In patients with prerenal azotemia, the FE_{Na} is usually $< 1\%$ and in ATN it is usually $>1\%$. However, there are exceptions. For example, some patients with ATN caused by severe burns, radiocontrast nephropathy, and underlying liver disease have a $FE_{Na} < 1\%$. This is probably due to severe renal vasoconstriction with low tubular flow rate and heterogeneous damage to the tubules. In addition, FE_{Na} is $< 1\%$ in some patients with glomerulonephritis as tubular function remains intact with increased, rather than decreased proximal tubular sodium reabsorption. Diuretic administration may confuse the interpretation of the FE_{Na}. For example, a patient with prerenal azotemia due to administration of a loop diuretic may have a $FE_{Na} > 1\%$. Therefore, the FE_{Na} should never be relied on as the sole means of determining the cause of ARF. Note also that if only a small amount of urine is available, the supernatant remaining after the spun sediment is examined may be sent for Urine [Na] and Urine [Cr] to permit calculation of the FE_{Na}.

Assessing Urine Output

Knowledge of the urine output is important not only from the standpoint of etiology but also and most importantly from the standpoint of management and outcome. Oliguria is defined as a 24-hour urine output between 100 and 400 mL/day. Anuria is defined as a urine output ≤ 100 mL/day. Nonoliguric renal failure occurs with a urine output > 400 mL/day. In patients with suprapubic discomfort and an obviously distended bladder or in patients with a history of declining urine output or documented oliguria, a bladder catheter should be placed temporarily to relieve or rule out bladder outlet obstruction. Patients with oliguric renal failure are easier to manage and have a lower overall

TABLE 2
Differential Diagnosis of ARF: Urinalysis, Water, and Sodium Metabolism

Diagnosis	Urinalysis	Water metabolism		Sodium handling	
		U/P Osm	U/P Cr	Na	FE_{Na}
Prerenal	Normal, or hyaline casts	≥ 1	>40	<20 mEq/L	$<1\%$
Intrarenal					
Tubular necrosis	Granular and epithelial cell casts	≤ 1	<40	>20 mEq/L	$\geq 1\%$
Interstitial nephritis	Pyuria, hematuria, mild proteinuria, granular and epithelial cell casts, eosinophils	≤ 1	<40	>20 mEq/L	$\geq 1\%$
Glomerulonephritis	Hematuria, marked proteinuria, RBC casts, granular casts	≥ 1	<40	>20 mEq/L	$<1\%$
Vascular disorders	Normal or hematuria, mild proteinuria	≥ 1	<40	>20 mEq/L	$<1\%$
Postrenal	Normal or hematuria, granular casts, pyuria	≤ 1	<40	>20 mEq/L	$\geq 1\%$

U, urine; P, plasma; Osm, osmolality; Cr, creatinine; Na, sodium; FE_{Na}, fractional excretion of sodium.

mortality rate than oliguric or anuric patients (see discussions on management and survival in accompanying sections). Measurement of subsequent daily urine output is an important feature of management of patients (see Chapter 41).

Fluid Challenge

In patients with suspected prerenal azotemia from significant intravascular volume depletion, an intravenous infusion of normal saline, colloid (such as albumin or dextran), or blood products may be helpful. If volume depletion is present, the fluid challenge should improve renal blood flow and result in increased urine output and correction of renal failure. This maneuver usually consists of an infusion of 1 to 2 L of normal saline administered over a 2 to 4-hour period depending on the clinical judgment of the treating physician. Close and careful bedside monitoring of vital signs, physical examination, and urine output are essential. Failure of this maneuver to improve the vital signs and urine output can help to point to intra- or postrenal causes of renal failure. Caution must be exercised during fluid challenge because of the potential for producing pulmonary edema in patients with congestive heart failure or intrinsic failure that do not respond to volume expansion.

Renal Imaging

Ultrasound

Renal ultrasonography is particularly useful for evaluating the urinary collecting system, including the calyces, pelvis, and bladder, for obstruction. The test is readily available, noninvasive, accurate, reliable, and reproducible. Technically it is easy to perform in most patients; however, difficulty visualizing the kidney does occur in obese patents, in patients with distention from abdominal gas, and in some patients with massive ascites and retroperitoneal fluid collections. Typically, obstructive uropathy is manifest by dilatation of the collecting system and ureters (see Chapter 6, Fig. 1, and Chapter 54, Fig. 2). However, in some cases of early obstruction or ureteral encasement by tumor or fibrosis, ureteral and renal pelvis dilatation may not be detected by ultrasound. The parenchymal pattern on ultrasound may be abnormal with increased echogenicity in the presence of intrinsic renal disease. However, this finding is nonspecific and cannot be used to determine the etiology of intrinsic renal failure. Moreover, in most cases of biopsy-proven ATN, the renal parenchymal pattern on ultrasound appears completely normal.

Doppler Scans

Doppler scans are used to evaluate renal parenchymal blood flow. However, because reduced renal blood flow occurs in both prerenal and intrarenal causes of renal failure, this test is of little diagnostic value in patients with ARF. One exception is the patient with thrombotic obliteration of the renal circulation, as the absence of flow to the kidneys can easily be discerned by this technique.

Nuclear Scans

Radionuclide imaging with ^{99m}Tc-DTPA or ^{131}I-hippuran can be used to assess renal blood flow and tubular function in ARF. However, the utility of such testing is similar to that of Doppler flow studies. Unfortunately, a marked delay in tubular excretion of radionuclide occurs in both prerenal and intrarenal diseases, and this technique is therefore of little value in most patients with ARF.

Magnetic Resonance Imaging

MRI may have some utility in diagnosing intrinsic renal failure. For example, increase in T_2-weighted signal may occur in patients with inflammatory renal disease such as acute tubulointerstitial nephritis and glomerulonephritis. Whether it is cost effective in the setting of ARF remains to be determined.

Renal Angiography

A renal angiogram is helpful in patients with ARF due to vascular disorders including renal artery stenosis with ARF from angiotensin-converting enzyme inhibition, renal artery emboli, aortic atherosclerosis with acute aortorenal occlusion, and in cases of systemic necrotizing vasculitis such

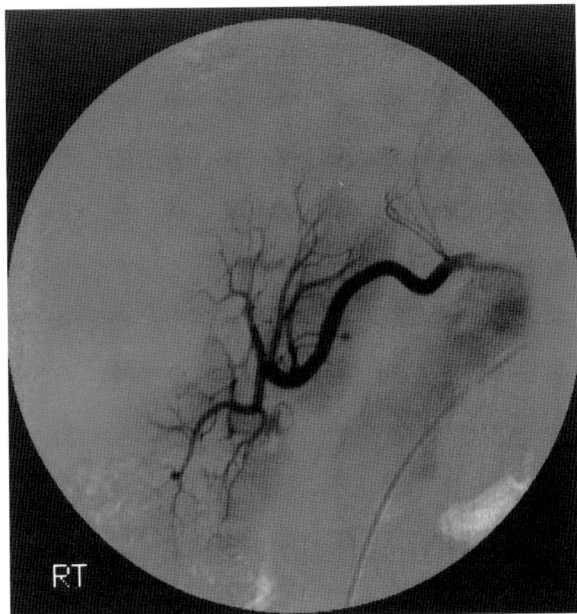

FIGURE 2 Renal angiogram in a patient with acute renal failure caused by systemic necrotizing vasculitis. The early phase of this selective injection of the left renal artery shows marked attenuation of cortical blood flow and multiple aneurysms of medium-sized arcuate arteries.

as polyarteritis nodosa and Takayasu's arteritis (Fig. 2). The latter can affect the distal aorta and present with advanced renal failure.

Renal Biopsy

Renal biopsy is the only diagnostic test that can establish the cause of intrinsic renal failure with absolute certainty. Furthermore, several studies have shown that biopsy in the setting of acute renal failure often (up to 40% of the time) reveals unexpected findings. Therefore, renal biopsy should be considered in any patient with ARF in whom the etiology is unknown and histologic diagnosis is important from a therapeutic perspective. For instance, patients presenting with the clinical syndrome of rapidly progressive glomerulonephritis should undergo renal biopsy unless there is an overt contraindication since effective renal preserving therapy is available and should be instituted as soon as possible. The biopsy is also particularly useful in cases of suspected interstitial nephritis from drugs. For example, in a febrile patient with endocarditis receiving broad spectrum antibiotic coverage, it may be impossible to distinguish between glomerulonephritis and acute tubulointerstitial nephritis on clinical grounds alone. The empiric use of glucocorticoids to treat suspected allergic interstitial nephritis could be considered without a biopsy, but their risk would be high in this setting. In most instances, a biopsy can be carried out safely despite ARF. Clinical judgment is important in determining candidates for biopsy and routine precautions should always be taken. Imaging with sonogram, CT, or MRI reduce the risk of biopsy complications in patients who are acutely ill.

Bibliography

Abuelo JG: Diagnosing vascular causes of renal failure. *Ann Intern Med* 123: 601–614, 1995.

Alkhunaizi AM, Schrier RW: Management of acute renal failure: New perspectives. *Am J Kidney Dis* 28: 315–328, 1996.

Barrett BJ: Contrast nephrotoxicity. *J Am Soc Nephrol* 5: 125–137, 1994.

Davda RK, Guzman NJ: Acute renal failure. Prompt diagnosis is key to effective management. *Postgrad Med* 96: 89–92, 1994.

Fogazzi GB: Crystalluria: A neglected aspect of urinary sediment analysis. *Nephrol Dial Transplant* 11: 379–387, 1996.

Hock R, Anderson R: Prevention of drug-induced nephrotoxicity in the intensive care unit. *J Crit Care* 10: 33–43, 1995.

Hou SH, Bushinsky DA, Wish JB, Cohen JJ, Harrington JT: Hospital-acquired renal insufficiency: A prospective study. *Am J Med* 74:243–8, 1983.

Liano F, Pascual J: Epidemiology of acute renal failure: A prospective, multicenter community-based study. Madrid acute renal failure study group. *Kidney Int* 50:811–8, 1996.

Pascual J, Liano F, Ortuno J: The elderly patient with acute renal failure. *J Am Soc Nephrol* 6:144–153, 1995.

Porter GA: Contrast-associated nephropathy: Presentation, pathophysiology and management. *Miner Electrolyte Metab* 20: 232–243, 1994.

36

RENAL FAILURE CAUSED BY THERAPEUTIC AGENTS

THOMAS M. COFFMAN

Compounds used for diagnostic and therapeutic purposes are common causes of renal insufficiency. The kidney is a frequent target for toxic injury because it is a major route of excretion for a variety of drugs. As a part of the excretory process, these materials may be greatly concentrated in the urinary space and within renal tubular cells, enhancing their potential to cause local toxicity. Also, the rate of blood flow per gram of tissue weight in the kidney is relatively high, resulting in exaggerated exposure of renal endothelial cells and glomeruli to circulating substances. Since most renal functions are dependent on tightly regulated blood flow patterns, agents that impair these hemodynamic relationships may interfere with the ability of the kidney to maintain normal homeostasis.

Drug toxicity in the kidney is manifested through the same clinical syndromes that are associated with kidney diseases of other causes. As depicted in Table 1, these include acute and chronic renal failure, and nephrotic syndrome. Moreover, a single agent may have more than one effect on kidney functions. The particular clinical manifestation of nephrotoxicity is determined by the dose and duration of exposure, chemical properties of the agent, as well as factors within the individual patient such as age, volume status, and genetic background. This chapter describes a general approach to nephrotoxicity and, reviews the renal effects of some common causative agents. More detailed discussions of individual agents or syndromes associated with toxic renal injury can be found in other chapters (see Chapters 31, 40, 42, and 49).

DIAGNOSIS

The possibility of drug-induced nephrotoxicity should be considered when the serum creatinine concentration rises during administration of a therapeutic agent. Because of the nonlinear relationship between serum creatinine and glomerular filtration rate (GFR), a substantial reduction in GFR is necessary before toxic injury can be appreciated clinically. This point is particularly important to consider in the context of agents that may cause chronic nephropathy. In this case, kidney injury may not be detected until 40 to 50% of kidney function has been irreversibly lost. While a number of potential diagnostic markers, such as urinary excretion of various tubular enzymes, have been evaluated as indicators of renal toxicity that might be more

sensitive and specific than serum creatinine, none of these have yet found widespread clinical application.

The clinical syndromes caused by drugs mimic those associated with kidney diseases of other causes. Thus, when the etiology of renal failure is being investigated, the possible role of therapeutic agents should always be considered and a detailed medication history is an extremely important part of the clinical evaluation. Temporal associations between the appearance of a kidney abnormality and medication changes must be documented. In patients who are receiving compounds known to be nephrotoxic, the plan for clinical management should include careful monitoring of renal function, avoidance of clinical risk factors and, in some cases, monitoring of serum drug levels. Also, the role of nephrotoxins in exacerbating renal failure from other causes should be considered. For example, in the hospitalized patient with acute tubular necrosis, the potentially additive detrimental effects of aminoglycosides, radiocontrast, or other nephrotoxins must be recognized. Moreover, renal clearance of some drugs will be substantially reduced in such patients and doses must be lowered appropriately (see Chapter 43).

Acute Renal Failure from Therapeutic Agents

In approaching any patient with acute kidney dysfunction, a potential causative role for therapeutic agents should always be considered. As illustrated in Table 1, mechanisms of acute renal failure related to drugs can be roughly categorized as prerenal/hemodynamic, intrarenal, or postrenal/obstructive syndromes. As described in Chapter 35, this separation can be extremely helpful in identifying the etiology and directing management of patients with acute renal failure (ARF) from any cause.

Prerenal Azotemia: Hemodynamically Mediated Renal Insufficiency Associated with Drugs

As shown in Table 1, several classes of therapeutic agents including cyclosporine, tacrolimus, radiocontrast, nonsteroidal anti-inflammatory drugs (NSAIDS), and angiotensin converting enzyme (ACE) inhibitors can cause a syndrome of abnormal kidney function that resembles prerenal azotemia. Similar to prerenal azotemia from other causes, hemodynamic renal dysfunction caused by drugs can be associated with low urine sodium excretion. While such renal

TABLE I
Renal Syndromes Caused by Therapeutic Agents

Clinical syndrome	Causative agents
Acute renal failure	
Prerenal/hemodynamic	Cyclosporine, tacrolimus, radiocontrast, amphotericin B, ACE inhibitors, NSAIDs
Intrarenal	
Acute tubular necrosis	Aminoglycosides, amphotericin B, cisplatin, certain cephalosporins
Acute interstitial nephritis	Penicillins, cephalosporins, sulfonamides, rifampin, NSAIDs, interferon, interleukin-2
Postrenal/obstructive	Acyclovir, analgesic abuse, methylsergide
Chronic renal failure	Lithium, analgesic abuse, cyclosporine, tacrolimus, cisplatin, nitrosoureas
Nephrotic syndrome	Gold, NSAIDs, penicillamine, captopril, interferon

Note: This is a representative, but not exhaustive list of etiological agents. Please refer to individual *Primer* chapters for more complete listings.

ACE inhibitors, angiotensin converting enzyme inhibitors; NSAIDs, nonsteroidal anti-inflammatory drugs.

dysfunction is usually reversible when the offending agent is discontinued, ischemic damage may result if the insult is prolonged or particularly severe.

Drugs can cause hemodynamically mediated renal dysfunction through several mechanisms. Agents such as cyclosporine, tacrolimus, radiocontrast, and amphotericin cause intense vasoconstriction in the kidney that reduces renal blood flow and glomerular perfusion. These compounds do not seem to affect vascular tone directly but may stimulate production of other vasoconstrictors such as endothelin or thromboxane A_2. Cyclosporine, tacrolimus, and amphotericin can produce renal insufficiency in normal subjects who have no underlying renal circulatory abnormalities.

In contrast, hemodynamic kidney dysfunction associated with NSAIDs generally occurs in patients with preexisting compromise of renal perfusion. NSAIDs inhibit the cyclooxygenase isoenzymes (also called PGH synthases 1 and 2), turning off the synthesis of prostaglandins. In normal subjects, renal prostaglandin production is low and administration of NSAIDs has very little effect on renal function. However, as an adaptive mechanism, production of vasodilator prostaglandins increases in situations in which renal perfusion is threatened. Inhibiting production of these vasodilator compounds by NSAIDs can cause precipitous declines in renal blood flow and GFR. This syndrome is most often seen in patients with volume depletion, heart failure, and preexisting renal disease (see Chapter 42).

Similarly, acute renal failure following administration of ACE inhibitors usually occurs in patients with underlying abnormalities of the renal vasculature and circulation. This syndrome is most commonly seen in patients with congestive heart failure on diuretics, in patients with severe bilateral renal artery stenosis, patients with critical renal artery stenosis in a single functioning kidney, and in patients with vascular disease and nephrosclerosis. ACE inhibitors lower blood pressure by inhibiting the conversion of angiotensin I to angiotensin II. Angiotensin II is a potent vasoconstrictor that acts to increase peripheral resistance. It also induces preferential constriction of efferent arterioles within the glomerulus helping to maintain GFR when renal blood flow is compromised. In the clinical settings described above, ACE inhibitors cause ARF by reducing systemic blood pressure while simultaneously reducing transglomerular pressure due to the fall in postglomerular, efferent arteriolar resistance. As with other forms of drug-induced hemodynamic renal insufficiency, kidney function usually returns to baseline when the ACE inhibitor is discontinued. Based on their pharmacology, the new type 1 (AT1) angiotensin receptor blockers would be expected to have similar effects in susceptible patients.

Intrarenal ARF: Acute Tubular Necrosis and Acute Interstitial Nephritis Caused by Drugs

Drug-induced acute renal failure from intrarenal mechanisms can be divided into two entities with distinct clinical and pathophysiologic characteristics: acute tubular necrosis (ATN) and acute interstitial nephritis (AIN). ATN is associated with drug administration shares many of the clinical features of ATN from other causes. This form of ARF can be seen following administration of agents that are primarily excreted by the kidney, such as aminoglycoside antibiotics, amphotericin B, and chemotherapeutic agents such as cisplatin. Nephrotoxicity often results from direct toxic effects of the compound on renal tubular cells although other hemodynamic mechanisms may play a role. In this setting, the onset of ARF is often nonoliguric and may be slow to develop. If nephrotoxicity is not detected and administration of the causative agent is continued, oliguric ARF may develop. The urinalysis is characteristically bland and may show modest proteinuria, tubular epithelial cells, and noncellular casts. Generally, tubular toxicity will abate when the offending agent is discontinued although there may be a lag before complete recovery of renal function occurs. An exception to this may occur following repetitive exposure to tubular toxins that can result in chronic, irreversible renal impairment.

In AIN, drug exposure causes ARF through a syndrome of intrarenal inflammation. This disorder is described in detail in Chapter 40 and is characterized by inflammatory cell infiltration of the renal interstitium with reduced GFR and renal blood flow. Systemic signs of hypersensitivity, including rash, arthralgias, and fever, may also occur. The urinalysis reflects active renal inflammation and usually contains red cells, white cells, and occasional cellular casts with nonglomerular levels of proteinuria. Eosinophiluria can also be observed but is not pathognomonic. Common causative agents include penicillins, cephalosporins, sulfonamide analogs, rifampin, and NSAIDs. AIN usually resolves after the offending agent is removed, although some have recommended a limited course of corticosteroids to hasten recovery.

Obstructive Nephropathy Associated with Therapeutic Agents

Drug-associated obstruction can occur at several anatomic sites: intratubular, intraureteral, and extrinsic ureteral obstruction from retroperitoneal fibrosis. These obstructive syndromes have been associated with specific causative agents. For example, the antiviral agent acyclovir can cause ARF due to the precipitation of the drug, which is relatively insoluble, within renal tubular lumens. In analgesic-associated nephropathy (discussed in Chapter 42), patients may present with symptoms of acute ureteral obstruction due to sloughing of necrotic renal papillary tissue. Methylsergide has been associated with retroperitoneal fibrosis causing obstructive nephropathy. In one survey, however, drug-induced retroperitoneal fibrosis made up less than 3% of cases of patients with this unusual syndrome.

Chronic Renal Failure from Therapeutic Agents

Chronic renal failure caused by drugs is usually manifested as a chronic tubulointerstitial process. This syndrome of chronic interstitial nephropathy has been associated with a number of structurally diverse agents, including lithium, analgesics, cyclosporine, cisplatin, and nitrosureas. Chronic interstitial disease caused by a drug most often presents as an elevation in serum creatinine, which may be slowly progressive. However, abnormalities of renal tubular function may be a predominant feature. Such abnormalities include renal tubular acidosis, concentrating defects, defective potassium secretion, and tubular proteinuria. On histologic examination, interstitial fibrosis, tubular atrophy, and infiltration of the renal interstitium with chronic inflammatory cells are observed. The urinalysis may contain white cells and red cells with modest levels of proteinuria. While patients with drug-induced chronic interstitial nephropathy may progress to end stage renal disease requiring renal replacement therapy, the course of the disease can usually be stabilized or reversed if the offending agent is identified and discontinued.

Nephrotic Syndrome Associated with Therapeutic Agents

Glomerulopathy with proteinuria may be caused by several drugs, including gold, penicillamine, and NSAIDs. Affected patients often present with proteinuria, edema, and hypoalbuminemia. Pathologically, membranous nephropathy has been associated with all of the agents listed above, whereas minimal change nephropathy has been seen in patients taking certain NSAIDs and penicillamine. In most cases, proteinuria remits when the agent is discontinued. However, in a few cases, renal injury has progressed after the drug is stopped.

SPECIFIC AGENTS WHICH CAUSE RENAL FAILURE

Antibiotics

As a class of drugs, antibiotics are the most common cause of clinically recognized drug-induced renal failure.

Within this group, aminoglycosides are responsible for the majority of episodes of nephrotoxicity in hospitalized patients. Aminoglycosides most commonly cause an ATN picture, while other antibiotics such as penicillins, rifampin, and sulfonamide more commonly produce AIN. In practice, antibiotics are often administered to patients who are severely ill with other coexistent processes that can independently affect renal function or may aggravate and potentiate nephrotoxicity. Thus, in an individual patient, a specific causative role for an antibiotic may be difficult to discern.

Aminoglycosides

Aminoglycosides are amphophilic, cationic antibiotics that are used to treat serious gram-negative bacterial infections. They are by far the most common cause of antibiotic-associated renal insufficiency in hospitalized patients. Depending on the criteria used for defining nephrotoxicity, the reported incidence of nephrotoxicity ranges between 7 and 36% of patients receiving aminoglycosides. Serum protein binding of aminoglycosides is minimal, they are freely filtered at the glomerulus, and renal excretion is the major route of elimination. Aminoglycosides accumulate within the renal cortex reaching saturation within the first 3 days of treatment. Accumulation of drug within cortical tubular cells probably causes toxicity, although the specific cellular mechanisms of aminoglycoside-induced ARF have not been completely defined. Evidence of tubular cell abnormalities and injury may be seen by both light and electron microscopy.

The usual clinical presentation of aminoglycoside nephrotoxicity is a rising BUN and creatinine that typically appears 5 to 7 days into the antibiotic course. Renal insufficiency may occur earlier in the presence of risk factors. Frank azotemia may be preceded by the development of a concentrating defect manifested as polyuria and the urinalysis most commonly shows modest proteinuria with noncellular casts and occasional tubular epithelial cells. Characteristically, renal function deteriorates progressively but the process is reversible if the diagnosis is suspected and the aminoglycoside is discontinued. However, there may be a lag time before renal function begins to improve. This is probably related to the kinetics of accumulation of aminoglycosides in renal cortical tissue, since urinary excretion of aminoglycosides has been detected for days to weeks after administration is discontinued.

While virtually every patient who receives aminoglycosides is at some risk of developing renal toxicity, there is a positive association between the dose and duration of therapy and the risk of developing renal failure. Tailoring aminoglycoside doses to maintain drug levels within a defined therapeutic range serves to minimize the risks of toxicity while maintaining bactericidal concentrations of antibiotic. Single daily dose regimens have been advocated by some authors as an approach to avoid aminoglycoside nephrotoxicity, but the benefits of these regimens have not been clearly demonstrated. Because aminoglycosides are primarily excreted by the kidney, increased aminoglycoside levels can be both a cause and a marker of nephrotoxicity. Monitoring peak and trough drug levels along with serum creatinine every 2 to 3 days is prudent, but daily monitoring may be required in the unstable patient with a serious infection and fluctuating level of renal function.

Several risk factors for aminoglycoside nephrotoxicity have been identified and are illustrated in Table 2. When aminoglycoside therapy is being initiated, these characteristics may be used to identify patients at high risk of developing toxicity for more intensive monitoring and to modify factors such as volume status and electrolyte abnormalities. When possible, alternative antibiotic choices might also be considered in high-risk patients. All members of the aminoglycoside family can potentially cause nephrotoxicity. While gentamicin is the most extensively utilized, tobramycin has a similar bactericidal profile and exhibits less nephrotoxicity, at least in animal models. Amikacin probably has an intermediate potential for nephrotoxicity between gentamicin and tobramycin.

Cephalosporins

Cephalosporins are semisynthetic β-lactam derivatives that have broad spectrum bactericidal activity. While they are generally tolerated well by patients, renal insufficiency is an infrequent but well-defined complication of cephalosporin therapy. Two forms of renal failure have been described with cephalosporins: ATN and AIN. A profile of tubular toxicity has been best documented with cephaloridine and cephalothin especially when higher doses are used. A rank order potential for cephalosporins to produce proximal tubular toxicity has been defined in animal studies as cephaloglycin > cephaloridine >> cefaclor > cephazolin > cephalothin >>> cephalexin and ceftazidime. Combination therapy with aminoglycosides or furosemide may increase the risk for cephalosporin-associated ATN.

Amphotericin B

Amphotericin B is a polyene antibiotic that is the treatment of choice for the majority of serious fungal infections. Unfortunately, this agent produces a number of side effects, with nephrotoxicity being the most clinically problematic. In some series, the degree of nephrotoxicity is roughly proportional to the total cumulative dose received. At least two mechanisms mediate the adverse effects of amphotericin in the kidney. First, the drug causes acute renal vasocon-

TABLE 2

Risk Factors for the Development of
Aminoglycoside Nephrotoxicity

Prolonged course of treatment (>10 days)
Volume depletion
Sepsis
Preexisting renal disease
Hypokalemia
Elderly patient
Combination therapy with certain cephalosporins (particularly cephalothin)
Concomitant exposure to other nephrotoxins (i.e., radiocontrast, amphotericin B, cisplatinum)
Gentamicin > amikacin > tobramycin

striction with a hemodynamically mediated reduction in GFR. Second, amphotericin is highly bound to cell membranes and causes damage that affects membrane integrity and permeability. In the kidney, this membrane injury is thought to be the basis for the potassium and magnesium wasting, inability to maximally concentrate urine, and distal tubule acidification defects that are characteristic of amphotericin nephrotoxicity. These abnormalities, along with an abnormal urine sediment, usually precede the development of clinically apparent azotemia. Renal failure is usually nonoliguric and progressive, but will slowly abate when the amphotericin is discontinued. However, high doses and repetitive exposure to amphotericin can cause permanent kidney damage and chronic renal failure. Volume depletion potentiates nephrotoxicity and it has been suggested that sodium loading and volume expansion may prevent or ameliorate renal injury.

Acyclovir

Acyclovir is an effective and relatively nontoxic antiviral agent that is widely used to treat herpes virus infections. When given by the oral route, acyclovir is essentially devoid of significant renal toxicity. However, nephrotoxicity has been described in a small number of patients who have received intravenous courses of acyclovir, particularly at high doses (>500 mg/m^2). Acyclovir undergoes tubular secretion in the kidney and renal tissue levels increase substantially during treatment. The mechanism of ARF is thought to be precipitation of the relatively insoluble drug within tubular lumens causing obstructive nephropathy. The urine sediment may contain red cells and white cells with needle-shaped birefringent crystals. Renal failure generally resolves when the acyclovir is discontinued. Risk factors for toxicity are volume depletion and bolus administration of drug. However, ARF has been observed despite adequate fluid repletion and the use of continuous infusion protocols.

Vancomycin

Vancomycin is a glycopeptide antibiotic developed in the 1950s for use against penicillin-resistant gram-positive infections. Recently, usage of vancomycin has increased because of changes in resistance profiles as well as its favorable pharmacokinetics in patients on dialysis. Vancomycin is also used frequently to treat methicillin-resistant *Staphylococcus aureus* infections and as primary treatment for pseudomembranous colitis caused by *Clostridium difficile*. In the early years of its use, azotemia was reported in up to 25% of patients who received this agent. However, this was probably related to impurities present in the early commercial preparations of the drug. Recent series suggest that the incidence of nephrotoxicity is <7% with modern vancomycin preparations. Clinical and animal studies suggest that coadministration of vancomycin with aminoglycosides may enhance the risk of developing nephrotoxicity.

Pentamidine

Approximately 25% of patients treated with pentamidine may experience a fall in GFR that is reversible when the drug is discontinued. Nephrotoxicity with pentamidine may be more common in AIDS patients and has been associated with significant hyperkalemia. Although the incidence of renal problems is reduced with inhaled preparations, renal insufficiency has been reported in association with aerosolized pentamidine use. However, a specific role for pentamidine is often difficult to identify due to the presence of other drugs or comorbid conditions that might also affect renal function.

Radiocontrast

The administration of radiocontrast is a relatively common cause of ARF in hospitalized patients. However, the reported incidence of contrast nephropathy from published studies is quite variable. This variation relates to differences in criteria for defining the syndrome, the period of observation after the contrast administration, and the prevalence of risk factors in the population studied. Preexisting renal insufficiency is the most important and best-documented risk factor and contrast-induced nephrotoxicity is rare in patients with normal renal function. Other potential risk factors are listed in Table 3. While animal studies suggested that low osmolality, nonionic contrast agents are less nephrotoxic than conventional high osmolality, ionic agents, prospective clinical studies have failed to demonstrate differences in nephrotoxicity in patients treated with ionic vs nonionic contrast.

The pathogenesis of radiocontrast nephropathy results from the vasoactive effects of radiocontrast. In animals, contrast injection initially causes vasodilatation of the renal circulation, followed by intense and persistent vasoconstriction. The etiology of this vasoconstrictive phase is not clear, but may include reduced production of vasodilator prostaglandins or changes in intracellular calcium. Patients with contrast nephrotoxicity typically develop a rise in their serum creatinine within 24 hours after the radiocontrast study, sometimes associated with oliguria. The urinary sediment is unremarkable and the fractional excretion of sodium is typically very low, consistent with the hemodynamic etiology of renal impairment.

Renal impairment is usually transient, although occasional patients will require support with acute dialysis. The clinician's efforts should be directed toward prevention

TABLE 3
Risk Factors for the Development of Acute Renal Failure Following Radiocontrast Administration

Preexisting renal dysfunction
Diabetic nephropathy
Severe congestive heart failure
Volume depletion
Elderly patient
Multiple myeloma
Large volumes of radiocontrast
Concomitant treatment with ACE inhibitors, NSAIDs, or exposure to other nephrotoxins

ACE inhibitors, angiotensin converting enzyme inhibitors; NSAIDs, nonsteroidal anti-inflammatory drugs.

of contrast nephropathy by avoiding unnecessary studies, particularly in patients with risk factors. If contrast administration is unavoidable, the high-risk patient should be given 0.45% saline intravenously at a rate of 1 mL per kilogram of body weight per hour beginning 12 hours before the procedure and continued for an additional 12 hours afterward. This regimen was found to provide better protection against acute decreases in renal function induced by radiocontrast than hydration plus mannitol or furosemide, which in the past had been suggested to be helpful in this setting. Concomitant administration of other nephrotoxic agents should be avoided and the amount of contrast used during the study should be kept to a minimum. As noted above, low osmolality, nonionic agents exert no clear benefit in preventing nephrotoxicity.

Immunosuppressive Drugs

Cyclosporine

Cyclosporine is an unusual cyclic peptide compound that inhibits early events involved in T cell activation and is extremely effective in suppressing transplant rejection. Since its introduction in 1983, cyclosporine has become the primary component of immunosuppressive regimens administered to patients with virtually every type of organ graft. In addition, cyclosporine has demonstrated efficacy in the treatment of autoimmune disorders such as psoriasis and uveitis. However, the clinical applications of cyclosporine have been limited by the frequent occurrence of nephrotoxicity and especially concern over the potential for developing chronic, irreversible renal injury.

Cyclosporine nephrotoxicity can be manifested by three distinct clinical syndromes: acute reversible renal dysfunction, chronic interstitial nephropathy, and thrombotic microangiopathy. Acute cyclosporine nephrotoxicity is the predominant renal abnormality seen within the first 6 to 12 months after initiating treatment and is characterized by an acute or subacute reduction in renal function that is often dose dependent. Generally, renal dysfunction is nonprogressive and reverses when the dose is lowered or the drug is discontinued. Virtually every patient who receives therapeutic doses of cyclosporine will experience a component of persistent, reversible reduction in GFR and renal blood flow. The mechanism of acute cyclosporine nephrotoxicity is hemodynamic and results from the ability of cyclosporine to induce intense renal vasoconstriction. NSAIDs may enhance acute effects of cyclosporine on renal hemodynamics. Cyclosporine does not cause renal vasoconstriction directly, but may act through stimulating production of other vasoconstrictor compounds such as thromboxane A_2, endothelin, or leukotrienes.

In renal transplant recipients within the first year after transplant, it is often difficult to clinically differentiate acute cyclosporine nephrotoxicity from acute rejection. A stable or slowly progressive increase in serum creatinine that reverses when the cyclosporine dose is reduced suggests nephrotoxicity. Renal biopsy can be helpful in this setting since aggressive inflammatory cell infiltrates are usually absent in acute cyclosporine nephrotoxicity and their presence in a biopsy specimen would suggest ongoing rejection.

In addition, prominent vacuolization of proximal tubular epithelial cells has been described in acute cyclosporine toxicity. While serum cyclosporine levels are frequently used to monitor therapeutic efficacy and to prevent toxicity, there is only a rough correlation between serum levels and clinical events.

Chronic cyclosporine nephrotoxicity is defined by the development of interstitial fibrosis with reduced levels of GFR in patients receiving long-term cyclosporine treatment. Generally, 6 to 12 months of treatment are required before signs of chronic nephropathy become apparent. Because of the irreversible nature of the morphologic abnormalities, this form of toxicity is more ominous than the acute form. Histologically, chronic cyclosporine nephrotoxicity is characterized by focal or striped medullary interstitial fibrosis. Often these changes are accompanied by tubular atrophy and obliterative arteriolar changes. In more advanced cases, diffuse interstitial fibrosis with focal and segmental glomerular sclerosis can be seen. In renal transplant patients, these changes may be difficult to differentiate from the typical features of chronic rejection. While the mechanism of chronic cyclosporine nephrotoxicity is not known, it is likely that cumulative dose, arterial hypertension, and immunologic injury contribute to the development of the lesion. In addition, animal studies suggest that severe sodium depletion may potentiate the development of renal fibrosis associated with cyclosporine administration.

In a small number of patients who have been treated with cyclosporine, fulminant ARF occurs with thrombocytopenia, consumptive coagulopathy, and thrombotic microangiopathy. This syndrome has been described in both kidney and bone marrow allograft recipients. In renal transplants, the histologic changes resemble those of hemolytic-uremic syndrome and the occurrence of this disorder carries a poor prognosis for kidney graft survival. However, patients usually recover when the cyclosporine is discontinued and some of these patients have been successfully retransplanted using other immunosuppressives. The mechanism of this devastating syndrome is not known but imbalances of vasoconstrictor to vasodilator eicosanoids have been suggested to play a role.

Cyclosporine is metabolized primarily through the action of hepatic P450 microsomal enzymes. Thus, agents that influence the activity of this enzyme system can cause significant changes in cyclosporine metabolism. Generally, drugs that reduce the rate of cyclosporine metabolism, such as erythromycin, ketoconazole, and verapamil, produce increased serum levels and potentiate toxicity. On the other hand, agents that increase the rate of cyclosporine metabolism, such as phenytoin, phenobarbital, and rifampin, may reduce serum levels and thus may blunt therapeutic efficacy.

Tacrolimus

Tacrolimus (formerly known as FK506) is a macrolide antibiotic with profound immunosuppressive properties. Despite its complete lack of structural similarity with cyclosporine, the effects of tacrolimus on cytokine expression and T lymphocyte activation are identical to those of cyclosporine. The molecular target for both tacrolimus and cyclosporine is calcineurin, a protein phosphatase that is required for signaling by the T cell receptor. However, tacrolimus is more than 100 times more potent than cyclosporine in inhibiting this pathway. In view of its enhanced potency, the efficacy of tacrolimus has been compared to cyclosporine in a series of clinical trials. In these studies, tacrolimus reduced the incidence of rejection; however, patient and graft survival were not prolonged. Moreover, the side effects of tacrolimus, including nephrotoxicity, were similar to and, in some cases, more severe than those in cyclosporine-treated patients. Both acute and chronic nephrotoxicity have been described with tacrolimus, but it has been suggested that hypertension occurs less frequently, which, if confirmed, would be a major clinical advantage. The observation that these chemically dissimilar compounds have in vivo effects that are essentially identical underscores the key role for calcineurin inhibition in both the efficacy and toxicities of tacrolimus and cyclosporine.

Bibliography

Appel GB, Given DB, Levine LR, Cooper GL: Vancomycin and the kidney. *Am J Kidney Dis* 8:75–80, 1986.

Bennett WM: The nephrotoxicity of immunosuppressive drugs. *Clin Nephrol* 43(Suppl 1):S3–57, 1995.

Branch RA: Prevention of amphotericin B-induced renal impairment. *Arch Intern Med* 148:2389–2394, 1988.

Humes HD, Weinberg JM, Knauss TC: Clinical and pathophysiologic aspects of aminoglycoside nephrotoxicity. *Am J Kidney Dis* 2:5–25, 1982.

Kaloyanides GJ: Antibiotic-related nephrotoxicity. *Nephrol Dial Transplant* 9(Suppl 4):130–134, 1994.

Kopp JR, Klotman PE: Cellular and molecular mechanisms of cyclosporin nephrotoxicity. *J Am Soc Nephrol* 1:162–179, 1990.

Parfrey PS, Griffiths SM, Barrett BJ, et al.: Contrast-material induced renal failure in patients with diabetes mellitus, renal insufficiency, or both: a prospective controlled study. *N Engl J Med* 320:143–149, 1989.

Sawyer MH, Webb DE, Balow JE, Straus SE: Acyclovir-induced renal failure. *Am J Med* 84:1067–1071, 1988.

Schwab SJ, Hlatky MA, Pieper KS, et al.: Contrast nephrotoxicity: A randomized controlled trial of a nonionic and an ionic radiographic contrast agent. *N Engl J Med* 320:149–153, 1989.

Solomon R, Werner C, Mann D, D'Elia J, Silva P: Effects of saline, mannitol, and furosemide on acute decreases in renal function induced by radiocontrast agents. *N Engl J Med* 331:1416–142, 1994.

Tune BM, Hsu C-Y, Fravert D: Cephalosporin and carbacephem nephrotoxicity: Roles of tubular cell uptake and acylating potential. *Biochem Pharmacol* 51(4):557–561, 1996.

US Multicenter FK506 Liver Study Group. A comparison of tacrolimus (FK506) and cyclosporine for immunosuppression in liver transplantation. *N Engl J Med* 331:1110–1115, 1994.

Welty TE, Copa AK: Impact of vancomycin therapeutic drug monitoring on patient care. *Ann Pharmacother* 28:1335–1339, 1994.

Whelton A. Therapeutic initiatives for the avoidance of aminoglycoside toxicity. *J Clin Pharmacol* 25:67–81, 1985.

Zager RA: Endotoxemia, renal hypoperfusion, and fever: Interactive risk factors for aminoglycoside and sepsis-associated acute renal failure. *Am J Kidney Dis* 20(3):223–230, 1992.

37

ACUTE RENAL FAILURE DUE TO METABOLIC DERANGEMENTS

CHRISTOF WESTENFELDER

Acute renal failure (ARF) can complicate acute elevations of (1) *uric acid*, causing *uric acid nephropathy;* (2) *calcium*, causing *hypercalcemic nephropathy;* and (3) *phosphate*, causing *hyperphosphatemic nephropathy*. Most patients with tumor lysis syndrome or with myoglobinuric ARF present with both severe hyperuricemia and hyperphosphatemia. All three complications can occur when patients with malignancy-induced hypercalcemia receive chemotherapy.

ACUTE URIC ACID NEPHROPATHY

Uric acid nephropathy (UAN) is a reversible form of ARF that develops when intraluminally precipitated uric acid (UA) and monosodium urate (UR) crystals cause extensive obstruction of renal collecting ducts. This occurs most commonly as part of the tumor lysis syndrome, i.e., when patients with myelo- or lymphoproliferative malignancies receive chemotherapy. The syndrome may also occur spontaneously, when tumor burden is high and cell turnover rapid. The high rate of nucleic acid breakdown leads to grossly augmented UA production, hyperuricemia, and hyperuricosuria. Reversal or prevention of UAN is successful in approximately 95% of patients.

Pathology

On gross examination, the papillae contain yellow, linear striations that outline the course of collecting ducts obstructed by precipitated UA and UR. On microscopic examination, the tubular lumens contain needle-shaped birefringent crystals. Proximal tubules may be dilated due to obstruction. The glomeruli are spared, except for mild dilatation of Bowman's space. If acute uric nephropathy is unresolved, acute and chronic inflammatory cells, tubulointerstitial granulomas, edema, and medullary microtophi appear.

Pathogenesis

Critical to the development of UAN is the extensive obstruction of collecting ducts by UA and UR crystals, which occurs when the distal tubular solubility of these purines is exceeded. Such an increase is observed in patients with severe hyperuricemia and, less commonly, in markedly dehydrated patients, in whom serum UA levels may be normal. With dehydration, UA solubility can be exceeded because the urine in the distal tubule is hyperconcentrated. Urinary acidification by the collecting duct is another factor that contributes to the development of UAN. With a decrease in urinary pH, UR is converted to the less soluble purine UA. In most patients with UAN, all three pathogenic mechanisms are contributory.

Homeostasis and Renal Handling of Uric Acid (UA)

Uric acid is the xanthine oxidase-dependent end product of endogenous and dietary nucleoproteins. The UA pool in the adult is 1 g and the daily turnover 500 to 700 mg. Of the latter, 80% appears in the urine and 20% is metabolized by colonic bacteria. Eighty percent of the UA pool is derived from the catabolism of endogenous nucleic acids and nucleotides, the remainder from the diet.

In the kidney, UR and UA are subjected to (1) glomerular filtration, (2) almost complete proximal tubular reabsorption, (3) proximal tubular secretion, and (4) proximal and a minor degree of distal tubular "postsecretory" reabsorption. The fractional excretion of UR is 10%, which corresponds to the 24-hour urinary excretion of 500 to 700 mg. Volume expansion and some organic acids, e.g., salicylates in high doses or probenecid, reduce UR reabsorption. Volume contraction, on the other hand, enhances UR reabsorption and causes hyperuricemia. Hyperuricemia also develops when proximal tubular secretion of UR via the organic acid transporter is inhibited by competing organic acids, e.g., salicylates in low doses, probenecid, pyrazinamide, lactate, and ketoacids. Finally, UR excretion increases as glomerular filtration decreases and BUN and serum creatinine rise. As a consequence, plasma UR levels in patients with end-stage renal disease plateau at 12 to 13 mg/dL.

Clinical Presentation

Predictably, marked hyperuricemia (> 20 mg/dL), particularly when combined with dehydration or acidemia, causes acute UAN. A sudden fall in urine output, complete anuria, and rarely flank pain or ureteral colic may be noted. When severe, the acute loss in renal function leads to progressive azotemia, symptoms of uremia, volume overload, hyperkalemia, hyperphosphatemia, and metabolic acidosis. Unless pretreated with allopurinol and adequate volume expansion, up to 90% of patients who receive chemo- or radiation therapy for an advanced myelo- or lymphoproliferative malignancy (see Table 1) will develop hyperuricemia and secondary UAN. At least 30% of these develop severe hyperkalemia and hyperphosphatemia, both major complications of the tumor lysis syndrome. Since marked hyperphosphatemia per se can cause ARF and severe hypocalcemia, patients with tumor lysis require particularly aggressive and prompt therapy. On rare occasions, dehydration alone has been found to precipitate UAN in patients with breast, gastric, or myelo- or lymphoproliferative malignancies.

Patients with the rare *Lesch-Nyhan syndrome* develop recurrent episodes of UAN, severe hyperuricemia, gout, and encephalopathy with self-mutilation. These complications result from a complete, X-linked deficiency of hypoxanthine-guanine-phosphoribosyltransferase. Overproduction of UR due to other genetic disorders is an uncommon cause of UAN. Occasionally, uricosuric agents such as salicylates and probenecid can precipitate UAN. A purine-rich diet per se does not cause UAN.

Diagnosis

Typically, patients with suspected UAN present with ARF and severe hyperuricemia as chemotherapy for a myelo- or lymphoproliferative malignancy is initiated. A

TABLE I
Metabolically Induced Acute Renal Failure

Uric acid nephropathy
  Hyperuricosuria (>600 mg/24 h) with hyperuricemia
    Myelo-, lymphoproliferative malignancies with tumor lysis
    Metastatic cancers of breast, lung, stomach with tumor lysis
    Rhabdomyolysis, crush injury, seizures, thyrotoxicosis
    Lesch-Nyhan syndrome
  Hyperuricosuria (>600 mg/24 h) without hyperuricemia
    Uricosuric drugs: High-dose salicylates, probenecid
    Fanconi syndrome, acquired, genetic

Hypercalcemic nephropathy
  Malignancies: Squamous cell carcinoma of lung, lymphoma, multiple myeloma, kidney, breast
  Primary hyperparathyroidism
  Sarcoidosis, granulomatous diseases
  Vitamin D or A intoxication
  Milk-alkali syndrome, immobilization

Hyperphosphatemic nephropathy
  Myelo-, lymphoproliferative malignancies with tumor lysis
  Metastatic cancers of breast, lung with tumor lysis
  Rhabdomyolysis, crush injury, seizures, thyrotoxicosis, bowel necrosis
  In renal insufficiency: PO₄ enemas, PO₄ laxatives, TPN with PO₄

serum urate level greater than 20 mg/dL should suggest the diagnosis because values are seldom this high in other causes of renal failure. Similarly, a urine urate:creatinine excretion ratio greater than 1 (calculated from concentrations expressed in mg/dL) may be helpful as it suggests that the hyperuricemia results from overproduction and is associated with hyperuricosuria. In contrast, volume depletion and other states that cause hyperuricemia by reducing urate excretion tend to be associated with low ratios. Diuretics induce volume contraction and compete with urate for secretion as do other organic acids, such as salicylates, probenecid, lactate, and ketoacids. A high ratio is not an invariable finding in UAN. UA crystalluria occurs frequently, but it is neither a constant nor pathognomonic finding.

Hyperphosphatemia, hypocalcemia, and hyperkalemia are features of the tumor lysis syndrome that may accompany UAN. However, due to muscle destruction, these findings and hyperuricemia may also occur with rhabdomyolysis. In rhabdomyolysis-induced ARF, plasma CK and myoglobin levels are elevated. Other distinguishing features of this disorder are discussed in Chapter 39.

The diagnosis of UAN may be more difficult if spontaneous tumor lysis is the presenting feature of the malignancy. In addition, other causes of cancer-associated ARF such as direct renal infiltration with tumor, ureteral obstruction, sepsis, and administration of nephrotoxic antibiotics or chemotherapeutic agents must be considered. The diagnosis is usually made clinically and a kidney biopsy is generally not indicated.

Therapy and Outcome

With appropriate therapy, recovery of renal function in UAN approaches 100%, and attendant morbidity and mortality are mostly a function of the underlying disease. Prevention of UAN in high-risk patients with myelo- and lymphoproliferative malignancies is successful in more than 95% of cases. The duration of UAN depends on the age of the patient and other complicating factors. These include the presence of underlying renal disease or renal insufficiency, pyelonephritis, vascular disease, the concomitant use of nephrotoxic antibiotics, and the hemodynamic and nutritional status.

Prophylaxis
Patients with myelo- and lymphoproliferative malignancies or with extensive solid tumors are at greatest risk for UAN. In these, baseline 24-hours UR excretion is frequently >1000 mg/24 hr, while serum UA levels may be misleadingly normal. When dehydration or acidemia occurs, UAN develops. The situation is similar in HGPRT deficiency, and rarely occurs with gout. Allopurinol, maintenance of euvolemia, a high urine output (>2.5 L/day), and normal acid–base balance are effective preventive measures. The same principles apply when such a patient is to undergo cancer therapy; volume deficits must be corrected with parenteral normal saline and oral fluids, and a urine output of >2.5 L/day established. Furosemide may

be added once hydration is assured. Optimally, the urine is alkalinized to a pH >7.0, using iv sodium bicarbonate, or Shohl's solution, and, if needed, additional acetazolamide. Since the latter measures can cause hypokalemia, serum potassium levels must be monitored and corrected. Allopurinol is begun 1 to 3 days prior to cancer therapy. When renal function is impaired, the allopurinol dose must be reduced. Allopurinol raises plasma and urinary hypoxanthine and xanthine levels, occasionally causing ARF due to intrarenal xanthine precipitation, i.e., *xanthine nephropathy.*

Established UAN

Once oligoanuric UAN has developed, uremic symptoms and other complications develop as in any patient with severe ARF. Conservative therapy, as described above, may suffice if renal clearance is above 30 ml/min. Daily hemodialysis is highly effective in reducing the UR pool and in treating uremic and other complications. With severe hyperphosphatemia (>10 mg/dL), a low calcium dialysate must be used to prevent soft tissue calcification and ARF due to intrarenal $CaPO_4$ precipitation. The latter can also occur when patients with high $CaPO_4$ products, as seen in tumor lysis, receive bicarbonate for the purpose of urinary alkalinization.

HYPERCALCEMIC NEPHROPATHY

Hypercalcemic nephropathy results from the effects of acute or chronic hypercalcemia, which, in 50% of the patients, is the consequence of an underlying malignancy (Table 1). In addition to acute renal failure the renal complications of hypercalcemia include tubular defects such as renal tubular acidosis and nephrogenic diabetes insipidus, as well as nephrocalcinosis and nephrolithiasis. The severity of renal insufficiency depends on the duration and magnitude of hypercalcemia and concurrent hyperphosphatemia and hyperuricemia. Unless renal insufficiency is advanced, correction of hypercalcemia improves kidney function, reverses nephrocalcinosis, and reduces kidney stone formation.

Acute hypercalcemia decreases creatinine clearance via intrarenal vasoconstriction. In addition, high calcium levels reduce the reabsorption of Na, K, Mg, and H_2O, potentially lead to volume contraction, prerenal azotemia, hypernatremia, polydipsia, polyuria, and, in 20 to 30% of patients, hypokalemia and hypomagnesemia. Acute and severe hypercalcemia (>15 mg/dL), especially with concomitant hyperphosphatemia, can precipitate reversible ARF by causing renal vasoconstriction and distal tubular $CaPO_4$ precipitation.

Chronic hypercalcemia produces calcification and subsequent necrosis of collecting duct cells. Cellular debris and $CaPO_4$ crystals cause distal obstruction and proximal tubular dilatation. Nephron loss results from tubular atrophy, interstitial scarring, diffuse nephrocalcinosis, and stones. Furthermore, evolving distal renal tubular acidosis may aggravate nephrocalcinosis and kidney stone formation.

Once GFR is 30 mL/min or less, hyperphosphatemia develops and serum calcium falls.

More than 50% of patients with hypercalcemia develop hypertension due to increased peripheral vascular resistance and high cardiac output. Passage of a kidney stone may be the first manifestation of hypercalcemia. With severe hypercalcemia, oliguria, hypovolemia, confusion, lethargy, and muscle weakness develop.

The diagnosis of hypercalcemic nephropathy rests on the simultaneous demonstration of renal insufficiency and hypercalcemia. The urinalysis may show cellular casts, RBCs, and calcium phosphate or oxalate crystals. Nephrocalcinosis, stones, and obstruction are diagnosed radiographically, or by ultrasonography.

Correction of acute hypercalcemia and attendant volume deficits promptly improves renal function by reversing renal vasoconstriction and tubular obstruction. Whenever renal function allows, volume expansion with normal saline and furosemide are employed to increase urinary calcium excretion. Patients with poor renal function require intensive hemodialysis with a low calcium bath. This will effectively reduce serum calcium levels and correct uremic and other electrolyte abnormalities. For other calcium-lowering therapies see Chapter 14.

The prognosis of hypercalcemic nephropathy depends on the underlying disorder. Primary hyperparathyroidism and most other benign causes of hypercalcemia are eminently treatable and recovery from hypercalcemic nephropathy should be expected. The prognosis is more guarded when the hypercalcemia is due to malignancy.

HYPERPHOSPHATEMIC NEPHROPATHY

Extreme hyperphosphatemia (>20 mg/dL) is commonly complicated by soft tissue calcifications, hypocalcemia, and ARF. In general, hyperphosphatemia is a prominent finding of tumor lysis seen in patients who receive chemotherapy for malignancies such as Burkitt's lymphoma, lymphoblastic leukemia, metastatic small cell lung carcinoma, and adenocarcinoma of the breast. In addition, hyperphosphatemia can complicate rhabdomyolysis, malignant hyperthermia, and extensive bowel necrosis (Table 1). Release of cellular PO_4, K, nuclear proteins, and LDH produces hyperphosphatemia, hyperkalemia, hyperuricemia, and markedly elevated LDH levels. In addition, excessive PO_4 administration to patients with renal insufficiency causes symptomatic hyperphosphatemia.

ARF results from $CaPO_4$ precipitation in collecting ducts and renal interstitium, impairing renal function by obstruction and interstitial inflammation. Renal histology is similar to that seen in hypercalcemic nephropathy. Rhabdomyolysis may cause myoglobinuric ARF. Hyperphosphatemic patients are also at high risk for the development of UAN and may thus undergo urinary alkalinization. In the presence of profound hyperphosphaturia, alkalinization may lead to additional $CaPO_4$ precipitation and a further deterioration of renal function. In patients with a creatinine clearance >50 mL/min, volume expansion with normal saline, modest urinary alkalinization, and acetazolamide diuresis will rapidly lower plasma PO_4 levels and improve renal function. Glucose and insulin can be used to induce a transient intracellular shift of PO_4 and K. With poor renal function and uremic manifestations, intensive dialysis is required.

Bibliography

Benabe JE, Martinez-Maldonado M: Hypercalcemic nephropathy. Arch Intern Med 138:777–779, 1978.

Cohen LF, Balow JE, Magrath IT, Poplack DG, Ziegler JL: Acute tumor lysis syndrome: A review of 37 patients with Burkitt's lymphoma. *Am J Med* 68:486–491, 1980.

Conger JD: Acute uric acid nephropathy. *Semin Nephrol* 1:69–74, 1981.

Emmerson BT, Thompson L: The spectrum of hypoxanthine-guanine phosphoribosyltransferase deficiency. *Q J Med* 166:423–440, 1973.

Hande KR, Noone RM, Stone WJ: Severe allopurinol toxicity: Description and guidelines for prevention in patients with renal insufficiency. *Am J Med* 76:47–56, 1984.

Jones DP, Mahmoud H, Chesney RW: Tumor lysis syndrome: Pathogenesis and management. *Pediatr Nephrol* 9:206–212, 1995.

Kelly WN: Pharmacologic approach to the maintenance of urate homeostasis. *Nephron* 14:99–115, 1975.

Kelton J, Kelley WN, Holmes EW: A rapid method for the diagnosis of uric acid nephropathy. *Arch Intern Med* 138:612–615, 1978.

Kjellstrand CM, Campbell DC, von Haritzsch B, Buselmeier TJ: Hyperuricemic acute renal failure. *Arch Intern Med* 133:349–359, 1974.

Klinenberg JR, Kippen I, Bluestone R: Hyperuricemic nephropathy: Pathologic features and factors influencing urate deposition. *Nephron* 14:88–98, 1975.

Lins LE: Reversible renal failure caused by hypercalcemia: A retrospective study. *Acta Med Scand* 203:309–314, 1978.

Rieselbach RE, Bentzel CJ, Cotlove E, Frei E, Freireich EJ: Uric acid excretion and renal function in the acute hyperuricemia of leukemia: Pathogenesis and therapy of acute uric acid nephropathy. *Am J Med* 37:872–884, 1964.

Rieselbach RE, Steel TH: Influence of the kidney upon urate homeostasis in health and disease. *Am J Med* 56:665–675, 1974.

Simmonds HA, Cameron JS, Morris GS, Davies PM: Allopurinol in renal failure and the tumor lysis syndrome. *Clin Chim Acta* 160:189–195, 1986.

Stryer L: Biosynthesis of nucleotides. In: *Biochemistry,* 3rd ed. Freeman New York, pp. 601–621, 1988.

Tungsanga K, Boonwicht D, Lekhakula A, Sitprija V: Urine uric acid and urine creatinine ratio in acute renal failure. *Arch Intern Med* 144:934–937, 1984.

Zusman J, Brown DM, Nesbit ME: Hyperphosphatemia, hyperphosphaturia and hypocalcemia in acute lymphoblastic leukemia. *N Engl J Med* 289:1335–1340, 1973.

CHOLESTEROL ATHEROEMBOLIC RENAL DISEASE

ARTHUR GREENBERG

Cholesterol atheroembolic renal disease results when cholesterol crystals and other debris separate from atheromatous plaques, flow downstream, and lodge in small renal arteries, producing luminal occlusion, ischemia, and renal dysfunction. Depending on the source and distribution of emboli, renal disease may be the sole or predominant manifestation or simply one feature of a systemic illness characterized by multiorgan ischemia or infarction.

Early, autopsy-derived descriptions of renal atheroembolism overemphasized a catastrophic presentation with irreversible renal failure, intestinal infarction, and death from intra-abdominal sepsis. Recently, atheroembolism

has been recognized as a cause of occult or reversible renal failure. Recovery of renal function may follow extended survival on renal replacement therapy.

PATHOLOGY

The initial lesion in cholesterol atheroembolism is obstruction of a medium-sized or small artery by atheromatous debris. Arterioles and capillaries are less commonly affected. Lesions may occur in any organ. Cholesterol dissolves in formalin used to process tissue for routine histologic examination; crystals are not seen in tissue sections

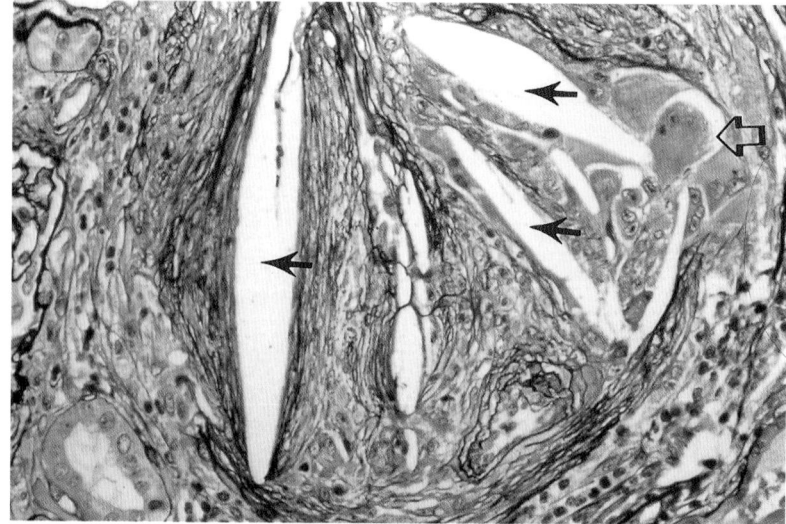

FIGURE I   Cholesterol atheroembolus occluding the lumen of an interlobular renal artery. Needle-like clefts (solid arrows) are present along with a macrophage/multinucleated giant cell reaction (open arrow) (methenamine silver-trichrome stain, 450X). (Courtesy of Dr. S.I. Bastacky.) Reproduced with permission from *Am J Kidney Dis* 29:334–344, 1997.

unless special fixatives are used. However, a characteristic cleft marks the space where the needle-like crystals had been (Fig. 1). The size of the artery affected is typically around 200 μm, but may range from 55 to 900 μm. The earliest lesion consists of cholesterol crystals and thrombus. After dissolution of the thrombus, macrophages engulf the cholesterol, but the predominant reaction is endothelial. New endothelium covers the crystals. If the vessel wall is eroded by the crystals, an intense perivascular inflamma-

tory response with giant cells is established (Fig. 1). As a late finding, concentric fibrosis, particularly involving the adventitia, occurs. Finally, there is recanalization of small vascular channels. Crystals may reach the glomerular capillary loops (Fig. 2). Crystal dissolution in vivo is slow; in experimental models, cholesterol clefts persist for long as 9 months after embolization. The main glomerular finding is that of ischemia, with glomerular collapse and basement membrane wrinkling. In some patients, focal segmental

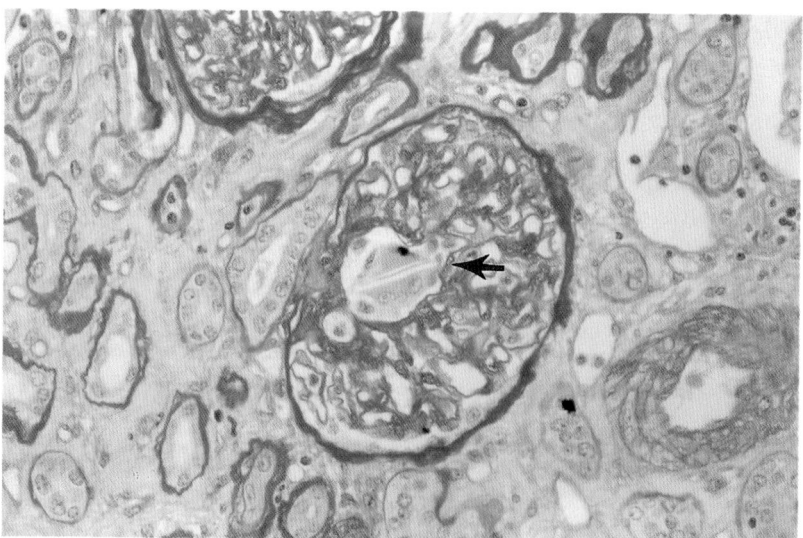

FIGURE 2   Glomerular findings in cholesterol atheroembolism. A distended glomerular capillary loop adjacent to the glomerular hilum contains a multinucleated macrophage with two cholesterol clefts (arrow) (hematoxylin-eosin stain, 150X). (Courtesy of Dr. Dennis Borochovitz.)

glomerulosclerosis with glomerular collapse and epithelial cell prominence occurs. This finding accounts for some of the cases associated with nephrotic range proteinuria.

PATHOGENESIS

The classic autopsy description by Flory noted cholesterol atheroembolism solely in patients with erosive plaques. The prevalence of atheroembolism paralleled the severity of aortic disease. Less severe atherosclerotic lesions or plaques covered by thrombus do not pose a risk of atheroembolism.

Embolization may be spontaneous—particularly with severe aortic disease—but mechanical disruption of plaque during angiographic or surgical procedures usually precedes it. Table 1 lists predisposing factors. Regardless of the area primarily targeted for imaging, passage of a catheter along the ascending or descending aorta proximal to the renal arteries confers a risk of embolization to the kidneys. Renal artery angioplasty may be a particular risk. The site of any concurrent nonrenal embolization depends on the path of the catheter.

Thrombus overlying atheromatous plaque may bind and immobilize friable debris. Anticoagulation or thrombolysis removes this protective covering; atheroembolism has been reported after heparin, warfarin, or thrombolytic therapy without angiography.

CLINICAL FEATURES

As expected of a process that complicates severe atherosclerosis, risk factors for atherosclerosis as well as evidence of disseminated atherosclerotic disease are commonly present. The incidence is higher in smokers. Up to 75% of patients are male. The mean age at diagnosis is in the mid-seventh decade. Fewer than 5% of patients are below age 50. Table 2 lists other accompanying or predisposing features. Notably, diabetes mellitus is not commonly observed.

Cholesterol atheroembolism is notable for its highly variable severity. Its manifestations depend on both the extent of renal involvement and the extrarenal sites affected. Mas-

TABLE 2

Associated Findings in 221 Patients with Cholesterol Atheroembolism[a]

Finding	% of cases
Hypertension	61
Coronary artery disease	44
Aortic aneurysm	25
Cerebrovascular disease	21
Congestive heart failure	21
Diabetes mellitus	11

[a] From Fine MJ, Kapoor W, Falanga V: *Angiology* 38:769–784, 1987.

sive and widespread embolization in the multiple cholesterol emboli syndrome presents catastrophically with fever, stroke, acute renal failure, abdominal pain and gastrointestinal bleeding due to bowel infarction, intra-abdominal sepsis, and death. The frequency of organ involvement is summarized in Table 3.

Autopsy reports are skewed toward patients with severe involvement. Recently, milder disease, with predominant renal and cutaneous involvement, has been recognized. Typically, the renal course is characterized by slowly deteriorating renal function. The daily increase in serum creatinine may be as little as 0.1 to 0.2 mg/dL and progression to end stage disease may occur over 30 to 60 days or even longer. Patients may also present over many months with the insidious development of renal insufficiency. Occasional patients present with heavy proteinuria—with or without associated clinical features of atheroembolism.

Skin involvement includes livedo reticularis of the lower extremities due to occlusion of small arteries as well as cyanosis of the toes. This classic "blue toes" lesion occurs in spite of preservation of distal pulses (Chapter 35, Fig. 1A). Digital ulceration may occur along with severe pain. Cutaneous involvement may be overlooked unless specifically sought.

Features of gastrointestinal involvement include abdominal pain, anorexia, weight loss, and bleeding that can range from a positive stool test for occult blood to brisk hemorrhage. Infarction and sepsis may occur. Central nervous system involvement includes stroke or diffuse cortical dysfunction due to widespread embolization as well as the scotomata, field cuts, or blindness that accompany the classic, but rare, retinal Hollenhorst plaque.

DIAGNOSIS

The diagnosis of atheroembolism relies on a high index of suspicion in patients at risk. During the acute phase, leukocytosis and an elevated erythrocyte sedimentation rate may be present. Eosinophilia is observed in approximately one half of affected individuals; hypocomplementemia occurs rarely. Hyperamylasemia suggests pancreatic involvement. Although nephrotic range proteinuria may

TABLE I

Risk Factors for Cholesterol Atheroembolic Renal Disease

Iatrogenic

Surgery on the aorta proximal to the renal arteries
  Aortic aneurysm repair
  Coronary artery bypass grafting
  Cardiac valve surgery
  Other

Angiography or angioplasty

Intra-aortic balloon pump circulatory augmentation

Anticoagulation or thrombolytic therapy

Spontaneous

Severe ulcerating atherosclerosis

TABLE 3

Histologic Involvement at Autopsy[a]

	% of cases
Kidney	75
Spleen	52
Pancreas	52
Gastrointestinal tract	31
Adrenal glands	20
Liver	17
Brain	14
Skin	6

[a] From Fine MJ, Kapoor W, Falanga V: *Angiology* 38: 769–784, 1987.

occur, proteinuria is typically modest and the urine sediment nonspecific.

Principal differential diagnostic considerations include radiocontrast-induced acute renal failure, ischemic acute tubular necrosis, systemic vasculitis, allergic interstitial nephritis, cryoglobulinemia, myeloma, hypertensive nephrosclerosis, and renal artery stenosis. Radiocontrast nephropathy (see Chapter 36) is readily distinguished from atheroembolism by its more rapid course. In dye nephropathy, renal failure occurs immediately, with renal function reaching a nadir within 3 or 4 days, and substantial recovery usually occurring over a similar period. In atheroembolism, the onset of renal failure may be delayed and progression is slower. Recovery occurs late—if at all.

Most instances of cholesterol atheroembolism are diagnosed clinically. If a tissue diagnosis is deemed necessary, biopsy of an area of livedo reticularis is the least invasive approach. A muscle biopsy may also be used. Although renal biopsy showing cholesterol atheroemboli is definitive, alternative means of diagnosis should be considered first.

THERAPY AND OUTCOME

Spontaneous atheroembolism occurs only in patients with more severe vascular involvement. Shedding of atheromatous debris often continues with a progressively declining course. In patients with atheroembolism after vascular surgery or angiography, embolization may be limited to the initial episode. Stabilization and gradual improvement may follow as small vessel inflammation subsides and re-

canalization with restoration of blood flow occurs. A typical patient will have gradually lessening anorexia and abdominal and digital pain with subsequent healing of digital ischemic lesions. Management focuses on supportive measures with local care of digital ischemia, analgesia for pain, and digital amputation if tissue is not viable. Anticoagulation should be stopped and repeat angiographic procedures avoided. Hemodialysis or peritoneal dialysis may be successfully employed. Some patients recover sufficient renal function to permit discontinuation of dialysis; in others, renal failure is irreversible. Recent reports note that abdominal or transesophageal ultrasonography may be used to localize diseased areas of aorta. Cholesterol atheroembolism occurs in an elderly population with extensive atherosclerotic disease and a high prevalence of hypertensive cardiovascular disease. Such patients present a formidable surgical risk; the role of endarterectomy or resection of diseased aortic segments has not been established.

Bibliography

Colt HG, Begg RJ, Saporito JJ, Cooper WM, Shapiro AP: Cholesterol emboli after cardiac catheterization. Eight cases and review of the literature. *Medicine* 67:389–400, 1988.

Fine MJ, Kapoor W, Falanga V: Cholesterol crystal embolization: A review of 221 cases in the English literature. *Angiology* 38:769–784, 1987.

Flory CM: Arterial occlusions produced by emboli from eroded aortic atheromatous plaques. *Am J Pathol* 21:549–565, 1945.

Greenberg A, Bastacky SI, Iqbal A, Borochovitz D, Johnson JP: Focal segmental glomerulosclerosis associated with nephrotic syndrome in cholesterol atheroembolism: Clinicopathologic correlations. *Am J Kidney Dis*, 29:334–344, 1997.

Kasinath BS, Corwin HL, Bidani AK, Korbet SM, Schwartz MM, Lewis EJ: Eosinophilia in the diagnosis of atheroembolic renal disease. *Am J Nephrol* 7:173–177, 1987.

Kassirer JP: Atheroembolic renal disease. *N Engl J Med* 280:812–818, 1969.

Mannesse CK, Blankestijn PJ, Man in 't Veld AJ, Schalekamp MADH: Renal failure and cholesterol crystal embolization: A report of 4 surviving cases and a review of the literature. *Clin Nephrol* 36:240–245, 1991.

McGowan JA, Greenberg A: Cholesterol atheroembolic renal disease. Report of 3 cases with emphasis on diagnosis by skin biopsy and extended survival. *Am J Nephrol* 6:135–139, 1986.

Thadhani RI, Carmago CA, Xavier RJ, Fang LST, Bazari H: Atheroembolic renal failure after invasive procedures. Natural history based on 52 histologically proven cases. *Medicine* 74:350–358, 1995.

Tunick PA, Perez JL, Kronzon I: Protruding atheromas in the thoracic aorta and systemic embolization. *Ann Intern Med* 115:423–427, 1991.

39

PIGMENT NEPHROPATHY

JAMES P. KNOCHEL

Pigment nephropathy is a term describing acute renal failure caused by rhabdomyolysis with myoglobinuria or hemolysis with hemoglobinuria.

RHABDOMYOLYSIS

Rhabdomyolysis results from injury to muscle cells, causing leakage of their contents into the blood and urine. Trauma or recurrent attacks of cramps or pain during exercise and excretion of cola-colored urine are classic events in rhabdomyolysis. Although some patients experience few symptoms, most demonstrate tender, stiff, or firm muscles. Severe weakness or even paralysis may occur due to extensive necrosis or hyperkalemia. Serum creatine phosphokinase (CK) is virtually always elevated in rhabdomyolysis. Idiopathic muscle necrosis in patients with diabetes mellitus is a rare exception.

Causes

Exertional and Traumatic Rhabdomyolysis
Normal subjects can develop rhabdomyolysis after intense exercise. Violent, repetitive activities or a grand mal seizure are good examples. Presumably, exhaustive exercise may not only directly injure structural components of muscle cells, but also deplete energy stores and disrupt cellular transport, thereby allowing calcium to accumulate in the cell. Calcium overload in turn activates proteolytic enzymes that result in cell death. Many factors lower the threshold for injury. These include poor physical condition or preexistent injury, typified by alcoholic myopathy. For any given unit of work, women unexplainably show much less rhabdomyolysis than men. Volume depletion and exercise in the heat, perhaps by causing overheating of muscle and reduced blood flow, are potentiating factors. Eccentric muscle contractions (running downhill) are more likely to cause rhabdomyolysis than concentric contractions (running uphill). Fasting lowers the threshold presumably by limiting substrates for muscle contraction. Finally, associated illnesses that primarily affect skeletal muscle, typified by influenza, reduce the threshold for injury induced by exercise. Death in cases of crush syndrome is often related to the complications of rhabdomyolysis.

Inherited Metabolic Myopathies
A number of specific enzyme derangements are responsible for exertional rhabdomyolysis. Classic examples are myophosphorylase deficiency (McArdle's syndrome) and carnitine palmityl transferase deficiency.

Acquired Metabolic Myopathies
Potassium deficiency is a typical example of an acquired metabolic myopathy. Potassium deficiency impairs glycogen synthesis in muscle. Since glycogen is a major energy substrate during anaerobic work, physical work performed by a potassium deficient individual can result in rhabdomyolysis. Potassium deficiency also interferes with the normal increase of muscle blood flow with exercise. This can impose damage by ischemia.

Hypoxia/Ischemia
Carbon monoxide poisoning, by causing hypoxia because of carbon monoxyhemoglobin formation, is a recognized cause of acute rhabdomyolysis. Severe congestive heart failure may cause modest rhabdomyolysis.

Drugs
Many drugs cause subtle muscle cell injury or frank rhabdomyolysis. Although hundreds of drugs have been implicated, those of major concern include cocaine, heroin, amphetamines, HMG-CoA inhibitors, and fibric acid derivatives used as cholesterol-lowering agents, especially when given in conjunction with cyclosporine, nicotinic acid, or erythromycin. The combination of lovastatin and gemfibrozil may also cause rhabdomyolysis. Drugs that appear to interfere with key glycolytic enzymes—such as isoniazide hydrazide, which impairs activity of glycogen phosphorylase—may also be implicated.

Special Causes
A number of substances are directly myotoxic. These include clostridial toxin in gas gangrene, the proteolytic enzymes in snake venom, or the myotoxin that accumulates in skeletal muscle of the quail when it ingests sweet parsley seeds. Hypothyroidism consistently causes elevated CK and sometimes causes frank rhabdomyolysis.

Laboratory Diagnosis
The CK-MM is the dominant isoform in skeletal muscle and the most sensitive test to confirm the diagnosis. Without ongoing necrosis, CK peaks at 12 to 36 hours and has

a half life of about 48 hours (Fig. 1). The CK-MB isoform, commonly employed to detect myocardial injury, may constitute 5% of total CK in skeletal muscle of highly trained athletes. Healthy persons undergoing training exercises often show CK enzyme elevations as high as 10,000 IU/L. Patients who are seriously ill from a variety of causes commonly show elevated CK-MM levels ranging from normal to 10,000 IU/L. These include congestive heart failure with hypoxia, sepsis, and a variety of acute infections. However, in rhabdomyolysis of clinical importance, elevations of this enzyme are higher, commonly reaching levels of 100,000 IU/L or higher. In extreme cases, CK may approach 3.0 million IU/L. Measurements of other muscle enzymes in rhabdomyolysis such as aldolase, lactic dehydrogenase, or transaminases provide no additional useful information.

A transient elevation of serum creatinine disproportionate to the elevation of BUN is commonly seen in acute rhabdomyolysis. This results from release of creatine phosphate from muscle which is spontaneously dehydrated to creatinine. The usual ratio of urea nitrogen to creatinine in serum is 10:1. Ratios of five or less shortly after onset suggest acute rhabdomyolysis. Uric acid in serum may exceed 40 mg/dL. Purines released from injured muscle are converted to urate in the liver. Hyperuricemia of this magnitude is seldom seen in other conditions, even acute tumor lysis induced by chemotherapy. Leukocytosis is common in rhabdomyolysis of any etiology. Hypoalbuminemia is an ominous sign and implies major capillary damage with leakage of plasma components out of the vascular space. On rare occasions, capillary damage may be so extensive that erythrocytes also escape into interstitial tissues. This results in shock with an acute reduction of hematocrit in the absence of bleeding or hemolysis. A urine sodium concentration above 20 mEq/L suggests tubular injury. However, the urine sodium concentration may be low in cases

of myoglobinuria and, accordingly, this finding in pigment nephropathy may be less helpful than in other oliguric settings. Hyperkalemia is often observed as a consequence of potassium release from damaged muscle cells. Profound hypocalcemia, with serum calcium values below 3.0 mg/dL, may result from hyperphosphatemia and trapping of calcium in injured muscle. Transient resistance to parathyroid hormone followed by hypercalcemia during the recovery phase may be observed. Glucose may be detected in the urine despite a normal glucose concentration in serum. This apparently represents proximal tubular injury as a result of pigment damage to the tubular epithelium. Finally, pigmented casts may be seen in the urine.

HEMOLYSIS AND HEMOGLOBINURIA

Visible hemoglobinemia and hemoglobinuria occur only in instances of major intravascular hemolysis. In extravascular hemolysis, hemoglobin released into tissues is promptly metabolized to bilirubin and the only pigment found in the urine will be increased quantities of urobilinogen.

Transfusion with mismatched blood is the most common cause of hemoglobin-induced nephropathy. Mycoplasma infection appears to be the most common cause of hemolysis mediated by infection-associated immunologic mechanisms. Patients undergoing transurethral resection of the prostate may develop major intravascular hemolysis as a result of absorption of glycine solution from the prostatic bed. Saline is not used in the perfusate because of the hazards of electrical conduction by ionic solutions when cautery is employed. The glycine is metabolized, allowing electrolyte-free water to induce hemolysis. An example of red cell oxidant injury is that mediated by application of copper sulfate to white phosphorus burns. The term "black water fever" refers to hemoglobinuria and acute renal failure in patients with falciparum malaria. Recent evidence suggests that drugs used to treat malaria in addition to the disease itself may be responsible for hemolysis or, alternatively, that some cases represent frank myoglobinuria as a result of rhabdomyolysis associated with the malarial infection. Laboratory findings in patients with intravascular hemolysis include elevations of lactic dehydrogenase which may be striking, slight hyperbilirubinemia, and in some instances hyperkalemia and hyperphosphatemia. Plasma hemoglobin levels will be markedly elevated. After hemolysis, haptoglobin levels will be abnormally low. The urine, similar to that from patients with rhabdomyolysis, may show pigmented casts as well as free hemoglobin or its product, hematin.

DISPOSITION OF HEME PIGMENTS IN PLASMA

There is a fundamental difference between the fate of hemoglobin and that of myoglobin after their release into plasma. Free hemoglobin in plasma saturates haptoglobin at a concentration of approximately 100 mg/dL. Because the hemoglobin haptoglobin complex is a large molecule, it is not filtered by the glomerulus. Accordingly, hemoglo-

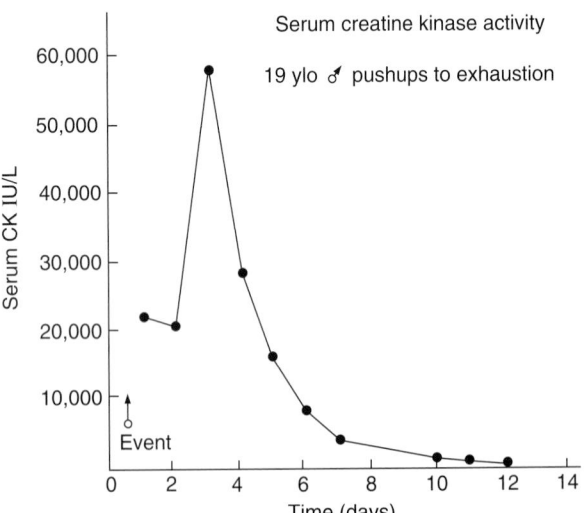

FIGURE I The course of serum CK activity in a 19-year-old healthy man who developed rhabdomyolysis of the deltoid and triceps muscles as a result of performing pushups to the point of absolute exhaustion.

bin will not appear in the urine until plasma haptoglobin becomes saturated and total hemoglobin exceeds 100 mg/dL. Hemoglobin becomes visible at a concentration of 100 mg/dL. In contrast to hemoglobin, myoglobin has no specific binding protein. Any myoglobin entering plasma is readily filtered by the glomerulus. Thus, the presence of stained serum suggests hemolysis, not rhabdomyolysis. Accordingly, if heme pigment is present in the urine, a clear serum suggests rhabdomyolysis and myoglobinuria. Because dipstick tests are exquisitely sensitive for detection of heme pigment in the urine, there is no practical need to perform more sophisticated and expensive tests to either detect or differentiate myoglobin or hemoglobin.

MECHANISMS OF PIGMENT NEPHROPATHY

When acute renal failure complicating crush injury was described shortly after World War II by Bywaters and Beall, it was recognized that when pigmenturia occurs in a setting of hypotension, decreased renal perfusion, and an acid urine, acute tubular necrosis is likely to follow. Subsequent experimental studies showed that if arterial volume, blood pressure, and renal perfusion were intact before the event, infusion of muscle extracts, myoglobin, or hemoglobin had no adverse effects on renal function. Experimental studies also showed that infusion of saline, bicarbonate solutions, or mannitol before pigmenturia was induced protected against acute renal failure.

The classic pathological findings in pigment nephropathy include proximal tubular necrosis and distal tubular obstruction by pigmented casts. The mechanisms underlying proximal tubular injury have been explored in detail. Once the myoglobin or hemoglobin molecule is filtered by the glomerulus and enters the proximal tubular fluid, it probably enters the proximal tubular cell by endocytosis. Hypothetically, the intact heme pigment molecule then is taken up by lysosomes. The pH of the lysosomes is sufficiently low that the heme pigment splits into its globin and ferrihemate components. Ferrihemate is then transported out of the tubular cell, requiring expenditure of ATP. In the presence of renal ischemia, hypoxia, and a critical reduction of ATP stores incident to active transport, the cell becomes injured. Distal tubular obstruction by casts appears to increase the amount of heme pigment absorbed by the proximal tubular cells and, accordingly, increases its toxicity. In addition, the iron portion of the ferrihemate molecule may generate toxic superoxide radicals. Cytochrome P450 may be a source of iron that catalyzes formation of these products. Pigment-induced nephrotoxicity is attenuated by substances, such as deferoxamine that scavenge free oxygen radicals. Experimentally, the kidney itself induces increased formation of heme oxygenase to protect against continued or repeated exposures to heme proteins. Heme pigments may also bind endogenous nitric oxide and thereby cause vasoconstriction. Another theory holds that intracellular stores of glutathione become exhausted and this source of protection against oxidation damage is lost. Although mannitol may be a free hydroxyl scavenger, its major effect is to act as a diuretic and dilute the concentra-

tion of heme proteins within the tubular lumen, thus possibly decreasing their nephrotoxicity. In addition, mannitol may enhance excretion of heme proteins, especially if they have been solubilized by alkalinization of the urine with bicarbonate. Unfortunately, no study has conclusively shown that either mannitol or bicarbonate exerts protection if given after the pigment is administered. Clearly, gelification of heme proteins in the distal tubule, a process requiring interaction with Tamm-Horsfall proteins, would be ameliorated by any intervention that decreases their concentration or renders them less likely to form gels. Accordingly, infusion of bicarbonate to alkalinize the urine has been recommended for 50 years. Nevertheless, it has not been clearly shown whether the prophylactic effect of bicarbonate is related to alkalinization or simply its osmotic diuretic effect. Recent evidence suggests that intestinal endotoxins may be absorbed under several conditions, such as in exhaustive exercise, trauma, or sepsis, thereby generating a cascade of cytokines (tumor necrosis factor and other interleukins) that might also play a role in the pathogenesis of tubular injury. This could be of particular importance in patients who sustain massive rhabdomyolysis as a result of a heavy exertion in the heat. Finally, renal tubular cell injury has also been related to accumulation of calcium in the cytoplasm which activates destructive proteases or phospholipases. The cytoprotective effect of drugs that prevent calcium entry in the cells as well as several amino acids that either protect against the harmful effects of heme-pigments (glycine) or promote their excretion (lysine) have also been reported.

TREATMENT OF PIGMENT NEPHROPATHY

In severe rhabdomyolysis, it is critical to correct hypovolemia and shock by infusion of blood or crystalloid to maintain perfusion of vital organs. Although its use is controversial, most physicians advocate mannitol in a single intravenous dose of 12.5 or 25 g over 15 to 30 minutes. A total of 12.5 g or 70 mmol of mannitol (MW = 180) infused into a total body water of 40 L results in only a trivial increase of plasma osmolality, extracellular, or intra-arterial volume. If this substance results in increased renal perfusion and more rapid clearance of the heme pigment from the kidney, its use is clearly justifiable. A single dose of furosemide is also recommended to reduce sodium transport and oxygen utilization by the kidney, thus theoretically preserving vital energy stores in the renal tubular cells. Its diuretic effect possibly reduces the concentration of heme proteins in the distal nephron. At the same time, because of the potential of increasing solubility of heme proteins, one should administer sodium bicarbonate to alkalinize the urine. In some patients, it is extremely difficult to achieve adequate urinary alkalinization because of the severity of the associated metabolic acidosis.

Hyperkalemia potentially causes arrhythmias, a fall in cardiac output, cardiac arrest, muscle paralysis, or respiratory failure if untreated. In severe rhabdomyolysis, even modest hyperkalemia may cause cardiotoxicity because of the simultaneous hypocalcemia that nearly always occurs.

Calcium ions electrically oppose the cardiotoxic effects of potassium. A serum potassium value of only 6.5 mEq/L may be cardiotoxic when serum calcium is profoundly decreased. For this reason, the serum level of potassium should not be relied upon as the sole marker of the severity of cardiotoxicity; rather, the electrocardiogram itself must be followed. Acute cardiotoxicity is most quickly and effectively treated by infusing calcium chloride, which produces instantaneous improvement in the electrocardiogram. Unfortunately, infused calcium salts are rapidly deposited in injured tissue so that their effect is transient. In addition, calcium infusions do not lower serum potassium concentration. Specific maneuvers to reduce serum potassium concentration must be introduced simultaneously. These include glucose and insulin infusions and therapy with potent β-sympathetic agonists such as albuterol. By convention, sodium bicarbonate infusions are also employed to shift potassium into cells. However, the efficacy of bicarbonate for treatment of hyperkalemia has been questioned. It should be kept in mind that injured muscle cells are less likely to take up potassium and these therapies may be less effective than expected. Thus, in some cases of hyperkalemia, despite treatment, potassium ions are released at such a rapid rate from injured muscle cells that dialysis becomes mandatory. If possible, 20% sorbitol containing the sodium potassium exchange resin disodium polystyrene disulfonate should be administered as soon as possible, by either the oral or the rectal route, or both. Although this measure is not effective as an acute treatment of hyperkalemia, it will help to blunt the rise of potassium over the next 2 or 3 days. Hypocalcemia per se does not usually require treatment unless calcium salts must be given for hyperkalemia or for a hypocalcemia-induced decrease in cardiac output. Despite hypocalcemia, tetany is very rare in these patients, probably because of the muscle injury and the antitetanic effect of metabolic acidosis. In those patients given large quantities of calcium salts intravenously, subsequent mobilization of calcium from injured tissue during the diuretic phase may result in potentially fatal hypercalcemia. Accordingly, calcium salts should not be used unless necessary. Hyperphosphatemia should be treated by administration of phosphate binding antacids, debridement of necrotic tissue in trauma cases, or dialysis.

Some authorities have advocated plasma exchange to remove heme proteins and other proteinaceous components of destroyed cells from the circulation. However, this is not an established form of treatment because of the rapid clearance of pigment from plasma by the liver and spleen. One must be vigilant for infection in any patient with acute renal failure. Other complications seen include disseminated intravascular coagulation and thrombocytopenia. In most instances, this complication clears spontaneously within a few days but may require fresh frozen plasma or specific components to facilitate blood clotting. Adult respiratory distress syndrome (ARDS) and multiple organ failure are also important complications.

One must be alert for development of fascial compartment compression syndromes. This is most apt to involve muscles of the lateral thigh, the gastrocnemius, the anterior tibial, and the gluteus maximus. Almost any muscle can be involved. When muscle injury occurs, protein components of muscle cells decompose and form powerful osmotic forces that pull water into the muscle cell. If the muscle is in a fascial compartment, the pressure rapidly increases and will soon exceed arterial pressure. Ischemia and necrosis follow. This can account for a secondary rise of CK in serum or the appearance of irreversible nerve damage. Measurement of tissue pressure in such locations can accurately predict the occurrence of a compartment syndrome. Prophylactic treatment by fasciotomy can prevent secondary tissue necrosis. Current investigations suggest that mannitol may also be helpful toward preventing the compartment syndrome.

Bibliography

Baliga R, Zhang Z, Baliga M, Shah SV: Evidence for cytochrome P-450 as a source of catalytic iron in myoglobinuric acute renal failure. *Kidney Int* 49:362–369, 1996.

Better OS, Stein JH: Early management of shock and prophylaxis of acute renal failure in traumatic rhabdomyolysis. *N Engl J Med* 322:825–829, 1990.

Bywaters EG, Beall D: Crush injuries with impairment of renal function. *Br Med J* 1:427–432, 1941.

Curry SC, Chang D, Connor D: Drug- and toxin-induced rhabdomyolysis. *Ann Emerg Med* 18:1068–1084, 1989.

Gabow PA, Kaehny WD, Kelleher SP: The spectrum of rhabdomyolysis. *Medicine* 61:141–149, 1982.

Haller RG, Knochel JP: Metabolic myopathies. In: Johnson RT, Griffin JW (eds) *Current Ther. Neurol. Dis.*, Decker, pp. 397–402, 1993.

Knochel JP: Catastrophic medical events with exhaustive exercise: White collar rhabdomyolysis. *Kidney Int* 38:709–719, 1990.

Knochel JP: Hematuria in sickle cell trait. *Arch Intern Med* 123:160–165, 1969.

Knochel JP: Hypophosphatemia and rhabdomyolysis. *Am J Med* 92:455–457, 1992.

Knochel JP: Mechanisms of rhabdomyolysis. *Curr Opin Rheumatol* 5:725–731, 1993.

Knochel JP: Potassium deficiency and rhabdomyolysis. *J Mol Cell Cardiol* 27:241–249, 1995.

Miller JH McDonald RK: The effect of hemoglobin on renal function in the human. *J Clin Invest* 30:1033–1040, 1951.

Nath KA, Balla G, Vercollotti GM, et al.: Induction of heme oxygenase is a rapid and protective response in rhabdomyolysis in the rat. *J Clin Invest* 90:267–270, 1992.

Umpierrez GE, Stiles RG, Kleinbart J, Krendel DA, Watts NB: Diabetic muscle infarction. *Am J Med* 101:245–250, 1996.

Wakabayashi Y, Kikuno T, Ohwada T, Kikawada R: Rapid fall in blood myoglobin in massive rhabdomyolysis and acute renal failure. *Inten Care Med* 20:109–112, 1994.

Zager RA: Rhabdomyolysis and myohemoglobinuric acute renal failure. *Kidney Int* 49:314–326, 1996.

40

ACUTE INTERSTITIAL NEPHRITIS

CATHERINE M. MEYERS

Primary interstitial nephropathies constitute a diverse group of diseases that elicit interstitial inflammation associated with renal tubular cell damage. This process typically spares both glomerular and vascular structures. Traditionally, interstitial nephritis has been classified morphologically and clinically into acute and chronic forms. Acute interstitial nephritis (AIN) generally induces rapid deterioration in renal function, and elicits marked interstitial inflammatory responses characterized by interstitial edema with varying degrees of tubular cell damage, as well as mononuclear cell infiltrates consisting primarily of lymphocytes (Fig. 1). Eosinophils, macrophages, plasma cells, and neutrophils may also be apparent within these infiltrates. In some cases of AIN, interstitial granuloma formation is also observed. Most commonly this form of granulomatous interstitial nephritis is associated with either drug- or infection-induced renal inflammation. By contrast, chronic tubulointerstitial disease follows an indolent course, characterized by tubulointerstitial fibrosis and atrophy associated with interstitial mononuclear cell infiltration. AIN is not an uncommon cause of renal dysfunction, and should always be considered in the differential diagnosis of acute renal failure (ARF). Moreover, estimates from recent large clinical studies suggest that AIN comprises approximately 10 to 15% of reported cases of ARF.

PATHOGENESIS

Despite the varied inciting factors of tubulointerstitial nephritis in humans (Table 1), the striking similarity of induced interstitial lesions, which consist primarily of T cell lymphocytes, suggests that immune-mediated mechanisms are important either in initiating the interstitial damage or in amplifying primary interstitial injury from nonimmune causes. Studies from experimental models of interstitial disease suggest that both humoral and cell-mediated immune mechanisms are relevant effector pathways for inducing interstitial injury. Cell-mediated events likely play a prominent role in most forms of human disease, in view of the preponderance of T cell lymphocytes ($CD4^+$ and $CD8^+$) present within interstitial infiltrates, generally in the absence of antibody deposition. Immunohistochemical studies conducted on biopsies obtained in drug-induced AIN also indicate the importance of cell–cell interactions in intrarenal inflammation, as there is a significant increase in interstitial expression of cellular adhesion molecules. In AIN, increased expression of LFA-1 and VLA-4 cell surface receptors, as well as their respective ligands ICAM-1 and VCAM-1, is generally observed in areas of mononuclear cell infiltration. Recent studies have extended these observations by examining the role of monocyte chemotactic peptide-1 (MCP-1), a potent chemoattractant and activating factor for monocytes, in interstitial nephritis. Renal expression of MCP-1 is markedly upregulated in AIN and correlates directly with the level of monocyte infiltration and interstitial damage. Further support for the cell-mediated hypothesis is also derived from the observation of in vivo (delayed-type hypersensitivity responses) and in vitro (lymphoblast transformation) activation on repeat exposure to specific inciting agents.

Humorally mediated events may also be important in eliciting some forms of tubulointerstitial injury as biopsies in occasional patients with drug-induced lesions (rifampin, methicillin, and phenytoin) have shown IgG and complement deposition along the tubular basement membrane (TBM). Circulating anti-TBM antibodies have also been reported in such settings.

One hypothesis concerning immune recognition of the interstitium suggests that portions of infectious particles or drug molecules may cross-react with or alter endogenous renal antigens. An immune response directed against these inciting agents would therefore also target the interstitium. Although it is tempting to speculate on the relevance of these cross-reactive antigens in interstitial disease, the nephritogenic potential of such a response has not been tested within an experimental system.

CLINICAL FEATURES

AIN occurs in four distinct clinical settings (Table 1). It may occur as a result of drug therapy, systemic or local infection, immunologic disease, or an idiopathic lesion without an apparent precipitating cause. AIN is observed in all age groups; however, older patients appear predisposed to developing ARF. Systemic manifestations of a hypersensitivity reaction, such as fever, rash, and arthralgias, are nonspecific findings that may accompany AIN. In such cases, an erythematous maculopapular rash involves the trunk and proximal extremities. Hypertension and edema are not characteristic of AIN, although they have been noted with specific drug-induced lesions. Other non-

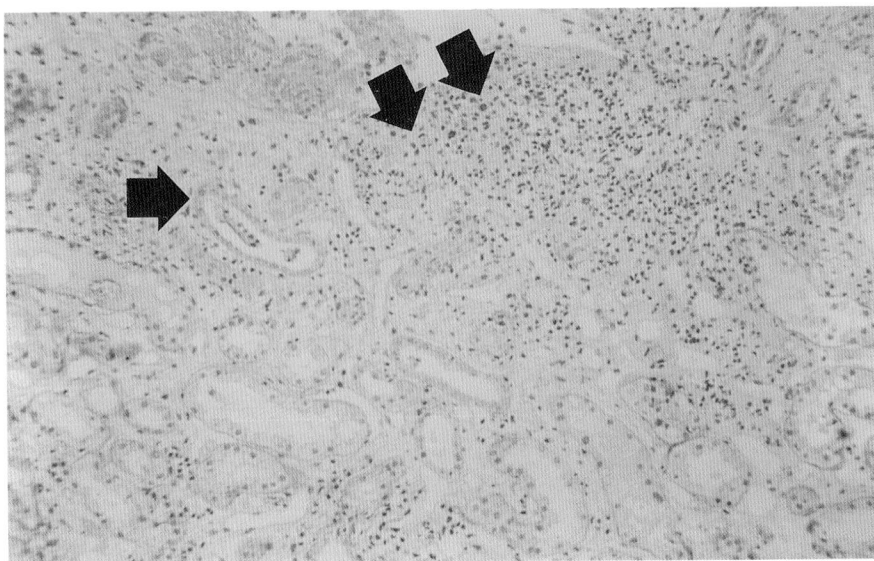

FIGURE 1   Acute interstitial nephritis. Light microscopic findings demonstrate the loss of normal tubulointerstitial architecture with a dense mononuclear cell infiltrate (double arrows) and some evidence of tubular dilatation and atrophy (single arrow). Note that the renal tubules are displaced by infiltrating mononuclear cells, edema, and mild interstitial fibrosis. (Courtesy of Dr. Michael P. Madiao, University of Pennsylvania, Philadelphia, PA.)

specific constitutional symptoms, as well as flank pain with gross hematuria, have been variably reported.

The spectrum of urinary abnormalities (Table 2) comprises microscopic hematuria that at times may be macroscopic, sterile pyuria, and white blood cell casts. Red blood cell casts have also been reported, albeit rarely, in AIN. Eosinophiluria, with more than 1% of urinary leukocytes positive by Hansel's stain, is suggestive evidence of AIN, but can be seen in other forms of renal injury and inflammation. In a recent single-center study, the diagnostic accuracy of eosinophiluria in AIN was examined. Fifty-one patients with various renal diseases, including 15 individu-

als with a confirmed diagnosis of AIN, were evaluated in this study. The sensitivity of eosinophiluria in this setting was 40% and the specificity was 72%, with a positive predictive value of only 38%. These data illustrate the association of eosinophiluria with various morphologic forms of renal inflammation and demonstrate that it is not a reliable indicator of AIN.

Mild proteinuria, generally less than 1 g/day, is frequently observed in AIN. Nephrotic range proteinuria with acute disease has been reported, however, with nephropathies induced by nonsteroidal anti-inflammatory drugs (NSAIDs), and rarely by ampicillin, rifampin, and interferon-α ther-

TABLE 1

Acute Interstitial Nephritis

Drugs
    Antibiotics (especially penicillin analogs, cephalosporins, sulfonamides, and rifampin)
    Nonsteroidal anti-inflammatory drugs
    Diuretics (especially thiazides and furosemide)

Infections
    Direct infection of renal parenchyma
    Associated with a systemic infection

Immunologic disorders
    Systemic lupus erythematosus
    Sjögren's syndrome
    Mixed essential cryoglobulinemia
    Acute allograft rejection

Idiopathic

TABLE 2

Laboratory Findings in Acute Interstitial Nephritis

Urinary sediment	Erythrocytes, leukocytes (eosinophils), leukocyte casts
Urinary protein excretion	<1 g/day, rarely >1 g/day (NSAIDs)
Fractional excretion of sodium	Usually >1
Proximal tubular defects	Glucosuria, bicarbonaturia, phosphaturia, aminoaciduria, proximal RTA
Distal tubular defects	Hyperkalemia, sodium wasting, distal RTA
Medullary defects	Sodium wasting, urine-concentrating defects

RTA, renal tubular acidosis.

apy. Serologic studies, such as anti-DNA antibodies, antinuclear antibodies (ANA), and complement levels, are typically normal in AIN, unless it occurs in the setting of a systemic autoimmune disorder. Recent case reports also note the presence of antineutrophil cytoplasmic antibodies (ANCA), a serologic marker for systemic vasculitis, in some patients during the acute phase of interstitial nephritis. Elevated pANCA titers have been observed in drug-induced AIN (omeprazole, ciprofloxacin) and cANCA in the tubulointerstitial nephritis and uveitis (TINU) syndrome. Of note, two cases of ciprofloxacin-induced AIN also had evidence of necrotizing vasculitis on renal biopsy. The clinical relevance of ANCA titers in AIN is unclear, however, as the overall incidence, antigen specificity, and pathogenicity of these antibodies have not been established.

Urinary fractional excretion of sodium is greater than 1 in many patients with AIN, but is not a reliable diagnostic indicator. Biochemical abnormalities (Table 2) reflective of the tubular damage induced by the inflammatory process are also observed in these patients. The pattern of tubular dysfunction observed varies with the principal site of injury. Lesions affecting the proximal tubule result in renal glucosuria, aminoaciduria, phosphaturia, uricosuria, and proximal renal tubular acidosis (type 2 RTA). Distal tubular lesions result in an inability to acidify urine (type 1 RTA), secrete potassium, and regulate sodium balance. Medullary lesions interfere with maximal urinary concentration and promote polyuria. A considerable degree of overlap in these proximal and distal abnormalities, however, may be apparent clinically. Renal ultrasound in affected patients typically reveals normal or enlarged kidneys, depending on the degree of interstitial edema. Renal gallium scanning has been advocated in some centers to distinguish AIN from other causes of ARF, primarily acute tubular necrosis, but this test is neither sensitive nor specific. In view of the nonspecific nature of many of these clinical feature of AIN, a definitive diagnosis can only be made through renal biopsy.

CLINICAL COURSE AND THERAPY

The spectrum of renal dysfunction in AIN ranges from mild, self-limited disease to oliguric renal failure requiring dialysis therapy. As this renal lesion is generally reversible, even when it presents with severe renal impairment, the overall prognosis is quite favorable. Recovery of renal function may occur over weeks to several months. Some patients have persistent tubular defects or residual renal impairment, or both. Progression to end-stage renal disease, however, has been reported with all forms of AIN. Moreover, a rapidly progressive fibrosing interstitial nephritis has recently been described in clusters of patients in weight loss programs who ingested Chinese herbal preparations tainted with nephrotoxic plants (*Aristolochia fangchi*). Renal disease in all affected individuals was irreversible, with many patients requiring dialysis therapy within 1 year of presentation.

Clinical studies suggest that a less favorable prognosis in AIN correlates with extensive interstitial infiltrates, interstitial fibrosis, tubular atrophy, and interstitial granuloma formation on renal biopsy. Other factors that correlate with persistent renal disease are advanced patient age, preexisting renal disease, and a protracted course of oliguric ARF (>3 weeks). In the recent literature, chronic renal insufficiency following a bout of AIN is most commonly induced by NSAIDs.

The therapy of AIN consists primarily of supportive measures, after possible inciting factors such as drugs or infections have been eliminated. The role of corticosteroids in treating AIN has not been clearly elucidated. Rapid improvement and complete recovery of renal function following steroid therapy in several drug-induced lesions have suggested their therapeutic utility in this disorder. Two empirically derived steroid regimens have been employed in drug (primarily antibiotic)-induced AIN. One protocol consists of parenteral methylprednisolone (0.5 to 1.0 g) administration for 1 to 4 days, and the other, more commonly employed regimen, consists of high-dose prednisone therapy (1 mg $\cdot$ kg^{-1} $\cdot$ day^{-1}) given daily for 7 to 14 days. Some clinical investigators have not corroborated the steroid responsiveness of this renal lesion, however, and randomized controlled studies have not been conducted. Steroids are not employed in infection-related AIN, but may be useful in the treatment of nephritogenic responses in systemic immunologic disorders. Although experimental models have suggested a disease-protective role for cyclophosphamide and cyclosporine in interstitial nephritis, similar studies have not been conducted in human disease.

DISTINCT CAUSES OF AIN

Drug-Induced AIN

The list of drugs that reportedly induce AIN is quite extensive (Table 3). Many of these cases of AIN are reports of single cases, however, and have developed in patients exposed to a number of different medications. Drug-induced AIN is a rare idiosyncratic reaction that occurs in a small subset of patients exposed to a particular medication. It is not dose dependent, and typically recurs on repeat exposure to the same or closely related drug. As seen in Table 3, implicated drugs have diverse chemical structures, although within a class of related drugs, structural similarity can lead to cross-reactive sensitivities. This has been observed particularly with β-lactam drugs, in that penicillin-induced nephropathies have been exacerbated with cephalosporin therapy. A few drugs, most notably penicillins, rifampin, NSAIDs, and sulfonamide derivatives, account for the majority of reported cases of AIN, and their characteristic features will be discussed below.

Penicillins

The β-lactam antibiotics, predominantly the penicillins, are the most common cause of drug-induced AIN. The

TABLE 3
Drug-Induced Acute Interstitial Nephritis

Antibiotics
  Penicillin analogs
    Methicillin, ampicillin, penicillin, nafcillin, carbenicillin,
      oxacillin, amoxicillin, mezlocillin, flucloxacillin
  Cephalosporins
    Cephalothin, cefotetan, cephradine, cephalexin, cefoxitin,
      cefazolin, cefaclor, cefotaxime
  Sulfonamide derivatives
    Sulfamethoxazole, cotrimoxazole
  Other antibiotics
    Rifampin, gentamicin, kanamycin, vancomycin, acyclovir,
      ciprofloxacin, aztreonam, erythromycin, azithromycin,
      ethambutol, tetracyclines, nitrofurantoin
Nonsteroidal anti-inflammatory drugs
  Fenoprofen, ibuprofen, naproxen, indomethacin, tolmetin,
    zomepirac, diflusinal, sulindac, phenylbutazone, aspirin,
    phenacetin, mefenamic acid, 5-aminosalicylic acid
Diuretics
  Thiazides, furosemide, triameterene, chlorthalidone
Miscellaneous Medications
  Phenytoin, allopurinol, cimetidine, ranitidine, phenobarbital,
    azathioprine, cyclosporine, aldomet, carbamazepine,
    diazepam, phenylpropanolamine, captopril, clolfibrate, anti-
    interferon, interleukin 2, anti-CD4 monoclonal antibodies,
    ticlopidine, quinine, propylthiouracil, omeprazole,
    streptokinase, Chinese herbs

Note: Drugs reported with greatest frequency are shown in italics.

largest number of cases occurred with methicillin, which is no longer used in clinical practice. AIN has been reported with most of the penicillin analogs more routinely prescribed (Table 2), although with much lower incidences than with methicillin. Renal failure in this setting has been observed most commonly in older children and young adults. The classic hypersensitivity triad of fever, rash, and eosinophilia in the setting of ARF may occur in up to 30% of patients with β-lactam-induced AIN. Oliguric renal failure has been reported in approximately 30% of these patients. Clinical studies suggest a beneficial role for steroids in this patient population, although as previously stated, randomized controlled studies have not been performed. AIN has developed during treatment of a variety of infections, such as endocarditis, osteomyelitis, pneumonia, cellulitis, and abscesses. An underlying infection is clearly not requisite for inducing this reaction, however, as several patients given prophylactic antibiotics have subsequently developed AIN.

NSAIDs

NSAIDs are among the most widely prescribed medications in clinical practice. They mediate a number of adverse renal side effects, largely as a result of their inhibition of renal prostaglandin synthesis, and are extensively discussed in Chapter 42 of this text. AIN is a less commonly observed side effect of these medications. Propionic acid derivatives appear to cause a disproportionate number of cases (two thirds of cases have been attributed to fenoprofen, ibuprofen, and naproxen), although AIN has been reported with most NSAIDs currently available (Table 3). Unlike other drug-induced reactions, AIN occurs following long-term exposure to the medication, and has been reported 2 weeks to 18 months after initiation of therapy. Patients tend to be nonoliguric females older than 60 years of age, who generally lack systemic manifestations of a hypersensitivity reaction. They may present with hypertension, edema, and nephrotic range proteinuria (up to 80% of cases). Interesting histologic features of induced interstitial lesions are the associated minimal change glomerulopathy and occasional interstitial granuloma formation apparent on renal biopsy. Renal disease generally improves after the drug is discontinued, with or without steroid therapy, although chronic renal insufficiency and end stage renal disease are not infrequent complications.

Rifampin

Numerous cases of rifampin-induced AIN have occurred during treatment of tuberculosis. Most of these cases have developed with intermittent therapy or upon restarting rifampin after a lapse in uneventful daily therapy. Patients typically complain of flu-like symptoms such as fever, chills, malaise, and headache. Unlike other drug-induced lesions, flank pain and hypertension are common in this form of AIN. Moreover, oliguric ARF occurs frequently, and dialysis is required in approximately two thirds of affected patients. In many cases, this reaction has occurred within hours of a single dose of rifampin. Some patients have developed thrombocytopenia, hemolysis, or abnormalities in liver function in addition to AIN. Histologically, evidence of acute tubular necrosis may be apparent along with AIN. In a few cases, an associated proliferative glomerulonephritis has also been observed. Circulating antirifampin antibodies, as well as IgG deposition along the TBM, have been reported in some affected patients. As AIN has developed in patients receiving concurrent rifampin and prednisone therapy, there is no evidence to suggest that steroids play a therapeutic role in this disease.

Sulfonamide Derivatives

Drug-induced AIN was first described in the setting of sulfonamide administration. The majority of cases of sulfonamide derivative-induced AIN occur with combination sulfamethoxazole and trimethoprim therapy. Thiazides and furosemide have also been associated with a few cases of AIN, some of which have developed in patients with preexisting renal disease. The associated hypersensitivity triad of fever, rash, and eosinophilia with renal dysfunction is variably present in affected patients. In addition to the characteristic histologic features of AIN, some biopsies have revealed a predominance of eosinophils within interstitial infiltrates, as well as interstitial granuloma formation.

Isolated case reports have suggested beneficial effects of steroid therapy in treating this variant.

Infections

AIN was first described in the preantibiotic era in the setting of diphtherial and streptococcal infections. It is now apparent that AIN complicates the clinical course of a number of bacterial, viral, fungal, and parasitic infections, as listed in Table 4. This inflammatory response within the kidney may occur as a result of direct renal infection, i.e., pyelonephritis, or as a reaction to a systemic infection. Pyelonephritis, the most common cause of acute infectious interstitial nephritis, typically presents with fever, costovertebral tenderness, dysuria, pyuria, bacteriuria, and leukocytosis. Renal function is unimpaired unless complicated by urinary tract obstruction. Characteristic renal parenchymal lesions consist of focal areas of neutrophils throughout the interstitium. Pyelonephritis responds well to antibiotic therapy and is discussed more extensively in Chapter 57 of this text. In contrast to pyelonephritis, other infection-associated interstitial processes occur in the absence of urinary tract infection. Interstitial infiltrates are frequently perivascular and comprised of mononuclear cells, predominantly T cell lymphocytes. As previously discussed, the pathogenesis of such immune targeting in these infections is not well understood, although cross-reactive determinants may play a role in immune recognition of interstitial structures. Infection-associated interstitial nephritis is generally transient and renal function improves with appropriate therapy of the systemic illness; however, chronic progression of renal insufficiency has been reported.

Immune Disorders

Although glomerulonephritis is the most common renal manifestation of systemic immunologic disorders, predominant interstitial pathology can be seen in systemic lupus erythematosus, Sjögren's syndrome, and mixed essential cryoglobulinemia. Most affected patients present with nonoliguric renal failure, and biochemical evidence of tubular dysfunction. In addition to the typical pathological features of AIN, biopsies from many of these patients also reveal immune-complex and complement deposition along the TBM, and occasionally within interstitial vessels. Concurrent glomerular pathology may also be apparent. Standard therapeutic modalities in these immunologic disorders consist of corticosteroids and cytotoxic agents. Acute renal allograft rejection, a distinct subset of immunologic disorders, also induces acute interstitial inflammation. These lesions are characterized by marked interstitial mononuclear infiltrates, consisting of recipient T cell lymphocytes. Allograft rejection is treated with high-dose (pulse) steroids, as well as antibody therapy targeting activated recipient T cells, and is discussed further in Chapter 75 of this text.

Idiopathic

In approximately 10 to 20% of biopsy-proven cases of AIN, no precipitating cause is detected. Systemic manifestations of a hypersensitivity reaction are generally absent in the majority of these idiopathic cases, which often present with nonoliguric renal failure. One subset of these apparently idiopathic lesions, the TINU syndrome, has been described in approximately 30 adolescent or adult females since 1975. Anterior uveitis can precede, accompany, or follow AIN. Bone marrow granuloma formation may be another common feature of this syndrome. Although the cause of TINU syndrome is not known, an autoimmune nature is suggested by occasional positive serologies, such as cANCA, rheumatoid factor, and ANA, in affected patients. Both renal and ocular changes respond to a brief course of steroid therapy, although a few patients have developed progressive renal disease.

TABLE 4
Infections Associated with Acute Interstitial Nephritis

Bacterial infections
  Streptococcus, diptheria, brucella, legionella, pneumococcus, *tuberculosis*

Viral Infections
  Epstein–Barr virus, *cytomegalovirus, BK virus, Hantaan virus,* measles (rubeola), human immunodeficiency virus, herpes simplex virus type 1

Fungal Infections
  Candidiasis, histoplasmosis

Other Infections
  Toxoplasmosis, leishmaniasis, schistosomiasis, *Rocky Mountain spotted fever,* ehrlichiosis, malaria, mycoplasma, *leptospirosis,* syphilis, ascaris lumbricoides

Note: Infections associated with direct renal infection are shown in italics.

Bibliography

Cameron JS: Immunologically mediated interstitial nephritis: primary and secondary. *Adv Nephrol* 18:207–248, 1989.

Colvin RB, Fang LST: Interstitial nephritis. In: Tisher CC, Brenner BM (eds) *Renal Pathology with Clinical and Functional Correlations.* Lippincott, Philadelphia, pp. 728–776, 1989.

Dodd S: The pathogenesis of tubulointerstitial disease and mechanisms of fibrosis. *Curr Topics Pathol* 88:51–67, 1995.

Heptinstall RH: Interstitial nephritis. A brief review. *Am J Pathol* 83:214–236,1976

Jones CL, Eddy AA: Tubulointerstitial nephritis. *Ped Nephrol* 6:572–586, 1992.

Kannerstein M: Histologic kidney changes in the common acute infectious diseases. *Am J Med Sci* 203:65–73, 1942.

Kida H, Abe T, Tomosugi N, et al.: Prediction of the long-term outcome in acute interstitial nephritis. *Clin Nephrol* 22:55–60, 1984.

Kleinknecht D: Interstitial nephritis, the nephrotic syndrome, and chronic renal failure secondary to nonsteroidal anti-inflammatory drugs. *Sem in Nephrol* 15:228–235, 1995.

Magil AB, Tyler M: Tubulointerstitial disease in lupus nephritis: A morphometric study. *Histopathology* 8:81–87, 1984.

Neilson EG. Pathogenesis and therapy of interstitial nephritis. *Kidney Int* 35:1257–1270, 1989.

Pusey CD, Saltissi D, Bloodworth L, et al.: Drug associated acute interstitial nephritis: Clinical and pathologic features and the response to high-dose steroid therapy. *Q J Med* 52:194–211, 1983.

Ruffing KA, Hoppes P, Blend A, et al.: Eosinophils in urine revisited. *Clin Nephrol* 41:163–166, 1994.

Shih DF, Korbet SM, Rydel JJ, et al.: Renal vasculitis associated with ciprofloxacin. *Am J Kidney Dis* 26:516–519, 1995.

Simon AHR, Alves-Filho G, Ribeiro-Alves MAVF: Acute tubulointerstitial nephritis and uveitis with antineutrophil cytoplasmic antibody. *Am J Kidney Dis* 28:124–127, 1996.

Vanherweghem JL, Depierreux M, Tielemans C et al.: Rapidly progressive interstitial renal fibrosis in young women: Association with slimming regimen including chinese herbs. *Lancet* 341:387–391, 1993.

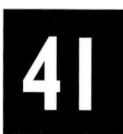

MANAGEMENT OF ACUTE RENAL FAILURE

FLORENCE N. HUTCHISON

Morbidity and mortality from acute renal failure (ARF) have improved significantly over past decades due in large part to improved supportive care and early dialysis. Since the kidney usually recovers from an episode of ARF within days or weeks, the goal of management of ARF is to prevent the consequences of the loss of kidney function and to prevent further renal injury. To develop a rational management plan, it is important to understand the normal function of the kidney because the symptoms and complications of renal failure derive from the loss of these functions. Homeostasis refers to the process by which the internal body milieu is maintained in a constant state despite marked changes in the external environment and variations in the intake of solute, water, and food. The normal kidney is critical to the maintenance of body homeostasis, particularly with regard to volume homeostasis, electrolyte balance, acid–base balance, and excretion of nitrogenous products of protein metabolism. Loss of these functions can result in the pulmonary edema, hyperkalemia, acidosis, and uremia which characterize severe renal failure. Although the causes of ARF are myriad, and specific interventions may be indicated for certain types of ARF, the consequences of ARF can be prevented in most cases by good conservative management, regardless of the etiology.

Therapy of ARF should be initiated as soon as renal injury has been detected. Thus, the first step in management is early recognition that renal failure is present. Since the relationship between serum creatinine concentration and glomerular filtration rate (GFR) is not linear, but exponential, an increase in serum creatinine will not become clinically evident until the GFR is reduced to less than about 50 mL/min. Many episodes of ARF with less severe renal dysfunction are not recognized and do not represent clinically significant events. However, the relationship between GFR and serum creatinine also implies that *any* increase in serum creatinine above the value previously determined for a given patient represents significant loss of renal function. This point is particularly pertinent in cachectic or elderly patients whose baseline serum creatinine may be only 0.8 mg/dL because of the smaller amount of creatinine generated from a reduced muscle mass. With an increase to 1.5 mg/dL the serum creatinine may still be within the range of normal values for most clinical laboratories, but this represents a significant increase in serum creatinine for this patient and indicates that ARF has occurred. It is also critical to determine the cause of renal dysfunction and to identify reversible causes of renal insufficiency such as prerenal azotemia or urinary tract obstruction. The differential diagnosis of acute renal insufficiency is detailed in Chapter 35.

MANAGEMENT OF VOLUME HOMEOSTASIS

Successful volume homeostasis permits maintenance of a constant internal circulatory and extracellular volume despite consumption of varying quantities of water and salt and varying insensible loss of water. The presence of pedal or sacral edema, or overt pulmonary edema in the setting of ARF implies that water and/or salt intake has exceeded the capacity of the injured kidney to excrete the water and salt load. This situation can be easily anticipated in the oliguric (<400 mL/day of urine) or anuric (no urine output) patient, but frequently complicates nonoliguric ARF as well.

Most patients with ARF lose the ability to either concentrate or dilute the urine and will excrete a constant volume of urine regardless of fluid intake. Likewise, the ability to excrete a sodium load may be severely curtailed. As a result, urine output and sodium excretion will rarely match spontaneous fluid and salt intake and either volume overload or volume depletion can result. A typical example is a patient with acute tubular necrosis whose urine output is fixed at 1200 mL/day. If he receives parenteral nutrition at a rate of 2000 mL/day along with intravenous antibiotics, he will gradually develop volume overload and edema unless adjustments are made to the volume of fluid administered. If parenteral nutrition is withheld and he is unable to eat, he will become volume depleted unless parenteral fluids are administered.

Management of volume homeostasis requires that the patient be examined daily to assess the volume status. This is accomplished by measurement of supine and standing blood pressure and pulse to note orthostatic changes suggestive of volume depletion, examination of skin turgor and hydration of mucous membranes, auscultation of the lungs for evidence of pulmonary congestion, a general exam for edema, detailed review of daily input and output records, and accurate measurement of serial daily weight changes.

Each patient with ARF should have a specific individualized prescription for fluid and sodium intake. As a general rule, the patient who is euvolemic on exam should be provided with a volume of fluid equal to daily urine output with an additional 300 to 500 mL/day to replace insensible water losses. A sodium intake of 2 g/day or less should be prescribed. Patients with increased insensible fluid loss such as those with severe diarrhea and large burns will have a much larger fluid requirement. Since insensible fluid loss cannot be accurately measured, it is imperative that a patient's volume status be assessed on a daily basis and the fluid prescription modified as necessary. All oral fluid intake as well as intravenous fluids and medications should be included in the patient's fluid prescription. The patient with clinical evidence of volume overload should be restricted to a fluid intake less than the daily urine output. A trial of diuretics is worthwhile since some cases of oliguric ARF may be converted to a nonoliguric state. Low-dose dopamine infusion ($0.3\ \mu g \cdot kg^{-1} \cdot min^{-1}$) has also been advocated to increase urine output in oliguric ARF, but it has not been shown to be efficacious in controlled trials. Patients with clinical evidence of volume depletion should be provided additional volume to achieve a euvolemic state. It should be emphasized that the goal of volume management is to maintain euvolemia. If a patient is allowed to remain hypovolemic because of concern that pulmonary edema may occur, the sustained hypovolemia may worsen renal injury or delay recovery from renal failure. Increased

fluid administration may be required during the polyuric recovery phase of ARF.

Hypernatremia and hyponatremia are observed frequently in patients with ARF. Since abnormal serum sodium concentrations are caused by disorders of water metabolism, prevention of hypo- or hypernatremia is linked to volume management. The capacity to modify water excretion is impaired in ARF, as demonstrated by the finding of a persistantly isosmotic urine. Hyponatremia is most common and results from an excess of free water relative to solute, while hypernatremia results when free water intake is inadequate. Although excessive oral intake of water can result in hyponatremia in the patient with ARF and inadequate oral intake will produce hypernatremia, the most common cause of either disorder in hospitalized patients with ARF is incorrect administration of intravenous fluids. Hypotonic saline solutions are frequently selected to avoid volume overload, but provide a large proportion of electrolyte free water. For example, administering 1000 mL of 0.45% saline is equivalent to giving 500 mL of isotonic (normal) saline and 500 mL of electrolyte free water. In contrast, 1000 mL of 0.9% saline is isotonic and provides no electrolyte free water. Most parenteral antibiotics are administered in 5% dextrose in water; their full volume is electrolyte-free water. Another source of excess free water intake is from enteral and parenteral feeding solutions, which are formulated with a low sodium concentration. Although prepared enteral solutions may be isosmotic or hypertonic, the solute consists predominantly of carbohydrates and protein that are taken up by cells and metabolized leaving electrolyte free water behind. Parenteral nutritional solutions are usually hyperosmotic when administered, but again the osmoles consist mainly of dextrose and amino acids which are metabolized leaving a large quantity of solute-free water.

The volume of free water required for an individual patient to maintain osmolar balance must be determined empirically and will vary considerably depending on the type and quantity of insensible fluid losses. For example, burn injuries induce large volumes of insensible fluid loss, but the fluid is isosmotic. In contrast, insensible losses from diarrhea and perspiration contain little solute and may dramatically increase the patient's electrolyte free water requirements. In the absence of abnormally high insensible fluid loss, a patient should be provided either orally or intravenously with 300 to 500 mL/day of electrolyte free water as part of the total volume prescription. In patients receiving hypotonic enteral nutritional solutions, the serum sodium concentration should be monitored regularly. If it decreases in the absence of volume overload, sodium can be added to the enteral solution as table salt.

In the intensive care unit, clinical assessment of a patient's volume status may be confounded by surgical wounds, severe pneumonia, or edema due to altered capillary permeability. In this setting, measurements of central venous pressure and pulmonary capillary wedge pressure are important adjuncts to monitor the patient's volume status. Frequently these patients are receiving multiple parenteral medications and parenteral nutrition which constitute a large obligatory volume load. Most parenteral medications can be given slowly in a concentrated solution to minimize the volume administered and the parenteral nutrition prescription should be written to provide optimal calories and protein in a minimum volume. Attention should also be given to the solution in which drugs are administered. Most drugs can be administered in normal saline rather than dextrose and water if hyponatremia is a problem.

MANAGEMENT OF ELECTROLYTE HOMEOSTASIS

Hyperkalemia can be a serious consequence of ARF. Normally serum potassium concentration is very tightly regulated by the shifts of potassium between the intra- and extracellular compartments. The kidney contributes to overall potassium homeostasis by excreting into the urine the approximately 100 mEq of potassium that is ingested in the average diet so that total body potassium remains constant. Although shifts between intra- and extracellular potassium may contribute to hyperkalemia in ARF, the main cause of hyperkalemia in renal failure is excessive intake of potassium relative to the injured kidney's reduced excretory capacity.

Prevention of hyperkalemia in the patient with ARF can usually be accomplished by restriction of potassium intake. Since certain types of foods, such as fruits, chocolate, and nuts, contain large quantities of potassium, eliminating these foods from the diet is often adequate to prevent hyperkalemia. The potassium content of the diet should be routinely specified for the patient with ARF and typically should be limited to less than 50 mEq/day. Potassium should be omitted from parenteral fluids. It is important not to overlook other nondietary exogenous sources of potassium. These include drugs such as potassium penicillin G, saturated solution of potassium iodide (SSKI), and potassium phosphate, dietary additives such as salt substitutes, which contain potassium chloride or citrate, and intravenous fluid such as lactated Ringer's and parenteral nutrition solutions, which typically are formulated with potassium chloride or potassium phosphate. Finally, drugs that impair renal potassium excretion, such as potassium-sparing diuretics, nonsteroidal anti-inflammatory agents, and angiotensin-converting enzyme inhibitors, should be avoided.

If dietary restriction of potassium is inadequate to prevent hyperkalemia, potassium binding resins such as sodium polystyrene sulfonate (Kayexalate) can be utilized. The binding resin is usually administered orally as 15 to 30 g in a solution of 20% sorbitol. It exchanges sodium for potassium in the bowel, there by increasing intestinal excretion of potassium. Potassium binding resins can also be administered rectally as a retention enema. This is particularly valuable if an ileus is present; the time of onset of action will be faster by this route. Although the resin is quite effective in removing potassium, it should not be considered a substitute for dietary potassium restriction. Since sodium is exchanged for potassium, chronic use of these compounds delivers a large sodium load and can

worsen volume overload or hypernatremia. Additionally, the binding resin causes constipation and should not be used orally in patients with intestinal ileus or obstruction. Diarrhea is a predictable consequence when the binding resin is administered repeatedly with sorbitol and may complicate acidosis by causing intestinal bicarbonate loss. The diarrhea may be intolerable to the patient.

Hyperkalemia that develops despite effective restriction of potassium intake and that cannot be easily corrected with potassium binding resin is an indication for dialysis, but should also be a cue to initiate an investigation for the source of the potassium. If diet or drugs cannot be implicated, one should consider endogenous causes of hyperkalemia such as hyperglycemia and insulinopenia, severe acidosis, hemolysis, rhabdomyolysis, ischemic tissue injury, or other causes of myonecrosis (see Chapter 13). Since potassium-lowering therapies, including dialysis, have only a transient effect, appropriate management of hyperkalemia requires identification and specific treatment of the cause of hyperkalemia.

Hypocalcemia frequently complicates ARF, but clinically significant hypocalcemia is rare, as is hypomagnesemia. However, failure to recognize these disorder can produce life-threatening tetany and cardiac arrhythmias. Most reported cases of symptomatic hypocalcemia in patients with ARF have been attributed to hypomagnesemia caused by urinary magnesium wasting in association with cisplatin, amphotericin B, or aminoglycosides. Although decreased synthesis of 1,25-dihydroxyvitamin D by the injured kidney may contribute to hypocalcemia by reducing intestinal calcium absorption, hypomagnesemia inhibits synthesis and release of parathyroid hormone and functional hypoparathyroidism is a primary mechanism responsible for hypocalcemia. Hypocalcemia may also result as a consequence of transfusion of large quantities of blood products preserved in citrate or as a consequence of phosphorus administration. Prevention and management of this problem can be accomplished by generous supplementation of both electrolytes. Calcium may be supplemented orally, usually 3 to 4 g/day in divided doses, but symptomatic hypocalcemia should be treated with parenteral calcium. Calcium gluconate and calcium chloride are available as 10% solutions containing approximately 10 and 28 mg/mL, respectively. Either solution should be diluted in saline or dextrose in water and administered slowly through a peripheral vein to avoid cardiac toxicity. Magnesium can be repleted orally as magnesium oxide or parenterally as intramuscular magnesium sulfate, usually 2 g as a single dose.

Phosphorus ingested in the diet and in drugs accumulates in renal failure and may result in hyperphosphatemia. In patients with ARF this is rarely of clinical consequence except when very high serum phosphorus levels contribute to hypocalcemia, as in rhabdomyolysis, tumor lysis syndrome, and hypercatabolic states. Hyperphosphatemia can be effectively prevented by dietary protein restriction as described below and by oral administration of aluminum hydroxide gels or calcium carbonate or calcium acetate with meals.

MANAGEMENT OF ACID–BASE HOMEOSTASIS

Consumption of a normal American diet by an individual weighing 70 kg produces 60 to 70 mEq of acid daily which must be excreted by the kidney to maintain normal acid–base balance. Accumulation of these acids in excess of the body's buffering capacity in patients with ARF can produce an anion gap acidosis. However, it is unusual for acidosis to be severe or to occur early in the course of ARF, and acidosis should not be attributed exclusively to ARF until other causes of acidosis have been eliminated, e.g., lactic acidosis, ketoacidosis. The presence of ARF may complicate acidosis of any cause if the kidney is unable to increase acid excretion in response to an acid load or is unable to reclaim bicarbonate filtered into tubular fluid. Acidosis not due specifically to ARF should be treated by removing the source of acid generation or bicarbonate loss as would be done in patients without ARF and is discussed in Chapter 9.

Since the majority of the ingested acid load is derived from protein metabolism, dietary protein restriction will slow the development of the acidosis of ARF. A diet containing approximately 0.8 g/kg body wt of good quality protein usually satisfies the nutritional requirement for protein and minimizes acid production. Restriction of nonprotein calories may worsen acidosis since body muscle proteins will be catabolized for the total energy requirement in the absence of other dietary energy sources. Many patients with ARF are anorexic yet have increased caloric requirements due to physiological stress, so inadequate calorie intake is common and should be assessed carefully. The assistance of a skilled dietitian can be invaluable in determining the patient's true calorie and protein requirements.

If acidosis develops despite dietary protein restriction or if protein restriction is not desired because of hypercatabolism with sepsis, burn, or a postoperative state, a base equivalent can be administered to buffer the acidosis. Sodium bicarbonate is most commonly used, but sodium acetate can also be used in parenteral solutions. Both compounds have the disadvantage of containing sodium and may worsen volume overload. Bicarbonate can be administered orally as tablets on a regular basis to compensate for continuing generation of acid. Parenteral bicarbonate should be administered as an isotonic solution. A solution containing approximately 150 mEq/L can be mixed by adding 3 ampoules of premixed hypertonic sodium bicarbonate (50 mEq/50 mL) to 1000 mL of 5% dextrose in water. Use of these ampoules, which contain 1000 mEq sodium bicarbonate/L without dilution, is not recommended unless serum pH is less than 7.1 and then only as a temporizing measure until the cause of the acidosis can be reversed or dialysis initiated since repeated administration will produce hypernatremia.

MANAGEMENT OF UREMIA

Uremia is a syndrome resulting from the accumulation of nitrogenous products of protein metabolism that are normally excreted by the kidney. Early symptoms of uremia are fatigue, lethargy, mental dullness, hiccups, anorexia, and nausea. It may be difficult to determine whether these symptoms are due to ARF or to intercurrent illness. More serious symptoms are myoclonus, confusion, delirium or coma, seizures, and pericarditis. The blood urea nitrogen (BUN) concentration correlates best with symptoms of uremia, but there is considerable variability among patients. As a general rule, few patients have symptoms when the BUN is less than 70 mg/dL and most patients will experience some symptoms when the BUN is greater than 100 mg/dL.

Since the accumulation of nitrogenous waste products is dependent on dietary protein intake, the degree of loss of renal function, and the duration of renal failure, it is not possible to predict which patients will develop uremic symptoms. In most cases the physican cannot alter either the degree of renal insufficiency or the duration of ARF, and must rely on protein restriction to prevent uremia and dialysis to ameliorate uremic symptoms. As noted previously, a protein intake of 0.6 to 0.8 g/kg body wt is considered the minimum amount adequate to supply nutritional requirements for protein.

NUTRITIONAL MANAGEMENT IN ARF

Most episodes of ARF occur as a complication of other serious illness or injury and studies have clearly demonstrated that adequate nutritional support substantially improves survival in patients in critical care units. Unfortunately, the dietary restrictions required for management of ARF, as well as the anorexia of uremia, may be counterproductive of efforts to optimize nutritional support. For example, very low protein diets (20 g protein/day) have been advocated to prevent uremia and avoid dialysis. However, the possible benefits of avoiding short-term dialysis by severe protein restriction must be weighed against the potential increase in morbidity and mortality due to impaired nutrition. This level of protein restriction is not recommended.

Parenteral nutrition is frequently necessary in seriously ill patients with ARF, but the composition of the parenteral solution must be modified in accordance with the loss of renal function. The minimum recommended protein intake in patients with ARF is 0.6 to 0.8 g · kg body · wt^{-1} · day^{-1} and may be considerably higher in very ill hypercatabolic patients. The assistance of an experienced nutritionist to calculate protein catabolic rate and calorie requirements is invaluable in estimating actual protein requirements so that excessive or inadequate amino acid administration can be avoided. Carbohydrate and lipid should be maximized with a target of providing 30 to 35 kcal · kg body wt^{-1} · day^{-1}. Provision of adequate carbohydrate and lipid calories will reduce protein requirements and limit symptoms of ARF. Since protein metabolism is the source of endogenous acid generation in renal failure, a base should be given in an amount adequate to buffer the acid generated from metabolism of the amino acids. Bicarbonate cannot be added to parenteral nutrition solutions without causing precipitation of calcium salts, so sodium acetate is used as a base equivalent. Since approximately 60 to 80 mEq of acid is generated each day, a similar amount of sodium acetate should be administered. Fluid volume should be limited to the minimum required to deliver adequate caloric intake. The sodium concentration (sodium chloride + sodium acetate) should be adjusted to provide approximately 300 to 500 mL as electrolyte-free water as discussed previously. For example, if a patient is given 2000 mL/day the total sodium concentration should be 100 mEq/L. This is approximately equivalent to 1500 mL of isotonic fluid and 500 mL of free water. If the patient is receiving 1000 mL/day, a sodium concentration of approximately 75 mEq/L will provide the equivalent of 500 mL of isotonic fluid and 500 mL of electrolyte-free water. In general, potassium, magnesium, and phosphorus should not be added to parenteral nutrition solutions in patients with ARF. If a deficiency of one of these electrolytes exists, it is better to replete that solute specifically than to administer potentially toxic solute on a continuous basis.

DIALYSIS IN ARF

In ARF, the role of dialysis is to prevent morbidity associated with complications of ARF and provide temporary support until the renal insufficiency resolves. The decision to initiate dialysis and the frequency of dialysis are based on the patient's clinical condition rather than a particular numerical value of BUN or serum creatinine concentration. Dialysis is indicated in ARF for management of specific problems. Pericarditis and other uremic symptoms can be resolved only with dialysis and are considered absolute indications for dialysis. Other problems, such as volume overload, hyperkalemia, and acidosis, are considered relative indications for dialysis; that is, dialysis should be instituted when conservative management has failed or is not practical. For example, an oliguric or anuric patient who requires mechanical ventilation for volume overload pulmonary edema should be dialyzed urgently since fluid restriction and diuretics will not be effective. The indications for dialysis are summarized in Table 1.

Since dialysis is a temporizing measure in this setting, the dialysis prescription may be considerably different from that typically used for a patient on chronic dialysis. For

example, in contrast to the chronic dialysis patient who receives 3 to 4 hours of hemodialysis three times a week, hypercatabolic oliguric ICU patients may require daily dialysis to limit uremic symptoms and to remove the fluid administered with parenteral nutrition and medications. Or a patient who presents with ARF and life-threatening hyperkalemia may require a single dialysis to correct the hyperkalemia and may then be maintained successfully with conservative management. The decision to initiate dialysis must be weighed against the risks associated with large bore dialysis catheter placement and dialysis. Bleeding, infection, and pneumothorax may complicate catheter placement, and dialysis may induce hypotension, mental confusion, and cardiac arrythmias, particularly in unstable critically ill patients.

The details of the dialysis prescription are beyond the scope of this discussion, but it is worthwhile to mention several variations on hemodialysis that are used routinely in patients with ARF. Conventional intermittent hemodialysis is most commonly used. Continuous renal replacement therapy may be preferred in patients whose major complication is volume overload, whose medical regimen requires ongoing administration of large volumes of fluid, or whose blood pressure is too unstable to permit hemodialysis. In its simplest form, this procedure provides volume removal only, but variants permit successful solute clearance (dialysis) as well. Peritoneal dialysis is also an effective modality for management of ARF and can provide both fluid removal and clearance of solute. Dialysis is discussed extensively in Chapters 63 and 64. The decision to initiate dialysis and the selection of the most appropriate mode of therapy requires the participation of a nephrologist experienced in these procedures.

DRUG MANAGEMENT IN ARF

Many frequently used drugs are eliminated through the kidney and doses must be modified in patients with ARF. In the setting of chronic renal failure, the physician can reliably estimate GFR on the basis of the patient's steady-state serum creatinine concentration and make adjustments in drug doses, but this is not the case with ARF. When GFR falls abruptly, the serum creatinine concentration rises as creatinine accumulates in the body until a new steady-state level is reached. Thus, in ARF, the rate of increase in serum creatinine concentration is a more accurate indicator of the severity of renal failure than the serum creatinine concentration on a given day. Serum creatinine is also dependent on body muscle mass, so an increase of $0.5 \text{ mg} \cdot \text{dL}^{-1} \cdot \text{day}^{-1}$ in an elderly patient with reduced muscle mass may indicate that GFR is <10 mL/min, but a similar rate of increase in serum creatinine concentration in a muscular young athlete may indicate that GFR is relatively well preserved at 30 to 40 mL/min.

A vital component of management of the patient with ARF is a review of all medications to identify those that are excreted in the urine and, especially, those that are toxic at high concentrations, such as digitalis compounds, or that may cause further renal injury, such as aminoglyco-

TABLE I

Indications for Dialysis

Absolute indications—Dialysis is the only possible treatment
  Uremic symptoms
  Uremic pericarditis
Relative indications—Dialysis will be required if conservative
  management of these abnormalities is unlikely to be
  successful or is contraindicated
  Volume overload
  Hyperkalemia
  Metabolic acidosis
  Other electrolyte abnormalities

TABLE 2
Guidelines to Management of Acute Renal Failure

1. What is the patient's volume status?
   Normal: Fluid intake = urine output + 300–500 mL/day
               Sodium intake = 2 g/day
   Overloaded: Fluid intake < urine output
               Sodium intake < 2 g/day
               Try loop diuretic
               Consider dialysis
   Depleted: Restore volume with isotonic saline, then
               prescribe fluid intake = urine output +
               300–500 mL/day
               Sodium intake = 2 g/day

2. Is the patient hyperkalemic?
   No: Potassium intake = 50 mEq/day
   Yes: Look for source of potassium
       Eliminate parenteral potassium
       Reduce dietary potassium intake to < 50 mEq/day
       Potassium binding resin
       Consider dialysis

3. Is the patient acidemic?
   No: Protein intake = $0.8 \text{ g} \cdot \text{k}^{-1} \cdot \text{day}^{-1}$, $30 \text{ kcal} \cdot \text{k}^{-1} \cdot \text{day}^{-1}$
   Yes: Look for cause of acidosis
       Reduce protein intake to $0.6 \text{ gm} \cdot \text{kg}^{-1} \cdot \text{day}^{-1}$; maintain
       $30 \text{ kcal} \cdot \text{kg}^{-1} \cdot \text{day}^{-1}$
       Oral bicarbonate or isotonic intravenous bicarbonate
       Consider dialysis

4. Is the patient uremic?
   No: Protein intake = $0.8 \text{ g} \cdot \text{kg}^{-1} \cdot \text{day}^{-1}$, $30 \text{ kcal} \cdot \text{kg}^{-1} \cdot \text{day}^{-1}$
   Yes: Reduce protein intake to $0.6 \text{ g} \cdot \text{kg}^{-1} \cdot \text{day}^{-1}$; maintain
       $30 \text{ kcal} \cdot \text{kg}^{-1} \cdot \text{day}^{-1}$
       Check for gastrointestinal bleeding
       Consider dialysis

5. Is the patient receiving medication?
   No: Check any new medications for toxicity and adjust doses
   Yes: Stop nephrotoxic drugs
       Adjust medication doses
       Check drug levels

6. Is the patient's nutrition adequate?
   No: Provide balanced nutrition with $30–35 \text{ kcal} \cdot \text{kg}^{-1} \cdot \text{day}^{-1}$ and $0.6–0.8 \text{ g} \cdot \text{kg}^{-1} \cdot \text{day}^{-1}$ protein
       Assess need for enteral or parenteral nutrition
   Yes: Reassess periodically

sides. Compounds containing magnesium and phosphorus are commonly used as antacids and cathartics and can induce hypermagnesemia and hypocalcemia in patients with

ARF. Aminoglycoside antibiotics and most vasopressor agents are removed with dialysis and dosing must be adjusted to compensate for dialytic losses. A variety of texts and handbooks provide modified dosing guidelines for specific drugs for use in patients with renal failure and in dialysis patients. Measurements of creatinine clearance using the average of the serum creatinine concentrations measured before and at the end of the urine collection and serum drug levels are also critical adjuncts to appropriate management. Drug prescribing in renal failure is discussed further in Chapter 43.

Table 2 is a checklist providing guidelines for basic management of the patient with ARF. Good management requires early recognition of renal failure, anticipation and prevention of potential problems, and ongoing evaluation of the patient's clinical condition.

Bibliography

Denton MA, Chertow GM, Brady HR: "Renal-dose" dopamine for the treatment of acute renal failure: Scientific rationale, experimental studies and clinical trials. *Kidney Int* 49:4–14, 1996.

Feld LG, Cachero S, Springate JE: Fluid needs in acute renal failure. *Pediatr Clin North Am* 37:337–350, 1990.

Gentric A, Cledes J: Immediate and long term prognosis in acute renal failure in the elderly. *Nephrol Dial Transplant* 6:86–90, 1991.

Kierdo H: Continuous versus intermittent treatment: Clinical results in acute renal failure. In: Siebert, HG, Mann, H, Stummvoll, HK (eds) *Continuous Hemofiltration*. Contrib. Nephrol., pp. 1–12, 1991.

Manian FA, Stone WJ, Alford RH: Adverse antibiotic effects associated with renal insufficiency. *Rev Infect Dis* 12:236–249, 1990.

Norton DF, Franklin SS: Acute renal failure in the critical care setting. *Acute Care* 13:127–156, 1987.

Pascual J, Orofino L, Liano F, et al.: Incidence and prognosis of acute renal failure in older patients. *J Am Geriatr Soc* 38:25–30, 1990.

Schetz M, Lauwers PM, Ferdinande P: Extracorporeal treatment of acute renal failure in the intensive care unit: a critical view. *Intensive Care Med* 15:349–357, 1989.

Schneeweiss B, Graninger W, Stockenhuber F, et al.: Energy metabolism in acute and chronic renal failure. *Am J Clin Nutr* 52:596–601, 1990.

Schrier RW, Gardenschwartz MH, Burke TJ: Acute renal failure: Pathogenesis, diagnosis, and management. *Adv Nephrol* 10:213–240, 1981.

Speigel DM, Ullian ME, Zerbe GO, Berl T: Determinants of survival and recovery in acute renal failure patients dialyzed in intensive-care units. *Am J Nephrol* 11:44–47, 1991.

SECTION 6

DRUGS AND THE KIDNEY

42

NONSTEROIDAL ANTI-INFLAMMATORY DRUGS AND THE KIDNEY

VARDAMAN M. BUCKALEW, JR.

The American public consumes billions of doses of over-the-counter (OTC) and prescription analgesics each year. These consist primarily of drugs from two distinct classes: (1) aspirin and other nonsteroidal anti-inflammatory drugs (NSAIDs) and (2) acetaminophen and other nonnarcotic analgesics. These analgesics are associated with adverse events involving a number of organs, including the kidney. Although the absolute event rate is probably low, the renal effects of these drugs are important because of the large numbers of individuals exposed to them.

Adverse renal events fall into two categories: those that occur acutely in individuals taking NSAIDs, and a chronic renal disease, analgesic nephropathy (AN), which occurs in individuals who consume analgesics habitually. This chapter discusses the epidemiology, pathophysiology, diagnosis, and treatment of these two types of adverse events.

ACUTE EFFECTS FROM NONSTEROIDAL ANTI-INFLAMMATORY DRUGS

Acute Renal Failure

Epidemiology

The incidence and prevalence of acute renal failure due to NSAIDs are not well documented. Available estimates vary widely depending on the methodology used, the setting in which the study was done, and the population observed. A search of a data base from a large health maintenance organization in which more than 100,000 outpatients were exposed to NSAIDs over an 11-year period revealed that none were hospitalized for any of their known renal complications. While the methodology used in this study would not have detected adverse events treated without hospitalization, these results indicate a very low overall rate of acute renal failure or any other serious complication, at least in this urban, largely middle-class population.

Two studies provide data on the incidence of acute renal failure in hospitalized patients. In a city hospital that serves primarily an indigent population, acute renal failure occurred in 343 of 1908 inpatients (18%) receiving ibuprofen. In most patients, there was a clinically insignificant rise in serum creatinine, and the incidence of severe acute renal failure was only 0.9%. Furthermore, acute renal failure was no more likely to occur in patients given NSAIDs than in a

control group given only acetaminophen. In a multivariate analysis, the only risk factors for NSAID-associated acute renal failure were age greater than 65 and coronary artery disease. In a study of an elderly population (mean age 87 years), 15 of 114 patients (13%) given NSAIDs developed a greater than 50% increase in serum urea nitrogen level (but no change in serum creatinine), which was reversible on stopping the drug. Multivariate analysis showed that concomitant use of loop diuretics and higher doses of drug correlated with acute renal failure.

Mechanism

Decreased Renal Blood Flow. The most common type of NSAID-induced acute renal failure is due to decreased synthesis of renal vasodilator prostaglandins (PGs) PGE_2 and PGI_2, leading to decreased renal blood flow and glomerular filtration rate (GFR). Renal blood flow is not dependent on these PGs in normal individuals. However, renal blood flow becomes dependent on their intrarenal production in certain clinical states, making these individuals susceptible to NSAID-induced acute renal failure (Table 1).

In volume depletion, including decreased effective volume in generalized edema, traumatic or septic shock, and general anesthesia, increased PG synthesis is probably stimulated by the renal vasoconstrictor effects of sympathetic nervous system and renin-angiotensin system activation. The stimulus for PG production is not so clear when renal mass is reduced, as occurs in renal transplantation and other renal diseases. Thus, patients with renal disease of any etiology may develop NSAID-induced renal failure, although those with immune-mediated glomerulonephritis and urinary obstruction may be particularly susceptible.

The well-known decrease in renal blood flow and GFR with age may underlie the increased susceptibility of the elderly to this condition. However, there may be other factors which have not yet been identified. The association of NSAID-induced acute renal failure with diuretic use may be related to the edema states for which these drugs are used or to their ability to stimulate vasodilator PG production. Triamterene may be a more potent stimulator of vasodilator PG production than other diuretics for reasons which are not clear, and its use with NSAIDs is not

TABLE I

Predisposing Factors for NSAID-Induced Hemodynamic Acute Renal Failure

Decreased effective blood volume
Congestive heart failure
Cirrhosis
Nephrotic syndrome
Anesthesia
Shock
Decreased absolute blood volume
Hemorrhage
Sodium and water depletion
Chronic renal failure
Acute renal failure due to contrast and obstruction
Drugs
Diuretics
Cyclosporine
Advanced age
Renal transplantation

recommended. Cyclosporine increases urinary excretion of vasodilator PGs, probably because of its renal vasoconstrictor effect. As a result, the drug increases the risk of NSAID-induced acute renal failure in renal and heart transplant patients as well as nontransplant patients receiving it.

In most cases of hemodynamic acute renal failure, the decrease in renal blood flow is purely functional and recovery is rapid on stopping the drug. In some cases, however, renal biopsy has demonstrated histologic changes of acute tubular necrosis, the presence of which may delay recovery.

Interstitial Nephritis (IN). This complication, which appears to be an idiosyncratic reaction, particularly to the propionic acid derivatives (ibuprofen, naproxen, and fenoprofen), is associated with the nephrotic syndrome in about 90% of cases. In contrast to acute interstitial nephritis (AIN) associated with other drugs, NSAID-induced AIN is associated with a low incidence of hypersensitivity symptoms, eosinophilia, and eosinophiluria and exhibits a predominance of lymphocytes rather than eosinophils in the renal interstitium. This latter phenomenon may explain why NSAID-induced IN is virtually the only type of IN that is accompanied by nephrotic syndrome since the glomerular lesion is thought to be due to inflammatory mediators such as leukotrienes produced by the interstitial lymphocytes.

In patients with the nephrotic syndrome, minimal change disease is usually found on renal biopsy. A few cases of minimal change glomerulopathy without interstitial nephritis have been observed after long-term (>3 months) use of NSAIDs. This entity has been reported with propionic acid and indoleacetic acid derivatives.

Causative Agents

Seven chemical classes of NSAIDs are available in oral form. At this time only the propionic acid derivatives are available OTC (ibuprofen, naproxen, and ketoprofen). All NSAIDs, including aspirin, have the potential for causing acute, hemodynamic renal failure. The likelihood of an individual drug causing acute renal failure is related to its potential for inhibiting renal PG synthesis. Of the commonly used agents, indomethacin is the most potent, and aspirin the least. Some studies have suggested that sulindac, an indoleacetic acid derivative, may have lower toxicity. This drug does have a unique metabolism, in that the active metabolite formed from the prodrug is inactivated by an intrarenal enzyme system. The renal sparing effect of sulindac, if it exists, is not absolute, however, and cases of acute renal failure have been reported. This has been explained as being due to individual differences in the rate at which the metabolite is inactivated or to high plasma levels of this metabolite which may occur after 10 days of therapy in patients with renal failure.

Alterations in Electrolyte and Water Excretion

NSAIDs may cause several alterations in water and electrolyte excretion. These effects are due either directly or indirectly to inhibition of PG synthesis.

Sodium Excretion

PGE_2 and PGI_2 increase renal sodium excretion by a variety of mechanisms, including renal vasodilation and direct inhibition of tubular sodium reabsorption. It is not surprising, therefore, that inhibition of PG synthesis by NSAIDs causes decreased renal sodium excretion. This effect, however, is relatively minor and is not often clinically significant. Because most diuretics stimulate vasodilator PG production, NSAIDs may interfere with the natriuretic effect of diuretics in both edema states and in hypertension. In the latter, this effect may cause blood pressure to be a few mmHg higher than usual.

Potassium Excretion

PGE_2 and PGI_2 increase renin release by a direct effect on the juxtaglomerular cells. Consequently, NSAIDs have been reported to cause hyperkalemia by inducing hyporeninemic hypoaldosteronism. A secondary mechanism for this effect may be a decrease in sodium delivery to the distal tubule and a decrease in urine flow. Risk factors for this adverse event include renal failure, preexisting hypoaldosteronism, advanced age, and the concomitant use of drugs that interfere with potassium excretion such as potassium-sparing diuretics and angiotensin-converting enzyme inhibitors.

Water Excretion

PGE_2 facilitates water excretion by decreasing Na^+ reabsorption in the loop of Henle and by inhibiting the hydroosmotic effect of vasopressin. Accordingly, NSAID administration may interfere with water excretion, causing the development of hyponatremia. Too few cases have been reported to identify the risk factors for this rare complication with certainty. However, two groups that may be at risk are the elderly and infants treated with NSAIDs for patent ductus arteriosus.

Management

In evaluating patients presenting with any of the adverse events listed above, NSAIDs should be suspected as an etiologic agent. It is important to remember that these drugs may be used either as self-medication or by prescription. The index of suspicion should be especially high in the groups at special risk, particularly the elderly and those with preexisting renal disease, congestive heart failure, and hepatic cirrhosis. A history of use of drugs known to increase the risk of NSAID complications should be sought. Individuals with predisposing factors should be discouraged from taking NSAIDs. Patients known to be taking NSAIDs regularly, especially those with increased risk and those taking large doses, should have their renal function checked frequently. The drugs should be discontinued with the appearance of any renal sids effects. Concomitant use of NSAIDs and an orally active PGE_1 analog, misoprostol, has been reported to blunt the decrease in renal blood flow in some patients with renal failure. Misoprostol has also been shown to reduce the renal vasoconstrictor effects of cyclosporine and could reduce the risk of NSAID-induced acute renal failure in transplantation. However, the place of this drug in the long-term management of these conditions remains to be determined.

Acute renal failure from hemodynamic factors should be differentiated from that due to interstitial nephritis. This can usually be done with a urinalysis, because 90% of patients with the latter have heavy proteinuria. Acute renal failure due to hemodynamic factors should reverse rapidly, usually within 3 to 5 days. Occasionally, recovery is delayed by the development of acute tubular necrosis, a condition that may be suspected on the basis of the typical urinary sediment. Recovery will also be slow when acute renal failure is due to interstitial nephritis. Steroids have been reported to improve this condition, but it may also remit spontaneously. No guidelines have yet been developed for steroid use. Renal biopsy may be indicated in patients whose renal failure does not respond quickly to cessation of the drug.

ANALGESIC NEPHROPATHY

It can be argued that the discipline of renal epidemiology began with the studies in the early 1950s of the association between regular consumption of analgesics mixtures and chronic renal failure. These studies suggested that the daily ingestion of analgesics containing aspirin and phenacetin caused a syndrome of chronic renal failure due to what was then called "chronic pyelonephritis" and which we now call "chronic tubulointerstitial nephropathy." Over the intervening 40 years, the literature on this entity has multiplied so that today there is general agreement among nephrologists and epidemiologists about its principal features. When the major offending agent was shown to be phenacetin, this popular analgesic was removed from the

market in most countries around the world. Despite this attempt to prevent analgesic nephropathy (AN), it continues to be a problem even in countries where phenacetin is no longer available, including the United States. This suggests that phenacetin was not the sole cause of the condition and indicates the need for further investigations and perhaps additional public health measures.

Epidemiology

The Syndrome of Habitual Analgesic Use

Numerous studies in many countries around the world have documented the existence of a population of individuals who habitually use OTC analgesics for a variety of self-diagnosed indications (Table 2). Estimates of the prevalence of habitual analgesic consumption, defined as daily ingestion for at least 1 year, vary widely geographically from as low as 2% to as high as 30%. The explanation for this wide variation is not clear. The highest prevalence is among industrial workers and hospital patients, and the lowest in community-based populations. Within these populations women are more likely to be habitual users than men. The nature of the preparations available has some influence, with the highest prevalence being in those areas where phenacetin was most popular. Inclusion of caffeine or codeine in the preparations may also increase habitual use. The effect of the recent changes in the pharmacopeia of OTC analgesics on habitual consumption has not yet been studied.

AN occurs in a subset of those who use analgesics habitually. Thus, the geographical variation in the prevalence of AN noted above is due mainly to the geographical variation in the prevalence of habitual analgesic use.

Which Analgesics Are Used Habitually?

The type of preparations available for OTC consumption vary with time and location. In the United States, two major changes have been made in the makeup of OTC analgesics: phenacetin was removed from the market in late 1983, and the first nonaspirin NSAID, ibuprofen, became available in 1984. These alterations have changed the prevalence of drugs used by habitual consumers (Table 3). The prevalence of aspirin use has declined, but that of total NSAID use (aspirin plus nonaspirin NSAIDs) has actually risen slightly. In addition, the increment in acetaminophen use is almost equal to the prevalence of phenacetin use when it was available.

The risk for developing AN currently must be evaluated in the light of this changing pattern of analgesic consump-

TABLE 2
Indications for Habitual Analgesic Use

Headache
Arthritis
Sleep aid
Backache
Don't feel well

TABLE 3

Prevalence of Habitual Use of Individual Analgesics in the
United States

	1978–1979 (%)	1980–1982 (%)	1991 (%)
Aspirin	55	38	39
NSAIDs	0	22	23
Acetaminophen	19	20	38
Phenacetin	26	20	0

TABLE 4

Risk of Renal Disease from Individual Analgesics

	Relative risk[a]	
Drug	ESRD	Chronic renal failure
Phenacetin	2.66–19.05 ($n = 5$)	5.11, 8.1 ($n = 2$)
Acetaminophen	2.1, 4.06 ($n = 2$)	3.21
Aspirin	1.0, 2.5 ($n = 2$)	1.3
NSAIDs	1.0	2.1

*Note: n = number of studies, if > 1.

[a] All risks greater than 1.3, adjusted for use of other analgesics, are statistically significant, except in one study in the phenacetin group wtih a risk of 4.

tion. Some authors have assumed, based on the decline in prevalence of AN observed in some countries following the removal of phenacetin from the market, that AN was due entirely to phenacetin and will therefore disappear. There is good reason to doubt this optimistic scenario.

The Relative Risk of AN

The relative risk, or odds ratio, of developing either chronic renal failure (CRF) or end-stage renal disease (ESRD) in habitual users of analgesics varied between 2.4 and 8 in eight studies from 1969 to 1992, when the makeup of OTC analgesic preparations was changing. In six of these eight, the risk of CRF or ESRD from individual analgesics could be estimated; phenacetin in five, acetaminophen in three, aspirin in three, and nonaspirin NSAIDs in two (Table 4).

The risk for developing ESRD from habitual phenacetin use varied from about 3 to 19, and for CRF from 5 to 8 with a cumulative threshold dose of about 0.5 to 1.0 kg. The risk of ESRD from habitual acetaminophen use varied from 2 to 4 in two studies and was 3.2 for CRF in one study. One study suggested consumption of as little as 360 pills containing acetaminophen (about 0.1 to 0.2 kg total dose) may increase risk of ESRD.

Of three studies of aspirin, one from the United States showed no risk of CRF and another showed no risk of ESRD. However, one study from Spain showed a significant risk of ESRD of 2.5. Two studies from the United States of nonaspirin NSAIDs have been reported—one in subjects with chronic renal failure and one with ESRD. In the study of CRF from North Carolina, the overall risk was slightly increased at 2.1; however, a risk of 16.6 was found in men over 65 years of age. In the study of ESRD from the mid-Atlantic area, there was no risk overall in subjects taking more than 360 but less than 5000 pills; however, in subjects taking more than 5000 pills lifetime the risk was 8.8.

These epidemiologic data suffer from the problem of accurately quantitating analgesic consumption by questionnaire or interview. In addition, case-control studies may overestimate risk if patients with renal disease have symptoms which might increase analgesic consumption, so-called "confounding by indication." Although these studies are not conclusive and further research is clearly needed, they do suggest the following tentative conclusions. First, habitual acetaminophen use increases the risk of renal disease at a total dose no higher than for phenacetin, but the risk appears to be somewhat less. A possible explanation

for this difference will be discussed below. Second, habitual NSAID use may increase the risk of renal disease, especially in the elderly, but the threshold dose is much higher than that for acetaminophen. Third, the risk of renal disease from habitual aspirin use, if any, must be lower than that for either acetaminophen or nonaspirin NSAIDs.

Mixtures vs Single Agents. A recent epidemiological study of AN from Europe suggests that AN occurs only in individuals consuming analgesic mixtures. Based on this and other evidence, the National Kidney Foundation recommended in a recent position paper that analgesic mixtures be made available by prescription only.

The hypothesis that only analgesic mixtures cause renal disease may explain the apparent lower risk of acetaminophen compared to phenacetin noted above. Phenacetin was always marketed as a mixture with other analgesics, usually aspirin plus caffeine, whereas acetaminophen is available both as a single agent and in mixtures with aspirin and other agents. Although the risks calculated from case control studies have been adjusted statistically for the use of other drugs, the question of whether habitual use of single analgesics increases risk of renal disease has not been answered.

Risk by Diagnosis. Classically, the nephropathy associated with analgesic use is a chronic interstitial nephritis. Nevertheless, two questionnaire-based studies show an increased risk of habitual acetaminophen consumption in patients with other renal diagnoses including hypertensive nephrosclerosis and diabetic nephropathy. Although these observations suggest that habitual acetaminophen use might contribute to the progression of established renal disease, confounding by indication is a particular problem in these studies because patients with known renal disease may consume acetaminophen preferentially. Nevertheless, the potential public health implications of these studies are important and further research is indicated.

The Prevalence of AN

The incidence and prevalence of AN in the dialysis population are reported periodically in ESRD registries in Europe, Australia, and now in the United States. In Europe, the average incidence of new cases starting dialysis was 2% in 1990, down from 3% in 1981. However, the rate, although declining, remains high in Switzerland (12%) and Belgium (11%). In Australia, the 1992 rate was 9%, down from over 20% in the early 1970s. The decline has been attributed to legislation limiting OTC availability of analgesic mixtures. The United States Renal Data System (USRDS) indicates that from 1989 to 1993, the diagnosis of AN was made in 0.8% of new dialysis patients. This rate was unchanged from the 1988 to 1991 data. The USRDS does not publish data on geographic variation; past reports indicated that AN was more common in the southeastern United States by a factor of about 5. In a recent population based study in the mid-Atlantic region (Maryland, northern Virginia, and the District of Columbia), the population-attributable risk for habitual acetaminophen use was 8 to 10%. This ten-fold discrepancy between the incidence of AN in the USRDS and that predicted from a community-based case control study could be due to geographical variation, or an underdiagnosis of AN by nephrologists, or to an overestimate of risk based on case-control methodology.

There are very few estimates of the incidence and prevalence of AN in the population of patients with chronic renal failure not on dialysis. During the phenacetin era in the 1970s, two studies estimated that 7% (in Philadelphia) and 13% (in northwest North Carolina) of patients with chronic renal failure had AN. It is likely that this figure is lower now than 20 years ago.

Pathogenesis

Concepts of the pathogenesis of AN are based primarily on studies in animal models. The results of studies in which single analgesics and various combinations have been fed to rats have, however, been somewhat controversial. In many cases, very large doses have been required to cause renal lesions. In general, combinations of analgesics, especially those which include aspirin, have been more nephrotoxic than single agents. In fact, aspirin is the most nephrotoxic of all analgesics studied in the rat. Most studies agree that dehydration increases the nephrotoxicity of these agents.

Chronic interstitial inflammation and papillary necrosis are the primary lesions of AN. This is probably due to the concentration of the offending agents, especially acetaminophen and salicylates, by the countercurrent mechanism. Acetaminophen is metabolized to toxic oxygen radicals by cytochrome P450 mixed-function oxidases located in the renal cortex and outer medulla and by prostaglandin endoperoxidase synthases in the renal papilla. Aspirin potentiates the toxicity of these radicals by depleting the kidney of reduced glutathione necessary for their detoxification.

A second proposed mechanism invokes a decrease in renal papillary blood flow in patients consuming analgesics containing aspirin or other NSAIDs that could inhibit renal PG production. In addition, a papillary microangiopathy of unknown pathogenesis which could interfere with the papillary circulation, has been demonstrated in autopsy

studies. A lipofuscin pigment in many tissues has been described in autopsies of humans dying with AN. It is thought to be an oxidized polymer of unsaturated fatty acids, probably arising from the effect of the aforementioned acetaminophen derived radicals. The role of this pigment in the pathogenesis of AN is not known.

Caffeine is present in many of the analgesic combinations taken by patients with AN., Its role in the pathogenesis of AN is not known. Most speculation has centered on the possibility that caffeine increases analgesic consumption by causing "caffeine withdrawal" headaches. However, caffeine may also play a role in the nephrotoxicity of acetaminophen as an adenosine antagonist. Adenosine diminishes the transport-associated respiration in the medullary thick ascending limb. Cell necrosis by oxygen radicals might be enhanced if respiration were stimulated by adenosine antagonism.

Urinary tract malignancies have been attributed most often to the N-hydroxylation metabolites of phenacetin. Because acetaminophen is also metabolized to potential carcinogens, it is not clear why the risk of urinary tract malignancies has been associated to date only with habitual use of phenacetin and not acetaminophen.

The Clinical Syndrome

History

The key to making the diagnosis is obtaining an accurate history of the type and amount of analgesic consumption. One-third or more of patients with AN will deny consuming analgesics and even those who admit taking them may underestimate the amount taken. The best approach to ascertaining that analgesics are used regularly is to question the patient about those chronic conditions for which analgesics might be taken (Table 2). Most patients with these conditions will readily describe them in detail but they may be reluctant to admit how much analgesic they take. The situation is not unlike that of obese patients underestimating the amount of food they eat. A frequently employed strategy to obtaining an accurate assessment of analgesic consumption is to ask family members. Another clue to the presence of habitual analgesic consumption is a history of peptic ulcer disease. Up to one third of patients with AN will have such a history.

Patients with AN may not be habitually consuming analgesics at the time they are seen by the nephrologist for CRF or ESRD. Not infrequently, the patient presenting with renal failure of unknown etiology will give a history of some chronic pain condition in the past which lasted for some significant period of time, but is no longer present, and for which analgesics had habitually been consumed.

An important criterion for making the diagnosis is the total dose of analgesic consumed. Most patients who admit to habitual analgesic use have a favorite preparation, the contents of which can be ascertained and a cumulative total dose estimated. Not all patients with AN habitually consume OTC preparations; some may be taking these preparations by prescription. It should also be kept in mind that patients with AN may also abuse other substances such as alcohol, sedatives, and perhaps other recreational drugs, and tobacco.

Physical Examination

The findings on physical examination in patients with AN are nonspecific. Some investigators have noted a typical personality type in women with this syndrome. They may be excessively dependent and passive-aggressive with a low threshold for pain and features of hypochondriasis. It has also been noted that women with this syndrome appear to be prematurely aged. Generalized atherosclerosis may be found, because this condition may occur with increased frequency in patients with AN compared to patients with other types of renal disease.

Laboratory Findings

The laboratory findings may be typically those of chronic tubulointerstitial nephritis as discussed in Chapter 48. Abnormalities found with increased frequency in patients with AN include sterile pyuria and bacteriuria. When the syndrome was caused by phenacetin, an anemia out of proportion to the degree of renal failure was frequently seen. This may not be observed in the syndrome caused by other analgesics.

Imaging of the kidney using ultrasonography, computed tomography (CT), or pyelography may show reduced renal size. The renal contour may have an irregular, wavy appearance described as "bumpy." Papillary necrosis may be manifest as renal medullary calcification. On ultrasound, this calcification is typically seen surrounding the central sinus and may appear as a complete or incomplete garland. However, renal contours may be difficult to discern on ultrasound in patients with advanced renal disease because of increased echogenicity. Furthermore, it is difficult to precisely localize renal calcium deposits on ultrasound, and papillary calcifications may be incorrectly diagnosed as vascular calcifications or renal calculi. A recent study from Europe explored the use of CT without contrast to evaluate

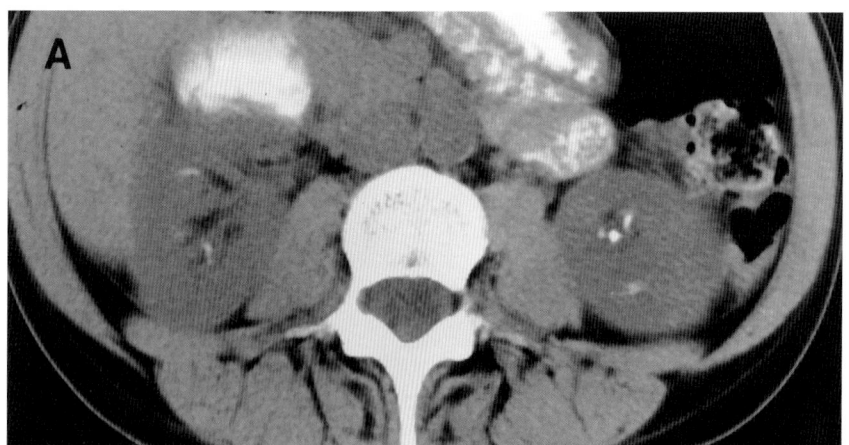

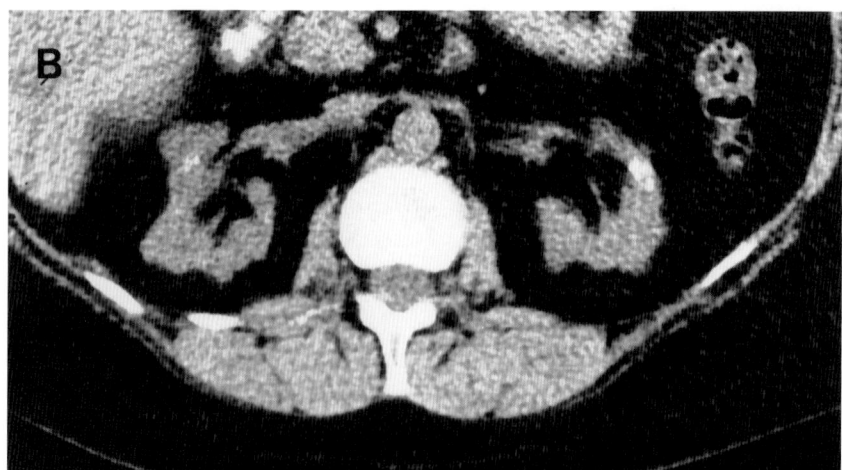

FIGURE 1 (A) CT scan without contrast in a 42-year-old female with a 20-year history of daily analgesic use for headache. Medullary calcifications are prominent without bumpy contours. (B) CT scan without contrast in a 56-year-old female with a 35-year history of habitual analgesic use for headaches. Bumpy renal contours and medullary calcifications are apparent. Renal volume was 61.3 mm on right and 59.2 mm on left (see text).

renal size, contour, and calcifications in subjects with AN. Renal size was measured as the sum of both sides of a rectangle enclosing the kidney at the level of the renal vessels. Renal volume was considered decreased if this sum was less than 103 mm in males and 96 mm in females. Renal contour was considered "bumpy" if three or more indentations were observed at the level where the most number of indentations were identified. Calcifications were localized as cortical, papillary, or central. The combination of reduced renal size and either bumpy contours or renal medullary calcification had a sensitivity and specificity of 90% for AN in patients with ESRD and 87% and 100% respectively in CRF without ESRD. These findings are illustrated in Fig. 1, which shows CT scans without contrast in two patients with CRF and a history of habitual analgesic ingestion.

An increased incidence of renal parenchymal, pelvic, and ureteral carcinoma has been documented in AN. However, this was probably due to phenacetin and may no longer be observed.

Diagnosis

Criteria for diagnosing AN, divided into major and minor categories, are summarized in Table 5. A high index of suspicion is indicated in those with CRF or ESRD of unknown etiology and two or three minor criteria, especially if there is a history of a chronic pain syndrome and peptic ulcer disease. Although always inferential, the diagnosis is indicated with a high degree of certainty if two or more major criteria are present, especially if accompanied by some of the minor criteria. In some cases, the diagnosis of AN only can be suspected when the patient has a chronic pain syndrome but denies heavy analgesic consumption.

Treatment

The successful treatment of AN depends on identifying habitual analgesic ingestion and either convincing the patient to discontinue the practice or to switch to a "safe" analgesic. Unfortunately, there may not be a completely

TABLE 5
Diagnostic Criteria for AN

Major
History of daily analgesic consumption >1 year
Small, bumpy kidneys and renal calcification on ultrasound
Decreased renal volume, bumpy contours, and medullary calcification on CT without contrast

Minor
Chronic pain syndrome
History of peptic ulcer disease
Dependent personality, hypochondriasis
Chronic tubulointerstitial nephritis
Sterile pyuria
Bacteriuria

safe analgesic that can be used habitually in patients with CRF. Aspirin taken alone may be the safest analgesic in these patients, but should not be given in combination with acetaminophen. Acetaminophen used alone is safe for episodic use, although, as noted above, this drug if used habitually may contribute to progression of renal failure in established renal disease of any cause. NSAIDs have been shown to decrease GFR in patients with CRF of any cause and therefore should probably be avoided. Propoxyphene taken alone is safe, but it should be used with caution in combination with acetaminophen. Tramadol (Ultram) is a new centrally acting analgesic with weak opioid activity and has no known renal toxicity. This drug can be tried in patients with renal disease with severe pain syndromes in whom habitual analgesics are needed. Nephrologists should monitor the type and amount of analgesic consumed by all patients with CRF, especially those whose renal failure is progressing.

Several studies have suggested that avoidance of nephrotoxic analgesics prevents progression of renal failure from AN. However, as with any type of renal disease, progression in AN may be affected by factors other than continued analgesic ingestion. Hypertension, if present, should be adequately controlled. The use of protein restricted diets in patients with chronic renal failure of any cause is discussed in Chapter 68. Patients with AN may develop acute papillary necrosis, urinary tract infections, or kidney stones. The treatment of these conditions is discussed elsewhere in this book.

Bibliography

Backris GL, Starke U, Heifets M, et al.: Renal effects of oral prostaglandin supplementation after ibuprofen in diabetic subjects: A double-blind, placebo-controlled, multicenter trial. *J Am Soc Nephrol* 5:1684–1688, 1995.

Beard K, Perera DR, Jick H: Drug-induced parenchymal renal disease in outpatients. *J Clin Pharmacol* 28:431–435, 1988.

Bennett WM, DeBroe ME: Analgesic nephropathy—a preventable renal disease. *N Engl J Med* 320(19):1269–1271, 1989.

Buckalew VM, Schey HM: Renal disease from habitual antipyretic analgesic consumption: an assessment of the epidemiologic evidence. *Medicine* 11(1):291–303, 1986

Elseviers MM, De Broe ME: Analgesic nephropathy in Belgium is related to the sales of particular analgesic mixtures. *Nephrol Dial Transplant* 9:41–46, 1994.

Elseviers MM, De Broe ME: A long-term prospective study of analgesic abuse in Belgium. *Kidney Int* 48:1912–1919, 1995.

Elseviers MM, De Schepper A, Corthouts R, et al.: High diagnostic performance of CT scan for analgesic nephropathy in patients with incipient to severe renal failure. *Kidney Int* 48:1316–1323, 1995.

Gurwitz JH, Avorn J, Ross-Degnan D, et al.: Nonsteroidal anti-inflammatory drug-associated azotemia in the very old. *JAMA* 264:471–475, 1990.

Henrich WL (ed): Analgesic nephropathy. *Am J Kidney Dis* 28(Suppl. 1):S1–S70, 1996.

Johnson AG, Nguyen TV, Day, RO: Do nonsteroidal anti-inflammatory drugs affect blood pressure? *Ann Intern Med* 121:289–300, 1994.

Klag MJ, Whelton PK, Perneger TV: Analgesics and chronic renal disease. *Curr Opin Nephrol Hyperten* 5:236–241, 1996.

Murray MD, Brater DC, Tierney WM, et al.: Ibuprofen-associated renal impairment in a large general internal medicine practice. *Am J Med Sci* 299:222–229, 1990.

Palmer BF: Renal complications associated with use of nonsteroidal anti-inflammatory agents. *J Invest Med* 43:516–533, 1995.

Perneger TV, Whelton PK, Klag MJ: Risk of kidney failure associated with the use of acetaminophen, aspirin, and nonsteroidal antiinflammatory drugs. *N Engl J Med* 331:1675–1679, 1994.

Sandler DP, Burr R, Weinberg CR: Nonsteroidal anti-inflammatory drugs and the risk for chronic renal failure. *Ann Intern Med* 115(3):165–172, 1991.

Sandler DP, Smith JC, Weinberg CR, et al.: Analgesic use and chronic renal failure. *N Engl J Med* 320:1238–1243, 1989.

Toto RD, Anderson SA, Brown-Cartwright D, et al.: Effects of acute and chronic dosing of NSAIDs in patients with renal insufficiency. *Kidney Int* 30:760–768, 1986.

Warren GV, Korbet SM, Schwartz MM, et al.: Minimal change glomerulopathy associated with nonsteroidal antiinflammatory drugs. *Am J Kidney Dis* 13:127–130, 1989.

Incidence and causes of treated ESRD. U.S. Renal Data System, USRDS 1995 Annual Data Report, The National Institutes of Health, National Institute of Diabetes, Digestive and Kidney Diseases, Bethesda, MD. *Am J Kidney Dis* 26(Suppl. 2):S39–S50, 1995.

43

PRINCIPLES OF DRUG THERAPY IN RENAL FAILURE

ARASB ATESHKADI

Patients with either acute or chronic renal failure typically receive multiple drugs to manage the associated complications. On the average, patients with chronic renal failure receive more than seven drugs; nearly one-fourth take 10 or more. Patients with renal impairment suffer from a high incidence of adverse drug reactions. Hence, familiarity with principles of drug dosage adjustment for patients with renal impairment is of critical importance for any clinician responsible for prescribing and monitoring pharmacotherapy. The importance of this assertion is illustrated by a recent study which showed that as many as 44% of patients with an estimated creatinine clearance (C_{cr}) of less than 40 mL/min received excessive doses of drugs. The average dose was 2.5 times higher (range: 1.07 to 6.45) than the maximum recommended for the patient's degree of renal dysfunction.

Currently, the drug approval process in the United States requires drug dosing recommendations for patients with renal failure as part of the product labeling. For most marketed drugs, this requirement was not in effect at the time the drug was approved, and such information may not be part of the product package. Numerous sources are available for guiding dosage adjustment in renal failure. Unfortunately, much of the information contained in these guidelines is based on single-dose pharmacokinetic studies, rather than multiple-dose pharmacokinetic or pharmacodynamic investigations. Creatinine clearance, the marker used to estimate glomerular filtration rate (GFR), may grossly overestimate actual GFR (see Chapter 2). Therefore, it is recommended that the available sources always be interpreted with caution. When such guidelines are absent or inadequate, the clinician must use knowledge of the drug's pharmacokinetics and pharmacodynamics to decide on the need for, and the manner of, dosage adjustment.

Fortunately, most drugs follow a first-order elimination process (i.e., linear pharmacokinetics), which means that as the dose is doubled, serum concentration is also doubled. This makes the effect of dosage adjustment on serum concentration predictable. A few drugs, such as phenytoin and high-dose salicylate, exhibit nonlinear pharmacokinetics, which means that the doubling of the dose results in a disproportionate rise in plasma concentration of the drug. The dosing of such drugs is often a greater challenge.

EFFECT OF RENAL FAILURE ON PHARMACOKINETICS

Drugs used in clinical practice can be divided into three categories based on their route of elimination: (1) category

I drugs (e.g., aminoglycosides) are primarily eliminated by the kidneys; (2) category II drugs (e.g., ethanol, acetaminophen) are primarily eliminated by nonrenal routes; and (3) category III drugs (e.g., bumetanide, nafcillin, vancomycin) are eliminated by a combination of renal and nonrenal routes. The need for dosage adjustment is often more critical for category I drugs, but drugs that undergo nonrenal elimination may also require dosage adjustment in patients with renal failure.

To fully appreciate pharmacokinetic changes in renal failure, it is important to become familiar with some of the commonly used pharmacokinetic terminology. *Bioavailability* (expressed as a percentage) is the fraction of the dose absorbed from the site of administration (e.g., subcutaneous, oral/gastrointestinal). The *apparent volume of distribution* (V_d; expressed in liters) is a mathematical concept that relates the amount of a drug in the body to the serum concentration. It is important to note that V_d does not correspond to any specific anatomic space within the body. *Half-life* ($t_{1/2}$; expressed in hours) is the time required to decrease the serum concentration of the compound by half. For example, a volume-overloaded patient receiving an aminoglycoside antibiotic may exhibit a prolonged $t_{1/2}$, not only because of decreased renal function (i.e., decreased renal clearance, Cl_{renal}), but also due to an increase in the drug's V_d. Table 1 lists drugs whose $t_{1/2}$ and Cl are affected by end-stage renal disease (ESRD) and dialysis.

Effect of Renal Failure on Drug Absorption

In patients with renal failure, a number of factors can affect drug absorption: uremic gastroparesis, changes in gastric pH due to high concentrations of gastric ammonia, gut wall edema, and alterations in first-pass metabolism. The altered gastric pH affects the absorption of drugs such as ferrous sulfate, ketoconazole, itraconazole, and dapsone. Gut wall edema, which may occur during severe generalized edema, may affect the absorption of furosemide.

First-pass metabolism refers to the intestinal or hepatic metabolism and inactivation of a drug, often by the cytochrome P450 enzyme system. Drugs with a high first-pass metabolism include propranolol, verapamil, and lidocaine. Drugs with decreased bioavailability in renal failure include furosemide and pindolol. Drugs with increased bioavailability in renal failure include dextropropoxyphene, dihydrocodeine, oxprenolol, and propranolol. Before a decision is made to decrease the dose of a drug with increased bioavailability, it is also important to appreciate the pharmacodynamic changes that occur in renal failure. For example, because the sensitivity of β-receptors is decreased in

TABLE I

Effect of End-Stage Renal Disease, Hemodialysis, and Peritoneal Dialysis on the Clearance and Half-Life of Selected Drugs

| | $t_{1/2}$ (h) | | Effect of hemodialysis[a] | | Effect of peritoneal dialysis[b] | |
Drug	Normal	ESRD	$t_{1/2}$ (h)	Cl (mL/min)	$t_{1/2}$ (h)	Cl (mL/min)
Amikacin	1.6	39	3.8–5.5	30–36	18–26	6.7
Azlocillin	0.9	5.1	2.2	ND	2.5	ND
Aztreonam	2.0	7.0	2.7	43	7.0	2.1
Cefazolin	2.2	28.0	2.6–5.0	NR	32	NR
Cefoxitin	0.8	13–25	4	NR	NR	1.5
Cefuroxime	1.3	15–22	3.5	NR	11.8	4.7
Cefotaxime	0.9	2.5	1.9–3.4	14–40	2.9–4.4	NR
Ceftazidime	1.8	26.0	2.8	27–50	8.7	8.5
Ciprofloxacin	4.4	8.4–12	3.0–5.5	29.6–47	ND	ND
Clavulanic acid	1.0	4.3	NR	141	ND	ND
Clindamycin	2.2–3.3	1.9–3.4	1.6–3.1	NR	ND	ND
Erythromycin	2.1	4.0	0.8	28.5	ND	ND
Gentamicin	2.2	53	5.2–11.3	24–47	8.5	12.5
Imipenem	0.9	2.9	1.0	84	ND	ND
Metronidazole	7.9	7.7	2.8	58–125	5.6	15.8
Nafcillin	1.0	2.1	NR	0	ND	ND
Ofloxacin	5–8	28–38	NR	116	ND	ND
Piperacillin	1.2	3.9	1.3–2.4	74	ND	ND
Sulfamethoxazole	10	13.3	3.2–11.1	21–84	13–18	1.2
Ticarcillin	1.2	14.8	3.4	33	10.6	7.2
Tobramycin	2.5	58	4.3–6.7	31–70	25	4.7
Trimethoprim	14	26–40	5.0–9.4	29–66	17–24	5.1
Vancomycin	6.9	161	NR	16.1	30–43	2.3–14.2

[a] Effect during a conventional hemodialysis treatment.
[b] Effect during a CAPD exchange.
Note: $t_{1/2}$, terminal half-life; Cl, dialysis clearance (mL/min); ND, no data; NR, not reported; ESRD, end stage renal disease.

renal failure, the dose of propranolol may actually need to be increased, despite its increased bioavailability in such patients.

In addition to these effects on drug metabolism, it is important to note that certain drugs commonly used in renal failure, such as cationic preparations used as phosphate binders (aluminum and calcium products), may also reduce the absorption of certain drugs, such as ampicillin, digoxin, and isoniazid.

Effect of Renal Failure on Distribution

Several drug properties determine the extent to which a drug distributes throughout the body. These include the drug's molecular size, hydrophilicity, plasma protein binding, and tissue binding. Drugs that are hydrophilic (e.g., aminoglycosides) tend to distribute mostly to the intravascular space and as a result have a low V_d. Likewise, drugs that are highly protein bound (e.g., furosemide) mostly tend to stay in the intravascular space. Conversely, drugs that are lipophilic (e.g., quinidine) or highly tissue bound (e.g., digoxin, cyclosporine) have a high V_d because they distribute to larger areas of the body. Knowledge of the drug's V_d is important for the purpose of calculating a loading dose (see below). In renal failure, the V_d may change due to changes in body composition, and decreased plasma protein binding. The body composition may change because of uremia-induced malnutrition and excess fluid volume. Reduction in protein binding of drugs is clinically significant only for agents that are highly bound to albumin (i.e., acidic and neutral drugs) (Table 2), and may in patients with renal disease, occur for three main reasons: hypoalbuminemia; drug displacement from binding sites on albumin by accumulated organic acids; and diminished affinity of albumin binding sites for drugs. With reduced protein binding, a therapeutic free (active) serum concentration will occur at a lower total serum concentration. If the dose of the affected drug is not properly targeted to achieve a total serum concentration appropriate for pa-

tients with normal renal function, toxicity will occur (e.g., phenytoin).

Effect of Renal Failure on Drug Elimination

Effect on Hepatic Metabolism

Renal failure reduces the nonrenal elimination of drugs metabolized by the P450IID6 isoenzyme (e.g., debrisoquine, quinidine, metoprolol, codeine). This may be due to the presence of a circulating inhibitor that competes with the drug for P450 binding sites.

Renal failure may decrease hepatic deacetylation, acetylation, hydroxylation, O-demethylation, N-demethylation, conjugation, and sulfoxidation of drugs. Renal disease may affect reversible reactions such as conjugation, such that inactive conjugated metabolites that are not renally excreted are converted back to the parent compounds. Examples of drugs with decreased nonrenal (hepatic) clearance in ESRD are listed in Table 3.

Renal failure may also increase clearance of drugs like phenytoin and propranolol by hepatic oxidative pathways. Other drugs with increased hepatic clearance in ESRD include bumetanide and nafcillin. Of particular interest is the elimination behavior of nafcillin. In healthy individuals, nafcillin undergoes both renal (60%) and nonrenal (40%) elimination; however, in ESRD, nonrenal clearance of nafcillin increases to the extent that no dosage adjustment is required.

Effect on Renal Metabolism

Virtually all the polypeptide hormones are metabolized by the kidneys. Hence, the clearance of these substances (e.g., insulin, parathyroid hormone) is greatly reduced in renal failure. Renal tissues contain many of the enzymes found in the liver. Most of the mixed-function oxidases (i.e., P450 enzymes) are present in the renal cortex. How-

TABLE 2

Example of Drugs with Reduced Protein Binding in Renal Failure

Barbiturates
Cephalosporins (some)
Clofibrate
Diazoxide
Furosemide
Penicillins (some)
Phenytoin
Salicylate
Sulfonamides
Valproate
Warfarin

TABLE 3

Example of Drugs with Reduced Nonrenal Elimination in End Stage Renal Disease

Acyclovir
Aztreonam
Captopril
Cefotaxime
Cimetidine
Cortisone
Imipenem
Metoclopramide
Nimodipine
Prednisone
Procainamide
Procaine
Sulindac
Zidovudine

ever, the kidneys have only 15% of the metabolic activity of the liver, and drug clearance may not be significantly affected by renal disease.

Effect on Renal Excretion

Renal handling of drugs includes filtration at the glomerulus and reabsorption and secretion by the tubules. The extent of reduction in renal drug elimination depends on both the fraction of the drug excreted by the kidneys and the degree of renal insufficiency. When available, the serum concentration of the parent compound and any active or toxic metabolite may help guide dosing (e.g., procainamide and its active metabolite N-acetylprocainamide). Management of drug levels is essential for drugs with a narrow therapeutic index, such as digoxin and aminoglycosides.

EFFECT OF RENAL FAILURE ON PHARMACODYNAMICS

Patients with renal failure may exhibit alterations in the degree of response to some drugs, such as diuretics, benzodiazepines, and antihypertensive agents. While such pharmacodynamic alterations are sometimes explainable by changes in the drug's pharmacokinetics (e.g., reduced clearance), physiologic aberrations that occur during renal failure can also affect how a patient responds to the pharmacologic effects of a drug. Altered pharmacodynamics in renal failure is typically due to: (1) change in receptor sensitivity, as occurs with insulin and β-receptor antagonists; or (2) a more severe form of the disorder under treatment, such as hypertension and volume overload. Diuretic resistance is perhaps the most common form of renal failure-induced alteration in pharmacodynamics. Patients with renal disease commonly require much higher doses of diuretics to achieve a natriuretic response similar to that of healthy individuals. Other examples of altered pharmacodynamics in renal failure are increased sensitivity to alprazolam and reduced effect of normal doses of commonly used antihypertensive drugs because of fluid overload.

ADJUSTING DOSAGE FOR RENAL FAILURE

In deciding whether to adjust the dose of a drug in a patient with renal failure, it is also important to take note of the underlying renal disorder, because it may cause alterations in pharmacokinetics or pharmacodynamics of the agent. For example, the rate and extent of absorption of a drug may be decreased in a patient with diabetic nephropathy and diabetic gastroparesis.

In adjusting drug doses for patients with renal failure, clinicians should not rely excessively or exclusively on nomograms, because these do not take into account all the variability that may exist in patients. Nomograms may be used for initial therapy, but only with close monitoring of the patient, and careful consideration of the following questions:

1. What is the patient's estimated renal function? Is it changing?
2. What is the extent of the drug's renal elimination?

3. Are the drug's metabolites pharmacologically or toxicologically active? If so, do they accumulate in renal failure?
4. Should the loading dose of the drug be altered?
5. Should the maintenance dose of the drug be adjusted?
6. Is the patient on dialysis?
7. What is the mode of dialysis?
8. If the patient is receiving hemodialysis or hemofiltration, which filter is being used?
9. How often and how efficient is the dialysis?

Estimation of GFR

Creatinine clearance (C_{cr}) remains, despite its limitations, the method of choice for estimating GFR in the clinical setting. C_{cr} can be determined by direct measurement via urine collection (see Chapter 2). Alternatively, the Cockroft-Gault method is commonly used in the clinical setting to estimate C_{cr}. This equation, however, can be used only when renal function is stable,

$$C_{cr} = \frac{(140 - age) \times LBW\ (kg)}{72 \times [Cr]} \qquad (1)$$
(multiply by 0.85 for females),

where [Cr] is serum creatinine and LBW is lean body weight (kg), calculated as

$$LBW\ for\ males = 50\ kg + 2.3 \times inches > 5\ feet$$
$$LBW\ for\ females = 45.5\ kg + 2.3 \times inches > 5\ feet. \qquad (2)$$

Route of Drug Elimination

Information on the routes of drug elimination can be obtained from various sources, including drug monographs (e.g., product package insert), and reviews of drug dosing in renal failure (see bibliography). As a general rule, drugs with extensive renal elimination (category I) will require some degree of dosage adjustment, whereas drugs that are extensively metabolized extrarenally (category II) need no dosage adjustment. The need for dosage adjustment for drugs that fall in category III (dual routes of elimination) is based on clinical pharmacokinetic studies.

Metabolite Accumulation

Hepatic drug metabolism mostly leads to production of hydrophilic compounds, which are then excreted in the urine. Some of these accumulated metabolites may have pharmacologic and/or toxicologic activity (Table 4). For example, meperidine is metabolized to normeperidine. Although it has no narcotic effect, normeperidine can lower the seizure threshold as it accumulates in uremic patients. Another example is the class Ia antiarrhythmic agent (sodium channel blocker) procainamide. This drug is metabolized to N-acetylprocainamide, which accumulates in renal failure and acts as a class III antiarrhythmic agent (potassium channel blocker). For certain drugs, the inactive metabolite may accumulate in renal failure and be converted back to the active parent compound (e.g., diflunisal, ketoprofen, clofibrate).

TABLE 4
Example of Parent Compounds and Their Pharmacologically or Toxicologically
Active Metabolites

Parent drug	Metabolite	Metabolite activity
Allopurinol	Oxypurinol	Inhibitor of xanthine oxidase
Azathioprine	6-Mercaptopurine	Immunosuppressant
Cephalothin	Desacetylcephalothin	Antibacterial potency 50% of parent compound
Chlordiazepoxide	Oxazepam	Anxiolytic
Chlorpropamide	2-Hydroxychlorpropamide	Hypoglycemic
Clofibrate	Chlorophenoxyisobutyric acid	Hypolipidemic with direct muscle toxicity
Daunorubicin	Daunorubicinol	Cytotoxic
Diazepam	Oxazepam	Anxiolytic
Doxorubicin	Doxorubicinol	Cytotoxic
Meperidine	Normeperidine	Lowers seizure threshold; psychotic changes
Procainamide	N-acetylporcainamide	Class III antiarrhythmic with possible cardiac toxicity
Propoxyphene	Norpropoxyphene	Narcotic analgesic
Propranolol	4-Hydroxypropranolol	β-Receptor antagonist
Rifampin	Desacetylrifampin	Antimicrobial activity
Sulfadiazine	Acetylsulfadiazine	Nausea, vomiting, rash

Dosage Adjustment in Renal Failure

In many instances where dosage adjustment is required in renal failure, literature or product labeling recommendation suffices; however, as previously mentioned, these recommendations must always be interpreted and used with caution.

Drug dosage adjustment must be made on a case-by-case basis, after considering concomittant medical conditions, other administered medicines, and severity of renal failure. Some drugs require dosing based on LBW (e.g., aminoglycosides), whereas others are based on total body weight (e.g., heparin, vancomycin).

Nonrenal disease, which may require additional dosage adjustment (e.g., hepatic disease), should be identified. If a therapeutic drug concentration is rapidly needed, as may be the case for a severe infection or an arrhythmia, a loading dose is calculated

$$\text{Loading dose} = V_d \times C_{max}, \qquad (3)$$

where C_{max} is the desired peak serum concentration. As can be seen from this equation, the drug's V_d must be known. In renal failure, the V_d may increase (e.g., digoxin, aminoglycosides), decrease (e.g., phenytoin), or remain unchanged. Determining a maintenance dose is often more challenging and is established on the basis of: (1) desired peak and trough concentrations of the drug (if known) and (2) estimated or calculated individual pharmacokinetic parameters. Two methods are used individually or together to adjust the maintenance dose: dosage reduction and interval extension. With some cardiovascular drugs, maintenance of a steady concentration is important; hence, dosage reduction is used while maintaining normal intervals. Conversely, aminoglycoside antibiotics require high peak concentrations for efficacy and low trough concentrations to minimize toxicity; therefore, both dosage reduction and interval expansion are often needed.

For many drugs with a narrow therapeutic index for which determination of serum concentrations are clinically available (Table 5), therapeutic drug monitoring is necessary. To better interpret a serum or plasma concentration,

TABLE 5
Drugs Which Require Therapeutic
Drug Monitoring

Amikacin

Carbamazepine

Cyclosporin

Digoxin

Gentamicin

Lidocaine

Lithium

Methotrexate

Netilmicin

Phenobarbital

Phenytoin

Procainamide/N-acetylprocainamide

Quinidine

Theophylline

Tobramycin

Valproate

Vancomycin

the drug dose, and the route and time of administration must be known. It must be noted that toxicity can still occur while the serum drug concentration is maintained within the therapeutic range. The use of digoxin in patients with hypokalemia is one such example.

Dosage Adjustment in Dialysis

The degree to which a drug is removed via dialysis determines whether a supplemental dose is needed or not. Although the peritoneal membrane has larger pore sizes than standard hemodialysis membranes, drug clearance during peritoneal dialysis is usually much lower due to a substantially reduced dialysate flow rate (see Chapters 63 and 64).

Drug Dosing in Hemodialysis

The amount of drug removed by hemodialysis is approximately the product of drug concentration in the dialysate and the dialysate volume. This value divided by the total body stores of the drug prior to dialysis (product of predialysis serum concentration and volume of distribution) yields the actual fraction of drug removed by dialysis (FDR). In addition, the dialysis membrane can bind a certain fraction of the drug, which will not appear in the dialysate. Measurement of dialysate drug concentrations is not practical in the clinical setting. Hence, several methods to predict the FDR have been proposed (see bibliography). The FDR is an index of the relative dialyzability of the drug and has been used to determine whether dosage adjustment is needed.

Endogenous clearance of a drug in the period between dialyses (i.e., interdialytic period) may also affect drug dosing. Knowledge of the amount of drug removed both during and between dialysis treatments is often necessary to design an optimal therapeutic regimen. The clearance and half-life of several drugs both on and off dialysis are presented in Table 1. Patients may require postdialytic or interdialytic dosing when the maintenance of serum concentrations within a narrow range is necessary (e.g., aminoglycosides). Accurate information on the dialysis kinetics of drugs is not always readily available; hence, complicated pharmacokinetic equations have been developed to aid in dosing patients on hemodialysis. Although a trained pharmacotherapist is sometimes able to estimate the fraction of a dose removed based on the properties of both the drug and the dialysis procedure, most clinicians find it easier to follow standard guidelines for drug dosing. Such guidelines are available from the product package insert, and dosing tables and nomograms when such recommendations are absent or inadequate, the clinician must use knowledge of certain properties of the drug and the dialysis procedure to make an educated guess regarding how much of the drug has been removed. Factors that favor dialysis of drugs are listed in Table 6. Water-soluble drugs with molecular weights less than 500 Da and low plasma-protein binding can be expected to be removed by dialysis. The charge characteristic of some drugs favor their adsorption to the hemodialysis membrane. Such drugs are removed from the blood without appearing in the dialysate (e.g., aminoglyco-

TABLE 6
Factors That Increase Drug Dialyzability

Drug properties
Molecular weight <500 D$_9$[a]
High water solubility
Small volume of distribution
No erythrocyte partitioning
Low nonrenal elimination

Dialysis properties
Membrane composition and charge[a] (drug dependent)
Large membrane surface area (e.g., high efficiency)
Large membrane pore size (e.g., high flux)
High dialysate flow rate or volume[a]
High blood flow rate[a]
Dialysate composition (drug dependent)
High ultrafiltration rate
Long dialysis treatment times
Long dialysate dwell time[b]

[a] For hemodialysis.
[b] For peritoneal dialysis.

sides binding to polyacrylonitrile membrane). Drugs with smaller V_d are distributed mostly in the intravascular space and hence are more likely to be available for removal by dialysis. Conversely, drugs which partition to the erythrocytes (e.g., cyclosporine) are less available for dialysis removal. Perhaps the two most important dialyzer-related properties for drug removal are membrane pore size and surface area. The use of larger-pore (i.e., high-flux) and/or larger surface-area (i.e., high-efficiency) dialysis membranes increase the dialyzability of drugs. High-flux membranes may remove compounds with molecular weights ranging from 5000 to 20,000 Da. As a result, drugs that are not dialyzed by standard dialysis membranes will be dialyzed when high-flux membranes are employed. For example, vancomycin (molecular weight, 1442 Da) which has a $t_{1/2}$ of 180 hours with standard dialysis membranes, has a $t_{1/2}$ of 56 hours with high-flux, high-efficiency membranes (Fig. 1).

Drugs that are efficiently removed by hemodialysis are administered postdialysis in amounts equal to the amount lost during dialysis. For example, during a typical hemodialysis session approximately half of the total body amount of an aminoglycoside is removed, and a dose equal to 50% of the maintenance dose will be required postdialysis.

Drug Dosing in Continuous Ambulatory Peritoneal Dialysis (CAPD)

Factors that increase drug removal by peritoneal dialysis include a low molecular weight, low protein binding, a small V_d, a rapid rate of equilibration between tissue binding sites and blood, and a limited amount of nonrenal metabolism and excretion (Table 6). As a general rule, if the amount of drug removed by daily peritoneal dialysis is greater than

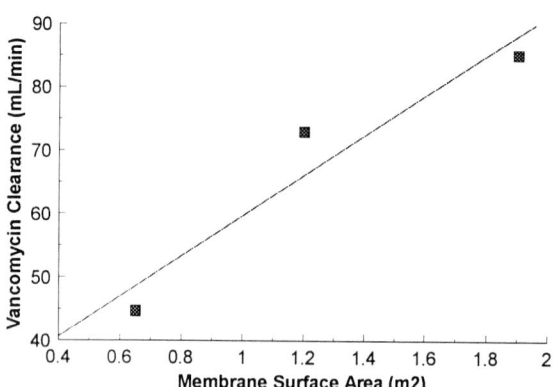

FIGURE 1   Effect of dialysis membrane surface area on extracorporeal clearance of vancomycin.

20 to 30% of the administered dose, larger doses must be administered. Example of drugs that require higher doses in CAPD include the aminoglycosides, most cephalosporins, and probably vancomycin (inconsistent data reported). Many other drugs do not require a dosing regimen different from those for a nondialyzed patient, because of their low clearance by CAPD. Drugs with a high V_d (e.g., digoxin), high nonrenal clearance (e.g., cimetidine), or high plasma protein binding (e.g., tricyclic antidepressants) are not cleared to any significant extent by CAPD.

Because fewer data are available on the effect of CAPD on pharmacokinetics of drugs, consideration of certain general principles allows for a reasonable prediction of whether dosing adjustment is required. Estimation requires the knowledge of several factors that influence drug movement across the peritoneal membrane (Table 6). These include the physicochemical and pharmacokinetic properties of the drug, the physiology and anatomy of the dialysis (peritoneal) membrane, and the dialysis regimen. To assess the amount of drug removed by CAPD, both the peritoneal clearance (Cl_{PD}) and the V_d of the drug must be known. Similar to calculating the total body clearance, Cl_{PD} can be calculated by dividing the total amount of drug recovered in the spent dialysate from one or more dwell periods by the area under the plasma concentration–time curve during the same period AUC_{0-t}. Alternatively, if at the end of each dwell period, equilibrium is reached between the drug concentrations in blood and the peritoneal cavity, and if there is no significant plasma protein binding, the Cl_{PD} is roughly equivalent to the dialysate flow rate. Given that in CAPD the dialysate flow rate rarely exceeds 5 to 7 mL/min, the amount of drug removed by CAPD is limited. In estimating the supplemental dose of a drug, the amount of drug or the fraction of the dose removed by CAPD (FDR_{PD}) may be determined from the formula

$$FDR_{PD} = \frac{Cl_{PD}}{Cl_{total} \times f_u}, \qquad (4)$$

where Cl_{total} is the systemic drug clearance and f_u is the unbound drug fraction. In this equation, Cl_{total} includes both the peritoneal (i.e., Cl_{PD}) and the endogenous (i.e., renal and nonrenal) clearances of the drug. The endogenous clearance may be estimated from the literature values for patients with ESRD. The unbound drug fraction is important, because plasma protein binding of the drug is the main limiting factor for diffusion of a drug into the peritoneal cavity. Ideally, f_u values from ESRD patients should be used. If not available, data from healthy subjects may be substituted. This equation does not take into account protein loss from the peritoneal cavity. Because the quantity of protein loss from the peritoneal cavity is small compared to the amount of protein in the systemic circulation, this loss does not substantially affect drug pharmacokinetics.

Pharmacokinetics of Intraperitoneally Administered Drugs

In patients on CAPD, intraperitoneal administration of drugs is the preferred route in at least three clinical situations: (1) for the administration of antibiotics in patients with CAPD peritonitis; (2) for the administration of insulin and (3) for the administration of deferoxamine in the treatment of aluminum overload. The intraperitoneal administration of a low-molecular-weight drug, such as most antibiotics, rapidly achieves a high local drug concentration within the peritoneal cavity. This concentration gradient leads to rapid diffusion of the drug from the peritoneal cavity into the systemic circulation. The reverse movement from the systemic circulation into the peritoneal cavity is much slower and restricted. As a result, intraperitoneal antibiotics used in the treatment of peritonitis (e.g., aminoglycosides, cephalosporins) are 50 to 80% bioavailable during a 6-hour dwell period. During bouts of peritonitis, the permeability of the peritoneal membrane increases, and as a result, both the rate and extent of intraperitoneal absorption of certain drugs (e.g., vancomycin, gentamicin, various β-lactam antibiotics) increase and remain so for days after the peritonitis episode.

Drug Dosing in Continuous Renal Replacement Therapy (CRRT)

Since dialysis is not employed during continuous hemofiltration, solute removal with CAVH or CVVH occurs exclusively via ultrafiltration (i.e., convective movement). CAVHD and COVHD rely on diffusion as well as convective clearance. As compared to standard hemodialysis, solute clearance per unit time may be lower during CRRT; however, due to its continuous nature, the overall clearance may be higher. For example, urea clearance during CRRT may be only 15 to 30 mL/min, versus approximately 200 mL/min for intermittent hemodialysis; however, because CRRT occurs 24 hours per day, the overall weekly clearance of urea for CRRT is 151 to 302 L vs. 48 L for intermittent hemodialysis. Drug removal during CRRT is affected by some of the same factors described above and listed in Table 6. Most of the hemofilters are the same as high-flux hemodialysis filters, and remove molecules with molecular weights of 5000 to 20,000 Da; hence, the molecular weight of the drug is usually not a rate-limiting factor for drug removal. As for hemodialysis, however, highly

TABLE 7
Total Clearance, Extracorporeal Clearance, and Adjustment Factor for Continuous Renal Replacement Therapy

Drug	Cl_{anuric} (mL/min)	$Cl_{extra} : Cl_{total}$	AF for ultrafiltration of 0.5 L/h
Amikacin	2	0.7–0.8	4–5
Atenolol	13	0.39	1.6
Carbenicillin	11	0.35	1.5
Cefalexin	15	0.32	1.5
Ceftazidime	12	0.38	1.6
Cefuroxime	8	0.47	1.9
Cisplatin	2	0.29	1.4
Fluconazole	6	0.55	2.2
Flucytosine	5	0.6	2.5
Ganciclovir	16	0.34	1.5
Gentamicin	4	0.6–0.7	3
Lamoxatam	10	0.33	1.5
Lithium	14	0.37	1.6
Methotrexate	9	0.33	1.5
Netilmicin	5	0.3–0.6	1–3
Phenobarbital	6	0.45	1.8
Sotalol	11	0.43	1.8
Tetracycline	15	0.31	1.4
Tobramycin	4	0.6–0.7	3

Cl_{anuric}, total clearance in anuric patients; $Cl_{extra} : Cl_{total}$, ratio of extracorporeal (CRRT) clearance to total endogenous clearance; AF, adjustment factor.

protein-bound drugs are not significantly removed by CRRT.

Limited data are available for drug dosing in CRRT. It should be further emphasized that the available literature values recommend dosing alterations based on various blood flow settings, filter types, and ultrafiltration rates, which may not be applicable to the specific patient. Because patients who receive CRRT are critically ill, drug dosing adjustments must be made with utmost care. When available, plasma or blood concentrations of drugs should be obtained and monitored, especially for drugs with a narrow therapeutic index (e.g., aminoglycosides, antiarrhythmics). In the absence of dosing guidelines, a trained pharmacotherapist may be consulted to calculate the amount of drug that may be removed, based on the drug's sieving coefficient (Si). The sieving coefficient of a substance is the relationship between drug concentration in the ultrafiltrate (C_{uf}) and the average drug concentration in the plasma or serum, as calculated from arterial (C_A) and venous (C_V) concentrations, and describes the ability of a drug to pass from the systemic circulation to the ultrafiltrate:

$$Si = \frac{C_{uf}}{(C_A + C_V)/2}. \quad (5)$$

Si values near 1.0 indicate free drug movement across the membrane, whereas Si values near 0 indicate complete lack of drug movement to the ultrafiltrate. Drugs with a high Si value include aminoglycosides, vancomycin, and some cephalosporins. If no data on Si are available, then the extent of the drug's plasma protein binding can provide a rough estimate, since there is a good correlation between f_u and Si. If the f_u value is to be used, ideally values from patients with acute renal failure should be used. If not available, data from with ESRD may be used.

Supplemental dosing may be required during CRRT if the ratio of extracorporeal clearance to endogenous clearance is greater than 0.25. If the nonrenal clearance is >60 mL/min, supplemental dosing during CRRT is not required.

In CRRT, the procedure for calculating a loading dose is identical to that described above for patients with renal failure. To calculate a maintenance dose, the dose recommended for anuric patients is multiplied by an adjustment factor (AF), as derived from the literature. Alternatively, the AF may be used to adjust the dosage interval,

$$\tau' = \frac{\tau}{AF}, \quad (6)$$

where τ' is the dosing interval for CRRT patients and τ is the dosing interval for anuric patients. Table 7 lists the total and extracorporeal clearances, as well as AF values for some commonly used drugs likely to be removed by CRRT.

Bibliography

Anders MW: Metabolism of drugs by the kidney. *Kidney Int* 18:636–647, 1980.

Anderson RJ. Drug prescribing for patients in renal failure. *Hosp Pract Off Ed* 18:145–149, 1983.

Ateshkadi A, Matzke GR: Dialysis therapy. In: Herfindal ET, Gourley DR (eds) *Textbook of Therapeutics: Drug and Disease Management*, 6th ed. Baltimore, Williams & Wilkins, pp. 429–464, 1996.

Bakris GL, Talbert R: Drug dosing in patients with renal insufficiency. A simplified approach. *Postgrad Med* 94:153–156, 1993.

Bennett WM: Guide to drug dosage in renal failure. *Clin Pharmacokinet* 15:326–354, 1988.

Bennett WM, Aronoff GR, Morrison G, et al.: Drug prescribing in renal failure: dosing guidelines for adults. *Am J Kidney Dis* 3:155–193, 1983.

Bjornsson TD: Nomogram for drug dosage adjustment in patients with renal failure. *Clin Pharmacokinet* 11:164–170, 1986.

Davis BB, Mattammal MB: Renal metabolism of drugs and xenobiotics. *Nephron* 27:187–196, 1981.

Gibson TP: Renal disease and drug metabolism: An overview. *Am J Kidney Dis* 8:7–17, 1986.

Keller E: Peritoneal kinetics of different drugs. *Clin Nephrol* 30(Suppl. 1):S24–528, 1988.

Lee CC: The assessment of fractional drug removal by extracorporeal dialysis. *Biopharm Drug Disposition* 3:163–173, 1982.

Reetze Bonorden P, Bohler J, Keller E: Drug dosage in patients during continuous renal replacement therapy. Pharmacokinetic and therapeutic considerations. *Clin Pharmacokinet* 24:362–379, 1993.

Swan SK, Bennett WM: Drug dosing guidelines in patients with renal failure. *West J Med* 156:633–638, 1992.

Talbert RL: Drug dosing in renal insufficiency. *J Clin Pharmacol* 34:99–110, 1994.

Touchette MA, Slaughter RL: The effect of renal failure on hepatic drug clearance. Ann *Pharmacother* 25:1214–1224, 1991.

Turnheim K: Pitfalls of pharmacokinetic dosage guidelines in renal insufficiency. *Eur J Clin Pharmacol* 40:87–93, 1991.

SECTION 7

HEREDITARY RENAL DISORDERS

SICKLE CELL NEPHROPATHY

JON I. SCHEINMAN

The recognized renal syndromes in sickle cell disease (SCD) include hematuria, (which may herald renal papillary necrosis) tubular dysfunction, and proteinuria associated with a sclerosing nephropathy (Table 1).

GROSS AND MICROSCOPIC HEMATURIA

Pathogenesis

Sickling in the renal medulla causes vascular obstruction, proximal congestion, and red blood cell (RBC) extravasation, resulting in hematuria. Specific conditions in the medulla predispose to sickling: the pO_2 of 35 to 40 mm Hg in the medulla is below the 45 mm Hg threshold for sickling; the very high osmolality causes water to move out of RBCs and concentrates the sickle hemoglobin, thereby aggravating sickling; and the low medullary pH also promotes sickling. In pathologic investigation, severe renal medullary vascular congestion is found in the kidneys of patients with gross hematuria. Diffuse microscopic extravasation occurs, and a specific bleeding point cannot be defined.

Renal papillary necrosis (RPN) may occur in some sickle cell patients with hematuria, both those patients with sickle cell disease and those with sickle cell trait. This RPN seems causally related to the medullary vascular congestion created by increased sickling induced by specific conditions in the medulla. When RPN has been studied in patients with hematuria, it appears as a diffuse fibrotic process with areas of active extravasation. Acute necrosis of large areas of the medulla is not observed. Collecting ducts appear within areas of amorphous collagenous scar, and vasa recta are selectively destroyed. The findings associated with RPN in sickle cell patients with hematuria resemble those in animal models with chemically induced RPN in which an initial dilatation and engorgement of vessels is followed by small, focal repeated infarctions in the papillae.

The pathologic findings of the RPN in SCD differ from those in analgesic abuse nephropathy or diabetes mellitus. In analgesic abuse nephropathy, the most serious fibrotic lesions are in the descending limbs of the loops of Henle and peritubular capillaries, and vasa recta are typically spared. In diabetes mellitus, massive infarction occurs with a sloughing of papillae that may cause obstruction.

Clinical Features

Gross hematuria can be one of the most dramatic clinical events in SCD. It can occur at any age, and its origin is usually unilateral, with greater propensity to be on the left. Gross hematuria can also be associated with sickle trait, and it has been shown to be more often associated with sickle cell trait than sickle cell anemia, postulated to be due to the associated greater genetic frequency of the sickle heterozygote in sickle trait. Thus, the workup of the patient with hematuria should include screening for sickle hemoglobin, especially in the absence of hypercalciuria or evidence of glomerular disease, and renal "sickle crisis" is the likely diagnosis when gross, painless hematuria occurs in a known HbSS or HbSA patient. Notably, severe pain makes the presumptive diagnosis of sickle hematuria less likely.

RPN has been postulated to have common etiologic factors with hematuria in sickle cell patients, but the clinical relationship of hematuria and necrosis is variable. Papillary necrosis may or may not be present in sickle cell patients with hematuria, and pain is not linked to either sickle cell hematuria or papillary necrosis. Papillary necrosis detected in sickle cell patients is usually without signs or symptoms. IVP surveys of patients without hematuria or pain have shown a higher prevalence of papillary necrosis in sickle cell patients than in those without hemoglobinopathy.

For the patient with known sickle cell hemoglobin presenting for the first time with gross hematuria, assays of coagulation parameters including platelets are appropriate. Renal and bladder ultrasound or intravenous pyelogram may reveal papillary necrosis (Fig. 1), but can also rule out bleeding from a tumor. Consideration of tumor is especially important in view of the recently described renal medullary carcinoma that appears almost exclusively in patients with sickle hemoglobin. Increased echo density of the medullary pyramids is common in sickle cell disease, even without papillary necrosis. A later finding in papillary necrosis is calcification of the medullary pyramids in a "garland" pattern surrounding the pelvis. A "shadowing" echo density seen in nephrocalcinosis is different from that resulting from other causes. It is probably unnecessary to perform contrast urography to visualize the renal architecture unless urinary obstruction is apparent by ultrasound. When urog-

TABLE I
Renal Findings in Sickle Cell Nephropathy

Hematuria
 Medullary congestion
 Renal papillary necrosis
 Medullary calcification
 Medullary carcinoma
Tubular dysfunction
 Concentration defect
 Increased sodium and phosphate reabsorption
 Decreased proton and potassium secretion
 Increased urate secretion
Glomerular sclerosis
 Hyperfiltration
 Glomerular hypertrophy
 Proteinuria/nephrotic sydnrome
 Focal segmental glomerulosclerosis

raphy is performed, the calyceal clubbing of RPN in SCD is not accompanied by cortical scarring, as is seen in pyelonephritic clubbing.

Treatment

Conservative management is appropriate in view of the benign pathology of sickle cell hematuria. Probably the most effective mode of conservative management is maintaining a high rate of urine flow by using hypotonic fluid intake (4 L/day) and diuretics (thiazide or loop diuretics such as furosemide). Diuresis can diminish medullary osmolarity and possibly alleviate sickling in the vasa recta, which in turn may also help prevent papillary necrosis. In addition, the high urine flow rate will promote clearance of clots from the bladder. Bed rest is often recommended, presumably to avoid dislodging clots, but there is little evidence to show that it is beneficial.

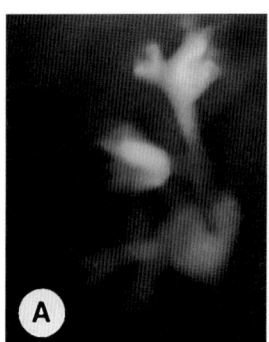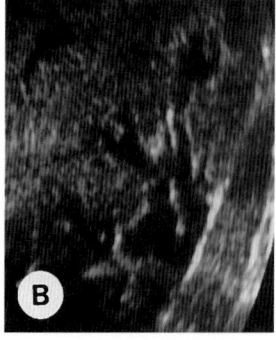

FIGURE I (A) Tomographic pyelography of an 18-year-old patient presenting with abdominal pain and hematuria. Papillary necrosis is evident from blunted medullary cavities. (B) Ultrasonographic visualization of the same kidney. The middle pole exhibits deep extensions into the papilla, likely sinus tracts, typical of the "papillary form" of renal papillary necrosis. The parenchyma adjacent to calyces is echodense, reflecting the fibrosis.

Another mode of conservative management is alkalinization of the urine with 8 to 12 g $NaHCO_3$ per day, which may reduce the tendency of the acid environment in the renal papillae to promote sickling. Alkalinizing the patient to increase hemoglobin O_2 affinity is theoretically helpful, but not of proven value.

Proceeding to less conservative treatments, transfusions may be necessary both to correct blood loss and, as in any other sickle crisis, to increase the proportion of normal HbAA cells.

Although ε-amino caproic acid (EACA) may be used in sickle cell hematuria to facilitate clotting in the urinary tract by inhibiting fibrinolysis, its use carries a risk of systemic thrombosis and is not advised unless other measures have failed. In one series, 4 of 12 cases required EACA after failures of treatment with volume and alkalinization. The effective adult dose of EACA is 8 g per day. Lower doses may be adequate to arrest hematuria. It may be worthwhile to start with 3 g and increase the dose until hemostasis occurs.

Other modes of treatment of sickle cell hematuria can be considered. In vitro, hyponatremia can induce swelling of RBCs, reduce the effective HbS concentration, and make cells less likely to sickle. Theoretically, a combination of vasopressin and hypotonic fluid administration could decrease plama osmolality and accomplish the same goals in vivo. However, because induced hyponatremia has not been proved safe or effective in humans and because other measures are usually sufficient, induced hyponatremia is not recommended. Experimental data suggest that angiotensin-converting enzyme (ACE) inhibition can induce a 50% increase in papillary blood flow, which could theoretically prevent RPN, but because increased blood flow could acutely aggravate hematuria, ACE inhibition is also not advised. Uncontrolled bleeding may be approached by arteriographic localization and local embolization of the involved renal segment. Pelvic irrigation with a sclerosing agent such as oxychlorosene has been used. Nephrectomy will be required only rarely.

TUBULAR DYSFUNCTION

Because the pathology in sickle cell disease primarily involves the medulla, the functions of the collecting ducts and juxtamedullary nephrons are most affected. Accordingly, a renal concentrating defect is the most commonly recognized renal problem in SCD.

Pathogenesis

Urinary Concentration and Water Reabsorption

Normally, the highest urine concentration is achieved by the collecting ducts of juxtamedullary nephrons which extend deepest into the medulla. The continued low-grade sickling and medullary congestion in SCD result in loss of the normal conditions for medullary water reabsorption and thus cause decreasing urine concentration. Vasopressin generation is normal in SCD, yet medullary damage results in a concentrating defect not responsive to vasopressin.

A maximum urinary osmolality in the range of 450 mOsm/kg is not a severe limitation for the SCD patient because this degree of concentration can be achieved by the outer medulla. Defective urinary concentration can often be restored in children with SCD by "hypertransfusion" therapy, presumably reversing the inner medullary congestion. However, in adults, the concentrating defect is not reversible; medullary fibrosis results in an irreversible destruction of collecting ducts.

The renal concentrating defect in SCD does not involve urinary diluting capacity, which normally depends on solute absorption in the ascending loop of cortical nephrons that leaves a dilute urine. The renal cortical area is relatively uninvolved in SCD, and urinary dilution is appropriate.

Tubular Secretion

Tubular secretion is altered in the kidneys of SCD patients. Effective renal plasma flow (ERPF) in SCD patients is increased, as indicated by increase in maximum hippurate tubular transport, a technique used because most hippurate is removed during a single pass through the kidney. Creatinine secretion in SCD is also increased, resulting in a creatinine clearance higher than expected for the glomerular filtration rate (GFR). Increased uric acid excretion likewise occurs, but a normal plasma uric acid level is maintained because urate production is increased in SCD patients.

Proximal Tubular Reabsorption

Proximal tubular reabsorption is also altered in SCD patients. Increased proximal sodium reabsorption is noted, causing less distal sodium delivery in response to saline infusion. The response to diuretics may be diminished because it is dependent on sodium delivery out of the proximal nephron. Phosphate reabsorption is similarly increased in the proximal tubules and may result in hyperphosphatemia during times of sickling and RBC destruction.

Acid and Potassium Excretion

Acid and potassium excretion are variably affected in SCD. Although it might be expected considering the severe involvement in SCD of the longer juxtamedullary nephrons where bicarbonate is normally most effectively reabsorbed, bicarbonate wasting or proximal renal tubular acidosis is not commonly seen in SCD. It is assumed that cortical nephrons are able to adequately compensate. Hydrogen ion (proton) secretion is performed by the "intercalated" collecting duct cells that are most prominent in the cortical segment of the collecting ducts. Because SCD does not typically involve this cortical area, a severe acidification defect is not usual. Still another factor in normal renal acid excretion, ammonium generation, is not affected by SCD. Titratable acid and ammonium generation in response to an ammonium chloride challenge in SCD patients are slightly decreased, but a maximal stimulus can produce normal acidification. Potassium excretion is impaired in SCD patients, but hyperkalemia is rare without renal failure. An observed decrease in acid and potassium excretion in SCD suggests that aldosterone deficiency is responsible, but renin and aldosterone values and their responses to volume depletion are normal. Electrolyte abnormalities resemble those in type IV renal tubular acidosis but actually result from an aldosterone independent end organ failure secondary to medullary fibrosis.

Possible Role of Prostaglandins in the Regulation of Renal Function in SCD

In general, decreased medullary transport and increased proximal activity have been ascribed to vasodilatory prostaglandin activity, possibly a compensation for defects in medullary sodium and water conservation. Data have come primarily from indomethacin inhibition of prostaglandin synthesis. Measurements of prostaglandin excretion are not demonstrably abnormal. In normal patients, indomethacin does not change GFR or ERPF. In SCD, both GFR and ERPF are decreased with indomethacin, suggesting that the high GFR and ERPF may be maintained by prostaglandins. Sodium retention is induced by indomethacin in both normals and SCD patients, but in normals, water reabsorption also increases, resulting in no change in serum osmolality. In SCD, water retention does not equally accompany sodium retention, and plasma osmolality increases. Compared to normals, SCD patients experience a greater fall in the fractional excretion of sodium after indomethacin. Urinary dilution in response to water loading, which is otherwise normal in SCD, is diminished by indomethacin but not in normals. Taken together, these findings are best explained by decreased delivery of sodium to the distal diluting segment.

Clinical Features

Clinically significant abnormalities in tubular function are more likely in patients developing renal insufficiency with failure of compensating mechanisms. The diagnosis of renal tubular abnormalities is evident from routine laboratory tests, which may show acidosis, hyperphosphatemia, hyperuricemia, and hyperkalemia.

Treatment

The tubular disorders in SCD usually require no treatment when renal function is normal. A failure of urinary concentration may result in increased susceptibility to dehydration. Early treatment of diarrhea or emesis will diminish that risk. Acidosis may require early treatment in the patient with SCD. Diuretics, especially the thiazides, may aggravate hyperuricemia. The edema accompanying severe anemia may be difficult to treat because of the diminished diuretic response. In the presence of renal insufficiency, potassium released from erythrocytes during severe hemolysis may exceed the patient's ability to excete potassium. β-Adrenergic blockade and ACE inhibition are potentially aggravating factors.

PROTEINURIA AND FOCAL SEGMENTAL GLOMERULOSCLEROSIS

Proteinuria is now recognized as the harbinger of progressive renal insufficiency in SCD. The incidence of renal failure has been estimated to be as great as 10 to 25% in HbSS or Hbc.

Pathogenesis

In sickle cell disease nephropathy, glomeruli are hypertrophied, and the hypertrophy correlates morphologically with ERPF and GFR. Proteinuria in SCD results from a functional "leak" in the size-dependent filtration barrier related to the high capillary flow in hypertrophied glomeruli. Hyperfiltration or increased GFR is common in young patients with SCD, and ERPF increases even more than GFR. Glomerular hypertrophy also relates to focal segmental glomerular sclerosis (FSGS) in SCD patients and is of greater magnitude than with idiopathic FSGS. The proteinuria of sickle cell nephropathy is closely associated pathologically with FSGS. The development of renal failure in SCD parallels the progression of FSGS and interstitial fibrosis.

Pathological lesions of SCD nephropathy vary. The earliest distinctive lesion in SCD glomerulopathy is a subendothelial zone lucency in the glomerular capillary loop. This may foreshadow either capillary collapse or a mesangial proliferative process. Focal tubulointerstitial fibrosis is present adjacent to sclerotic glomeruli. In addition to these findings, hemosiderin granules are seen in the tubular cytoplasm as a residual of hemolysis. There is little evidence of immune complex deposition in SCD patients with heavy proteinuria, suggesting that the proteinuria does not result from an inflammatory reaction.

Diagnosis

The upper limit of the normal GFR in SCD is never certain, whether determined with the "gold standard" inulin clearance or with the other clearance methods commonly used. In addition, an accurate measure of GFR is not necessary for most clinical purposes. However, a decrease over time in any measure of GFR in a patient with SCD, especially when accompanied by proteinuria, is ominous.

Proteinuria in a patient with SCD should be quantitated, and renal function should be assessed. Diseases other than sickle cell glomerulopathy should be ruled out, but biopsy will not often be needed in the SCD patient with insidious development of proteinuria. Sudden edema and massive proteinuria could indicate a process other than SCD. The presence of hypertension is unusual in SCD without nephropathy. Recent data suggest that patients who develop FSGS are more likely to be severely anemic but do not have greater frequency of sickle crises.

Treatment

Because it is likely that some aspect of the sickle cell condition predisposes to nephropathy, it is reasonable to attempt to minimize sickling—despite the finding that the nephropathy of SCD is not obviously related to frequency of sickle crises.

In treating SCD nephropathy, FSGS should also be addressed. Those factors of coexisting disease states that promote FSGS should be corrected to the extent possible. The development of FSGS in animal models is accelerated by a high protein intake, suggesting a treatment in humans with protein restriction. However, because restriction of protein intake may increase the risk of delayed growth and development that is already present in children with SCD, only the avoidance of an unusually high protein intake is advisable. It is uncertain whether alterations in hemodynamics can affect the progression of FSGS to renal insufficiency in SCD. Glomerular hyperperfusion and proteinuria may be mediated by increased glomerular capillary pressure. Although conventional antihypertensives decrease blood pressure, they do not appear to alter proteinuria. However, reduction of glomerular capillary pressure by ACE inhibition could protect the glomerulus from FSGS. The reduction of proteinuria and glomerular sclerosis by ACE inhibition in rats has prompted human trials. In a 2-week trial of enalapril therapy in 10 patients with mild SCD nephropathy, proteinuria diminished by 57% but rebounded after treatment withdrawal. Blood pressure and GFR did not change significantly. A long-term trial is needed to determine whether ACE inhibition is beneficial in preventing the progression of sickle cell nephropathy to renal failure.

Several therapies are available for advanced nephropathy in SCD patients. Treatment of renal failure should be considered even in the presence of a serious primary disease; dialysis can be undertaken, and renal transplantation has been as successful in SCD as in other diseases. Although the anemia in SCD patients with end stage renal disease is resistant to conventional doses of erythropoietin, larger doses may be necessary and appropriate. While it has been proposed that erythropoietin could increase the proportion of fetal hemoglobin, this has not been observed. However, if erythropoietin is administered in combination with hydroxyurea, the proportion of fetal hemoglobin appears to increase. Recently, bone marrow transplantation has been used for unusual cases of sickle cell anemia and may be relevant to treatment of SCD nephropathy.

Bibliography

Allon M: Renal abnormalities in sickle cell disease. *Arch Intern Med* 150:501–504, 1990.

Allon M, Lawson L, Eckman JR, Delaney V, Bourke E: Effects of nonsteroidal anti-inflammatory drugs on renal function in sickle cell anemia. *Kidney Int* 34:500–506, 1988.

Bakir AA, Hathiwala SC, Ainis H, et al.: Prognosis of the nephrotic syndrome in sickle glomerulopathy: A retrospective study. *Am J Nephrol* 7:110–115, 1987.

Bhathena DB, Sondheimer JH: The glomerulopathy of homozygous sickle hemoglobin (SS) disease: Morphology and pathogenesis. *J Am Soc Nephrol* 1:1241–1252, 1991.

Chatterjee SN: National study in natural history of renal allografts in sickle cell disease or trait: A second report. *Transplant Proc* 19:33–35, 1987.

Chauhan PM, Kondlapoodi P, Natta CL: Pathology of sickle cell disorders. *Pathol Ann* 18:253-276, 1983

deJong PE, Statius van Eps LW: Sickle cell nephropathy: New insights into its pathophysiology. *Kidney Int* 27:711–717, 1985.

Falk RJ, Scheinman JI, Phillips G, Orringer E, Johnson A, Jennette JC: Prevalence and pathologic features of sickle cell nephropathy and response to inhibition of angiotensin converting enzyme. *N Engl J Med* 326:910–915, 1992.

Mapp E, Karasick S, Pollack H, Wechsler RJ. Karasick D: Uroradiological manifestations of S-hemoglobinopathy. *Semin Roentgenol* 22:186–194, 1987.

Powars DR, Elliott-Mills DD, Chan L, et al.: Chronic renal failure in sickle cell disease: Risk factors, clinical course, and mortality. *Ann Intern Med* 115:614–620, 1991.

Sklar AH, Campbell HT, Caruana RJ, et al.: A population study of renal function in homozygous sickle cell anemia. *Int J Artif Organs* 13:231–236, 1990.

Tomson CRV: End stage renal disease in sickle cell disease: Future directions. *Postgrad Med J* 68:775–778, 1992.

45

POLYCYSTIC AND ACQUIRED CYSTIC DISEASES

PATRICIA A. GABOW

Renal cysts are a common, if dramatic, end point for a wide variety of renal insults. Renal cysts occur as part of both congenital and hereditary disorders or can be acquired later in life. Cysts can be single or multiple, replacing virtually all the renal parenchyma in some disorders; they can be clinically inconsequential or contribute to serious complications and sequelae.

CONGENITAL AND SYNDROMIC CYSTIC DISEASES

Congenital disorders occur in the course of fetal development but are not necessarily heritable. Numerous congenital or rare heritable syndromes include renal cysts (Table 1). These disorders are usually diagnosed *in utero* or early in life and are defined by a characteristic array of abnormalities. The diversity of these syndromes with cysts serves to underscore the nonspecific nature of renal cystic disease. In these disorders the renal cysts often do not pose the most significant clinical problem.

HEREDITARY RENAL CYSTIC DISEASES

The four important hereditary cystic renal diseases are autosomal recessive polycystic kidney disease (ARPKD), autosomal dominant polycystic kidney disease (ADPKD), von Hippel–Lindau disease, and tuberous sclerosis (TS).

The latter three have an autosomal dominant pattern of inheritance and the chromosomal location or locations of a putative gene have been identified.

Autosomal Recessive Polycystic Kidney Disease

ARPKD is a rare disease with incidence estimates ranging from 1:6000 to 1:40,000. A gene for this disease is located on chromosome 6. The diversity of phenotypic presentation in terms of age of onset and systemic manifestations had led some clinicians to question whether the disorder represents a single genetic disease. However, gene linkage analysis to date has not demonstrated genetic heterogeneity. The identification of the gene location has permitted prenatal diagnosis with gene linkage analysis in some families. The disorder can be diagnosed *in utero* in many fetuses after the 24th week of gestation by ultrasonography from the findings of large hyperechoic kidneys and often oligohydramnios. However, there is no definitive information on how frequently an affected fetus will have a noncharacteristic ultrasonogram. Although prenatal ultrasonography is appropriate in families with a previously affected child, it is not yet clear that a normal study excludes disease development later in life. Often the diagnosis of ARPKD is made after birth and is prompted by the finding of abdominal masses. Children with large kidneys *in utero*

From Gilberg-Barness EF, Opitz JM, Barness LA: In: Spitzer A, Avner ED (eds) *Inheritance of Kidney and Urinary Tract Diseases*. Kluwer Academic, Boston, pp. 327-400, 1990, with kind permission from Kluwer Academic Publishers.

TABLE I

Syndromes with Renal Cysts

Sporadic disorders
  Facioauricular–vertebral syndrome

Chromosomal abnormalities
  Trisomy 21, 18, 13, 9
  Triploidy
  Deletion of 17p, 4p
  Duplication of 10q, 3q, 1q
  Sex chromosome abnormalities 45,X; 47,XYY

X-linked recessive disorders
  Oculocerebrorenal syndrome of Lowe
  Orofacial–digital syndrome

Autosomal recessive disorders
  Meckel's syndrome
  Miranda's syndrome
  Smith Lemli–Opitz syndrome
  Lissencephaly type II
  Baret–Biedl syndrome
  Hydrolethalus syndrome
  Fryns syndrome
  Orofacial–digital syndrome type I
  Short-rib–polydactyl syndrome type I and II
  Acrocephalopolydactylous dysplasia
  Cerebrohepatorenal syndrome (Zellweger)
  Glutaric acidemia type II
  Neonatally lethal adrenoleukodystrophy
  Chondysplasia calcificans punctate, rhizomelic type

often have immediate respiratory distress from pulmonary hypoplasia and pneumothorax; these complications can result in perinatal death.

ARPKD is characterized by the development of renal cysts, or, more correctly, tubular ectasia of the collecting ducts, and congenital hepatic fibrosis. In older children, the kidneys appear large with increased echogenicity in the medulla and macrocysts on ultrasonograms. Pathologically the liver displays increased numbers of dilated bile ductules and fibrosis in the portal areas. Hepatic macrocysts are unusual. The clinical manifestations of the hepatic disease include cholangitis and portal hypertension with esophageal varices and gastrointestinal bleeding. The renal manifestations include hypertension, which is often severe, urinary tract infection, and, ultimately, renal failure.

Children who present early in life tend to show a predominance of renal abnormalities; those who present later in childhood tend to have a predominance of hepatic manifestations. Recent studies have shown a better prognosis than previously reported; children who survive the first month of life do quite well, with a 78% probability of surviving beyond 15 years of age. Early identification and aggressive treatment of the hypertension may improve the renal disease prognosis in these children. A few children with

ARPKD have successfully undergone simultaneous renal and liver transplantation.

The other major diagnoses to be considered in children who present with renal cysts are TS, ADPKD glomerulocystic disease, and the syndromes listed in Table 1. The presence of other characteristic phenotypic abnormalities and the pattern of inheritance provide valuable information that facilitates making specific diagnosis. Although ADPKD cannot be differentiated from ARPKD solely on the basis of ultrasonographic findings, the presence of discrete renal cysts, particularly in a fetus, favors ADPKD. The single most reliable means of differentiating between these two hereditary childhood cystic diseases is to perform renal ultrasonography in the parents. The diagnosis ARPKD is favored if neither parent has the characteristic findings of ADPKD. In some instances, a liver and/or renal biopsy in the affected child may be helpful. Although congenital hepatic fibrosis has also been reported in ADPKD, its virtual 100% occurrence in ARPKD and its rare occurrence in ADPKD strongly favor the diagnosis of ARPKD.

Autosomal Dominant Polycystic Kidney Disease

ADPKD is both the most common hereditary renal disease and one of the most common hereditary disease in this country. It affects 1 : 400 to 1 : 1000 Americans and is the fourth most common cause of end stage renal disease (ESRD). At least three different genes can produce the disorder. The ADPKD1 gene is responsible for approximately 90% of the disease in the white population of European ancestry. Recently cloned, this gene is located on the short arm of chromosome 16 and is a very complicated large gene. The gene product, polycystin, is thought to be a membrane glycoprotein involved in cell–cell or cell–matrix interactions. The ADPKD2 gene, which is on chromosome 4, has also been cloned. The chromosomal location of the ADPKD3 gene is yet to be determined. The frequency of the gene distribution in other racial and ethnic groups has not been defined.

The identification of the location of the ADPKD genes has added gene linkage analysis to the diagnostic armamentarium for this disease. This technique permits the diagnosis to be made *in utero* or in children or adults prior to the development of renal cysts if multiple family members can be tested. Blood samples from at least two affected family members are necessary to identify the DNA marker that is linked to the ADPKD gene. Commercially available probes make this technique applicable in most ADPKD1 families; probes are now available for ADPKD2 families. Nonetheless, gene linkage analysis is not generally needed to make the diagnosis. Ultrasonography remains the diagnostic test of choice because it is sensitive, relatively inexpensive, safe and able to provide information about the degree of structural renal involvement, while requiring only the participation of the individual wishing the information (Fig. 1). Recent studies have demonstrated that approximately 3 to 24% of individuals with ADPKD1 will have a normal renal ultrasonogram before 30 years of age. In children the percentage of false negative ultrasonograms

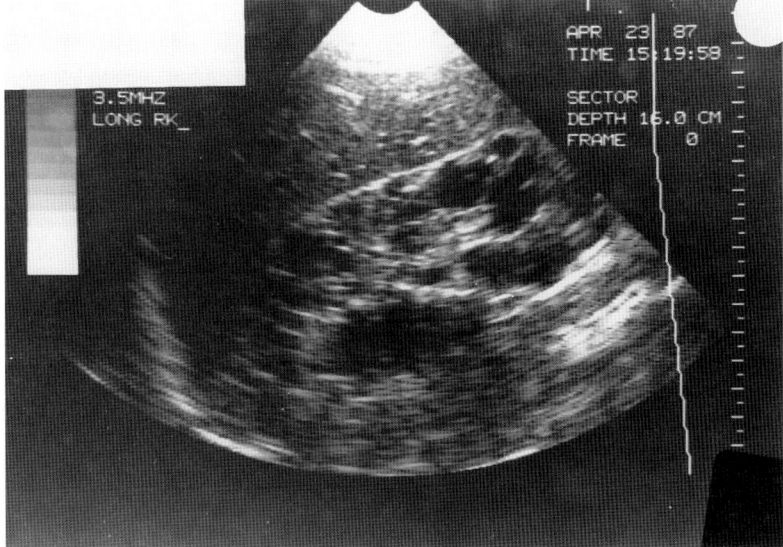

FIGURE I Renal ultrasonogram of a 44-year-old male with autosomal dominant polycystic kidney disease. The kidney is moderately enlarged and contains multiple cysts of
variable size.

is even higher, approaching 40% in children under age 5
years. Therefore, gene linkage analysis is likely to be of
value in establishing the gene status only in these individuals and in fetuses. However, there are caveats regarding
ADPKD screening of asymptomatic children and adults,
because it has the potential for adverse psychological consequences and can affect insurability. Moreover, genetic
screening of fetuses does not predict the course of the
disease. In contrast, children diagnosed *in utero* or in the
first year of life via a characteristic renal ultrasonogram
tend to have a more severe disease than individuals diagnosed later in life and have an approximately 27% chance
of renal failure or renal insufficiency before adulthood.

ADPKD is not only a renal disease; it is a systemic
disorder with a myriad of manifestations (Table 2). The
renal manifestations of clinical importance include hypertension, infection, nephrolithiasis, acute and chronic pain,
and renal failure. The renal cysts are responsible for many
of these complications (Fig. 2). Hypertension occurs in
about 30% of ADPKD children, 60% of adults prior to
ESRD, and about 80% of ADPKD patients with ESRD.
Hypertension is more common in individuals with more
severe cystic involvement and may be ameliorated at least
temporarily, in adults, by cyst decompression. It has been
suggested that the cysts alter the intrarenal circulation creating areas of renal ischemia with activation of the renin-
angiotensin-aldosterone system. Renin and aldosterone
levels are higher in ADPKD hypertensive patients than in
patients with a similar degree of essential hypertension.
Because of the role of the renin-angiotensin system in
ADPKD hypertension, angiotensin converting enzyme inhibitors are often the drug of choice in treating hypertension in these patients. However, there are no long-term
studies comparing the renal outcomes in patients treated
with different antihypertensive drugs.

TABLE 2

Manifestations of Autosomal Dominant Polycystic
Kidney Disease in Adults

Extrarenal manifestations
Gastrointestinal
Hepatic cysts
Cholangiocarcinoma[a]
Congenital hepatic fibrosis[a]
Pancreatic cysts
Diverticula
Cardiovascular
Cardiac valvular abnormalities
Intracranial aneurysms
Thoracic and abdominal aortic aneurysms (?)
Miscellaneous cysts
Ovarian cysts
Arachnoid cysts[a]
Pineal cysts[a]
Splenic cysts[a]
Renal manifestations
Anatomical
Renal cysts
Renal adenomas
Complications
Hypertension
Hematuria and/or hemorrhage
Acute and chronic pain
Urinary tract infection—bladder, interstitium, cysts
Nephrolithiasis
Nephromegaly
Renal failure

[a] Rare.

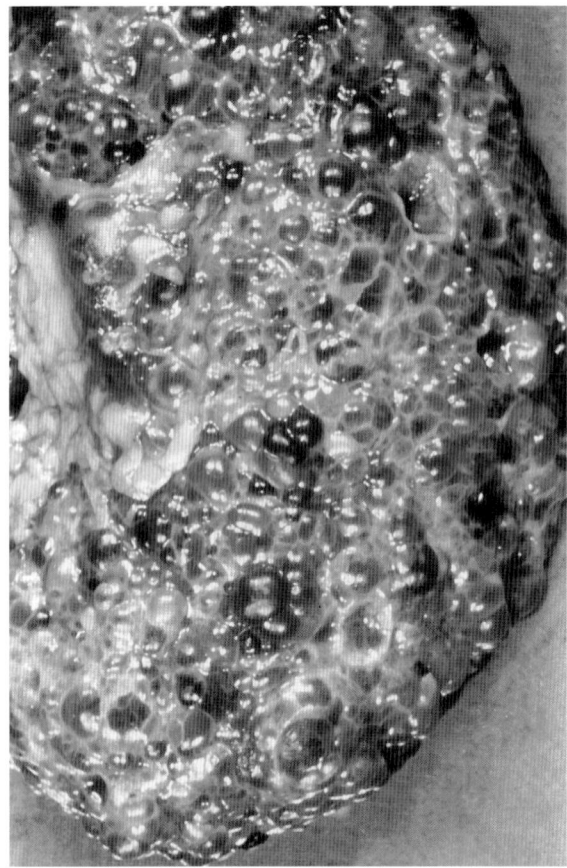

FIGURE 2   A nephrectomy specimen of a kidney from a patient with autosomal dominant polycystic kidney disease. The kidney appears moderately enlarged with cysts of varying size—some of which appear hemorrhagic. Reprinted by permission of *The New England Journal of Medicine*, Gabow PA: 329:332–342, 1993. *Massachusetts Medical Society*. All rights reserved.

Acute abdominal, flank, or back pain are common and can result from renal and extrarenal complications. One renal etiology of pain is infection in the interstitium or the cysts. ADPKD patients who appear to have simple cystitis or pyelonephritis can be treated as one would treat any other patients with these maladies. A patient with presumed pyelonephritis who fails to demonstrate an appropriate response should be considered to have a renal cyst infection. Renal cyst infections are also suggested by the presence of discrete renal tenderness, positive blood cultures, and absence of white blood cell casts. The failure of antibiotic therapy reflects the lack of cyst penetration of a majority of the antibiotics. Those antibiotics with good cyst fluid accumulation include trimethoprim-sulfamethoxazole, ciprofloxacin, and chloramphenicol; hence they are the antibiotics of choice for patients with presumed cyst infection.

Nephrolithiasis, which occurs in as many as 34% of ADPKD patients, can also present as an acute pain syndrome. Stone formation likely reflects both intrarenal urinary stasis due to cysts and metabolic abnormalities including decreased citrate excretion. Acute pain can also be caused by cyst hemorrhage; this is not always accompanied by hematuria. Diagnosis of this complication is usually possible by computed tomography.

Chronic disabling pain occurs in a small group of ADPKD patients. These patients can benefit from cyst decompression procedures, such as surgical unroofing of cysts, percutaneous or laparoscopic cyst decompression, and cyst drainage and alcohol sclerosis, which prevents rapid fluid reaccumulation.

Although renal failure is the most serious renal complication of ADPKD, it is not an invariable outcome. Only about 50% of ADPKD patients progress to ESRD before 60 years of age. The factors associated with a worse renal outcome include the ADPKD1 gene (in contrast to the ADPKD2 gene), male gender, African origin, sickle hemoglobin, earlier age of presentation, hypertension, episodes of gross hematuria, and urinary tract infections in males. Data on the effect of pregnancy on renal outcome are variable, but several studies suggest that more than three or four pregnancies, particularly in hypertensive women, is associated with a worse long-term renal outcome. In experimental models of renal cystic disease a variety of interventions including treatment with taxol, prednisone, sodium and potassium bicarbonate, and lovastatin as well as protein restriction have been shown to ameliorate the renal cystic disease. A few human studies have been performed, the largest being the Modification of Diet in Renal Disease (MDRD) study, which failed to show efficacy of protein restriction or rigorous control of blood pressure on renal disease progression. However, the patients had advanced renal disease and the study was of relatively short duration. Hence the efficacy of these interventions early in the course of disease remains undetermined.

Extrarenal cystic manifestations include hepatic cysts, perhaps ovarian cysts, and rarely, pancreatic, splenic, and arachnoid cysts. Hepatic cysts occur in about 60% of the overall ADPKD population. However, hepatic cysts are very rare in childhood. Their prevalence increases with age with a peak occurrence in the fifth to sixth decade. Massive hepatic cystic disease appears to be mainly a disorder of ADPKD women; pregnancy is a major correlate of hepatic cyst number and size. Although massive hepatic cystic disease can result in substantial abdominal distention and pain, it only very rarely affects hepatic function; other causes should always be sought for abnormal liver function tests in an ADPKD patient. Hepatic cysts can occasionally become infected; both antibiotics and drainage appear to be required for recovery. The other extrarenal cystic manifestations usually have no clinical sequelae.

Extrarenal noncystic manifestations include gastrointestinal, cardiovascular, and musculoskeletal abnormalities. Diverticular disease is more frequent and more severe among ADPKD patients with ESRD than in non-ADPKD ESRD patients and age-matched controls. One of the most common extrarenal manifestations is cardiac valvular abnormalities, particularly mitral valve prolapse which occurs in 26% of ADPKD patients compared to 2% of a non-

ADPKD control group. It is often accompanied by palpitations and atypical chest pain.

One of the most devastating manifestations of ADPKD is rupture of an intracranial aneurysm. About 5 to 10% of ADPKD patients have intracranial aneurysms. However, the risk may not be evenly distributed across all families; some data suggest that aneurysms cluster in certain ADPKD families. Although it is clear that aneurysms can be detected before rupture by noninvasive methods such as dynamic computed tomography or magnetic resonance angiography, screening of all ADPKD patients for aneurysms is not cost-effective. Therefore, the current recommendations are to screen only those patients who have a family history of aneurysm, those undergoing elective surgery with a high likelihood of developing hypertension during surgery, or those engaged in an activity in which sudden loss of consciousness would be associated with grave consequences to themselves or others. Of course, any patient with acute symptoms compatible with aneurysmal rupture requires immediate investigation. However, chronic headaches do not identify patients with aneurysms.

Von Hippel–Lindau Disease

This systemic disease is an uncommon autosomal dominant disorder which occurs in 1:36,000 live births. The defective gene is on chromosome 3. The eye, the central nervous system (CNS), the pancreas, the adrenal glands, the epididymis, and the kidney may be involved. The manifestations of the disease include retinal angiomas and cerebellar and spinal hemangioblastomas, pancreatic cysts and islet cell carcinomas, and pheochromocytomas. The latter may be bilateral. The epididymal abnormalities include cystic and solid epididymal masses. Renal cysts and renal cell carcinomas are observed. As many as 75% of patients with this disease will have renal cysts. These cysts pathologically are more like those in acquired cystic disease and less like simple cysts (see below) in that the cyst epithelium displays a histologic spectrum from normal-appearing single-layered epithelium to epithelial hyperplasia to renal cell carcinoma. It is estimated that between 38 and 55% of patients with Von Hippel–Lindau disease develop renal cell carcinoma which can be bilateral and multicentric in up to 60% of the cases. Renal cell carcinoma occurs on average in the fourth and fifth decade, considerably earlier than in the general population. It accounts for 20 to 50% of the deaths in these patients.

Because of the devastating CNS and renal complications, regular screening by imaging the brain and abdomen in at-risk family members has been recommended. Genetic screening permits limiting these studies to those family members who are found to be gene carriers.

Tuberous Sclerosis

TS is another autosomal dominant disease with similarities to ADPKD. As with ADPKD, different genes can produce the disease; these genes occur on chromosomes 9 and 16—very close to the ADPKD1 gene. TS is characterized by epilepsy, mental retardation, skin abnormalities including adenoma sebaceum and ash-leaf spots, and hamartomas of many organs including angiomyolipoma of the kidneys and renal cysts. Angiomyolipomas occur in 40 to 60% of patients with or without renal cysts, and renal cysts occur alone in about 18% of patients. In neonates or young children the occurrence of isolated renal cysts can lead to the misdiagnosis of ARPKD or ADPKD. Particularly in the presence of aggressive cystic disease, renal failure can occur. In fact, renal disease is the most common serious complication of this disease in patients over 30 years of age.

ACQUIRED CYSTIC DISEASES

There are several types of acquired cystic disease: simple renal cysts, hypokalemia-related cystic disease, and acquired cystic disease (ACD). Simple renal cysts increase with age, occurring in less than 0.1% of children and up to 20% of individuals over age 50. Although cysts are usually single and unilateral, they may be multiple and bilateral. However, the latter should raise the question of a polycystic renal disease. On ultrasonography simple cysts are smooth-walled without internal debris. As they are only very rarely malignant, they require no further evaluation, if these characteristic ultrasonographic features are present.

Multiple renal cysts have been described in patients with hypokalemia secondary to hyperaldosteronism. In some of these patients the renal cysts regressed after successful resection of the adrenal adenoma. The cellular proliferative stimulus of hypokalemia may be pathogenetic in this setting.

ACD refers to a specific disorder in which renal cysts develop in the kidneys of both adults and children with ESRD due to a noncystic renal disorder. Although its pathogenesis remains to be defined, abnormal cell proliferation and intratubular obstruction with oxalate crystals have been suggested. Risk factors for the development of ACD include the duration of renal insufficiency, including years on dialysis, and in some studies male gender and African ancestry. ACD occurs in 7 to 22% of patients with renal failure who are not on dialysis, 40% of patients who have been on dialysis for 3 years, and 80 to 90% of patients who have been on dialysis for 4 to 10 years. In some patients a successful renal transplant leads to the regression of ACD. In contrast, ACD may occur in the transplanted kidneys of patients with chronic rejection. Most ACD patients are asymptomatic; among symptomatic patients the most common manifestations are pain, hematuria, and fever. In addition, cyst hemorrhage and retroperitoneal bleeding (presumably from cyst rupture), erythrocytosis, hypercalcemia, and hypoglycemia have also been reported. Both benign and malignant renal neoplasms are common; the most serious sequela of ACD is renal cell carcinoma. This complication has been estimated to be 50 times more frequent in dialysis patients with ACD than in the general population. As with the disease itself, male gender and African ancestry appear to be risk factors for the development of malignancy. Although agreement on the metastatic potential of these tumors is lacking, it is clear that metastatic disease does occur in at least some ACD patients. The survival is similar to that of other patients with renal cell carcinoma. The occurrence of malignancy and its potential to metastasize has raised concern about the need for screening. Although some decision analysis data have suggested that screening is not cost-effective, many clinicians recommend a screening program. One guideline includes an ultrasonogram at the onset of dialysis and follow-up ultrasonography every 3 years thereafter. There is also rationale for opting to screen only males in good health who have been on dialysis for more than 7 years. Because metastatic potential appears to relate to tumor size, any tumor greater than 2 cm is a strong indicator for nephrectomy.

Acknowledgments

This work was supported by Grant 5 P01 DK34039, Human Polycystic Kidney Disease (PKD), awarded by the Department of Health and Human Services, Public Health Service, NIDDK, and the Clinical Research Center, Grant MORR-00051 from the General Clinical Research Centers Research Program of the Division of Research Resources, National Institutes of Health.

Bibliography

Chapman AB, Rubinstein D, Hughes R, et al.: Intracranial aneurysms in autosomal dominant polycystic kidney disease. *N Engl J Med* 327:916–920, 1992.

Choyke PL, Glenn GM, Walther MM, Patronas NJ, Linehan WM, Zbar B: von Hippel-Lindau disease: Genetic, clinical, and imaging features. *Radiology* 194:629–642, 1995.

Fick GM, Gabow PA: Hereditary and acquired cystic disease of the kidney (review). *Kidney Int* 46:951–964, 1994.

Fick GM, Duley IT, Johnson AM, Strain JD, Manco-Johnson ML, Gabow PA: The spectrum of autosomal dominant polycystic kidney disease in children. *J Am Soc Nephrol* 4:1654–1660, 1994.

Gabow PA, Johnson AM, Kaehny WD, et al.: Factors affecting the progression of renal disease in autosomal-dominant polycystic kidney disease. *Kidney Int* 41:1311–1319, 1992.

Gilbert-Barness EF, Opitz JM, Barness LA: Heritable malformations of the kidney and urinary tract. In: Spitzer A, Avner ED (eds) *Inheritance of Kidney and Urinary Tract Diseases.* Kluwer Academic, Boston, pp. 327–400, 1990.

Guay-Woodford LM: Autosomal recessive polycystic kidney disease: Clinical and genetic profiles. In: Watson ML, Torres VE (eds) *Polycystic Kidney Disease.* Oxford University Press, New York, pp. 237–266, 1996.

Harris PC, Ward CJ, Peral B, Hughes J: Polycystic kidney disease 1: Identification and analysis of the primary defect. *J Am Soc Nephrol* 6:1125–1133, 1995.

Huston J, Torres VE, Sulivan PP, Offord KP, Wiebers DO: Value of magnetic resonance angiography for the detection of intracranial aneurysms in autosomal dominant polycystic kidney disease. *J Am Soc Nephrol* 3:1871–1877, 1993.

Ishikawa I: Acquired cystic disease: Mechanisms and manifestations. *Semin Nephrol* 11:671–684, 1991.

Klahr S, Breyer JA, Beck GJ, et al.: Dietary protein restriction, blood pressure control, and the progression of polycystic kidney disease. *J Am Soc Nephrol* 5:2037–2047, 1995.

Linehan WM, Lerman MI, Zbar B: Identification of the von Hippel-Lindau (VHL) gene. *JAMA* 273:564–570, 1995.

Roach ES, Delgado MR: Tuberous sclerosis. *Dermatol Clin* 13:151–165, 1995.

Sarasin FP, Wong JB, Levey AS, Meyer KB: Screening for acquired cystic kidney disease: A decision analytic perspective. *Kidney Int* 48:207–219, 1995.

Torres VE, King BF, Holley KE, Blute ML, Gomez MR: The kidney in the tuberous sclerosis complex. *Adv Nephrol* 23:43–70, 1994.

ALPORT'S SYNDROME AND RELATED DISORDERS

MARTIN C. GREGORY

Alport's syndrome is a disease of collagen that affects the kidneys always, the ears often, and the eyes occasionally. Cecil Alport described the association of hereditary hematuric nephritis with hearing loss in a family whose affected males died in adolescence. Genetic advances have broadened the scope of the condition to include ocular defects, platelet abnormalities, late-onset renal failure, and normal hearing in some families. At least 80% of kindreds are X-linked and over half of those result from a mutation of COL4A5, the gene located at Xq22 that codes for the $\alpha5$ chain of type IV collagen. Autosomal recessive inheritance occurs in perhaps 5% of cases and autosomal dominant inheritance has been shown in a few kindreds with associated thrombocytopathy and in very rare kindreds with otherwise typical Alport's syndrome.

JUVENILE AND ADULT FORMS

This distinction is fundamental to the understanding of Alport's syndrome. Renal failure tends to occur at a similar age in all male hemizygotes in a given kindred, but this age can differ widely between kindreds. Uremia in males occurs in childhood or adolescence in some families, and in the late thirties in others. The families with early onset of renal failure in males are termed "juvenile" and those with renal failure in middle age are called "adult" type nephritis. Extrarenal manifestations tend to be more prominent in the juvenile kindreds. Moreover, because males in juvenile kindreds do not commonly survive to reproduce, these kindreds tend to be small and frequently arise from new mutations. Adult type kindreds are typically much larger and new mutations occur infrequently.

CLASSICAL GENETICS

In most kindreds inheritance is X-linked. This was suggested by classical pedigree analysis, strengthened by formal likelihood analysis, proved by extremely tight linkage to restriction fragment length polymorphic markers (RFLPs), and finally cemented by identification of mutations.

MOLECULAR GENETICS

Causative mutations of COL4A5, the gene coding for the $\alpha5$ chain of type IV collagen, appear consistently in many kindreds. Deletions, point mutations, and splicing errors occur. Deletions and splicing errors result in severe renal disease and severe hearing loss. Missense mutations may cause juvenile disease with hearing loss or adult disease with or without hearing loss. Deletions involving the 5' end of the COL4A5 gene and the 5' end of the adjacent COL4A6 gene occur consistently in families with esophageal and genital leiomyomatosis. Homozygotes or mixed heterozygotes for mutations of COL4A3 or COL4A4 can develop autosomal recessive Alport's syndrome. Some cases of autosomal recessive Alport's syndrome may be homozygotes for a COL4A4 mutation that causes benign familial hematuria.

IMMUNOCHEMISTRY

Patients with Alport's syndrome lack a component of the glomerular basement membrane (GBM). After transplantation, about 10% of Alport males develop anti-GBM nephritis, presumably because tolerance to this normal antigen has not been acquired. Recurrences of anti-GBM

nephritis are usual but not inevitable after retransplantation. The anti-GBM antibodies developing after transplantation are heterogeneous. All will stain normal GBM but only some stain epidermal basement membrane. In most kindreds with Alport's syndrome the GBM of affected males fails to stain in the normal fashion with anti-GBM sera, and the GBM of female heterozygotes stains in an interrupted fashion. Certain sera have in common activity against $\alpha3(IV)$ and also epidermal basement membrane. The "Alport antigen" that these sera recognize is a 26-kDa monomer belonging to the $\alpha3(IV)$ chain.

BIOCHEMISTRY

The open meshwork of interlocking molecules of type IV collagen that forms the framework of glomerular basement membrane is composed of heterotrimers of α chains. Most of these heterotrimers consist of two $\alpha1(IV)$ chains and one $\alpha2(IV)$ chain, but an important minority contain an $\alpha3(IV)$, an $\alpha4(IV)$, and an $\alpha5(IV)$ chain. The primary chemical defect in Alport's syndrome most commonly involves the $\alpha5(IV)$ chain, but faulty assembly of the $\alpha3,4,5$ heterotrimer produces similar pathology in glomerular, aural, and ocular basement membranes regardless of which α chain is defective. As an illustration of failure of normal heterotrimer formation, many patients whose genetic defect is in the gene coding for the $\alpha5(IV)$ chain lack demonstrable $\alpha3(IV)$ chains in GBMs.

PATHOLOGY

In young children light microscopy may be normal or near normal. An increased number of "fetal" glomeruli may be seen. As disease progresses, interstitial and tubular foam cells may become quite prominent, although they can also be found in many other conditions. Eventually progressive glomerular sclerosis and interstitial scarring develop (Fig. 1). Routine immunofluorescence examina-

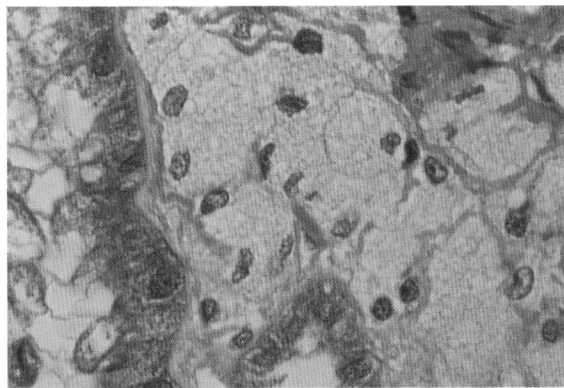

FIGURE 1 High-power photomicrograph of foam-filled tubular and interstitial cells in a renal biopsy from a patient with Alport's syndrome. Relatively normal proximal tubular cytoplasm stains red in the tubules on the left and at the top. The remaining cells appear "foamy" because of the spaces left where lipids have been eluted during processing.

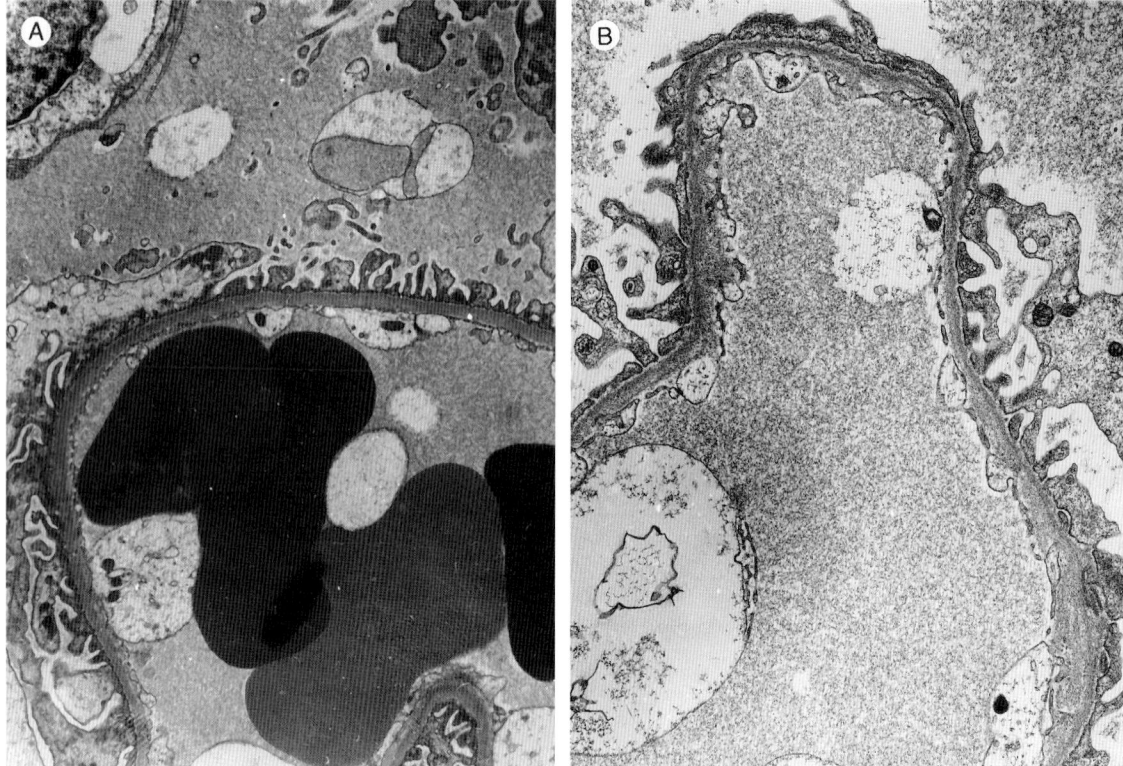

FIGURE 2 (A) Medium power electron micrograph of normal human glomerular basement membrane. The lamina densa of the basement membrane is of uniform density, texture, and thickness throughout its length. (B) Electron micrograph of glomerular basement membrane from a patient with Alport's syndrome at the same magnification as (A). The glomerular basement membrane varies in thickness. It is thinner than normal at the top left of the capillary loop. At middle left the lamina densa is split into two layers and at bottom right the basement membrane is very broad and frays into several lamellae. Electron micrographs kindly supplied by Dr. Daniel A. Terreros.

tion is negative. The characteristic features are seen by electron microscopy (Fig. 2). The GBM is thickened up to two or three times its normal thickness, split into several irregular layers, and frequently interspersed with numerous electron dense granules about 40 nm in diameter. In florid cases of juvenile types of disease the lamellae of basement membrane material may branch and rejoin in a complex "basket weave" pattern. Early in the development of the lesion, thinning of the GBM may predominate or may be the only abnormality visible. The abnormalities in children or adolescents with adult-type Alport's syndrome may be unimpressive or suggestive of thin basement membrane disease.

CLINICAL FEATURES

Renal Features

Uninterrupted microscopic hematuria is present from birth in affected males. Hematuria may become visible after exercise or during fever; this is more common in juvenile kindreds. Microscopic hematuria has a penetrance of approximately 90% in heterozygous females in adult-type kindreds. In juvenile kindreds, the penetrance of hematuria in females may be lower, but this has been studied

less extensively. Urinary erythrocytes are dysmorphic, and red cell casts can usually be found. Proteinuria is very variable; occasionally it reaches nephrotic levels.

Hemizygous males inevitably progress to end stage rend disease (ESRD). This occurs at widely variable ages that are fairly constant within each family. Heterozygous females are generally much less severely affected. Around one fifth of them will develop ESRD, usually after the age of 50, but renal failure in girls in their teens and even younger does occur.

In families with autosomal inheritance, females are affected as severely and as early as males. Renal failure often occurs before the age of 10 years in homozygotes with autosomal recessive Alport's syndrome.

Nonrenal Features

Hearing Loss

Bilateral high-frequency cochlear hearing loss is present in many but not all kindreds. Some authors do not use the term Alport's syndrome unless there is substantial hearing loss in the family. Regardless of terminology, the important clinical point is that X-linked nephritis progressing to ESRD can occur in families without overt hearing loss.

Expectation of hearing loss has resulted in many diagnoses being missed and has introduced a substantial ascertainment bias against those with normal hearing. In families with juvenile type disease, hearing loss is almost universal in male hemizygotes and common in severely affected female heterozygotes.

Hearing loss affects all frequencies but is maximal at 6 through 8 kHz. The loss is also severe at 8 to 20 kHz, but these frequencies are not covered by conventional audiometry. In adult-type Alport's syndrome with hearing loss, there is no perceptible deficit until age 20, but loss progresses to 60–70 dB at 6–8 kHz at ages over 40. Hearing loss occurs earlier in juvenile kindreds. The kinetics are not well established, but many gradeschoolers or adolescents require hearing aids.

Ocular Defects

These appear confined to juvenile kindreds. Myopia, arcus juvenilis, and cataracts occur but lack diagnostic specificity. Three changes that are present in a minority of kindreds but that are nearly diagnostic are anterior lenticonus, posterior polymorphous corneal dystrophy, and retinal flecks. Anterior lenticonus is a forward protrusion of the anterior surface of the ocular lens. It results from a weakness of the type IV collagen forming the anterior lens capsule. The resulting irregularity of the surface of the lens causes an uncorrectable refractive error. The retina cannot be clearly seen by ophthalmoscopy and with a strong positive lens in the ophthalmoscope the lenticonus can often be seen through a dilated pupil as an "oil drop" or circular smudge on the center of the lens. Retinal flecks are small yellow or white dots scattered around the macular or in the periphery of the retina. If sparse they may be difficult to distinguish from small hard exudates.

Leiomyomatosis

Several X-linked families show the precocious development of striking leiomyomas of the esophagus and female genitalia in association with Alport's syndrome. These tumors are frequently large and multiple. They may bleed or obstruct and their resection can be difficult. All families described so far have had a deletion at the 5' end of the COL4A5 gene that extends into the COL4A6 gene.

DIAGNOSIS

No single feature is pathognomonic. The diagnosis is made by finding hematuria in multiple family members, together with a history of renal failure in related males, and reinforced by a biopsy showing characteristic ultrastructural changes in the proband or a relative. Immunofluorescence examination of the biopsy should include staining with fluoresceinated anti-GBM antibody; this will help distinguish Alport's syndrome from familial thin GBM disease. In families with a previously defined mutation, molecular diagnosis of affected males and gene carrying females is possible. In relatively large families without a known mutation, segregation analyses can decide with near

certainty whether a particular individual carries a defective gene.

The key to diagnosis is to suspect the possibility of Alport's syndrome in any patient with otherwise unexplained hematuria, glomerulopathy, or renal insufficiency. In many cases the familial nature of the condition will not be immediately apparent. Inquiry into the family must be detailed and insistent. The patient is a usually a young male. Chances are that he knows little of his distant relatives, but his mother will likely know more of the family details. Male relatives linked to the patient through one or more females may have renal failure. Check a urine sample from the patient's parents, particularly his mother, for microscopic hematuria. Hearing loss is a helpful clue, but it is crucial to remember that hearing loss is neither a sensitive nor a specific marker of Alport's syndrome. Indeed, it is neither necessary nor sufficient for the diagnosis. Most patients with hearing loss and renal disease do not have Alport's syndrome, but rather a variety of other disorders most commonly glomerulonephritis and a banal cause for hearing loss such as noise exposure or aminoglycoside therapy.

TREATMENT

There is no specific treatment for Alport's syndrome. General measures to retard the progression of renal failure, such as effective treatment of hypertension and modest protein restriction appear warranted, but are unproved. As for other forms of progressive renal disease, angiotensin-converting enzyme inhibitors may offer a specific advantage. Males should wear hearing protection in noisy surroundings. Hearing aids improve but do not completely correct the hearing loss. Tinnitus is generally resistant to all forms of therapy; hearing aids may render it less disruptive by amplifying ambient sounds.

Retinal lesions do not appear to affect vision and thus need no therapy. The serious impairment of vision caused by lenticonus or cataract cannot be corrected with spectacles or contact lenses. Lens removal with reimplantation of an intraocular lens is standard and satisfactory treatment.

RELATED DISORDERS

Familial Thin Basement Membrane Disease

Familial thin basement membrane disease or benign familial hematuria is an autosomal dominant basement membrane glomerulopathy. Some cases result from mutations of the COL4A4 gene at 2q35–q37. Ultrastructurally the GBM is uniformly thinned to about half its normal thickness. There is no disruption or lamellation of the GBM, nor are any other abnormalities of the glomeruli, tubules, vessels, or interstitium visible by light, immunofluorescence, or electron microscopy. Renal insufficiency does not occur. Longevity is unaffected by this condition and survivors into the ninth decade are recorded. Minor degrees of lamellation of the GBM and hearing loss have been described in some families. The significance of these findings is uncertain in view of the ease with which adult-type Alport's syndrome can be mistaken for familial thin basement membrane disease.

Once the precise diagnosis is established the patient and family can be spared further invasive tests and an appropriate prognosis given to them and to insurers. Unfortunately, the distinction between Alport's syndrome and benign familial hematuria is not always easy to make. Intermediate forms appear to exist.

To be sure of the pattern of inheritance requires a large pedigree with accurate diagnoses in all the family members. A single mistaken diagnosis from incidental renal disease, inaccurate urinalysis, or incomplete penetrance may vitiate the conclusions about the pattern of inheritance in the entire pedigree. Even biopsy evidence is fallible. Early cases of Alport's syndrome may show ultrastructural changes indistinguishable from those of benign familial hematuria. This is particularly likely to occur if a child from an adult-type Alport's kindred is biopsied. Stability of serum creatinine for several years in this child is as compatible with adult-type Alport's syndrome as it is with benign familial hematuria. It is not clear whether lamellation is an occasional feature of thin GBM disease, or whether some families with adult-type Alport's syndrome were misdiagnosed as familial thin GBM disease. The interpretation is further clouded because in some families with familial thin GBM disease, homozygous individuals have Alport's syndrome. In these families, autosomal dominant thin GBM disease and autosomal recessive Alport's syndrome are caused by the same mutations.

Alport's Syndrome with Thrombocytopathy (Epstein's Syndrome)

This uncommon autosomal dominant variant of Alport's syndrome associates moderate thrombocytopenia with severe hearing loss and renal failure in both males and females. The platelets are much larger than normal (about 7 μm in diameter), and there is a mild or moderate bleeding tendency. In some families there are inclusion bodies (Fechtner granules) in leukocytes.

Autosomal Recessive Alport's Syndrome

A few children who develop severe renal disease before the age of 10 years have homozygous or mixed heterozygous mutations of the genes for the α3 or α4 chains of type IV collagen. Boys and girls are equally severely affected. The heterozygous parents may or may not show hematuria.

APPROACH TO THE PATIENT WITH HEREDITARY NEPHRITIS

Although Alport's syndrome is less common than polycystic kidney disease, it is probably more common than is generally appreciated. Important differential diagnoses of hematuria in young persons are IgA nephropathy or other glomerulonephritis, renal calculi, or medullary sponge kidney. The differential diagnosis of familial renal disease with

hematuria includes familial thin GBM disease and familial IgA nephropathy, and, of course, polycystic kidney disease. Familial renal diseases without hematuria that might be confused include polycystic kidney disease, medullary cystic disease, and some poorly defined forms of inherited glomerular and tubulointerstitial renal disease. If a patient with unexplained hematuria or renal insufficiency has a family history of hematuria or renal failure, the family history should be extended, concentrating particularly on the mother's male relatives. Finding hearing loss strengthens, and finding specific ocular lesions greatly strengthens, suspicion for Alport's syndrome. Renal biopsy will generally be indicated in one or two family members, but once the diagnosis of a hereditary basement membrane nephropathy is established in a family, it is hard to justify further biopsies unless there are features suggesting another diagnosis. The extent of investigation will be guided by your judgment and will relate inversely to the strength of the family history. For example, a young man on the line of descent of a known Alport family whose urine contains dysmorphic erythrocytes needs minimal investigation, perhaps nothing more than a serum creatinine unless there are additional clinical features suggesting a systemic disease. With an uncertain family history, an intravenous pyelogram or abdominal flat plate and renal sonogram, ANA, and possibly anti-GBM antibody, ANCA, and renal biopsy may be appropriate. Genetic testing is presently of very limited applicability in sporadic cases and small kindreds because most families have "private" mutations. Patients may wish to enroll in research studies that may eventually identify the mutation in their family. There are a dozen or more small families and two very large kindreds in the US with mutations for which specific mutation tests are available. In these families, direct mutation analysis can quickly establish whether an individual is a gene carrier. It is not yet clear whether the two common mutations are sufficiently widespread to justify screening for them in adults with unexplained renal failure or before undertaking a renal biopsy in an adult or child with hematuria.

Patients with any hereditary nephropathy should be informed of the nature of their disease and perhaps given a copy of the renal biopsy report in order to avoid unnecessary further investigation. Similar considerations apply to family members who are potentially gene carriers. Those with Alport's syndrome should be followed for elevation of blood pressure or serum creatinine. The frequency of follow-up will depend on the anticipated age of onset of renal deterioration in the family and will become closer as this age is approached. Those with familial thin basement membrane disease should be checked about every 2 years, because some may ultimately have Alport's syndrome.

Bibliography

Alport AC: Hereditary familial congenital haemorrhagic nephritis. *Br Med J* I:504–506, 1927.

Barker DF, Fain PR, Goldgar DE, et al.: High-density genetic and physical mapping of DNA markers near the X-linked Alport syndrome locus: Definition and use of flanking polymorphic markers. *Hum Genet* 88:189–194, 1991.

Barker DF, Hostikka SL, Zhou J, et al.: Identification of mutations in the COL4A5 collagen gene in Alport syndrome. *Science* 248:1224–1227, 1990.

Dische FE, Brooke IP, Cashman SJ, et al.: Reactivity of monoclonal antibody P1 with glomerular basement membrane in thin-membrane nephropathy. *Nephrol Dial Transplant* 4:611–617, 1989.

Epstein CJ, Sahud MA, Piel CF, et al.: Hereditary macrothrombocytopathia, nephritis and deafness. *Am J Med* 52:299–310, 1972.

Gleeson MJ: Alport's syndrome: Audiological manifestations and implications. *J Laryngol Otol* 98:449–465, 1984.

Govan JA: Ocular manifestations of Alport's syndrome: A hereditary disorder of basement membranes? *Br J Ophthalmol* 67:493–503, 1983.

Gregory MC, Atkin CL. Alport's syndrome, Fabry's disease, and nail-patella syndrome. In: Schrier RW, Gottschalk CW (eds) *Diseases of the Kidney*, 6th ed. Little, Brown, Boston, pp. 561–590, 1997.

Gregory MC, Terreros DA, Barker DF, et al.: Alport syndrome—Clinical phenotypes, incidence, and pathology. In: Tryggvason

K (ed) *Molecular Pathology and Genetics of Alport Syndrome.* Karger, Basel, pp. 1–28, 1996.

Hinglais, N, Grunfeld JP, Bois E: Characteristic ultrastructural lesion of the glomerular basement membrane in progressive hereditary nephritis (Alport's syndrome). *Lab Invest* 27:473–487, 1972.

Hostikka SL, Eddy RL, Byers MG, Hoyhtya M, Shows TB, Tryggvason K: Identification of a distinct type IV collagen alpha chain with restricted kidney distribution and assignment of its gene to the locus of X chromosome-linked Alport syndrome. *Proc Natl Acad Sci USA* 87:1606–1610, 1990.

Kashtan CE, Kleppel MM, Gubler M-C. Immunohistologic findings in Alport syndrome. In: Tryggvason K (ed) *Molecular Pathology and Genetics of Alport Syndrome.* Karger, Basel, pp. 142–153, 1996.

Lemmink HH, Nilleson WN, Mochizuki T, et al.: Benign familial hematuria due to mutation of the type IV collagen ;ga4 gene. *J Clin Invest* 98:1114–1118, 1996.

Tiebosch AT, Frederik PM, van Breda Vriesman PJ, et al.: Thin-basement-membrane nephropathy in adults with persistent hematuria. *N Engl J Med* 320:14–18, 1989.

MEDULLARY CYSTIC DISEASE

ELLIS D. AVNER

Medullary cystic disease is a renal cystic disorder characterized by tubular cystic lesions in corticomedullary regions of the kidney. It is an uncommon, genetically determined tubulointerstitial nephritis that presents in children and young adults and inexorably progresses to end stage renal disease.

DEFINITIONS AND EPIDEMIOLOGY

Medullary cystic disease is a distinct clinicopathological entity that is part of a group of congenital tubulointerstitial nephropathies known as the juvenile nephronophthisis medullary cystic disease (JN-MCD) complex (Table 1). Although genetically heterogeneous, all of the diseases of the JN-MCD complex share common morphologic and functional renal alterations, which lead to similar clinical features and clinical course. The gene responsible for autosomal recessive juvenile nephronophthisis has been localized by linkage analysis to chromosome 2p, but genes responsible for the other variants of the complex have not yet

been localized or identified. The nosology of the diseases comprising the JN-MCD complex has been quite confusing, and they have been presented under a variety of terms including uremic medullary cystic disease, cystic disease of the renal medulla, familial juvenile nephronophthisis, autosomal-recessive nephronophthisis, autosomal dominant nephronophthisis, Fanconi's nephronophthisis, salt-losing nephritis, and uremic sponge kidney. The overall incidence and prevalence of JN-MCD is unknown. The diseases appear to be uncommon, although more than 300 cases have been reported in the literature and JN has been reported to cause 10 to 30% of pediatric end stage renal disease in European centers. Pooled data demonstrate a much lower prevalence (less than 5%) in the North American pediatric end stage renal disease population.

PATHOLOGY AND PATHOGENESIS

In general, no significant differences in renal pathology have been demonstrated for the individual conditions that

TABLE I
The Juvenile Nephronophthisis-Medullary Cystic Disease (JN-MCD) Complex[a]

Variant	Genetics	Percentage of JN-MCD cases	Mean age at onset year	Associated features
Juvenile nephronophthisis	AR	50	10	
Renal-retinal dysplasia	AR	15–20	10	Hepatic fibrosis, cerebellar ataxia, neurocutaneous dysplasia, skeletal abnormalities
Medullary cystic disease	AD	15–20	28	Hyperuricemia, gouty arthritis
Nonfamilial sporadic	—	15	17	

Note: AR, autosomal recessive; AD, autosomal dominant.

[a] Modified from Bernstein J, Gardner KD: In: Contran RS, Brenner BM (eds) *Tubulointerstitial Nephropathies.* Churchill-Livingstone, New York, pp. 335–358, 1983; and Hildebrand F, Jugners P, Grunfeld J-P: In: Schrier RW, Gottschalk CW (eds) Diseases of the Kidney, 6th ed. Little, Brown, Boston, pp. 499–520, 1996.

comprise the JN-MCD complex. Early in the course of the disease, there are few renal structural changes which emphasize the functional nature of the renal tubular defects (see below). The characteristic feature of more advanced cases is severe tubular atrophy with interstitial fibrosis and inflammatory cell infiltration, tubular basement membrane thickening, periglomerular fibrosis, and patchy glomerular obsolescence. Ultrastructural analysis demonstrates thickening and loss of definition of tubular basement membranes. These changes progress to produce symmetrically small kidneys with severe, diffuse cortical atrophy.

A major feature of diseases of the JN-MCD complex is renal medullary cysts. Cysts measuring 1 to 2 mm in diameter are generally concentrated along the corticomedullary junctions, and have been localized by microdissection to the distal convoluted and medullary collecting tubules. Although the presence of characteristic cysts has been considered a diagnostic criterion, many cases have been identified in which cysts are absent or detected only late in the course of disease progression. Such cases are otherwise morphologically, genetically, and clinically identical to cases in which medullary cysts are a prominent feature, suggesting that medullary cysts are neither of primary importance in causing clinical manifestations or tubulointerstitial nephritis nor necessary for disease progression to renal failure.

The pathogenesis of tubulointerstitial nephritis and medullary cyst formation in JN-MCD remains unknown. The ultrastructural findings of irregularly thickened and lamellated tubular basement membranes, as well as the decreased or absent expression of certain tubular basement membrane antigens, have suggested a primary biochemical or ultrastructural abnormality of the tubular basement membrane. Studies in a murine model of JN-MCD suggest an immunopathogenic basis in which a defect in regulatory T-cell function leads to functional inactivation of suppressor T cells, loss of tolerance to tubular antigens, and facilitated expression of effector T cells that mediate tubulointerstitial injury. Further study into the genetics and pathophysiology of these diseases is required to validate or disprove these attractive hypotheses.

CLINICAL FEATURES

All variants of JN-MCD complex are characterized by the insidious onset of renal failure. The most common symptoms at presentation are polydipsia, polyuria, and enuresis. Additional symptoms include weakness and pallor. Short stature and failure to thrive may be prominent presenting symptoms in children.

Unless at-risk individuals with parents or siblings affected with JN-MCD are monitored for the early symptom of polyuria, most patients present with a reduced glomerular filtration rate (GFR). Anemia is present in most patients at the time of diagnosis and has been considered by some, but not all, investigators to be disproportionately severe relative to the degree of renal dysfunction. Impairment of urinary concentrating ability is the earliest pathophysiological feature of JN-MCD. It has been documented prior to any decrease in GFR and may be present with minimal histological abnormalities. In some families with autosomal recessive variants of the JN-MCD complex, obligatory heterozygotes have demonstrated similar decreases in urinary concentrating ability. Unfortunately, this is not a consistent finding and cannot be utilized to identify heterozygotes for the autosomal recessive conditions. Renal salt wasting is another characteristic feature of JN-MCD and has been reported in 20 to 60% of affected patients. Salt wasting presumably reflects the severity and distribution of histological changes, as it does in other tubulointerstitial nephropathies, and may occur with or without the presence of medullary cystic lesions. An additional characteristic clinical feature of JN-MCD is the paucity of urinary abnormalities. Proteinuria and hematuria are exceedingly rare and reported only in some individuals with autosomal dominant variants of the complex. Pyuria and documented urinary tract infection are also uncommon, as is hypertension prior to end-stage renal disease. The absence of these clinical features may help differentiate JN-MCD from the other genetically determined polycystic kidney diseases.

As noted in Table 1 one-fourth to one-third of all patients with autosomal-recessive JN-MCD have associated retinal changes and are clinically classified as the renal-retinal dysplasia variant. Retinal findings are characterized by progressive tapetoretinal degeneration, and visual impairment may be present in early infancy or childhood. Fundoscopic alterations are present in all patients with renal-retinal dysplasia by the age of 10 years, and the diagnosis can be confirmed with electroretinography. Some reported patients with this clinical variant also have hepatic fibrosis, cerebellar ataxia, neurocutaneous dysplasia, and various skeletal abnormalities. The sporadic nature of these associations, as well as the irregular clustering in some families, makes these associations difficult to further classify. Retinal findings as well as the noted multiorgan associations have not been reported in the autosomal dominant or nonfamilial sporadic variants of the JN-MCD complex.

The diagnosis of JN-MCD should be suspected in the child or young adult who presents with progressive renal failure and normal to small kidneys in association with the clinical and laboratory features noted above. The differential diagnosis may include renal hypoplasia-dysplasia, congenital obstructive uropathies, autosomal dominant or recessive polycystic kidney disease, bilateral impairment of the renal circulation, or other forms of chronic tubulointerstitial nephritis. A complete history, with particular attention to family history, physical examination, examination of the urinary sediment, and radiographic imaging (ultrasonography, with computed tomography and arteriography as indicated) will be adequate to establish the diagnosis of JN-MCD in most cases. In rare instances, a renal biopsy may be indicated to definitively establish a histopathological diagnosis. However, pathognomonic medullary cysts may not be apparent on needle biopsy specimens. The gene responsible for the autosomal recessive variant of JN-MCD has been linked to human chromosome 2p. Thus, in "genetically informative" families, diagnosis by genetic linkage analysis (pre- or postnatal) may be possible.

PROGNOSIS AND THERAPY

JN-MCD is characterized by variable, but inexorable progression to end-stage renal disease. No specific factors have been identified which modify the rapidity of progression or clinical course. Genetic counseling is a cornerstone of therapy for families with genetically defined variants of the complex. If affected individuals are identified prior to the development of end stage renal disease, adequate hydration and sodium supplementation are critical to avoid dehydration and superimposed prerenal insults. This is particularly true in infants and young children who are subject to episodic febrile illnesses and intercurrent episodes of gastroenteritis. Children with severe polyuria secondary to renal-concentrating defects and salt wasting may require nasogastric or gastrostomy tube feedings to maintain hydration and provide adequate nutrition. Anemia is treated with recombinant human erythropoietin and other manifestations of progressive uremia are treated in standard fashion. Ultimately, dialysis and renal transplantation are utilized to treat end-stage renal failure. JN-MCD has not, to date, been reported to recur in transplanted kidneys.

Bibliography

Antignac C, Kleinknecht C Habib R: Toward the identification of a gene for familial juvenile nephronophthisis (autosomal recessive medullary cystic kidney disease). *Adv Nephrol Necker Hosp* 24:379–33, 1995.

Avasthi PS, Erickson DG, Gardner KD: Hereditary renal-retinal dysplasia and the medullary cystic disease-nephronophthisis complex. *Ann Intern Med* 84:157–161, 1976.

Bernstein J, Gardner KD: Hereditary tubulo interstitial nephritis. In: Contran RS, Brenner BM, Stein JH (eds) *Tubulointerstitial Nephropathies.* Churchill-Livingstone, New York, pp.335–358, 1983.

Cohen AH, Hoyer JR: Nephronophthisis, a primary tubular basement membrane defect. *Lab Invest* 55:564–574, 1986.

Hildebrandt F, Jungers P, Grunfeld J-P: Medullary cystic and medullary sponge renal disorders. In: Schrier RW, Gottschalk CW (eds) *Diseases of the Kidney*, 6th ed. Little Brown, Boston, pp. 499–520, 1996.

Kelly CJ, Neilson EG: Medullary cystic disease: An inherited form of autoimmune interstitial nephritis? *Am J Kidney Dis* 10: 389–395, 1987.

Kleinknecht C, Habib R: Nephronophthisis. In: Cameron S, Davison AM, Grunfeld JP, Kerr D, Ritz E (eds) *Oxford Textbook of Clinical Nephrology*, Oxford Press, Oxford, pp. 2188–2197, 1992.

Mongeau JG, Worthen HG: Nephronophthisis and medullary cystic disease. *Am J Med* 43:345–355, 1967.

SECTION 8

TUBULOINTERSTITIAL NEPHROPATHIES AND DISORDERS OF THE URINARY TRACT

48

TUBULOINTERSTITIAL DISEASE

WILLIAM F. FINN

DEFINITION AND CLASSIFICATION

Chronic structural abnormalities involving the renal tubules and interstitum develop in two circumstances. In the first, tubulointerstitial nephritis is found as the primary lesion after prolonged exposure to various therapeutic or environmental agents or in association with a number of systemic illnesses (Table 1). Such primary chronic interstitial nephritis accounts for up to 15 to 30% of cases of end stage renal disease. In the second, tubulointerstitial changes occur as a result of progressive glomerular and vascular injury. This has come to be recognized as a significant determinant of the final outcome of these conditions.

HISTOLOGY

The characteristic lesion is composed of an interstitial inflammatory mononuclear cell infiltrate containing lymphocytes—mostly T cells—and occasional plasma cells. This acute cellular infiltrate is generally accompanied by interstitial edema, disruption of the tubular basement membrane, and dissolution of normal interstitial architecture. The transition to a chronic process occurs with the development of interstitial fibrosis, which is accompanied by tubular ectasia, tubular atrophy, and a marked increase in extracellular matrix. Eventually, glomerular and vascular structures are involved and fibrotic and sclerotic changes occur throughout the kidney.

CLINICAL MANIFESTATIONS

The manifestations of tubulointerstitial nephritis depend on the extent of injury (diffuse or focal), the tubular segments most severely involved (proximal or more distal), and the degree of compensation achieved by the less severely involved nephrons. When proximal tubules are damaged, such substances as sodium, glucose, amino acids, uric acid, and low-molecular-weight proteins, which are ordinarily reabsorbed or metabolized at this site, appear in the urine. A decrease in bicarbonate reabsorption may lead to proximal renal tubular acidosis. Damage to more distal structures, including the loop of Henle, the distal convoluted tubule, and the collecting duct, is accompanied by an inability to maximally concentrate and dilute the urine. The defect in the ability to concentrate the urine may result in polyuria. Damage in this area may decrease excretion of titratable acid and urinary ammonia excretion, leading to metabolic acidosis. This may be present in conjunction with a defect in the secretion of potassium and result in type IV renal tubular acidosis.

DIAGNOSIS

The clinical diagnosis of tubulointerstitial nephritis is often a diagnosis of exclusion, made when glomerular disease is absent. The histologic diagnosis of tubulointerstitial nephritis requires evidence of an inflammatory infiltrate accompanied by interstitial fibrosis. In the absence of other definable disease, presumptive evidence includes a history of significant exposure to an offending agent or the coexistence of a condition known to be associated with tubulointerstitial disease, the demonstration of abnormalities of tubular function out of proportion to the reduction in glomerular function, and a urinalysis marked by the absence of heavy proteinuria with a tendency for leukocyturia rather than hematuria.

Urinalysis

Evaluation of the urine in patients with chronic interstitial nephritis yields variable results, except that marked proteinuria in uncommon; by quantitative tests, a trace-to-1+ protein may be present; by qualitative analyses, usually less than 1 g of protein per 24 hours, and often less than 500 mg is found. Microscopic examination may disclose a preponderance of white blood cells and occasionally white cell casts and granular casts. A general estimate of integrated tubular function may be obtained by determining the capacity of the kidneys to concentrate or dilute the urine in response to water deprivation or administration, the ability to excrete an administered acid load, and the precision with which sodium balance is maintained.

Proteinuria

The normal values of the major urinary proteins are listed in Table 2. In contrast to the high-molecular-weight proteins, a finite amount of low-molecular-weight proteins is normally filtered and then reabsorbed by proximal tubular cells. When the reabsorptive capacity of the proximal tubular epithelium is disrupted, various low-molecular-weight proteins appear in the urine.

TABLE I
Causes of Chronic Tubulointerstitial Disease

Category	Examples
Therapeutic agents/ occupational or environmental agents	Analgesics
	NSAIDs
	Chemotherapeutic agents (cisplatin, nitrosoureas)
	Immunotherapeutic agents (cyclosporine, FK-506)
	Heavy metals (lead, cadmium)
	Lithium
Immunologic conditions	Renal allograft rejection
	Amyloid
	Vasculitis
	Cryoglobulinemia
	Sjögren's syndrome
	SLE
	Wegener's granulomatosus
Hematopoietic/neoplastic diseases	Sickle cell disease
	Multiple myeloma
	Light chain disease
	Dysproteinemias
	Lymphoproliferative disease
Mechanical disorders	Ureteral obstruction
Vascular diseases	Radiation
	Hypertension
	Atheromatous emboli
Hereditary/genetic	Karyomegalic interstitial nephritis
	Medullary cystic disease/ nephronophthis complex
	Polycystic kidney disease
	Hereditary nephritis
Miscellaneous conditions	Balkan nephropathy
	Chinese herb nephropathy
	Mycotoxins
	Sarcoidosis
Metabolic disorders	Hypercalcemia
	Hypokalemia
	Uric acid nephropathy
	Oxalate nephropathy
	Cystinosis
Infections	Systemic
	Local

SLE, systemic lupus erythomatosus.

High-Molecular-Weight Proteinuria

The distinction between "glomerular" proteinuria and "tubular" proteinuria is based on the quantity and quality of the proteins measured in the urine. The appearance in the urine of serum proteins with a molecular weight in excess of 40,000 to 50,000 Da is an early marker of glomerular damage. The commonly measured high-molecular-weight proteins include albumin, transferrin, and IgG.

Low-Molecular-Weight Proteinuria

In contrast, tubular proteinuria is due to excretion of low-molecular-weight proteins. The two most commonly

TABLE 2
Normal Values for Urinary Proteins in Humans

Urinary protein	MN (da)	Normal value
Tamm-Horsfall glycoprotein[a]		14.3 (5.1–25.5)
Albumin[a]	69,000	5.2 (2.8–15)
α_1-Microglobulin[a]	29–33,000	4.20 ± 6
IgG[a]	146,000	1.2 (0.35–2.7)
Transferrin[a]	77,000	0.17 (0.08–0.83)
Cystatin C	13,300	0.113 ± 0.125 mg/L
Protein 1[a]	18,700	0.092 (0.02–0.3)
β_2-Microglobulin[a]	11,800	0.062 (0.021–0.142)
Retinol-binding protein[a]	21,400	0.055 (0.03–0.13)
Lysozyme		0.015 (0.002–0.12) mg/L

[a] mg/g creatinine

mentioned as potential markers of renal tubular damage are β_2-microglobulin (β_2-m) and retinol binding protein. Other low-molecular-weight proteins include α_1-microglobulin (α_1-m), protein 1, amylase, lysozyme, ribonuclease, and cystatin C. Due to its molecular weight and small radius, β_2-m is readily filtered at the glomerulus. Approximately 99.9% is reabsorbed by the proximal tubular epithelial cells and ultimately catabolized. A very small amount appears in the urine. The urinary excretion of β_2-m is considerably increased in cases of renal tubular impairment. Since β_2-m undergoes degradation at urinary pH of 5.5 or less, accurate measurement demands alkalinization of the urine. Retinol-binding protein is a low-molecular-weight protein synthesized in the liver, where it binds to retinol. Once the retinol is released at peripheral sites, the binding protein is rapidly eliminated from plasma by glomerular filtration. It is then reabsorbed and catabolized by proximal tubular cells. Because of its stability in acid urine, the assay of urinary retinol binding protein is preferred over that of β_2-m.

Tamm–Horsfall Protein

Tamm-Horsfall glycoprotein is the most abundant protein of renal origin in normal urine and is the major constituent of urinary casts. Tamm–Horsfall glycoprotein is synthesized by cells of the thick ascending limb of the loop of Henle, and is excreted in the urine at a relatively constant rate. Urinary excretion can increase following injury to the distal tubule.

Enzymuria

The interpretation of urinary enzyme titers is founded on the premise that the sole source of high-molecular-weight enzymes is damaged tubular cells. However, it is hard to correlate specific disease states with the presence or absence of enzymuria. In addition, a relationship between the severity of cellular injury and the magnitude of enzymuria has been difficult to establish. This has been due in part to the observation that urinary enzyme activity is affected by various factors that are independent of cellular integrity, i.e., urinary pH, osmolarity, and the presence of various enzyme inhibitors or activators. However, in addition to normal cell shedding, enzymes also gain urinary access because of altered cell membrane permeability, increased rate of enzyme synthesis, and frank cell necrosis. Only a limited number of enzymes have been generally accepted as valuable urinary biomarkers. These include *N*-acetyl-β-D-glucosaminidase, alanine aminopeptidase, and intestinal alkaline phosphatase. It is important to emphasize that the measurement of these enzymes, while of considerable theoretical interest, is of limited clinical utility (Table 3).

N-Acetyl-β-glucosaminidase is found in both the straight (S3) segment of proximal tubular cells and the distal nephron as a lysosomal enzyme. In humans, it has its highest activity in the S3 segment, with less activity in the collecting duct. Elevated urinary levels accompany proximal tubular cell injury. It may also been found in the urine of patients with various forms of glomerular disease, obstructive uropathy, and nephrosclerosis. Other nonspecific increases in urinary activity that limit its usefulness as a diagnostic tool have been described.

Alanine aminopeptidase is restricted to the proximal tubule. Increased excretion has been reported in a variety of renal diseases including pyelonephritis, glomerulonephritis, urologic cancers and renal transplant rejection. In addition, increased excretion has been reported in association with many well-defined nephrotoxins. Although not specific in discriminating between glomerular and tubular disease, it is very sensitive to acute tubular injury.

Intestinal alkaline phosphatase and nonspecific tissue alkaline phosphatase are two urinary isoenzymes that have elicited interest as potential segment specific markers of

TABLE 3
Some Enzymes Used as an Index of Nephrotoxicity

Enzymes	Cellular location
Alanine aminopeptidase	Brush border
Alkaline phosphatase	
γ-Glutamyltransferase	
Maltase	
Trehalase	
Glutamic oxaloacetic transaminase	Cytosol
Glutamic pyruvic transaminase	
Lactate dehydrogenase	
Malate dehydrogenase	
N-Acetyl-β-D-glucosaminidase	Lysosome
Acid phosphatase	
β-Glactosidase	
β-Glucosidase	
β-Glucuronidase	
Glutamate dehydrogenase	Mitochondria

the human nephron. Intestinal alkaline phosphatase is expressed on the brush border of the tubuloepithelial cells of the S3 segment of the proximal tubule. The intestinal alkaline phosphatase released in urine has its origin in the kidney and is considered to be a specific and sensitive marker for alterations of the S3 segment. In the kidney, tissue alkaline phosphatase is localized on the brush border in all segments of the proximal tubule. By measuring both enzymes, judgments as to the involvement of S1-S2 vs. S3 segments can be achieved in experimental models.

Tubular Antigens

The urinary excretion of specific proximal tubular antigens is increased in a variety of renal diseases. Monoclonal antibodies to membrane and other cellular derived antigens are new, sensitive, specific, and readily available markers of renal cell injury. Increased excretion of tubular antigens occurs in exposure to cadmium, hydrocarbons, cisplatin, and radiographic contrast media. Monoclonal antibodies to human brush-border antigens have been produced and used in investigational studies. Their use may permit detection of site-specific renal damage.

MECHANISM OF FIBROGENESIS

Infiltrating cells stimulate fibrogenesis through the release of various cytokines and growth factors. In response, resident cells in the kidney undergo phenotypic changes and acquire smooth muscle and fibroblastic characteristics. Active in this process may be transforming growth factor-β (TGF-β), one of the more potent stimulators of collagen and noncollagen basement membrane components. Examples of the latter include proteoglycans and fibronectin. TGF-β also inhibits matrix degrading enzymes such as collagenase and metalloproteinases. The net result is that for a time the excessive deposition of extracellular matrix can be removed, but eventually complete resolution becomes unlikely. TGF-β also controls the interaction of cells with the extracellular matrix by regulating the expression of various cell adhesion molecules such as integrins. Platelet-derived growth factor also stimulates chemotaxis, influences the production of extracellular matrix, and regulates its subsequent metabolism. Added to this are the interleukins which modulate inflammatory and immune responses by regulating the growth, differentiation, and mobility of effector cells. In as yet unknown manner, angiotensin II may be linked to the irreversible changes of tubulointerstitial fibrosis.

PRIMARY VASCULAR AND GLOMERULAR RENAL DISEASE

In many forms of renal disease due to primary glomerular injury, there is a remarkable inverse correlation between the extent of tubulointerstitial damage and the glomerular filtration rate. This observation has directed attention to the important role of the tubulointerstitial compartment in the progression of renal disease.

The most obvious explanation to account for the tubulointerstitial injury that occurs with primary glomerular disease is that inflammatory glomerular lesions are accompanied by acute interstitial mononuclear cell infiltrates which later lead to chronic fibrotic changes by mechanisms described above. Other mechanisms have been suggested. For instance, it is clear that persistent high-grade proteinuria is associated with a progressive loss of renal function and the development of tubulointerstitial disease and renal fibrosis. With the loss of permselectivity that occurs with glomerular injury, various circulating plasma proteins—usually prevented from passing this barrier—may find their way into the glomerular filtrate and tubular fluid where they exert toxic effects on epithelial cells. Some of these proteins may precipitate within the tubular lumen, thereby forming casts and obstructing tubular fluid flow. Preglomerular vasoconstriction follows, with a decrease in peritubular capillary blood flow, eventual tubular atrophy and further interstitial inflammation. As tubular reabsorptive mechanisms are stimulated, lysosomal degradative enzymes may spill into the cytosol and cause damage. Alternatively, filtered low-molecular-weight cytokines may bind to tubular epithelial cells and lead to activation of the alternate complement pathway.

Without question, immunologic processes involving either the cell-dependent or the humoral pathway may be responsible for the ongoing damage. A release of chemotactic lipids may further the inflammatory response. In addition, changes in tubular oxidative metabolism leading to an increase in renal ammoniagenesis and the generation of reactive oxygen species may contribute to the progressive lesions. Ammonia may interact with the third component of complement with activation of the alternate complement cascade and subsequent immunologic cellular injury. Cytokine-induced generation of nitric oxide and the transferrin-related release of iron with accumulation in tubular cell lysosomes may be associated with oxidative cellular injury. Finally, arachidonic acid metabolites, particularly thromboxane A_2, may stimulate extracellular matrix protein formation and in this way contribute to the progression of renal disease.

Bibliography

Eddy AA: Experimental insights into the tubulointerstitial disease accompanying primary glomerular lesions. *J Am Soc Nephrol* 5:1273–1287, 1994.

Dodd S: The pathogenesis of tubulointerstitial disease and mechanisms of fibrosis. *Curr Top Pathol* 88:117–143, 1995.

Jones CL, Eddy AA: Tubulointerstitial nephritis. *Pediatr Nephrol* 6:572–586, 1992.

Nath KA: Tubulointerstitial changes as a major determinant in the progression of renal damage. *Am J Kidney Dis* 20:1–17, 1992.

Sedor JR: Cytokines and growth factors in renal injury. *Semin Nephrol* 12:428–440, 1992.

LITHIUM-INDUCED RENAL DISEASE

GREGORY L. BRADEN

Lithium is the best treatment for manic–depressive illness, but therapy with this drug has been associated with side effects in many body systems, including the kidneys. Lithium is freely filtered at the glomerulus, reabsorbed like sodium at several tubular sites, and concentrated in the renal medulla—circumstances that might favor lithium-induced renal disease. Although lithium initially was thought to produce only functional renal disorders, such as nephrogenic diabetes insipidus (NDI), additional disorders now attributed to lithium include renal tubular acidosis, chronic interstitial nephritis, and nephrotic syndrome.

NEPHROGENIC DIABETES INSIPIDUS

Polydipsia occurs in up to 40% and polyuria greater than 3 L/day occurs in up to 20% of patients treated with lithium. Despite the high prevalence of polyuria, urine volume is rarely increased enough to require cessation of lithium therapy. Most humans with lithium-induced polyuria are unresponsive to the administration of exogenous antidiuretic hormone (ADH). This could occur either due to abnormalities in the medullary osmotic gradient that drives ADH-mediated water reabsorption or due to direct inhibition of the tubular hydroosmotic effects of ADH. Chronic administration of lithium diminishes the medullary and papillary osmolar gradients due to depletion of urea without affecting sodium chloride concentrations. However, lithium-induced polyuria is mainly due to direct inhibition of the ADH-dependent aspects of water conservation. Only one lithium-treated patient has been reported to have a defect in the pituitary release of ADH indicative of central diabetes insipidus.

Lithium impairs the hydro-osmotic response to ADH by several mechanisms. First, there is abundant physiological and biochemical evidence that lithium directly inhibits the adenylate cyclase system in the mammalian distal nephron, leading to decreased generation of the second messenger, cyclic adenosine $3',5'$-monophosphate (cAMP), the putative stimulus for transepithelial water movement. In addition, lithium has been shown to inhibit transepithelial water movement after the administration of exogenous cAMP, suggesting inhibition of water flow at a site distal to the generation of cAMP.

Although lithium-induced NDI usually improves after lithium withdrawal, some patients have persistent concentrating defects lasting for years. Amiloride has been shown to reduce urinary volume and enhance the concentrating ability of patients with lithium-induced NDI. Amiloride blocks distal tubular reabsorption of lithium, thus lowering the renal tissue lithium level. In addition, amiloride is a diuretic and the combination of dietary salt restriction and the natriuretic effect of the diuretic induces mild extracellular fluid volume depletion which decreases the glomerular filtration rate and lessens urinary volume. Thiazide diuretics have also been utilized for this purpose, but they may raise serum lithium levels. They are more useful in patients with symptoms that persist after lithium discontinuation. Interestingly, amiloride has been shown to be effective without inducing any changes in creatinine clearance or serum lithium levels, suggesting that the inhibition of lithium uptake in the distal nephron may be the most important factor for its efficacy. Indomethacin has been effective in a few patients, presumably by inducing a significant fall in the glomerular filtration rate. As with diuretics, this may lower urinary volume. In addition, indomethacin inhibits synthesis of urinary prostaglandins that inhibit the tubular action of ADH. As with thiazides, use of nonsteroidal anti-inflammatory drugs (NSAIDs) in patients still on lithium requires great caution and frequent monitoring of lithium levels. Finally, a few patients with severe NDI will require cessation of lithium and the substitution of either carbamazepine or valproic acid to treat the manic-depressive illness.

RENAL TUBULAR ACIDOSIS

Lithium impairs distal hydrogen ion secretion in at least 50% of treated patients. During administration of intravenous sodium bicarbonate, distal nephron bicarbonate delivery is increased. In normal humans, this stimulates hydrogen ion excretion by the distal nephron proton pumps. The additional protons are buffered by bicarbonate; the carbonic acid formed then dissociates and raises the urinary pCO_2 from 40 to 80 mm Hg or greater. This distal nephron response is impaired in lithium-treated patients; however, there is no evidence for renal bicarbonate wasting (such as in proximal renal tubular acidosis), and the excretion of the urinary buffer, ammonium, is normal. Despite this defect in urinary acidification, the serum bicarbonate and pH remain normal. Taken together, these studies indicate that lithium induces incomplete distal renal tubular acidosis. Thus, patients treated with lithium are prone to systemic acidosis during stressful conditions such as sepsis or catabolic states.

ACUTE RENAL FAILURE/LITHIUM INTOXICATION

Acute renal failure due to biopsy-proven acute tubular necrosis may occur in lithium-intoxicated patients. Nephrotic syndrome due to minimal change disease may occur concomitantly with acute tubular necrosis. Whether lithium can directly cause tubular necrosis or whether tubular necrosis in these patients is secondary to hemodynamic factors is unknown.

Lithium intoxication is classified into three grades of severity based on the blood level (mild, <2.5 mEq/L; moderate, 2.5 to 3.5 mEq/L; severe, >3.5 mEq/L). Toxic effects include nausea, ataxia, tremors, twitching, muscle rigidity, disordered consciousness, seizures, and coma. The pathophysiology of lithium intoxication may be due to its ability to induce dehydration and salt depletion secondary to its inhibitory effect on ADH action and the acute effects of lithium to induce a natriuresis, leading to extracellular fluid volume depletion, activation of the serum-angiotensin system, a decrease in glomerular filtration rate, and, in turn, increased serum lithium levels. In addition, angiotensin-converting enzyme inhibitors and NSAIDs may cause renal dysfunction leading to lithium intoxication, especially in patients on high therapeutic doses of lithium. Close monitoring of serum lithium levels is warranted after initiation of therapy with these agents.

Patients with lithium intoxication should be admitted to the hospital, since seizures can occur at any time. The drug should be discontinued and, if there is an acute ingestion, either gastric lavage or ipecac should be given. Restoration of depleted extracellular fluid volume should occur with the administration of intravenous 0.9% normal saline if there is no hypernatremia present. For those patients with mild intoxication with a serum level of 2.5 mEq/L or less, saline diuresis may be enough to enhance renal lithium clearance. If there is no history to preclude vigorous volume expansion, then up to 6 L of saline can be given daily until the lithium level decreases to the nontoxic range. With this therapy, the lithium level should fall approximately 1 mEq/day. However, patients who are euvolemic usually do not respond to saline and/or forced diuresis. For those patients with moderate or severe toxicity, hemodialysis is the therapy of choice and may need to be repeated if serum lithium levels rebound after the first hemodialysis treatment. Continuous renal replacement therapy may be employed at centers where hemodialysis is unavailable. This modality effectively removes lithium and is not complicated by post therapy rebound.

NEPHROTIC SYNDROME

Lithium causes nephrotic syndrome in a small number of patients. Renal biopsies have demonstrated minimal change disease in the majority of patients and focal segmental glomerulosclerosis in a smaller number. Several reports demonstrate that patients may undergo a complete remission of the nephrotic syndrome upon withdrawal of lithium. Minimal change disease may recur after readministration of lithium.

CHRONIC INTERSTITIAL NEPHRITIS

The association of lithium with chronic interstitial nephritis was first reported in 1977, when a renal biopsy study described an increase in interstitial fibrosis, focal nephron atrophy, or both, in lithium-treated patients compared to age-matched controls. In this study, 80% of the lithium-treated patients had decreased creatinine clearances. Subsequently, a number of retrospective and uncontrolled studies found the prevalence of renal insufficiency to range from 3 to 20% in patients treated long term with lithium, but other disorders causing renal insufficiency were not always excluded. In contrast, additional studies compared lithium-treated patients to a more suitable control group, i.e., psychiatric patients not receiving lithium, and found no differences in serum creatinine or creatinine clearance. Renal biopsies were not performed.

Prospective studies demonstrate that chronic lithium therapy in psychiatric patients can significantly impair the glomerular filtration rate compared to similarly matched psychiatric patients who never received lithium. Renal biopsies in lithium-treated patients have demonstrated increased interstitial fibrosis and a unique tubular lesion consisting of microcyst formation due to cystic dilatation of the tubules.

Taken together, these studies indicate that a small number of patients treated with lithium develop progressive renal damage associated with chronic interstitial nephritis. However, no patient has yet been reported to develop end stage renal failure from lithium use. Baseline renal function studies including serum creatinine, BUN, and creatinine clearance should be performed prior to the initiation of lithium therapy and thereafter measured yearly. Patients who demonstrate deterioration in renal function should have lithium therapy withdrawn and either carbamazepine or valproic acid initiated. For those patients who can only be managed on lithium, lithium therapy can probably be continued with careful monitoring of renal function over time while maintaining the serum lithium level within the therapeutic range.

Bibliography

Allen HM, Jackson RL, Winchester MD, Deck LV, Allon M: Indomethacin in the treatment of lithium-induced nephrogenic diabetes insipidus. *Arch Intern Med* 149:1123–1126, 1989.

Batlle D, Gaviria M, Grupp M, Arruda JAL, Wynn J, Kurtzman NA: Distal nephron function in patients receiving chronic lithium therapy. *Kidney Int* 21:477–485, 1982.

Batlle DC, von Riotte AB, Gaviria M, Grupp M: Amelioration of polyuria by amiloride in patients receiving long-term lithium therapy. *N Engl J Med* 312:408–414, 1985.

Boton R, Gaviria M, Batlle DC: Prevalence, pathogenesis, and treatment of renal dysfunction associated with chronic lithium therapy. *Am J Kidney Dis* 10:329–345, 1987.

Leblanc M, Raymond M, Bonnardeaux A, et al.: Lithium poisoning treated by high-performance continuous arteriovenous and venovenous hemodiafiltration. *Am J Kidney Dis* 27:365–372, 1996.

Lehmann K, Ritz E: Angiotensin-converting enzyme inhibitors may cause renal dysfunction in patients on long-term lithium treatment. *Am J Kidney Dis* 25:82–87, 1995.

Okusa MD, Crystal LJT. Clinical manifestations and management of acute lithium intoxication. *Am J Med* 97:383–389, 1994.

Tam VKK, Green J, Schwieger J, Cohen AH: Nephrotic syndrome and renal insufficiency with lithium therapy. *Am J Kidney Dis* 27:715–720, 1996.

Hestbech J, Hansen HE, Amdisen A, Olsen S: Chronic renal lesions following long-term treatment with lithium. *Kidney Int* 12:205–213, 1977.

Jorkasky DK, Amsterdam JD, Oler J, et al.: Lithium-induced renal disease: a prospective study. *Clin Nephrol* 30:293–302, 1988.

Walker RG, Bennett WM, Davies BM, Kincaid-Smith P: Structural and functional effects of long-term lithium therapy. *Kidney Int* 21:513–519, 1982.

50

LEAD NEPHROTOXICITY

WILLIAM F. FINN

HISTORY

The relationship between lead exposure and chronic interstitial nephritis was first recognized in 1862. Since then it has become widely appreciated that renal damage may occur in persons who have had a heavy exposure to lead over a number of years. Whether exposure to lead in the general population leads to impaired renal function is not known. Also of uncertain nature is the relationship between childhood plumbism and the later development of chronic lead nephropathy.

RISK FACTORS

Populations at Risk

Occupational exposure to lead occurs in smelters, miners, painters, and plumbers, and in workers involved in the manufacture of storage batteries, pottery, and pewter. Environmental exposure occurs through the use of inadequately glazed pottery, the consumption of "moonshine" whiskey, and the ingestion of lead-containing food or water. Lead pipes and soldered joints are important sources of lead in drinking water, while soil contaminated with lead from industrial activities is an important source of lead in foodstuffs. It should be noted that lead is most harmful to children under 6 years of age in that they absorb about 50% of the ingested lead. In comparison, adults absorb only 5 to 10%. For children, flaking lead-based paint and dust in old homes are important sources of lead. The removal of lead from gasoline and paint has significantly reduced the lead exposure in children and adults alike.

Markers of Susceptibility

In addition to the age at which exposure occurs, the amount of lead absorbed and the severity of the disease may be influenced by the amount of calcium in the diet, the presence of iron deficiency, and exposure to sunlight and vitamin D. Iron deficiency enhances lead-induced hepatic metallothionein synthesis and in this way may promote the accumulation of lead in the kidney.

Markers of Exposure

The most useful screening tests for excessive lead exposure are blood lead and erythrocyte protoporphyrin. Erythrocyte protoporphyrin becomes elevated when blood lead concentrations reach about $20\,\mu g/mL$ ($1.0\,\mu mol/L$), approximately twice the average blood level in the United States.

PATHOPHYSIOLOGY

Markers of Effect

Low lead exposure has little definable effect on the creatinine clearance (C_{cr}), whereas moderate exposure may be accompanied by a slight state of hyperfiltration. However, a negative correlation between blood lead and the C_{cr} has been found, such that a 10-fold rise in blood lead concentration was associated with as much as a 10 to 13 mL/min reduction in the C_{cr}. Thus, lead exposure may impair renal function in the population at large, although it is possible that renal impairment itself may lead to an increase in the blood lead concentration.

Proteinuria of either a low- or high-molecular-weight is an inconsistent finding. Albuminuria tends to occur only with advanced disease. With elevated blood lead levels, an increase in urinary retinol binding protein or β_2-microglobulin may be found. Likewise, elevated blood lead levels may be accompanied by an increase in urinary N-acetyl-β-D-glucosaminidase activity. Lower urinary excretion of 6-keto-PGF$_{1\alpha}$ and an enhanced excretion of thromboxane (TxB$_2$) have been found, but no deleterious effect on renal function has been identified.

Mechanism of Toxicity

The nephrotoxicity is due in part to the fact that urinary elimination is a major route of lead excretion from the body. Nuclear inclusion bodies in proximal tubule epithelial cells that have a high sulfhydryl group content probably include a lead-binding protein that sequesters intracellular lead. A major toxic effect involves the inhibition of cellular respiration and energy production as a result of the accumulation in mitochondria and the ensuing defects in mitochondrial structure and function. Interaction with membranes and enzymes disrupts calcium metabolism, glucose homeostasis, and ion transport processes.

CLINICAL MANIFESTATIONS

Three forms of lead intoxication occur: (1) acute inorganic lead poisoning from the inhalation of lead oxide,

(2) lead poisoning caused by inhalation or absorption through the skin of tetraethyl lead, and (3) chronic inorganic lead poisoning from inorganic lead in the form of lead oxide, lead carbonate, or similar compounds. Initially, the highest concentrations can be found in the kidney. The lead concentration is 50 times greater in the cortex than in the medulla. From the kidney, lead is excreted in the urine or redistributed to other tissues, most notably bone. The rate of urinary excretion of lead depends on the duration of exposure as well as on the absolute body burden.

At least two types of renal impairment may be found in association with lead poisoning. In the first and more acute form, generalized defects in proximal tubular function result in the Fanconi syndrome with amino-aciduria, glycosuria, and phosphaturia. Serum uric acid levels are generally elevated because of a specific defect in its tubular secretion. Occasionally, the urine contains cells with eosinophilic intranuclear inclusions composed of lead and protein. These abnormalities most often occur in children following several months of heavy lead ingestion. Although this impairment is generally rapidly reversible, it is likely that some cases go on to develop chronic lead nephropathy.

Chronic lead nephropathy, the second type of renal impairment associated with lead poisoning, is an indolent disease difficult to separate from other forms of chronic, slowly progressive renal insufficiency. In the absence of a history of acute lead nephropathy, the diagnosis is suspected when the course of the renal disease is protracted, without definable cause, and associated with symmetrical contraction of both kidneys. Urine protein excretion tends to be less than 1 g/24 h and is marked by the presence of low-molecular-weight proteins such as β_2-microglobulin or retinol-binding protein. Evidence of excessive lead absorption is supplied by determining urinary lead excretion after administration of the calcium disodium salt of ethylene diamine tetraacetic acid (EDTA), a lead chelator, as described below. Chronic lead nephropathy is generally considered to be irreversible.

Hypertension

A weak positive association exists between blood pressure and lead exposure. Some have found an increase in mobilizable lead in hypertensive patients with normal renal function. At least one large epidemiological study has shown that blood lead levels correlate directly with diastolic blood pressure. Chronic lead exposure suppresses plasma renin concentration, blunts the renin response to sodium deprivation, and may be the cause of hyporeninemic hypoaldosteronism in hypertensive patients.

Saturnine Gout

Chronic lead toxicity is associated with saturnine gout. Since gout is unusual in other forms of chronic renal failure, chronic lead nephropathy should be considered a patient with chronic renal failure and symptomatic gout. This is particularly true in women, as there is an overwhelming male predominance of idiopathic gout. Indeed, "gouty

nephopathy" is more likely to be a manifestation of lead nephropathy rather than urate nephropathy.

Renal Cancer

There is a relationship between lead-induced chronic renal disease and renal adenocarcinoma. In fact, an increased incidence of renal cancer occurs among lead-exposed workers even without a statistically increased rate of chronic renal disease. Variability in individual susceptibility may be explained by differences in lead-binding proteins among lead-exposed persons.

PATHOLOGY

With acute lead nephropathy, alterations in mitochondrial structure and cytosolic and acid-fast intranuclear inclusion bodies can be seen. With chronic lead nephropathy, a nonspecific focal interstitial nephritis predominates with tubular atrophy resulting in shrunken kidneys. The characteristic inclusion bodies are often absent. The histopathology is virtually indistinguishable from that of nephrosclerosis. The finding of a variety of immunoglobulin deposits in glomerular capillaries and tubular basement membranes, suggests that immune mechanisms may be involved in these changes.

DIAGNOSIS

The most useful screening tests for excessive lead exposure in adults are blood lead levels and erythrocyte protoporphyrin. Blood lead levels represent recent exposure along with some degree of equilibration with lead present in soft tissues and bone. Erythrocyte protoporphyrin provides evidence of impaired heme synthesis from lead toxicity. Erythrocyte protoporphyrin concentrations are not useful in screening for low-level exposure to lead, and thus blood lead levels should be used as the primary screening method for children and newborns.

In cases with chronic low-level lead exposure, a lead mobilization test may provide evidence of excessive lead absorption. The test is performed by measuring urinary lead excretion following the administration of EDTA. After baseline determinations, 1 g of EDTA is given twice, 8 to 12 hours apart. During this time, a 24-hour urine specimen is collected. An excessive body lead burden is indicated by excretion of more than 1000 μg of lead per day. Alternatively, 1 g of EDTA in 250 mL of 5% glucose solution may be given intravenously over the course of 1 hour. Urine is collected at 24-hour intervals for 3 consecutive days or longer depending on the level or renal function. Excretion of more than 600 μg is indicative of excess body lead.

Often, the diagnosis of chronic lead nephropathy rests on clinical evidence of indolent, slowly progressive renal failure marked by shrunken kidneys and histologic evidence of renal cortical atrophy, tubular fibrosis, and proliferation of the interstitial tissue. The finding of low-molecular-weight proteinuria, the de novo appearance of gout, and an appropriate history of environmental or occupational exposure to lead further support the diagnosis.

TREATMENT

Community prevention measures are necessary for all children with blood lead levels ≥10 µg/dL, nutritional intervention for levels ≥15 µg/dL, medical and environmental intervention for levels ≥20 µg/dL, chelation therapy for levels ≥45 µg/dL, and immediate intervention for levels ≥70 µg/dL. In adults with blood lead levels between 40 and 80 µg/dL, symptoms or findings consistent with lead intoxication require treatment. Workers with blood lead levels >50 µg/dL must be removed from occupational lead exposure until their blood lead levels fall below 40 µg/dL. Workers whose blood lead exceeds 70 to 80 µg/dL may require chelation therapy.

In the absence of marked interstitial fibrosis, patients who have been demonstrated to have an excessive body burden of lead may be treated with long-term, low-dose chelation therapy, 1 g $CaNa_2EDTA$ (with procaine) intramuscularly three times a week. $CaNa_2EDTA$ is not nephrotoxic when administered at an appropriate dosage even in patients with compromised renal function. Normalizing the EDTA lead mobilization test defines the end point of therapy, although actual documentation of improved renal function is limited.

Bibliography

Bernard AM, Vyskocil A, Roels H, Kritz J, Kodl M, Lauwerys R: Renal effects in children living in the vicinity of a lead smelter. *Environ Res* 68:91–95, 1995.

Fowler BA: Mechanisms of kidney cell injury from metals. *Environ Health Perspec* 100:57–63, 1993.

Kim R, Rotnitsky A, Sparrow D, Weiss S, Wager C, Hu H: A longitudinal study of low-level lead exposure and impairment of renal function. The Normative Aging Study. *JAMA* 275:1177–1181, 1996.

Moel DI, Sachs HK: Renal function 17 to 23 years after chelation therapy for childhood plumbism. *Kidney Int* 42:1226–1231, 1992.

Nolan CV, Shaikh ZA: Lead nephrotoxicity and associated disorders: biochemical mechanisms. *Toxicology* 73:127–146, 1992.

Payton M, Hu H, Sparrow D, Weiss ST: Low-level lead exposure and renal function in the Normative Aging Study. *Am J Epidemiol* 140:821–829, 1994.

Rosello J, Gelpi E, Mutti A, De Broe M, Stolte H: Nephron target sites in chronic exposure to lead. *Nephrol Dial Transplant* 9:1740–1746, 1994.

Staessen JA, Lauwerys RR, Buchet JP, et al.: Impairment of renal function with increasing blood lead concentrations in the general population. The Cadmibel Study Group. *N Engl J Med* 327:151–156, 1992.

Verberk MM, Williams TE, Verplanke AJ, De Wolff FA: Environmental lead and renal effects in children. *Arch Environ Health* 51:83–87, 1996.

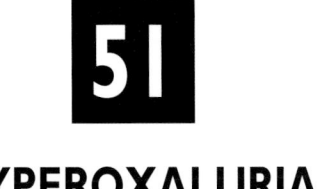

HYPEROXALURIA

DAWN S. MILLINER

The pathologic properties of oxalate result from the relative insolubility of calcium oxalate in body fluids and tissues. Calcium oxalate crystals form readily in supersaturated urine and lead to urolithiasis. Seventy-five percent of stones formed in the upper urinary tract are composed of calcium oxalate. In certain circumstances such as primary hyperoxaluria, oxalate-induced renal tubular and parenchymal injury leads to compromise of renal function followed by calcium oxalate deposition in multiple organ systems and severe multisystem disease. Idiopathic hyperoxaluria associated with urolithiasis is the most common hyperoxaluric state. Metabolic overproduction of oxalate, as in the primary hyperoxalurias, accounts for the most severe consequences of hyperoxaluria. Secondary forms of hyperoxaluria, including enteric hyperoxaluria and ingestion of drugs and toxins, are also encountered but have variable clinical manifestations.

PHYSIOLOGY OF OXALATE

Oxalate is an end product of metabolism and is not degradable by any known biologic system of humans. Elimination of oxalate depends almost entirely on renal excretion. The daily balance among absorption, metabolic production, and excretion is such that plasma oxalate levels in healthy individuals are much lower than urine covalues and are on the order of 2.5 μmol/L. Endogenous metabolic production accounts for 80 to 90% of the oxalate excreted in the urine. Conversion of precursors to oxalate occurs in the liver, and the relevant metabolic pathways are only partially understood (Fig. 1). Primary substrates include glycine and ascorbate. However, exogenous ascorbic acid, even in large amounts, does not result in substantial increases in oxalate production in normal individuals. Hepatic peroxisomal alanine glyoxylate aminotransferase (AGT) is important in converting glyoxylate to glycine, thereby diverting glyoxylate from oxalate production. Pyridoxine acts as a cofactor in the AGT pathway and can sometimes be used to therapeutic benefit. Glycerate dehydrogenase is also believed to play an important role, although its specific site in the enzyme pathway is not as well understood.

Ten to twenty percent of oxalate in the urine derives from dietary intake. Oxalate is a constituent of many foods, particularly those of plant origin. Estimates of the oxalate content of the average Western diet range from 80 to 175 mg/day. In healthy subjects, only 2 to 14% of ingested oxalate is absorbed. Bioavailability for absorption varies considerably depending on other dietary constituents. Dietary calcium binds to oxalate in the lumen of the intestinal tract and has a large effect on the proportion of dietary oxalate absorbed. Availability of dietary oxalate for absorption may also be influenced by oxalate degrading bacteria residing in the intestinal tract. Concentrations of these bacteria of up to 10^8/g of stool have been demonstrated. The quantitative importance and role of oxalate degrading bacteria has yet to be established.

Absorption of oxalate under normal conditions can occur across gastric mucosa and all segments of the intestine, although most oxalate from food is absorbed in the small bowel. Patients with total colectomy appear to absorb and excrete the same amount of oxalate as individuals with an intact colon. Oxalate absorption does occur across the normal large intestine, and it is at this site that enhanced oxalate absorption occurs in patients with enteric hyperoxaluria. Absorption of dietary oxalate occurs early after a meal as demonstrated by increases in urine oxalate occurring within 2 to 4 hours following ingestion of high oxalate foods.

Data regarding renal handling of oxalate are limited. There is general agreement that oxalate is freely filtered and then undergoes bidirectional transport along the renal tubule. In humans, the proximal tubule appears to play a major role in both absorption and secretion. The proximal tubule secretion of oxalate exhibits some of the characteristics of an active, carrier-mediated transport process. Oxalate is one of many anions secreted by the proximal tubule. Although it has been speculated that oxalate shares a common secretory pathway with other organic anions such as urate or PAH, recent studies of isolated membrane vesicles have suggested that the oxalate transporters are distinct but may share common partners such as sodium with other transporters. Whether overall tubular handling of oxalate results in net secretion or reabsorption remains controversial. Studies in healthy subjects suggest net reabsorption, while those in patients with disorders of high oxalate production suggest net secretion.

The upper limit of normal for urinary oxalate excretion is approximately 0.5 mmol/24 hours. Normal values vary somewhat depending on the assay method employed. Enzymatic and ion chromatographic techniques are the most reliable. There is no difference in urine oxalate excretion between males and females, and during adult life there is no difference by age. In growing children and adolescents, urine oxalate excretion normalized to body surface area, is the same as for adults. Acidification of the urine to a pH of less than 2 with HCl during or immediately after the collection is important to ensure accurate results. Acidification prevents precipitation of oxalate and also prevents in vitro autoconversion of excreted ascorbate to oxalate.

Colonic excretion of oxalate has been demonstrated in animal models of chronic renal failure, and there have been

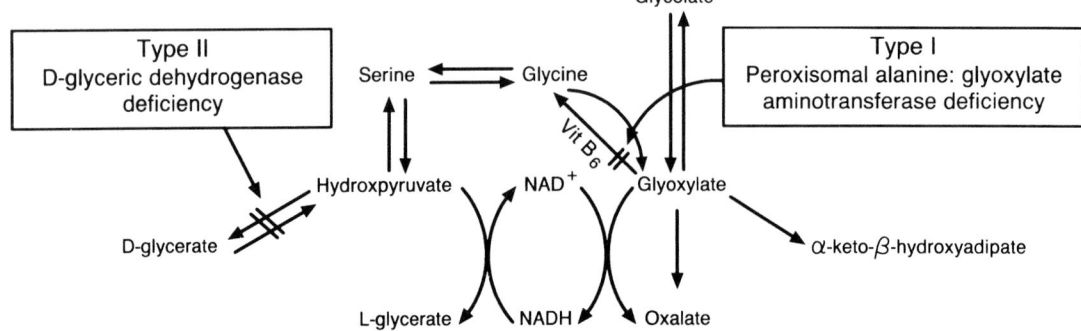

FIGURE 1   Pathways of glyoxylate and hydroxypyruvate metabolism in primary hyperoxaluria. Reproduced with permission of Lippincott Raven Publishers from Smith LH: Urolithiasis. In: Schrier RW, Gottschalle CW (eds.) *Diseases of the Kidney,* 4th ed., Little Brown, and Company, Boston, MA, pp. 785–813, 1988.

preliminary observations of increased concentrations of oxalate-degrading bacteria in the large intestine of patients with chronic renal failure. A role for intestinal secretion of oxalate in chronic renal failure is suggested but remains to be established.

METABOLIC OVERPRODUCTION OF OXALATE

The Primary Hyperoxalurias

Two types of primary hyperoxaluria (PH) have been well described. Both are inherited as autosomal recessive disorders. In type I PH (PH-I), a deficiency or mistargeting of hepatic peroxisomal AGT results in accumulation of glyoxylate which is then converted to oxalate and glycolate (Fig. 1). Patterns of enzyme expression in patients with PH-I are varied and include absence of both immunoreactive AGT and AGT catalytic activity (approximately 30% of PH-I patients), presence of immune reactive AGT but absence of enzymatic activity (approximately 25% of PH-I), and presence of immunoreactive AGT and present but reduced enzymatic activity (approximately 40%). In patients with reduced AGT enzymatic activity, the AGT is most often selectively mistargeted from the peroxisomes to the mitochondria. When located in mitochondria, the AGT is ineffective in glyoxylate metabolism. Hepatic enzyme profiles do not correlate well with clinical severity and have been of limited prognostic usefulness to date. The gene encoding AGT is located at the tip of the long arm of chromosome 2. A number of mutations and polymorphisms have been identified, corresponding to enzymatic phenotypes.

Patients with PH-I most often present clinically with urolithiasis and demonstrate active stone formation. The diagnosis is strongly suggested by a 24-hour urine oxalate value of greater than 1.2 mmol (105 mg)/1.73 m^2 and an elevated urine glycolate. In patients with typical features and no other identifiable causes of hyperoxaluria, these findings may be sufficient to establish the diagnosis. As many as 20 to 25% of patients with PH-I will have normal urine glycolate excretion. In this circumstance, liver biopsy for AGT analysis is needed to confirm PH-I. Some patients with PH-I first come to medical attention with end stage renal failure and have no antecedent history of urolithiasis. Due to the low GFR, urine studies may not be helpful, but the diagnosis is suggested by elevated plasma oxalate and plasma glycolate concentrations. Interpretation of plasma oxalate values in dialysis patients is complicated by the high plasma values seen in patients with renal failure of other causes. In hemodialysis patients, predialysis plasma oxalate levels often range from 30 to 70 μmol/L and are difficult to distinguish from the values of 40 to 120 μmol/L typically seen in PH patients on dialysis. Most patients with end stage renal disease due to PH will have dense nephrocalcinosis demonstrable on a plain film of the kidneys (Fig. 2). Since this is rarely seen in other clinical settings, it is a valuable clue to the diagnosis. Abundant oxalate deposits will be evident on kidney biopsy (Fig. 3). If renal failure has been present for more than a few

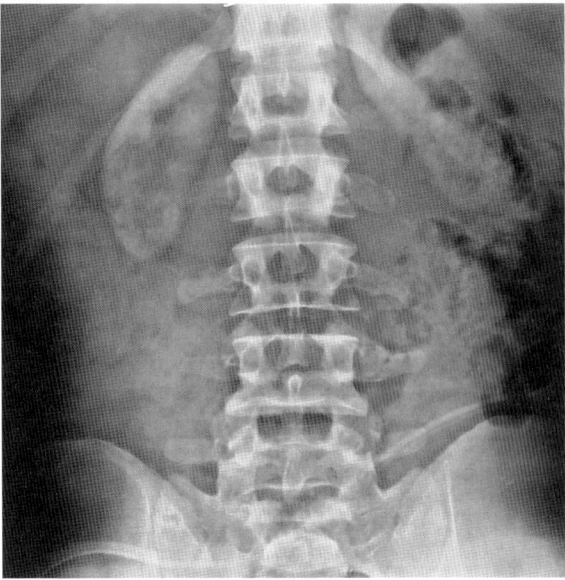

FIGURE 2 Abdominal radiograph showing dense nephrocalcinosis in a patient with primary hyperoxaluria and end stage renal disease.

months, bone marrow examination may be helpful in detecting oxalate deposits. Due to the difficulty in interpreting laboratory results, most patients with end stage renal disease and suspected PH require liver enzyme analysis to confirm the diagnosis, differentiate between PH-I and PH-II, and provide a basis for decisions regarding renal replacement therapy.

The diagnosis of PH-I is most often made during the first or second decade of life, although the disease may remain unrecognized in some patients until the third or fourth decade. As long as renal function is well preserved, the excess oxalate is excreted by the kidneys, the plasma oxalate level remains normal or only mildly elevated, and the primary clinical problem is urolithiasis. With time, pro-

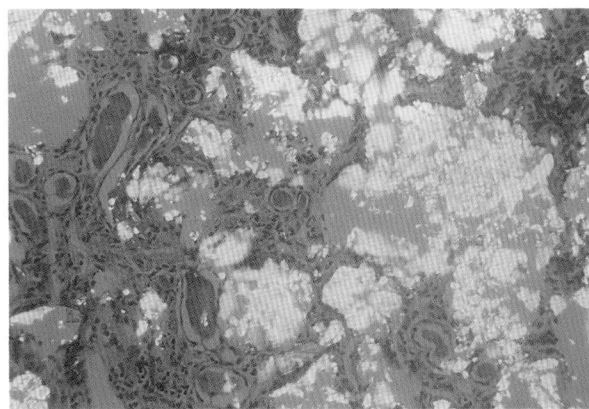

FIGURE 3 Histologic section of a kidney of a patient with end stage renal disease due to PH-I. Note the extensive oxalate deposits in the tubules and interstitium.

gressive damage to kidneys occurs as a result of parenchymal deposition of calcium oxalate as well as urolithiasis, infection, urologic procedures for stone removal. When the GFR declines to 20 to 30 mL · min^{-1} · 1.73 m^{-2}, plasma oxalate concentration increases, setting the stage for systemic calcium oxalate deposition. Bone marrow, trabecular bone, myocardium, the cardiac conduction system, the vascular system, retina, and soft tissues are the most frequently affected. Most dialysis regimens cannot keep pace with daily production. Patients maintained on dialysis almost always continue to accumulate oxalate in multiple organ systems. Prior to the implementation of aggressive treatment regimens, including transplantation, nearly all patients died before the third decade of life. Even with intensive dialysis or transplantation, patients with systemic oxalosis are very ill and pose substantial management challenges.

Treatment strategies for PH-I must take into account individual patient characteristics, including renal function. Twenty to thirty percent of patients with PH-I respond to pharmacologic doses of pyridoxine (a cofactor in the AGT enzyme pathway) with a reduction in oxalate production to normal or near normal. Accordingly, all patients suspected of having PH-I should receive a trial of pyridoxine of 5 to 10 mg · kg^{-1} · day^{-1} for a minimum of 3 months. In patients with adequate renal function, serial urine oxalate determinations will confirm a response. In patients with advanced renal failure, assessment of pyridoxine responsiveness is difficult, though plasma oxalate and glycolate are sometimes helpful. When the response is uncertain, pyridoxine should be continued. Most pyridoxine responsive patients require no more than 5 to 7 mg · kg^{-1} · day^{-1}. A few appear to respond only to very high-dose pyridoxine (up to a gram per day in adult patients). Peripheral neuropathy can occur with long-term use of very high-dose pyridoxine (>10 mg · kg^{-1} · day^{-1}). Although it has not been reported in PH-I patients. The risk of neuropathy due to high-dose pyridoxine in this population is unknown.

High oral fluid intake to maintain a urine volume of 3 to 6 L daily (depending on individual oxalate production) is a mainstay of management in all patients other than those with end stage renal failure. Orthophosphate at 30 to 40 mg · kg^{-1} · day^{-1} of elemental phosphorus (in divided doses) has been shown to decrease calcium oxalate crystalluria, decrease calcium oxalate supersaturation, and increase inhibitors of calcium oxalate crystal formation in the urine of patients with PH-I. Orthophosphate also appears to be beneficial with regard to long-term preservation of renal function. Phosphate therapy should be considered in all patients with adequately preserved renal function (i.e., GFR >30 mL · min^{-1} · 1.73 m^{-2}). It should be used with caution at lower GFRs and is contraindicated in patients with end stage renal disease due to the risk of hyperphosphatemia. Citrate may be beneficial in patients with PH-I as well. Magnesium has been advocated, but to date there have been no intermediate or long-term studies to substantiate its effectiveness. Low oxalate diets are of limited benefit in primary hyperoxaluria since metabolic overproduction accounts for nearly all the oxalate excreted.

Patients with advanced renal insufficiency pose particular problems, and management is best individualized, ideally with assistance from someone who has expertise in this disorder. Since the majority of patients progressively accumulate tissue oxalate while on dialysis, the goal should be early transplantation, ideally at a GFR of approximately 20 mL · min^{-1} · 1.73 m^{-2} and before a large oxalate tissue burden develops. If there is a delay in transplantation, daily hemodialysis or a combination of hemodialysis 3 to 4 days per week along with daily peritoneal dialysis is necessary to minimize oxalate tissue deposition. Pyridoxine responsive patients and those with minimal tissue oxalate may be best served by kidney transplantation alone. This is particularly true if a living donor is available and transplantation can be done expeditiously. Other patients may benefit more from combined liver and kidney transplantation. Loss of renal allografts due to rapid oxalate deposition continues to be a major problem with both kidney and combined liver/kidney transplantation. This is due to large tissue oxalate stores that typically accumulate before transplantation and continue to be mobilized and excreted for months to years after transplantation. Patients with PH require intensive posttransplant monitoring and treatment interventions specifically directed to minimize damage to the allograft. A transplant center experienced in the management of PH-I patients is preferred.

Type II primary hyperoxaluria (PH-II) is a rare disorder that is due to deficiency of hepatic glycerate dehydrogenase. The cause of increased oxalate production is unclear. Hydroxypyruvate accumulation may indirectly increase oxalate synthesis from glyoxylate. The reduction of hydroxypyruvate to L-glycerate enhances the oxidation of glyoxylate to oxalate in a coupled reaction catalyzed by lactic dehydrogenase (Fig. 1). The resulting increase in glycerate production appears to account for the hyperglyceric aciduria characteristic of PH-II.

Patients with PH-II typically present in the first two decades of life with urolithiasis. Urine oxalate excretion tends to be lower in PH-II patients than PH-I but is usually greater than 1.0 mmol (88 mg) · 1.73 m^{-2} · 24 h^{-1}, and there is considerable overlap in the amount of oxaluria and in clinical features in types I and II. The diagnosis is suggested by a markedly elevated urine oxalate without an identifiable secondary cause, elevated urine glycerate, and normal urine glycolate. The diagnosis can be confirmed by hepatic enzyme analysis. Treatment consists of a high oral fluid intake and, in most patients, orthophosphate therapy. Oral citrate and/or magnesium may be considered. Stone formation is easier to control, and there is better preservation of renal function over time in PH-II patients when compared with PH-I.

The term type III primary hyperoxaluria has been used by some authors to describe atypical hyperoxaluria syndromes. The small number of patients described to date have heterogeneous features, and some were evaluated before reliable assays were available for oxalate, glycolate, and glycerate and before hepatic enzyme analysis was available. Until such patients can be well characterized and diagnostic criteria developed, the use of this term is best avoided.

Oxalate Precursors: Drugs and Toxins

Intake of drugs or toxins that are metabolized to oxalate causes marked hyperoxaluria and can result in acute renal failure. Ethylene glycol (found in antifreeze) ingestion is encountered more frequently than others. Epidemics of acute renal failure due to diethylene glycol contamination of paracetamol elixirs have occurred in recent years in Bangladesh, Nigeria, and Haiti. Ethylene glycol ingestion should be considered in unexplained acute renal failure accompanied by a severe anion gap metabolic acidosis not attributable to other causes. The acidosis is caused by the accumulation of glycolic acid. The glycolic acid is further metabolized to oxalic acid and formic acid. The symptom complex may include central nervous system changes, cardiovascular instability, and respiratory insufficiency. As little as 100 mL of ethylene glycol can be lethal. Since the initial metabolic degradation step involves alcohol dehydrogenase, early intravenous infusion of ethanol can slow the metabolic degradation and is of therapeutic benefit. Hemodialysis is effective in clearing the ethylene glycol as well as the toxic metabolites and should be initiated promptly. Measurement of blood ethylene glycol concentration is valuable if obtained before metabolic conversion to glycolic acid. Ethylene glycol ingestion is suggested by calcium oxalate crystalluria and can be confirmed by a urine oxalate level or, if the patient is anuric, by measuring the plasma oxalate. A renal biopsy will show characteristic deposition of calcium oxalate crystals in tubules and interstitium.

Other agents metabolized to oxalate include methoxyflurane anesthetics and xylitol. Mild hyperoxaluria has also been observed in premature infants on parenteral nutrition. There has been controversy regarding the potential for ingested ascorbic acid to undergo endogenous metabolism to oxalate. Recent studies suggest that reports of high urine oxalate under such circumstances represent in vitro autoconversion of ascorbate to oxalate rather than in vivo metabolism. Oral doses of up to 2 g/day of ascorbic acid do not produce an increase in urine oxalate.

INCREASED ABSORPTION OF OXALATE

Enteric Hyperoxaluria

Enteric hyperoxaluria has now been recognized in a variety of clinical circumstances including small bowel resection, small bowel bypass for obesity, primary small bowel disease with malabsorption, chronic pancreatitis, and liver diseases such as primary biliary cirrhosis and chronic cirrhosis of other causes. The common feature is intestinal malabsorption of other substances with a resultant increased absorption of oxalate in the colon. Factors responsible for the enhanced oxalate absorption include: (1) Increased delivery of malabsorbed bile acids to the colon thereby increasing colonic permeability to oxalate; (2) complexing of calcium in the lumen of the intestine with malabsorbed

fatty acids, freeing oxalate to be absorbed; and (3) increased permeability of the colon to oxalate due to fatty acids. All of these factors are influenced by diet composition. A high oxalate diet, especially if dietary calcium is low or fat content is high, will be particularly disadvantageous and can have a pronounced effect on the amount of oxalate absorbed. Patients with enteric hyperoxaluria often have very active stone formation, and some patients have developed renal calcium oxalate deposition and renal failure. The hyperoxaluria is moderate, most often 0.8 to 1.1 mmol $(70–97\,mg) \cdot 1.73\,m^{-2} \cdot 24\,h^{-1}$. In adults, enteric hyperoxaluria is by far the most common cause of moderate hyperoxaluria.

The most effective treatment is to attenuate or eliminate the malabsorption. A low fat diet can be very helpful for patients with steatorrhea. Cholestyramine should be considered in patients with bile acid malabsorption. A low oxalate, high calcium diet should be prescribed. Occasionally, calcium supplements are recommended. Increased oral fluid intake as tolerated is important in improving the solubility of oxalate in the urine. Malabsorption can cause increased lithogenicity of the urine by a variety of mechanisms. Hyperoxaluria is typically only one component. Others include increased urine osmolality due to fluid loss in the gastrointestinal tract, hyperuricosuria, hypomagnesemia, and hypocitric aciduria. The multifactorial aspects of urinary tract stone formation in patients with malabsorption should be taken into account and treatment regimens individualized. Some patients with difficult stone problems and persistently low urine pH may benefit from citrate or bicarbonate administration. Potassium or magnesium supplements may be needed.

Dietary Factors

In normal subjects, an increase in dietary animal protein from 55 to 89 g/day results in an increase in urinary oxalate of up to 24%. This is because meat proteins contain amino acids that are partially metabolized to oxalate. Low calcium diets result in higher oxalate excretion due to reduced binding of oxalate to calcium in the intestinal lumen, with increased absorption of the unbound oxalate. The contribution of dietary oxalate to urine oxalate excretion is less than that of either protein or calcium but can be a significant factor when the diet is also low in calcium.

HYPEROXALURIA IN IDIOPATHIC UROLITHIASIS

Twenty to thirty percent of patients with idiopathic urolithiasis have hyperoxaluria. Due to the high prevalence of urolithiasis in the general population, this form of hyperoxaluria accounts for a large majority of the patients with hyperoxaluria encountered in any clinical practice. The degree of idiopathic hyperoxaluria is modest (typically in the range of 0.5 to 0.8 mmol (44 to 70 mg) $\cdot 1.73\,m^{-2} \cdot 24\,h^{-1}$) but has an effect on urinary supersaturation of calcium oxalate that exceeds equivalent increases in urine calcium concentrations. There may be more than one cause for the hyperoxaluria in this condition. Enhanced gastrointestinal absorption of oxalate, an abnormality of cellular oxalate transport, and alterations in glyoxylate metabolism may all play a role.

Enhanced absorption of dietary oxalate (up to 16 to 20% of ingested oxalate) has been found in a number of studies of patients with idiopathic urolithiasis. However, most studies involved manipulations of dietary calcium, and it is unclear whether the increased absorption of dietary oxalate was a primary feature or was a byproduct of the lower calcium content of the study diets.

Abnormalities of cellular transport of oxalate may occur in idiopathic urolithiasis and have implications for intestinal absorption and excretion and for renal tubular secretion of oxalate. An abnormal transmembrane flux rate of oxalate in red blood cells is characteristic of patients with idiopathic calcium oxalate stone disease and is not present in patients with secondary forms of calcium urolithiasis. This trait has been shown to be autosomal, monogenic, and dominant with complete penetrance but variable expressivity. It has now been described in several ethnic groups. Renal cortical and papillary epithelial cells and colonic epithelial cells share many features of oxalate transport with RBCs. The increased RBC oxalate flux found in patients with idiopathic calcium oxalate stone disease is associated with faster intestinal absorption and a higher renal clearance of oxalate. Some patients with idiopathic hyperoxaluria have an increased fractional excretion of oxalate that can exceed 1. Identification of this transport abnormality may have implications for treatment, since the transport is returned to normal by thiazide diuretics. To date, however, there have been no reports of the effect of thiazides on the urine oxalate in patients with this RBC transport abnormality.

Elevations of urine glycolate have been observed in a small number of patients thought to have idiopathic hyperoxaluria suggesting increased metabolic production of oxalate. Administration of pyridoxine has been reported to reduce both the oxalate and glycolate to normal in these circumstances. Additional studies are needed to more fully characterize glyoxylate metabolism in such patients.

Patients with idiopathic hyperoxaluria are most effectively managed with a high oral fluid intake to reduce the concentration of oxalate in the urine and a low oxalate diet that contains an adequate amount of calcium. Foods and beverages with high oxalate bioavailability such as peanuts, almonds, pecans, chocolate, spinach, rhubarb, tea, and colas should be avoided. If these measures are insufficient to control stone formation, additional treatment is warranted. Neutral phosphate and potassium citrate have been shown to be effective in idiopathic calcium oxalate urolithiasis. If there is concomitant hypercalciuria, addition of a thiazide may be considered.

Bibliography

Allison MJ, Cook HM, Milne DB, et al.: Oxalate degradation by gastrointestinal bacteria from humans. *J Nutr* 116:455, 1986.

Brinkley LJ, Gregory J, Pak CYC: A further study of oxalate bioavailability in foods. *J Urol* 144:94–96, 1990.

Chlebeck PT, Milliner DS, Smith LH: Long-term prognosis in primary hyperoxaluria type II (L-Glyceric Aciduria). *Am J Kidney Dis* 23:255–259, 1994.

Cochat P, Schärer K: Should liver transplantation be performed before advanced renal insufficiency in primary hyperoxaluria type 1? *Pediatr Nephrol* 7:212–218, 1993.

Danpure CJ, Rumsby G: Enzymology and molecular genetics of primary hyperoxaluria type 1. Consequences for clinical management. In: Khan SR (ed) *Calcium Oxalate in Biological Systems.* CRC Press, New York, pp. 189–205, 1995.

Danpure CJ, Smith LH: The primary hyperoxalurias. In: Coe FL, Favus MJ, Pak CYC, Parks HJ, Preminger GM (eds) *Kidney Stones: Medical and Surgical Management.* Lippincott-Raven, Philadelphia, pp. 859–881, 1996.

Hanif M, Mobarak MR, Ronan A, et al.: Fatal renal failure caused by diethylene glycol in paracetamol elixir: The Bangladesh epidemic. *Br Med J* 311:88–91, 1995.

Hatch M, Freel RW: Oxalate transport across intestinal and renal epithelia. In: Khan SR (ed) *Calcium Oxalate in Biological Systems.* CRC Press, New York, pp. 217–238, 1995.

Hillman RE: Primary hyperoxalurias. In: Scriver CR, Beaudet AL, Sly WS, Valle D (eds) *Metabolic Basis of Inherited Diseases,* 6th ed., McGraw-Hill, New York, pp. 933–944, 1989.

Johnson CM, Wilson DM, O'Fallon WM, et al.: Renal stone epidemiology: A 25-year study in Rochester, Minnesota. *Kidney Int* 16:624–631, 1979.

Lindsjö M: Oxalate metabolism in renal stone disease with specific reference to calcium metabolism and intestinal absorption. *Scand J Urol Nephrol* 119:1–53, 1989.

Marangella M, Fruttero B, Bruno M, et al.: Hyperoxaluria in idiopathic calcium stone disease: Further evidence of intestinal hyperabsorption of oxalate. *Clin Sci* 63:381–385, 1982.

Marangella M, Petrarulo M, Vitale C, et al.: Plasma and urine glycolate assays for differentiating the hyperoxaluria syndromes. *J Urol* 148:986–989, 1992.

Milliner DS, Eickholt JT, Bergstralh E, et al.: Primary hyperoxaluria: Results of long-term treatment with orthophosphate and pyridoxine. *N Engl J Med* 331:1553–1558, 1994.

Mitwalli A, Ayiomamitis A, Grass L, et al.: Control of hyperoxaluria with large doses of pyridoxine in patients with kidney stones. *Int Urol Nephrol* 20:353–359, 1988.

Robertson WG: Epidemiology of urinary stone disease. *Urol Res* 18(1):S3–S8, 1990.

Smith LH: Enteric hyperoxaluria and other hyperoxaluric states. In: Coe FL, Brenner BM, Stein JH (eds) *Contemporary Issues in Nephrology.* Churchill Livingstone, New York, pp. 136–164, 1980.

Wilson DM, Liedtke RR: Modified enzyme-based colorimetric assay of urinary and plasma oxalate with improved sensitivity and no ascorbate interference: Reference values and sample handling procedures. *Clin Chem* 37:1229–1235, 1991.

MEDULLARY SPONGE KIDNEY

ELLIS D. AVNER

Medullary sponge kidney (MSK) is a renal cystic disorder characterized by tubular cystic lesions in the inner medullary regions of the kidney. Medullary sponge kidney is a common, and in most instances, nonheritable, disorder in which ectasia and cyst formation localized to intrapyramidal or intrapapillary segments of renal collecting tubules are generally asymptomatic unless complicated by nephrolithiasis, hematuria, or urinary infection.

DEFINITIONS AND EPIDEMIOLOGY

MSK is a relatively common renal development abnormality in which ectasia and cyst formation of medullary collecting ducts give rise to a sponge-like appearance of the renal medulla. The frequency of MSK in the general population is estimated to be between 1:5000 and 1:20,000, although its true prevalence is unknown because patients are asymptomatic unless their course is complicated by nephrolithiasis, hematuria, or infection. MSK has been detected in 0.5 to 10% of unselected patients being studied with intravenous pyelograpy for urological disease.

Most cases of MSK are believed to be sporadic, nonheritable, developmental abnormalities. However, familial clustering has been reported, and pedigrees in which the disease is transmitted in an autosomal-dominant fashion have been described. Since MSK is frequently asymptomatic and difficult to diagnose in mildly affected individuals, the number of heredofamilial cases may be underreported.

PATHOLOGY AND PATHOPHYSIOLOGY

MSK is characterized pathologically by ectasia and cyst formation localized to the intrapyramidal or intrapapillary segments of renal medullary collecting tubules. The disease may be asymmetrical and focal, with one or more renal pyramids demonstrating dilated collecting tubules and multiple small cysts measuring 1.0 to 7.5 mm in diameter. Microdissection studies have revealed the cysts may communicate with each other, with ectatic collecting tubules, or directly with the minor calyces. Extensive changes can lead to overall enlargement of affected pyramids and calyces.

The etiology of tubular ectasia and cyst formation in MSK is unknown. Proposed theories, such as fetal collecting tubular obstruction or structural alteration secondary to hypercalciuria, are unsubstantiated and have little scientific basis. The failure of structural lesions to progress, the pres-

ence of remnants of embryonal tissue in some cases, and the reported association with other congenital abnormalities suggest that MSK is a congenital disorder of abnormal collecting duct development.

CLINICAL FEATURES

In the absence of complications, MSK is a benign asymptomatic condition in which glomerular filtration rate is normal and structural changes in medullary collecting tubules are associated with mild impairments of urinary concentration or defects in acidification that are of no clinical concern. Proteinuria, other abnormalities of the urinary sediment, and hypertension are not seen in the absence of complications.

MSK may present symptomatically with nephrolithiasis, hematuria, or urinary tract infection during the second or third decades of life, although symptoms have been reported in children as young as 2 years of age. Five to twenty-one percent of patients with nephrolithiasis have underlying MSK. In such patients, metabolic studies reveal a high incidence of hypercalciuria (40 to 50%), which may lead to mild secondary hyperparathyroidism in some patients. It is believed that hypercalciuria, in combination with increased urinary pH due to mild urinary acidification defects and urinary stasis in ectatic tubules leads to stone formation in MSK. Increased urinary oxalate and decreased urinary citrate reported in some patients may also contribute to nephrolithiasis. Stones in MSK are generally composed of calcium oxalate and apatite, although concurrent infection with urease producing organisms can lead to aggressive struvite stone formation.

Gross hematuria has been reported in 10 to 20% of patients with MSK and intermittent microscopic hematuria is present in the majority. Hematuria may be unrelated to stones or infection and may be secondary to hypercalciuria or increased fragility of ectatic or cystic tubules that may bleed with minor or inapparent trauma.

Urinary tract infection may also frequently complicate the course of MSK in the presence or absence of nephrolithiasis. Patients may initially present with urinary tract infections, and more than two infections occur in 35% of female and 5% of male patients with MSK. Older reports reveal chronic pyelonephritis in 10 to 15% patients with MSK, although the current prevalence is probably much lower due to improvements in diagnosis and treatment of urinary tract infections over the past two decades. No studies have actually documented an increased incidence of urinary tract infections in uncomplicated MSK when compared to control populations, and there is no reported increase of risk factors for renal infection (such as vesicoureteral reflux, bladder dysfunction, or bladder outlet obstruction) in affected patients. However, in MSK complicated by obstructing stones, urinary stasis probably represents a risk factor for renal infection.

MSK has been associated with a variety of developmental abnormalities of the kidneys and other organ systems, including congenital hemihypertrophy and, less frequently, the Ehlers-Danlos syndrome, congenital pyloric stenosis, Marfan syndrome, Caroli disease, cardiac malformations, Beckwith-Wiedemann syndrome, congenital anodontia, polycystic kidney disease, horseshoe kidney, and renal malrotation or duplication. The common embryopathic basis of these associations is unknown.

MSK is diagnosed by intravenous pyelography. The dilated collecting tubules, when opacified by contrast medium, appear as linear striations leading to a "blush-like" pattern of the renal medulla or as spherical cysts leading to a "bunch of grapes" or "bouquet of flowers" pattern (Fig. 1). The dilated collecting tubules fill poorly (or not at all) by retrograde pyelography. With severe involvement, the renal pyramids and corresponding calyces as well as the entire kidney, may be enlarged. With superimposed nephrolithiasis, dense clusters of stones in the dilated and cystic medulla are often appreciated. Mild or asymptomatic cases may be difficult to diagnose and identification depends on optimal opacification of the pelvocalyceal system with good visualization of each individual calyx and infundibulum. There is generally no role for sonography, computerized tomography, or arteriography in the diagnosis of MSK.

The characteristic pyelogram in an asymptomatic individual or in association with nephrolithiasis, hematuria, or urinary tract infection is generally diagnostic of MSK. Mild or localized disease may present a radiographic differential diagnosis of autosomal-recessive polycystic kidney disease, calyceal diverticuli, renal tuberculosis, renal papillary necrosis, or other causes of nephrocalcinosis (such as distal renal tubular acidosis). However, these conditions are readily differentiated from MSK on clinical grounds.

PROGNOSIS AND THERAPY

Unless complicated by nephrolithiasis, hematuria, or infection, MSK is an asymptomatic condition which is not associated with any increased morbidity or mortality. Asymptomatic patients should be regularly screened for hypercalciuria and bacteriuria. Hematuria in MSK is a benign condition which resolves spontaneously and requires no specific therapy in the absence of nephrolithiasis or infection. It is unclear whether treatment of hypercalciuria, if present, will reduce the incidence of hematuria in MSK. Nephrocalcinosis is treated with standard regimens of fluid intake and, if hypercalciuria is present, thiazide diuretics. Inorganic phosphates have also been reported to be particularly effective in treating nephrolithiasis for patients with MSK. Urinary tract infections are treated with standard antimicrobial regimens. Low-dose urinary tract antimicrobial prophylaxis is recommended for patients with recurrent infections.

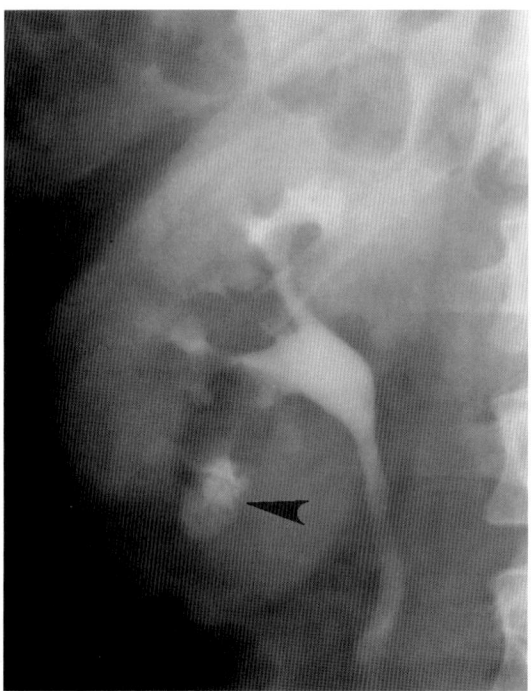

FIGURE 1 Intravenous pyelogram of a patient with MSK. The classical medullary pyramidal "blush" is demonstrated (arrowhead) in the lower pole. (Figure kindly provided by W. Bush, M.D. and W. Winters, M.D., Department of Radiology, University of Washington.)

Bibliography

Abehouse BS, Abehouse GA: Sponge kidney: A review of the literature and a report of five cases. *J Urol* 84:252–267, 1960.

Hildebrandt F, Jungers P, Grunfeld J-P: Medullary cystic and medullary sponge renal disorders. In: Schrier RW, Gottschalk CW (eds) *Diseases of the Kidney*, 6th ed. Little Brown, Boston, pp. 499–520, 1996.

O'Neil M, Breslav NA, Pak CY: Metabolic evaluation of nephrolithiasis in patients with medullary sponge kidney. *JAMA* 245:1233–1236, 1987.

Osther PJ, Mathiasen H, Hansen AB, Nissen HM: Urinary acidification and urinary excretion of calcium and citrate in women with bilateral medullary sponge kidney. *Urol Int* 52(3):126–130, 1994.

Palubinskas AJ: Renal pyramidal structure opacification in excretory urography and its relation to medullary sponge kidney. *Radiology* 81:963–970, 1963.

Yendt ER: Medullary sponge kidney. In: Gardner KD, Bernstein J (eds) *The Cystic Kidney*. Kluwer, Dordrecht, pp. 379–392, 1990.

53

RENAL PAPILLARY NECROSIS

GARABED EKNOYAN

Necrosis of the renal parenchyma may affect the cortex or the medulla. Unlike cortical necrosis which is an acute and often catastrophic event, necrosis of the medulla is a chronic event which generally pursues an insidious course and is often localized to the inner zone of the medulla and more specifically the papilla. Renal papillary necrosis (RPN) occurs in a relatively limited number of individuals afflicted with an apparently disparate group of diseases (Table 1).

PATHOGENESIS

Restriction of the necrotic lesions to the papilla can be ascribed to the unique structural and functional features of this region. The first is the blood supply to the papilla. The rich vascular plexus formed by the descending and ascending vasa rectae is principally devoted to the counter-current exchange mechanism necessary to maintain medullary hypertonicity. The small fraction of medullary blood flow that serves a nutrient function is provided by capillaries that branch off for this purpose. Hence, total medullary blood flow cannot be equated with tissue supply. Additionally, the size of the vessels and their intercommunications and branching nutrient capillaries gradually decrease during the course of their descent to the inner zone such that the tip of the papilla has only small terminal vessels with sparse intercommunications. As there is a three- to fourfold increase in interstitial mass in the inner zone of the medulla as compared to that of the cortex and medulla, the net effect is a relatively poor blood supply to the parenchyma of the papilla compared with the remainder of the kidney. Conditions associated with occlusive lesions of the small blood vessels of the kidney (diabetes mellitus, sickle hemoglobinopathy, transplanted kidney) therefore predispose to ischemic necrosis of the renal papilla. Furthermore, over 50% of RPN cases are observed in individuals greater than 60 years of age (except in sickle hemoglobinopathies). The propensity of the elderly to arteriosclerosis has been implicated as a further cause of reduced medullary blood flow. Another feature of the papillary vasculature that predisposes it to papillary necrosis is its apparently greater dependence on vasodilator prostanoids. On a mole per tissue weight basis the ratio of prostaglandin synthetase activity of the papilla to that of the medulla and cortex is 100:10:1. Agents that inhibit cyclooxygenase activity [nonsteroidal anti-inflammatory drugs (NSAIDs)] could compromise blood flow sufficiently to result in ischemia of this relatively underperfused region.

A second factor predisposing the papilla to necrosis is the ability of the tubule to concentrate solute to in this region. Although necessary to promote water reabsorption, this has a deleterious effect when potentially nephrotoxic agents are concentrated in the medulla, with the greatest accumulation being in the papillary tip. This explains the prevalence of renal papillary necrosis in individuals who abuse analgesics (phenacetin, acetaminophen, salicylates). While the coadministration of these agents provides a biochemical basis of their cytotoxicity, by producing an oxidant stress and blocking its reduction, it is their concentration in the medulla that localizes the initial and major injury caused by analgesic abuse to the papilla. Experimental studies have demonstrated that abolition of medullary hypertonicity by water diuresis results in a reduction in the concentration of analgesics in the papilla and provides protection from RPN.

Another aspect of medullary hypertonicity relevant to papillary necrosis may be its detrimental effect on the normal phagocytic function of polymorphonuclear leukocytes, which may predispose to infection. Urinary tract infection was once considered a principal cause of papillary necrosis. However, while urinary tract infection is present in most patients with papillary necrosis, it is not a uniform finding. It may be a secondary complication superimposed on necrotic foci, particularly when the necrotic tissue interferes with the normal outflow of urine, i.e., obstruction occurs. Independent of infection, obstruction of the urinary tract can cause RPN, because of reduced medullary blood flow. Following acute obstruction, an initial period of vasodilatation and increased blood flow is followed by significant vasoconstriction with a decline in blood flow that persists for the duration of obstruction. These changes in blood flow appear to be mediated by cytokines released by infiltrating monocytes which invade the interstitium shortly after obstruction. That this monocyte-mediated vasoconstriction should exert its most detrimental effect in the papilla is not unexpected given the sparse blood flow of this region and its dependence on vasodilatory prostanoids.

In the clinical conditions which have been associated with papillary necrosis more than one causative factor (obstruction, infection, diabetes, analgesic abuse, and NSAID use) is present in over half of the patients who develop

TABLE I

Clinical Conditions Associated with Renal Papillary Necrosis

Condition	Frequency
Diabetes mellitus	50–60%
Urinary tract obstruction	10–40%
Analgesic abuse	15–20%
Sickle hemoglobinopathy	10–15%
Renal allograft rejection	<5%
Pyelonephritis	<5%

Note: The figures indicate the frequency with which each cause has been noted in major reviews of RPN cases.

RPN. As such, although each of these clinical conditions (Table 1) alone may cause papillary necrosis, the coexistence of more than one predisposing condition increases the risk of papillary necrosis. Thus, the diabetic who abuses analgesics would be more prone to develop medullary injury. To the extent that the region injured by diabetes now produces less vasodilatory prostanoids it is more prone to further vascular injury (due to NSAIDs). Additionally, the necrotic focus can become the nidus of an infection; should it slough it could cause obstruction. Once established, a vicious cycle of vasospasm, vascular occlusion, infection, and obstruction may lead to full-blown papillary necrosis. Thus, papillary necrosis may be considered to be the result of an overlap phenomenon where multiple detrimental factors operate in concert to produce medullary injury.

COURSE AND CLINICAL MANIFESTATIONS

The necrotic process may be localized to one papilla or involve several. Both kidneys are involved in 65–70% of cases. Patients who have a unilateral lesion at the time of initial diagnosis will often develop papillary necrosis in the other kidney as well. The process begins with foci of coagulative necrosis, consistent with ischemic necrosis, which coalesce and extend to involve the rest of the tissue. Depending on the localization of the initial necrotic process it may assume the medullary form, in which the necrosis is in the innermost medullary region while the fornices and papillary tip are viable, or the papillary form, in which the fornices and papillary tip are destroyed. The medullary form is more common in sickle cell hemoglobinopathies.

The necrotic lesions have a well-demarcated sharp border and proceed to form a sequestrum which may either calcify, slough, or be resorbed leaving a sinus tract or cavity at its site. Cavity and sinus formation is more common in the medullary form while calcification and sloughing is more common in the papillary form. The sloughing is generally associated with hematuria, which can be massive. The passage of sloughed necrotic tissue may be associated with lumbar pain and ureteral colic which is clinically similar to that of nephrolithiasis. The necrotic tissue or the stagnant urine in the cavities may be the nidus of a urinary tract infection that can either be chronic, smoldering and recurrent, or present in an acute, fulminant form. With the advent of antibiotics and improved management of urinary tract infection, the central role once attributed to infection in the development and course of RPN has diminished considerably.

The course of papillary necrosis is variable. Occasionally, it will present as an acute disease with septicemia and rapidly progressive renal failure. Sometimes, it will pursue a protracted but symptomatic course with recurrent episodes of urinary infection or renal colic. More commonly, the lesions will remain totally asymptomatic, with the papillary RPN detected as an incidental finding on urography or unexpected discovery at postmortem examination.

The level of renal insufficiency which develops depends on the number of papillae involved. While some loss of renal reserve is expected to result from any renal parenchymal necrosis, renal failure does not always occur. Even when the lesions are bilateral, if they affect only a few of the papillae on each side, sufficient unaffected nephrons remain to maintain adequate renal function. Even when several papillae are affected, localization of the necrosis to the papillary tips results in the loss of only the juxtamedullary nephrons whose loops descend to the papillary tip while the cortical nephrons, which terminate in the outer zone of the medulla, are spared leaving sufficient functioning nephrons to maintain homeostasis. As more of the papillae necrose and cortical scarring develops renal failure will ultimately occur.

Because the deep nephrons are primarily affected, an inability to concentrate the urine maximally is an early manifestation. Consequently, polyuria and nocturia are common and may be a presenting complaint, can be elicited in the history, or may be demonstrated by appropriate testing.

Proteinuria is common (70 to 80% of cases) but is usually only modest (<2 g/day). Pyuria is also common (60 to 80% of cases). Microscopic hematuria (20 to 40%) and gross hematuria (20%) are less common.

DIAGNOSIS

In symptomatic patients, the diagnosis can be made on finding portions of necrotic tissue in the urine, the pathologic examination of which establishes their papillary origin. A deliberate search for papillary fragments should be made by straining the urine through a filter.

In the absence of a tissue diagnosis excretory urography has been the best method to establish a diagnosis. Unfortunately, the radiologic changes do not become apparent until the lesions are advanced and the papillae are shrunk or sequestered (see Fig. 1). Ultrasonography and computerized tomography are less sensitive but, on occasion, can be helpful in patients with poor renal function where excretory urography cannot visualize the outflow tracts and is associated with increased susceptibility to dye-induced nephropathy.

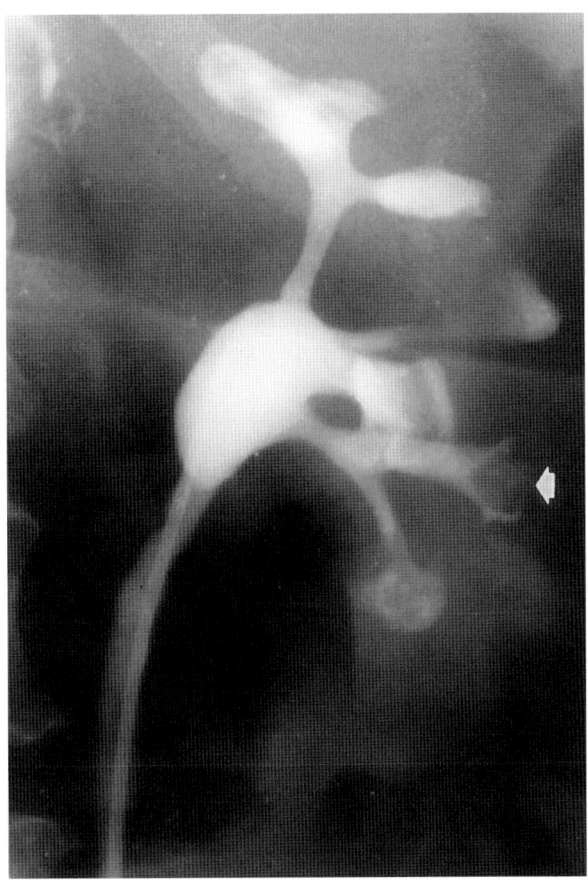

FIGURE I   Retrograde pyelogram of a diabetic patient with papillary necrosis. The calyces are all blunted. One (arrow) demonstrates a sloughed papilla nearly encircled by contrast—the "ring" sign. (Courtesy Dr. William L. Campbell.)

THERAPY

In the absence of a causative factor which can be avoided (analgesics) or surgically corrected (obstruction), therapy is directed toward associated complications. Control and/ or eradication of urinary infection is essential. The blood sugar of diabetics should be well controlled. NSAID should be avoided. Control of hypertension, as in any other renal disease, is important. Anti-hypertensive agents which reduce renal blood flow (β-blockers, thiazides) are best avoided. Volume depletion, which compromises renal blood flow, and dehydration, which increases blood viscosity, should be prevented.

Bibliography

Bach PH, Hardy TL: Relevance of animal models to analgesic-associated renal papillary necrosis. *Kidney Int* 28:605–613, 1985.

Eknoyan G, Qunibi WY, Grissom RT, Tuma SN, Ayus JC: Renal papillary necrosis: An update. *Medicine* 61:55–73, 1982.

Griffin MD, Bergstralh EJ, Larson TS: Renal papillary necrosis—A sixteen year clinical experience. *J Am Soc Nephrol* 6:248–256, 1995.

Groop L, Laasonen L, Edgren J: Renal papillary necrosis in patients with IDDM. *Diabetes Care* 12:198–202, 1989.

Lagergren C, Ljungqvist A: The intrarenal arterial pattern in renal papillary necrosis. *Am J Pathol* 41:633–643, 1962.

Russell GI, Bing RF, Thurston H, Swales JD: Haemodynamic consequences of experimental papillary necrosis in the rat. *Clin Sci* 72:599–604, 1987.

Sabatini S, Eknoyan G (eds): Renal papillary necrosis. *Semin Nephrol* 4:1–106, 1984.

Shyan-Yih C, Porush JG, Faubert PE: Renal medullary circulation: Hormonal control. *Kidney Int* 37:1–13, 1990.

OBSTRUCTIVE UROPATHY

STEPHEN M. KORBET

INTRODUCTION

Obstructive uropathy refers to the structural or functional interference with normal urine flow anywhere along the urinary tract from the renal tubule to the urethra. The resultant increase in pressure within the urinary tract proximal to the obstruction contributes to a number of structural and physiologic changes. Hydronephrosis, dilatation of the calyces and renal pelvis, is the anatomic outcome of an obstructive process that affects the collecting system distal to the renal pelvis (Fig. 1). Hydroureter (the term applied to ureteral dilatation) can accompany hydronephrosis when the level of obstruction is distal to the ureteropelvic junction. The functional and pathologic changes of the kidney that often ensue are referred to as obstructive nephropathy.

In 1993, almost 400,000 patients were discharged from the hospital with a diagnosis of obstructive uropathy. The overall prevalence of obstructive uropathy based on the presence of hydronephrosis at autopsy is approximately 3%, with men and women affected equally. This obviously underestimates the true incidence of the disorder, as temporary conditions such as nephrolithiasis would not be included. The frequency and causes of obstruction vary among males and females and with age. Up to the age of 20 years, the frequency of obstruction is similar in males and females. Strictures of the urethra or ureter and neurologic abnormalities account for most causes of obstruction identified at autopsy in those patients ≤10 years of age. The obstruction rate is higher in women between age 20 and 60, primarily because of obstruction from pregnancy and gynecologic cancers. Above age 60 years, obstructive uropathy is more common in males due to benign prostatic hypertrophy or prostate cancer.

If left untreated, urinary tract obstruction can result in progressive, irreversible loss of renal function and end stage renal disease if both kidneys are affected or if only a solitary kidney is present. However, obstructive uropathy is one of the few potentially curable forms of renal disease. It should therefore be considered in the differential diagnosis of any patient presenting with unexplained acute or chronic renal failure. Since the overall success of therapeutic intervention is directly linked to the duration and degree of obstruction, early identification is crucial.

CLASSIFICATION, CLINICAL AND LABORATORY MANIFESTATIONS

Urinary tract obstruction is often classified according to the duration, location, and degree of the obstructive process. The duration of obstruction is described as acute (hours to days), subacute (days to weeks) and chronic (months to years). The location (Tables 1–3) can be anywhere from the renal tubule to the urethral meatus and thus can affect one (unilateral obstruction) or both (bilateral obstruction) collecting systems. Finally, the degree of obstruction may be partial or complete.

These basic attributes of the obstructive process ultimately determine the clinical and laboratory manifestations with which a patient presents. Patients with an acute obstruction typically present with the abrupt onset of pain. With unilateral obstruction at the level of the pelvis or ureter, severe flank pain results, often described as colicky in nature when due to an intraluminal process such as nephrolithiasis or papillary necrosis. If obstruction occurs at the level of the bladder outlet, suprapubic pain and fullness may be experienced. It may be accompanied by urinary frequency and urgency if the outlet obstruction is partial, or anuria if it is complete. Flank tenderness on percussion or a suprapubic mass may be present on physical examination in patients with outlet obstruction. Laboratory manifestations of unilateral obstruction are often limited to an abnormal urinalysis if the patient has two kidneys. With intrinsic forms of obstruction, microscopic or gross hematuria may be observed, and with either intrinsic or extrinsic processes, secondary infection may result in pyuria and bacteriuria. In conditions leading to bilateral obstruction (or unilateral obstruction in patients with a solitary kidney), laboratory features of acute renal failure will be observed.

The presenting clinical features associated with subacute or chronic obstruction are generally more subtle and insidious in nature. Patients may be asymptomatic. Instead of severe pain, the development of vague symptoms such as flank or suprapubic fullness may be described, depending on the location of the obstruction. In addition, patients

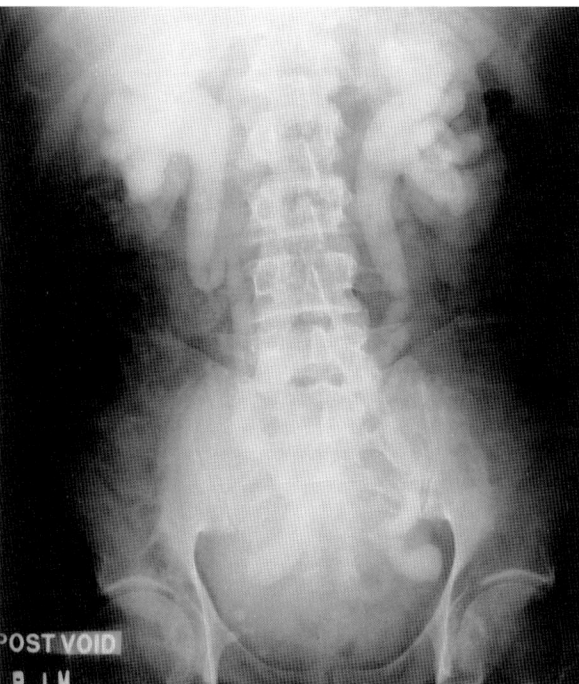

FIGURE 1 Intravenous pyelogram demonstrating bilateral, severe dilatation of the renal pelvis, calyces, and ureter in an elderly male with prostate cancer.

TABLE I
Acquired, Intrinsic Causes of Obstructive Uropathy

Intraluminal
  Intrarenal
    Tubular precipitation of crystals or proteins
      Acyclovir
      Bence Jones proteins
      Methotrexate
      Sulfonamides
      Uric acid
  Extrarenal
    Blood clots
    Fungus balls
    Nephrolithiasis
    Papillary necrosis
Intramural
  Anatomic
    Tumors (benign or malignant)
      Renal pelvis
      Ureter
      Bladder
      Urethra
    Strictures (ureteral or urethral)
      Granulomatous disease
      Infections
        Gonococcal urethritis
        Nongonococcal urethritis
          Chlamydia trachomatis
          Ureaplasma urealyticum
        Schistosomiasis haematobium
        Tuberculosis
      Instrumentation or trauma
      Radiation therapy
  Functional
    Cerebrovascular accident
    Diabetes mellitus
    Multiple sclerosis
    Parkinson's disease
    Spinal cord abnormalities or injury
    Drugs: Anticholinergic agents, disopyramide, levodopa

may experience frequency, polyuria, or nocturia. They may also have difficulty initiating or stopping urination along with urgency if bladder outlet obstruction is present. The physical findings may include a flank mass from a hydronephrotic kidney or a suprapubic mass extending to the umbilicus, due to a greatly distended bladder. Laboratory evaluation of the urine can be similar to that seen in acute obstruction but may include proteinuria (usually less than 2 g/24 hr). Impairment in renal function will also be observed in patients with bilateral disease, as evidenced by laboratory features of chronic renal failure, hyperkalemia, renal tubular acidosis, and an inability to concentrate urine.

The differential diagnosis of obstructive uropathy is extensive (Tables 1–3). In addition to the features described above, clinical and laboratory characteristics unique to the individual disorders should be considered and pursued in the evaluation of a patient with obstructive uropathy.

ETIOLOGY

Acquired Obstructive Uropathy

The acquired forms of obstructive uropathy (Tables 1 and 2) are often classified based on the location of the obstructive process as intrinsic (obstruction occurring within the urinary tract) or extrinsic (obstruction resulting from external compression of the urinary tract).

Intrinsic disorders leading to obstruction are divided into intraluminal and intramural processes. Intraluminal obstruction may be the result of renal tubular obstruction,

otherwise referred to as intrarenal obstruction. This is most often identified with acute renal failure in multiple myeloma from the precipitation of Bence-Jones proteins in the tubules (myeloma kidney) and in the tumor lysis syndrome (generally with a lymphoma) where spontaneous cell turnover or chemotherapy-induced malignant cell lysis leads to the massive production and subsequent precipitation of uric acid crystals within the tubules (see Chapter 31). A number of drugs are also associated with intrarenal obstruction due to precipitation or crystal formation within the renal tubules including sulfadiazine, sulfamethoxazole, acyclovir, and methotrexate. The predisposition for obstruction in these conditions is enhanced in the setting of volume contraction with the excretion of a concentrated, acidic urine. Of the extrarenal causes of obstruction, nephrolithiasis is the most common, particularly in young men. The most common form of stone is composed of calcium,

TABLE 2
Acquired, Extrinsic Causes of Obstructive Uropathy

Reproductive system
  Females
    Uterus
      Pregnancy
      Prolapse
      Tumors
        Cervical carcinoma
        Fibroadenoma
        Uterine carcinoma
    Ovary
      Abscess
      Cysts
      Tumor
    Tubules
      Pelvic inflammatory disease
  Males
    Prostate
      Adenocarcinoma of the prostate
      Benign prostatic hyperplasia
Gastrointestinal system
  Appendicitis
  Colorectal carcinoma
  Crohn's disease
  Diverticulitis
  Pancreatitis
Vascular system
  Arterial aneurysms
    Abdominal aortic
    Iliac
  Venous
    Ovarian vein thrombophlebitis
    Retrocaval ureter
Retroperitoneal diseases
  Fibrosis
    Idiopathic
    Drug related
    Inflammatory
  Hemorrhage
  Iatrogenic complication of surgery
  Infection
  Pelvic lipomatosis
  Radiation therapy
  Tumor
    Primary (lymphoma, sarcomas)
    Metastatic (cervix, bladder, breast, prostate, etc.)

TABLE 3
Congenital Causes of Obstructive Uropathy

  Ureter
    Ureteropelvic junction obstruction
    Ureteroceles
    Ectopic ureter
    Ureteral valves
    Megaureter
  Bladder
    Myelodysplasias (neurogenic)
    Bladder diverticula
  Urethra
    Prune-belly syndrome
    Urethral diverticula
    Posterior urethral valves

most often calcium oxalate (see Chapter 56). Papillary necrosis can lead to ureteral obstruction and may be seen in sickle cell disease, diabetes mellitus, amyloidosis, and analgesic abuse. In addition, gross hematuria with blood clots resulting from any cause, especially renal trauma, polycystic kidney disease, IgA nephropathy, or sickle cell trait may lead to extrarenal obstruction. Intramural obstruction can be divided into anatomic or functional causes. Of the anatomic abnormalities that lead to urinary obstruction (tumors and strictures), transitional-cell carcinomas of the renal pelvis and ureter account for the highest proportion. Of particular note is that patients with analgesic ne-

phropathy are at increased risk for the development of transitional cell carcinoma of the urinary tract. Ureteral or urethral strictures may result from infection, trauma, or postradiation therapy for pelvic tumors. Worldwide, schistosomiasis haematobium infection is a considerable problem affecting nearly 100 million people. Ova deposited in the walls of the distal ureter and bladder cause inflammation which leads to ureteral stricture and fibrosis and contracture of the bladder in 50% of chronically infected patients. The incidence of bladder cancer is also increased in these patients. Rarely, obstructive uropathy may result from ureteral strictures due to granulomatous disease or urethral stricture due to gonococcal and nongonococcal infections. Functional obstruction results from an abnormality (neuromuscular), leading to an alteration in the normal dynamic response of the urinary tract. In neurologic disorders resulting in injury to upper motor neurons, involuntary bladder contraction (spastic bladder) results; with lower motor neuron injury, the bladder becomes flaccid and atonic. Either condition may lead to abnormalities in the forward flow of urine and an increase in residual urine volume that can result in obstructive uropathy with vesicoureteral reflux. Almost 90% of patients with multiple sclerosis develop bladder dysfunction, which is also common in patients with long-standing diabetes mellitus. It may complicate Parkinson's disease as well as cerebrovascular accidents. Medications that are known to alter the neuromuscular activity of the bladder can result in decreased contractility or tone and thus urinary retention, with an incidence as high as 10% with some drugs (levodopa and disopyramide). The use of these agents may be particularly problematic when a preexisting obstructive condition such as benign prostatic hyperplasia is present.

The most common cause of extrinsic obstruction in women is pregnancy (see Chapter 60). In up to 90% of pregnant women, some degree of ureteral dilatation will be observed by the third trimester. This has been attributed to pressure by the gravid uterus on the pelvic brim and affects the right ureter more than the left. However, ureteral dilatation may be seen as early as the first trimester, possibly as a result of hormonal (progesterone) effects on peristalsis. This process is often asymptomatic and resolves spontaneously after delivery. Rarely, bilateral ureteral obstruction during pregnancy can lead to acute renal failure. The second most common cause of urinary obstruction in women is carcinoma of the cervix, with obstruction seen in 30% of patients, usually a result of direct extension. In older women, uterine prolapse can lead to hydronephrosis, and this may occur in up to 80% of patients if there is total prolapse. In these women the ureters are trapped between the levator muscles and the fundus of the prolapsed uterus. Endometriosis occasionally leads to pelvic inflammation with fibrosis and ureteral obstruction. Pelvic inflammatory disease is associated with significant obstruction in up to 40% of patients if a tubo-ovarian abscess is present.

Benign prostatic hyperplasia is the most common cause of obstructive uropathy in older men, resulting in symptoms of outlet obstruction in 50 to 75% of males over age 50 and significant hydronephrosis in 10%. Overall, adenocarcinoma of the prostate is second only to carcinoma of the cervix as the leading form of extrinsic obstruction due to tumor. Obstruction from prostate cancer (or any pelvic malignancy) can be due either to direct extension of tumor to the bladder outlet or ureters, or to metastases to the ureters or surrounding lymph nodes.

In addition to colorectal carcinomas (ureteral metastases), a number of gastrointestinal disorders are associated with obstruction (often unilateral) resulting from local infection and/or inflammatory processes. Vascular diseases, the most common of which is abdominal aortic aneurysm, will lead to obstruction from retroperitoneal fibrosis (inflammatory aneurysms) or from direct pressure of the expanding aneurysm. Rarely, systemic diseases associated with vasculitis (systemic lupus erythematosus, polyarteritis nodosa, Wegener's granulomatous, and Henoch-Schönlein purpura) have been associated with obstruction.

A number of conditions involving the retroperitoneal space may result in ureteral obstruction by fibrosis or direct invasion and compression. Periureteral fibrosis can be observed postradiation, trauma, surgery, granulomatous disease, or infection and is associated with obstruction from some abdominal aneurysms. Retroperitoneal fibrosis has been linked to the use of a number of drugs, including methysergide, bromocriptine, and β-blockers. Idiopathic retroperitoneal fibrosis occurs in some patients without an obvious cause. It is predominantly a disease of men (3:1) in the fifth and sixth decades of life. Dull, non colicky flank pain of insidious onset is the presenting symptom in 80% of patients. Fever, weight loss, and nonspecific gastrointestinal complaints may also be present. On intravenous pyelography, medial deviation of the ureters is a characteristic feature. Although the etiology of this entity is unknown, the histologic findings are those of an inflammatory process involving collagen and fibrosis. Surgical release of the ureters (ureterolysis) is often successful in relieving obstruction and pain symptoms. The fibrous tissue appears to extends out from the aorta, encasing and drawing the ureters medially, and may be up to 6 cm thick. Primary tumors involving the retroperitoneal space that are frequently associated with obstruction include lymphoma (Hodgkin's disease) and reticulum-cell sarcoma. In addition, metastatic

spread to the retroperitoneum of a number of carcinomas, most commonly cervix (30%) and bladder (20%), but including breast, prostate, colon, and ovary, can also result in ureteral obstruction. The most likely cause of obstruction in patients who have undergone pelvic irradiation for malignancy is recurrent tumor if obstruction occurs within 2 years of therapy and radiation fibrosis thereafter.

Congenital Obstructive Uropathy

Of the congenital causes of obstructive uropathy (Table 3), ureteropelvic junction obstruction and posterior urethral valves are the most common. If severe enough, obstruction may have its onset in utero and lead to major renal abnormalities in the developing fetus. Early in development, obstruction results in a kidney that appears dysplastic. Obstruction later leads to a kidney with cortical cysts and a reduced nephron mass. Those fetuses in whom obstruction develops late in gestation have features similar to those seen postnatally, such as hydronephrosis and renal parenchymal thinning. In some cases, obstruction may not manifest itself until childhood. Ureteropelvic junction (UPJ) obstruction is considered the most common cause of hydronephrosis in infancy and early childhood. In childhood, the majority of patients are males, whereas in adults females predominate. In infancy, UPJ obstruction is bilateral in 30% of cases—an uncommon finding in adults. The presentation in children is that of an abdominal mass with flank pain or abdominal pain and failure to thrive. In adults, the pain is episodic and often precipitated by high urine flow rates. Abnormal peristalsis due to a derangement in the smooth muscles of the renal pelvis has been proposed as a primary mechanism for UPJ obstruction. Additionally, a hyperdistensible renal pelvis, incapable of draining completely, has been proposed in some cases. Less often, UPJ obstruction may result from crossing blood vessels, fibrous bands, or strictures. Posterior urethral valves, leading to outlet obstruction, are seen strictly in males and best diagnosed by a voiding cystourethrogram. Presentation in infancy consists of a palpable bladder and kidneys with marked renal insufficiency. Older children will often present with urgency or enuresis. One of the more unusual causes of obstructive uropathy is the prune-belly syndrome. Predominantly seen in males, this consists of the triad of deficiency of abdominal muscles (resulting in loose, wrinkled, redundant skin over the abdomen appearing like a "prune"), cryptorchidism, and hydroureteronephrosis. The obstruction is bilateral, with abnormal ureteral peristalsis and prostatic hypoplasia implicated as possible mechanisms.

Nonobstructive Urinary Tract Dilatation

Dilatation of the urinary tract may occur without evidence of obstruction. However, if the underlying cause is chronic, impaired renal function and atrophy of renal parenchyma may result. This can be seen with vesicoureteral reflux, acute pyelonephritis, and high flow states (such as diabetes insipidus or psychogenic polydipsia). The ureteral dilatation characteristic of pregnancy occurs as early as the first trimester and involves the right collecting system more often than the left. In the majority of cases, the ureteral dilatation is thought to result from decreased peristalsis, rather than mechanical obstruction, due to the muscle relaxant effects of progesterone. The dilatation resolves within a few weeks of delivery and therefore does not result in functional or pathologic renal impairment unless complicated by infection.

PATHOPHYSIOLOGY

Our understanding of the consequences of urinary tract obstruction on renal function are primarily derived from the effects of short-term (24 hours) complete obstruction in experimental animals. The alterations in renal function that result are divided into those that affect either glomerular function or tubular function.

Glomerular Function

Glomerular filtration rate (GFR) declines progressively after complete obstruction. Within the first few hours of acute ureteral obstruction, there is an increase in proximal tubular pressure, the magnitude of which is partially dependent on hydration status (greater with increased hydration). This results in a decrease in net glomerular filtration pressure (net glomerular filtration pressure = glomerular filtration pressure − intratubular pressure) and thus a decrease in GFR. Simultaneously, an increase in the production of prostacyclin and PGE_2 leads to afferent arteriolar dilatation (vasodilative phase) and an increase in renal blood flow which increases glomerular filtration pressure. However, since the increase in glomerular filtration pressure is not proportional to that of the intratubular pressure, a decrease in net glomerular filtration pressure persists, resulting in a GFR that is 80% of the preobstruction value.

At 4 to 5 hours after obstruction, intratubular pressure begins to decline due to ongoing reabsorption of sodium and water by the nephron, dilatation of the collecting system, and lymphatic absorption of solute and water. A decrease in renal blood flow due to an increase in afferent arteriolar resistance (vasoconstrictive phase) also ensues, leading to a decrease in glomerular filtration pressure. Since glomerular filtration pressure declines at a faster rate than the intratubular pressure, a further decrease in net glomerular filtration pressure occurs and GFR continues to decline. Thus, the relatively higher intratubular pressure remains a significant factor responsible for the ongoing decrease in GFR which can be as low as 20% of normal by 24 hours.

The vasoconstrictive phase is mediated by angiotensin II (AII), thromboxane A_2, antidiuretic hormone (ADH), and a decrease in endothelium-derived relaxing factors (EDRF) or nitric oxide production. The increase in intrarenal production of AII is a consequence of decreased delivery of sodium and chloride to the macula densa and the effects of vasodilating prostaglandins on renin release. The source for the increased synthesis of thromboxane in the obstructed kidney appears to be not only intrinsic glomerular cells, but leukocytes (macrophages and T lymphocytes) which infiltrate soon after obstruction. In addition to their effects on vascular resistance, AII and thromboxane A_2 alter GFR by producing mesangial contraction, which leads to a decrease in the ultrafiltration coefficient. It is of interest that pretreatment with angiotensin-converting enzyme (ACE) inhibitors and inhibitors of thromboxane A_2 synthesis has been shown to counteract the effects on GFR and renal plasma flow in experimental models of obstruction.

The degree of improvement in GFR after release of obstruction in animals is related to the duration of obstruction. Complete recovery of GFR is observed after obstruction of up to 7 days, 70% recovery with 14 days of obstruction, 30% recovery with 28 days of obstruction, and essentially no recovery of renal function after obstruction of 56 days.

Tubular Function

Abnormalities in reabsorption of sodium and water and excretion of potassium and hydrogen ions are characteristic of obstructive nephropathy. In the acute phases of obstruction, there is an initial increase in sodium and water reabsorption secondary to underperfusion of the distal nephron. This is evident by reductions in urinary sodium concentration, fractional excretion of sodium, and free water clearance. In clinical practice, this results in urinary indices that can have a prerenal appearance with a urinary sodium of <20 mEq/L, fractional excretion of sodium of <1%, and a urine osmolality of >500 mOsm. With more prolonged or chronic obstruction, subsequent alterations in tubular function result in a decrease in sodium and water reabsorption which is characterized by a urinary sodium of >20 mEq/L, fractional excretion of sodium of >1%, and a urine osmolality of <350 mOsm.

After the release of chronic (≥24 hour) obstruction, there is decreased sodium reabsorption by the nephrons, leading to an increased fractional excretion of sodium. The decrease in sodium reabsorption results from a reduction in Na,K-ATPase activity in the nephron. Additionally, an associated increase in excretion of calcium, phosphate, and magnesium parallels sodium excretion. The ability to concentrate urine is impaired after release of obstruction and results in an increased fractional excretion of water. The concentrating defect is due to multiple factors, including (1) decreased medullary tonicity from washout of solute due to an increase in medullary blood flow and decreased sodium chloride reabsorption at the thick ascending limb of Henle, (2) decreased response to ADH, and (3) a decrease in the number of functional juxtamedullary nephrons. The greater natriuresis and diuresis observed after release of bilateral ureteral obstruction (BUO) compared with unilateral renal obstruction (UUO) are attributed to the accumulation of sodium and water, urea retention, retention of other impermeable solutes, and higher levels of atrial natriuretic peptide which occur in BUO but not UUO.

Abnormalities in potassium and hydrogen excretion are common in obstructive uropathy. Hyperkalemia disproportionate to the degree of renal dysfunction results as the fractional excretion of potassium is lower in obstructive uropathy than in other forms of renal disease. The decrease in potassium secretion is attributed to a reduction in the secretion or response of the distal tubule to aldosterone or a combination of both. Hyperkalemic-hyperchloremic acidosis is also frequently seen in patients with obstructive uropathy. Explanations include a defect in hydrogen ion secretion and maximal urine acidification (distal renal tubular acidosis), or a defect in secretion of aldosterone secondary to a decrease in renin production (hyporeninemic aldosteronism or type IV renal tubular acidosis). A decrease in sodium reabsorption in the distal nephron has been suggested as an additional factor. By reducing the degree of intraluminal negativity this would decrease the voltage-dependent secretion of both potassium and hydrogen. Finally, reduced levels of in H^+-ATPase (a major transport pathway) in the cortical and medullary collecting ducts have been observed in obstructive uropathy and may further explain the diminished hydrogen ion excretion. The acidifying defect is usually reversible but may persist.

RENAL PATHOLOGY

The pathology of hydronephrosis is similar, irrespective of the underlying cause of obstruction. In early hydronephrosis the kidney is enlarged and edematous with an increase in the renal pelvic cavity and blunting of the renal papilla. Later, there are retraction and dimpling of the papilla, which is most evident at the upper and lower poles. Microscopically, the renal cortex appears normal but the tubules may be dilated and Tamm-Horsfall protein is present in Bowman's space. A principal lesion in the medulla and papilla is ischemic atrophy associated with flattening and atrophy of tubular epithelium and interstitial fibrosis. As the hydronephrosis advances, the atrophy becomes even more pronounced. The kidney essentially transforms into a fluid-filled sac with loss of papillae and marked thinning of the cortex and medulla. With progressive sclerosis and fibrosis, few recognizable renal features remain.

The morphologic changes in obstructive nephropathy are primarily attributed to the ischemia from the marked reduction in renal blood flow. However, another contributing factor is invasion of the interstitium early on in obstruction by macrophages and T lymphocytes. Beginning 4 to 12 hours after obstruction, the number of interstitial macrophages increases. Chemoattractants, such as monocyte chemoattractant peptide-1 and osteopontin, appear to be released from tubular epithelial cells in response to the increase in intratubular pressure from ureteral obstruction. Fibrogenic cytokines, such as transforming growth factor-β (TGF-β), produced by the invading macrophages and T lymphocytes become central in the progressive fibrosis observed in obstructive nephropathy. TGF-β increases matrix synthesis by interstitial fibroblasts and decreases matrix degradation by downregulating the production of matrix degradation proteins and promoting the generation of proteinase inhibitors. Vasoactive compounds such as angiotensin II may directly stimulate the production of TGF-β by tubular epithelial cells. The use of ACE inhibitor in the experimental setting significantly decreases the degree of tubulointerstitial fibrosis seen in obstruction, suggesting a potential role for ACE inhibitors in the clinical treatment of obstructive uropathy.

DIAGNOSIS

When the diagnosis of obstructive uropathy is suspected, a careful history, complete physical, and appropriate laboratory evaluation (including biochemistry profile and urinalysis) are essential. Findings from these evaluations are invaluable in establishing the presence and functional severity of obstruction, and in determining its etiology. Dilatation of urinary tract is the radiographic finding characteristically used to confirm the presence of obstruction (Fig. 1). The diagnostic approach may vary depending on whether acute or chronic obstruction is suspected.

In acute obstruction, such as in nephrolithiasis, there may not be sufficient time for identifiable dilatation of the collecting system to occur. In this setting, the intravenous pyelogram (IVP) has been considered the procedure of choice or "gold standard." Whether the use of simpler and less invasive technology such as ultrasound (US) can replace the IVP in detecting acute urinary tract obstruction has been an area of intense interest (Fig. 2a and 2b), as the contrast required for performing the IVP carries a small but definite risk. The success of ultrasound in diagnosing acute obstruction varies substantially (sensitivity reported to be as low as 50% and as high as 90%). In part, the variable success of US is attributed to its subjective nature. It is highly operator dependent with most false negatives due to cases of grade 1 hydronephrosis (mild dilatation of the renal sinus central-echo complex) or nondilated obstructive uropathy (i.e., retroperitoneal fibrosis). Since nephrolithiasis is the leading cause of acute renal colic and obstruction, and >90% of renal stones are radiopaque, combining plain abdominal radiography (kidney, ureter, bladder-KUB) with US increases the sensitivity for detecting obstruction to >95%. Finally, the use of duplex doppler US, to demonstrate the presence of a high resistive index (>70%) from increased vascular resistance in obstruction, has been shown to further reduce the false-negative results associated with US in both acute and chronic obstruction. Thus, in situations where obtaining an IVP may be difficult or the use of contrast a major concern or contraindicated, the combination of US and KUB may provide a viable alternative. A limitation of US remains its inability to determine the level and the cause of obstruction as compared to IVP. Recent enthusiasm is mounting for the use of unenhanced helical (spiral) computed tomography (CT) in the evaluation of acute renal colic. The scan can image the top of kidney to the base of the bladder and does not require contrast. Furthermore, it is more sensitive than combined KUB and US in identifying causes of renal colic and allows visualization of the obstructive lesion.

A chronic form of obstruction, UPJ obstruction, is often associated with symptoms that are acute in nature and reproduced only during periods of high urine flow rates.

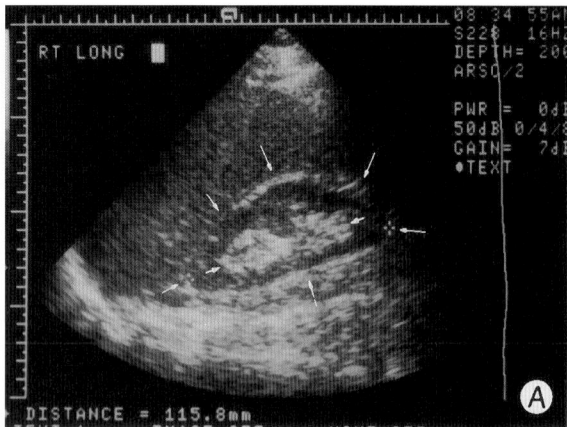
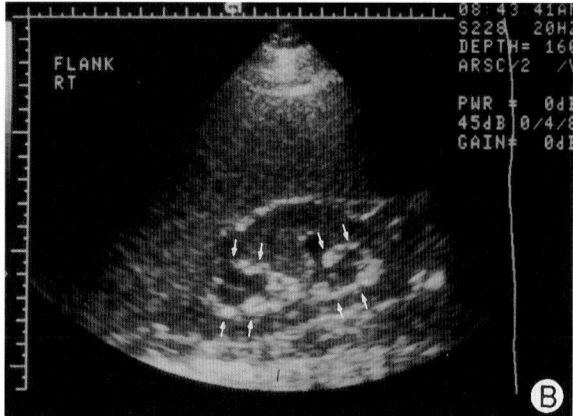

FIGURE 2 (A) Ultrasound of the right kidney, long axis (outlined by long arrows), demonstrating the normal echo-dense central area, the renal sinus central echo-complex (between short arrows). (B) Repeat ultrasound of the right kidney, long axis, in the same patient 3 weeks later after presentation with a 3-day history of right flank pain. Note hydronephrosis (pyelocalyceal dilatation) as demonstrated by a marked separation of the renal sinus central echo-complex (between short arrows).

Often a diagnosis of UPJ obstruction requires the use of diuresis urography, which combines the use of intravenous furosemide with an IVP in order to evaluate for dilatation and abnormal emptying of the upper urinary tract during a state of high urine flow. A similar evaluation can be obtained with diuresis renography using radionuclides.

In chronic obstruction, sufficient time for dilatation of the urinary tract has transpired, and if the obstruction is bilateral, renal insufficiency may be present. In this setting, the use of intravenous pyelogram contrast is best avoided and ultrasonography is the procedure of choice with a sensitivity of 98% and a specificity of 75%. A false-negative US evaluation should be extremely rare in the evaluation of chronic obstruction. CT is also an accurate technique for the detection of urinary tract dilatation and may be more likely than US to identify the obstructing lesion. However, with conventional CT, contrast is often required. Whether unenhanced helical (spiral) CT will prove beneficial in the evaluation of chronic obstruction is undetermined. Ultimately, antegrade or retrograde pyelography may be required to further define the site and cause of obstruction. Retrograde pyelography may be of particular value when a nondilated obstructive uropathy is suspected. Although these studies can be useful when intravenous contrast is contraindicated due to allergy or renal failure, the risk of urinary tract infection is of concern, particularly with retrograde pyelography. To evaluate causes of lower urinary tract obstruction, cystoscopy and urodynamic studies may be utilized. Urodynamic studies are most worthwhile when a functional abnormality of the bladder (neurogenic bladder) is suspected.

Nonobstructive urinary tract dilatation may be differentiated from that due to obstruction by means of diuresis renography or urography. Diuresis renography utilizes radionuclide imaging and evaluates the pattern of radionuclide elimination by each kidney before and after intravenous furosemide. Prolonged retention of radioactivity or contrast after diuresis is consistent with obstruction. In nonobstructed dilatation, however, there is a rapid "washout" of marker with the furosemide-induced diuresis.

TREATMENT

The treatment of obstructive uropathy is dictated by the underlying cause and its location. It should be obvious that acute or chronic renal failure resulting from urinary tract obstruction (obstructive nephropathy) warrants emergent attention as the potential for permanent renal damage increases with the duration of obstruction. The urgency and aggressiveness with which obstructive uropathy must be treated are also determined by the severity of symptoms as well as by the presence of infection.

Nephrolithiasis, the most common cause of acute unilateral obstruction, can most often be treated with conservative measures such as intravenous fluids and pain medications. As 90% of stones less than 5 mm pass spontaneously with increased urine flow alone, often no additional treatment is required. However, with increasing stone size, the likelihood of spontaneous passage diminishes, and the need for more aggressive measures arises. The urological management of nephrolithiasis is discussed in Chapter 56. Rarely, chronic or recurrent unilateral obstruction of any cause may lead to advanced hydronephrosis associated with severe pain, recurrent pyelonephritis, or pyonephrosis, in which case a nephrectomy may be indicated, especially if the renal function of the affected kidney is minimal.

The initial treatment approach for patients presenting with bilateral urinary tract obstruction and renal failure is primarily dictated by the location of the obstruction. In patients with a neurogenic bladder or disorders involving the bladder outlet, the placement of a urethral catheter will often suffice. For patients in whom a urethral catheter cannot be passed into the bladder, a suprapubic cystostomy may be required. Lesions obstructing the ureters result in the need for cystoscopy and stent placement. If a stent cannot be passed beyond the ureteral obstruction in a retrograde fashion, a percutaneous nephrostomy tube can be placed and antegrade placement of a stent can be attempted. Placement of a percutaneous nephrostomy is successful in more than 90% of patients, resulting in clinical improvement in up to 70% of cases. Major complications (abscess, sepsis, hematomas) occur in less than 5% of patients.

Once acute relief of the obstruction has been achieved, specific treatment of the underlying disease becomes the primary focus. For example, in neurogenic disorders of the bladder, voiding regularly and pharmacologic agents may be useful. In patients with a spastic bladder, the anticholinergic agents oxybutynin and propantheline bromide are employed. Particularly in patients with bladder atony, however, intermittent catheterization of the bladder (four times daily) is required. For men with prostatic hyperplasia the long-term treatment approach depend on the severity of the outlet obstruction. If symptoms are minimal, and not associated with infection or upper urinary tract abnormalities, close observation is appropriate. Cases with mild to moderate symptoms of prostatism can be managed medically with either alpha antagonists or 5-α-reductase inhibitors. Alpha antagonists (doxazosin or terazosin) act by relaxing the smooth muscle of the prostate and bladder neck, thus decreasing urethral pressure and outlet obstruction. Hormonal therapy with a 5-α-reductase inhibitor (finasteride) inhibits the conversion of testosterone to the active dihydrotestosterone and thereby leads to a reduction in prostate size. The combined use of these agents may be beneficial in some patients, as the agents are thought to act synergistically. For patients with hyperplasia of the prostate resulting in signs and symptoms of severe obstruction (significant urinary retention or renal failure), surgical intervention with transurethral resection of the prostate (TURP) or transurethral incision of the prostate (TUIP) is generally required.

In disease processes that lead to irreparable damage of the lower urinary tract (as in bladder, cervical, or prostate cancer), a diversion procedure such as an ileal conduit or percutaneous nephrostomy will be needed. In patients with obstructive nephropathy secondary to malignancy, percutaneous nephrostomy has relieved the obstruction in >75% of cases and resulted in a significant increase in survival (>6 months in 50%) as well as an increase in number of days spent at home compared to patients in whom the procedure was not performed. Thus, selected patients can benefit from this aggressive approach.

The likelihood of regaining renal function postobstruction is dependent on the degree and duration of obstruction. In general, complete recovery of renal function is anticipated in patients with acute uncomplicated obstruction of short duration ($\leq$1 to 2 weeks), and little to no

improvement occurs after severe, complete or partial obstruction of a prolonged duration (>12 weeks). However, recovery of renal function in patients has been recorded after obstruction for up to 70 days. Radionuclide renography performed several weeks after relief of obstruction has been proposed as one method to predict recovery.

Release of bilateral obstruction can result in marked polyuria (postobstructive diuresis). A number of factors—physiologic and pathologic—lead to development of this condition. Physiologic factors contributing to the diuresis include excess sodium and water retention, accumulation of urea, and other nonreabsorbable solutes that act as osmotic diuretics, and accumulation of atrial natriuretic peptide. Pathologic factors include decreased tubular reabsorption of sodium, inability to maximally concentrate urine due to a decreased medullary concentrating gradient and decreased response to ADH, and increased tubular flow reducing equilibration time for absorption of sodium and water. Once excess sodium and water have been excreted, the potential for severe volume contraction as well as hypokalemia exists if patients are not carefully monitored and given appropriate fluid and solute replacement. Urinary output should be measured frequently during the diuresis (at least every 6 hours and in cases with large urine outputs, hourly). Once the patient has diuresed enough to become euvolemic, fluid replacement (intravenous plus oral) should be given as needed to prevent volume contraction. A suitable method is replacement of 75% of the urine losses with intravenous fluids having a solute composition similar to what is excreted (0.45% normal saline), but careful monitoring to avoid over- and underhydration is essential. Serum electrolyte levels should be monitored closely during the diuresis, at least daily if not more often, and replaced as needed. The postobstructive diuresis is self-limited, resolving over several days to a week. Persistence of the polyuria is often due to overzealous hydration which perpetuates the solute and water diuresis.

Bibliography

Cronan JJ: Contemporary concepts for imaging urinary tract obstruction. *Urol Radiol* 14:8–12, 1992.

Curhan GC, Zeidel ML: Urinary tract obstruction. In: Brenner BM (ed) *The Kidney,* 5th ed. W.B. Saunders, Philadelphia, pp. 1936–1958, 1996.

Davidson AJ, Hartman DS: The dilated pelvocalyceal system. In: Davidson AJ, Hartman DS (eds) *Radiology of the Kidney and Urinary Tract,* 2nd ed. W.B. Saunders, Philadelphia, pp. 571–780, 1994.

Diamond JR: Macrophages and progressive renal disease in experimental hydronephrosis. *Am J Kidney Dis* 26:133–140, 1995.

Haddad MC, Sharif HS, Shahed MS, et al.: Renal colic: Diagnosis and outcome. *Radiology* 184:83–88, 1992.

Harrington KJ, Pandha HS, Kelly SA, Lambert HE, Jackson JE, Waxman J: Palliation of obstructive nephropathy due to malignancy. *Br J Urol* 76:101–107, 1995.

Hill GS: Calcium and the kidney, nephrolithiasis, and hydronephrosis. In: Heptinstall RH (ed) *Pathology of the Kidney,* 4th ed. Little, Brown, Co., Boston, pp. 1563–1629, 1992.

Hoffman LM, Suki WN: Obstructive uropathy mimicking volume depletion. *JAMA* 236:2096–2097, 1976.

Katz DS, Lane MJ, Sommer FG: Unenhanced helical CT of ureteral stones: Incidence of associated urinary tract findings. *AJR* 166:1319–1322, 1996.

Klahr S: Pathophysiology of obstructive nephropathy: A 1991 update. *Semin Nephrol* 11:156–168, 1991.

Klahr S: New insight into the consequences and mechanisms of renal impairment in obstructive nephropathy. *Am J Kidney Dis* 18:689–699, 1991.

Klahr S, Purkerson ML: The pathophysiology of obstructive nephropathy: The role of vasoactive compounds in the hemodynamic and structural abnormalities of the obstructed kidney. *Am J Kidney Dis* 23:219–223, 1994.

Klahr S, Ishidoya S, Morrissey J: Role of angiotensin II in the tubulointerstitial fibrosis of obstructive nephropathy. *Am J Kidney Dis* 26:141–146, 1995.

Spital A, Spataro R: Nondilated obstructive uropathy due to a ureteral calculus. *Am J Med* 98:509–511, 1995.

Suki W, Eknoyan G, Rector FC Jr, Seldin DW: Patterns of nephron perfusion in acute and chronic hydrinephrosis. *J Clin Invest* 45:122–131, 1966.

Vehmas T, Kivisaari L, Mankinen P, et al.: Results and complications of percutaneous nephrostomy. Ann Clin Res 20:423–427, 1988.

55

VESICOURETERAL REFLUX AND REFLUX NEPHROPATHY

JORGE A. VELOSA

DEFINITIONS

Vesicoureteral reflux (VUR) is the abnormal retrograde flow of urine from the bladder into the upper urinary tract. *Primary* VUR is a common congenital abnormality of the vesicoureteric junction. *Secondary* VUR results from an anatomic or functional obstruction at any level in the urinary tract, (including inflammatory disorders affecting the vesicoureteral junction, bladder neck obstruction, surgery on the ureteric orifice, paraurethral diverticulum, posterior urethral valves, ureteropelvic junction obstruction, ureteral duplications, hypospadias, and ureteroceles). *Intrarenal reflux* is the retrograde flow or urine into the ducts of Bellini (pyelotubular backflow). The term reflux nephropathy refers to renal scarring associated with VUR. It is a major cause of end-stage renal disease in children and adolescents, accounts for 5 to 15% of cases of end stage renal disease in adults less than 50 years of age.

PATHOGENESIS

Vesicoureteral Reflux

The anatomic features of the normal valve mechanism of the ureterovesical junction are the oblique insertion of the ureter into the bladder and an adequate length of the intramural segment of the ureter. As a result of these anatomic characteristics, the intravesical portion of the ureter is compressed by the bladder musculature when it contracts during micturition. Primary VUR may result from congenitally anomalous shortening of the intravesical portion of the ureter with resultant valve dysfunction. The intravesical ureter lengthens with growth, increasing the competence of the valve mechanisms; reflux, therefore, tends to diminish or disappear with increasing age.

Little evidence supports the notion that occult VUR occurs in asymptomatic normal individuals. Studies of the urinary tract conducted in humans without urinary tract complaints or infection showed that only 0.4% had VUR. However, 50% of children in whom a urinary tract infection developed before age 1 year and 38% of children with urinary tract infection before age 12 years were noted to have VUR. In adults with urinary tract infection, the prevalence is approximately 5%. There is a high familial incidence of VUR, which suggests a hereditary abnormality. Prospective studies of siblings of patients with VUR showed an incidence of VUR of 32 to 45%. Sixty percent of the affected siblings had no previous symptoms to suggest urinary tract infection, and 56% had severe VUR. Race influences the incidence of VUR. The Southwest Pediatric Nephrology Study Group reported only 8 African-American children of a total of 113 with VUR.

VUR may be unilateral or bilateral, and its severity is variable. Voiding cystography—a standardized technique—is frequently used to determine the severity of reflux (Table 1).

The incidence of renal scarring has been related to the severity of the VUR. By use of the International Classification, renal scarring was identified in 85% of patients with grade V, 37 to 64% with grade IV, 25% with grade III, and 6 to 14% with grade II VUR. To put these numbers in perspective, mild and moderate grades of VUR occurred more often than severe VUR, 70 and 30%, respectively.

Scar Formation

Scar development usually represents the combined effects of VUR, intrarenal reflux, and infection. Two studies document the importance of infection in the development of new scars. In one study, 75 children were given low-dose prophylactic antibacterial therapy; after 15 years of follow-up, only two fresh scars were documented. In the other, children from various institutions were treated for symptomatic urinary tract infections, but in many, treatment of infection was delayed. New scars developed in 87 of 148 kidneys in the study.

Sterile Reflux and Urodynamic Factors

There is support for the suggestion that high-pressure VUR and intrarenal reflux in the infant kidney can produce damage because of urodynamic factors in the absence of bacterial infection (sterile reflux). Severe obstructive uropathy with high intrapelvic pressures may be necessary to produce renal damage, such as in children with posterior urethral valves or other obstructive congenital anomalies. However, there is still controversy regarding the frequency with which such damage occurs clinically. This is in contrast to the overwhelming evidence that VUR in the presence of bacterial infection leads to renal scarring in children.

TABLE I
Grading System Adopted by the International Reflux Study Committee

Grade I	Reflux up the ureter only
Grade II	Reflux up the ureter, pelvis, and calices with no dilatation and normal caliceal fornices
Grade III	Same as grade II plus mild or moderate dilatation and tortuosity of the ureter; no blunting of the fornices
Grade IV	Moderate dilatation or tortuosity or both of the ureter and moderate dilatation of the pelvis and calices; complete blunting of fornices
Grade V	Gross dilatation and tortuosity of the ureter, pelvis, and calices. Absent papillary impressions in the calices

Reflux Nephropathy and Progressive Renal Failure

Progressive renal insufficiency associated with VUR and reflux nephropathy occurs in two circumstances. In the most severe cases of bilateral reflux, coarse scar formation may lead to renal insufficiency. More frequently, however, the progression to renal insufficiency in patients with reflux nephropathy is related to complicating factors such as proteinuria and hypertension associated with glomerulosclerosis.

Hypertension

The most common cause of hypertension in children and adolescents is reflux nephropathy; it is a cue for the investigation of reflux in these patients. The risk of development of hypertension increases with the severity of the reflux nephropathy and renal scarring. In a study of adults and children, 32 of 41 patients with reflux nephropathy who progressed to advanced renal insufficiency had hypertension.

Proteinuria and Glomerulosclerosis

Several studies have documented the association of proteinuria due to glomerulosclerosis with reflux nephropathy. In patients with glomerulosclerosis, progressive renal insufficiency develops even if VUR is corrected or urinary tract infections or hypertension are absent. The characteristic clinical feature of these patients is persistent proteinuria; the pathologic correlate is focal and segmental glomerulosclerosis involving unscarred segments of the kidney.

In a long-term follow-up of adults with reflux nephropathy, 294 patients over 15 years of age were studied with regard to renal function, hypertension, and proteinuria. At presentation, (mean age 17 years), 8.5% had hypertension, 4.8% proteinuria, and 2% renal insufficiency. At follow-up (mean age 34 years), 38% had hypertension, 31% proteinuria, and 24% renal insufficiency. Proteinuria and renal insufficiency were significantly more frequent in those with severe bilateral reflux nephropathy. In another study of patients with VUR and an abnormal serum creatinine at presentation, all 34 patients progressed to end-stage renal disease.

The degree of proteinuria correlates with the presence and extent of glomerular lesions. In a study of 94 adult patients with primary bilateral VUR, all patients with progressive renal insufficiency had significant proteinuria (≥ 1.5 g/24 h) at the time of the initial evaluation, and there was a significant negative correlation between the 24-hour urine protein excretion and the simultaneous determination of renal function. It is now accepted that the occurrence of proteinuria in patients with reflux nephropathy indicates the development of a focal segmental sclerosing glomerulopathy and the likelihood of progressive renal insufficiency even in the absence of further scarring.

The pathogenesis of VUR related glomerulopathy is still unclear. The most attractive explanation is that it results from compensatory intrarenal hemodynamic changes and single nephron hyperfiltration in response to the decrease in renal mass caused by scarring. Although this hypothesis is compatible with the clinical course of many patients with reflux nephropathy, a small number of patients with only mild scarring may have significant proteinuria and glomerulosclerosis. Moreover, all patients with severe scarring develop proteinuria and progressive renal insufficiency. It is possible that other factors play a role in the pathogenesis of the glomerulopathy associated with reflux nephropathy.

CLINICAL MANIFESTATIONS

Diagnosis and Evaluation

Urinary tract infections are the most common manifestations of VUR and reflux nephropathy in infants and children. Current practice requires that children with urinary tract infection be evaluated for VUR after the first infection has been treated successfully. However, the type of studies to be performed and the age limits for follow-up remain controversial. Prospective studies may settle these important issues.

Several techniques have been used to demonstrate the presence of VUR: voiding cystourethrography, radionuclide cystography, excretory urography, and cystoscopy. Voiding cystourethrography is the most precise method available for demonstrating VUR; the use of low-dose fluoroscopic technique decreases the radiation exposure. Radionuclide voiding cystography is gaining wide acceptance for assessment and management of patients with VUR and may be more sensitive than a standard contrast voiding cystourethrogram. Important limitations of this technique are the inability to distinguish accurately the grade of reflux and to evaluate the urethra at voiding. Cystoscopic evaluation of the bladder and urethra is used less often than in the past.

Investigations of the upper urinary tract to demonstrate reflux nephropathy include intravenous urography and radionuclide scanning; ultrasonography also has been used. Intravenous urography with nephrotomography is the traditional imaging technique for demonstrating reflux nephropathy because it gives the best anatomic detail. The radiologic hallmarks of reflux nephropathy are the irregularly scarred surface of the kidney and the clubbing of the underlying calyx, indicating full-thickness scarring of a renal lobe, most frequently seen in the polar regions (Fig. 1). This is the most common form of reflux nephropathy. In patients wtih the most severe reflux nephropathy, the renal damage is diffuse, and there is marked and generalized reduction of renal mass, with uniform papillary change. The main limitations of intravenous urography are its failure to demonstrate focal scarring in some patients (particularly at the upper poles) and its inability to provide information regarding renal function. For these reasons, technetium-99 is now widely used as a complementary investigation (Fig. 2). Technetium-99 scanning [technetium-99 dimer-captosuccinic acid (DMSA)] is the most sensitive method for estimating early renal damage. Reflux nephropathy can also be detected by ultrasonography, but this

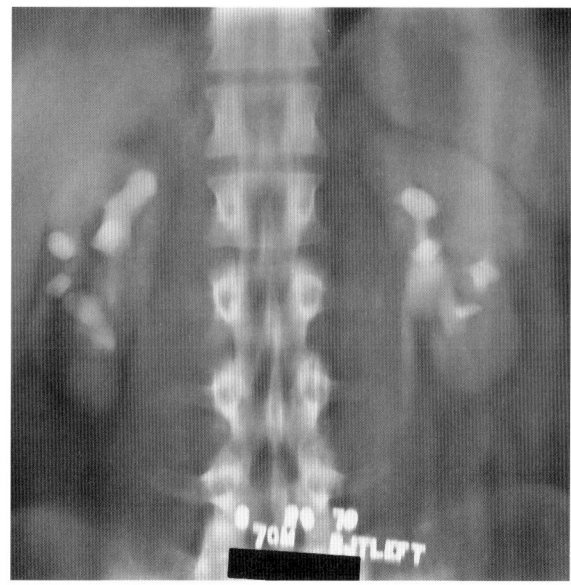

FIGURE 1   The midcortex of the left kidney shows a scar interrupting the smooth outline of the kidney due to parenchymal loss. The right kidney shows severe scarring with blunting and deformed calices.

method is operator dependent, has several limitations, and does not provide information on renal function, either.

In summary, an intravenous urogram and voiding cystourethrogram or radionuclide cystography are indicated in children younger than 5 years with urinary tract infection. The initial evaluation in older children with urinary tract infection includes intravenous urography or DMSA. In

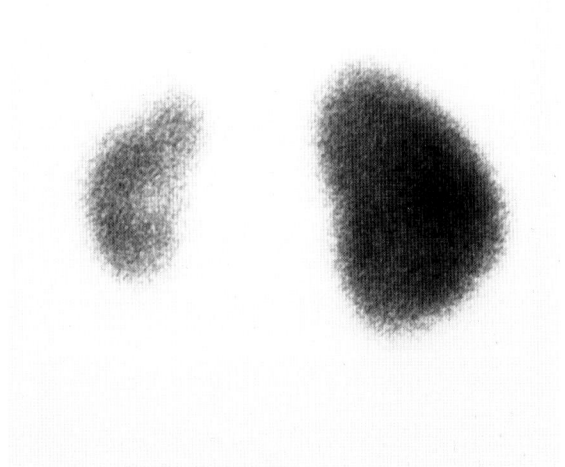

FIGURE 2   DMSA scan demonstrates decreased size of the right kidney with irregular contour of the upper pole consistent with scarring. The left kidney has a normal contour. Calculated function: 80% on the left kidney and 20% on the right kidney.

adults with recurrent pyelonephritis or complicated urinary tract infections, intravenous urography is the technique of choice complemented with DMSA when information regarding differential renal function is deemed necessary. Preadolescent siblings of patients with VUR should have a screening cystogram for VUR because 30 to 50% of this population has demonstrated abnormalities.

MANAGEMENT OF VESICOURETERAL REFLUX

Despite many publications and several controlled trials, either completed or under way, there is no universal agreement among nephrologists and urologists regarding management of patients with VUR. It is, however, generally agreed that the main objective in children with VUR is to prevent reflux nephropathy. To this end, urinary tract infections must be recognized promptly, confirmed by culture, and treated aggressively and appropriately with antibiotics. Elimination of bacteriuria with treatment should be documented by follow-up culture of the urine 48 to 72 hours after treatment initiation. Patients with VUR should have annual voiding cystography by contrast or radionuclide study until the VUR disappears. Resolution of VUR should be documented with two consecutive cystograms. If the kidney imaging studies at the time of diagnosis of VUR are normal, but the clinical picture is suspicious for VUR, a second study after 2 years is recommended. Adolescents with no scars or hypertension who had previous VUR are at minimal risk and require no further surveillance. As adult patients with reflux seldom form new scars, surveillance imaging studies are not necessary. The majority of adult patients with VUR have multiple episodes of urinary tract infections, although some have a history of a single episode and some no history of urinary tract infections. In adult patients with multiple urinary tract infections, prophylactic therapy with trimethoprimsulfamethoxazole or trimethoprim alone is indicated. In young adults with frequent episodes of acute pyelonephritis, antireflux surgery is an acceptable alternative to many years of chronic prophylactic therapy. Patients with hypertension, proteinuria, or decreased renal function and history of VUR need attention to these problems. It is possible that progressive glomerular injury may be minimized by treatment of angiotensin converting enzyme inhibitors and perhaps protein restriction, but formal studies are not available. In women with VUR, the risks of hypertension and urinary tract infection increase during pregnancy; they require renal function monitoring, control of the hypertension, and early treatment of urinary tract infections. Given the familial nature of VUR, prenatal or neonatal ultrasonographic screening of the fetus for pelvic dilatation is recommended.

There is general agreement regarding the aggressive treatment of infection in patients with VUR. Antibiotic prophylaxis and the treatment of asymptomatic bacteriuria are the current standards of care, but there is no general agreement on this issue. The prospective controlled trials used daily antimicrobial therapy with trimethoprim-sulfamethoxazole, trimethoprim alone, or nitrofurantoin;

the treatment was continued until puberty or the reflux spontaneously disappeared. The option of screening for bacteriuria rather than antibiotic prophylaxis seems reasonable in the setting of vigilant attention and prompt access to medical care. Periodic urine cultures every 2 to 3 months are indicated.

Comparison of Conservative vs Surgical Treatment

As a rule, surgery is of no benefit if the patient has proteinuria, renal insufficiency, or hypertension. There is still considerable disagreement concerning the indications for antireflux surgery in very young children because in many children refluxing will stop spontaneously and because once renal damage occurs, neither conservative nor surgical treatment reliably prevents hypertension or deterioration of renal function.

Results from prospective controlled trials comparing conservative and surgical treatment are now setting the standard for management of VUR. The Birmingham Reflux Study Group compared conservative management with surgical correction of moderate and severe VUR in patients younger than age 15 years. After 5 years of follow-up, the incidence of urinary tract infections was not different between the two groups: 50% of patients treated conservatively had no VUR and 7% had new renal scars compared with 5% new renal scars in the surgically treated group. In the International Reflux Study in Children, patients younger than age 11 years with grades III and IV VUR were allocated randomly to conservative and surgical treatment. After 5 years of follow-up, new renal scars developed in 12% of children treated medically compared to 13% of children treated surgically. No significant difference in outcome was found between conservative and surgical management in terms of the development of new renal lesions or the progression of established renal scars. These studies demonstrate that conservative and surgical treatment yield comparable results regarding prevention of further renal injury in patients with severe VUR. The Southwest Pediatric Nephrology Study Group investigated the evolution of milder forms of VUR: grades I, II, and III. Children younger than age 5 years and without evidence of renal scarring were treated conservatively and followed for 5 years. In an interim report, after 3 years of observation, fewer than 10% of kidneys showed definitive scars, whereas 25% showed renal parenchymal thinning. Publication of further follow-up data from these two important studies should be available in the near future.

Studies of adults in our institution treated medically or surgically showed outcomes similar to those in children. A group of 27 adults with VUR treated medically was compared with 67 adults with VUR treated surgically during the same interval. After 13 years of follow-up, renal function was similar, irrespective of the method of management and appeared to be determined by the severity of renal scarring, level of renal function at the initial evaluation, and presence of proteinuria. However, 93% of the patients treated surgically experienced a decrease in the rate of acute pyelonephritis. The presence or absence of proteinuria is of prognostic value in adults with reflux nephropathy. Urinary protein levels of more than 1.5 g/24 h, especially when associated with severe renal scarring and depressed renal function, indicate progressive reflux nephropathy.

In summary, the treatment of choice for children with stage I or II VUR is medical therapy. The treatment for severe reflux may be either medical or surgical, and the choice of treatment depends on the clinical circumstances. Surgical correction of VUR may be indicated in the following clinical settings: (1) children or adults with recurrent symptomatic pyelonephritis difficult to control medically, (2) the presence of gross reflux and ureteral dilatation in a young child, and (3) patient and family considerations, in particular those that limit compliance with medical treatment.

Bibliography

Arant BS Jr: Vesicoureteric reflux and renal injury. *Am J Kidney Dis* 17:491–511, 1991.

Arant BS: Medical management of mild and moderate vesicoureteral reflux: Follow-up studies of infants and young children. A preliminary report of the Southwest Pediatric Nephrology Study Group. *J Urol* 148(Pt 2):1683–1687, 1992.

Birmingham Reflux Study Group. Prospective trial of operative versus non-operative treatment of severe vesicoureteric reflux in children: five years' observation. *Br Med J* 295:237–241, 1987.

Dick PT, Feldman W: Routine diagnostic imaging for childhood urinary tract infections: A systematic overview. *J Pediatr* 128:15–22, 1996.

Hodson CJ, Cotran RS: Vesicoureteral reflux, reflux nephropathy, and chronic pyelonephritis. *Contemp Issues Nephrol* 10:83–120, 1983.

Linshaw, M: Asymptomatic bacteriuria and vesicoureteral reflux in children. *Kidney Int* 50:312–329, 1996.

Neves RJ, Torres VE, Malek RZ, et al.: Vesicoureteral reflux in the adult. IV. Medical vs. surgical management. *J Urol* 132:882–885, 1984.

Smellie JM, Tamminen-Möbius T, Oilbing H, et al.: Five-year study of medical or surgical treatment in children with severe reflux: radiological renal findings. The International Reflux Study in Children. *Pediatr Nephrol* 6:223–230, 1992.

Torres VE, Velosa JA, Holley KE, et al.: The progression of vesicoureteral reflux nephropathy. *Ann Intern Med* 92:776–784, 1980.

Zhang Y, Bailey RR: A long term follow up of adults with reflux nephropathy. *NZ Med J* 108:142–144, 1995.

56

NEPHROLITHIASIS

ALAN G. WASSERSTEIN

Nephrolithiasis has an annual incidence of 7 to 21 cases per 10,000 persons and accounts for 7 to 10 of 1000 hospital admissions in the United States. Men are affected about four times as often as women. The lifetime prevalence of kidney stones in white men is about 10% and in excess of 25% in parts of the "stone belt" in the southeastern United States. The predominant age of onset is the third to fifth decade. Incidence has increased in the developed countries in the 20th century, probably as a consequence of increased dietary animal protein intake. In underdeveloped countries nephrolithiasis is relatively uncommon and bladder stones predominate.

The most common clinical consequence of nephrolithiasis is stone passage with acute renal colic. Flank pain radiating to the groin, abrupt in onset and extreme in severity, is typical. Gross or microscopic hematuria, dysuria or frequency, and nausea, vomiting, and occasionally ileus can accompany stone passage. Stones that are associated with nephrocalcinosis (primary hyperparathyroidism, renal tubular acidosis) or with staghorn formation (struvite, cystine) can cause renal failure, but the majority of stones cause renal failure only if associated with bilateral urinary obstruction or obstruction in a solitary kidney.

Classification and characteristics of renal calculi are given in Table 1. Most stones are mixed calcium oxalate/calcium phosphate or pure calcium oxalate and their pathogenesis is idiopathic. Predominant calcium phosphate stones usually reflect alkaline urine and have specific causes such as primary hyperparathyroidism, renal tubular acidosis, alkali therapy, or milk-alkali syndrome.

TABLE I

Classification and Characteristics of Renal Calculi

Type	Frequency (%)	Sex	Crystals	Radiography
Calcium oxalate	75	M	Envelope	Round, radiodense
Uric acid	10–15	M = F	Diamond	Round or staghorn, radiolucent
Struvite	15–20	F	Coffin-lid	Staghorn, radiodense
Cystine	1	M = F	Hexagon	Staghorn, intermediate

TABLE 2

Urinary Risk Factors for Calcium Nephrolithiasis

Crystalloid Concentration
  Hypercalciuria
  Hyperoxaluria
  Low urine volume
Promoters
  Hyperuricosuria
  Alkaline pH
Inhibitor Deficiency
  Hypocitraturia
  Hypomagnesuria
  Macromolecules
    Nephrocalcin
    Uropontin
    Tamm-Horsfall protein

Stone disease tends to recur. After a first calcium stone 40% of untreated patients have another stone within 5 years, and an additional 40% within the next 25 years. Patients who lack renal calcifications on plain abdominal film are less likely to have recurrent stone formation. Stone formers show decreased stone formation and decreased need for urological procedures after they begin medical follow-up (the "stone clinic effect"); this observation may be due to regression to the mean or to increased fluid intake (see below).

PATHOGENESIS

Stone formation can be attributed to increased urinary concentration of crystalloids, decreased inhibitors, or increased promoter substances (Table 2). Stone formation begins with nucleation, the association of small amounts of crystalloid to form submicroscopic particles. Nucleation generally occurs on existing surfaces (heterogeneous nucleation), such as papillary epithelium. Urine must be saturated—the concentration product of constituent crystalloids must exceed the solubility product—to permit such association. Greater supersaturation (higher concentrations of calcium and/or oxalate) favors nucleation. Submicroscopic particles would ordinarily wash out in the urine; but they either are attached to the urothelial surface of the papilla, or associate rapidly to form larger particles too large to wash away (aggregation). Stone growth occurs by aggregation, or by crystal growth, the orderly movement of ions out of solution onto growing crystal.

Urinary saturation with respect to calcium oxalate is frequent in the general population. Hence the role of inhibitors must be crucial. Citrate and magnesium form soluble complexes with calcium and oxalate, respectively. These complexes do not participate in nucleation. Nephrocalcin is a highly acidic protein of renal tubular origin containing the amino acid γ-carboxyglutamic acid. It binds to the crystal surface and inhibits nucleation, aggregation, and crystal growth; some calcium stone formers have abnormal nephrocalcin that lacks γ-carboxyglutamic acid. Tamm-Horsfall protein inhibits only aggregation; some calcium stone formers have abnormal Tamm-Horsfall protein that self-aggregates and loses inhibitory activity. These large inhibitor proteins may have a major if not predominant role in stone formation, but they are not as yet measured in clinical practice.

Not all stone disease can be attributed to metabolic risk factors. Several conditions predispose to stone formation because of anatomical derangements, including polycystic kidney disease, horseshoe kidney, and medullary sponge kidney. Medullary sponge kidney is a congenital condition in which the collecting ducts undergo cystic dilatation, predisposing to calcium stones and recurrent urinary tract infection (but not renal insufficiency). Its characteristic urographic appearance is papillary striation or brush effect. Medullary nephrocalcinosis may be extensive.

METABOLIC EVALUATION OF NEPHROLITHIASIS

Two kinds of stone activity should be distinguished: anatomic activity, the movement of an existing stone (usually into the pelvis or ureter) to cause symptoms; and metabolic activity, the formation of a new stone, growth of an existing stone, or formation and passage of multiple tiny stone fragments ("gravel"). Much as in the evaluation of a pulmonary nodule by comparison with prior chest radiographs, serial abdominal films are needed to determine metabolic activity. Figure 6 in Chapter 6 shows an anatomically active stone. It is highly desirable that stones be recovered and analyzed: The discovery of uric acid, struvite, pure calcium phosphate, or cystine can transform the diagnostic approach. Urine should be strained during acute stone passage and after extracorporeal shock wave lithotripsy (ESWL). A first stone requires limited evaluation beyond stone analysis: urinalysis, serum calcium, phosphate, uric acid, creatinine, and blood urea nitrogen. Recurrent stone formers should have, in addition, 24-hour urine collections for measurement of calcium, phosphate, oxalate, citrate, uric acid, creatinine, volume, pH, urea nitrogen, and sodium, preferably on several occasions. These collections are done during usual dietary intake; medications that could interfere with urinary determinations (e.g., NSAIDs, diuretics, calcium supplements, antacids) should be avoided if possible. Analysis of a diet diary for animal protein, calcium, and oxalate is also useful. The metabolic evaluation and treatment of calcium and uric acid stones is summarized in Table 3.

RISK FACTORS FOR CALCIUM NEPHROLITHIASIS

Calcium oxalate stones are the consequence of a wide variety of urinary abnormalities, including low urinary volume, hypercalciuria, hyperoxaluria, hypocitraturia, and hyperuricosuria; usually more than one is present in an individual case.

Low Urinary Volume

Some patients have habitually low fluid intake. Controlled studies have not generally detected low urinary volumes in stone formers, possibly because stone formation and/or hypercalciuria impair urinary concentrating ability. Epidemiological studies suggest that calcium stone formation rises sharply when urinary volume falls below 1100 ml daily. Saturation of urine with regard to relevant crystalloids falls as water is added to urine, whether *in vitro* or by increased oral intake. Universal advice to increase fluid intake may account for the so-called stone clinic effect. Patients who continued to form stones in a stone clinic setting were those who, retrospectively, increased urine output by an average of 50 mL daily; those who formed no further stones were those who

increased urine output by 500 mL daily. Stone formers should strive to excrete at least 2 L of urine daily. A useful prescription is two eight-ounce glasses of water every four hours by the clock while awake; dilute apple juice may be substituted, but high oxalate beverages such as tea, colas, and citrus juices should not constitute the bulk of ingested fluid.

Hypercalciuria

Hypercalciuria is defined as daily excretion of more than 300 mg in men or 250 mg in women or 4 mg/kg in either sex. Distribution of calcium excretion is not normal, and 10% of the stone-free general population has excretion above these limits. Desirable calcium excretion (to limit stone formation) is probably significantly lower, in the range of 200 mg daily.

Hypercalciuria, usually idiopathic, occurs in about 60% of calcium stone formers. A small proportion (5%) has primary hyperparathyroidism. Renal tubular acidosis, sarcoidosis, and various familial hypercalciuric syndromes are rare causes of hypercalciuria. Primary hyperparathyroidism affects predominantly middle-aged and older women. Hypercalciuria is due to excess renal production of 1,25-dihydroxyvitamin D under the influence of parathyroid hormone. The degree of hypercalcemia is usually mild to moderate. So-called subtle or normocalcemic hyperparathyroidism occurs when serum calcium fluctuates into the high–normal range; diagnosis depends on repeated blood determinations of calcium and parathyroid hormone (PTH), documenting simultaneous elevation. Some "normocalcemic" hyperparathyroidism is due to an inappropriate normal range: The true upper limit of normal serum calcium in women (10.1 mg/dL) is lower than that in men.

TABLE 3
Metabolic Evaluation and Treatment of Nephrolithiasis

Abnormality	Evaluation	Treatment
Calcium stones	Measure serum and urine calcium, urine oxalate, citrate, uric acid, magnesium, creatinine, and volume on self-selected diet	
Hypercalciuria	Urine sodium and urea nitrogen	Dietary salt and protein restriction, thiazides, neutral phosphate
Hypercalcemia	PTH and ionized serum calcium	Parathyroidectomy
Hyperoxaluria	Assess dietary oxalate and calcium, vitamin C, artificial sweetener (xylitol), ileal disease or bypass	Dietary oxalate restriction, magnesium supplements, pyridoxine, calcium supplements (enteric)
Hypocitratria	Acid load (if severe) Serum K, creatinine, urine culture	Alkali (potassium citrate)
Hyperuricosuria	Assess dietary purine intake	Dietary purine restriction, allopurinol
Low urine volume	Measure 24-hour urine volume	Scheduled fluid intake 16 oz. q 4 hr while awake
Uric acid stones	Measure urinary uric acid and postprandial urine pH	
Acid urine	R/o chronic diarrhea or gout	Alkali (potassium citrate)
Hyperuricosuria	Assess dietary purine	Dietary purine restriction, allopurinol

Some patients with normal total serum calcium may have elevations of the ionized fraction. In general, the diagnosis of primary hyperparathyroidism need not be considered unless the serum calcium is high (or high–normal); on the other hand, stone formers with hypercalcemia are overwhelmingly likely to have primary hyperparathyroidism. Presence of nephrocalcinosis and stone composition exclusively of calcium phosphate should also heighten suspicion of primary hyperparathyroidism. Parathyroid adenoma is responsible for primary hyperparathyroidism in 85% of cases, parathyroid hyperplasia for the remainder. Parathyroid exploration is indicated in all stone formers with primary hyperparathyroidism, regardless of the level of the serum calcium.

Idiopathic hypercalciuria is predominantly a disease of men in the third to fifth decade. It is associated with obesity, hypertension, and possibly affluence, and it is familial. Intestinal calcium absorption is high, PTH levels normal or low, and fasting urine calcium excretion elevated in 40%. Increased serum 1,25-dihydroxyvitamin D levels could explain these findings but are not invariably present. Increased nonparathyroid hormone-mediated bone resorption could explain low–normal PTH levels and high fasting calcium excretion, as well as reduced bone mineral content and the tendency to negative calcium balance on low-calcium diet in idiopathic hypercalciuria; but bone resorption does not account for high intestinal calcium absorption or high serum 1,25-dihydroxyvitamin D levels. A group of patients has been described in which osteoporosis and hypercalciuria were apparently due to IL-1-mediated bone resorption. Phosphate depletion could account for elevated 1,25-dihydroxyvitamin D production and consequent abnormalities including low PTH and high fasting calcium excretion, but hypophosphatemia is found only in a fraction of patients. In clinical practice there is not a pressing need to delineate the pathogenesis of idiopathic hypercalciuria. Pak has suggested that absorptive hypercalciuria (type 2) is corrected by low-calcium diet alone and that reduced bone mineral density is not found in these patients; but concern about future development of low bone density should temper use of low-calcium diet even in this group.

There are several dietary factors that exacerbate idiopathic hypercalciuria. The most important of these is dietary sodium, which is easily assessed by measuring 24-hr urinary sodium excretion. Dietary sodium increases renal calcium excretion; proximal tubular sodium reabsorption is reduced, as is the reabsorption of moieties handled in parallel with sodium, such as calcium. Another factor is dietary protein, which can be assessed by diet diary or by urine urea nitrogen. Dietary animal protein exacerbates calciuria by multiple mechanisms: acid load increases urine calcium excretion; protein increases glomerular filtration rate and filtered load of calcium; sulfate in dietary protein binds to calcium and inhibits tubular reabsorption; and hormonal factors stimulated by dietary protein, such as insulin, glucagon, and prostaglandins, are calciuric. Dietary animal protein has been convincingly associated with nephrolithiasis in epidemiological studies, but dietary protein restriction has not been proven to ameliorate stone formation in prospective trials. A third factor is dietary calcium. In normal persons, only 6% of dietary calcium appears in the urine; hypercalciuria from dietary calcium excess alone is therefore unusual. In patients with idiopathic hypercalciuria the proportion of ingested calcium that is absorbed in the intestine is higher, but intestinal oxalate absorption in such patients rises disproportionately during dietary calcium restriction. Since urinary oxalate may be at least as important as urinary calcium in the genesis of nephrolithiasis, dietary calcium restriction may be deleterious even in patients with hypercalciuria. In a large prospective study of patients without nephrolithiasis, the risk of developing kidney stones was inversely related to dietary calcium intake, perhaps because of the inverse relation between dietary calcium and urinary oxalate. Regardless of the presence of hypercalciuria, patients with nephrolithiasis should be counseled to maintain at least a moderate calcium intake (two to three servings daily) because of the twin risks of increased urinary oxalate and loss of bone mineral. An even higher level of dietary calcium may be desirable, but optimum calcium intake in calcium stone-formers has not been defined. Refined carbohydrates and possibly alcohol are also calciuric, and high dietary fiber is hypocalciuric. Dietary measures should be tried before drug therapy in the treatment of idiopathic hypercalciuria: moderate sodium (100 to 125 mEq), moderate protein (60 to 70 g/day), moderate calcium (two dairy servings daily), high fiber, and low refined carbohydrates.

If metabolic activity is present despite high fluid intake and dietary modification, drug treatment is indicated. Thiazides work by two mechanisms: first, by causing ECF volume depletion and thereby increasing proximal tubular calcium absorption; second, by stimulating calcium reabsorption directly in the early distal convoluted tubule. A low-salt diet is essential in order that ECF volume contraction be maintained. Several recent double-blind trials have confirmed the efficacy of thiazides in reducing stone formation. Tachyphylaxis to thiazide treatment may occur after several years of successful treatment.

Another treatment that inhibits calciuria and stone formation is neutral orthophosphate. It works at multiple sites to inhibit calciuria and stone formation: reduced intestinal calcium absorption, increased tubular calcium absorption, reduced bone resorption, and increased urinary levels of pyrophospate, an inhibitor of calcium phosphate nucleation. A potassium preparation of neutral or alkaline pH is preferred, as acid or sodium increase calciuria. Phosphate should be given with meals, as it blunts protein-induced calciuria. Orthophosphate can cause diarrhea, and it is contraindicated in renal insufficiency and infection stones. Compared to thiazides it has fewer metabolic side effects, but it has not yet been proven efficacious in a controlled prospective study. Cellulose phosphate is a nonabsorbed form of phosphate that binds calcium in the gut. Its use should be avoided, as it increases urine oxalate excretion and risks bone mineral loss.

Hyperoxaluria

Oxalate is an end product of metabolism that forms a poorly soluble complex with calcium. Normal excretion is 15 to 40 mg daily, the bulk derived from endogenous synthesis. Physicochemical considerations suggest that a small increment in urinary oxalate has a larger effect on calcium oxalate saturation than a relatively greater increase in urinary calcium. Hyperoxaluria may be due to increased synthesis or increased intestinal absorption. Increased synthesis can be due to congenital enzyme deficiencies (primary hyperoxaluria types I and II), which produce extreme elevations of urinary oxalate, dense nephrocalcinosis, and renal failure in early adulthood (see Chapter 51). High vitamin C intake (2 g daily) in susceptible persons can also increase oxalate production, as can pyridoxine deficiency. Increased absorption can be due to high oxalate diet, intestinal malabsorption (enteric hyperoxaluria), or calcium restriction (or cellulose phosphate) in patients with idiopathic hypercalciuria. Enteric hyperoxaluria occurs particularly in Crohn's disease and ileal surgery; an intact colon is required. Three mechanisms have been proposed: (1) intestinal calcium is bound in soaps and unavailable for calcium oxalate complex formation, so free oxalate is hyperabsorbed in the colon; (2) poorly absorbed bile salts stimulate increased colonic transport of oxalate; and (3) poorly absorbed bile salts inactivate an oxalate-metabolizing bacterium (*Oxalobacter formigenes*) and thereby promote oxalate absorption. Dietary calcium restriction in patients with idiopathic hypercalciuria presumably enhances oxaluria by a similar mechanism, reducing luminal calcium and calcium-oxalate complexation and thereby increasing free oxalate absorption. Hyperoxaluria is treated by reducing dietary oxalate (tea, citrus juices, colas, spinach, rhubarb, peanuts, and chocolate) and adding magnesium supplements with meals (which bind intestinal oxalate). Pyridoxine is sometimes effective in rare cases of oxalate overproduction. Enteric oxaluria is treated with calcium supplements, which also bind intestinal oxalate; urinary calcium excretion is low and hypercalciuria is not a concern.

Hypocitraturia

Normal citrate excretion is 300 to 900 mg daily. Citrate acts as an inhibitor of nucleation by forming insoluble complexes with calcium. Urinary citrate is higher in premenopausal women than in men; it is also higher in pregnancy, teleologically a useful response as pregnancy markedly increases urinary calcium excretion. Idiopathic hypocitraturia is found in 10 to 40% of stone formers. Hypocitraturia also may be due to any cause of intracellular acidosis, including potassium deficiency, renal failure, distal (type I) renal tubular acidosis (RTA), chronic diarrheal states and malabsorption, or acetazolamide. In urinary tract infection, bacteria may metabolize citrate and reduce its urinary excretion.

Distal RTA causes a profound reduction of urinary citrate excretion, usually to less than 50 mg daily; it also causes hypercalciuria and persistently alkaline urine, but hypocitraturia is the most important contributor to stone diathesis. Measurement of urinary citrate is a useful alternative to acid loading to establish the diagnosis of distal RTA. Nephrocalcinosis and renal failure may occur. The alkali requirement to correct hypocitraturia (4 mEq · kg^{-1} · day^{-1} or more) may be higher than that required to correct systemic acidosis or hypokalemia (1 to 2 mEq · kg^{-1} · day^{-1}). Hypocitraturia may be the relevant guide to alkali dosage in these patients.

Potassium citrate is the treatment of choice of idiopathic hypocitraturia and of distal RTA, either in sustained release capsules or in liquid form. Sodium citrate or bicarbonate are less desirable, as their sodium content tends to increase calciuria. Thiazides reduce urinary citrate, presumably because of potassium depletion. Potassium citrate is the potassium supplement of choice in calcium stone formers.

Uric Acid

Hyperuricosuria is a risk factor for calcium stone formation, probably because uric acid acts as a surface for heterogeneous nucleation. Dietary purine restriction should suffice to ameliorate hyperuricosuria, which is usually due to high purine consumption. Allopurinol has been shown to reduce calcium stone formation in patients with isolated hyperuricosuria.

OTHER TYPES OF NEPHROLITHIASIS

Uric acid stones occur in two circumstances: excessive urinary uric acid and persistently acid urine. Only 20% of patients with uric acid stones have hyperuricosuria. Excessive urinary uric acid is due, with rare exceptions, to dietary purine overconsumption. Persistently acid urine, due to deficient renal ammoniagenesis, is a feature of gout and of idiopathic uric acid stones and of chronic diarrheal disease, because of loss of alkali equivalent in the stool. Uric acid is 10 to 20 times more soluble at pH 7 than at pH 5. Hence urine alkalinization is an effective treatment for most patients with uric acid stones; indeed it is more effective than allopurinol, which generally reduces uric acid excretion by about half. Target urine pH is 6.5 to 7.0, monitored by the patient with nitrazine paper; higher urine pH should be avoided because of the risk of calcium phosphate stones. Allopurinol can be added if uric acid production is excessive (over 1200 mg daily) and if dietary purine restriction is unsuccessful. Unlike calcium stones, uric acid stones dissolve during alkali therapy (if they are not secondarily calcified).

Infection stones are the most severe form of nephrolithiasis: they can cause progressive renal failure, urosepsis or perinephric abscess, intractable urinary tract infection, pain, and bleeding. Infection stones consist of struvite (magnesium ammonium phosphate) and apatite (calcium phosphate). They form only during urinary infection with urease-positive bacteria, usually *Proteus* or *Providencia* species, almost never *Escherichia coli*. These bacteria cleave urea to ammonia, elevating the urine pH to 8 or more and favoring precipitation of struvite and apatite. Bacterial infection is difficult to clear, as the organisms are inaccessible in stone interstices.

Approximately 40% of patients with struvite stones have an underlying metabolic abnormality; this abnormality (e.g., primary hyperparathyroidism) is presumed to be the original cause of nephrolithiasis. Secondary infection then causes formation of struvite stones. This pathogenesis is more likely if patients have had stone passage; patients with primary struvite stone formation and no other abnormality have large staghorn calculi and usually do not pass stones.

Treatment consists first of antibiotics, usually penicillin or ampicillin. Sterile urine is achieved in only about 20% of patients. Because of the large stone burden, stone removal usually requires combined percutaneous and extracorporeal lithotripsy. Infusion of acidifying solutions directly into the kidney can help to dissolve stones and clear fragments. If stone removal is complete, cure may be hoped for. If not, residual fragments are a nidus for intractable infection and recurrent stone formation, and antibiotic suppression is continued indefinitely. The urease inhibitor acetohydroxamic acid can help to prevent stone formation if urinary tract infection persists. However, it has been associated with hemolytic anemia, thrombophlebitis, and migraine.

Cystine stones result from an unusual inherited disorder in which renal tubular reabsorption of cystine, ornithine, arginine, and lysine (COAL) is reduced. Cystine is the disulfide reduction product of cysteine. The solubility of cystine is 250 to 300 mg/L. In patients with relatively low levels of cystinuria, high urine volume (4 L/day) will be sufficient to reduce the concentration of cystine below this threshold. It is particularly important to continue high fluid intake throughout the night, as there is disproportionate cystine excretion at that time. Those with more severe cystinuria require pharmacotherapy. Penicillamine or tiopronin react with cystine to form a soluble mixed cysteine disulfide; they also reduce cystine production. These agents are also indicated for stone dissolution.

UROLOGICAL MANAGEMENT OF STONES

Most symptomatic renal calculi (90%) pass spontaneously. The probability of spontaneous passage depends on width, length, and location of stone. Ureteral stones 4 mm or less in width are likely (more than 70%) to pass within 1 year; stones 8 mm or more in width are unlikely (less than 10%) to pass. Length of stone is less critical than width in determining rate of stone passage, presumably because stones orient lengthwise as they pass down the ureter. For example, a stone 6 mm in length has the same chance of spontaneous passage (85%) as a stone 3 mm in width. Stones that come to clinical attention in the lower ureter are twice as likely to pass as upper ureteral stones. Stones that are judged to be likely to pass and that are not associated with pain or obstruction are managed expectantly for

as long as 1 year. Indications for urological intervention for ureteral stones include obstruction, pain, fever, and observed or anticipated failure of spontaneous passage. On the basis of incomplete animal data, it is believed that complete obstruction requires relief within 2 weeks and partial obstruction within 4 to 6 weeks (depending on severity of hydronephrosis) to avoid permanent renal injury. Fever requires emergency decompression of the obstructed urinary tract with retrograde stent or percutaneous nephrostomy; definitive stone removal is deferred until infection resolves. Stones in the renal pelvis or upper ureter are treated with extracorporeal shock wave lithotripsy (ESWL); stents are placed in cases where large stone burden increases the risk of obstruction by pulverized material (Steinstrasse) after ESWL. Lower ureteral stones can also be treated with ESWL but the rate of success is only 70 to 80%; ureteroscopy with basket retrieval or ultrasonic or laser lithotripsy (for impacted stones) is successful in 98 to 99%. Recommendations for use of ESWL for asymptomatic intrarenal calculi are conflicting. With calyceal stones we reserve ESWL for the classic indications of pain, obstruction, or bleeding. However, a stone of 5 mm or more in the renal pelvis generally should have ESWL to prevent obstruction. ESWL requires that the distal urinary tract be free of obstruction so that fragmented material can pass; ESWL is contraindicated in obstruction, pregnancy, and aortic or renal artery aneurysm. In pregnancy, an obstructing stone can be managed with a retrograde stent till after delivery, when ESWL can safely be performed. The success of ESWL begins to diminish as stones exceed 1 cm and is poor with stones above 2 cm. In these cases, percutaneous lithotripsy is combined with ESWL. Cystine stones are relatively refractory to ESWL and percutaneous techniques may be necessary. ESWL and percutaneous techniques have dramatically reduced the need for open surgical treatment of nephrolithiasis; the latter accounts for less that 5% of urological interventions. ESWL and percutaneous lithotripsy are not without complications. Loss of renal function (particularly in the medulla where juxtamedullary nephrons may be involved), bleeding and hematoma, and urosepsis may occur even in the best centers. All patients undergoing either procedure should be screened with a urine culture and treated with appropriate antibiotics prior to the procedure. Patients should also be counseled that delayed hypertension may result, although this remains controversial.

Bibliography

Coe FL, Parks JH, Asplin JR: Pathogenesis and treatment of kidney stones. *N Engl J Med* 327:1141–1152, 1992.

Consensus Conference: Prevention and treatment of kidney stones. *JAMA* 260:977–981, 1988.

Curhan GC, Willett WC, Rimm EB, Stampfer MJ: A prospective study of dietary calcium and other nutrients and the risk of symptomatic kidney stones. *N Engl J Med* 328:833–838, 1993.

Goldfarb S: Dietary factors in the pathogenesis and prophylaxis of calcium nephrolithiasis. *Kidney Int* 34:544–555, 1987.

Hosking DH, Erickson SB, van den Berg CJ, Wilson DM, Smith L: The stone clinic effect in patients with idiopathic calcium urolithiasis. *J Urol* 130:1115–1158, 1983.

Lemann J: Composition of the diet and calcium kidney stones. *N Engl J Med* 328:880–882, 1993.

Lerner SP, Malachy JG, Griffith DP: Infection stones. *J Urol* 141:753–758, 1989.

Mulley AG, Carlson KJ, for the Health and Public Policy Committee, American College of Physicians: Lithotripsy. *Ann Intern Med* 103:626–629, 1985.

Nakagawa Y, Abram V, Kezdy FJ, Kaiser ET, Coe FL: Purification and characterization of the principal inhibitor of calcium oxalate

monohydrate crystal growth in human urine. *J Biol Chem* 256:3936–3944, 1981.

Pahira JJ: Management of the patient with cystinuria. *Urol Clin North Am* 14:339–346, 1987.

Pak CYC, Fuller C: Idiopathic hypocitraturic calcium-oxalate nephrolithiasis successfully treated with potassium citrate. *Ann Intern Med* 104:33–37, 1986.

Uribarri J, Oh MS, Carroll HJ: The first kidney stone. 111:1006–1009, 1989.

Wasserstein AG: Kidney stones: Advice on preventing first episodes and recurrences. *Consultant* 26:81–104, 1986.

URINARY TRACT INFECTIONS

WALTER E. STAMM

Urinary tract infections can be classified as uncomplicated or complicated. Due to their very different etiology, pathogenesis and management, uncomplicated and complicated urinary tract infections will be discussed separately.

UNCOMPLICATED URINARY TRACT INFECTION

Definition

Uncomplicated urinary tract infections (UTI) occur in patients without physiologic or anatomic abnormalities of the urinary tract and in the absence of recent urological surgery or instrumentation. They are community-acquired. Laboratory evidence of infection typically includes bacteriuria and pyuria; in some cases, hematuria may be present. Uncomplicated urinary tract infections can be further divided into acute cystitis (lower tract infection) and acute pyelonephritis (upper tract infection).

Etiology and Incidence

Almost all acute uncomplicated urinary tract infections occur in women, especially between the ages of 18 and 40. Infections occasionally occur before menarche but the incidence increases markedly in late adolescence and during the second and third decades of life. In the United States, an estimated 6 to 7 million cases of acute cystitis involve young women in this age range annually. At least

250,000 cases of acute pyelonephritis occur annually. Uncomplicated infections of the urinary tract are rare in males. Recent studies suggest that uncircumcised infants and adult homosexual males may be at increased risk. In young males, uncomplicated urinary tract infection may occasionally spread from the bladder to the prostate (acute prostatitis) or the epididymis (acute epididymitis), but such cases are also infrequent.

Uncomplicated urinary tract infections are caused by a very narrow spectrum of microbes. Eighty percent are due to *Escherichia coli. Staphylococcus saprophyticus* causes 10 to 15% of uncomplicated urinary tract infections in young women, especially during the summer and fall months. *Proteus mirabilis* and *Klebsiella* are occasional causes (2 to 5%).

Pathogenesis

Uncomplicated urinary tract infections in women are caused by fecal *E. coli* that migrate from the perianal skin to colonize the vaginal introitus and urethra. The organisms then ascend through the urethra into the bladder and, in cases of acute uncomplicated pyelonephritis, from the bladder to the kidney via the ureters. Both bacterial and host factors are important in predisposing to acute uncomplicated urinary tract infection. Sexual intercourse appears to facilitate migration of bacteria from the periurethral zone into the bladder. Diaphragm–spermicide use and spermicide use alone have also been linked to an increased risk, probably via spermicide-mediated alterations in the vaginal flora that result in overgrowth with *E. coli.* Some women may be predisposed to recurrent urinary tract infections because their uroepithelial cells have increased number of receptors for *E. coli,* a trait that may be genetically determined. Behavioral factors such as not voiding after intercourse or postponing voiding also appear to increase risk of infection. Uropathogenic *E. coli* (particularly those *E. coli* strains that cause urinary tract infection) appear to possess specific virulence determinants such as fimbriae or production of hemolysin or aerobactin that enable them to colonize and infect the urinary tract more efficiently than strains lacking these virulence factors.

Clinical Manifestations

Typical symptoms of acute uncomplicated cystitis include dysuria, frequency, urgency, voiding of small urine volumes, and suprapubic or lower abdominal pain. Up to one-third of patients may develop gross hematuria, and many patients describe foul-smelling or cloudy urine. On examination, suprapubic tenderness may be present. Fever and costovertebral angle tenderness are generally absent.

Acute pyelonephritis characteristically presents with localized flank, low-back, or abdominal pain accompanied by fever, chills, sweats, headache, nausea, vomiting, and malaise. Symptoms of lower tract infection may or may not be present. On examination, fever and flank tenderness are present. The severity of illness associated with acute pyelonephritis ranges from very mild to quite severe, including gram-negative septicemia and necrotizing intrarenal or perinephric abscesses. Approximately 20% of patients with acute uncomplicated pyelonephritis have positive blood cultures.

Differential Diagnosis

Acute bacterial cystitis must be distinguished from other common genital infections that produce dysuria, most commonly, vulvovaginitis due to yeast, trichomonas, or bacterial vaginosis, or sexually transmitted infections that involve both the urethra and cervix (*Chlamydia trachomatis, Neisseria gonorrhoeae,* or herpes simplex virus infection). Typically, bacterial cystitis is sudden in onset and produces multiple urinary symptoms (dysuria, urgency, frequency, and gross hematuria), while urethritis due to sexually transmitted pathogens causes milder symptoms, is more gradual in onset, and is often characterized by dysuria without other urinary symptoms. Signs of cervicitis may also be present in these women. Although dysuria may be the presenting complaint, on further questioning most women with vaginitis have other symptoms suggesting that diagnosis, including vaginal discharge, vaginal odor, or dyspareunia. The presence of hematuria (gross or microscopic) strongly suggests bacterial cystitis since women with vaginitis or urethritis caused by STD agents seldom have hematuria.

Acute pyelonephritis must be differentiated from other intraabdominal conditions seen in young women, most importantly pelvic inflammatory disease, appendicitis, ectopic pregnancy, or ruptured ovarian cyst.

Diagnosis

The suspected diagnosis of acute uncomplicated lower urinary tract infection can be readily confirmed by microscopic examination of the urine and by urine culture. Essentially all women with acute cystitis have associated pyuria if a careful microscopic examination of unspun urine is performed. Additionally, up to 50% may have microscopic hematuria. The leukocyte esterase dipstick can also be used to rapidly screen a urine specimen for pyuria but is less sensitive than a microscopic exam. Culture of midstream urine will generally demonstrate the etiologic bacterial agent in concentrations $\geq 10^5$ cfu/mL. However, in about one-third of cases, colony counts will range from 10^2 to 10^4 colony-forming units per milliliter. The Gram stain of unspun urine will demonstrate the etiologic agent in cases with $\geq 10^5$ cfu/mL of bacteria, but will be negative in cases with lower bacterial counts. Thus, a negative urine Gram stain does not rule out acute bacterial cystitis in those cases characterized by low colony counts.

In acute pyelonephritis, urinalysis nearly always demonstrates pyuria, and in 80% of cases, bacteriuria can be seen on the Gram stain of unspun urine. About 20% of cases have colony counts $<10^5$/mL and thus negative Gram stains. Urine culture will almost always confirm the presence of the infecting organism, and blood cultures are positive in 20% of patients. The presence of leukocyte casts in a freshly voided specimen of urine strongly supports the diagnosis, but casts are demonstrable in only 20 to 40% of cases.

Treatment

Women with acute uncomplicated cystitis should generally be treated with 3-day course of trimethoprim, trimethoprim-sulfamethoxazole, or a fluoroquinolone such as norfloxacin, ciprofloxacin, ofloxacin, lomefloxacin, or enoxacin (Table 1). Single-dose therapy results in higher recurrence rates and is thus not recommended. The frequent occurrence of *in vitro* resistance to ampicillin, amoxicillin, and first-generation cephalosporins among *E. coli* strains causing uncomplicated infections, plus the propensity of these agents to foster recurrences, argues against their routine use. These agents, however, are the agents of choice for treatment of cystitis during pregnancy, and should generally be given for 7 days. Patients who recur after an initial 3-day course of therapy should be treated with a 7-day course with one of the above antimicrobials. Women with multiple recent infections, with symptoms longer than 7 days, who are pregnant, or who have other complicating factors should also be treated initially with a 7-day regimen.

Patients with acute uncomplicated pyelonephritis can be safely treated in the outpatient setting if they have no nausea or vomiting, no evidence of septicemia, are reliable, are not pregnant, and have a clear-cut diagnosis. Fourteen

TABLE I
Treatment Regimens for Bacterial Urinary Tract Infections

Condition	Characteristic pathogens	Mitigating circumstances	Recommended empirical treatment[a]
Acute uncomplicated cystitis in women	*E. coli, S. saprophyticus, P. mirabilis, Klebsiella pneumoniae*	None	3-day regimens: oral trimethoprim-sulfamethoxazole, trimethoprim, norfloxacin, ciprofloxacin, ofloxacin, lomefloxacin, or enoxacin[b]
		Diabetes, symptoms for >7 days, recent urinary tract infection, use of diaphragm, age >65 yr	Consider 7-day regimen: oral trimethoprim-sulfamethoxazole, trimethoprim, norfloxacin, ciprofloxacin, ofloxacin, lomefloxacin or enoxacin[b]
		Pregnancy	Consider 7-day regimen: oral amoxicillin, macrocrystalline nitrofurantoin, cefpodoxime proxetil, or trimethoprim-sulfamethoxazole[b]
Acute uncomplicated pyelonephritis in women	*E. coli, P. mirabilis, K. pneumoniae, S. saprophyticus*	Mild-to-moderate illness, no nausea or vomiting—outpatient therapy	Oral[c] trimethoprim-sulfamethoxazole, norfloxacin, ciprofloxacin, ofloxacin, lomefloxacin, or enoxacin for 10–14 days
		Severe illness or possible urosepsis—hospitalization required	Parenteral[d] trimethoprim-sulfamethoxazole, ceftriaxone, ciprofloxacin, ofloxacin, or gentamicin (with or without ampicillin) until fever gone; then oral[c] trimethoprim-sulfamethoxazole, norfloxacin, ciprofloxacin, ofloxacin, lomefloxacin, or enoxacin for 14 days
		Pregnancy—hospitalization recommended	Parenteral[d] ceftriaxone, gentamicin (with or without ampicillin), aztreonam or trimethoprim-sulfamethoxazole until fever gone; then oral[c] amoxicillin, a cephalosporin, or trimethoprim-sulfamethoxazole for 14 days
Complicated urinary tract infection	*E. coli,* proteus species, klebsiella species, pseudomonas species, serratia species, enterococci, staphylococci	Mild-to-moderate illness, no nausea or vomiting—outpatient therapy	Oral[c] norfloxacin, ciprofloxacin, ofloxacin, lomefloxacin, or enoxacin for 10–14 days
		Severe illness or possible urosepsis—hospitalization required	Parenteral[d] ampicillin and gentamicin, ciprofloxacin, ofloxacin, ceftriaxone, aztreonam, ticarcillin-clavulanate, or imipenem-cilastatin until fever gone; then oral[c] trimethoprim-sulfamethoxazole, norfloxacin, ciprofloxacin, ofloxacin, lomefloxacin, or enoxacin for 14–21 days

[a] Treatments listed are those to be prescribed before the etiologic agent is known (Gram's staining can be helpful); they can be modified once the agent has been identified. The recommendations are the authors' and are limited to drugs currently approved by the Food and Drug Administration, although not all the regimens listed are approved for these indications. Fluoroquinolones should not be used in pregnancy. Trimethoprim-sulfamethoxazole, although not approved for use in pregnancy, has been widely used. Gentamicin should be used with caution in pregnancy because of its possible toxicity to eighth-nerve development in the fetus.

[b] Multiday oral regimens for cystitis are as follows: trimethoprim-sulfamethoxazole, 160–800 mg every 12 hr; trimethoprim, 100 mg every 12 hr; norfloxacin, 400 mg every 12 hr; ciprofloxacin, 250 mg every 12 hr; ofloxacin, 200 mg every 12 hr; lomefloxacin, 400 mg every day; enoxacin, 400 mg every 12 hr; macrocrystalline nitrofurantoin, 100 mg four times a day; amoxicillin, 250 mg every 8 hr; and cefpodoxime proxetil, 100 mg every 12 hr.

[c] Oral regimens for pyelonephritis and complicated urinary tract infection are as follows: trimethoprim-sulfamethoxazole, 160–800 mg every 12 hr; norfloxacin, 400 mg every 12 hr; ciprofloxacin, 500 mg every 12 hr, ofloxacin, 200–300 mg every 12 hr, lomefloxacin, 400 mg every day; enoxacin, 400 mg every 12 hr, amoxicillin, 500 mg every 8 hr; and cefpodoxime proxetil, 200 mg every 12 hr.

[d] Parenteral regimens are as follows: trimethoprim-sulfamethoxazole, 160–800 mg every 12 hr; ciprofloxacin, 200–400 mg every 12 hr; ofloxacin, 200–400 mg every 12 hr; gentamicin, $1 \text{ mg} \cdot \text{kg}^{-1} \cdot \text{body}^{-1}$ every 8 hr; ceftriaxone, 1–2 g every day; ampicillin, 1 g every 6 hours; imipenem-cilastatin, 250–500 mg every 6–8 hr; ticarcillin-clavulanate, 3.2 g every 8 hr; and aztreonam, 1 g every 8 to 12 hr.

days of trimethoprim-sulfamethoxazole, trimethoprim alone, or a fluoroquinolone are preferred regimens (Table 1). For inpatients, parenteral therapy should be used initially. Depending on the local antimicrobial sensitivity pat-

terns of uropathogens causing acute uncomplicated pyelonephritis, preferred regimens include trimethoprim-sulfamethoxazole, gentamicin, a fluoroquinolone, or a third-generation cephalosporin which should be given intravenously until defervescence and signs of clinical improvement occur. In 80% of patients, improvement occurs within 72 hours, at which time oral therapy can be provided for the remainder of the treatment course. Extension of the period of therapy is not required solely because a patient had positive blood cultures. Routine use of ultrasound or CT scanning in hospitalized cases of acute uncomplicated pyelonephritis has not apparent benefit, but failure to improve after 72 hours of appropriate antibiotic therapy indicates the need to seek evidence of obstruction or an abscess.

Prognosis

Acute uncomplicated cystitis responds to effective initial therapy in over 90% of cases. The remainder respond either to a second treatment course or more prolonged therapy. Twenty percent of women with acute uncomplicated cystitis develop a pattern of frequent recurrences characterized by episodes occurring as often as once per month or once every other month. Episodes of cystitis, even when they recur frequently, do not appear to produce long-term sequelae.

Acute uncomplicated pyelonephritis also responds to antimicrobials in over 90% of cases. Failure to respond to initial antimicrobial therapy should suggest a drug-resistant strain, an anatomic abnormality, or urinary obstruction. Acute pyelonephritis generally heals without significant renal scarring and without impairment of renal function. Some women with acute pyelonephritis develop intranephric or perinephric abscesses that do not respond to antimicrobial therapy and require either percutaneous drainage or surgical intervention along with prolonged antibiotic administration. Intranephric or perinephric abscesses should be suspected if a pyelonephritis-like illness does not respond to appropriate antimicrobial therapy or in patients with fever and unilateral flank pain for 2 or more weeks. Other risk factors for abscess formation include diabetes mellitus and nephrolithiasis. Renal ultrasound or a CT scan will establish the presence of intrarenal and perinephric abscesses.

In women prone to frequent recurrent episodes of cystitis, low-dose antimicrobial prophylaxis reduces the incidence of recurrent infections to nearly zero and can be used safely for long periods. Successfully used regimens include daily or thrice weekly trimethoprim (100 mg), trimethoprim-sulfamethoxazole ($\frac{1}{2}$ single-strength tablet daily), or nitrofurantoin (100 mg daily). Women who can temporally relate their recurrent infections to intercourse can use these same regimens after intercourse rather than on a regular basis. Voiding soon after intercourse also reduces the likelihood of recurrent urinary tract infections. In diaphragm–spermicide users who develop recurrent urinary tract infections, use of an alternative contraceptive may be warranted. In postmenopausal women with frequently recurring uncomplicated cystitis, topically applied intravaginal estrogen may also be an effective means of prevention.

COMPLICATED URINARY TRACT INFECTIONS

Complicated urinary tract infections occur in patients with obstruction, anatomic, or functional disorders of the urinary tract. Instrumentation, calculi, and catheterization also predispose to complicated infection, as does pregnancy which induces hydroureter, bladder enlargement, and urinary stasis (Table 2).

Etiology and Incidence

Complicated urinary tract infections occur most frequently at the extremes of life. Urinary infections in newborns or infants often indicate an underlying anatomic abnormality in the urinary tract. While such infections occur in fewer than 2% of infants, their occurrence should prompt the use of appropriate urological studies to seek an underlying anatomic abnormality. The vast majority of complicated urinary tract infections occur in older men and women. In men, the occurrence of urinary tract infections is less than 1% until the fifth to sixth decade, at which time prostatic hypertrophy and obstruction occur, leading to urological instrumentation. With aging, hospitalization for other illnesses often leads to urinary catheterization and acquisition of nosocomial urinary tract infections. Over 10% of hospitalized patients have urinary catheters placed, and approximately 10 to 15% of them develop subsequent bacteriuria. Catheter-associated urinary tract infections account for 40% of all nosocomial infections, over one million infections annually. In addition, urosepsis secondary to catheter-associated bacteriuria is the most common source of gram-negative bacteremia in hospitalized patients.

The spectrum of bacterial species causing complicated and hospital-acquired urinary tract infections is much broader than that seen in community-acquired infections. While *E. coli* remains the most common organism, many other gram-negative bacilli cause complicated urinary infections, including *Proteus mirabilis,* other proteus species, providencia, serratia, klebsiella, and pseudomonas. These organisms generally exhibit more antimicrobial resistance than those causing uncomplicated urinary infection. In addition, enterococci and pseudomonas are far more frequent in this setting than in uncomplicated urinary tract infections, and *Staphyloccus aureus* causes complicated infections as well. Increasingly, yeast (candida) infections are

TABLE 2
Factors Associated with Complicated Urinary
Tract Infections

Indwelling or intermittent urinary catheter
Urinary instrumentation or urological surgery
Postvoid residual urine (>100 mL)
Urinary obstruction
Vesicoureteral reflux
Urologic anatomic abnormality
Azotemia, renal dysfunction
Renal transplantation
Neurogenic bladder
Pregnancy
Male patient
Nephrolithiasis
Diabetes

being seen in catheter-associated infections, in diabetics, and in immunosuppressed patients.

Pathogenesis

As in uncomplicated infections, most bacteria causing complicated UTI invade the urinary tract in an ascending manner. Rarely, the kidney is infected secondary to bacteremia. Obstruction to urine flow or other functional abnormalities of the urinary tract impair the normally efficient ability of the bladder to eliminate bacteria. Instrumentation of the urinary tract, particularly catheterization, provides a portal of entry for bacteria and also makes it more difficult to eradicate bacteriuria with antimicrobial agents. Vesicoureteral reflux may facilitate the ease with which bladder bacteria can ascend to the kidney, producing pyelonephritis. Interestingly, most of the bacteria causing complicated urinary infection lack the specific urovirulence determinants characteristic of strains causing uncomplicated UTI, suggesting that their pathogenicity relates mainly to host impairment.

Clinical Manifestations

The clinical manifestations produced by complicated urinary tract infection range widely from asymptomatic bacteriuria to gram-negative septicemia. Most catheter-associated urinary tract infections, for example, remain asymptomatic and do not produce clinical manifestations. Similarly, asymptomatic bacteriuria without an associated catheter is common in elderly patients. In some patients, complicated urinary tract infections will present with either the syndrome of acute cystitis or acute pyelonephritis as outlined above. The hallmark of such episodes in the complicated setting is their lesser responsiveness to antimicrobial therapy and their tendency to recur after treatment. In hospitalized patients who develop fever, hypotension, and signs of septicemia, the urinary tract should be suspected as a possible source despite the absence of urinary symptoms, especially in patients with recent instrumentation or catheterization.

Differential Diagnosis

The considerations outlined for uncomplicated urinary tract infections apply in the setting of complicated urinary tract infections as well. In patients with septicemia, urosepsis must be differentiated from other potential sources of bacteremia. The presence of recent instrumentation, catheterization, and evidence of bacteriuria and pyuria strongly suggests urosepsis.

Diagnosis

In symptomatic patients, urinary microscopy and culture should be used to confirm the presence of infection as described for uncomplicated UTI. In asymptomatic bacteriuria, at least two successive cultures growing the same organism in quantities greater than or equal to 10^5/mL should be obtained to confirm the diagnosis.

Since by definition, complicated UTIs occur in patients with abnormal urinary tract anatomy or function, determining which patients should undergo further study is a key issue. The yield of anatomic evaluation in women with no risk factors is low and anatomic evaluation in this population should be reserved for women with frequent recurrences or slow response to treatment. Men are much more likely to have anatomic defects, in particular bladder outlet obstruction from prostate enlargement, and appropriate evaluation is in order after a first UTI. Patients presenting with hypotension or other features of sepsis should also be evaluated since prompt drainage of obstruction is essential. Evaluation for reflux or other anatomic defects should be strongly considered in children, particularly those younger than 5 years of age, with a first or second UTI.

Depending on the clinical circumstance, computed tomography scanning, ultrasound, or intravenous pyelography may be useful in demonstrating the nature of the urologic abnormality or obstruction. These procedures may also be useful in identifying focal infections such as a perinephric or intranephric abscess or nephrolithiasis.

Treatment

Asymptomatic bacteriuria in the patient with a urinary catheter, as well as in the elderly noncatheterized patient, should ordinarily not be treated. Treatment in such patients should be instituted if clinically apparent infection arises or in special circumstances such as patients who are neutropenic or have a renal allograft. Asymptomatic bacteriuria should always be treated in pregnancy due to the markedly increased risk of ascending infection with attendant complications for both mother and child.

Selection of antimicrobials for treatment of symptomatic complicated urinary tract infections should take into account the relatively broad array of bacterial species that cause such infections and the degree of illness in the patient (Table 1). For septicemia in hospitalized patients, parenteral therapy with broad spectrum agents must be used initially until the infecting organism is identified. Initial therapy should provide an effective antimicrobial spectrum that includes activity against the enterococcus and pseudomonas. Acceptable regimens include ampicillin plus gentamicin, imipenem-ciliastatin, or a third-generation cephalosporin with antipseudomonal activity. Once the etiologic agent is known, therapy can be specifically targeted to the infecting agent. In patients with complicated urinary tract infection who have lesser degrees of illness and can be managed in the outpatient setting, fluoroquinolones can be given orally. The duration of therapy for complicated urinary tract infections ranges from 7 to 21 days, depending on the clinical circumstance. Prolonged therapy may be needed in patients with urinary calculi. In catheterized patients with candiduria, amphotericin bladder washes may be effective, especially if the catheter can be removed. Oral fluconazole can also be used. The relative efficacy of these therapeutic approaches has not been established.

Prognosis

Complicated urinary tract infections often recur unless the underlying anatomic or functional defect can be corrected. Infection usually cannot be eradicated in patients with nephrolithiasis without removal of the calculi, either by surgical means (in the case of larger or staghorn calculi) or by lithotripsy (in the case of smaller stones). Patients with indwelling catheters will continue to develop episodes of infection despite treatment of individual episodes as they arise. Infections caused by pseudomonas and enterococci are especially prone to recurrence. Chronic and recurrent infections of the urinary tract may lead to suppurative sequelae or to loss of functioning renal tissue with subsequent impaired renal function.

Prevention

Urinary catheters should not be used unless they are medically indicated. Sterile insertion and maintenance of a closed catheter system can reduce the incidence of catheter-associated urinary tract infections. Condom catheters may be an alternative. As the prevalence of infection increases with the duration of catheterization, catheters should always be removed as soon as possible. In particular, the junction between the distal catheter and the collecting system should remain closed, downhill gravity drainage should be maintained at all times, and sterile technique should be used whenever urine is drained from the collecting bag. Detailed guidelines for prevention of catheter-associated infections have been published elsewhere. Antimicrobial prophylaxis has no value in chronically catheterized patients or in most patients with intermittent asymptomatic

bacteriuria. Antimicrobial prophylaxis should be provided to patients undergoing prostatic surgery or other urological procedures since such prophylaxis prevents postoperative urinary tract infection and urosepsis. All pregnant women should be screened for bacteriuria in the first trimester and treated if positive.

Bibliography

Hooton TM, Scholes D, Hughes JP, et al.: A prospective study of risk factors for symptomatic urinary tract infections in young women. *N Engl J Med* 355:468–474, 1996.

Johnson JR, Stamm WE: Urinary tract infections in women: Diagnosis and treatment. *Ann Intern Med* 11:906–912, 1989.

Lipsky BA: Urinary tract infections in men: Epidemiology, pathophysiology, diagnosis, and treatment. *Ann Intern Med* 110:138–150, 1989.

Schaeffer AJ, Jones JM, Dunn JK: Association of in vitro Escherichia coli adherence to vaginal and buccal epithelial cells with susceptibility of women to recurrent urinary tract infections. *N Engl J Med* 304:1062–1066, 1981.

Stamm WE: Catheter-associated urinary tract infections: Epidemiology, pathogenesis, and prevention. *Am J Med* 91(Suppl 3B):65S–71S, 1991.

Stamm WE, Hooton TM, Johnson JR, et al.: Urinary tract infections: From pathogeneis to treatment. *J Infect Dis* 159:400–406, 1989.

Stamm WE, Hooton TM: Management of urinary tract infections in adults. *N Engl J Med* 329:1328–1334, 1993.

Strom BL, Collins M, West SL, Sreisberg J, Weller S: Sexual activity, contraceptive use, and other risk factors for symptomatic and asymptomatic bacteriuria. *Ann Intern Med* 107:816–823, 1987.

RENAL AND URINARY TRACT NEOPLASIA

ROBERT R. BAHNSON

It is estimated that in 1996, approximately 83,000 individuals will be diagnosed with cancer of urinary organs (bladder, kidney, and other urinary) and roughly 24,000 deaths from urinary neoplasia will occur. In addition, more than 317,000 men will be diagnosed with cancer of the prostate and more than 41,000 will die from this common malignancy (Table 1). Neoplasms of the kidney, renal pelvis, ureter, bladder, and prostate will be discussed separately highlighting their etiology, pathology, diagnosis, staging, and treatment.

RENAL NEOPLASMS

Etiology

The most common cancer of the kidney is renal cell carcinoma. The tumor is more common in men, with a male : female ratio of roughly 2 : 1. It is generally a tumor of adults, with peak incidence between the fifth and seventh decades of life. A recessive oncogene located on chromosome 3p (short arm) is associated with the formation of

TABLE I

	Estimated new cases of urinary organ cancer			Estimated deaths from urinary organ cancer		
	Bladder	Kidney and other urinary	Prostate	Bladder	Kidney and other urinary	Prostate
Men	38,300	18,500	317,000	7800	7300	41,400
Women	14,600	12,100		3900	4700	
Total	52,900	30,600		11,700	12,000	

both sporadic and familial renal cell carcinoma. This observation is supported by findings of loss of chromosome 3p alleles in renal cell carcinomas from patients with von Hippel-Lindau (VHL) disease. VHL syndrome is a hereditary disease characterized by spinal and cerebellar hemangioblastomas, retinal angiomas, pheochromocytomas, renal and pancreatic cysts, cystadenomas of the epididymis, and renal cell carcinomas. From 28 to 45% of VHL patients will develop renal cell carcinomas of the clear cell type. The tumors in these patients occur early in life (mean age at diagnosis is 39 years) and are frequently multiple and bilateral. No definite causal relationship between environmental carcinogens and the development of renal cell carcinoma has been documented.

Patients with chronic end stage renal disease (ESRD) often develop acquired cystic disease of the kidney (ACDK). Approximately 1 to 4% of these patients develop renal carcinoma. This rate is roughly three to six times greater than that of the general population.

Pathology

The proximal tubular cell has been identified by electron microscopy and monoclonal antibodies as the origin of renal cell carcinoma. The tumor is generally composed of four common histologic types: clear cell, granular cell, tubulo papillary, and sarcomatoid. These cells grow in solid sheets, trabecular patterns, or less commonly in papillary configurations. The sarcomatoid renal cell carcinoma is also known as the bone-metastasizing variant because of its predilection for bony metastases. This histologic subtype is characterized by aggressive clinical behavior and a poor prognosis.

Diagnosis

Renal cell carcinoma has often been called the internist's tumor due to the variety of its presentation and the uncommon number of systemic syndromes that have been reported to occur in patients with the disease (Table 2). The classic triad of flank pain, palpable mass, and hematuria is present in only 10% of patients and is often an indication of advanced disease. The majority of clinically confined renal tumors are now discovered serendipitously by ultrasound, computed tomography (CT), and magnetic resonance imaging (MRI). As an initial radiologic test, ultrasound can distinguish cystic, solid, and complex renal masses. Any mass that does not meet the criteria for simple

cyst should be further evaluated by CT. As a single diagnostic imaging study, CT scanning is probably the best method to evaluate a suspected renal mass lesion as it gives fairly reliable information about the local extension of tumor, lymph node involvement, and presence of tumor thrombus in the renal vein or inferior vena cava. Renal arteriography is seldom necessary unless required for the planning of parenchyma sparing surgery.

The issue of screening for renal cell carcinoma in VHL and ACKD is controversial (see Chapter 45). Since renal involvement in VHL occurs in 28 to 66% of patients and bilateral renal cell cancers develop in 63 to 75% of those with renal lesions it has been recommended by some that such lesions be followed by annual CT examinations. ACKD increases significantly in frequency after 3 years of dialysis. As in VHL, CT is probably the best imaging technique. Clearly any patient with VHL or ACKD with symptoms or hematuria should undergo a complete imaging evaluation.

Staging

Staging of kidney carcinoma is best performed using the tumor, node, metastases (TNM) classification agreed on by the International Union Against Cancer and the American Joint Committee on Cancer (Table 3). Cost effective clinical staging of patients can be accomplished with a history and physical exam, chest X ray, liver function tests, and serum calcium determination. The most frequent sites of metastases in decreasing order of frequency are lymph nodes, lung, liver, and bone. Patients with a palpable liver or abnormalities of liver functions should have further radiographic or radionuclide imaging of the liver. Symptoms of skeletal involvement or an increase in serum calcium or alkaline phosphatase should prompt a radionuclide bone scan.

Treatment

The only successful treatment for patients with localized renal cell carcinoma is surgical extirpation. Radial nephrectomy, removal of the kidney with its surrounding fascial envelope (Gerota's) and the ipsilateral adrenal gland, is the preferred surgical approach. The 5-year survival of patients with node negative tumors without metastases ranges from 47 to 82%. The presence of positive lymph nodes or distant metastasis augurs poorly for survival beyond 2 years. Regrettably, radiation therapy and chemo-

TABLE 2

Incidence of Systemic Syndromes in Patients
with Renal Cell Carcinoma

Syndrome	%
Raised erythrocyte sedimentation rate	55.6
Hypertension	37.5
Anemia	36.3
Cachexia, Weight loss	34.5
Pyrexia	17.2
Abnormal liver function	14.4
Raised alkaline phosphatase	10.1
Hypercalcemia	4.9
Polycythemia	3.5
Neuromyopathy	3.2
Amyloidosis	2.0

therapy have been of limited value in this disease. Several studies have failed to confirm an advantage to treated patients who received either pre- or postoperative radiotherapy. Multiple, single agent, and combination chemotherapy trials have proven that renal cell carcinoma is highly resistant to commonly employed cytoxic agents. The single most active drug appears to be vinblastine, but objective response rates are too low to justify its routine use.

The most promising therapy of metastatic renal cell carcinoma in the past decade has been immunotherapy. Nonspecific active, systemic immunotherapy with bacillus Calmette-Guerin (BCG) or *Cornybacterium parvum* has shown only modest success. Cytokine therapy utilizing interferons has shown response rates reported in the 15 to 20% range. Most patients who respond have undergone nephrectomy, have an excellent pretreatment performance status, and have limited pulmonary metastases. Rosenberg and colleagues at NCI have used adoptive immunotherapy with lymphokine-activated killer (LAK) cells and interleukin-2 (IL-2). They reported a 35% objective response rate in 72 patients with renal cell carcinoma. Since then, efforts of this group have focused on using genetically altered tumor infiltrating lymphocytes (TIL) which are grown from single-cell tumor suspensions cultured in IL-2. Response rates of 0 to 33% have been reported in five trials of combination IL-2/TIL in patients with metastatic renal cell carcinoma.

Other Renal Tumors

Renal Oncocytoma

Oncocytomas constitute approximately 5% of solid renal neoplasms and invariably pursue a benign course. Microscopically these tumors are composed of polygonal cells with intense eosinophilia, granular cytoplasm, and abundant mitochondria. Grossly, on cut section, these tumors have brown pigmentation and are often associated with a central scar. The origin of these tumors is thought to be the distal collecting tubule. Because preoperative diagnosis is difficult and because oncocytomas can coexist with renal

cell carcinoma, the treatment of choice is radical nephrectomy.

Angiomyolipoma

Angiomyolipomas are hamartomas composed of blood vessels, adipocytes, and abundant smooth muscle. They are seen commonly in patients with tuberous sclerosis and have a tendency to multiplicity and bilaterality. The fat content of these lesions often permits radiographic diagnosis with CT imaging. Asymptomatic tumors under 4 cm may be observed with radiographic monitoring. Symptomatic lesions can often be treated with angioinfarction. If surgery is required, excision of the lesion using renal parenchymal sparing techniques should be attempted because of the tendency toward multiplicity and bilaterality.

Sarcomas

Sarcomas represent less than 5% of all malignant tumors of the kidney. The most common sarcoma is leiomyosarcoma. Others include osteogenic sarcoma, liposarcoma, carcinosarcoma, fibrosarcoma, rhabdomyosarcoma, and malignant fibrous histiocytoma. The treatment of choice for all of these tumors is radical nephrectomy, if possible.

Metastatic Tumors

Because of their rich vascularity, the kidneys are frequently the site of metastatic spread. These tumors are often asymptomatic and discovered only at autopsy. Lymphoma is probably the most common metastatic neoplasm of the kidney; it may involve the renal parenchyma diffusely. With the exception of lymphomatous involvement which may respond to systemic therapy, treatment is usually unnecessary since the patient's prognosis from their primary tumor is almost uniformly poor.

RENAL PELVIC AND URETERAL TUMORS

Epithelial tumors of the upper urinary tract are uncommon. They show a male to female predominance of roughly 2:1 and are more common among whites than African-Americans. Tumors of the upper urinary tracts are common in patients with Balkan nephropathy and are more frequently bilateral. These upper tract tumors are commonly associated with bladder tumors which occur in 40 to 75% of patients at some point in time. Patients with bladder tumors have a slight (2 to 13%) chance of developing ureteral or renal pelvic tumors.

Etiology

An increased risk of renal pelvic and ureteral tumors has been reported for patients who smoke, abuse analgesics (particularly phenacetin), and who have been occupationally exposed to chemicals, petrochemicals, plastics, coke, coal, asphalt, and tar. Among these, cigarette smoking is the major risk factor for carcinoma of the upper urinary tract.

Pathology

Transitional cell carcinoma accounts for more than 90% of all upper tract urothelial tumors. The remaining 10%

TABLE 3
The Staging of Kidney Cancer

Primary tumor (T)				
TX	Primary tumor cannot be assessed			
TO	No evidence of primary tumor			
T1	Tumor 2.5 cm or less in greatest dimension, limited to the kidney			
T2	Tumor more than 2.5 cm in greatest dimension, limited to the kidney			
T3	Tumor extends into major veins or invades adrenal gland or perinephric tissues, but not beyond Gerota's fascia			
	T3a Tumor invades adrenal gland or perinephric tissues, but not beyond Gerota's fascia			
	T3b Tumor grossly extends into renal vein(s) or vena cava			
T4	Tumor invades beyond Gerotas fascia			

Regional lymph nodes (N)

The regional lymph nodes are the abdominal para-aortic, paracaval, and renal hilar. Laterality does not affect the N classification. The significance of the regional lymph node metastasis in staging kidney cancer lies in the number and size and not in whether unilateral or contralateral.

NX	Regional lymph nodes cannot be assessed
N0	No regional lymph node metastasis
N1	Metastasis in a single lymph node, 2 cm or less in greatest dimension
N2	Metastasis in a single lymph node, more than 2 cm but not more than 5 cm in greatest dimension, or multiple lymph nodes, none more than 5 cm in greatest dimension
N3	Metastasis in a lymph node more than 5 cm in greatest dimension

Distant metastasis (M)

MX	Presence of distant metastasis cannot be assessed
M0	No distant metastasis
M1	Distant metastasis

AJCC/UICC stage grouping

Stage I	T1	N0	M0
Stage II	T2	N0	M0
Stage III	T1	N1	M0
	T2	N1	M0
	T3a	N0	M0
	T3a	N1	M0
	T3b	N0	M0
	T3b	N1	M0
Stage IV	T4	Any N	M0
	Any T	N2	M0
	Any T	N3	M0
	Any T	Any N	M1

consists of adenocarcinoma, squamous cell carcinomas, and inverted papillomas. Nonurothelial tumors are exceedingly rare.

Diagnosis

The most common presentation of upper tract tumors is gross, total (i.e., bloody throughout micturition), painless hematuria. The presence of string-like clots is suggestive of an upper tract origin of the bleeding. The diagnosis is confirmed by radiologic imaging, most often with excretory or retrograde urography. At the time that retrograde pyelography is undertaken, saline barbotage and/or brush biopsy of the lesion can be performed. Cellular material obtained by such maneuvers can be examined cytopathologically to confirm the diagnosis.

Staging

Metastatic evaluation is best performed utilizing CT scanning to assess the presence and degree of local, regional, and distant disease. Staging is illustrated in Table 4.

Treatment

The treatment of upper tract urothelial tumors almost always involves surgical excision. Neither radiotherapy nor chemotherapy has been shown in large series to have a substantial impact on response or survival. Renal pelvic tumors are treated by nephroureterectomy with bladder cuff excision because the risk of ipsilateral ureteral or bladder tumor recurrence is high (30 to 75%). Upper and mid-ureteral tumors are best treated by segmental resection if the tumors are solitary or low grade, and by nephroureter-

TABLE 4
Staging Systems of Upper Tract Urothelial Tumors

Finding	Grabstald-Cummings Stage	1987 UICC Stage
Carcinoma in situ	I	Tis
Noninvasive papillary tumor	I	Ta
Tumor involving submucosa	II	T1
Muscle-invasive tumor	III	T2
Tumor invading renal parenchyma	III	T3
Tumor invading peripelvic or periureteral soft tissue	III	T3
Invasion of contiguous organs	IV	T4
Lymph node metastases	IV	(N1–3)
Distant metastases	IV	M1

ectomy if they are multiple or high grade. Distal ureteral tumors are most effectively treated with distal ureterectomy and ureteroneocystostomy.

BLADDER NEOPLASMS

Bladder cancer is a common urologic tumor that is broadly divided into two biologically meaningful subtypes. The first is superficial low grade transitional cell carcinoma which has as its greatest risk a tendency for frequent recurrence within the bladder. The second is invasive high grade cancer which often presents in advanced stages and is associated with substantial mortality.

Etiology

Bladder tumors are more frequent in men than women (approximately 3 : 1) and in older patients. The peak incidence of the disease is the seventh decade of life. Environmental carcinogens have been postulated as the major causative factor in this cancer. There is a clear causal relationship between cigarette smoking and bladder cancer. Smokers have at least a fourfold increased risk of developing bladder tumors, and it is estimated that smoking is responsible for the development of one third of all bladder tumors. Occupational exposure to aromatic amines is similarly known to predispose a patient to the development of bladder cancer. In particular, a high prevalence of bladder tumors has been shown in individuals exposed to aniline dyes. Other occupations linked to bladder cancer development include truck driving, painting, and leather working, as well as others in which there has been chronic exposure to volatile chemicals such as dry cleaning. Similar to upper tract urothelial cancers, analgesic abuse is associated with an increased risk of bladder tumors. Other putative carcinogens include radiation therapy and cyclophosphamide chemotherapy.

Bladder irritation from chronic infection or a long-term indwelling foley catheter is associated with the development of squamous cell carcinoma. From 2 to 10% of paraplegics with chronic indwelling catheters develop bladder cancer, and approximately 80% are of squamous histology.

In the Nile River Valley, schistosomal infestation of the bladder (bilharziasis) is associated with the development of squamous cell carcinoma.

Pathology

The overwhelming majority of bladder tumors are transitional cell carcinomas. Although most bladder tumors arise de novo, a number of proliferative lesions of the bladder have been identified. These include atypical hyperplasia, Von Brunn's nests, cystitis cystica, cystitis follicularis, cystitis glandularis, inverted papilloma, nephrogenic adenoma, squamous metaplasia, and leukoplakia.

Both uroepithelial dysplasia and carcinoma in situ (CIS) of the bladder have been documented as preneoplastic lesions. Dysplasia is characterized as mild, moderate, and severe, and is intermediate between normal uroepithelium and carcinoma in situ. CIS is a term reserved for poorly differentiated transitional cell carcinoma confined to the surface uroepithelium. It may be asymptomatic or associated with symptoms of bladder irritability such as frequency, urgency, or dysuria. At cystoscopy, it often appears as a velvety patch of erythematous mucosa. CIS is frequently (20 to 75%) noted to coexist (in adjacent or distant mucosa) with muscle invasive transitional cell carcinomas of the bladder. Although the natural history of this disease is not fully known, it is of interest that 20% of patients who underwent cystectomy for treatment of carcinoma in situ were found to have microscopically invasive cancer. At present, the treatment of choice for CIS is intravesical instillation of BCG which produces complete regression in approximately 50 to 65% of patients.

As mentioned previously, more than 90% of bladder cancers are transitional cell carcinoma. These tumors arise most commonly at the bladder neck and lateral bladder walls. Roughly 70% are low-grade superficial tumors. While the majority of patients will develop a recurrence, only a small percentage of these tumors (10 to 15%) will progress to the more serious muscle invading tumors. Unfortunately, 80 to 90% of the patients with muscle invasive tumors have the diagnosis made at their first presentation. Even more sobering is the fact that nearly 50% of this group will already have occult distant metastases.

Much less common are squamous cell carcinoma and adenocarcinomas. Squamous cell carcinomas are frequent in Egypt because of chronic infection with *Schistosoma haematobium*. In the United States they constitute 3 to 7% of tumors and afflict patients with chronic irritation from infection, stones, or indwelling catheters. Treatment consists of radical cystectomy, since radiation and chemotherapy are ineffective. Adenocarcinomas represent less than 2% of bladder tumors and are most often seen in patients born with extrophic bladders or in urachal tumors that invade the dome of the bladder. Adenocarcinomas respond poorly to radiotherapy or cytotoxic chemotherapy and are best treated by exenterative surgery.

Diagnosis

Patients with carcinoma of the bladder usually (85%) present with gross painless hematuria. Although conventional cytology, flow cytometry, and quantitative fluorescent image analysis have all been utilized to diagnose bladder tumors, the diagnosis is most reliably confirmed by cystoscopy and biopsy. Excretory urography is used to rule out involvement of the upper tracts by tumor and to detect ureteral obstruction which is almost always a sign of muscle invasive cancer.

Early detection studies have reported the favorable experience of using chemical reagent strips to test for hematuria. Approximately 20% of the population was positive and 8 to 22% of those further evaluated were found to have urinary malignancies. Two thirds of the detected tumors were bladder cancers. Further studies are necessary before screening can be recommended.

Staging

Clinical staging of bladder patients is essential for planning therapy. The most important information is the pathologic evaluation of the transurethral bladder tumor resection. Grade and depth of penetration of the tumor into the bladder wall determine if the patient has a low-grade, superficial or high-grade, infiltrating tumor. Superficial tumors do not require further staging evaluation. Muscle infiltrating tumors are best staged with CT scanning to rule out lymph node or visceral metastases. Chest radiography and serum chemistries should also be performed and if the alkaline phosphatase is elevated a bone scan should be considered. The most accurate means of detecting lymph node metastases is pelvic lymphadenectomy but this is usually performed at the same time as radical cystectomy. The TNM classification of bladder tumors is best utilized for staging and is illustrated in Table 5.

Treatment

Patients with superficial tumors can be managed effectively by transurethral resection. Patients should have follow-up cystoscopy at 3 month intervals for 2 years, then every 6 months for 2 years and annually thereafter. This can usually be performed in the office using flexible cystoscopes. The troublesome feature of superficial tumors is their 70% recurrence rate.

Patients who are judged to have a high risk of recurrent tumor because of increased grade or stage, multiple tumors, or a history of recurrence can be treated with intravesical chemotherapy or immunotherapy. Thiotepa, doxorubicin, and mitomycin C are cytotoxic agents commonly employed in patients with superficial transitional cell carcinoma. They have been shown to reduce recurrence rates to 30 to 44%. Intravesical BCG has been shown in prospective trials to be highly effective in reducing recurrence rates (0 to 41%), and is currently the favored method of prophylaxis.

Patients who present with muscle invasive bladder cancer can be treated with surgery, radiation therapy, or chemotherapy. At present, the most effective local therapy is radical cystectomy. Pelvic recurrence rates are 10 to 20%, compared to 50 to 70% with radiation therapy, chemother-

apy, or combination of both. The disadvantage of radical surgery is the loss of normal bladder function. Radical cystectomy in men consists of removal of the pelvic lymph nodes, bladder, and prostate. If the tumor is associated with diffuse CIS of the bladder or involvement of the prostate, total urethrectomy is included. In women the operation is commonly called an anterior exenteration and includes excision of pelvic lymph nodes, bladder, urethra, ovary, fallopian tubes, uterus, and the anterior wall of the vagina. Bladder reconstruction usually consists of a ileal conduit or a continent urinary reservoir. The continent diversions may be cutaneous, or in eligible men, brought down to the urethra. The morbidity of radical cystectomy and bladder reconstruction is 25 to 35% and mortality rate is 1 to 2%. Five-year survivals of 75% have been reported for patients with T2, T3a disease, 44% for T3a, T3b tumors, and 36% for T4 lesions.

Radiation as monotherapy has not been shown to have high cure rates in patients with invasive disease. Five-year survival rates have averaged 20 to 35%. Bladder sparing protocols utilizing chemotherapy with cisplatin, methotrexate and vinblastine (CMV), and radiation therapy (4000 cGy) have been reported. If the patients have a complete response from this treatment, further radiotherapy to a total dose of 6480 cGy is given. Patients with only a partial response are advised to have a cystectomy.

Chemotherapy has been utilized primarily in metastatic disease but more recently has been used as an adjunct to surgery or radiotherapy. Cisplatin is the single most active agent, but combination chemotherapy with methotrexate, vinblastine, doxorubicin, and cisplatin (M-VAC) has been shown in patients with metastatic disease to be superior in a multicenter randomized trial. However, the complete response rates are still low and of relatively short duration.

Chemotherapy prior to planned surgery (neoadjuvant) has been advocated to reduce the risk of disease recurrence after cystectomy. Proponents of this approach argue that; (1) micrometastases may be present at the time of diagnosis; (2) micrometastases are eliminated most efficiently when the volume of tumor is small (3) downstaging of the tumor prior to surgery can occur, and (4) there may be a reduction in the chemotherapy access to tumor as a consequence of surgery. As yet, there is no evidence from properly designed trials to favor this approach. Similarly, no well-designed properly executed trials have been performed which show a definite advantage to the use of adjuvant chemotherapy following surgery. Nevertheless, the increased effectiveness of combination chemotherapy makes the concept of adjuvant therapy appealing and some studies suggest a potential advantage for patients at high risk for disease recurrence who are treated with adjuvant chemotherapy.

Other Bladder Tumors

Besides the more common transitional, adeno, and squamous cell carcinomas, other epithelial tumors include small cell carcinoma and carcinosarcoma. Small cell neoplasms

TABLE 5
Staging for Urinary Bladder Carcinoma

Primary tumor (T)

The suffix "m" should be added to the appropriate T category to indicate multiple tumors.

The suffix "is" may be added to any T to indicate the presence of associated carcinoma in situ.

TX	Primary tumor cannot be assessed
TO	No evidence of primary tumor
Ta	Noninvasive papillary carcinoma
Tis	Carcinoma in situ: "flat tumor"
T1	Tumor invades subepithelial connective tissue
T2	Tumor invades superficial muscle (inner half)
T3	Tumor invades deep muscle (outer half) or perivesical fat

    T3a Tumor invades deep muscle (outer half)
        i.   microscopically
        ii. macroscopically (extravesical mass)

T4   Tumor invades any of the following: prostate, uterus, vagina, pelvic wall, abdominal wall

    T4a Tumor invades any: prostate, uterus, vagina
    T4b Tumor invades pelvic wall and/or abdominal wall

Regional lymph nodes (N)

Regional lymph nodes are those within the true pelvis; all others are distant nodes.

NX	Regional lymph nodes cannot be assessed
N0	No regional lymph node metastasis
N1	Metastasis in a single lymph node, 2 cm or less in greatest dimension
N2	Metastasis in a single lymph node, more than 2 cm but not more than 5 cm in greatest dimension, or multiply lymph nodes, none more than 5 cm in greatest dimension
N3	Metastasis in a lymph node more than 5 cm in greatest dimension

Distant Metastasis (M)

MX	Presence of distant metastasis cannot be assessed
M0	No distant metastasis
M1	Distant metastasis

AJCC/UICC stage grouping

Stage 0	0a	Ta	N0	M0
	0is	Tis	N0	M0
Stage I		T1	N0	M0
Stage II		T2	N0	M0
Stage III		T3a	N0	M0
		T3b	N0	M0
Stage IV		T4	N0	M0
		Any T	N1	M0
		Any T	N2	M0
		Any T	N3	M0
		Any T	Any N	M1

are thought to arise from neuroendocrine cells and stain positively for neuroendocrine markers using immunohistochemistry. Carcinosarcomas are tumors which contain both epithelial and mesenchymal elements. Both of these aggressive tumors are treated with radical surgery.

Nonepithelial bladder tumors are quite uncommon and consist of sarcomas such as neurofibroma, leiomyosarcome, angiosarcoma, and rhabdomyosarcoma. These tumors are best treated with surgery. In addition to these tumors, pheochromocytomas, lymphomas, and malignant melanoma have all been reported in the bladder. Surgical excision is preferred except for lymphoma which can be treated effectively with radiation therapy.

PROSTATE CANCER

Etiology

Prostate cancer is the most common cancer occurring in adult American men and the second leading cause of cancer

TABLE 6
Staging for Prostate Carcinoma

Primary tumor (T)
TX	Primary tumor cannot be assessed
T0	No evidence of primary tumor
T1	Clinically inapparent tumor not palpable nor visible by imaging
T1a	Tumor incidental histologic finding in 5% or less of tissue resected
T1b	Tumor incidental histologic finding in more than 5% of tissue resected
T1c	Tumor identified by needle biopsy (e.g., because of elevated PSA)
T2	Tumor confined within prostate
T2a	Tumor involves half of a lobe or less
T2b	Tumor involves more than half of a lobe, but not both lobes
T2c	Tumor involves both lobes
T3	Tumor extends through the prostatic capsule
T3a	Unilateral extracapsular extension
T3b	Bilateral extracapsular extension
T3c	Tumor invades seminal vesicle(s)
T4	Tumor is fixed or invades adjacent structures other than seminal vesicles
T4a	Tumor invades any of: bladder neck, external sphincter, rectum
T4b	Tumor invades levator muscles and/or is fixed to pelvic wall

Regional lymph nodes (N)
The regional lymph nodes are the nodes of the true pelvis.
NX	Regional lymph nodes cannot be assessed
N0	No regional lymph node metastasis
N1	Metastasis in a single lymph node, 2 cm or less in greatest dimension
N2	Metastasis in a single lymph node, more than 2 cm but not more than 5 cm in greatest dimension, or multiple lymph node metastases, none more than 5 cm in greatest dimension
N3	Metastasis in a lymph node more than 5 cm in greatest dimension

Distant metastasis (M)
MX	Presence of distant metastasis cannot be assessed
M0	No distant metastasis
M1	Distant metastasis
M1a	Non-regional lymph node(s)
M1b	Bone(s)
M1c	Other site(s)

AJCC/UICC stage grouping
Stage 0	T1a	N0	M0	G1
Stage I	T1a	N0	M0	G2, 3–4
	T1b	N0	M0	Any G
	T1c	N0	M0	Any G
	T1	N0	M0	Any G
Stage II	T2	N0	M0	Any G
Stage III	T3	N0	M0	Any G
Stage IV	T4	N0	M0	Any G
	Any T	N1	M0	Any G
	Any T	N2	M0	Any G
	Any T	N3	M0	Any G
	Any T	Any N	M1	Any G

death. African-Americans and men with a family history of carcinoma of the prostate are at increased risk of developing the disease. A diet high in fat may predispose to the development of prostate cancer as well.

Pathology

More than 95% of the prostate cancers are acinar adenocarcionmas. Most are multifocal and arise from the peripheral zone of the prostate.

Diagnosis

Low stage prostate cancer usually is clinically silent. Asymptomatic tumors are most often discovered by digital rectal examination during a routine physical or by an elevation of serum prostate specific antigen (PSA). Screening for cancer of the prostate should be performed annually beginning at age 50, or in the case of African-Americans or those with a positive family history, at age 40. Suspicious digital rectal exam or increased PSA should prompt confirmatory diagnostic needle biopsy of the prostate. This is most often performed conjointly with transrectal ultrasound.

Staging

Prostate cancers are best staged using TNM classification (Table 6). The most frequent sites of metastasis are the lymph nodes and bone. It is no longer cost effective to perform routine bone scans in patients with PSA levels <10 ng/mL. CT and MRI studies are not sensitive or specific for evaluating either T or N stage, and their routine use should be discouraged. Recently, careful retrospective study has confirmed the utility of nomograms utilizing clinical stage, Gleason score, and serum PSA to accurately predict pathologic stage in patients with clinically localized carcinoma of the prostate. Tumor-derived PSA appears more likely to circulate in plasma in a protein-bound form than PSA originating in benign tissue. Preliminary data suggest that a low ratio of free to bound PSA may discriminate prostate cancer from benign prostate hypertrophy (BPH). However, these findings require further validation.

Treatment

The treatment of patients with carcinoma of the prostate is controversial. The debate has been engendered by the observation that men with carcinoma of the prostate often are older and die of other diseases before the cancer causes serious morbidity or mortality. Thus, therapeutic decisions involve an assessment of a patient's general health and life expectancy. For patients with clinically localized tumors and a life expectancy of 10 years or more, radical prostatectomy or external beam radiotherapy are the best options. Other acceptable strategies include observation or androgen deprivation therapy. Androgen deprivation can be accomplished by bilateral orchiectomy or by the use of LHRH agonists with or without oral antiandrogens. Patients with metastatic disease are best treated with androgen deprivation since nearly 80% of those men will have a favorable response to therapy.

Bibliography

Catalona WJ: Urothelial tumors of the urinary tract. In: Walsh, Retik, Stamey, Vaughn (eds) *Campbell's Urology,* 6th ed. W.B. Saunders, Philadelphia, pp. 1094–1158, 1992.

deKernion JB, Belldegrun A: Renal tumors. In: Walsh, Retik, Stamey, Vaughn (eds) *Campbell's Urology,* 6th ed. W.B. Saunders, Philadelphia, pp. 1053–1093, 1992.

Garnick M, Fair WR: Prostate cancer: Emerging concepts. Part I. *Ann Intern Med* 125:118–125, 1996.

Garnick MB, Fair WR: Prostate cancer: Emerging concepts. Part II. *Ann Intern Med* 125:205–212, 1996.

Motzer RJ, Bander NH, Nanus D: Renal-cell carcinoma. *N Engl J Med* 335:865–875, 1996.

Vogelzang NJ, Scardino PT, Shipley WU, Coffey DS: *Comprehensive Textbook of Genitourinary Oncology.* Williams & Wilkins, Baltimore, 1996.

Rosenberg SA: Karnofsky memorial lecture: The immunotherapy and gene therapy of cancer. *J Clin Oncol* 10:180, 1992.

SECTION 9

THE KIDNEY IN SPECIAL CIRCUMSTANCES

59

THE KIDNEY IN INFANTS AND CHILDREN

R. ARIEL GOMEZ

ANATOMICAL DEVELOPMENT OF THE KIDNEY

In humans, the metanephric or definitive kidney appears during the fifth week of gestation. Nephrogenesis terminates by 32 to 36 weeks of gestation. Renal function and urine production begin about 10 weeks into embryonic life. The kidneys can be detected by ultrasound by the 18th week of gestation. Term infants are born with a full complement of nephrons. However, because deeper glomeruli develop earlier than superficial ones (centrifugal maturation), juxtamedullary glomeruli are larger and more mature than outer cortical ones. The glomeruli become equal in size by the 14th postnatal month and reach adult size (200 um) at 3 1/2 years of age. The proximal tubule continues to increase in length well into adult life.

FUNCTIONAL DEVELOPMENT OF THE KIDNEY

Glomerular Filtration Rate

In newborn babies, glomerular filtration rate (GFR) correlates with gestational age. The GFR increases postnatally and doubles by 2 weeks of age. When corrected for surface area, the GFR reaches adult values at 1 to 2 years of age. The normal values of GFR for infants and children are shown in Table 1. Factors responsible for the increase in GFR with maturation include: increase in arterial pressure, increase in renal blood flow, increase in glomerular permeability, and increase in filtration surface area.

Creatinine clearance can be used to measure the GFR after 1 month of age providing that urinary creatinine excretion is between 15 and 25 $mg \cdot kg^{-1} \cdot day^{-1}$. However, in infants it is difficult to obtain 24-hour urine collections. Shorter collections are not adequate because of variations in creatinine excretion throughout the day. The following formula permits estimation of GFR ($mL \cdot min^{-1} \cdot 1.73\ m^{-2}$) without the need for urine collections,

$$GFR = K\ L/S_{cR},$$

where K is a constant (0.33 in preterm, 0.45 in term neonates, 0.55 in children and adolescent girls, and 0.70 in adolescent boys), L. is the length of the infant in cm, and S_{cr}. is serum creatinine (mg/dL). Although this formula is clinically useful, inulin clearance or iothalamate clearance should be obtained if a more accurate value of GFR is needed. Along with changes in GFR, serum creatinine levels vary with age and degree of maturity. During the first 48 hours after birth, creatinine levels are similar to the maternal values. A week after birth, the full-term neonate should have a creatinine below 1 mg/dL. These levels should continue to decrease to about 0.3 mg/dL by 3 months of postnatal life. In preterm infants, however, creatinine levels can be high (about 1.5 mg/dL) during the first few weeks of postnatal life. These levels progressively decrease to 0.4 to 0.8 mg/dL by 3 to 6 months of postnatal life. When evaluating a neonate with a high creatinine, serial measurements are more meaningful than a single determination; creatinine levels should progressively decrease. An increase in serum creatinine indicates a reduction in GFR, regardless of the gestational age. The normal values for creatinine during childhood are shown in Fig. 1.

Urine Concentration

In human fetuses, urine flow rate increases from 0.1 mL/min at 20 weeks of gestation to 1.0 mL/min at 40 weeks of gestation. In neonates, urine flow rate decreases again to around 0.1 mL/min. Fetal urine flow correlates with (and may be modulated by) fetal arterial pressure. The fetal urine is hypotonic (100 to 200 mOsm/L), unless stress such as hypoxemia or volume depletion develops. Nevertheless, the urinary concentrating ability is lower in the fetus than in the adult. Several factors contribute to the decreased urinary concentrating ability. In the fetus, the organization and anatomical development of the medulla is delayed with respect to glomerular development. Short loops of Henle and reduced NaCl transport in the ascending loops of Henle are also important factors. In addition, preferential blood flow to the inner portions of the cortex dissipates an already low intrarenal concentration gradient. Although AVP is secreted properly in response to volume and osmolar challenges, decreased AVP receptor number or coupling to cAMP generation likely contribute to the decreased concentrating ability found in infants.

Maximal urinary concentration increases progressively throughout the first year of life (Table 2). In premature neonates, maximal urine osmolality is about 400 to 500 mOsm/L. Later in life, infants born prematurely are able to concentrate their urine to levels found in term infants of similar postnatal age. This is probably due to a rapid maturation of the concentration gradient in the premature infant.

TABLE 1

Normal Values of GFR[a] (ml · min⁻¹ · 1.73 m⁻²)

Preterm (25–28 weeks)	
1 week	11.0 ± 5.4
2–8 weeks	15.5 ± 6.2
Preterm (29–34 weeks)	
1 week	15.3 ± 5.6
2–8 weeks	28.7 ± 13.8
Term	
5–7 days	50.6 ± 6.8
1–2 months	64.6 ± 5.8
3–4 months	85.8 ± 4.8
5–8 months	87.7 ± 11.9
9–12 months	86.9 ± 8.4
2–12 years	133 ± 27

[a] From Schwartz et al.: *Pediatr Clin North Am* 34: 571–590, 1987 and Greene MG: *The Harriet Lane Handbook. A Manual for Pediatric House Officers,* 12th ed. Mosby, St. Louis, pp. 1–434, 1991.

TABLE 2

Maximal Urine Osmolality (mOsm/L)

3 days	515 ± 172
6 days	663 ± 133
10–30 days	896 ± 179
10–12 months	1118 ± 154
14–18 years	1362 ± 109

Means ± SD.

Sodium

Sodium metabolism in the newborn period is characterized by: (1) a progressive increase in renal reabsorptive capacity, (2) positive balance in the term infant, and (3) an inability to promptly excrete a solute and volume load.

About 30% of the dietary sodium is retained by the healthy infant receiving formulas containing different sodium concentrations. Although sodium intake varies widely, positive sodium balance is usually maintained, thus allowing the conservation of sodium which is a necessary requirement for somatic growth. However, premature infants excrete more sodium than full-term infants. In fact, sodium excretion is negatively correlated to gestational age. The fractional excretion of sodium at 31 weeks of gestation is approximately 5% and declines to less than 1% by 2 months after birth. Thus, in contrast to full-term healthy newborns that are able to conserve sodium and maintain a positive sodium balance, preterm infants are at risk of developing a negative sodium balance during the first weeks of life. It is believed that the high sodium excretion in the premature baby is due to a relative inability of the distal tubule to respond to aldosterone. Newly born preterm infants who receive human breast milk or formulas with a composition similar to that of breast milk containing relatively low sodium concentrations continue to excrete large amounts of sodium in the urine and eventually develop a negative sodium balance and hyponatremia. The hyponatremia can be prevented by the addition of supplemental sodium chloride to the formula.

Although sodium retention in the maturing individual is essential for growth, the counterpart of this chronically enhanced sodium reabsorption is that newborns have difficulty in rapidly excreting an acute load of sodium and water.

The renal excretory response to a sodium load increases progressively during infancy and is fully developed by the

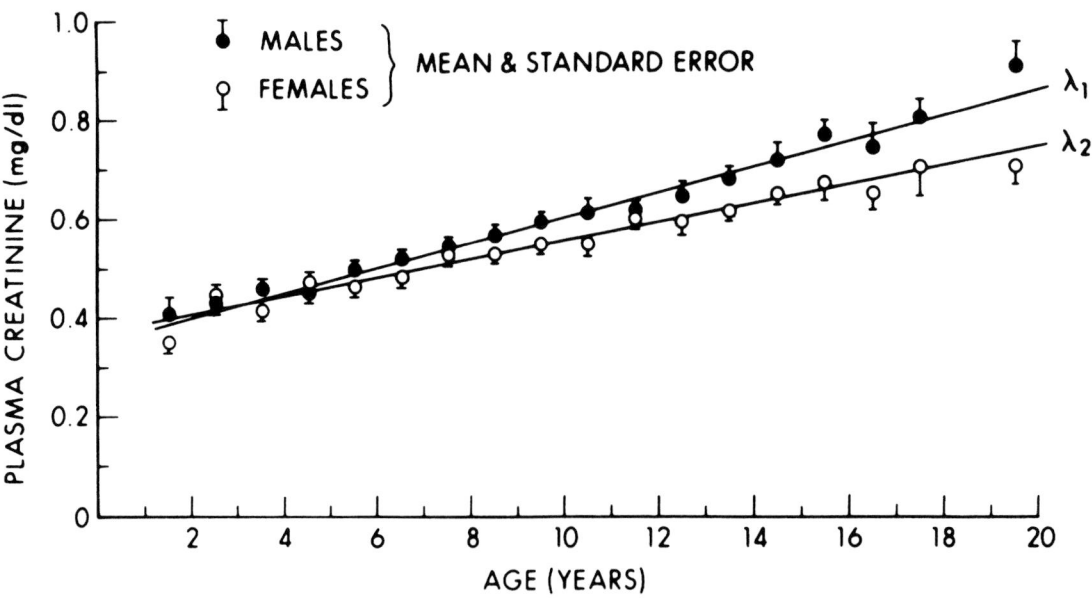

FIGURE 1   Values of plasma creatinine in normal males and females. From Schwartz et al.: *J Pediatr* 88:828–830, 1976. With permission.

first year of life. In addition to the low GFR, enhanced distal tubular sodium reabsorption is responsible for the retention of sodium.

Based on the information described above, the sodium requirements for a term newborn range from 1 to 1.5 mEq $\cdot$ kg^{-1} $\cdot$ day^{-1}, whereas the requirements for a preterm neonate range from 3 to 5mEq $\cdot$ kg^{-1} $\cdot$ day^{-1}. The sodium content of breast milk is appropriate for the feeding of the healthy term infant. It should be remembered, however, that if excess sodium is given, such as feeding undiluted cow's milk, there is a risk of inducing sodium and water retention with extracellular volume expansion and sometimes clinically evident edema.

Oliguria

Most neonates void within the first 24 hours after birth. Any newborn baby, whether term or premature, who has not urinated within the first 24 hours of life should be evaluated for renal disease. Oliguria in infancy is defined as urine flow rate less than 1 mL $\cdot$ kg^{-1} $\cdot$ hr^{-1}. This is based on the usual renal solute load (7 to 15 mOsm $\cdot$ kg^{-1} $\cdot$ day^{-1}) contributed by feedings and a maximal urinary osmolality of 500 mOsm/kg. To maintain solute balance, the newborn will therefore need to urinate about 30 mL $\cdot$ kg^{-1} $\cdot$ day^{-1} (1.25 mL $\cdot$ kg^{-1} $\cdot$ hr^{-1}). In infants, oliguria can be easily evaluated by calculating the fractional excretion of sodium (FE$_{Na}$) (see Chapter 2).

Determination of the FE$_{Na}$ is convenient because it does not require a timed urine collection. The FE$_{Na}$ is particularly helpful in distinguishing oliguria due to a prerenal (low FE$_{Na}$) etiology from that due to a renal (high FE$_{Na}$) cause. In the oliguric term neonate, a FE$_{Na}$ higher than 2.5% indicates a renal cause (such as acute tubular necrosis), whereas a FE$_{Na}$ of less than 2.5% suggests prerenal causes such as dehydration, hypovolemia, hypoalbuminemia, or decreased effective plasma volume. As mentioned above, premature babies normally have higher FE$_{Na}$ (around 5%) and, therefore, the cutoff of 2.5% is not useful until after 10 days of postnatal life. In the child as in adults a FE$_{Na}$ of 1% is utilized as the break point.

Calcium

Fetal calcium levels are higher than maternal values because of active calcium transport across the placenta toward the fetal side. The fractional reabsorption of calcium by the loop of Henle increases with maturation. Therefore, infants excrete more calcium in the urine than older children. Most commonly, hypercalciuria in the newborn is

seen in neonates with bronchopulmonary dysplasia who have received calciuric drugs such as furosemide or glucocorticoids. Hypercalciuria, in turn, can lead to nephrocalcinosis, urolithiasis, and decreased renal function. When possible, a thiazide diuretic that reduces urine calcium excretion should be used instead of furosemide. Phosphate depletion in preterm infants can also lead to hypercalciuria. With the use of new formulas richer in phosphate, hypercalciuria, and other complications of phosphate depletion such as osteopenia are less frequently observed.

Urine calcium excretion in the neonate can be estimated by calculating the calcium/creatinine ratio in a random urine sample. A ratio above 0.8 in preterm and 0.4 in full-term infants is considered hypercalciuria. In older children, a ratio above 0.2 or a calcium excretion in a timed urine sample of 4mg $\cdot$ kg^{-1} $\cdot$ 24 hr^{-1} are used to diagnose hypercalciuria.

Newborn infants are also prone to hypocalcemia, especially when they are sick. Contributing factors include decreased responses to PTH, high serum phosphate levels, and the rapid bone mineralization characteristic of the newborn period. The normal range for calcium levels in infants and children are shown in Table 3.

Phosphate

Serum phosphate concentration is normally higher in the neonate than in the adult (Table 4). Any neonate with a serum phosphate below 4 mg/dL should be evaluated for tubular wasting of phosphate. This can be easily done by calculating the tubular reabsorption of phosphate (TRP) after measuring the concentrations of creatinine and phosphate both in urine and plasma:

$$TRP = [1-(U_{PO4}/P_{PO4})/(U_{cr}/P_{cr} \times 100\%$$

where U_{PO4} and P_{PO4} are the urinary and plasma concentrations of phosphate (mg/dL), (respectively and P_{cr} and U_{cr} are the plasma and urinary concentrations of creatinine (mg/dL), respectively. It should be remembered that the normal TRP varies with age. After the first week of postnatal life, the TRP should exceed 95% in full-term and 75% in preterm neonates. After the first month of postnatal life and throughout adulthood, the TRP should be above 85%. Values below those mentioned above should suggest Fanconi's syndrome, hyperparathyroidism, or chronic renal failure.

Potassium

The total body potassium (K$^+$) in infants is 40 mEq/kg, compared with the adults of 50 mEq/kg. Growing infants

TABLE 3
Calcium Levels According to Age

	(mg/dL)
Premature (<1 week)	6–10
Full-term (<1 week)	7–12
Child	8.0–10.5
Adult	8.5–10.5

TABLE 4
Normal Phosphorus Levels

	(mg/dL)
Newborn	4.2–9.0
1 year	3.8–6.2
2–5 yr	3.5–6.8
Adult	3.0–4.5

maintain a positive K+ balance which is necessary for growth. Conservation of K+ during infancy is reflected also by higher serum K+ values (Table 5). The newborn has a low basal rate of K+ excretion and a decreased ability to rapidly excrete a K+ load, in comparison with the adult (Table 5). The fractional excretion of K+ in the newborn is about half of that in the adult (Table 5). This may be due to reduced K+ secretion by the cortical collecting duct, the main site for K+ excretion. The factors that limit urinary K+ excretion by the principal cells during early life are: (1) unfavorable electrochemical gradient (low cellular K+ concentration, decreased Na, K-ATPase activity and transepithelial voltage), (2) limited membrane permeability to K+, (3) low tubular fluid flow rates, and (4) decreased sensitivity to mineralocorticoids. Also, enhanced K+ absorption by intercalated cells of the medullary collecting ducts may be a contributory factor. In fact, medullary collecting tubules (which reabsorb K+) mature earlier than the principal cells of the cortical collecting duct (which secrete K+), a factor that may be important in the decreased ability to excrete K+ during early life. Also, as GFR increases with maturation, fluid delivery to the cortical collecting duct increases promoting K+ secretion. Under normal conditions, the reduced ability of the neonate to excrete K+ is not manifested clinically. However, hyperkalemia can develop if the neonate is exposed to excessive exogenous or endogenous (i.e., cell breakdown) K+ loads.

Acid–Base Balance

Infants have lower blood pH and HCO_3^- than older children and adults (Table 6). Overall, the newborn kidney is capable of maintaining normal acid–base status. However, infants are prone to the development of acidosis when they are sick or receive inadequate nutrition or in response to an exogenous acid load. The plasma concentration of HCO_3^- increases with age, due to an increase in the renal threshold of HCO_3^- with maturation. The approximate renal threshold of HCO_3^- is 18 mEq/L in the premature and 21 mEq/L in the term neonate. Adult values (24 to 26 mEq/L) are reached by 1 year of life. Several factors seem to be responsible for the low renal HCO_3^- threshold observed in infancy: low activity of carbonic anhydrase, extracellular fluid volume expansion contributing to proxi-

TABLE 6
Acid-Base Measurements as a Function of Age[a]

Age	pH	$paCO_2$ (mm Hg)	HCO_3^- (mEq/liter)
Preterm (1 week)	7.34 ± 0.06	31 ± 3*	17.2 ± 1.2*
Preterm (6 weeks)	7.38 ± 0.02	35 ± 6	21.9 ± 4.4*
Term (birth)	7.24 ± 0.05*	49 ± 10*	20.0 ± 2.8*
Term (1 hr)	7.37 ± 0.05	34 ± 9	19.0 ± 2.3*
3–6 months	7.39 ± 0.03	36 ± 3	22.0 ± 1.9*
21–24 months	7.40 ± 0.02	35 ± 3	21.8 ± 1.6*
3.5–5.4 years	7.39 ± 0.04	37 ± 4	22.5 ± 1.3*
5.5–12 years	7.40 ± 0.03	38 ± 3	23.1 ± 1.2*
12.5–17.4 years	7.38 ± 0.03	41 ± 3	24.0 ± 1.0*
Adult males	7.39 ± 0.01	41 ± 2	25.2 ± 1.0

[a] From Schwartz GJ: General principles of acid–base physiology. In: Holliday MA, Barrett TM, Avner E (eds). *Pediatric Nephrology,* 3rd ed. Williams and Wilkins, Baltimore, pp. 222–246, 1993.

Mean ± 1 *SD.* * Significantly different from adult males ($p <$ .05) by Tukey's test.

mal HCO_3^- wasting, immaturity of luminal Na-H+ exchange, and imbalance between filtration and reabsorption of HCO_3^- in newly formed nephrons. Also, HCO_3^- reabsorption in the distal nephron may not compensate for HCO_3^- that escapes the proximal tubule.

Infants have a decreased ability to acidify the urine when compared to adults under basal conditions. Maximal titratable acid and ammonium excretion increase with age and achieve adult values (when corrected by GFR) by 2 months of age. Several factors are responsible for the relative inability of the newborn to excrete an acid load including a limited availability of urinary buffers such as phosphate and ammonium. The low GFR and high tubular reabsorption of phosphate (TRP) prevailing in the neonatal period markedly limit the phosphate available as a urinary buffer. Prior to 2 months of age, ammonia generation and secretion are also limited. Immaturity of the collecting ducts (fewer intercalated cells, fewer proton pumps per cell) and immaturity of carbonic anhydrase activity could also limit distal acidification. In addition to this impairment in renal excretion infants have an increased exogenous and endogenous proton load in comparison to adults. In prematures, endogenous acid production can be as high as 2 to 3 mEq · kg^{-1} · day^{-1}. A large amount of acid is generated during the metabolism of proteins. Accretion of calcium into the growing bone results in the release of 0.5 to 1.0 mEq · kg^{-1} · day^{-1} of H+ that needs to be excreted by the kidney or neutralized by HCO_3^- absorbed through the gastrointestinal tract. For this reason is during episodes of gastroenteritis, infants are susceptible to metabolic acidosis.

Blood Pressure

The normal blood pressure values vary with age, gender, stature, and degree of maturation. Accepted normal values are based on demographic studies. The reader should consult the report of the "Second Task Force on Blood Pres-

TABLE 5
Plasma Levels and Excretion of Potassium in Normal Infants and Children[a]

Age (years)	Plasma (K) (mEq/liter)	K Clearance (ml · min^{-1} · 1.73 m^{-2})	FE_K (%)
0–0.3	5.2 ± 0.8	5 ± 3	8.5 ± 3.8
0.4–1.0	4.9 ± 0.5	14 ± 6	14.6 ± 5.0
3–10	4.2 ± 0.5	20 ± 11	14.5 ± 8.9
11–20	4.3 ± 0.3	21 ± 8	16.2 ± 8.2

[a] From Jones DL and Chesney RW: Tubular function. In: Holliday MA, Barrett TM, Avner ED (eds). Pediatric Nephrology, 3rd ed. Williams and Wilkins, Baltimore, pp. 117–147, 1993.

TABLE 7

Classification of Hypertension by Age Group[a]

Age group	Significant hypertension	Severe hypertension
Newborn		
7 days	Systolic ≥ 96 mm Hg	Systolic ≥ 106 mm Hg
8–30 days	Systolic ≥ 104 mm Hg	Systolic ≥ 110 mm Hg
Infant (< 2 yr)	Systolic ≥ 112 mm Hg	Systolic ≥ 118 mm Hg
	Diastolic ≥ 74 mm Hg	Diastolic ≥ 82 mm Hg
Children (3–5 yr)	Systolic ≥ 116 mm Hg	Systolic ≥ 124 mm Hg
	Diastolic ≥ 76 mm Hg	Diastolic ≥ 84 mm Hg
Children (6–9 yr)	Systolic ≥ 122 mm Hg	Systolic ≥ 130 mm Hg
	Diastolic ≥ 78 mm Hg	Diastolic ≥ 86 mm Hg
Children (10–12 yr)	Systolic ≥ 126 mm Hg	Systolic ≥ 134 mm Hg
	Diastolic ≥ 82 mm Hg	Diastolic ≥ 90 mm Hg
Adolescents (13–15 yr)	Systolic ≥ 136 mm Hg	Systolic ≥ 144 mm Hg
	Diastolic ≥ 86 mm Hg	Diastolic ≥ 92 mm Hg
Adolescents (16–18 yr)	Systolic ≥ 142 mm Hg	Systolic ≥ 150 mm Hg
	Diastolic ≥ 92 mm Hg	Diastolic ≥ 98 mm Hg

[a] From the Report of the Second Task Force on Blood Pressure Control in Children: *Pediatrics* 79(1):1–25, 1987.

sure Control in Children—1987" which provides normative data and guidelines for detection of children with hypertension. A child is considered hypertensive if the systolic or diastolic blood pressure is above the 95th percentile for age and sex on at least three occasions. The classification of hypertension by age group is shown in Table 7. The etiology of hypertension varies with the age of the patient. As a rule, the younger the patient, the more likely it is for hypertension to be secondary. In the newborn period, renal artery thrombosis, congenital renal malformations, coarctation of the aorta, and bronchopulmonary dysplasia are the most common causes. In children between infancy and 6 years of age, renal parenchymal diseases, renal artery stenosis, and coarctation of the aorta are leading cause. Between 6 and 10 years of age, renal parenchymal diseases, renal artery stenosis, and essential hypertension are frequently found. In the adolescent, essential hypertension and renal parenchymal diseases are the two most prominent causes.

Bibliography

Al-Dahhan J, Haycock GB, Nichol B, Chantler C, Stimmler L: Sodium homeostasis in term and pre-term neonates. III. Effect of salt supplementation. *Arch Dis Child* 59:945–950, 1984.

Chevalier RL: Developmental renal physiology of the low birth weight pre-term newborn. *J Urol* 156:714–719, 1996.

Ekblom P: Embryology and prenatal development. In: Holliday MA, Barrett TM, Avner E (eds) *Pediatric Nephrology*, 3rd ed. pp. 2–20, Williams & Williams, Baltimore, 1993.

Gomez RA: Postnatal regulation of water and electrolyte excretion. In Brace RA, Ross MG, Robillard JE (eds) *Reproductive and Perinatal Medicine, Vol. XI. Fetal and Neonatal Body Fluids: The Scientific Basis for Clinical Practice.* Perinatology Press, New York, pp. 307–318, 1989.

Greene MG: *The Harriet Lane Handbook. A Manual for Pediatric House Officers.* 12th ed. Mosby-Year Book, St. Louis, pp. 1–434, 1991.

Jones DP, Chesney RW: Tubular function. In Holliday MA, Barrett TM, Avner ED (eds), Pediatric Nephrology, 3rd ed. Williams & Wilkins, Baltimore, pp. 117–147, 1993.

Mathew OP, Jones AS, James E, Bland H, Groshong T: Neonatal renal failure: Usefulness of diagnostic indices. *Pediatrics* 65:57–60, 1980.

Polacek E: The osmotic concentrating ability in healthy infants and children. *Arch Dis Child* 40:291, 1965.

Report of the Second Task Force on Blood Pressure Control in Children—1987. *Pediatrics* 79(1): 1–25, 1987.

Schwartz GJ, Brion LP, Spitzer A: The use of plasma creatinine concentration for estimating glomerular filtration rate in infants, children and adolescents. *Pediatric Clin North Am* 34:571–590, 1987.

60

THE KIDNEY IN PREGNANCY

SUSAN H. HOU

CHANGES IN RENAL FUNCTION DURING PREGNANCY

Dramatic changes in renal function occur during pregnancy. Renal plasma flow increases to 50 to 70% above normal during the first two trimesters and remains 40% above normal in the third trimester. An increase in glomerular filtration rate (GFR) begins by the fourth week of gestation and peaks at 150% of normal at 13 weeks (Fig. 1). An appreciation of this change is essential for evaluation of renal disease in pregnant women, because the average BUN for pregnancy is 9 mg/dL and the average serum creatinine is 0.7 mg/dL. A BUN of 14 mg/dL or higher or a serum creatinine of 0.9 mg/dL or higher is indicative of abnormal renal function. GFR varies with position, particularly late in pregnancy when it may be 20% lower in the supine position than in the lateral recumbent position. The increased GFR leads to increased clearance of uric acid and a decrease in serum uric acid levels—the mean being 3 mg/dL. Tubular function also changes. The threshold for reabsorption of glucose increases, and glycosuria may occur without hyperglycemia. The osmostat is reset such that thirst is experienced at a level 10 mOsm below the nonpregnant normal and serum sodium is about 5 mEq/L below nonpregnant normal.

Anatomical changes occur in the kidney during pregnancy as well. Renal length is increased by 1 to 1.5 cm. A physiologic dilatation of the ureters occurs, giving rise to hydronephrosis. Stasis of the urine in the ureters predisposes to urinary tract infection and complicates timed urine collections.

Urinary Tract Infection

Urinary tract infection is the most common renal disease occurring during pregnancy. Asymptomatic bacteriuria, which occurs in 5% of pregnancies, has been associated with small for gestational age babies and some argue that it plays a role in hypertension and anemia. If left untreated, 30% of women with asymptomatic bacteriuria develop pyelonephritis. Treatment of asymptomatic bacteriuria reduces the incidence of pyelonephritis in this group to 3%. Pyelonephritis is a serious disease in pregnant women. Ten percent are bacteremic and a transient decrease in GFR is common. Pyelonephritis has been associated with premature labor and intrauterine fetal death. Asymptomatic bacteriuria should be treated with a 10-day course of antibiotics

and followed by monthly screening urine cultures. All patients with symptomatic pyelonephritis should be hospitalized and treated with intravenous antibiotics. They should receive intravenous antibiotics until they have been afebrile for 24 hours at which time they can be switched to oral antibiotics. Single, large-dose therapy with an antibiotic which may be effective in nonpregnant patients should not be used in pregnant women. Chronic suppressive therapy should be used for the duration of the pregnancy after recovery from acute pyelonephritis.

Hypertension

In normal pregnancy, blood pressure drops in the first two trimesters as a result of the combination of arterial vasodilatation mediated by the production of vasodilatory prostaglandins, and by refractoriness to the pressor effects of angiotensin. Hypertension in pregnancy is defined as any rise in systolic blood pressure of greater than 30 mm Hg or any rise in diastolic blood pressure greater than 15 mm Hg above baseline, or by the use of antihypertensive medications. The blood pressure may rise by 10 mm Hg in the third trimester in normal pregnancy, but a blood pressure of greater than 140/85 is abnormal even in the third trimester. Blood pressures greater than 125/75 before 32 weeks gestation have been associated with an increase in the frequency of adverse fetal outcome.

The Joint National Committee on Detection, Evaluation and Treatment of High Blood Pressure defines four types of hypertension in pregnancy: preeclampsia-eclampsia, chronic hypertension, chronic hypertension with superimposed preeclampsia, and transient hypertension (Table 1). Hypertension can also complicate pregnancy in women with virtually any type of preexisting renal disease.

Preeclampsia is a disease that occurs only in pregnancy. It includes the triad of hypertension, proteinuria, and edema and occurs after the 20th week of gestation. Hyperreflexia is characteristic of the disease. Most affected women have a mild to moderate decrease in GFR with serum creatinine levels inappropriately high for pregnancy. Serum uric acid levels are elevated and hematocrit may rise as a result of hemoconcentration. Pathologically, preeclampsia is characterized by swelling of glomerular epithelial cells termed glomerular endotheliosis (Fig. 2). It occurs primarily in first pregnancies and biopsy studies have found that 75% of the multiparous women given the diagnosis of

388

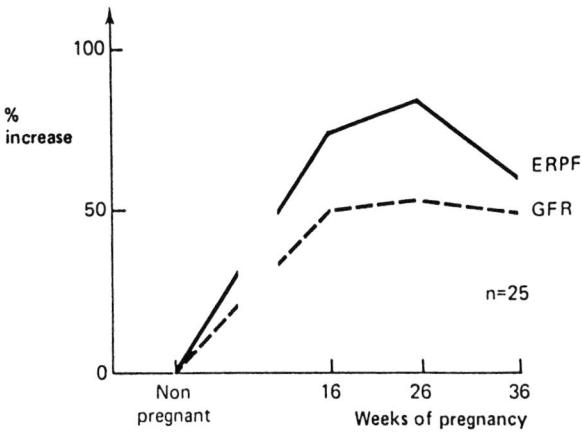

FIGURE 1 Increase in glomerular filtration rate and effective renal plasma flow during pregnancy. From Davison JM: *Am J Kidney Dis* **9:** 248, 1987. With permission.

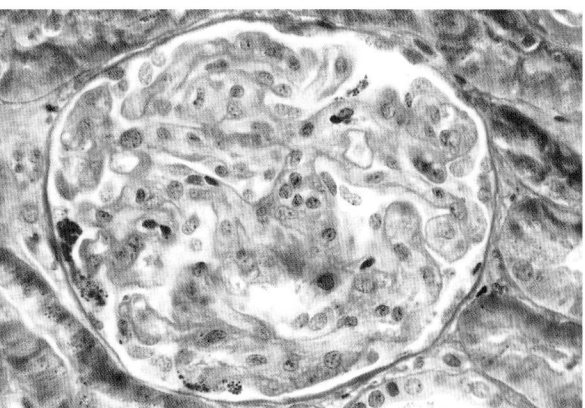

FIGURE 2 Glomerulus from a 29-year-old. woman in the 22nd week of pregnancy who had developed 3.6 g/24 hr proteinuria and hypertension (preeclampsia). The glomerulus has endotheliosis with obliteration of most capillary lumens by swollen endothelia cells (Masson trichrome stain). Courtesy of Dr. J. Charles Jennette.

TABLE 1
Hypertensive Disorders of Pregnancy

Preeclampsia
  Primigravida
  Onset after 20 weeks gestation
  Proteinuria
  Generalized edema
  Patients at extremes of childbearing years
  Hyperreflexia
  Vasospasm on fundoscopic exam
  Multisystem involvement
  No ↑ hypertension at follow-up

Chronic hypertension
  May occur in any pregnancy
  Before or anytime during pregnancy
  No proteinuria
  May have mild pretibial edema
  More common in older age group
  May have eye ground changes of essential hypertension
  Normal reflexes
  ↑ risk of placental separation
  Hypertension at follow-up

Chronic hypertension with superimposed preeclampsia
  30% of women with chronic hypertension
  Hypertension before or early in pregnancy
  ↑ 30 mm Hg systolic, 15 mm Hg diastolic after 20 weeks
    gestation
  Proteinuria
  May occur in any pregnancy
  More common in older age group
  Hyperreflexia
  Generalized edema
  Hypertension at follow-up

Transient hypertension
  No hypertension prior to pregnancy
  Third trimester or 24 hours postpartum
  No proteinuria
  No hyperreflexia
  Predicts hypertension later in life

preeclampsia on clinical grounds have some other renal disease.

The acronym HELLP (hemolysis, elevated liver enzymes, low platelets) syndrome has been used to describe severe preeclampsia with manifestations of multisystem involvement. In addition to its hepatic and hematologic manifestations, HELLP syndrome may be complicated by disseminated intravascular coagulation, acute renal failure, cerebrovascular accident, retinal detachment or heart failure (Table 2). The most serious complication of this condition is eclamptic seizures which may result in maternal death. Anticonvulsant and antihypertensive medication may be used to protect the mother while preparing for delivery. Magnesium sulfate has recently been shown to

TABLE 2
Clinical Manifestations of HELLP Sydrome[a,b]

Maternal complications	
Disseminated intravascular coagulopthy	21%
Abruptio placentae	16%
Acute renal failure	8%
Severe acites	8%
Pulmonary edema	6%
Cerebral edema	1%
Retinal detachment	1%
Laryngeal edema	1%
Subcapsular hematoma of the liver	1%
Adult respiratory distress syndrome	1%
Laboratory findings	
Platelet count (no/mm^3)	7000–99,000
Serum aspartate amino transferase (U/L)	70–6193
Lactic dehydrogenase (U/L)	564–23,584
Total bilirubin (mg/dL)	0.5–25.5
Serum creatinine (mg/dL)	0.6–16.0

[a] Data derived from Sibai et al.: *Am J Obstet Gynecol* 169: 1002–1003, 1993.
[b] n = 442.

be more effective than phenytoin in preventing seizures in preeclamptic women. Intravenous hydralazine and labetolol are effective and safe for treatment of severe hypertension. However, delivery is the definitive treatment, although the manifestations of preeclampsia may appear or worsen for several days postpartum.

The major mechanism by which preeclampsia causes tissue damage is intense vasoconstriction. Normal pregnancy is characterized by resistance to the pressor effects of angiotensin. This resistance is lost in preeclampsia. The production of both the vasodilatory prostaglandin prostacyclin and the vasoconstrictor thromboxane by vascular endothelial cells are increased in pregnancy. In normal pregnancy, the effects of prostacyclin predominate. In preeclampsia the ratio of the two shifts toward thromboxane and vasoconstriction results. There is evidence in small studies of women at high risk for preeclampsia that low-dose aspirin prevents its development by inhibiting thromboxane formation. This finding has not been confirmed in several prospective randomized studies in large numbers of women. Preeclampsia occurs primarily in first pregnancies.

Chronic hypertension can be diagnosed when hypertension is present before pregnancy or before 20 weeks gestation. Occasionally the diagnosis is difficult when a woman first seeks prenatal care after 20 weeks gestation or when hypertension is masked by the pregnancy associated drop in blood pressure which occurs in the first trimester. Thirty percent of women with essential hypertension experience such a drop. Signs such as left ventricular hypertrophy or hypertensive eye ground changes support the diagnosis of chronic hypertension. In the absence of superimposed preeclampsia, pregnant women with chronic hypertension do not have proteinuria. If proteinuria appears in a woman with essential hypertension, she should be presumed to have superimposed preeclampsia. Women who develop hypertension for the first time during pregnancy should be screened for pheochromocytoma. Although rare, pheochromocytoma carries a 50% maternal mortality rate if the diagnosis is not made.

There is debate about the effect of chronic hypertension on pregnant women and their infants and about the target blood pressure. Most physicians aim for systolic blood pressures below 140 and diastolic blood pressures between 90 and 100. Nonpharmacologic treatment should include bed rest and avoidance of alcohol. Salt restriction is not indicated and weight loss is contraindicated.

When pharmacologic treatment is needed, the most commonly used drugs include methyldopa, a variety of β-blockers, labetolol, and hydralazine. The use of calcium channel blockers is increasing. Methyldopa in doses up to 3 g/day in divided doses has been used for 35 years; no serious problems have been identified in children exposed to the drug in utero in intensive follow-up testing. Labetolol and β-blockers are the other first-line drugs. Early reports of fetal growth restriction and inability to tolerate anoxic stress in the infants of mothers treated with β-blockers have not been born out by widespread use. If these first-line drugs are ineffective in controlling blood pressure, hydralazine in doses up to 200 mg bid can be added to the regimen. Clonidine has been shown in a single controlled trial to be as effective as methyldopa. Although calcium channel blockers have been widely used, there are a few reservations. In some studies, fetal loss rate has been high, although pregnancy outcome is better than predicted by previous obstetric history in the same patients. Nifedipine may result in profound hypotension when used in conjunction with magnesium sulfate in women with preeclampsia.

Angiotensin converting enzyme (ACE) inhibitors should not be used in pregnancy. In animal studies, captopril has been associated with 80 to 93% fetal loss. The use of ACE inhibitors in humans has been associated with oligohydramnios resulting in neonatal death from hypoplastic lungs and neonatal anuria resulting in death or the need for dialysis.

Superimposed preeclampsia may complicate pregnancy in women with chronic hypertension. The woman with chronic hypertension should be monitored every week after the 20th week to look for the development of worsening hypertension, proteinuria, hemoconcentration, elevated transaminases, thrombocytopenia, elevated uric acid, and decreased serum albumin. If it appears that she is developing superimposed preeclampsia, she should be hospitalized and delivered for the same indications as women with simple preeclampsia.

Transient hypertension develops in the third trimester and resolves postpartum. It is not accompanied by any of the other manifestations of preeclampsia and is a strong predictor of chronic hypertension later in life.

CHRONIC RENAL DISEASE IN PREGNANCY

Hypertension

The most serious problem complicated pregnancy in women with renal disease is hypertension, which can be seen even in the absence of severe renal insufficiency. In a 1980 report of 121 pregnancies in 89 women with a wide variety of renal disease and moderately well-preserved renal function, 35% of pregnancies were complicated by a blood pressure of > 140/90. In more than half of the hypertensive pregnancies, diastolic blood pressure exceeded 110 mm Hg. Hypertension was more common in women with glomerular diseases and hypertensive nephrosclerosis than in women with interstitial diseases.

Conception is less common in women with severe renal insufficiency, but enough data are available to determine that hypertension is common in this group as well. A 1996 report contain information on 82 pregnancies in 67 women with serum creatinine 1.4 mg/dL or greater at conception or in the first trimester. Forty-eight percent had a mean arterial blood pressure greater than 105 mm Hg in the third trimester, compared to 28% in the first trimester. Hypertension occurs in approximately 60% of pregnancies in dialysis patients. In six reports of pregnancies in renal transplant recipients, there were 46 instances of hypertension in 135 pregnancies. Although none of these studies report any maternal death from hypertension, there are reports of progression of preeclampsia to eclampsia.

The approach to the control of hypertension during pregnancy in women with renal disease is similar to the approach to treatment of women with chronic hypertension, except that the hypertension of renal disease has a component of volume overload which may require salt restriction, the judicious use of diuretics, or, in severe renal insufficiency, dialysis. Occasionally, volume status can be uncertain enough that central pressure monitoring is necessary.

Women with renal disease and hypertension are at risk for superimposed preeclampsia, but the recognition of this complication may be difficult. Even in pregnancies in women without known renal disease, discrepancies between clinical diagnosis and pathological findings frequently occur. In the setting of renal disease, many clinical signs and symptoms occur that simulate preeclampsia, thus further complicating the diagnostic process. For example, as discussed below, proteinuria is expected to increase in women with glomerular disease. Plasma uric acid levels may be elevated in women with decreased GFR, obscuring the development of preeclampsia. Even worsening of hypertension or decrease in GFR an occur in the absence of preeclampsia. In this context, the development of hyperreflexia is useful in making the distinction as it does not generally develop except in preeclampsia. The occurrence of elevated liver enzymes, thrombocytopenia, and microangiopathic changes on the peripheral blood smear, which almost certainly signal the development of preeclampsia, are late signs. However, it is hoped that diagnosis and delivery will not be delayed until these signs develop. The diagnostic and therapeutic dilemma is usually resolved if blood pressure cannot be adequately controlled. In these circumstances, the pregnancy is usually terminated. Unfortunately in some series which did not specifically address women with renal disease, eclampsia occurred with a diastolic blood pressure as low as 80 mm Hg. Because the use of magnesium sulfate is dangerous in women with severe renal insufficiency, an alternative anticonvulsant should be used. If magnesium is used, the loading dose should be given in two separate infusions with measurement of serum magnesium level between the two infusions. Serum magnesium should be measured every 2 hours, and additional magnesium given only when the level falls below 4 mg/dL. Continuous infusion should not be used with moderate renal insufficiency, and measurement of serum magnesium every 2 hours is necessary in women even with mild decrements in GFR.

Proteinuria

Pregnancy in women with all types of renal disease is associated with an increase in proteinuria. Nephrotic syndrome frequently develops in women who excreted only a small amount of protein prior to pregnancy, particularly in women with glomerular diseases. The increased proteinuria is thought to result from an increased filtered load of protein, a change that occurs to a lesser extent in normal pregnant women. Heavy proteinuria by itself, without hypertension or worsening renal function, is not associated with poor pregnancy outcome. When heavy proteinuria develops, salt restriction may decrease edema formation. Massive edema frequently develops and may be disabling for the mother. Even in this situation, diuretics are best avoided. The risk of low doses of diuretics is relatively low in the absence of preeclampsia. High doses are generally required in women with nephrotic syndrome, and little is known about the effect of high doses of diuretics on the fetus. Diuresis may aggravate intravascular volume contraction in the mother and increase the risk of thromboembolic events. If bed rest is required in a woman with nephrotic syndrome, low-dose heparin should be used because of the increased risk of thromboembolic disease.

PREGNANCY IN WOMEN WITH RENAL DISEASE AND GOOD RENAL FUNCTION

The most important determinant of whether renal function declines during pregnancy is renal function at conception. If renal function is normal at the time of conception, pregnancy does not accelerate the progression of renal disease. A 1995 study reported the effect of pregnancy on the progression of renal disease in 171 women with glomerulonephritis who became pregnant after the diagnosis of renal disease as compared to 189 women of childbearing age with glomerulonephritis who did not conceive after the onset of renal disease. There was no difference in the risk of progression to end stage renal disease between the two groups. Hypertension and certain histological subgroups were at increased risk for progression to renal failure, but in no subgroup did pregnancy increase the risk. If renal function is well preserved, women with renal disease can undertake pregnancy without increased risk of progression to end stage renal disease, but other complications such as hypertension and increased proteinuria are common.

The outcome for infants is somewhat worse than for the general population. Twenty percent of infants are born prematurely and approximately 10% of pregnancies which continue beyond the second trimester end in stillbirth or neonatal death.

PREGNANCY IN WOMEN WITH CHRONIC RENAL INSUFFICIENCY

Women who conceive when the serum creatinine is greater than 1.4 mg/dL have an increased risk that their renal function will deteriorate more rapidly than if they do not become pregnant. In 43% of the 82 pregnancies in women with moderate to severe renal insufficiency mentioned above there was a pregnancy associated decline in renal function. In 31% of pregnancies, deterioration in renal function persisted 6 months after pregnancy, and in 10% there was a deterioration between 6 weeks and 6 months postpartum. At 12 months postpartum, eight women, seven of whom had had a pregnancy associated decline in renal function, had reached end stage renal disease. Deterioration in renal function was more common in women who were hypertensive during the third trimester, but the pressure of a normal blood pressure did not guarantee preservation of renal function. A greater degree of renal insufficiency at conception was associated higher with a likelihood of acceleration of disease during pregnancy.

Despite maternal complications, fetal survival was good (93%). Other studies indicate that even in women with renal failure severe enough to require the initiation of dialysis during pregnancy, fetal survival is 74%.

DIABETIC NEPHROPATHY

The effect of pregnancy on diabetic nephropathy depends on renal function at the time of conception as it does in other renal diseases. Two studies including 57 pregnancies in women with diabetic nephropathy found no evidence that pregnancy accelerates the course of the disease. However, these studies included only a handful of women with seriously impaired renal function. A 1996 report of pregnancies in 11 women with diabetic nephropathy and serum creatinine equal to or greater than 1.4 mg/dL found an acceleration in the progression to end stage renal disease when compared to the rate of decline of renal function prior to pregnancy and when compared to a control group.

LUPUS NEPHRITIS

Lupus nephritis is most common in women of childbearing age. Few diseases are capable of producing such fulminant but potentially treatable renal failure. Approximately half of 365 women with preexisting lupus nephritis in 19 reports suffered an exacerbation of their lupus during pregnancy. While lupus flares are less common in women who have been in remission for more than 6 months, one third of women in this group suffer exacerbations of their lupus during pregnancy. When lupus is active at the time of conception, the risk of renal failure is higher. Lupus flares are less common in women with mesangial proliferation on biopsy than in women with diffuse proliferative disease. Despite its more indolent course in patients who do not become pregnant, membranous lupus is as likely to give rise to a flare during pregnancy as is diffuse proliferative disease. Prednisone and azathioprine can be used in pregnancy with the same precautions that apply to transplant recipients. Cyclophosphamide is teratogenic when used during the first trimester. Later in pregnancy, there is concern about the risk of fetal bone marrow suppression. There have been a few case reports of thyroid cancer in children exposed to cyclophosphamide in utero. Therapeutic abortion is advisable if cyclophosphamide must be used during the first trimester.

Termination of pregnancy is often recommended in women with renal failure from lupus nephritis. Although therapeutic abortion is not accompanied by an increase in lupus flares when it is done before the exacerbation of disease, it does not carry any guarantee of controlling the disease once it has become active. If lupus itself or high-dose steroid therapy gives rise to uncontrollable hypertension, it may be necessary to terminate the pregnancy to facilitate blood pressure control. Fetal loss reaches about 50% in women with lupus nephritis and renal insufficiency.

Fetal loss may occur because of hypertension, renal failure, or placental vasculopathy. If the fetus is beyond 34 weeks gestation when a severe lupus flare or renal failure occurs, the baby should be delivered, because fetal distress and demise may occur so rapidly that they are not anticipated by antenatal testing. The fetus that is viable but not yet mature should be monitored on a daily basis with non stress tests and biophysical profiles and delivered if evidence of fetal distress develops. The infants should be monitored for several manifestations of neonatal lupus. Skin rashes and thrombocytopenia may occur because of antibodies that cross the placenta. These usually resolve over weeks to months as maternal antibodies are lost. Permanent congenital heart block can develop as a result of antigen antibody deposition in the conducting system of the fetus.

PREGNANCY IN DIALYSIS PATIENTS

Infertility is the rule in chronic dialysis patients. Approximately 0.5% of women of childbearing age treated with chronic dialysis conceive each year. Although it is common to increase the total amount of dialysis in women who become pregnant, the benefit of this practice has not yet been demonstrated and is currently under investigation. Experience with more than 300 pregnancies in dialysis patients in the US has shown no advantage of one dialysis modality over another. Pregnancy in dialysis patients is accompanied by worsening anemia. Although recombinant human erythropoietin has been used without ill effects in a handful of pregnant dialysis patients the dose must be increased to maintain the prepregnancy hematocrit. The most serious complication faced by the pregnant dialysis patient is hypertension, which can be life threatening. Intensive monitoring and aggressive antihypertensive treatment is necessary for the safety of the mother. The only category of antihypertensive drugs clearly contraindicated in pregnancy is ACE inhibitors which are associated with neonatal anuria and neonatal death from hypoplastic lungs.

Thirty to forty percent of pregnancies in women who conceive after starting dialysis result in surviving infants. Twenty percent of pregnancy losses result from second trimester spontaneous abortions. The children born to dialysis patients are almost always premature and frequently are small for gestational age. The best chance for successful pregnancy in women with end stage renal disease is renal transplantation.

PREGNANCY IN RENAL ALLOGRAFT RECIPIENTS

Fertility is often restored in renal transplant recipients and there have been more than 6000 pregnancies reported in women with renal transplants. Nonetheless, there are numerous problems associated with such pregnancies.

Transplant patients are generally advised to wait 1.5 to 2 years after successful transplantation and then to undertake pregnancy only if renal function is stable with a serum creatinine of 2 mg/dL or less. Other favorable conditions are the absence of hypertension, significant proteinuria, renal pelvocaliceal distension, or evidence of graft rejection and the requirement for only low doses of immunosuppressives. Women whose graft function is impaired at the time of conception have a substantial risk of worsening renal function. There are occasional instances where irreversible loss of graft function has occurred in women with good stable renal function and normal blood pressure prior to and throughout pregnancy.

When renal function deteriorates in a transplant recipient during pregnancy, the differential diagnosis includes cyclosporine or tacrolimus toxicity, rejection, recurrence of the primary disease and preeclampsia, as well as other pregnancy-related causes of renal failure. Cytomegalovirus infection may be related to graft dysfunction.

Exposure in utero to immunosuppressive drugs is a concern in the infants of transplant recipients. Ideally, women should wait to conceive until the prednisone dose is 15 mg/day or lower. Maternal blood levels of prednisolone are ten times the levels in cord blood. Nonetheless, adrenal insufficiency occasionally occurs in the infant— Even in infants who appear to be stable should be monitored in a high-risk nursery for several days after birth. Steroid doses should be reduced at the same rate as would be done in a nonpregnant patient. High-dose steroids can safely be used for the treatment of rejection.

Azathioprine requires conversion in the liver to its active metabolite, 6-mercaptopurine, and then to 6-thiosinic acid. During the first trimester when organogenesis is taking place, the fetus lacks the enzyme inosinate pyrophosphorylase necessary for this conversion, thus affording the fetus some protection from the effects of the drug. The frequency of congenital anomalies is only slightly increased in women taking azathioprine, if at all. It has been found empirically that the risk of fetal leukopenia can be minimized by keeping maternal leukocyte count over 8500 mm^{-3}. Azathioprine may contribute to growth retardation in the 20 to 50% of infants who are small for gestational age.

Cyclosporine crosses the placenta easily. Although it has not been associated with congenital anomalies, it does appear to cause more severe growth retardation than azathioprine. The serum creatinine at conception is generally higher in women taking cyclosporine than in women taking only prednisone and azathioprine, and hypertension is worse in these women. Cyclosporine levels may vary unpredictably during pregnancy and should be monitored on a weekly basis.

Although pregnancy in transplant recipients is complicated, the fetal outcome is good, with 92% surviving infants in pregnancies that go beyond the first trimester.

ACUTE RENAL FAILURE IN PREGNANCY

Acute renal failure (ARF) remains an unusual but life-threatening complication of pregnancy. ARF requiring dialysis occurs in less than 1 in 10,000 to 15,000 pregnancies in industrialized countries, whereas the frequency of milder degrees of renal insufficiency is higher. The greatest risk of pregnancy-related ARF is late in pregnancy. At one time, sepsis following illegal abortion accounted for a large proportion of obstetric ARF, making renal failure more common early in pregnancy. Sepsis following illegal abortion remains a common cause of renal failure in countries with poor access to health care. While many organisms have been implicated in causing postabortal sepsis, *Clostridium welchii* accounts for a disproportionate number of the cases of acute renal failure, because it produces a toxin which causes hemolysis and renal failure.

Obstruction

Although obstruction is uncommon as a cause of ARF in pregnancy, it must be considered when ARF occurs in any setting because of its reversibility. Renal stone formation is not increased during pregnancy, despite an augmentation of calcium absorption from the gut and calcium excretion by the kidney. However, when severe abdominal pain occurs during pregnancy, renal calculi should be considered. Stones can lead to renal failure if they are bilateral or occur in a solitary kidney.

Ureteral obstruction by the gravid uterus is unique to pregnancy. The description of this problem is still limited to a number of case reports. Polyhydramnios is a common feature, and several episodes of renal failure have occurred in patients with a solitary kidney. Ultrasound for the diagnosis of obstruction is difficult to interpret because of the normal physiologic dilatation of the collecting system. Intravenous or retrograde pyelography may be necessary to make the diagnosis despite the radiation exposure to the fetus.

Preeclampsia-Eclampsia

Renal insufficiency with a mild increase in serum creatinine above normal for pregnancy is common in preeclampsia. In most instances, renal function returns to baseline quickly after delivery. Persistent renal dysfunction and frank ARF occur in a minority of cases, and then only when the disease is very severe prior to delivery. Although ARF is an uncommon complication of preeclampsia, preeclampsia is common enough that it accounts for a substantial percentage of the cases of pregnancy-associated ARF. The course is similar to the course of acute tubular necrosis (ATN) from other causes, and recovery of renal function is the rule.

Acute Tubular Necrosis and Cortical Necrosis

Common causes of ARF are major obstetric complications including hemorrhage, abruptio placentae, amniotic fluid embolism, and retained dead fetus. In many series, obstetric patients have a better prognosis for survival than other patients with ATN.

Although ATN is the most common pathologic finding, most series report a greater frequency of cortical necrosis in obstetric patients than in other patients with ARF. Obstetric patients account for more than half of the cases of cortical necrosis. With improved obstetric care, this entity has become extremely rare.

Both arteriogram and renal biopsy have been used to distinguish between ATN and cortical necrosis. In patients with cortical necrosis, biopsy shows fibrin thrombi in the glomerular capillaries with widespread necrosis of the glomeruli, sometimes sparing the juxtamedullary glomeruli. Re renal arteriogram in cortical necrosis shows an inhomogeneous or absent cortical nephrogram. As there is no specific treatment for cortical necrosis, establishing diagnosis is useful only for prognostic purposes. Permanent renal failure and partial recovery are common.

Hemolytic Uremic Syndrome

The hemolytic uremic syndrome (HUS, see chapter 32) is an unusual cause of renal failure. Its usual occurrence is several days to 10 weeks after a normal pregnancy. Severe renal failure is associated with microangiopathic hemolytic anemia, thrombocytopenia, and variable neurological symptoms. It is part of a spectrum of diseases that includes thrombotic thrombocytopenic purpura in which neurological symptoms predominate and renal failure is usually less severe. Both pregnancy and oral contraceptives have been associated with HUS. The primary event in the development of the disease appears to be endothelial damage. Many of the factors which have been identified as inciting events for HUS cause endothelial cell damage in tissue culture. Endothelial cell damage in turn leads to the disruption of the cell processes which prevent thrombogenesis, with the result being the formation of microthrombi in the vessels of many organs.

The prognosis for postpartum HUS is poor with a high mortality rate from central nervous system disease or uncontrollable bleeding. Permanent renal failure is the rule in survivors. The observation that prognosis is improved in TTP with plasma exchange has led to its use in HUS and there are anecdotal reports of a return of function.

Acute Fatty Liver of Pregnancy

Acute fatty liver of pregnancy is an unusual complication of pregnancy, usually presenting in the third trimester. It most often presents as liver failure with incidentally noted ARF. The renal failure is a variant of hepatorenal syndrome but it is usually reversible. Approximately 80% of patients recover with early cesarean section and supportive care. The availability of liver transplant should further improve the prognosis, but the 80% recovery rate makes it important not to perform a liver transplant prematurely. Treatment for the renal failure is supportive. It is generally mild, but oliguric ATN may occur if there are septic complications.

FOLLOW UP OF WOMEN DEVELOPING RENAL ABNORMALITIES DURING PREGNANCY

Preeclampsia, even when severe, does not predict hypertension in later life. These women need careful follow-up until all the manifestations of preeclampsia have resolved. They can then be treated as healthy women, although they should be regarded as high-risk patients during subsequent pregnancies. Those with newly discovered essential hypertension require ongoing treatment and those with transient hypertension are likely to develop essential hypertension in later life. A woman who develops new onset proteinuria during pregnancy should be followed until the proteinuria resolves, If it persists, a renal biopsy should be conducted at 6 weeks postpartum. Women who have had ARF should be evaluated carefully to determine the completeness of recovery. If there is persistent renal insufficiency, treatment for the specific disease should be presented if available, along with general measures to prevent the progression of renal disease.

Bibliography

Benigni A, Gregorini G, Frulska T, et al.: Effect of low dose aspirin on fetal and maternal generation of thromboxane by platelets in women at risk for pregnancy induced hypertension. *N Engl J Med* 321:357–362, 1989

Davison JM: Pregnancy in renal allograft recipients: prognosis and management. *Clin Obstet Gynaecol (Bailliere's)* 8: 501–525, 1994.

Dunlop W, Davison JM: Renal haemodynamics and tubular function in human pregnancy. *Clin Obstet Gynaecol (Bailliere's)* 1: 769–787, 1987.

Gallery EDM, Brown MA: Volume homeostasis in normal and hypertensive human pregnancy. *Clin Obstet Gynaecol (Bailliere's)* 1: 835–851, 1987

Hou SH: Peritoneal and haemodialysis in pregnancy. *Clin Obstet Gynaecol (Balliere's)* 8: 481–500, 1994

Joint National Committee on Detection, Evaluation and Treatment of Hypertension: National high blood pressure education program working group report on high blood pressure in pregnancy. *Am J Obstet Gynecol* 163: 1689–1712, 1990.

Jones DC, Hayslett JP: Outcome of pregnancy in women with moderate or severe renal insufficiency. *N Engl J Med* 335: 226–232, 1996.

Jungers P, Houillier P, Forget D, et al.: Influence of pregnancy on the course of primary chronic glomerulonephritis. *Lancet* 346:1122–1124, 1995.

Kass EH: Infectious diseases and perinatal morbidity. *Yale J Biol Med* 55: 231–237, 1982

Katz AL, Davison JM, Hayslett JP, Singson E, Lindheimer MD: Pregnancy in women with kidney disease. *Kidney Int* 18: 192–206, 1980.

Mochizuki M, Morikawa H, Yamasaki M, et al.: Vascular reactivity in normal and abnormal gestation. *Am J Kidney Dis* 17:139–143, 1991.

Remuzzi G: HUS and TTP: Variable expression of a single entity. *Kidney Int* 32: 292–308, 1987

61

THE KIDNEY IN AGING

JEROME G. PORUSH

ANATOMY OF THE KIDNEY

Aging is associated with numerous anatomical and functional renal alterations (Table 1). Much like other organs, the kidneys undergo involutional changes with age (Table 2). There is a gradual decline in kidney weight starting in the fifth decade, with the most marked decrease occurring between the seventh and eighth decades. The progressive loss of kidney mass appears to affect the renal cortex more than the medulla. Up to age 40 the normal human kidney has 600,000 to 1,200,000 glomeruli. Thereafter, there is a progressive decrease of 30 to 50% in the number of glomeruli. Below age 50, 95% of the normal population have less than 10% of sclerotic glomeruli. After age 50, the percent of sclerotic glomeruli increases, making the distinction between involutional and disease-related sclerosis unclear. The outer cortical glomeruli are, in general, more extensively involved than the deeper glomeruli.

In addition to glomerular sclerosis, there is a gradual increase in interstitial fibrosis in the medulla primarily, with little inflammatory response. Tubular length decreases and proximal tubular volume of individual nephrons decreases from a mean of 0.076 mm^3 at 20 to 39 years to a mean of 0.050 mm^3 at 80 to 100 years. Since the loss of glomerular mass is proportional to the loss of tubular mass, glomerular balance is usually well preserved. Lastly, there is an increase in reduplication and an increase in focal thickening of both glomerular and tubular basement membranes, probably due to the accumulation of type IV collagen.

The increase in the fraction of sclerotic glomeruli has been attributed to the protein-rich diet characteristic of western society. In the rat, this diet induces a state of chronic glomerular hyperfiltration and hyperperfusion, contributing to progressive glomerulosclerosis and age-related decrease in glomerular filtration rate. An increase in the function of residual intact nephrons would be expected to lead to an increase in nephron size; however, no significant correlation is found between glomerular area and glomerulosclerosis. Another possible explanation for the progressive increase in sclerotic glomeruli is glomerular ischemia secondary to an age related decrease in renal blood flow (see below), since it has been shown that both age and vascular disease correlate independently with the percentage of hyalinized glomeruli in the aged.

The mechanism for the decrease in renal blood flow does not appear to be related to a decrease in cardiac output, and may be explained by changes in the vasculature. The interlobar arteries usually become tortuous and spiraling, and fibroelastic hyperplasia of arcuate arteries and arterioles is seen progressively with age. The changes are more pronounced in the cortical vessels, so that perfusion pressure is relatively well maintained in the juxtamedullary nephrons.

RENAL BLOOD FLOW AND GLOMERULAR FILTRATION RATE

In cross-sectional and longitudinal studies, a gradual decrease in renal blood flow (RBF) and glomerular filtration rate (GFR) is noted with age (Tables 3 & 4). RBF declines progressively at a rate of approximately 10% per decade, starting after the fourth decade. After the age of 30, there is a 7.5 to 8 mL/min decline in the GFR per decade. An age-adjusted derived creatinine clearance can be determined for males with the formula:

creatinine clearance (mL·min^{-1}·1.73m^{-2}) =
$$133 - (0.64 \times age).$$

For females, multiply the result by 0.93. For instance, a 60 kg, 90-year-old male is expected to have a creatinine clearance of $133 - (0.64 \times 90) = 75.4$ mL·min^{-1}·1.73m^{-2}. It should be noted that the result of this formula is only an estimate, and the error inherent can be substantial since some subjects will maintain stable renal function while aging (approximately one third of the population), while a small number will even have an increase in GFR. Serum creatinine is the most commonly used marker of kidney function (GFR) in clinical medicine. The decrease in creatinine clearance occurring with age is attended by a parallel reduction in daily creatinine excretion so that there is frequently no change in the serum creatinine (Table 5). Lean body mass declines by 12 kg in males and by 5 kg in females by age 65 to 70, so that the decrease in creatinine excretion probably reflects a decrease in muscle mass and creatinine production. Also, because a significant number of the elderly suffer from chronic, debilitating diseases, including neurogenic diseases, muscle atrophy is quite prevalent. Thus, an estimate of renal function based solely on the serum creatinine may be deceptive in the elderly. For a more meaningful evaluation of kidney function, a creatinine clearance or other measurement of GFR is essential.

TABLE I

Renal Changes in the Elderly

Diminished renal mass
  Dropout of functioning nephrons
  Glomerular sclerosis
  Increased medullary interstitial fibrosis

Decreased GFR

Decreased RPF

Diminished creatinine production

Impaired sodium conservation

Diminished plasma renin and aldosterone levels

Increased prevalence of hyperkalemia

Impaired ammoniagenesis

Impaired maximal urinary concentration

Impaired maximal water excretion

GFR, glomerular filtration rate; RPF, renal plasma flow.

Measurement of creatinine clearance requires a timed urine collection (which is notoriously inaccurate in the elderly because of bladder emptying problems). A formula developed by Cockcroft and Gault obviates this problem as it allows calculation of the creatinine clearance from the subject's age, weight, and serum creatinine:

Creatinine clearance (C_{cr}) (mL/min) = ((140-age)
    $\times$ weight in kg) $\div$ (72 $\times$ serum creatinine in mg/dL).

For females, multiply the result by 0.85. This formula is applicable as long as the patient has stable kidney function and is without severe chronic debilitating disease. In general, this formula overestimates the creatinine clearance in females, the malnourished, and the debilitated. For these subjects, another formula can be used:

for males, $C_{cr} = (19 \times$ serum albumin in g/dL + 32)
    $\times$ weight (kg) $\div$ 100 $\times$ serum creatinine (mg/dL);

for females, $C_{cr} = (13 \times$ serum albumin + 29)
    $\times$ weight $\div$ 100 $\times$ serum creatinine.

Filtration fraction tends to increase with age (Table 3), due to the fact that GFR falls proportionally less than RPF, and because there is a higher percentage of functioning deep cortical nephrons in the elderly.

As noted earlier, advancing age is associated with fibroelastic hyperplasia and hyalinization of small arteries and arterioles. It has also been found that blood pressure increases with age. The obvious question is whether the decline in renal function with age is mainly a reflection of the increasing blood pressure. At a mean arterial pressure (MAP) less than 107 mm Hg, no correlation is found between C_{cr} and blood pressure. For pressures above that level, however, there appears to be a negative correlation between C_{cr} and MAP. Thus, the progressive decline in GFR with the associated anatomical changes are a function of age per se, but increasing the blood pressure appears to accelerate the decline.

Infusion of amino acids in the elderly is associated with an increase in GFR, similar to that seen in younger individuals. The renal plasma flow response, however, is blunted and less predictable in the elderly and might be due to the structural changes rather than an alteration in the response to vasodilators such as prostacyclin and nitric oxide, both of which have been found to contribute to the renal vasodilatory response to amino acids. Finally, patients over 60 years of age can undergo compensatory hypertrophy to the same extent as younger patients as early as 7 months after unilateral nephrectomy.

TUBULAR FUNCTION

As noted earlier, the anatomical changes affecting the glomeruli are associated with changes in the tubules, so that glomerular–tubular balance is generally adequately maintained in the elderly.

TABLE 2

Anatomical Changes in the Kidney in Various Age Groups[a]

Age in year	Under 39	40–49	50–59	60–69	70–79	Above 80
Wt. of kidneys (g) (144)	432 ± 36 (12)	388 ± 24 (23)	366 ± 20 (20)	355 ± 14 (35)	327 ± 11 (32)	295 ± 18 (22)
Size of glomeruli[b] (μm) (182)	190 ± 1 (12)	199 ± 1 (25)	192 ± 1 (35)	191 ± 1 (43)	189 ± 1 (42)	185 ± 1 (25)
Cell number of glomerular tufts (181)	156 ± 4 (12)	133 ± 3 (25)	142 ± 2 (36)	125 ± 2 (42)	121 ± 2 (42)	106 ± 2 (25)
No. of epithelial cells of convoluted tubules in a given area (125,600 μm^2) (100)	178 ± 6 (6)	159 ± 4 (15)	152 ± 4 (17)	127 ± 3 (23)	121 ± 3 (23)	118 ± 3 (16)
Size of epithelial cell nuclei[b] (μm) (100)	7.1 ± 0.1 (7)	6.9 ± 0.1 (14)	7.1 ± 0.1 (17)	7.0 ± 0.1 (24)	7.2 ± 0.1 (22)	7.3 ± 0.1 (16)

[a] From Tauchi H, Tsubi K, Okutomi J: *Gerontology* 17:87–97, 1971. With permission.
[b] Square root of value area.
Note: Number of kidneys examined is indicated in parentheses.

TABLE 3

Changes in GFR and RPF with Age[a]

Age (yr)	Insulin clearance (mL · min^{-1} · 1.73m^{-2})	Effective renal blood flow (mL · min^{-1} · 1.73m^{-2})	Filtration fraction (%)
50–59	99.3 ± 14.6	849 ± 123	21 ± 3
60–69	96.0 ± 25.5	775 ± 139	22 ± 3
70–79	89.0 ± 19.9	589 ± 133	26 ± 8
80–89	65.3 ± 20.4	475 ± 141	23 ± 4

[a] From Davies DF, Schock NW: *JCI* 29:496–507, 1950. With permission.

SODIUM BALANCE

Low Sodium Diet

In general, the elderly do not conserve sodium as well as younger patients when placed on a low sodium diet. When routine sodium balance studies are performed, they are nor always conclusive. However, if one determines the rate at which balance is achieved, it is evident that the elderly do not conserve sodium normally. From age 30 to 60 years, dietary sodium restriction is associated with a half-time for renal sodium conservation of 23.4 ± 1.1 hours compared to 30.9 ± 2.8 hours for subjects over 60 years of age.

The underlying mechanism for this difference is not clear, and is undoubtedly, multifactorial. There is experimental evidence that during salt restriction both proximal and distal parts of the nephron participate in the increased sodium reabsorption. The decrease in activity of the autonomic nervous system with age might contribute to the inability of the elderly subject to conserve salt normally since this system is known to contribute to the increased proximal sodium reabsorption noted during salt restriction. Despite a reduction in nephron number and cortical blood flow in the elderly, medullary flow is well preserved. As a result of this disparate blood flow, medullary washout might occur, reducing the efficacy of the countercurrent system and, thereby, decreasing the amount of sodium removed by the ascending limb of deep nephrons. Furthermore, as GFR decreases, the solute load per surviving nephron increases, producing a solute diuresis, which may impair the tubular ability to conserve sodium.

Plasma renin activity and plasma aldosterone have been measured in different age groups during unrestricted (120 mEq Na/day) and low sodium (<10 mEq Na/day) diets in the supine and standing position. Both plasma renin activity and plasma aldosterone decrease progressively with each decade of life, starting after the fourth decade. The same pattern persists whether subjects are on unrestricted or restricted sodium diets, supine or standing. The reduced renin levels may be due to the decreased sympathetic activity in the elderly or to a possible decrease in their ability to activate prorenin to renin. The lower basal plasma aldosterone level may be explained by a decrease in adrenal responsiveness to circulating angiotensin. Following salt restriction, plasma aldosterone rises appropriately in the elderly, however, so that it is unlikely that the level, per se, is responsible for impaired sodium conservation.

Whatever the explanation, the diminished ability of the elderly to conserve sodium when challenged with a low sodium diet makes the defense of extracellular volume precarious. Therefore, sodium restriction should be undertaken with caution in the elderly in order to prevent volume contraction which may lead to acute reductions in renal function or symptomatic orthostatic hypotension. The latter is particularly a problem in the elderly because of their impaired baroreceptor response to the upright position.

Volume Expansion

Subjects over the age of 40 excrete a saline load slower than younger subjects. This may be explained, in part, by the decrease in filtered load, as GFR decreases with age. Compared to younger subjects, the elderly excrete sodium, potassium, and total solutes at a proportionately higher rate at night. The baseline plasma level of atrial natriuretic peptide, a substance that participates in the natriuresis associated with volume expansion, increases with age, possibly due to a decrease in its catabolic rate. As saline loading in the elderly results in a significant rise in atrial natriuretic peptide, the blunted natriuresis after saline loading cannot be attributed to an inappropriate response.

POTASSIUM BALANCE

The low plasma renin activity and plasma aldosterone levels in the elderly contribute to their tendency to develop hyperkalemia, particularly when receiving potassium supplementation. The incidence of hyperkalemia complicating

TABLE 4

Age and Creatinine Clearance[a]

Age (yr)	Creatinine clearance (mL · min^{-1} · 1.73m^{-2})
45–54	128 ± 2
55–64	122 ± 2
65–74	110 ± 3
75–84	97 ± 3

[a] From Rowe JW, Andres R, Tobin JD, et al: *J Gerontol* 31:155–163, 1976. With permission.

TABLE 5
Relationship between Serum and Urine Creatinine and Creatinine Clearance[a]

Age (yr)	Serum creatinine (mg/dL)		Urine creatinine (mg · kg⁻¹ · 24h⁻¹)		Creatinine clearance (mL · min⁻¹ · 173m⁻²)	
	(male)	(female)	(male)	(female)	(male)	(female)
40–49	1.10	1.00	19.7	17.6	88	81
50–59	1.16	0.99	19.3	14.9	81	74
60–69	1.15	0.97	16.9	12.9	72	63
70–79	1.03	1.02	14.2	11.8	64	54
80–89	1.06	1.05	11.7	10.7	47	46
90–99	1.20	0.91	9.4	8.4	34	39

[a] From Kampman M, Siersback-Nielson K, Kirstensen M, et al: *Acta Med Scand* 196:517–520, 1974. With permission.

diuretic therapy with potassium supplementation is reported to be 0.5% in patients under the age of 50, 4.0% in those 50-60 years, and even higher in older subjects. The use of drugs that interfere with the distal tubular secretion of potassium, such as potassium-sparing diuretics, angiotensin converting enzyme inhibitors, angiotensin receptor blockers, nonsteroidal antiinflammatory drugs, and β-adrenergic antagonists necessitates careful monitoring of serum potassium in elderly patients.

ACID–BASE BALANCE

Blood pH and bicarbonate levels do not change significantly with age. With advancing age, the kidneys maintain their ability to maximally acidify the urine in the presence of appropriate stimuli. Unfortunately, bicarbonate reabsorption by the proximal tubule has not been studied under different loads. However, since plasma bicarbonate remains unchanged despite a gradual decrease in GFR with age, it appears that glomerular–tubular balance for this ion is well maintained. Nevertheless, one would expect the elderly to excrete a bicarbonate load slower than younger subjects, making them more prone to the development of metabolic alkalosis. Under normal circumstances, the excretion of titratable acid and ammonium is similar among different age groups. However, after a 2 mmol/kg ammonium chloride load, urinary excretion of net acid is significantly lower in elderly subjects. This defect is accounted for solely by a decrease in ammonium excretion, since titratable acid excretion is not altered with age. This impairment of ammonium excretion represents a reduction in the maximum capacity of the nephron to synthesize ammonia.

URINARY CONCENTRATION

Aging is associated with a diminished capacity to maximally concentrate the urine. The results of one study of 12 hours of water deprivation showed that the elderly (mean age = 68 years) achieve a mean urine osmolality of 882 mOsm/kg compared to 1051 mOsm/kg in a group of middle-aged subjects (mean age = 49 years) and 1109 mOsm/kg H_2O in a younger group of subjects (mean age = 33). To achieve maximal urine concentration the following features should prevail:

1. A normally functioning hypothalamic-hypophyseal axis. If anything, it has been shown that there is a significant age-related increase in osmoreceptor sensitivity. For the same osmolar stimulus, elderly subjects tend to release twice as much antidiuretic hormone (ADH) as younger subjects.

2. Adequate solute delivery to the distal nephron. Although GFR decreases with age, no significant relationship has been found between creatinine clearance and urine osmolality, suggesting that solute delivery to the distal nephron is not a limiting factor.

3. A collecting tubule responsive to ADH. Although the maximum urine osmolality following infusion of large doses of vasopressin is decreased in the elderly undergoing a water diuresis, urine osmolality responds normally to stepwise incremental doses of vasopressin, insufficient to maximally concentrate the urine, ruling out any significant impairment in the ability of the collecting duct to respond to vasopressin.

4. A normally functioning ascending limb of Henle. There are suggestions of a defect in sodium reabsorption in the ascending limb of Henle's loop in elderly subjects. This defect, coupled with the previously noted state of medullary washout, leads to a significant reduction in medullary tonicity, and consequently the maximum urinary concentration. The age-related decrease in urinary concentrating ability and the defective thirst mechanism in the elderly further increases their susceptibility to volume depletion when placed on a low Sodium diet.

URINARY DILUTION

During water loading, the minimum urine osmolality achieved by the elderly has been found to be higher than that of younger subjects by some, but not all investigators. However, the hourly free water clearance is consistently lower in the elderly. The recovery of serum osmolality to baseline is slower, and the average osmolar clearance lower in the elderly during water loading. The observed delayed water excretion may be explained by the loss of nephrons and subsequent increase in solute load per nephron. It may also be related to the reduction in the renal synthesis of prostaglandins seen with aging, which may be associated with enhanced ADH responsivness. Whatever the specific mechanism, this inability to normally handle a water load makes the elderly susceptible to hyponatremia.

TUBULAR REABSORPTION OF GLUCOSE

The maximum rate of renal tubular reabsorption of glucose decreases linearly with age. However, because GFR decreases as well, glycosuria at normal plasma glucose levels is not seen.

Bibliography

Agarwal BN, Cabebe FG: Renal acidification in elderly subjects. *Nephron* 26: 291–295, 1980.

Brenner B, Meyer TW, Hostetter TH: Dietary protein intake and the progressive nature of kidney disease: The role of hemodynamically mediated glomerular injury in the pathogenesis of progressive glomerular sclerosis in aging, renal ablation and intrinsic renal disease. *N Engl J Med* 307:652–659, 1982.

Cockcroft DW, Gault MH: Prediction of creatinine clearance from from serum creatinine. *Nephron* 16:31–41, 1976.

Epstein M, Hollenberg NK: Age as a determinant of renal sodium conservation in normal men. *J Lab Clin Med* 87: 411–417, 1976

Helderman JH, Vestal RE, Rowe HW, et al.: The response of arginine vasopressin to intravenous ethanol and hypertonic saline in man: The impact of aging. *J Gerontol* 33:39–47, 1978

Hollenberg NK, Adams DF, Solomon HS, et al.: Senescence of the renal vasculature in normal man. *Circ Res* 34:309–316, 1974

Kaplan C, Pasternack B, Shah H, et al.: Age-related incidence of sclerotic glomeruli in human kidneys. *Am J Pathol* 80:227–234, 1975.

Kasiske BL: Relationship between vascular disease and age associated changes in the human kidney. *Kidney Int* 31: 1153–1159, 1987.

Lindeman RD, Tobin J, Shock NW: Longitudinal studies on the rate of decline in renal function with age. *J Am Gerontol Soc* 33: 278–285, 1985

Miller JH, Shock NW: Age differences in the renal tubular response to antidiuretic hormone. *J Gerontol* 8: 446–450, 1953

Porush JG, Faubert PF: *Renal Disease in the Aged.* Little, Brown, & Co, Boston, 1992.

Rowe JW, Andres R, Tobin JD, et al.: The effect of age on creatinine clearance in man: A cross-sectional and longitudinal study. *J Gerontol* 31: 155–163, 1976.

Rowe JW, Andres R, Tobin JD, et al.: Age-adjusted standards for creatinine clearance. *Ann Intern Med.* 84:567–559, 1976.

Rowe JW, Shock NW, DeFronzo RA: The influence of age on the renal response to water deprivation in man. *Nephron* 17: 270–278, 1976

Sanaka M, Takano K, Shimakura K, Koike Y, Mineshita S: Serum albumin for estimating creatinine clearance in the elderly with muscle atrophy. *Nephron* 73: 137–144, 1996.

Tauchi H, Tsuboi K, Okutomi J: Age changes in the human kidney of the different races. *Gerontologia* 17: 87–97, 1971.

SECTION 10

CHRONIC RENAL FAILURE AND ITS THERAPY

62

THE UREMIC SYNDROME

R. VANHOLDER

INTRODUCTION

The uremic syndrome is characterized by the deterioration of biochemical and physiologic functions that occurs with the progression of renal failure. It results from the retention of substances that are ordinarily removed by the healthy kidneys; the intake of precursors, mainly via nutrition, also plays a role. The uremic syndrome also results from derangements of hormonal and enzymatic homeostasis. The quest for "the" uremic toxin has been overemphasized. Some researchers and nephrologiots consider one specific toxin or group of toxins as responsible (e.g., urea, parathormone, β_2-microglobulin, the group of "middle" molecules with molicular weight, from 300 to 12,000 Da), not taking into account the uremic syndrome as the cumulative result of retention of innumerable compounds and deficiency of others. This chapter reviews the current knowledge about the uremic syndrome, its clinical and biochemical characteristics, and the factors playing a role in its development.

CLINICAL CHARACTERISTICS

The uremic syndrome is characterized by a quantitative and qualitative overall deterioration of performance, affecting the cardiovascular, neurologic, hematologic, immunologic, and other systems. In addition, malnutrition and acidosis may play an important pathophysiologic role. Full-blown uremic syndrome results in a complex clinical picture consisting of fatigue, anorexia, weight loss, itching, muscle cramps, pericarditis, sensory and concentration disturbances, and thirst. It may eventuate in stupor, coma, and death (Table 1).

Cardiovascular Anomalies

One or more cardiovascular anomalies such as hypertension, congestive heart failure, valvular stenosis or insufficiency, accelerated athero-sclerosis and uremic pericarditis, occur commonly during the progression of renal failure. Myocardial dysfunction is related to increased myocardial calcium content, especially in patients undergoing chronic dialysis. Increased cytosolic Ca^{2+} which is observed in many uremic patients has been associated with an increase of peripheral vascular resistance, resulting in hypertension.

It should be stressed, however, that hypertension in the uremic patient may result from a host of other causative factors, such as enhanced renin and angiotensin production due to decreased blood delivery to the kidneys, sodium retention, and fluid overload.

Apart from changes in systolic contractility, a decrease in diastolic compliance of the heart also plays a major role. The basic mechanism is an increase of the interstitial component of heart tissue. As a consequence, the heart shows a decreased capability to relax during diastole, hence decreasing the margin between fluid overload and hypovolemia. Consequently, patients will develop hypotension when minor quantities of fluid are removed from the body by dialysis procedures. It is especially near the end of the interval between dialyses that they will easily develop hypertension and pulmonary edema. Heart disease in dialysis patients is also discussed in Chapter 70.

Uremic Encephalopathy and Peripheral Neuropathy

These disorders may develop alone or in combination. The spectrum of central neuropathy is variable and ranges from subtle cognitive impairment to coma. Sleep disorders, mainly sleep-apnea syndrome from upper airway obstruction are among the major causes. Dialysis prevents encephalopathy, so that this complication is encountered only in exceptional circumstances, such as patients who do not seek medical help until late in their course, or when dialysis is abandoned because of grave disease.

Severe peripheral polyneuropathy has also become unusual today, although less pronounced forms still persist, even in patients treated by apparently adequate dialysis. Neuroleptic manifestations of renal failure are discussed in Chapter 71.

Anemia

Until the introduction of genetically engineered recombinant erythropoietin, uremic anemia was one of the major reasons for the impaired physical condition of renal failure patients. This hypoproliferative anemia is mainly due to inadequate erythropoietin production by the failing kidneys and, to a lesser extent, by defective body iron stores, vitamin deficiency, hemolysis, and erythrocyte fragility. The causative role of inhibitors of erythropoiesis remains a matter of debate. Two proven inhibitors of in vitro hematopoiesis found in uremic plasma are the polyamines sper-

TABLE I
The Uremic Syndrome: Clinical Alterations

Nervous system

Stupor, coma	Polyneuritis
Fatigue	Convulsions
Dementia	Motor weakness
Malaise	Concentration disturbances
Insomnia	Drowsiness
Headache	Irritability
Restless legs	Cramps
Flapping tremor	

Gastrointestinal system

Stomatitis	Pancreatitis
Gastritis	Gastrointestinal ulcers
Anorexia	Nausea, vomiting

Hematological system

Anemia	Bleeding

Cardiovascular system

Pericarditis	Hypertension
Atheromatosis	Cardiomyopathy
Edema	Hypotension
Decreased diastolic compliance	

Pulmonary system

Pleuritis	Pulmonary edema
Uremic Lung	

Skin

Pruritus	Melanosis
Retarded wound healing	Nail atrophy

Bone disease

Osteodystrophy	Amyloidosis (β2M)
Hyperparathyroidism	Calcitriol metabolism defect

Miscellaneous

Thirst	Uremic foetor
Weight loss	Hypothermia
Impotence, diminished libido	

mine and spermidine. Anemia and other hemologic feature of uremics are discussed in Chapter 72.

Disturbances of Coagulation

Disturbances of coagulation may include a varied spectrum of abnormalities ranging from a bleeding tendency to hypercoagulability. Uremic bleeding tendency has a multifactorial origin: platelet related alterations (adherence, aggregation), uremic anemia, and hyperparathyroidism. In earlier studies dating from the 1970s, urea and the guanidines were held responsible for defective coagulation. Recent studies have not confirmed these findings because coagulation disturbances could only be demonstrated at concentrations of these compounds that were much higher than those currently observed today with uremia. Recent data incriminate nitric oxide (NO) as an important inducer of defective coagulation in uremia. Hemodialysis patients also receive regular systemic heparinization.

Immune Deficiency

Susceptibility to infection, increased incidence of cancer, and inadequate production of antibodies, e.g., against hepa-

titis B, all point to immune deficiency in uremia. The problem here is not entirely due to toxins, since bioincompatibility of dialyzer membranes, vitamin D deficiency, and anatomical lesions (e.g. dialysis fistula and peritoneal catheters which predispose to infection) may contribute as well. The circulating number of white blood cells is not altered, but their function is abnormal.

The factors responsible for the depression of immune function in uremia have not been identified. Candidates include a lack of circulating opsonins (e.g., fibronectin), iron overload, uremic anemia, and accumulation of circulating substances with immune suppressant effect (endomorphins, phenols, indoles, parathyroid hormone, high and middle molecular weight compounds).

Endocrine Dysfunction

The endocrine dysfunction of uremia (see also Chapter 73) affects carbohydrate metabolism, and thyroid, growth, and reproductive hormones, resulting in a progressive catabolic state. In addition to disturbances in hormonal states, other causes of negative nitrogen balance are insufficient food intake due to medication side effects, gastrointestinal disease, central nervous system dysfunction, enhanced tissue breakdown from an apparent chronic low grade inflammatory state, and urinary protein losses. Acidosis inhibits many metabolic functions, including protein synthesis. Dialysis treatment, although life-saving, may result in a further enhancement of catabolic status and of nitrogen losses as amino acids are abnormal in hemodialysis and peritoneal dialysis and albumin is lost directly during peritoneal dialysis.

Changes in carbohydrate metabolism consist of alterations of glucose metabolism, pancreatic glucose-induced insulin secretion, and target organ sensitivity to insulin. Together, these abnormalities result in abnormal glucose tolerance. Normal to mildly elevated fasting glucose and high insulin levels are usually found.

Levels of T3 and T4 may be low normal or depressed, the pituitary responsiveness being abnormal, in spite of a euthyroid appearance.

Basal levels of growth hormone are elevated in uremia, in proportion to the degree of renal impairment. Nevertheless, growth retardation is a major problem in uremic children. Contributing factors are malnutrition, acidosis, renal osteodystrophy, inadequate gonadotropic hormone secretion, and increased concentrations of growth hormone binding protein.

Advanced renal failure results in reproductive abnormalities in both males and females, related to hormonal disturbances. In uremic women, follicular stimulating hormone (FSH), progesterone, and estradiol levels are similar and luteinizing hormone (LH) levels tend to be higher than those observed in the follicular phase of the menstrual cycle in normal women. Uremic men may be infertile or impotent, in association with increased LH and decreased testosterone levels. Spermatogenesis is compromised, because of increased FSH levels. Prolactin levels may be elevated, inducing galactorrhea and amenorrhea in women and impotence in men. Gynecomastia may occur in men.

Uremic Bone Disease

Hyperparathyroidism, aluminum toxicity, vitamin D deficiency and resistance, and accumulation of β_2-microglobulin, all contribute to development of renal osteodystrophy. In addition, uremic retention solutes may induce a general resistance to the metabolic effects of $1,25(OH)_2VitD_3$. This topic is covered in Chapter 69.

Pruritus

Pruritus is a disturbing epiphenomenon of uremia, with unclear pathophysiologic mechanisms. Several different factors have been incriminated: increased levels of serum vitamin A, hyperparathyroidism, high skin contents of divalent cations, mast cell proliferation with increased release of histamine, and abnormal cutaneous innervation. Responsible toxins, if any, have not been incriminated, apart from parathormone.

Malnutrition

A substantial proportion of uremic patients are undernourished. Protein–calorie malnutrition is associated with an increase in morbidity and mortality. Contributing factors include anorexia, nausea, vomiting and the subsequent decreased nutrient intake, hormonal and metabolic derangements, and catabolic factors related to the uremic status as well as the dialytic treatment of uremia (see Chapter 68).

Acidosis

Acidosis results from the accumulation of protons and bicarbonate wasting, although the relative contribution of both factors to uremic acidosis may differ from patient to patient. Bicarbonate wasting and retention of chloride result in hyperchloremic acidosis. If phosphate and organic acid (uric acid, hippuric acid, lactic acid) retention is sufficient, an increased anion gap will occur.

Acidosis leads to a host of metabolic alterations, hyperventilation, anorexia, headache, stupor, decreased cardiac inotropic response, catabolism, and hyperkalemia. This complication of uremia can easily be corrected by the administration of extra alkali or removal of acid by dialysis.

BIOCHEMICAL ALTERATIONS

Enzymatic and Metabolic Dysfunction

A host of enzymatic and metabolic functions are depressed: gluconeogenesis, lactate dehydrogenase activity, mitochondrial storage of calcium and oxygen consumption, alkaline phosphatase isoenzyme activity, insulin degradation, Na,K-ATPase activity, tubular anion transport, production and metabolic clearance of calcitriol, and DNA repair ability.

Changes in Drug Protein Binding

Two protein binding defects are seen in uremia. One group of mostly acidic drugs shows decreased binding, which leads to an increase in the free, active fractions of the drugs in plasma. Because, for most drugs, total plasma (bound plus unbound) concentrations are monitored, therapeutic free levels are achieved at a lower than normal total concentration. At conventional normal levels, toxic side effects should be expected. Examples of drugs include theophylline, phenytoin, methotrexate, diazepam, digoxin, and salicylate. Basic drugs, e.g., propranolol, cimetidine, clonidine, imipramine, have increased protein binding. This causes a decrease in the plasma free concentration, diminishing the therapeutic effect. Higher plasma total concentrations are usually required for these drugs.

Attempts to identify the ligands responsible for decreased protein binding have been scant. Several studies suggest that hippuric acid would be one of the main contributing compounds, but its relative importance remains undefined. Other potential competitors are indoxyl sulfate, derivates of furanpropanoic acid and other furancarboxylic acids, and indole-3-acetic acid. It should be stressed that alterations in drug protein binding are not the only pharmacologic changes in uremia. Decreased renal clearance or metabolism and changes in distribution volume may also alter drug effect. In addition, accumulation of active drug metabolites may augment drug potency or toxicity (see Chapter 43).

UREMIC SOLUTE RETENTION

Current knowledge indicates that each metabolic or physiologic change in uremia may be attributed to certain solutes that are retained as a result of renal failure. Some substances that are not toxic may be used as markers of retention.

Under normal conditions, molecules with molecular weights up to approximately 58,000 Da are cleared by the glomerular filter. Uremic retention products have been arbitrarily subdivided in several groups, according to their molecular weight: low molecular weight MW (<300 Da), e.g., urea (MW: 60), creatinine (MW: 113 Da); middle MW (300 to 15,000 Da), e.g., parathormone (MW: 9424 Da), β_2-microglobulin (MW: 11,818 Da); and high-molecular-weight molecules (>15,000 Da) e.g., myoglobin (MW: 18,800 Da).

A listing of some currently known uremic retention solutes with their molecular weights is given in Table 2. In the following discussion, the most important organic compounds and their presumed toxicity will be reviewed.

Urea

Urea is responsible for the elevated concentration of hemoglobin A1C observed in nondiabetic uremics, due to carbamylation of the protein. Other proteins probably undergo structural changes in a similar manner. It is accepted that in general, urea produces acute clinical symptoms only at higher concentrations than those usually encountered nowadays. Given the extensive number of toxicity studies to which urea has been submitted, the number of proven toxic effects is disappointingly limited. Nevertheless, some toxic effects such as inhibition of platelet

TABLE 2
The Most Currently Known Uremic Solutes with Their Molecular Weights

Compound	MW	Compound	MW
Nitric oxide	30	Guanidinoacetate	177
Urea	60	Hippurate	179
Methylguanidine	73	myo-Inositol	180
Phenol	94	ADMA/SDMA	202
Phosphate	96	Dimethylarginine	202
p-Cresol	108	Spermine	202
Creatinine	113	CMPF	240
Hypoxanthine	136	Pseudouridine	244
Spermidine	145	Indoxyl sulfate	251
Xanthine	152	Phenylacetylglutamine	264
Urate	168	β-Endorphin	2465
Guanidinosuccinate	175	Parathormone	9425
Indole-acetate	175	β_2-Microglobulin	11818

CMPF, carboxymethylpropylfuranpropionic acid; ADMA, asymmetric dimethylarginine; SDMA, symmetric dimethylarginine.

aggregation and Na,K-ATPase have been demonstrated. Conceivably, urea may exert some chronic toxicity even at the lower concentrations encountered currently. Even in the absence of any toxicity, urea has been recognized as a useful marker of uremic solute retention and elimination in dialysis patients. Careful multicenter studies by the U.S. National Cooperative Dialysis Study (NCDS) revealed a direct correlation between urea kinetics and morbidity of patients on hemodialysis, which resulted in a number of practical and objective indices of dialysis efficiency, allowing better patient management (see Chapter 63).

Methylguanidine and Other Guanidines

Guanidinosuccinic acid and methylguanidine accumulate in uremic serum at levels that are potentially toxic. Methylguanidine, when injected to healthy dogs, causes symptoms of heavy intoxication. Guanidinosuccinic acid has been shown to interfere with platelet function and with the production of calcitriol from its precursors in the rat. Guanidines may also contribute to uremic neuropathy.

Indoxyl Sulfate

Indoxyl sulfate has been held responsible for decreased binding of drugs to plasma proteins, and to defects of cellular organic acid transport, especially in the renal cortical tubules. Reduction of serum indoxyl sulfate concentration, by intraintestinal absorption of the precursor indole, reduces uremic itching. Indoxyl sulfate is not removed effectively during hemodialysis, due to its high protein binding. Removal by CAPD is more effective.

Due to its substantial protein binding (about 100% in normals, and 90% in uremics), indoxyl sulfate's intradialytic behavior does not correspond to that of other small, water soluble compounds such as urea and creatinine.

Hippuric Acid

Hippuric acid inhibits the transport of a variety of organic acids, especially in the renal proximal tubule, the chorioid plexus of the brain, the ciliary body of the eye, the thyroid, the liver, and erythrocytes. It also interferes with the protein binding of acidic drugs, such as phenytoin and theophylline, and with glucose tolerance. Hippuric acid (MW: 179 Da) also behaves like a larger molecule, due to its protein binding.

Peptides

Concentration changes of vasoactive peptides may play a role in the regulation of blood pressure in uremic patients. Endothelin is retained in uremic patients. Atrial natriuretic factor (ANF-atriopeptide) may be elevated in uremia, especially during states of expanded extracellular fluid volume, e.g., before the start of hemodialysis. The effect of hemodialysis on vasoactive peptide concentration has recently been evaluated. Whereas endothelin decreased only with high flux dialyzers, atriopeptide decreased with all types of dialyzers, irrespective of their pore size, due to the decrease in intravascular volume that occurred during dialysis.

Parathormone (PTH), a middle molecule with a MW of approximately 9000 Da, is oversecreted during uremia to correct for hypocalcemia and hyperphosphatemia. PTH causes glucose intolerance, inhibition of human platelet function, cardiomyopathy, inhibition of erythropoiesis, altered red cell osmotic resistance, altered B cell proliferation, synaptosome and T-cell dysfunction, and defects of fatty acid oxidation.

The molecular weight of PTH makes it a classical middle molecule. Although PTH removal by dialysis has a rather weak influence on its plasma concentration, serum PTH serves as one of the indirect parameters of long-term adequacy of dialysis, since its production is correlated with long-term phosphate accumulation.

β_2-Microglobulin (β_2M) (MW approximating 11,000 Da), a breakdown product of the major histocompatibility complex, is also a middle molecule. Amyloidosis, frequently observed in long-term dialysis patients (see Chapter 69), is caused by deposition of β_2M in various sites. It is not entirely clear whether this disorder is related to accumulation as such, or other factors such as the enhanced release of the protein or a result of membrane or dialysate contact during hemodialysis.

Dialysis-related amyloidosis, is characterized by the deposition of β_2M amyloid in bone, causing cysts that may be painful, and in the tendons, tendon rupture and carpal tunnel syndrome. The latter results in nerve and motor dysfunction of the hands.

The intradialytic plasma concentration of β_2M is determined by both removal and hemoconcentration. Plasma β_2M levels often increase during dialysis using membranes with small pores because the proteins are not removed and also because removal of water causes hemoconcentration. Removal of β_2M is, however, achieved during dialysis using dialyzers with large pores, but even removal by these membranes cannot keep pace with the daily generation of β_2M. Patients treated exclusively with polyacrylonitrile (AN69) membranes with large pore size have less bone amyloidosis than those treated with small pore size cellulosic membranes. Breakdown products of larger proteins such as β_2M are also potentially deleterious. Two polypeptides extracted from uremic plasma ultrafiltrate, one with structural homology with a part of β_2M, have immunosuppressive effects.

Organic Phosphates

A high level of organic phosphates may cause uremic itching. Accumulation of organic phosphates stimulates parathyroid activity, resulting in hyperparathyroidism. Phosphates are primarily derived from protein intake and catabolism as well as other dietary sources. Dialytic phosphate removal is followed by a marked rebound, suggesting multicompartmental behavior which does not correlate with urea elimination.

At high concentrations, organic phosphates complex with calcium and are deposited in the tissue as phosphate-calcium complexes; this causes metastatic calcification in many tissues, inducing functional disturbances besides itching and conjunctivitis.

FACTORS INFLUENCING PLASMA CONCENTRATION OF UREMIC SOLUTES

Numerous factors influence the plasma concentration of uremic solutes, such as protein intake, general metabolic status, residual renal function, dialysis performance, protein binding, and multicompartimental distribution. Elimination via the urine remains important even after dialysis has been started. For example, at a clearance of 5 mL/min, the kidneys still clear 50 L/week, to be compared with a clearance of 15 to 150 L/week (depending on the specific solute) through artificial kidneys.

CONCLUSIONS

The uremic syndrome results from the accumulation of multiple toxins rather than of one single substance, and from the deficiency of certain substances. Clinically employed markers of uremia, such as urea and creatinine, do not play a major role in the development of the clinical uremic syndrome.

The source of these uremic toxins is only related in part to protein breakdown. Whereas urea and organic phosphates are products of protein catabolism, and creatinine and the guanidines from muscle breakdown, the origin of many other uremic toxins is less clear. For some, such as hippuric acid, their origin is a specific amino acid together with non protein sources. Others have completely different origins, as is the case for indoxyl sulfate, β_2M, and PTH.

Calculations based on urea removal are often used to guide the dialysis prescription, because urea is a small, water-soluble non-protein-bound compound that is generated from protein and easily measured. However, the removal and generation of many of the putative uremic toxins

discussed above are not readily predicted from the behavior of urea, because they are hydrophobic, protein bound, or not products of protein catabolism.

Depending on the renal replacement strategy, there may be a dissociation between the removal of small water soluble markers such as urea and creatinine as compared to toxic retention compounds with a higher molecular weight (e.g., β_2M, PTH) or lipophilicity (e.g., phenols, p-cresol). Substantial improvement in artificial kidney technology awaits a more thorough understanding of both the basic metabolic disturbances that occur in uremia and the toxic compounds responsible.

Bibliography

Fraser CL, Arieff AI: Nervous system complications in uremia. *Ann Intern Med* 109, 143–153, 1988.

Haas T, Hillion D, Dongradi G: Phosphate kinetics in dialysis patients. *Nephrol Dial Transplant* 6 (Suppl 2), 108–113, 1991.

Hörl WH, Haag-Weber M, Georgopoulos A, Block LH: Physicochemical characterization of a polypeptide present in uremic serum that inhibits the biological activity of polymorphonuclear cells. *Proc Natl Acad Sci USA* 87, 6353–6357, 1990.

Hsu CH, Patel SR, Young EW, Vanholder R: The biological action of calcitriol in renal failure. *Kidney Int* 46, 605–612, 1994.

Kushner D, Beckman B, Nguyen L, et al.: Polyamines in the anemia of end-stage renal disease. *Kidney Int* 39, 725–732, 1991.

Lowrie EG, Laird NM, Parker TF, Sargent JA: Effect of the hemodialysis prescription on patient morbidity. *N Engl J Med* 305, 1176–1181, 1980.

Mall G, Rambausek M, Neumeister A, Kollmar S, Vetterlein F, Ritz E: Myocardial interstitial fibrosis in experimental uremia: implications for cardiac compliance. *Kidney Int* 33, 804–811, 1988.

Niwa T, Fujishiro T, Uema K, et al.: Effect of hemodialysis on plasma levels of vasoactive peptides: endothelin, calcitonin-gene related peptide and human atrial natriuretic peptide. *Nephron* 64, 552–559, 1993.

Noris M, Benigni A, Boccardo P, et al.: Enhanced nitric oxide synthesis in uremia: implications for platelet dysfunction and dialysis hypotension. *Kidney Int* 44, 445–450, 1993.

Parfrey PS, Harnett JD, Barre PR. The natural history of myocardial disease in dialysis patients. *J Am Soc Nephrol* 2, 2–12, 1991.

Piafsky KM: Disease-induced changes in the plasma binding of basic drugs. *Clin Pharmacokin* 5, 246–262, 1980.

Ringoir S, Schoots A, Vanholder R. Uremic toxins. *Kidney Int* 33 (Suppl 24), S4–S9, 1988.

Ritz E, Matthias S, Seidel A, Reichel H, Szabo A, Hörl WH: Disturbed calcium metabolism in renal failure: pathogenesis and therapeutic strategies. *Kidney Int* 42 (Suppl 38), S37–S42, 1992.

Vallance P, Leone A, Calver A, Collier J, Moncada S: Accumulation of an endogenous inhibitor of nitric oxide synthesis in chronic renal failure. *Lancet* 339, 572–575, 1992.

Vanholder R, Ringoir S: Adequacy of dialysis: a critical review. *Kidney Int* 42, 540–558, 1992.

Vanholder R, Ringoir S: Infectious morbidity and defects of phagocytic function in end-stage renal disease: a review. *J Am Soc Nephrol* 3, 1541–1554, 1993.

Vanholder R, Patel S, Hsu CH: Effect of uric acid on plasma levels of 1,25 (OH)$_2$D in renal failure. *J Am Soc Nephrol* 4, 1035–1038, 1993.

Vanholder R, De Smet R, Waterloos MA, et al.: Mechanisms of uremic inhibition of phagocyte reactive species production: characterization of the role of p-cresol. *Kidney Int* 47, 510–517, 1995.

HEMODIALYSIS AND HEMOFILTRATION

ALFRED K. CHEUNG

STRUCTURE OF HEMODIALYZERS AND HEMOFILTERS

Extracorporeal therapy for renal failure refers to the process in which fluid and solutes are removed from or added to the patient's blood outside the body. During this process, blood from the patient is continuously circulated through a hemodialyzer or hemofilter containing an artificial semipermeable membrane and then returned to the patient.

A typical modern hemodialyzer is composed of several thousand parallel hollow fibers. The wall of these fibers is the semipermeable membrane separating the blood in the fiber lumen from the dialysate outside. The total internal surface area of all the fibers is usually between 0.5 and 2.0 m^2. Less commonly, the membranes are in the form of flat sheets rather than hollow fibers. Regardless of the membrane geometry, blood from each parallel flow path is channelled into the single inlet and single outlet of the plastic casing. There is also an inlet and an outlet for the dialysate compartment in which the dialysate is usually circulated in a single-pass fashion countercurrent to the blood flow. Hemofiltration employs no dialysate; hemofilters have an inlet and an outlet for blood and a single outlet for the ultrafiltrate compartment.

TYPES OF EXTRACORPOREAL THERAPY FOR RENAL FAILURE

Among the numerous modalities of extracorporeal renal therapy outlined in Table 1, "conventional hemodialysis" and "high efficiency hemodialysis" are most commonly used, although "high flux hemodialysis" is gradually gaining popularity. Dialysis removes solutes by *diffusion*, based on concentration gradients of solutes between the blood and dialysate across the semipermeable membrane (Fig. 1A). For example, urea diffuses from the blood to the dialysate compartment, thereby decreasing the total urea mass in the body as well as the urea *concentration* in the plasma. Conversely, the concentration gradient of bicarbonate usually favors the diffusion of this ion from the dialysate to the blood compartment. Fluid movement is not a prerequisite for solute transport in this modality, although fluid loss from the patient is often desirable. High efficiency hemodialysis refers to hemodialysis using high blood flow rates and/or large surface area membrane dialyzers in order to remove urea and other small solutes (such as urea and potassium) more rapidly than during conventional

hemodialysis. High flux hemodialysis utilizes membranes with large pores in order to rapidly remove water and solutes that are substantially larger than urea ("middle molecules") (see Chapter 62). For chronic renal failure patients, maintenance hemodialysis is usually performed intermittently, for example, 3 to 5 hours three times a week either at home or in-center at a dialysis unit.

Hemofiltration is another form of extracorporeal therapy which removes fluid by *convection*, i.e., movement of water across the large pore hemofiltration membrane into the ultrafiltrate compartment drags along the solutes which are dissolved in the water (Fig. 1B). A crucial distinction between hemodialysis and hemofiltration is that fluid must be removed in hemofiltration for solute removal. Removal of fluid with its accompanying solutes results in a loss in the total body *mass* of the solute, but not a decrease in the plasma *concentration*. In order to achieve a substantial decrease in the concentration, "clean" replacement fluid is infused intravenously to approximately replace the large volume of plasma fluid removed in the hemofilter. This modality is analogous to the glomerulus, which also removes plasma solutes by convection. In the case of the glomerulus, however, the replacement fluid is the water and electrolytes that are selectively reabsorbed from the renal tubules (Fig. 1C). Hemodiafiltration refers to the combination of hemodialysis and hemofiltration operating simultaneously using a large pore membrane, i.e., solutes are removed by both diffusion as well as convection. Hemofiltration and hemodiafiltration are used in the United States primarily for acute renal failure. Under these circumstance, they are applied continuously for days to weeks, usually in the intensive care unit, and are therefore termed "continuous renal replacement therapy." In Europe and Japan, hemofiltration and hemodiafiltration are also utilized on an intermittent basis to treat chronic renal failure. During a 4-hour session of maintenance hemofiltration, 16 to 20 L of body fluid is typically exchanged.

Hemoperfusion is the removal of solutes (usually toxins) from blood by adsorption onto materials, such as charcoal or resins, in the extracorporeal circuit. Hemoperfusion is primarily used to treat acute poisoning.

HEMODIALYSIS AND HEMOFILTRATION MEMBRANES AND MACHINES

Transport and, to a lesser extent, biocompatibility are two characteristics of dialysis membranes that are of inter-

408

TABLE I

Glossary of Various Types of Extracorporeal Therapy for Renal Failure

Hemodialysis (HD)

    Conventional hemodialysis—hemodialysis using a conventional low flux (small pore size) membranes. Solute removal is primarily by diffusion.

    High efficiency hemodialysis—hemodialysis using a low flux (small pore size) membrane with high efficiency (K_oA) for removal of small solutes. Typically achieved by using a larger surface area membrane.

    High flux hemodialysis—hemodialysis using a high flux (large pore size) membrane. It is more efficient in removing larger solutes, but may or may not be more efficient than conventional hemodialysis in removing small solutes.

Hemofiltration (HF)

    Continuous arteriovenous hemofiltration (CAVH)—removal of small and larger solutes using a high flux membrane and convection rather than diffusion. Blood is accessed from an artery and returned to a vein with the driving force deriving from the systemic arterial pressure. Because it is performed continuously (usually in the intensive care setting), it is also very effective in removing large amount of fluid.

    Continuous venovenous hemofiltration (CVVH)—similar to CAVH except that blood is accessed from a vein and returned to another vein using a blood pump.

    Intermittent hemofiltration—hemofiltration performed on an intermittent basis for chronic renal failure.

Hemodiafiltration (HDF)

    Continuous arteriovenous hemodiafiltration (CAVHD)—similar to CAVH in that solutes are removed by convection using a high flux membrane in an acute setting. In addition, dialysate flows continuously through the dialysate compartment in order to enhance solute removal by diffusion, i.e., it is a combination of hemodialysis and hemofiltration.

    Continuous venovenous hemodiafiltration (CVVHD)—similar to CAVHD except that blood is accessed from a vein and returned to another vein using a blood pump.

    Intermittent hemodiafiltration—hemodiafiltration performed on an intermittent basis for chonic renal failure.

Hemoperfusion (HP)—removal of solutes by adsorption to charcoal or resin, primarily for treatment of acute poisoning.

est to clinical nephrologists. Although there are exceptions, hemodialysis membranes that are made from cellulose usually have small pores which restrict the movement of large solutes, and to some extent, the movement of water. In contrast, high flux hemodialysis membranes, which can also be used for hemofiltration, are usually made from synthetic polymers with large pores that facilitate transport of water and middle molecules. Modern hemodialysis machines contain ultrafiltration control devices that precisely regulate the flow of fluid across these porous membranes, thereby preventing an excessively rapid decrease in intravascular volume. Because of their high hydraulic permeability (or ultrafiltration coefficient, see below), high flux membranes can only be used with machines that are equipped with these devices.

Biocompatibility of dialysis membranes refers to the interactions that occur as a result of contact of blood with the membrane. Examples of such interactions include the activation of proteins of the coagulation and complement system, as well as various peripheral blood cells. Biocompatibility is relative, since all dialysis membranes induce reactions to a certain extent which can manifest, for example, as thrombosis in the dialyzer and, rarely, acute anaphylactoid reactions. Recent studies have suggested that patients with acute renal failure who were dialyzed with membranes that activate less complement and neutrophils had more rapid recovery of renal function and lower mortality rates than patients who were dialyzed with membranes that activate complement and neutrophils more intensely.

The dialysis machine incorporates many important features including, a pump to deliver blood to the dialyzer at a constant rate, monitors to ensure that the pressures inside the extracorporeal circuit are not excessive, a detector for leakage of red blood cells from the blood compartment into the dialysate compartment, an air detector and shut-off device to prevent air from entering the patient, a pump to deliver dialysate, a proportioning system to properly dilute the dialysate concentrate, a heater to warm the dialysate to approximately body temperature, and conductivity monitors to check dialysate ion concentrations. These devices ensure the proper, safe, and reliable delivery of blood and dialysate to the dialyzer where exchange of water and solutes occurs. Machines employed for intermittent hemofiltration are similar to those for hemodialysis, with the additional requirements for precise ultrafiltration and fluid replacement coordination and control.

In contrast, continuous arteriovenous hemofiltration (CAVH) does not require any machinery. Blood is delivered to the hemofilter from an artery, such as the femoral artery, via a large bore (~14–15 gauge) catheter and returned to a large vein, with the driving force derived directly from the heart rather than a mechanical pump. Unfortunately, blood flow and therefore ultrafiltration rates are sometimes erratic in CAVH. Machines have been developed which pump blood from a vein through the hemofilter and back to a vein—a technique known as continuous venovenous hemofiltration (CVVH). The machines for CVVH are usually simpler in design than conventional

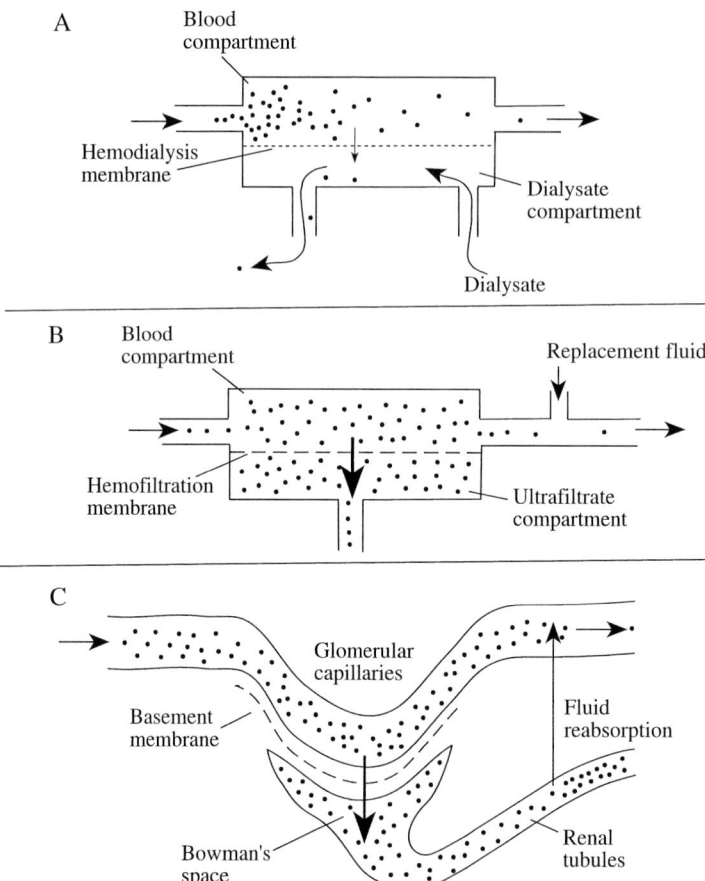

FIGURE 1 Schematic representation of solute and fluid transport across the semipermeable membranes. (A) Hemodialyzer. The plasma concentration of small solutes (solid circles) in the blood inlet is high. Because of the diffusive loss across the semipermeable hemodialysis membrane (dotted line), the plasma concentration in the blood outlet is much lower. The thin arrow across the dialysis membrane represents a small amount of fluid loss (which is not necessary for solute removal). High dialysate flow rate is necessary to maintain the concentration gradient across the dialysis membrane. (B) Hemofilter. Plasma concentration of small solutes in the blood compartment remains unchanged as blood travels the length of the fiber, and is similar to their concentrations in the ultrafiltrate. The hemofiltration membrane (broken line) has relatively large pores, which allow the necessary removal of large volume of fluid (heavy arrow). Replacement fluid is infused into the blood outlet in order to lower the plasma concentration of solutes and compensate for the fluid loss. (C) Glomerulus. Analogous to hemofiltration, plasma concentration of small solutes remains unchanged throughout the length of the glomerular capillary and is similar to that in Bowman's space. Fluid removal across the glomerular basement membrane (broken curve) is large (heavy arrow). Reabsorption of fluid from the renal tubules lowers the plasma concentration of the solutes.

hemodialysis machines, because dialysate production and many other devices are absent. One disadvantage of CAVH and CVVH is that they are less efficient than hemodialysis in removing urea, potassium, and other small solutes because there is no dialysate to permit diffusion. In order to improve solute clearance, continuous dialysate flow is sometimes added to these systems—techniques known as continuous arteriovenous hemodiafiltration (CAVHD) and continuous venovenous hemodiafiltration (CVVHD).

Unfortunately, the addition of dialysate also adds complexity to these systems.

WATER TRANSPORT AND SOLUTE CLEARANCE PROFILES

The effectiveness of water transport across a dialysis membrane is measured as the ultrafiltration coefficient, which is sometimes imprecisely called the ultrafiltration rate. Ultrafiltration coefficients for conventional hemodialysis membranes are usually 2 to 5 mL · hr^{-1} Hg^{-1}. With a transmembrane pressure of 200 mm Hg, a dialyzer with a coefficient 2.5 mL · hr^{-1}. Hg^{-1} will remove 0.5 L of fluid per hour or 2 L in 4 hours. Ultrafiltration coefficients for high flux dialysis or hemofiltration membranes are much higher, at 15 to 60 mL · hr^{-1} · mm Hg^{-1}.

The solute transport properties of dialysis membranes are usually expressed as the mass transfer-area coefficient, which is the product of the mass transfer coefficient (K_o) and membrane surface area (A). The mass transfer coefficient of a dialysis membrane is similar to its diffusivity. The clearance profile of solutes by conventional analysis membranes presented in Fig. 2 reflects primarily the K_oA of the membranes and only provides a rough estimation of what might be achieved clinically. The actual solute clearances depend also on the blood flow rate, dialysate flow rate, and removal. Diffusive clearance of solutes by hemodialysis decreases rapidly with increasing molecular size. For small solutes such as urea, however, removal per unit time by hemodialysis is more efficient than that by the native kidneys. Urea clearance is typically between 180 and 220 mL/min for hemodialysis, which is two times the value for the glomeruli in two kidneys (often 90 to 110 mL/min for adults). Because of the limited number of hours (usually 9 to 15) that the patient actually spends on hemodialysis per week, the total weekly clearance of urea by hemodialysis is

far lower than that achieved by native kidneys (168 hours/week).

Clearance of larger solutes, such as β_2-microglobulin (12,000 Da), by conventional hemodialysis is much lower than that for urea. Because of the diffusive nature of transport, clearance by high flux membranes also decreases rapidly with molecular size, albeit less rapidly compared to conventional low flux dialysis membranes. In contrast, clearance by hemofiltration, even using the same membranes as for high flux hemodialysis, is maintained for solutes up to ~1000 Da. This is because the mode of transport in hemofiltration is convection, which is governed by the membrane sieving coefficient (defined as ultrafiltrate to plasma concentration ratio) of the solute rather than its diffusivity, and the sieving coefficient remains near 1.0 up to ~1000 Da. For higher molecular weight solutes, however, the sieving coefficients, and hence clearances, also decline.

DIALYSATE

The dialysate creates solute concentration gradients to drive diffusion across the dialysis membrane. The typical composition of dialysate is shown in Table 2. Sodium is removed primarily by convection such that ultrafiltration of 4 L of isotonic fluid results in ~560 mEq or 13 g of sodium removal without a change in plasma sodium *concentration*. In fact, dialysate sodium is usually kept at concentrations similar to or higher than that in plasma to avoid a decrease in plasma sodium concentration. In contrast, dialysate potassium concentration is often kept low in order to decrease plasma potassium concentration. Because dialysis patients are generally acidemic, base in the form of either bicarbonate or acetate is offered. Acetate dialysate is slightly less expensive but has the disadvantages of inducing hypoxemia and a transient worsening of metabolic acidosis because of the initial loss of bicarbonate from the plasma. It also causes intradialytic hypotension and an ill sensation in some patients. Proportioning systems in modern ma-

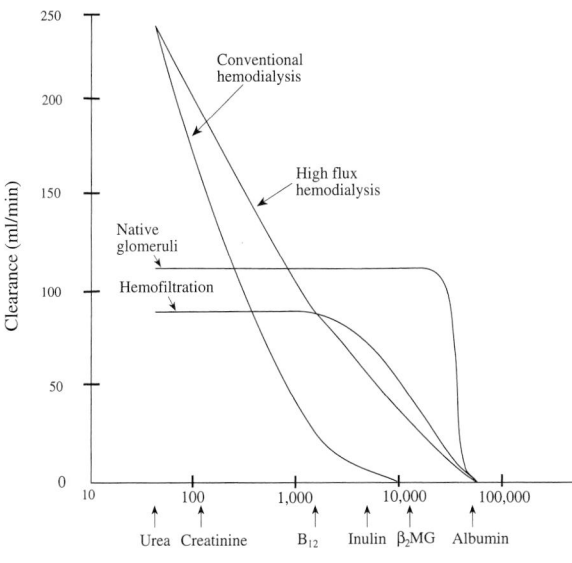

FIGURE 2 Solute clearance profile of various modalities. The curves are constructed based partially on data and partially on theroretical projection. The actual values may vary depending on the surface area of the membrane and operating conditions, such as blood flow rate. Native glomeruli refer to the summation of all the glomeruli in two normal kidneys. "Glomeruli" instead of "kidneys" are used because tubular reabsorption lowers the renal clearance of certain solutes (e.g., urea and glucose) substantially. B$_{12}$, vitamin B$_{12}$; β_2MG, β_2-microglobulin.

TABLE 2
Composition of Dialysate Commonly Used in Clinical Hemodialysis

Ions	Concentrations
Na$^+$	132–145^a mEq/L
K$^+$	0–4.0 mEq/L
Cl$^-$	103–110 mEq/L
HCO$_3^-$	0–40 mEq/L
Acetate^b	2–37 mEq/L
Ca^{2+}	0–3.5 mEq/L
Mg^{2+}	0.5–1.0 mEq/L
Glucose	0–200 mg/dL

^{a} Higher dialysate sodium concentration is sometimes used at the beginning of the dialysis session ("sodium modeling").

^{b} Either HCO$_3^-$ or acetate is used primarily as buffer.

chines have made delivery of bicarbonate dialysate a relatively easy task. Calcium concentration in the dialysate varies depending on the specific need of the patient. Dialysate magnesium concentration is sometimes lowered so that the patient can take oral magnesium-containing phosphate binders. Glucose is usually provided at 200 mg/dL to maintain the plasma glucose level stable for both diabetic and nondiabetic patients.

VASCULAR ACCESS

An adequate vascular access for hemodialysis should permit blood flow to the dialyzer of 200 to 500 mL/min in adults, depending on the size of the patient. For acute hemodialysis, a large vein, such as the femoral vein, is often cannulated with a double-lumen catheter. One lumen is for extracting the blood from the patient (so-called "arterial" side even though it may come from the patient's vein), and the other returns blood to the patient ("venous" side). Femoral catheters are seldom left in place for more than one dialysis session unless the patient is nonambulatory, because they are prone to kinking, dislodgement, and infection.

For usage of one to several weeks, an indwelling double-lumen catheter is often placed in an internal jugular or subclavian vein percutaneously. These catheters can be infected, dislodged, or occluded by thrombi. In addition, catheters at these sites predispose the vessels to stenosis. Stenosis of these vessels can cause outflow obstruction and severe swelling of the ipsilateral arm, especially if a permanent arteriovenous fistula, with arterialized venous pressure and augmented blood flow, is present in that arm. Subclavian veins appear to be more likely to develop stenosis than internal jugular veins and therefore should be avoided if at all possible. Stiff catheters are incriminated more frequently than softer ones. Softer catheters with anchoring cuffs offer a good alternative. These catheters are usually tunneled subcutaneously in the upper thorax before entering a proximal vessel or, rarely, inserted via the groin into the femoral vein. They may be used for several weeks to over a year. Thrombosis of these semipermanent catheters can be resolved with local instillation of thrombolytic agents. The original form of temporary vascular access was the Scribner shunt, a plastic conduit placed outside the skin with the two internal ends inserted and anchored to an artery and a vein, respectively. The disadvantage of this shunt is that it often destroys a potential site for a future permanent access. Scribner shunts are also prone to infection and carry the potential danger of rapid blood loss if one or both ends are dislodged. They are sparingly used nowadays but their high blood flow rate is an advantage in selected patients.

Long-term vascular access for hemodialysis is usually established by the creation of an arteriovenous (AV) fistula in an upper extremity, although a lower extremity or even an axillary vessel may sometimes be employed. A fistula is established by connecting an artery to a nearby vein either by direct surgical anastomosis of the native vessels or with an artificial vascular graft, for example, one made of polytetrafluoroethylene (PTFE). Native fistulae are pre-

ferred over PTFE grafts because of their relative longevity (approximately 80% vs 50% patency in 3 years) and lower susceptibility to infection. The disadvantages are a need for sufficiently large native veins and a 4 to 8-week maturation period during which the wall of the fistula thickens and the lumen enlarges before the fistula is ready for use. PTFE grafts can be used earlier, occasionally at one week or less, but they tend to elicit acute transient local inflammatory reactions manifested by pain, swelling, and redness which usually subside spontaneously within a few weeks. PTFE grafts are also more prone to thrombosis and infection, but the convenience that they offer has made them a popular choice among many dialysis personnel and more common than native fistulae in the United States. Declotting of AV fistulae can be accomplished surgically, with local infusion of thrombolytic agents, or, more recently, with mechanical devices inserted percutaneously to break up the clot.

Stenosis at the outflow tract of AV fistulae occurs frequently. Partial obstruction impedes the flow of cleansed blood from the dialyzer back to the patient; as a result, the blood recirculates back to the "arterial" (afferent) limb of the fistula and decreases the amount of fresh systemic blood that can be delivered to the dialyzer. Hence, the overall efficiency of the dialysis process is diminished. Plasma urea concentration obtained from the arterial (afferent) and venous (efferent) tubings of the dialyzer, as well as that obtained from a peripheral vessel have been used to calculate the degree of blood recirculation in the dialysis circuit. Obstruction of the fistula outflow tract also leads to an increase in pressure inside the venous (efferent) tubing during hemodialysis, which has been used as a clue to the presence of fistula outflow stenosis. The reliability of both the urea recirculation method and the venous pressure method in detecting fistula stenosis has recently been questioned. Instead, other techniques involving noninvasive devices and the dilution principle have been developed to assess the total blood flow through AV fistulae. Monitoring changes in total fistula flow rates over time allows earlier detection of stenosis. An angiogram (also called "fistulogram" in this context) with the injection of contrast dye (or carbon dioxide for patients who are allergic to contrast) remains the gold standard for the confirmation and anatomical definition of AV fistula stenosis. Fistula stenosis is treated surgically by replacing or bypassing the stenotic segment. Alternatively, stenosis may be relieved by angioplasty with or without the placement of a stent to keep the lumen open. If left untreated, most stenotic fistulae eventually become totally occluded by thrombi. AV fistulae can be infected by both Gram positive, especially Staphylococcus, and Gram negative bacteria. Mild infection can be treated with antibiotics; more severe infection is treated by resection of the fistula. Although they are more difficult to treat conservatively, infected artificial grafts do not invariably require surgical removal.

Blood flow through the AV fistula often exceeds 1 L/min and occasionally 2 L/min, accounting for 20 to 40% of cardiac output, although the blood flow through the dialysis needles inserted into the fistula is considerably lower. This diversion of cardiac output from the capillary beds can cause distal ischemia, i.e., steal syndrome. In addition, it can precipitate or exacerbate congestive heart failure in certain patients. Abandonment or decreasing the luminal diameter of the fistula surgically is sometimes necessary.

Early planning and placement of a permanent native AV fistula before the chronic renal failure patient requires dialysis is the preferred approach. For patients with poor veins, artificial grafts will have to be used. When early placement of an AV fistula is not accomplished, surgical placement of a semipermanent soft catheter in the proximal internal jugular vein is a good alternative while waiting for the AV fistula to mature. For patients with a short life expectancy or when sites for placement of fistula are no longer available, these semipermanent catheters are sometimes used indefinitely. If percutaneous temporary catheters are used, they should be placed with minimal trauma to the vessel during insertion. The internal jugular vein on the contralateral side of the planned AV fistula is preferrable. The temporary catheter should be removed as soon as the permanent access becomes functional. Repeat catheterization of femoral veins for individual dialysis sessions, especially for short periods, is a reasonable alternative.

Anticoagulation

Exposure of blood to the extracorporeal circuit activates the clotting mechanisms. Heparin is used commonly as the anticoagulant in clinical hemodialysis. It is often given as an intravenous bolus of 1000 to 5000 U at the beginning of the session, followed by either continuous infusion or intermittent boluses at ~500 to 2000 U/hr up until the last hour of dialysis. In some dialysis units, the activated clotting time or partial thrombin time is measured periodically for determining heparin requirement and monitoring for individual patients. In patients in whom bleeding is likely or potentially disastrous, for example, immediate postoperative patients, lower dose heparin (termed by some "tight" heparin or "minimum" heparin) is used with careful observation of the extracorporeal circuit for clotting. Hemodialysis can sometimes be performed without using any anticoagulants. Underlying coagulation defects, high blood flow rates, and periodic flushing of the blood compartment with saline help prevent clotting under these circumstances.

Regional heparinization involves infusion of heparin into the arterial blood entering the dialyzer, and neutralizing the heparin effect by infusion of protamine sulfate in the venous line. Regional citrate is a similar technique except that citrate and calcium are used to produce and reverse anticoagulation, respectively. These procedures are relatively cumbersome and are employed infrequently, although some have advocated their use in patients with a high risk of bleeding in the acute setting. The antiplatelet agent prostacyclin has also been used sucessfully by a few centers as a systemic anticoagulant during clinical hemodialysis. Hypotension can be a significant side effect of this medication.

INDICATIONS FOR HEMODIALYSIS AND HEMOFILTRATION

Acute hemodialysis is primarily performed for renal failure and drug overdose. Indications for emergency dialysis

in the acute renal failure setting include fluid overload, hyperkalemia, metabolic acidosis, and uremic signs and symptoms (see Chapter 41 for more details). Initiation of dialysis prior to onset of these problems is preferable. If reversal of the acute renal failure does not appear to be imminent, prophylactic dialysis is often instituted when the BUN is around 70 to 80 mg/dL or estimated glomerular filtration rate is 5 to 10 mL/min, although some have advocated the initiation of dialysis even earlier. Maintenance dialysis for chronic renal failure is usually started at similar glomerular filtration rates, unless the clinical condition dictates earlier intervention. Although hemofiltration is more effective in removing larger solutes than hemodialysis, the clinical indications for this form of therapy on a chronic intermittent basis have not been precisely defined.

Continuous extracorporeal therapies, such as CAVH and CVVH, are particularly useful for patients in the intensive care unit whose cardiovascular status is too unstable for rapid fluid removal, as may occur during intermittent hemodialysis. They are also used in patients from whom removal of substantial amounts of fluid on a continuous basis is desired, e.g., patients with multiple trauma receiving parenteral nutrition, blood products, and various intravenous medications. Clearances of urea and potassium by CAVH and CVVH are sometimes inadequate to maintain plasma concentrations of these solutes in the desirable range. Under these circumstances, continuous dialysate flow is added to the system, i.e., CAVHD or CVVHD is employed. Preliminary results from a randomized trial have suggested that the employment of continuous extracorporeal therapies is associated with a greater rate of kidney recovery from acute renal failure and shorter hospitalization stay than intermittent hemodialysis, although there was no difference in mortality rates. Peritoneal dialysis is another form of continuous therapy that can be used in patients suffering from acute renal failure with unstable hemodynamics, but for technical reasons it has been largely replaced by continuous extracorporeal modalities in this setting.

QUANTITATION OF HEMODIALYSIS

The amount of chronic hemodialysis that should be delivered to patients has not been well defined. Not infrequently, an arbitrary duration, blood flow rate, and size of the dialyzer are used based on the experience and intuition of the nephrologist. Removal of fluid to keep the patient euvolemic, or slightly hypovolemic, after dialysis is often desirable, but this so-called "dry weight" for individuals is often defined arbitrarily as the weight below which the patient develops symptomatic hypotension or muscle cramps. There are, of course, many imprecisions associated with this approach. For example, the likelihood of developing hypotension depends not only on the amount of fluid removed, but also on the rate of fluid removal.

Normalization of plasma electrolytes, such as potassium and hydrogen ions, is obviously important. Guidelines for removal of other uremic toxins are, however, more difficult to establish. Urea has been widely used as a marker to guide dialysis because it is an index of the production and accumulation of all nitrogenous waste products derived from protein metabolism. In addition, the removal of urea by hemodialysis appears to correlate with clinical outcome. In urea kinetic modeling, the index Kt/V is often used for quantitation of the dose of dialysis therapy; K is the hemodialyzer clearance, t is the duration of the dialysis session, and V is the volume of distribution of urea in the body. A Kt/V value of 1.2 is currently considered to be the minimum amount. Because Kt/V is tedious to determine precisely, some have simply used the decrease in BUN during dialysis as an alternative guide. A postdialysis to predialysis BUN ratio of 0.35 or a "urea reduction ratio" [calculated as (predialysis BUN minus postdialysis BUN) divided by predialysis BUN] of 65% is roughly equivalent to a Kt/V of 1.2. There are some suggestions that a larger dose of hemodialysis, for example, a Kt/V value of 1.6 to 1.8, is beneficial, although definitive data supporting this notion are lacking. Delivery of large doses of hemodialysis requires an adequate vascular access to provide high blood flow rates, a highly efficient dialyzer, and/or the willingness of the patient to endure longer dialysis sessions. It must be emphasized that the use of urea kinetics does not substitute for frequent and diligent clinical evaluation of the patient. Increasing the amount of dialysis should be considered if the patient exhibits uremic symptoms, regardless of the Kt/V value. In fact, urea kinetics are not used as the principal guide for hemodialysis therapy in some centers in Europe, although they are gradually gaining popularity. The clinical impact of removal of larger solutes (middle molecules) is at present unclear, although limited data suggest that they are also important.

Quantitation of acute hemodialysis is even more empirical. The dosage of dialysis provided for the treatment of exogenous toxins, for example, salicylates and lithium, is often guided by the plasma levels of the toxin and the clinical status. Dosage of dialysis for acute renal failure has been guided by the plasma chemistry, such as BUN, potassium, and bicarbonate, body fluids, and other clinical status, with the objective of maintaining the BUN below ~80 mg/dL most of the time. Recently, some nephrologists have advocated the quantitation of hemodialysis for acute renal failure using urea kinetics as well, although it is unclear if Kt/V values similar to those targeted for chronic dialysis are also appropriate in the acute setting. The significance of middle molecule removal in acute renal failure has not been carefully studied.

COMPLICATIONS OF HEMODIALYSIS

Although hemodialysis is nowadays a relatively safe procedure, Several complications may still arise. Some are inherent side effects of the normal extracorporeal circuit; some result from technical errors, and others are due to abnormal reactions of patients to the procedure. Intradialytic hypotension is common and has been attributed variably to body volume depletion, shifting of fluid from extra- to intracellular space as a result of decrease in serum osmolality induced by dialysis, impaired sympathetic activity,

vasodilation in response to warm dialysate, as well as splanchnic pooling of blood while eating during dialysis. Treatments include avoiding large interdialytic fluid gain, administration of normal saline, hypertonic saline, hypertonic glucose, mannitol, or colloids, decreasing dialysate temperature to produce vasoconstriction, and avoidance of eating during dialysis. Isolated ultrafiltration, which removes fluid in the absence of dialysate and therefore does not reduce the plasma osmolality, and "sodium modeling", which tailors dialysate sodium concentrations (135 to 160 mEq/L) throughout the dialysis session, are sometimes useful to minimize hypotensive events. Cardiac arrhythmias may occur as a result of rapid electrolyte changes, especially in patients taking digitalis and dialyzed against very low potassium dialysate (0 to 1 mEq/L). Arrhythmias can induce or aggravate hypotension and overt or silent myocardial ischemia.

Muscle cramps, nausea, and vomiting occur commonly during hemodialysis, and are often a result of rapid fluid removal. Too rapid removal of urea and other small solutes may lead to acute dysfunction of the central nervous system, sometimes referred to as disequilibrium syndrome (see Chapter 71). These patients may experience headache with nausea and vomiting, altered mental status, seizures, coma, and death. The pathophysiology of this symptom complex has not been well defined. Current evidence suggests that it may at least be partially attributed to the rapid decrease in plasma urea concentration and osmolality, with consequential fluid shifts into the intracranial compartment that cause cerebral edema. Severe disequilibrium syndrome is rare nowadays because hemodialysis is usually initiated at an early stage when the BUN is still not very high, and the efficiency of solute removal is often deliberately limited during the first treatment session.

Anaphylactoid reactions during hemodialysis are rare. They are manifested by various combinations of hypertension or hypotension, pulmonary symptoms, chest and abdominal pain, vomiting, fever, chills, flushing, urticaria, and pruritus. Cardiopulmonary arrest and death occasionally follow. The etiologies are probably multifactorial and may involve activation of the plasma complement or kinin systems by dialysis membranes, administration of angiotensin converting enzyme inhibitors concomitant to dialysis using membranes that intensely activate kinins, or the release of noxious materials that have contaminated the dialyzers during the manufacturing or sterilization process. Treatment for these anaphylactoid reactions is largely symptomatic. Preventive measures include thorough rinsing of the dialyzer before use and avoidance of the type of dialyzer and/or medications to which a particular patient is hypersensitive. Dialyzers or dialysates that are contaminated with microorganisms or their toxins can rarely cause fever and infection. Hepatitis B was prevalent in the 1970s, whereas hepatitis C infection is more common in hemodialysis units nowadays. The mode of transmission of hepatitis C in dialysis units has not be well established.

Hypoxemia occurs commonly during hemodialysis when acetate (instead of bicarbonate) is used as the dialysate buffer. The primary mechanism appears to be the initial loss of bicarbonate and carbon dioxide by diffusion into the dialysate, with subsequent hypoventilation. Dialysis membrane bioincompatibility may play a role by releasing mediators that impair gas exchange in some instances. A decrease in systemic partial oxygen pressure of 10 to 12 mm Hg is not uncommon, which could be deleterious for patients with underlying cardiopulmonary disease.

An array of technical errors associated with hemodialysis has been described, but fortunately they occur rarely. Inadequate purification of city water prior to use may result in high levels of contaminants in the dialysate, resulting in, for example, aluminum or calcium intoxication. Dialysate contaminated with chloramine and improper proportioning or overheating of dialysate by the dialysis machine also lead to hemolysis. Rupture of the dialysis membrane causes blood loss into the dialysate and entry of microorganisms from the dialysate into the blood. Defective blood circuit and monitoring devices may result in air embolism. Difficult or improper puncture with the dialysis needle may cause a local hematoma around the vascular access or external bleeding, which can be aggravated by intradialytic administration of heparin.

DIALYZER REUSE

Hemodialyzers can be reused repeatedly on the same patient after thorough cleansing and sterilization, employing various agents such as formaldehyde, glutaraldehyde, sodium hypochlorite (bleach), and the combination of hydrogen peroxide and peroxyacetic acid. The blood compartment must be thoroughly rinsed to remove all the sterilants prior to the next use, because residual sterilants infused into the body can be harmful. Inadequate sterilization, on the other hand, has been associated with infection by microorganisms. In general, reused dialyzers can clear small solutes as effectively as new dialyzers unless a substantial portion of the hollow fibers is occluded by clotted blood; in contrast, middle molecule clearance is sometimes impaired even when small solute clearance is maintained. Fiber bundle volume is checked after each processing, and the dialyzer is discarded if the volume is below 80% of that of a new dialyzer. Other contraindications to reuse include a disrupted dialyzer casing and hepatitis B infection. Reports on the effect of reuse on long-term clinical outcome are conflicting. Because of the economic benefits and lack of definite harmful effects when practiced properly, dialyzer reuse is popular in the United States.

CHOICE OF HEMODIALYZERS

There are several considerations when choosing a hemodialyzer for clinical use. One important consideration is the capacity (K_oA) of the membrane to clear urea, because urea removal by dialysis has been shown to correlate positively with patient survival and United States federal regulations have set criteria for the minimum urea removal.

Increasing amounts of data suggest that the removal of middle molecules is also beneficial. Biocompatibility characteristics of dialysis membrane are taken into account by some, albeit not all nephrologists. Therefore, high flux dialysis membranes, which are more effective in removing middle molecules and are in general more biocompatible, have gained popularity in recent years. Purchase cost and reusability of the dialyzer are additional concerns.

DRUG USAGE IN HEMODIALYSIS

Hemodialysis removes certain medications which are intended for therapeutic use. The removal of a drug depends on the properties of the drug as well as the conditions of the dialysis procedure (see Chapter 43). Guidelines for dosing medications in renal failure with or without dialysis have been published. It is imperative to refer to these publications for individual drugs if the physician is unfamiliar with their use in these settings. For example, different types of pencillins behave differently and the clearance of a drug by hemodialysis can be substantially different from that by peritoneal dialysis. It is also important to remember that these publications provide only a rough guideline. The information might be derived from conventional hemodialysis and might not be applicable to high flux dialysis. Finally, the efficacy of the particular dialysis session must be take into account. A short and inefficient dialysis because of vascular access problems would remove only small amount of aminoglycosides and the postdialysis supplemental dose should be adjusted accordingly. Frequently, monitoring of drug levels is required.

Bibliography

A symposium on practical issues in the use of continuous renal replacement therapies. *Sem in Dialysis* 9:79–223, 1996.

Ahmad S, Blagg CR, Scribner BH: Center and home chronic hemodialysis. In: Schrier RW, Gottschalk CW (eds) *Diseases of the Kidney,* 5th ed. Little, Brown, Boston, pp. 3031–3068, 1993.

Cheung AK, Leypoldt JK: The hemodialysis membranes: A historical perspective, current state and future prospect. *Sem in Nephrol,* 17:196–213, 1997.

Current concepts in the creation, maintenance, and preservation of hemodialysis access. *Sem in Dialysis* 9(suppl 1):S1–S54, 1996.

Feldman HI, Kobrin S, Wasserstein A: Hemodialysis vascular access morbidity. *J Am Soc Nephrol* 7:523–535, 1996.

Hakim RM, Wingard RL, Parker RA: Effect of the dialysis membrane in the treatment of patients with acute renal failure. *N Engl J Med* 331:1338–1374, 1994.

Held PJ, Port FK, Wolfe RA, et al.: The dose of hemodialysis and patient mortality. *Kidney Int* 50:550–556, 1996

Lowrie EG, Laird NM, Parker TF, Sargent JA: Effect of hemodialysis prescription on patient morbidity: Report from the National Cooperative Dialysis Study. *N Engl J Med* 305:1176-1181, 1981.

Nissenson AR, Fine RN, Gentile DE (eds): *Clinical Dialysis,* 3rd ed. Appleton & Lange, Norwalk, 1995.

Suki WN, Massry SG (eds): *Therapy of Renal Diseases and Related Disorders,* 2nd ed. Kluwer Academic Publishers, Boston, 1991.

Vanholder RC, Ringoir SM: Adequacy of dialysis: A critical analysis. *Kidney Int* 42:540–558, 1992.

64

PERITONEAL DIALYSIS

BETH PIRAINO

Peritoneal dialysis (PD) is a form of dialysis in which dialysate (content shown in Table 1) is instilled in the peritoneal cavity, periodically drained, and replaced with fresh solution via a catheter. The forms of PD are listed in Table 2. With continuous ambulatory peritoneal dialysis (CAPD), the patient manually exchanges the dialysate four to five times each day, as shown in Fig. 1. With continuous cycler peritoneal dialysis (CCPD), the patient connects the catheter to the cycler at bedtime. The cycler delivers a set number of exchanges over 8 to 10 hours, the last fill constituting the long day dwell. In the morning the patient disconnects the catheter from the cycler. The increasing popularity of CCPD (35% of all PD utilization in the United States in 1995) may be due to the convenience of performing the dialysis connections only twice per day and to the new cycler models which are smaller and more attractive to patients.

PERITONEAL MEMBRANE

Dialysis involves the movement of small solutes and water across a semipermeable membrane. The peritoneal membrane is the dialyzing surface in peritoneal dialysis. The visceral peritoneal membrane covers the abdominal organs, while the parietal peritoneum lines the abdominal cavity. The peritoneal membrane consists of a single layer of mesothelial cells overlying an interstitium in which the blood and lymphatic vessels lie. The mesothelial cells are covered by microvilli that markedly increase the 2 m^2 surface area of the peritoneum. The normal peritoneum is only a few millimeters in thickness.

During PD, solutes, such as urea nitrogen, creatinine, and potassium, move from the peritoneal capillaries across the peritoneal membrane to the peritoneal cavity, whereas other solutes, such as bicarbonate and calcium, move from the dialysate into the peritoneal capillaries. Clearance is achieved by both diffusion and convection. Small solute movement is mainly by diffusion and is thus based on the concentration gradient of the solute between dialysate and blood. Thus, substances with a low molecular weight such as creatinine, urea, and potassium, which are not in the infused dialysate, are effectively removed by PD. With increasing dwell time, the ratio of dialysate to serum urea levels approaches one (Fig. 2). Because the peritoneal membrane has a negative charge, negatively charged solutes such as phosphate will move across it more slowly than positively charged solutes such as potassium. Macromolecules such as albumin cross the peritoneum by mechanisms not completely understood, but probably via lymphatics and through large pores in the capillary membranes.

Dialysate contains a high concentration of dextrose. Thus, the dialysate is hyperosmolar compared to the serum, causing ultrafiltration, or fluid removal, to occur. The volume of ultrafiltration depends on the dextrose solution used for each exchange (Fig. 3), the length of the dwell, and the individual patient's peritoneal membrane characteristics (see below). With increasing dwell time, transperitoneal glucose absorption diminishes the dialysate glucose concentration and the osmotic gradient. Ultrafiltration is therefore decreased with long dwell times, for example with the overnight exchange on CAPD or the daytime exchange on CCPD. As the glucose concentration gradient falls during a dwell, the hydrostatic pressure created by the dialysate within the abdominal cavity overcomes the osmotic gradient, resulting in fluid reabsorption into the systemic circulation. In addition, continuous lymphatic absorption diminishes net fluid removal. A newer osmotic agent, icodextrin, which is a high molecular weight compound allowing continuous ultrafiltration for up to a 12-hour dwell time, appears promising as an alternative to dextrose, but is not yet commercially available.

The rate of movement of small solutes such as creatinine between dialysate and blood differs from one patient to another. Peritoneal function characteristics have been quantified in the peritoneal equilibration test (PET). In this standardized test, 2 L of 2.5 g/dL dextrose exchange are infused and the dialysate:plasma creatinine ratio at the end of a 4-hour dwell (D/P_{cr}) is measured. Using this test each patient's peritoneal membrane can be categorized as having high ($D/P_{cr} > 0.81$), high average (0.65 to 0.81), average (0.65), low average (0.50 to 0.65) or low (<0.5) peritoneal transport. Patients with a high D/P_{cr} have rapid clearance of small molecules but poor ultrafiltration due to dissipation of the concentration gradient between dialysate and blood by glucose absorption. Patients with a low D/P_{cr} have lower clearances and generally require increased numbers of dialysis exchanges and/or increased volume per exchange to avoid uremia once residual renal function is lost. Ultrafiltration in this category of patient is usually excellent. The majority of patients have high average, average, or low average peritoneal transport and do well on either CAPD or CCPD.

TABLE I

Composition of Peritoneal Dialysis Fluid

Sodium (mEq/L)	132
Chloride (mEq/L)	102, 96, or 95
Lactate (mEq/L)	35 or 40
Calcium (mEq/L)	2.5 or 3.5
Magnesium (mEq/L)	0.5 or 1.5
Dextrose (g/dL)	1.5, 2.5, or 4.25

PERITONEAL CATHETERS

The access for PD is a catheter, which is inserted into the abdominal cavity by either a surgeon or a nephrologist, generally using local anesthetic with sedation. Although there are numerous newer catheter designs, none offers a significant advantage over the original double-cuffed silastic Tenckhoff catheter which is still used most often. The intra-abdominal portion of the catheter has multiple perforations through which dialysate flows. With the deep cuff placed in a paramedian position in the rectus muscle, the catheter is tunneled through the subcutaneous tissue to exit laterally and downward. The subcutaneous superficial cuff is located about 3 cm from the exit site of the catheter. PD can be initiated immediately if exchange volumes are small and the patient is kept recumbent. Alternatively, PD may be deferred until the insertion site is well healed, at which time the patient is trained to perform CAPD or CCPD. Hemodialysis can be used if necessary as a temporary measure until PD is initiated.

Several potential catheter-related problems exist. A dialysate leak usually presents as clear fluid draining from the exit site. The leak can be confirmed by a strongly positive dipstick for glucose. CAPD is discontinued and hemodialysis used temporarily. Edema of the perineum, penis, scrotum, or abdominal wall generally indicates a subcutaneous dialysate leak. The location of the leak can usually be identified using CT with intra-abdominal contrast, following which the defect can be surgically closed. Inadequate flow in a catheter may be due to constipation (which responds to laxatives), catheter obstruction with fibrin or omentum, or poor catheter position. Ideally the catheter tip should be in the patient's pelvis. A poorly positioned catheter can sometimes be manipulated using a wire or via

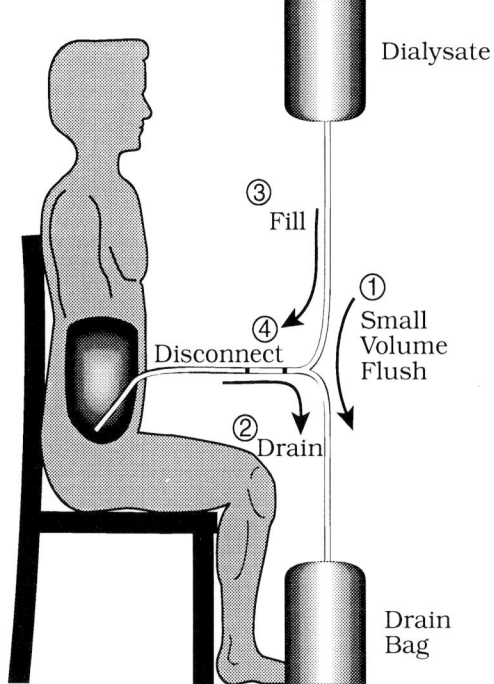

FIGURE I Diagram of a CAPD exchange using the Y-set. Between exchanges, the abdomen contains dialysate and only a short, capped extension tubing attached to the peritoneal catheter is present. The Y-set consists of tubing with a full bag of dialysate at one end (hanging at top in the picture) and an empty drainage bag which is placed on the floor. Clamps on the tubing direct the flow of fluid by gravity. To begin the exchange, the patient connects the Y tubing to the short exchange tubing attached to the catheter. The patient flushes air from the tubing (Step 1) by opening the clamp to the full dialysate bag and the drainage bag (keeping the peritoneal catheter clamped) for a count of 10. In Step 2, the clamp to the full bag is closed, and the clamp on the peritoneal catheter opened to allow the spent dialysate to flow into the drainage bag. This takes approximately 10 minutes. In Step 3, the patient closes the clamp to the drainage bag and opens the clamp on the tubing leading to the filled dialysate bag, thus allowing fresh dialysate to drain into the abdomen. The final step is to close the clamp on the peritoneal catheter extension tubing, disconnect the Y tubing, and cap the short extension tubing.

TABLE 2

Forms of Peritoneal Dialysis

Manual procedures	
Continuous ambulatory peritoneal dialysis (CAPD)	Three to four day time dwells plus a long bedtime exchange
Daytime peritoneal dialysis (DPD)[a]	Four short day dwells, no night dwell
Automated procedures	
Continuous cycling peritoneal dialysis (CCPD)	One to two long day dwells, three to four short nighttime exchanges
Nocturnal intermittent peritoneal dialysis (NIPD)[a]	No day dwell, multiple short nighttime exchanges
Intermittent peritoneal dialysis (IPD)[a]	Rapid cycling on an intermittent basis (usually three to four times per week), no dialysis between treatments

[a] Clearance inadequate unless the patient has a highly permeable membrane (high D/P_{cr}) and/or significant residual renal function.

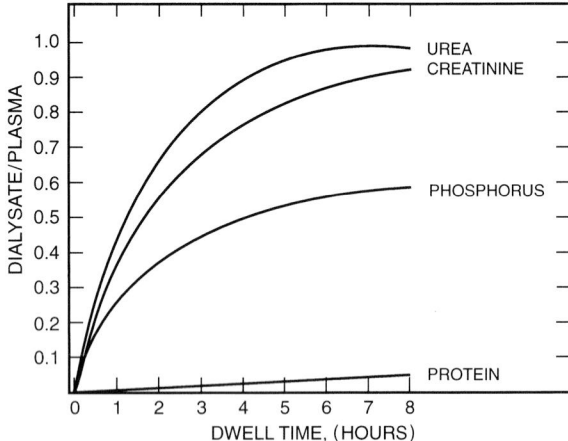

FIGURE 2 Dialysate to serum ratio over the period of a dwell using 1.5 g/dL dextrose, 2 L volume. From Popovich RP, Moncrief JW, Nolph KD, et al.: Continuous ambulatory peritoneal dialysis. *Ann Intern Med* 88:453, 1978; and Nolph KD, Twardowski ZJ, Popovich RP, Rubin J: Equilibraton of peritoneal dialysis solutions during long dwell exchanges. *J Lab Clin Med* 93:246–256, 1979. Reproduced with permission of Mosby–Year Book, Inc., St. Louis, and American College of Physicians, Philadelphia.

laparoscope to a better position, but catheter replacement may be required.

Peritoneal catheter infections include infections of the exit site (erythema or purulent drainage from the exit site) and tunnel infections (edema, erythema, or tenderness over the subcutaneous pathway). *Staphylococcus aureus* is responsible for the majority of catheter infections. *S. aureus* exit site infections are difficult to treat (Table 3), with frequent progression to tunnel infections and peritonitis, in which case catheter removal is required for resolution. *S. aureus* nasal carriage is associated with an increased risk of *S. aureus* catheter infections. Treatment of nasal carriers with intranasal mupirocin twice a day for 5 days each month, mupirocin applied daily to the exit site, or oral

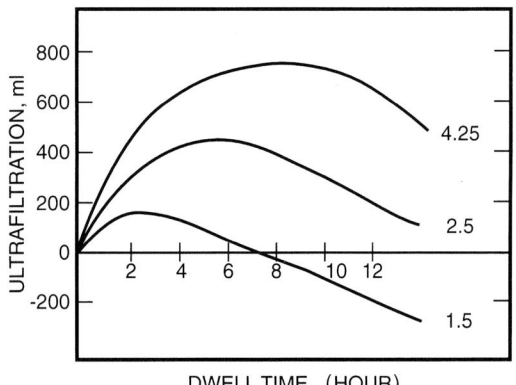

FIGURE 3 Ultrafiltration with 1.5, 2.5, and 4.25 g/dL dextrose dialysate, 2 L volume. From Twardowski ZJ, Khanna R, Nolph KD: *Nephron* 42:93–101, 1986. Reproduced with permission of S. Karger AG, Basel.

rifampin 600 mg every day for 5 days every 12 weeks are all effective in reducing *S. aureus* catheter infections. *Pseudomonas aeruginosa* catheter infections are also difficult to resolve and frequently relapse. Ciprofloxacin is used to treat *P. aeruginosa* catheter infections, but if *P. aeruginosa* peritonitis develops, the catheter must be removed to resolve the infection.

PERITONITIS

Peritonitis is defined as cloudy dialysate in which there are 100 white blood cells/mm^3, more than 50% of which are polymorphonuclear. The patient generally has abdominal pain, but may or may not have fever, nausea, or vomiting. Bacteremia is rare. Gram stain of the effluent is seldom helpful, except for fungal peritonitis, but cultures are generally positive. In many centers, 20% of peritonitis episodes result in no growth, predominately due to inadequate culture techniques. The etiologies of peritonitis are given in Table 4.

Peritonitis remains an important cause of hospitalization, catheter loss, and transfer to hemodialysis. Peritonitis rates, originally very high, have decreased to less than 1.0 episodes per dialysis year due to improvements in the procedure for performing the dialysis connections, which have decreased the risk of peritonitis due to contamination (Fig. 1). Because the flush and drain occur after the connection to the catheter, small numbers of bacteria present because of touch contamination at the connection site (predominately *S. epidermidis;* Table 3) may be flushed into the drain bag instead of into the patient's abdominal cavity. As a result, peritonitis rates due to *S. epidermidis* have decreased, and *S. aureus* and enteric organisms account for a larger proportion of peritonitis episodes than before. Because patients with these organisms are more symptomatic than those with *S. epidermidis* peritonitis, peritonitis has become a less frequent, but more severe complication, often requiring hospital admission. The catheter removal rate for peritonitis depends on the infecting microorganism. Peritonitis with *S. epidermidis* is less likely to result in catheter loss than peritonitis due to *S. aureus* or *P. aeruginosa*. Fungal peritonitis generally requires catheter removal.

The initial treatment of peritonitis is empiric and designed to cover both Gram positive cocci and Gram negative bacilli. A first-generation cephalosporin, such as cefazolin or cephalothin, may be used in conjunction with an aminoglycoside or a third-generation cephalosporin, with subsequent therapy tailored to the culture and sensitivity results. A listing of antibiotics and the dosing schedule is given in Table 5. Because of the concern about the emergence of vancomycin-resistant organisms, vancomycin use should be restricted to treatment of methicillin-resistant organisms or for patients allergic to cephalosporins.

PERITONEAL DIALYSIS PRESCRIPTION AND DETERMINATION OF ADEQUACY

Adequacy of PD is determined by both clinical assessment and clearance measurements. The well-dialyzed pa-

TABLE 3
Treatment of Exit Site and Tunnel Infections

Gram positive catheter infections	
Cephalexin	250–500 mg po qid, or
Oxacillin	250–500 mg po qid, or
Trimethoprim/sulfamethoxazole	160/800–320/1600 mg po qd
Add rifampin if slow to resolve[a]	300 mg po bid
Gram negative catheter infections[b]	
Ciprofloxacin	500 mg bid
Fleroxacin	800 mg po, then 400 mg po qd
Ofloxacin	400 mg po, then 200 mg po qd
Add ceftazidime if slow to resolve[c]	500 mg/L, then 125 mg/L in each exchange

[a] For *Staphylococcus aureus*.

[b] Cephalexin or trimethoprim/sulfamethoxazole may also be options. Choice based on sensitivities; quinolones will be needed for pseudomonas infections. Antacids will interfere with the absorption of quinolones.

[c] For *Pseudomonas aeuruginosa*.

tient has a good appetite, no nausea, minimal fatigue, and feels well. In contrast, the uremic patient is anorectic with dysgeusia, nausea, and complains of fatigue. In addition to these clinical parameters, urea and creatinine clearances based on 24-hour collections of effluent and urine are used as laboratory measures of adequacy (Table 6). The clearance of urea nitrogen divided by the urea distribution volume (V) is termed Kt/V. Kt is obtained by multiplying the effluent : blood urea nitrogen concentration ratio by the 24-hour effluent drain volume. (Note that the t in Kt refers to time and is a carryover from hemodialysis in which the urea nitrogen clearance is multiplied by the time of the hemodialysis treatment. This is not applicable to a continuous form of dialysis, but the term Kt/V continues to be frequently used in continuous peritoneal dialysis to represent K/V). Renal urea nitrogen clearance is added to this. The daily value is multiplied by 7 to provide a weekly value. V can be estimated as 60% of weight in males and 55% of weight in females. The creatinine clearance is also obtained from a 24-hour collection of dialysate, to which is added the average of the renal creatinine and urea nitrogen clearance (since creatinine clearance overestimates glomerular filtration rate due to the tubular secretion of creatinine). An adjustment for body surface area is also required The current recommendations are given in Table 6. These recommendations are still preliminary and will no doubt be revised as more research is done in this area.

Clearance of small molecules such as urea nitrogen and creatinine is dependent on the patient's peritoneal membrane characteristics, the length of the dwell time, and the

TABLE 4
Causes of Peritonitis

Contamination at the time of an exchange
Catheter tunnel infection
Transmural, across bowel wall
Bacteremia (rare)
Vaginal (rare)

volume of effluent drained per unit time. Many CAPD patients are prescribed 4 exchanges of 2 L volumes per day. Four 2 L CAPD exchanges per day with 2 L of ultrafiltration per day represents a drain volume of 70 L/week, which is inadequate in the absence of renal function for most patients. Initially, most patients have residual renal function contributing to the total clearance. As renal function is lost, patients require larger exchange volumes (2.5 or 3 L) and may also need 5 daily exchanges to avoid uremic symptoms and reach the target values of Kt/V and creatinine clearance. The fifth exchange may be provided by use of a device that will deliver a middle-of-the-night exchange. Larger patients should be started on 2.5 or 3 L exchange volumes. To achieve adequate clearances on cycler PD, one or two day dwells are needed in addition to three to four nocturnal exchange volumes of 2.5 to 3 L.

ULTRAFILTRATION FAILURE

PD is an extremely effective method for fluid removal for most patients. The continuous nature of CAPD allows a more liberal intake of sodium and water than is possible for patients on intermittent forms of therapy such as hemodialysis. The patient adjusts ultrafiltration by chosing the correct concentration of dextrose dialysate dependent on fluid intake and volume status.

Poor ultrafiltration occurs in patients who have a high dialysate : serum creatinine ratio, as previously described, due to rapid dissipation of the glucose concentration gradient. These patients are best managed with frequent short dwells and elimination of long dwells, such as with either diurnal or nocturnal PD (Table 2). Mortality in this group is higher than in other patients on PD and transfer to hemodialysis may be necessary.

Some patients initially have normal ultrafiltration but after a period of time develop ultrafiltration failure due to changes in the peritoneal membrane. A severe form of ultrafiltration failure occurs in sclerosing encapsulating peritonitis, a misnomer because this pathologic condition is not actually peritonitis, but characterized by marked

TABLE 5
Antibiotic Doses Used to Treat Peritonitis[a]

Antibiotic	Initial dose (mg/L)	Subsequent doses mg/L continuously (each exchange)	Subsequent doses mg/L intermittently (one exchange per day)
Ampicillin	125	125	No data
Aztreonam	1000	250	1000 qd
Cefazolin or cephalothin	500	125	500 qd
Ceftazidime	250	125	1000 qd
Fluconazole	200 mg po		200 mg po qd
Gentamicin, netilmicin, tobramycin[a]	0.6 mg/kg	4	0.6 mg/kg/qd or 20 mg/L qd
Metronidazole	500 mg po/iv		500 mg po/iv tid
Vancomycin	15–30 mg/kg	25	15–30 mg/kg q 5–7 d

[a] Intraperitoneal unless otherwise indicated. Patients with residual renal function may require higher doses or more frequent dosing than once daily. Limited data on use of aminoglycosides in PD patients.

thickening of the peritoneum. Sclerosing peritonitis occurs in 1 to 2% of the chronic PD population. Multiple etiologies for sclerosing peritonitis have been identified including chlorhexidine (used at one time to sterilize connection sites), acetate (as opposed to the currently used dialysate which contains lactate), practolol (an antihypertensive medication), and infectious peritonitis, especially episodes occurring late in the course of PD. Once sclerosing peritonitis develops, PD can no longer be continued successfully.

NUTRITION IN THE PERITONEAL DIALYSIS PATIENT

Forty percent of PD patients are protein malnourished. This is in part due to losses of amino acids and protein in the dialysate, the latter generally 8 to 10 g/d. Peritonitis markedly increases dialysate protein losses. The patient's appetite may be suppressed from the absorbed dialysate dextrose as well as from uremia. Both Kt/V and weekly creatinine clearance correlate, albeit weakly, with protein intake, suggesting that a certain minimum dose of dialysis is required for adequate protein intake. The serum albumin level is inversely related to both mortality and hospitalization in PD patients. A protein intake of at least $1.2 \text{ g} \cdot \text{kg}^{-1} \cdot \text{day}^{-1}$ is recommended for PD patients, but many patients ingest only 0.8 to $1.0 \text{ g} \cdot \text{kg}^{-1} \cdot \text{day}^{-1}$. Amino acid dialysate (in which amino acids replace the dextrose) has been used on a limited basis as a means of correcting protein malnutrition, but proof of its long-term efficacy is so far lacking.

The calories absorbed from dialysate glucose depend on the dextrose concentration used (1.5, 2.5, 4.25 g/dL), as well as on the patient's membrane permeability. The development of obesity, therefore, is not unusual in PD patients, especially those already overweight at the start of dialysis. In addition, glucose absorption frequently results in hyperlipidemia, which may contribute to cardiovascular disease.

DIABETICS ON PERITONEAL DIALYSIS

Diabetic glomerulosclerosis is the most common cause of renal failure in CAPD/CCPD patients. The vast majority of diabetic patients require insulin on CAPD/CCPD, even

if they did not require insulin prior to the initiation of PD. This is partly due to glucose absorption from the dialysate and the associated weight gain. Insulin can be given to CAPD patients via the intraperitoneal route, the subcutaneous route, or a combination of both. If given intraperitoneally, the patient checks a fingerstick glucose at the time of each exchange and adds regular insulin to the exchange based on a sliding scale. Patients on CCPD generally require long-acting subcutaneous insulin (with or without intraperitoneal regular insulin) for adequate glucose control. The use of intraperitoneal insulin has not been shown to increase the risk of peritonitis.

OUTCOME IN PERITONEAL DIALYSIS PATIENTS

The death rate of PD patients in the United States from 1991 to 1993 was 30 per 100 dialysis years at risk. The leading causes of death are cardiovascular disease and infections. In the United States, patients over age 55 had a greater risk of death on PD compared to hemodialysis, but these results have not been seen in other countries such as Italy and Canada, whose PD patients have lower mortality rates than those in the US. Risk factors for death on PD include increasing age, the presence of cardiovascular disease and/or diabetes mellitus, decreased serum albumin level, poor nutritional status, and inadequate dialysis. For CAPD patients, a decrease in the Kt/V by 0.1 U/week increases mortality by 6%, while a decrease in creatinine clearance by $5 \text{ L} \cdot \text{week}^{-1} \cdot 1.73 \text{ m}^{-2}$ increases mortality by 7%.

A high proportion of patients transfer off PD to hemodialysis for a multitude of reasons including peritonitis or exit site infection, catheter malfunction, inability to perform the dialysis procedure, and inadequate clearance or ultrafiltration (particularly with loss of residual renal function). In many cases the patient who loses a catheter due to either peritonitis or a catheter infection may elect to remain on hemodialysis permanently. The increasing use of the disconnect systems is associated with improved technique survival on CAPD, primarily due to lower peritonitis rates.

TABLE 6
Adequacy Measures in Peritoneal Dialysis

Solute	Adjusted to size	Minimum weekly goal
Urea nitrogen clearance	V, distribution of urea	$Kt/V = 2.1$
Creatinine clearance	Body surface area	$C_{cr}/1.73 \text{ m}^2 = 60\text{–}70 \text{ L}$

Transplantation is the goal for most patients on dialysis. The allograft and patient survivals of PD patients who are transplanted are similar to those of transplanted hemodialysis patients. If the transplant does not initially function, PD can be continued, as long as the peritoneal cavity was not entered. The peritoneal catheter is generally left in place for 2 to 3 months until the graft is functioning well.

PERITONEAL DIALYSIS FOR ACUTE RENAL FAILURE

Intermittent peritoneal dialysis (IPD) may be succesfully used to manage patients with acute renal failure. In this case, the peritoneal catheter is often inserted percutaneously using a stylet, without a subcutaneous tunnel (which, however, increases the risk of a leak). Rapid exchanges are done to maximize small solute clearance, often 1 to 2 exchanges per hour, using a cycler. The patient may be kept on the cycler for 48 hours or even longer, or IPD may be performed daily for 10 to 12 hours. Although extremely effective for volume control and better tolerated in the hemodynamically unstable patient than hemodialysis, clearance of small solutes may be inadequate in catabolic patients or patients on total parenteral nutrition receiving large protein loads. In addition, in the ICU setting there is considerable risk of peritonitis. For these reasons, IPD has been largely replaced by hemodialysis and continuous hemodiafiltration for the management of acute renal failure.

Bibliography

Bloembergen WE, Port FK, Mauger EA, et al.: A comparison of mortality between patients treated with hemodialysis and peritoneal dialysis. *J Am Soc Nephrol* 6:177–183, 1996.

CANADA-USA Peritoneal Dialysis Study Group. Adequacy of Dialysis and Nutrition in Continuous Peritoneal Dialysis: Association with Clinical Outcomes. *J Am Soc Nephrol* 7:198–207, 1996.

Davies SJ, Bryan J, Phillips L, et al.: Longitudinal changes in peritoneal kinetics: the effects of peritoneal dialysis and peritonitis *Nephrol Dial Transplant* 11:498–506, 1996.

Gokal R, Ash SR, Helfrich GB, et al.: Peritoneal catheters and exit-site practices: Toward optimum peritoneal access *Perit Dial Int* 13:29–39, 1993.

Golper TA, Brier ME, Bunke M, et al.: Risk factors for peritonitis in long term peritoneal dialysis: The network 9 peritonitis and catheter survival studies *Am J Kidney Dis* 28:428–436, 1996.

Holley JL, Bernardini F, Piraino B.: Infecting organisms in continuous ambulatory peritoneal dialysis patients on the Y-set. *Am J Kidney Dis* 23:569–573, 1994.

Keane WF, Alexander SR, Bailie GR, et al.: Peritoneal dialysis-related peritonitis treatment recommendations 1996 Update. *Perit Dial Int* 16:557–573, 1996.

Khanna R and Nolph KD. The physiology of peritoneal dialysis *Am J Nephrol* 9:504–512, 1989.

Lupo A, Tarachini R, Cancarini G, et al.: Long-term outcome in continuous ambulatory peritoneal dialysis: A 10-year survey by the Italian Cooperative Peritoneal Dialysis Study Group *Am J Kidney Dis* 24:826–837, 1994.

Piraino B, Bernardini J, Sorkin M: Catheter infections as a factor in the transfer of continuous ambulatory peritoneal dialysis patients to hemodialysis *Am J Kidney Dis* 13:365–369, 1989.

Pollock CA, Ibels LS, Caterson RJ, Mahony JF, Waugh DA, Cocksedge B: Continuous ambulatory peritoneal dialysis: Eight years of experience at a single center. *Medicine* 68:293–308, 1989.

Twardowski ZJ: Clinical value of standardized equilibration tests in CAPD patients current concepts of CAPD. *Blood Purification* 7:95–108, 1989.

U.S. Renal Data System, USRDS 1996 Annual Report. VI. Causes of Death. *Am J Kidney Dis* 28 (Suppl 2):S93–S102, 1996.

Young GA, Kopple JD, Lindholm B, et al.: Nutritional assessment of continuous ambulatory peritoneal dialysis patients: An international study. *Am J Kidney Dis* 17:462–471, 1991.

65

OUTCOME OF END STAGE RENAL DISEASE THERAPIES

WENDY E. BLOEMBERGEN

The availability of dialysis and transplantation or renal replacement therapies has allowed the survival of patients with end stage renal disease (ESRD), previously a fatal illness. However, the expected outcomes of an ESRD patient remain inferior to the general population. This chapter includes an overview of ESRD patient outcomes, assessed in terms of mortality, but also morbidity, technique survival, quality of life, rehabilitation, and cost. The availability of the United States Renal Data System (USRDS), a national database of all Medicare-treated ESRD patients (93% of the U.S. ESRD population), and large cohort studies allows the description of many of these outcome measures.

MORTALITY

The mortality of the ESRD population is high relative to the general population. In 1993, the crude mortality rate of the US ESRD population was 17.6 deaths per 100 patient years. For the dialysis population only the rate was 23.3 deaths per 100 patient years. The expected remaining lifetime of a patient with ESRD is one third to one fifth that of the general population for all age and race categories. Figure 1 shows that the diagnosis of ESRD carries with it a prognosis between that for colon and lung cancer. For example, a healthy 45- to 54-year-old person can expect to live about 30 more years. The expected remaining lifetime would be 10 years if this person developed colon cancer, 7 years with ESRD, or 3 years with lung cancer.

The failure of currently available "renal replacement" therapies to provide ESRD patients with expected survival similar to the general population is likely due to the high prevalence of comorbid conditions among the ESRD population (many of which are already present as patients start ESRD therapy), the inability of dialysis to fully replace all of the functions of native kidneys, and adverse consequences or side effects of the "replacement therapy," dialysis, or transplantation.

Causes of Death

Characterization of causes of death helps to better understand the high mortality of the ESRD population. National data on reported cause of death is published by the USRDS. Figure 2 shows the reported causes of death for the ESRD population over age 20 from 1991 to 1993. Cardiac causes combined account for 48% of all deaths. Infection, cerebrovascular disease, and malignancy account for 15%, 6%, and 4%, respectively.

The predominant cause of cardiac deaths is reportedly cardiac arrest or sudden death, accounting for 39%, followed by acute myocardial infection (MI; 24%), arrhythmia (14%), cardiomyopathy (10%), and atherosclerotic heart disease (9%) (Fig. 3). A high prevalence of both coronary artery disease and left ventricular hypertrophy, which is already present among patients starting ESRD therapy, contributes to these cardiac deaths.

Disruption of the skin barrier by the vascular access in hemodialysis patients and the peritoneal catheter in peritoneal dialysis patients are factors which are partly responsible for the high risk of death due to infection. Comorbid conditions such as peripheral vascular disease also contribute to infectious deaths. In addition, there is laboratory evidence that patients with ESRD have defects in cellular immunity, neutrophil function, and complement activation. Figure 3 also shows the reported breakdown of infectious causes. Septicemia due to the vascular access and due to peritonitis were each reported to account for 8% of deaths. It is possible that other access infections present as blood borne infections in other organs and may be misclassified.

Factors Associated with Mortality

Demographics

Several demographic factors have been shown to be associated with mortality in the ESRD population. Increasing age, white race, and male gender are associated with higher mortality. Cause of ESRD is also an important predictor (Fig. 4). Patients with diabetes as the cause of ESRD have approximately twice the mortality risk as patients with ESRD due to glomerulonephritis. Patients with ESRD due to hypertension have mortality rates between those for patients with ESRD due to glomerulonephritis and diabetes.

Comorbidity

The prevalence of various comorbid conditions that are shown to be associated with worse survival is high among

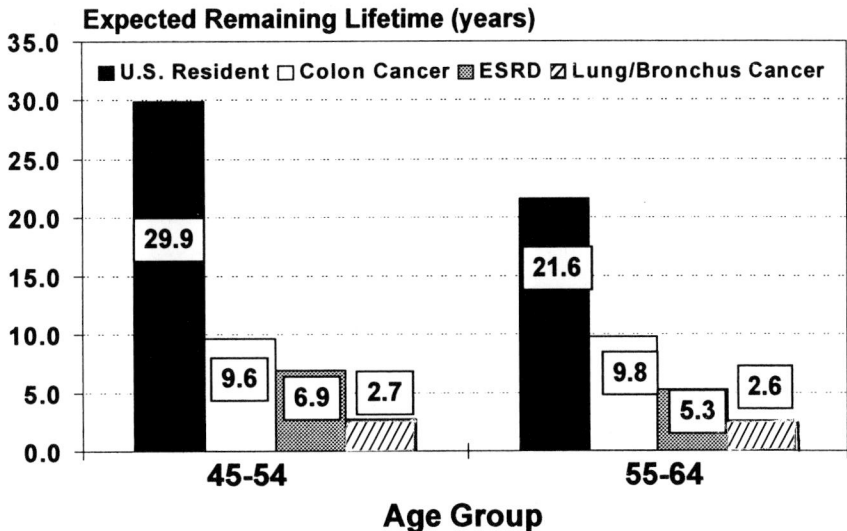

FIGURE 1 Expected remaining lifetime for age groups 45 to 54 and 55 to 64 for U.S. resident population (1990), and selected subpopulations with chronic disease, including colon cancer population (1983–1989), ESRD population (1992), and lung/bronchus cancer population (1983–1989). From the U.S. Renal Data System 1995 Annual Data Report. National Institutes of Health, National Institute of Diabetes and Digestive and Kidney Diseases, Bethesda, MD, 1995.

patients treated for ESRD (Table 1). For example, by chart review, 45% of patients in a national random sample of hemodialysis patients had coronary artery disease (CAD; defined as prior history of CAD, MI, abnormal angiogram, angioplasty, or coronary artery bypass graft), which is associated with a 44% higher risk of mortality compared to those without CAD, adjusted for demographics and other comorbid conditions. As the table indicates, patients with a history of congestive heart failure, arrhythmia including

atrial fibrillation, peripheral vascular disease, cerebrovascular disease, chronic obstructive lung disease and neoplasm have higher independent risks of death than patients without these conditions. In a recent study, an ankle-arm blood pressure index of less than 0.9, a sensitive and specific measure of peripheral vascular disease, was shown to be present among 35% of hemodialysis patients and was associated with more than a sevenfold risk of cardiovascular mortality. In another study, echocardiograms performed

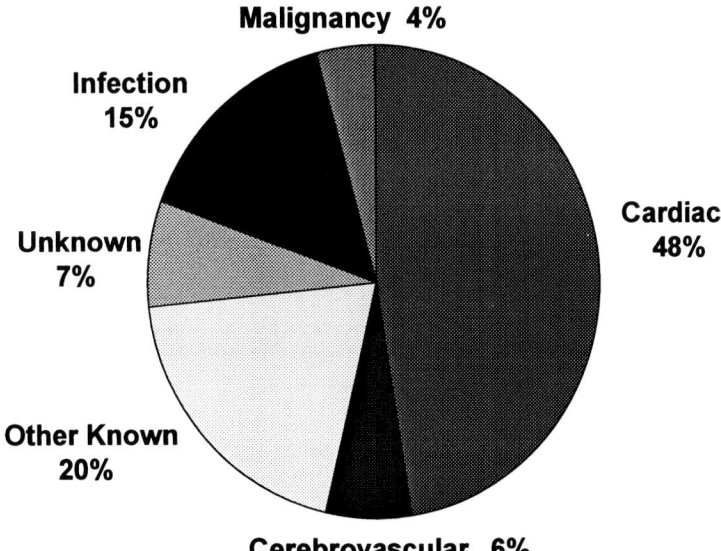

FIGURE 2 Percent distribution of causes of death for ESRD patients over age 20 (1991 to 1993). Data from The 1996 USRDS Annual Data Report. National Institutes of Health, National Institute of Diabetes and Digestive and Kidney Diseases, Bethesda, MD, 1996.

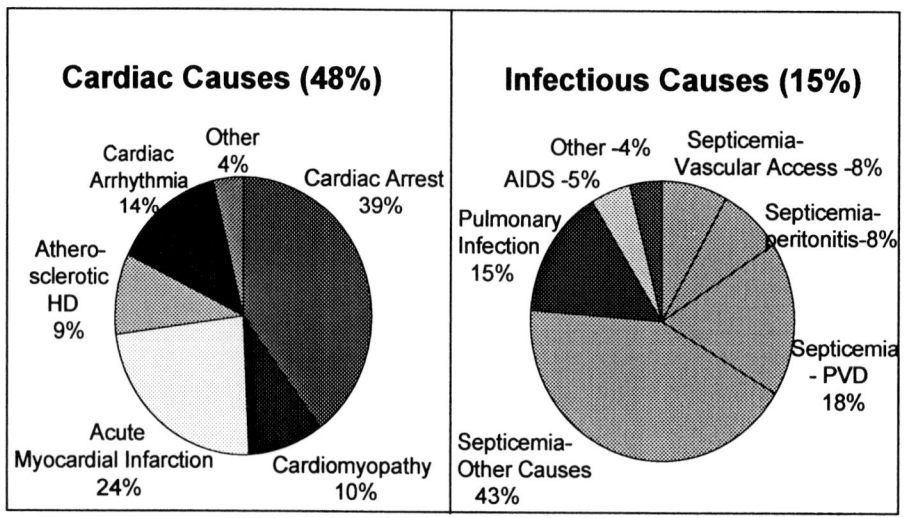

FIGURE 3 Percent distribution of specific cardiac causes of death among all cardiac causes and of specific infectious causes of death for all infectious deaths for ESRD patients. Data from The 1996 USRDS Annual Data Report. National Institutes of Health, National Institute of Diabetes and Digestive and Kidney Diseases, Bethesda, MD, 1996.

on a cohort of 433 patients starting dialysis found the presence of left ventricular hypertrophy in 74%, which was associated with a higher risk of mortality.

Among patients starting dialysis, low serum albumin has consistently been shown to be a strong predictor of mortality. Although it is too simplistic to equate albumin with nutritional status since many other factors affect its concentration, other measures of nutrition have also been predictive of mortality among ESRD patients. In a national random sample of 3400 patients starting hemodialysis, 14% were undernourished (as indicated in the medical records). Those who were undernourished had a 26% higher risk of mortality. Worsened nutritional status as measured by subjective global assessment and percentage lean body mass was associated with an increased relative risk of death among a large cohort of patients starting continuous ambulatory peritoneal dialysis (CAPD) who were followed prospectively. Low serum creatinine, also thought to be a measure of reduced muscle mass possibly due to malnutrition, has been shown to be predictive of elevated mortality risk.

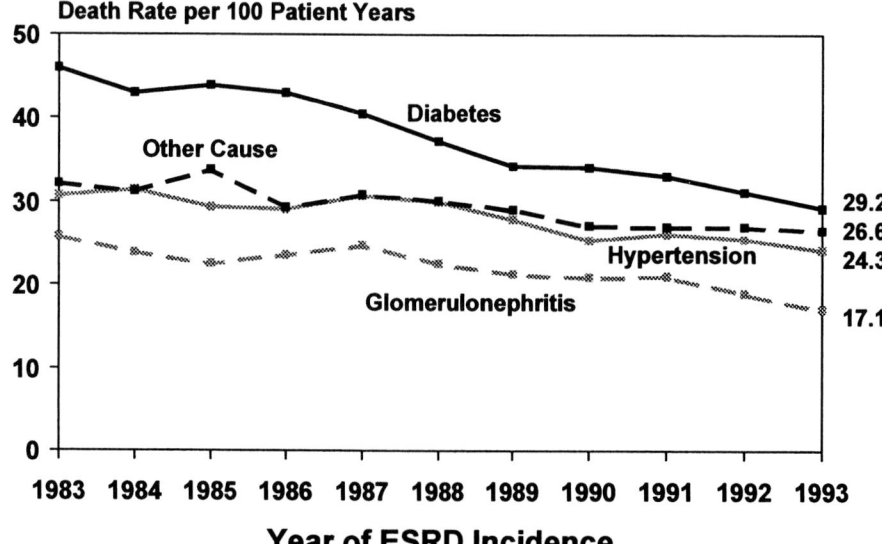

FIGURE 4 Death rates by diagnosis and year of incidence, adjusted for age, race, and sex. From the U.S. Renal Data System 1996 Annual Data Report. National Institutes of Health, National Institute of Diabetes and Digestive and Kidney Diseases, Bethesda, MD, 1996.

TABLE I

Prevalence and Relative Mortality Risk of Comorbid
Conditions among US Hemodialysis Patients (1991)

Comorbid conditions	Prevalence (%)	Relative mortality risk
Coronary artery disease	45	1.44
Congestive heart failure	42	1.62
Arrhythmia	31	1.51
Peripheral vascular disease	22	1.62
Cerebrovascular disease	16	1.31
Chronic obstructive lung disease	12	1.62
Neoplasm	9	1.32

These data suggest that greater attention to nutritional therapy may be beneficial to patients with ESRD, although it may be the case that a patient's nutritional status is simply a measure of other comorbidity and is not necessarily modifiable by nutritional interventions.

Socioeconomic Status

Socioeconomic factors have also been shown to predict mortality. Previous studies have found higher mortality to be associated with (1) lower income, (2) lack of family support and (3) patients who live alone.

Modality

A patient who develops end stage renal failure must choose between several end stage renal replacement therapy options. Broadly classified these include two main types of dialysis [hemodialysis (HD) and peritoneal dialysis (PD)], and transplantation. Several factors should be considered when choosing a treatment modality including coexistent disease, the patient's social or living circumstances, as well as preferences and beliefs regarding the treatment options. Relative outcomes are also important in the decision process.

Survival rates for transplanted patients are better than for dialysis patients. However, patient selection obviously plays a role because patients too ill to be referred for transplantation remain on dialysis. A recent study comparing survival of transplanted patients to those who were receiving dialysis after being included on the transplant waiting list found substantially better survival among transplanted patients. This study is the best to date to address this question as the issue of selection bias has been reduced.

Recipients of cadaveric transplants have lower survival than those of living related transplants. From 1992 to 1993, 1 year survival was 95.5% for living related transplants and 91% for cadaveric transplants. Among transplanted patients, there has been an overall trend to improved survival over the past decade (see Chapters 74 and 75).

Although most comparative studies of hemodialysis and peritoneal dialysis published prior to the 1990s showed no consistent difference in mortality, several recent studies have found higher mortality associated with peritoneal dialysis among some specified patient groups in the US. For example, one study comparing randomly selected patients new to ESRD (3376 HD and 681 PD) found higher mortality for those treated with PD compared to HD among diabetics, but not among nondiabetics after adjustment for comorbidity differences. Another study using national data compared mortality among prevalent patients receiving HD or PD (170,000 years of follow-up) and found a 19% higher mortality risk among PD-treated patients. This risk was increasingly large and significant for ages > 55 years and was accentuated in diabetics and females although it was also present in nondiabetics and males. An evaluation of causes of death found that the risk of death was increased among PD patients for all major cause of death categories except malignancy. It is not clear if these mortality differences are due to differences in dose of dialysis, compliance, patient selection, medical quality of care, or a true adverse treatment effect. The pilot study of a large multinational randomized clinical trial comparing outcomes of PD and HD is currently being performed. If the full-scale study is deemed feasible and proceeds it should provide definitive answers to questions regarding comparative outcomes of PD and HD.

Treatment Parameters

There are several treatment parameters which, in epidemiologic studies, have been shown to be associated with mortality. In several studies, lower dose of dialysis as measured by either Kt/V or urea reduction ratio (URR) among HD-treated patients and weekly Kt/V or creatinine clearance among PD-treated patients (see Chapters 63 and 64) was associated with higher mortality. In hemodialysis, dialyzer reuse has been associated with higher mortality in subgroups of dialysis patients. The use of unmodified cellulosic membranes has also been associated with higher mortality than modified cellulosic or synthetic membranes. However, to date, no clinical trials have been done to sort out if these treatment factors rather than other confounding factors (e.g., dialysis facility quality) are responsible for the worse outcomes. A large multicenter NIH-sponsored clinical trial comparing high vs. conventional dose dialysis is currently in progress.

In the area of transplantation, the use of cyclosporine has been shown to be associated with improvements in patient survival.

Standardized Mortality Ratio

The standardized mortality ratio (SMR) is a method which has been used in the ESRD community to compare mortality for a dialysis facility relative to the national norm. It is a ratio of the observed number of deaths divided by the number of deaths which would be expected given the specific age, race, gender, and causes of ESRD at the individual facility.

MORBIDITY

There are relatively few US studies available which comprehensively quantitate and characterize the occurrence of morbid events among the ESRD population in a prospective fashion. Descriptions have more frequently been retrospective and have used number of hospital admissions, length of admission, or total number of hospitalized days per calendar year as measures of morbidity. To date, most published reports are not cause-specific and therefore also do not differentiate, for example, between a hospitalization for access surgery as compared to a complication of ESRD. Limitations imposed by Medicare eligibility rules, health insurance, and geographic location must also be considered.

USRDS data indicates that on average, the morbidity of the dialysis population is substantial. In 1993, dialysis patients ages < 65 were admitted to hospital a mean of 1.3 times per year and were confined to hospital for 11.5 days/year. Forty-two percent of patients had no admissions. However 8% had five admissions or more, showing the great degree of variability. Eleven percent were admitted for more than 30 days/year. Overall, however, there has been a trend toward decreasing hospitalization rates.

One study of more than 500 hemodialysis patients that did report cause-specific hospitalization found that more than 25% of admissions were access related (vascular access declotting, replacement, infection, or PD catheter placement). The second most frequent reason for admission was cardiac/circulatory followed by gastrointestinal/metabolic disorders. The remainder were due to a variety of less frequent causes. In another study of Canadian ESRD patients the probability of requiring hospitalization for an MI infarction or angina was approximately 10% per year. There was a similar probability of developing pulmonary edema requiring hospitalization or ultrafiltration.

Hospitalization rates increase by patient age, as expected. Females have consistently been shown to have higher hospitalization rates than males. African-Americans are hospitalized more than whites at younger ages, whereas the reverse occurs for older age groups. Native Americans have the highest rates in general, whereas Asians have the lowest. Rates for diabetics are higher than those for nondiabetics in all age groups. There are also substantial differences in hospitalization by geographic region, with the highest rates in the South Central, Middle Atlantic, and Northeast regions. The factors responsible for these observed differences are not clear.

As one would expect, the presence of comorbid conditions including angina, congestive heart failure, peripheral vascular disease, low serum albumin, and decreased activity level have been associated with increased hospital utilization. Hospitalization rates have been shown to be higher among PD treated compared to HD-treated patients in all age groups except for patients ≥ 65. However, hospitalization rates have been steadily falling for PD patients, whereas those for HD patients have remained relatively stable. Patients with arteriovenous fistulas also have fewer hospitalizations than those with PTFE grafts.

TECHNIQUE SURVIVAL

The probability of failure of the chosen modality for renal replacement therapy may be an important factor in a patient's modality decision. Among dialytic techniques, there is a substantially higher failure rate among patients treated with PD compared to HD. Among patients treated with HD, less than 5% will have switched to PD at 2 years whereas among patients initially treated with PD, approximately 15% will have switched to HD. Failure on PD is most frequently due to peritonitis, and exit site or tunnel infections, but can also be due to other CAPD-related complications, inadequate dialysis, or social reasons.

Among patients who receive a transplant, renal allograft survival is dependent on donor source. In 1993, 1-year graft survival for living related transplants was 91%, and for cadaveric transplants was 83% (Fig. 5). Five year graft survival was 73% and 56% for living related and cadaveric transplants, respectively. Graft survival has improved steadily over the past decade. Factors which have been identified as predictors of worse graft survival include donor age over 55 or less than 10 years, prolonged cold ischemic time, older recipient age, HLA mismatch, and female donor. The use of cyclosporine or FK506 has enhanced survival rates. Post-transplantation factors which predict worse graft survival include absence of first day diuresis, dialysis at 1 week, rejection at discharge, and elevated discharge serum creatinine.

QUALITY OF LIFE

Quality of life, a more refined outcome measure than morbidity and mortality, is emerging as an important factor in the assessment of various treatment choices among patients with ESRD. Interest in factors affecting how best to improve quality of life has increased tremendously in the past several years, partly because the quality of life experienced by ESRD patients, as among patients with many other chronic illnesses, such as arthritis and chronic obstructive lung disease, is often significantly compromised. The renal failure itself, the underlying disease responsible for the renal failure and the high degree of associated comorbidity, are likely contributing factors. Patients on dialysis often complain of fatigue, lack of energy, anorexia, depression, decreased libido, musculoskeletal symptoms, and pruritus. HD is usually required three times a week for 3 to 4 hours, and can be accompanied by various physical discomforts, nausea, dizziness, headaches, and lack of energy during or after dialysis. Dietary restrictions are strict and involvement in work, social, and recreational activities is frequently reduced. PD requires frequent dialysate exchanges and may be complicated by peritonitis or catheter tunnel infections. Renal transplant patients may experience side effects of immunosuppressive therapy including infection, acne, hirsutism, and weigh gain. Medical complications, financial pressures, marital discord, sexual dysfunction, emotional stress, and anxiety about loss or death are common, regardless of modality.

The measurement of quality of life—the self-assessed value of an individual's health experiences—is a complex, multidimensional concept typically measured by a number of domains including physical functioning, social functioning, psychological/emotional well-being, physical symp-

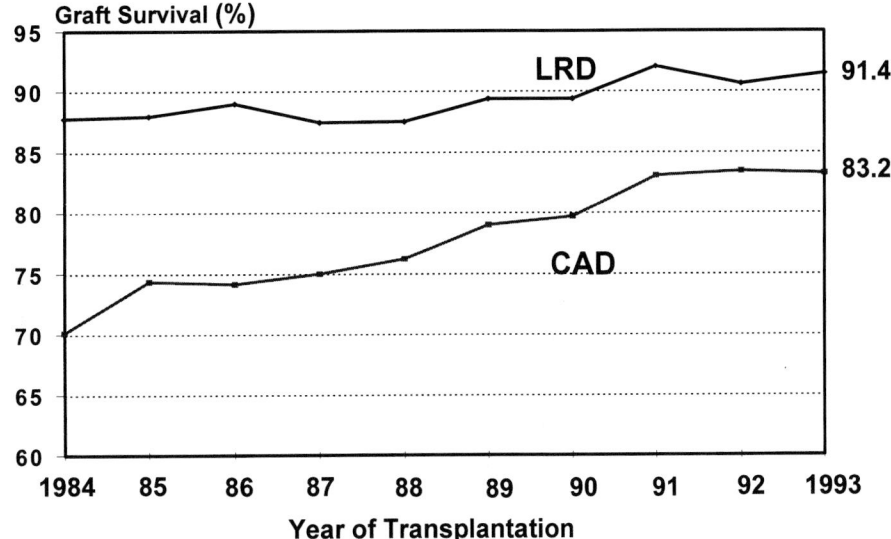

FIGURE 5 One year graft survival by donor type and year, adjusted for age, sex, race, first transplants only. LRD, living related renal transplant; CAD, cadaveric renal transplant. From the U.S. Renal Data System 1996 Annual Data Report. National Institutes of Health, National Institute of Diabetes and Digestive and Kidney Diseases, Bethesda, MD, 1996.

toms, cognitive function, vocational functioning, and over-all satisfaction with health. It has been measured by both generic and ESRD specific quality of life instruments among this population. Numerous studies have documented poor quality of life in patients with ESRD. For example, from 30 to 50% of patients on chronic dialysis are reported to have impaired physical performance capacity, and up to 70% have moderate to severe levels of stress. Studies have suggested that among the ESRD population, quality of life varies by demographic factors, comorbidity, underlying disease, and mode of treatment. It is inferior among patients with comorbid conditions and those with diabetes as a cause of renal failure. Among the ESRD modality choices, transplantation appears to offer substantially better quality of life than hemodialysis as shown by two recent prospective studies which compared quality of life of dialysis patients while on the transplant waiting list and the same patients after transplantation. Data on which dialysis modality type offers the best quality of life are less conclusive. Various cross-sectional or small studies comparing quality of life by dialysis type have generally found highest quality of life among patients treated with home hemodialysis, followed by PD, and in-center dialysis. However due to study design, these observations may be partly explained by patient selection. Large longitudinal studies and the pilot study for a clinical trial aimed to compare quality of life by dialysis modality are currently in progress.

Both longitudinal studies and a randomized clinical trial have found superior quality of life among dialysis patients treated with recombinant human erythropoietin.

REHABILITATION

When Medicare coverage for ESRD began in 1973, the expectation was that many of those whose lives were pro-

longed would contribute to society through work and taxes. However, since then the patient population has changed dramatically with the acceptance of older and sicker patients, and now the majority of patients do not work. Consequently, rehabilitation no longer can be judged by employment alone, but must address the patient's level of function before ESRD and their return to a comparable status.

Efforts to maintain employment should be made for patients who work, and vocational counseling should be provided to unemployed patients who are capable of working. The nephrologist plays a crucial role in the motivation of patients toward these goals. Participation in an exercise program has been advocated to enhance rehabilitation outcome for all patients. To the extent possible, transplantation should be encouraged among suitable patients. In a recent prospective study, the proportion of ESRD patients employed increased from 30% before transplantation (on dialysis) to 45% 2 years post-transplantation. This is probably because a more flexible schedule allowed patients to engage in employment, as well as because of improved physical and mental abilities. As healthcare costs rise, the vocational and functional rehabilitation of patients undergoing dialysis or transplantation is receiving more attention by Congress and the public.

COST

In 1972, Congress elected to cover the cost of ESRD therapy for eligible patients with ESRD through amendments to Medicare. Currently, approximately 93% of ESRD patients have their treatment covered by Medicare. The estimated total monetary cost of treating ESRD in the US in 1994 was $11.13 billion, of which the portion paid by Medicare was $8.31 billion. This includes the cost of dialysis and hospitalizations (each approximately 40% of total cost), as well as supplies, covered medications, physician fees, etc. (remaining 20% of total cost). Average Medicare spending per patient year was $36,900. On average, the total cost per patient (Medicare, other insurance, patient obligations, etc.) is approximately 20 to 25% higher. There is substantial variation by modality. Annual Medicare costs for HD averages $44,200, $39,400 for PD, and $17,600 for transplanted patients. In a prospective study assessing the cost utility of renal transplantation compared with dialysis in Canada, the cost of dialysis care pretransplant and the cost of the first year after transplant was similar. At 2 years, transplantation was clearly associated with better quality of life and was less costly than dialysis among all subgroups.

Annual costs for all ESRD patients rise steadily with age, an observation primarily attributable to the decline in transplantation with increasing age. Diabetic patients are considerably more costly to treat than nondiabetics. Average medicare payments are slightly higher for females than males in most age categories. Payments for African-Americans are higher than for whites among patients less than 65, again partly due to lower transplantation rates.

Acknowledgments

Some of the data reported here have been supplied by the USRDS. The interpretation and reporting of these data is the responsibility of the author and in no way should be seen as an official policy or interpretation of the U.S. Government.

Bibliography

Bloembergen WE, Port FK, Mauger EA, Wolfe RA: A comparison of mortality between patients treated with hemodialysis and peritoneal dialysis. *J Am Soc Nephrol* 6:177–183, 1995.

Canada-USA (CANUSA) Peritoneal Dialysis Study Group: Adequacy of dialysis and nutrition in continuous peritoneal dialysis: Association with clinical outcomes. *J Am Soc Nephrol* 198–207, 1996.

Canadian Erythropoietin Study Group. Association between recombinant human erythropoietin and quality of life and exercise capacity of patients receiving haemodialysis. *Br Med J* 300:573–578, 1990.

Churchill DN, Taylor DW, Cook RJ, et al.: Canadian hemodialysis morbidity study. *Am J Kidney Dis* 19:214–234, 1992.

Evans RW, Manninen DL, Garrison LP Jr, et al.: The quality of life of patients with end-stage renal disease. *N Engl J Med* 312:553–559, 1985.

Excerpts from U.S. Renal Data System 1996 Annual Data Report, Chapters on: Causes of Death; Patient Mortality and Survival; Hospitalization; Renal Transplantation: Access and Outcomes; The Economic Cost of ESRD and Medicare Spending for Alternative Modalities of Treatment. National Institutes of Health, National Institite of Diabetes and Digestive and Kidney Diseases, Bethesda, MD, 1996. *Am J Kidney Dis* 28:S1–S165, 1996.

Fishbane S, Young S, Flaster E, Adam G, Maesaka JK: Ankle-arm blood pressure index as a predictor of mortality in hemodialysis patients. *Am J Kidney Dis* 27:668–672, 1996.

Foley RN, Parfrey PS, Harnett JD, et al.: Clinical and echocardiographic disease in patients starting end-stage renal disease therapy. *Kidney Int* 47:186–192, 1995.

Habach G, Bloembergen W, Mauger EA, Wolfe RA, Port FK: Hospitalization among U.S. dialysis patients: Hemodialysis versus peritoneal dialysis. *J Am Soc Nephrol* 5:1940–1948, 1995.

Held PJ, Port FK, Wolfe RA, et al.: The dose of hemodialysis and patient mortality. *Kidney Int* 50:550–556, 1996.

Held PJ, Wolfe RA, Gaylin DS, Port FK, Levin NW, Turenne MN: Analysis of the association of dialyzer reuse practices and patient outcomes. *Am J Kidney Dis* 23:692–708, 1994.

Hakim RM, Held PJ, Stannard D, et al.: The effect of the dialysis membrane on mortality of chronic hemodialysis patients (CHD) in the U.S. *Kidney Int* 50:566–570, 1996.

Jones KR. Factors associated with hospitalization in a sample of chronic hemodialysis patients. *Health Serv Res* 26:671–699, 1991.

Laupacis A, Keown PA, Pus N, et al.: A study of the quality of life and cost utility of renal transplantation. *Kidney Int* 50:235–242, 1996.

Owen WF, Lew NL, Liu Y, Lowrie EG, Lazarus JM: The urea reduction ratio and serum albumin concentration as predictors of mortality in patients undergoing hemodialysis. *N Engl J Med* 329:1001–1006, 1993.

Port FK: Morbidity and mortality in dialysis patients. *Kidney Int* 46:1728–1737, 1994.

Port FK, Wolfe RA, Mauger EA, Berling EA, Jiang K: Comparison of survival probabilities for dialysis patients vs cadaveric renal transplant recipients. *JAMA* 270:1339–1343, 1993.

Rocco MV, Soucie JM, Reboussin DM, McClellan WM: Risk factors for hospital utilization in chronic dialysis patients. *J Am Soc Nephrol* 7:889–896, 1996.

Russell JD, Beecroft ML, Ludwin D, Churchill DW: The quality of life in renal transplantation—a prospective study. *Transplantation* 54:656–660, 1992.

Terasaki PI, Yuge J, Cecka JM, Gjertson DW, Takemoto S, Cho YW: Thirty-year tends in clinical transplantation. In: Terasaki PI, Cecka JM (eds) *Clinical Transplants 1993*, UCLA Tissue Typing Laboratory, Los Angeles, 1994.

Wolfe RA, Gaylin DS, Port FK, Held PJ, Wood CL. Using USRDS generated mortality tables to compare local ESRD mortality rates with national rates. *Kidney Int* 42:991–996, 1992.

66

PROGRESSION OF RENAL DISEASE

THOMAS H. HOSTETTER

Progression of renal insufficiency to end stage kidney failure is a process which extends over months to years in most cases. The term renal insufficiency refers to a reduction in glomerular filtration rate (GFR) but with sufficient residual filtration that the patient does not require dialysis or transplantation, the point at which kidney failure or end stage renal disease (ESRD) is said to occur. The circumstances in which the progression is more rapid are considered in other sections of this *Primer*. While a wide variety of renal diseases progress, the patterns of that progression have substantial clinical, laboratory, and pathological similarities. Indeed, the uremic state in which they culminate is generally considered as an almost generic entity, irrespective of the initial disease. Furthermore, over the last 15 years, the notion has arisen that common mechanisms underlie this progression at a pathophysiologic level.

THE COURSE OF PROGRESSION

While many functions of the kidney tend to fail in a roughly proportionate manner such that acidosis, anemia, disorders of bone and mineral metabolism, and more non-specific uremic symptoms develop concurrently, the course of progressive renal disease is charted principally by decline in GFR. Clinically, the trajectory of progressive renal disease is typically followed by the serum creatinine. The relation of serum creatinine level to creatinine clearance and GFR is, of course, inverse. Indeed, the decline in inverse serum creatinine (1/serum creatinine) has been used as a clinically expedient means of following the change in renal function. Without major interventions to alter the progression of renal disease or the supervention of additional renal damage, the 1/serum creatinine tends to decline in a relatively linear manner for individual patients. The use of the Cockcroft–Gault formula for calculation of creatinine clearance from serum creatinine, age, weight, and sex yields an approximate value for GFR which is satisfactory for most clinical indications. Rarely is it useful to perform multiple measurements of creatinine clearance by urinary collections or even more accurate measurements of GFR by infusion of exogenous filtration markers such as iothalamate or inulin. Rather, serum creatinine, interpreted as its inverse and in the light of body habitus, is sufficiently accurate for following the progression of disease in almost all cases (see also Chapter 2).

The rate of decline in GFR varies between patients and, to some extent, between diseases. Glomerular diseases, diabetic glomerulopathy, and hypertension tend to progress faster than tubulointerstitial diseases. However, data from one large study suggested that patients with polycystic kidney disease may also progress as rapidly as those with glomerular injury. The level of renal dysfunction at which one can predict that a specific patient is likely to progress to ESRD is uncertain. Clearly, the higher the level of serum creatinine when a patient is first encountered, the more likely the patient will progress to uremia. However, a small fraction of patients with renal insufficiency may remain relatively stable for protracted periods of time even without specific therapies. A number of clinical risk factors in addition to disease type associate with the likelihood of progression or higher rates of progression. Patients with proteinuria are more likely to suffer inexorable declines in renal function than those without proteinuria and the degree of proteinuria is a predictor of that likelihood. Those manifesting the highest rates of protein excretion generally demonstrate the most rapid, and certain, declines. Arterial hypertension also appears to be a risk factor for progression to ESRD; its therapy is discussed below. Finally, a number of factors have persistent but more modest effects on the propensity to progress. These include African-American descent, male sex, hypercholesterolemia, and smoking.

MECHANISMS OF PROGRESSION

Arterial hypertension is not only a primary cause of chronic renal failure, but also is a risk factor for the progression of renal disease initiated by other mechanisms such as diabetic nephropathy and chronic glomerulonephritis. In these latter settings, the systemic blood pressure appears to enhance the progressive decline in renal function. The pathways whereby hypertension arises after renal injury from some other primary insult likely involve a combination of sodium retention and persistent activation of various pressor systems including the sympathetic nervous system, the renin-angiotensin-aldosterone system, and local vascular mediators such as endothelin activation or nitric oxide suppression. Whatever the genesis of this increased perfusion pressure, many studies show a direct association between hypertension and the rate of progression. Furthermore, lowering blood pressure with antihypertensives mitigates the decline of filtration rates, as discussed below.

In addition to the deleterious effects of systemic hypertension, the compensations that nephrons undergo after surviving the initial insults of a primary renal disease seem to conspire with arterial hypertension to perpetuate injury. Before discussing these compensations, it is important to emphasize that most progressive renal diseases attack the kidney initially in a heterogeneous manner. For example, in the course of chronic glomerulonephritis, some glomeruli may be reduced to obsolescence relatively early in the disease course, whereas others are spared. The basis for this heterogeneity of injury is uncertain. An experimental model of these adapted surviving nephrons has been a reduction in nephron mass by simple surgical removal or infarctive ablation of renal tissue, often called the remnant kidney model. Studies of the residual units in this model demonstrate that they undergo a complex series of changes. Broadly, these changes have been termed compensatory hypertrophy and hyperfunction, and have been viewed as adaptive, allowing these nephrons to carry a greater filtration rate and other metabolic functions. The increase in filtration rate in the surviving nephrons compensates for the more severely damaged or destroyed nephrons and is driven largely by vasodilatation of the arterioles supplying those nephrons with increases in their plasma flow and glomerular capillary pressures. The combination of arterial hypertension and compensatory afferent vasodilation of residual nephrons sustains the elevated glomerular pressure. Capillary hypertension has also been demonstrated in a number of other experimental disease models, some even without systemic hypertension. Furthermore, a reduction of the capillary pressure by several maneuvers including dietary protein restriction and specific antihypertensive agents such as angiotensin converting enzyme (ACE) inhibitors has been associated with amelioration of structural and functional injury to surviving glomeruli. Thus the combination of systemic hypertension and this compensatory vasodilation of surviving glomeruli increases the risk for secondary injury along this presumed common pathway of progressive renal disease.

The remnant kidney model involves removal of function of more than one kidney. Simple unilateral nephrectomy leads to some of the above compensatory changes but they are not so great as seen with the larger degrees of ablation of the remnant model. Also, simple nephrectomy seems to cause little arterial hypertension and is not associated with initial scarring in the remaining kidney tissue as occurs in the remnant model. It is probably for these reasons—lesser compensatory structural and functional adaptations, absence of arterial hypertension and initial scarring—that simple nephrectomy is associated with considerably less injury in surviving nephrons. Indeed, long-term clinical follow-ups of patients undergoing nephrectomy due to trauma, cancer, or kidney donation, have found little damage accrued by the remaining kidney. Thus, this procedure does not seem to predispose to progressive injury very often, if ever, as long as arterial hypertension and other renal insults are not superimposed.

The cellular mechanisms whereby heightened glomerular pressures such as those seen in the remnant model and in diabetes lead to scarring and eventual occlusion of these capillary units are less certain than the fact that it occurs. In all likelihood, the microvascular hypertensive injury is multifactorial and includes pressure- or tension-induced increases in synthesis of mesangial matrix as well as mechanical disruption of the capillary wall, yielding permeability defects and proteinuria. Indeed, proteinuria itself may contribute to the progression of renal disease and, as noted above, is one of the strongest quantitative risk factors for progression of kidney injury. A large number of potential mechanisms have been ascribed to the relationship between proteinuria and progressive injury. The excessively filtered plasma proteins are, in part, reabsorbed by proximal tubular cells and, in that process, various small molecules and substances bound to the proteins are liberated. In particular, the removal of iron from transferrin may provide a catalyst for the synthesis of locally damaging reactive oxygen species. Small lipids bound to these filtered proteins and freed during protein reabsorption may also have inflammatory or chemotactic properties which would accentuate tubulointerstitial disease. Finally, the inspissation of filtered proteins due to water abstraction in the distal nephron may lead to cast formation and intrarenal obstruction.

In addition to the vascular adaptations of vasodilation and capillary hypertension, metabolic adaptations of the nephron, particularly the tubular epithelium, have been invoked as potentially deleterious factors in the progression of renal injury. A necessary consequence of increased filtration rates in the residual nephrons is an increase in tubular reabsorption. This increase in reabsorption of solutes necessitates increases in oxygen consumption and should generate damaging reactive oxygen species as byproducts of that heightened oxidative process. Ammonia production by residual nephrons is also augmented, even though total kidney ammonia production excretion eventually falls, accounting for uremic acidosis. The high levels of ammonia in the cortex can have inflammatory consequences by reacting with components of the complement system and producing both direct tissue injury and attraction of leukocytes. Elevations in the calcium-phosphorus product as well as serum oxalate levels may lead to deposition of these substances in the renal interstitium providing a nidus for inflammation and tissue destruction. Finally, disorders of circulating cholesterol and triglycerides are common in chronic renal disease, especially with proteinuria, and considerable attention has focused on the possibility that hyperlipidemia may induce injury in the renal microvasculature.

Together with the functional adaptations of residual nephrons, these units increase in size throughout their length from glomerulus through collecting duct. This process of compensatory growth is stimulated by circulating factors that are as yet unidentified. Roles for growth in the functional alterations and ultimately in progressive injury have been suggested. Specifically, increases in glomerular size may allow increased filtration but may also confer a mechanical disadvantage in that the increased capillary radii will augment wall tension, an effect that would be exaggerated by the heightened capillary pressures described above. In addition, enlargement of the glomerular capillary likely disrupts the permselectivity of the glomerulus. The podocytes covering the capillary and providing the fine definition of permeability are limited in their ability to proliferate and hence may become in a sense "overextended" on an enlarged capillary surface. Likewise, expansion of mesangial areas may adversely influence the normal clearance mechanisms of macromolecules that circulate through this region. Whether the enlargement of tubular epithelial cells also has untoward consequences, has yet to be examined.

In addition to the overall compensatory renal growth stimulated by as yet unidentified circulating factors, the production of a large number of locally acting specific growth, proliferative, and fibrogenic peptides play an important role in the sclerosis, scarring, and remodeling that occur as renal disease progresses. Although a very large number of these factors have been identified, the chief among those demonstrated to contribute to the progression of experimental and clinical renal disease has been transforming growth factor-β, platelet-derived growth factor, and endothelin. These factors emanate from both invading cells (such as monocytes) and native renal cells, including mesangial and epithelial cells, and interact in complex networks linking them with each other and yet other substances including components of the renin cascade. These latter factors, specifically angiotensin II and aldosterone, must have pivotal roles because drugs blocking their production and actions have striking effects in many models of chronic renal injury and act through pathways in addition to the classical hemodynamic or pressor ones. For example, the growth and fibrogenic actions of angiotensin II are mediated, in part, through transforming growth factor-β; however, links to endothelin, platelet-derived growth factor, reactive oxygen metabolites, and other mediators also exist. The nexus of these local factors has been a complex but evolving area of research in progressive renal injury.

TREATMENT OF PROGRESSION

Blood Pressure

Control of systemic hypertension is the most important therapeutic maneuver in slowing the progression of chronic progressive renal disease. Of course, no exact definition of acceptable control is available. However, more intensive control is justified than that applied in primary or essential hypertension. A mean arterial pressure of 90 to 95 mm Hg is a currently suggested guideline and derives from the Modification of Diet in Renal Disease (MDRD) study. The mean arterial pressure is calculated as the diastolic pressure plus one third the difference between systolic and diastolic pressure. Thus, an arterial pressure of 120/80 mm Hg corresponds to a mean arterial pressure of 93 mm Hg.

Considerable attention has focused on which drugs best controll hypertension in a patient with established renal disease. Experimental studies principally in models of diabetes and the subtotally ablated rat kidney indicate that

drugs interrupting the renin-angiotensin-aldosterone system are most efficacious. Specifically, ACE inhibitors and, more recently, angiotensin II type I receptor blockers have lessened injury more than other agents. Clinical trials comparing different antihypertensive regimens have generally confirmed that ACE inhibitors retard progression more effectively than comparable drugs. At present, the data for angiotensin receptor antagonists are not as extensive as for the ACE inhibitors. Furthermore, the bulk of the clinical evidence derives from studies of patients with diabetic nephropathy. Nevertheless, studies in other types of renal disease generally show the greater efficacy of ACE inhibitors for slowing the progression of renal disease. It should be noted that there are a rather limited number of studies comparing specific agents. However, some studies have suggested that calcium channel blockers may also retard progression. Diuretics are a particularly reasonable additional drug as they enhance the effects of the aforementioned classes and are often especially useful in patients with renal insufficiency whose hypertension has an important "volume" component. Beyond these choices, there are no strong rational bases on which to choose among the other classes of agents for maintaining blood pressure within the acceptable range.

The administration of ACE inhibitors and angiotensin receptor blockers in patients with renal insufficiency does have some hazards. Specifically, reductions in renal function may occur rather promptly, particularly in patients who have renovascular disease or intrarenal arterial damage. Severe and clinically significant worsening of renal function occurs in these settings. The fall in arterial perfusion pressure and glomerular pressure reduce filtration may actually exacerbate the functional effects of the vascular stenoses. Less severe diminutions in filtration rate may occur with any antihypertensive therapy in patients with renal insufficiency but without major renal vascular stenoses. Such declines in GFR are the result of imperfect autoregulation (the capacity to maintain constant blood flow and filtration over a range of arterial perfusion pressure) when renal disease afflicts the kidney. Although exact guidelines do not exist, a rise in serum creatinine of more than 1 mg/dL after starting ACE inhibitor therapy should in most instances lead to its discontinuation and consideration of underlying renal vascular disease. Lesser elevations in serum creatinine, if stable, can be accepted and followed without stopping therapy in most cases. Also, patients may develop hyperkalemia with these drugs due to suppression of aldosterone. Therefore, measurements of both serum creatinine and potassium should be obtained shortly after beginning these drugs in patients with established renal insufficiency. In most instances, these compounds are tolerated and have particularly beneficial effects.

Dietary Management

Dietary protein restriction has been recommended as a means of retarding the progression of renal disease. Several clinical trials have attempted to assess its role, but the results have often been confusing. However, at least one meta-analysis of multiple trials has suggested that dietary protein restriction does lessen progressive renal damage. It is difficult to specify the exact level of dietary protein that is both consistent with benefit and also consistent with stable nitrogen balance. In part, this difficulty resides in the fact that patients generally eat a greater level of protein than that they are prescribed, even in careful long-term clinical trials. In general, patients, including those with significant proteinuria, can maintain a neutral nitrogen balance with 0.6 of high biological value protein per kg body weight per day. Some data suggest that even more liberal protein intake (up to 0.75 g · kg^{-1} · d^{-1}) still provides benefit, but in all likelihood, patients would tend to eat yet more if prescribed higher protein diets and at some point the efficacy of protein restriction would be lost. This level of protein restriction (0.6 to 0.75 g · kg^{-1} ·d $^{-1}$) requires counseling of the patient by a qualified dietitian. Furthermore, for many patients this restriction represents a considerable change in their style of eating. If patients are begun on a protein-restricted diet, monitoring of their protein nutrition is required using follow-up of serum albumin. Although most patients will eat a greater amount of protein than prescribed, some will self restrict excessively or may have other catabolic events that lead to greater protein requirements. Notably, patients who are receiving glucocorticoid therapy will require higher levels of protein and, indeed, dietary protein restriction in such patients may not be worth the risk of protein malnutrition given the adverse effects of glucocorticoids on protein catabolism. Although the risks of protein malnutrition in general seem to be rather modest, it should be carefully avoided because protein depletion is a great liability for patients who enter the end stage therapies of dialysis or transplantation. While protein restriction may be a less powerful tool for retarding progression of renal disease than careful antihypertensive therapy as outlined and may be more cumbersome, it still should be offered to patients as yet another means of altering the course of their renal disease.

Other Therapies

Therapies designed to affect metabolic function such as acid production, calcium phosphorous metabolism, lipid levels, and reactive oxygen moieties in order to retard the progression of renal disease remain to be tested in any significant clinical trials. However, these therapies as well as those directed at specific intrarenal growth or fibroproliferative factors may be employed in the future.

Bibliography

Bakris GL, Copley JB, Vicknair N, Sadler R, Leurgans S: Calcium channel blockers versus other antihypertensive therapies on progression of NIDDM associated nephropathy. *Kidney Int* 50:1641–1650, 1996.

Benigni A, Remuzzi G: Glomerular protein trafficking and progression of renal disease to terminal uremia. *Semin Nephrol* 16(3):151–159, 1996.

Brenner BM, Lawler EV, Mackenzie HS: The hyperfiltration theory: a paradigm shift in nephtology. *Kidney Int* 49(6):1774–1774, 1996.

Cockcroft DW, Gault HW: Prediction of creatinine clearance from serum creatinine. *Nephron* 16:31–41, 1976.

Floege J, Johnson RJ: Multiple roles for platelet-derived growth factor in renal disease. *Miner Electrolyte Metab* 21(4-5):271–282, 1995.

Kasiske BL, Kalil RS, Ma JZ, Liao M, Keane WF: Effect of antihypertensive therapy on the kidney in patients with diabetes: a meta-regression analysis. *Ann Intern Med* 118(2):129–138, 1993.

Ketteler M, Noble NA, Border W. Transforming growth factor-beta and angiotensin II: the missing link from glomerular hyperfiltration to glomerulosclerosis? *Annu Rev Physiol* 57:279–295, 1995.

Klahr S, Levey AS, Beck GJ, et al.: The effects of dietary protein restriction and blood-pressure control on the progression of chronic renal disease. *N Engl J Med* 330:887–884, 1994.

Lewis EJ, Hunsicker LG, Bain RP, ct al.: The effect of angiotensin-converting enzyme inhibition on diabetic nephropathy. *N Engl J Med* 329:1456–1462, 1993.

Levey AS, Adler S, Caggiula AW, et al.: Effects of dietary protein restriction on the progression of advanced renal disease in the Modification of Diet in Renal Disease Study. *Am J Kidney Dis* 27(5):652–663, 1996.

Maschio G, Alberti D, Janin G, et al.: The effect of angiotensin converting-enzyme inhibitor benazepril on the progression of chronic renal insufficiency. *N Engl J Med* 334:939–945, 1996.

Nath KA. Tubulointerstitial changes as a major determinant in the progression of renal damage. *Am J Kidney Dis* 20(1):1–17, 1992.

Pedrini MT, Levey AS, Lau J, Chalmers TC, Wang PH: The effect of dietary protein restriction on the progression of diabetic and nondiabetic renal diseases: a meta-analysis. *Ann Intern Med* 124(7):627–632, 1996.

Rosenberg ME, Smith LJ, Correa-Rotter C, Hostetter TH: The paradox of the renin-angiotensin system in chronic renal disease. *Kidney Int* 45:403–410, 1994.

Zucchelli P, Zuccalà A, Borghi M, et al.: Long-term comparison between captopril and nifedipine in the progression of renal insufficiency. *Kidney Int* 42:452–458, 1992.

67

MANAGEMENT OF THE PATIENT WITH CHRONIC RENAL DISEASE

PAUL L. KIMMEL

STAGES OF CHRONIC RENAL DISEASE

The course of patients with chronic renal disease is generally progressive, comprises a continuum, and may be divided into four phases for convenience: loss of renal reserve, renal insufficiency, chronic renal failure, and uremia and end stage renal disease (ESRD) (Fig. 1). Each phase presents the clinician with different issues and management challenges.

Loss of renal reserve may not be clinically apparent. Although glomerular filtration rate (GFR) is within the normal range, the response to pregnancy, a dietary protein load, or other stimuli which usually enhance GFR is diminished.

Renal insufficiency is characterized by biochemically apparent diminution in renal function. The BUN and serum creatinine concentrations are increased and the creatinine clearance is decreased. Patients usually have no symptoms of renal disease. Homeostatic mechanisms adequately maintain circulating calcium, phosphorus, and potassium levels and balance. This phase of chronic renal disease may, however, be associated with changes in the levels of circulating hormones such as calcitriol, parathyroid hormone (PTH), and insulin.

Renal failure is associated with a marked decrease in renal function, but symptoms, if any, are mild. Patients may have abnormal calcium and phosphorus levels when compensatory mechanisms are no longer adequate. Normochromic, normocytic anemia may be present, especially when the GFR is less than $20 \text{mL} \cdot \text{min}^{-1} \cdot 1.73 \text{ m}^{-2}$.

As the patient progresses through these three stages, the clinician must establish the renal diagnosis, treat the specific disease, and initiate nonspecific therapy such as treatment of hypertension and the use of an appropriate diet. Control of serum phosphorus levels may be important to limit the development or extent of renal osteodystrophy. Evaluation and treatment of anemia related to chronic renal disease should be undertaken. Perhaps most importantly, preparation of the patient for renal replacement therapy should commence.

Uremia is characterized by the onset of symptoms of renal disease, including nausea, vomiting, malaise, pruritus, and mental lassitude and inability to concentrate. Treatment of uremic symptoms may involve initiation of perito-

neal dialysis or hemodialysis, or cadaver or living related renal transplantation. The uremic syndrome is discussed in detail in Chapter 62. The time when such therapy begins in a patient whose renal impairment is expected to be permanent and irreversible marks the onset of ESRD.

Clinical measurement of renal function uses creatinine, a normal product of muscle metabolism, as an endogenous marker of GFR. The serum creatinine concentration rises as the GFR falls, but it is an imperfect filtration marker. Creatinine is secreted as well as filtered by the kidneys, and its production rate depends on diet and muscle mass. The latter falls with advancing age or muscle wasting. In addition to observing changes in serum creatinine directly, the progression of renal disease may also be followed by plotting the reciprocal of the creatinine concentration over time. In many patients, a straight line can be fit to the serial changes. A change in the slope of such a plot may reveal a change in the course of progressive renal disease, such as the superimposition of acute renal failure upon chronic renal failure. Alternatively, such changes have been used to monitor the patient's course on a newly prescribed protein restricted diet.

TREATMENT OF THE PATIENT WITH CHRONIC RENAL DISEASE

Treatment involves at least five imperatives: (1) identification and elimination of factors which can reversibly decrease renal function, (2) institution of measures to slow the progression of renal disease, (3) maintenance of nutritional status while minimizing the patient's symptoms and accumulation of toxic waste products, (4) identification and treatment of complications of chronic renal disease, and (5) preparation of the patient for ESRD therapy.

Factors which may interfere with or reversibly decrease renal function in patients with chronic renal disease are outlined in Table 1. Patients with an unexpected increase in BUN and creatinine concentrations who exhibit signs of volume depletion may respond to volume repletion. Gastrointestinal bleeding should be excluded as a cause of volume depletion and increased renal insufficiency, particularly when the rise in BUN is proportionally greater than the rise in serum creatinine. Infection can result in volume

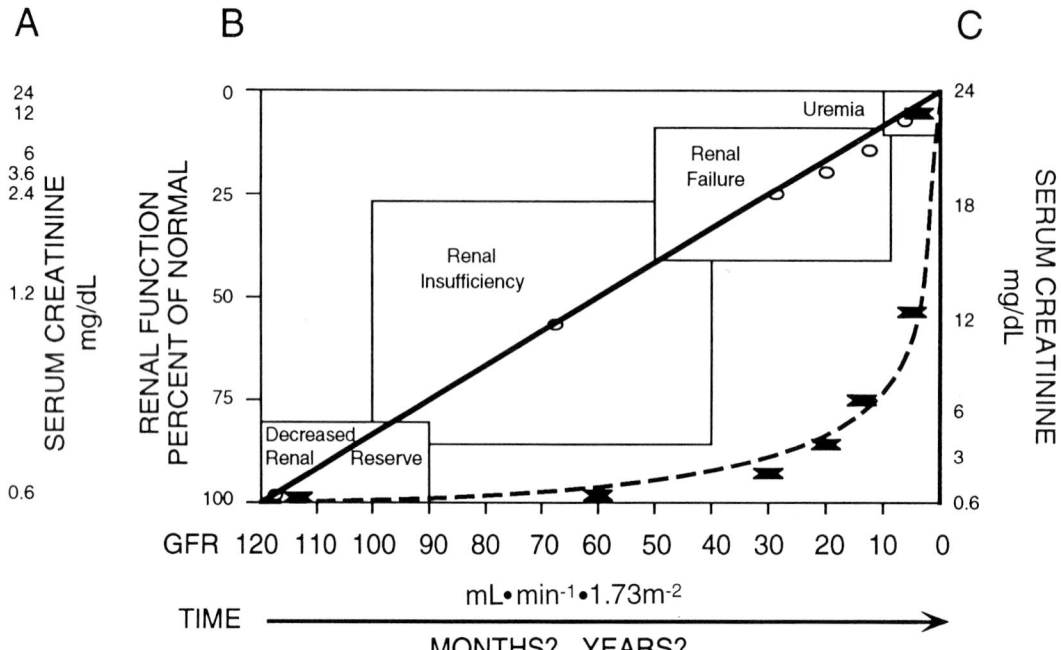

FIGURE 1 The course of progressive renal disease. The course of a patient who began with normal renal function, corresponding to a serum creatinine concentration of 0.6 mg/dL and GFR of 120 mL·min^{-1}·1.73 m^{-2}, is shown. *Y-axes*: The geometric serum creatinine ordinate at the extreme left (A), applies to the solid line of identity (open circles) and the rectangles depicting the various stages of progressive renal disease. The serum creatinine ordinate at the right side of the figure (C) should be used with the dashed curve (axe-heads) only. The central ordinate (B) which describes the percentage of renal function remaining applies generally. *Line of identity*: This line shows a decrease in function from 100 to 0% of normal, corresponding to the diminution in GFR from 120 to 0 mL·min^{-1}·1.73 m^{-2}. The matching creatinine scale (A) is geometric. *Dashed curve*: Since GFR = daily creatinine excretion/serum creatinine concentration and since the creatinine excretion is equal to daily production, which is constant, this equation is of the form $y = k/x$, which defines a hyperbola. This relationship remains valid over the course of chronic renal disease unless the creatinine production changes. The curve emphasizes that large changes in GFR may produce small and clinically imperceptible changes in serum creatinine concentration when overall renal function is near normal. Conversely, trivial changes in GFR produce large changes in serum creatinine concentration when the GFR is low. The rate of progression throughout the delineated stages depends on the nature of the underlying renal disease, host factors, treatment, and compliance with the medical regimen.

depletion if patients have anorexia or vomiting, have diarrheal illnesses, or lose water through insensible routes because of fever. Sepsis may result in the superimposition of acute renal failure on established chronic renal disease. Patients with congestive heart failure and renal disease may have diminution of renal blood flow as cardiac function worsens. Therapy directed at improving cardiac hemodynamics may in turn substantially improve renal hemodynamics. Optimizing volume status in patients with liver disease and ascites or the nephrotic syndrome may similarly improve renal hemodynamics. Diuretics, aldosterone antagonists and angiotensin-converting enzyme (ACE) inhibitors may play important roles in the management of such patients by counteracting hormonal factors which favor sodium retention and enhancing urinary sodium excretion.

The measurement of fractional excretion of sodium (FE$_{Na}$), a useful guide to renal responses to volume disorders in patients with oliguria, is less helpful in patients with chronic renal disease. This is the case since the fractional excretion of many solutes typically increases as renal function diminishes, a result predicated both by clinical findings and predictable from the mathematical definition of the fractional excretion of a given solute, x.

$$FE_x = \frac{\text{renal clearance of } x}{\text{GFR}}, \text{ or, in clinical settings,}$$

$$FE_x = \frac{\dfrac{[U]_x V}{[P]_x}}{\dfrac{[U]_{cr} V}{[P]_{cr}}} = \frac{\dfrac{[U]_x}{[P]_x}}{\dfrac{[U]_{cr}}{[P]_{cr}}}$$

Early in the course of chronic renal disease, solute balance and urinary solute excretion in patients are maintained, even as GFR falls. The combination of maintenance or increase in the numerator of the FE equation with the progressive decrease in its denominator dictates that the FE of a solute tends to increase during the course of the development of renal insufficiency and chronic renal failure.

The use of nephrotoxic drugs should be avoided, if possible, in patients with chronic renal disease. Patients with

TABLE I
Factors Which Can Interfere With Evaluation of or Decrease Marginal Renal Function

Volume disorders
  Volume depletion
    Poor nutritional intake
    Excessive salt restriction
    Excessive diuretic administration
    Vomiting or diarrhea
    Gastrointestinal bleeding
  Infection
    Volume depletion
    Septic vasodilatation
  Volume overload
    Congestive heart failure
    Ascites
    Nephrotic syndrome
Nephrotoxic agents
  Nephrotoxic drugs
    Aminoglycoside antibiotics
    Nonsteroidal antiinflammatory drugs
    Anesthetic agents
    Chemotherapeutic agents
  Radiographic contrast material
Infection
  Septic acute tubular necrosis; indirect effects
Uncontrolled hypertension
Hypotension
ACE inhibitors
Pericardial disease
Renal arterial disease
Urinary tract obstruction
Pregnancy
Hypercalcemia, hyperuricemia
Agents which interfere with tubular creatinine secretion[a]
  Cimetidine
  Trimethoprim

[a] These agents increase serum creatinine concentration without changing glomerular filtration rate.

diabetes mellitus, multiple myeloma, and preexisting renal insufficiency are at increased risk for the development of renal impairment from aminoglycoside antibiotics. Nonsteroidal anti-inflammatory drugs (NSAIDs) may decrease renal function by limiting renal blood flow in patients with chronic renal disease, especially in the setting of volume depletion (see Chapter 42). Administration of radiocontrast material can result in temporary, or rarely, permanent loss of renal function. Cimetidine and trimethoprim interfere with creatinine secretion by the renal tubules and decrease creatinine clearance, leading to a secondary increase in serum creatinine concentration. Although GFR is not affected, the use of such substances in patients with chronic renal disease may lead to confusion in interpreting clinical results.

ACE inhibitors are effective therapy for treating hypertension in patients with chronic renal dysfunction; they play an important role in limiting the progression of some forms of chronic renal disease. With advanced renal failure or renal artery disease, however, use of ACE inhibitors can result in deterioration of renal function. This can occur in selected patients as a result of excessive afferent and efferent renal arterioral vasodilatation, and subsequent decrease in the net glomerular hydrostatic pressure favoring filtration. A secondary decrease in circulating aldosterone levels may also result in the development of hyperkalemia.

Uremic patients may develop pericardial disease (Table 2). Pericarditis, pericardial effusion, or cardiac tamponade can interfere with renal blood flow and result in a precipitous drop in GFR in patients with already compromised renal function. Such events are indications for the initiation of dialytic therapy. Renal arterial disease may progress simultaneously with long-standing chronic parenchymal renal disease, and should be suspected in patients with a history of atherosclerotic vascular disease, smoking, or an unexpectedly swift loss of GFR, especially after treatment with ACE inhibitors. Consideration should be given to renal angiography, in spite of potential complications, in such clinical settings. Procedures which do not employ contrast, such as magnetic resonance imaging, may provide useful information in such cases, but rigorous comparative trials of their place in the management of patients with renal vascular disease and renal insufficiency are not available. Urinary tract obstruction should be considered, especially if the progression of the patient's renal dysfunction is unusually rapid, or if the history or physical examination suggest obstructive uropathy.

FORESTALLING THE PROGRESSION OF RENAL DISEASE TO ESRD

Hypertension is a common finding in patients with kidney disease, and may lead to progressive renal insufficiency by causing renal ischemia or increased glomerular pressure. It has been most often associated with volume overload secondary to the kidneys' limitation in excreting a daily ingested sodium load; but hormonal factors such as activation of the renin-angiotensin-aldosterone system may also play a role. Patients with chronic renal disease and volume

TABLE 2
Therapeutic Measures Employed to Treat the Progression of Chronic Renal Disease

Treatment of hypertension
  Systemic
    Treatment with ACE inhibitors
    Treatment with alternative antihypertensives
  Intraglomerular
    Treatment with ACE inhibitors
    Dietary protein restriction
Dietary protein restriction
Phosphorus restriction and treatment of hyperphosphatemia
Control of glucose metabolism in patients with diabetes mellitus
Treatment of hyperlipidemia?

overload can be appropriately treated with diuretics. Because of decreased renal blood flow, the doses may need to be increased to ensure desired pharmacologic effects. Treatment of hypertension, regardless of the specific antihypertensive regimen, is effective in forestalling the progression of renal disease (Table 2). Studies in patients with diabetes mellitus have suggested that control of hypertension, achieved by disparate medications, results in diminution of progressive loss of renal function. ACE inhibitors are effective in reducing proteinuria and the rate of loss of GFR in patients both with and without diabetic nephropathy, although the mechanism underlying such effects is not completely understood. Although some studies have suggested that ACE inhibitors exert their protective effects independent of effects on systemic blood pressure in patients with nondiabetic renal disease, this is currently controversial. Patients with chronic renal insufficiency taking ACE inhibitors must be monitored for the development of decreased GFR and hyperkalemia. Calcium channel blockers have also been used both to treat hypertension and in an attempt to slow the progression of renal disease. Nondihydropyridine calcium antagonists (e.g., diltiazem) may reduce proteinuria in patients with renal disease, while dihydropyridine agents (e.g., nifedipine, nicardipine, felodipine, amlodipine, isradipine) may be less effective. A meta-analysis suggested in diabetic patients with renal insufficiency that, compared with other antihypertensive agents, dihydropyridine calcium antagonists did not have the beneficial effects on renal function noted in nondiabetic patients with renal insufficiency. The risks and benefits of these calcium channel blockers must be evaluated in each individual patient, in light of the paucity of long-term data or well-designed large clinical trials evaluating their effects in patients with chronic renal insufficiency.

When treated aggressively with potent antihypertensives such as minoxidil and ACE inhibitors, some patients with advanced renal insufficiency and malignant hypertension regain enough function to forestall the need for dialysis. Occasionally patients who start dialytic therapy regain enough renal function after control of hypertension is established to discontinue dialysis.

Protein-restricted diets have been used over the last three decades to limit symptoms of uremia. Changes in dietary protein intake modulate glomerular hemodynamics and GFR in patients with chronic renal disease, as well as normal subjects. Some studies have demonstrated the efficacy of protein-restricted diets in preserving GFR in patients with chronic renal insufficiency. The separate roles of reduced protein intake and effective antihypertensive therapy in determining renal functional outcomes over time is currently a matter of investigation. The stage in the development of renal disease during which protein restriction should be prescribed, the degree of protein restriction to be employed, and the type of diet administered are currently under study. Extremely limited protein diets with ketoacid supplements have also been successfully employed in patients with chronic renal disease. Different protein restricted diets have been instituted in patients in studies at a level of GFR below 50 mL · min^{-1} · 1.73 m^{-2}

with beneficial results (see Chapter 66). It is important, however, to ensure that the patient maintains overall good nutritional status with adequate caloric intake while being treated with a protein-restricted diet (see Chapter 68).

COMPLICATIONS OF CHRONIC RENAL DISEASE

The complications of chronic renal disease are discussed in other chapters of the *Primer*. For convenience, they can be divided into fluid, electrolyte, and acid–base disorders, and disorders of metabolism and organ-system function associated with renal dysfunction (Table 3).

Sodium Balance

Sodium balance is usually maintained until approximately 90% of GFR is lost. As GFR falls, FE$_{Na}$ rises, a consequence of diminished renal tubular sodium reabsorption. Patients with chronic renal disease cannot readily respond physiologically to large and/or acute changes in sodium intake with appropriate changes in urinary sodium excretion—a result primarily of tubular dysfunction. A patient with renal insufficiency habitually ingesting a high sodium intake may continue to excrete relatively large amounts of sodium when placed on a low sodium diet. Inappropriate urinary sodium losses, sodium depletion, and worsening BUN and creatinine may result. Similarly, patients may develop volume depletion and oliguria, with increased levels of BUN and creatinine, because of over-

TABLE 3
Complications of Chronic Renal Disease

Fluid, electrolyte and acid–base complications
  Volume overload
  Volume depletion
  Water overload (Hyponatremia)
  Water depletion (Hypernatremia)
  Hyperkalemia
  Hypokalemia
  Hypocalcemia
  Hyperphosphatemia
  Hypermagnesemia
  Metabolic acidosis
  Metabolic alkalosis

Disorders of metabolism and organ-system function
  Hypertension
  Renal osteodystrophy
  Anemia
  Disordered lipid metabolism
  Coagulopathy
  Pericarditis
  Gastrointestinal Disorders
  Neuropathy and encephalopathy
  Sleep disorders
  Sexual dysfunction
  Psychological disorders
  Immune disorders
  Dermatologic complications

zealous diuretic use or when vomiting, fever, diarrhea, or gastrointestinal bleeding occur. Clues to such volume mediated superimposed renal insufficiency include clinical signs of volume depletion and orthostasis. Conversely, such patients may develop pulmonary edema when challenged with an intravenous sodium load, medications with high sodium content, or a high salt diet. In such cases, diuretics or sodium restriction may be effective. Treatment of congestive heart failure in patients with chronic renal disease may result in a fall in GFR if renal perfusion decreases. As cardiac and renal disease worsen, it becomes increasingly difficult to balance the need for diuresis to treat congestive heart failure with the requirement for adequate intravascular volume to maintain GFR.

Water Metabolism

The limited ability of diseased kidneys to excrete a concentrated or dilute urine may result in the development of hypernatremia or hyponatremia. The urinary concentrating mechanism is most affected by renal disease. Therefore, the response to volume depletion or water deprivation is affected more than the ability to excrete a water load. Thirst is usually an adequate guide to maintain a patient's plasma sodium concentration within the physiologic range. If a patient with chronic renal disease experiences a sudden change in mental status, and does not receive enough water, hypernatremia may result. Alternatively, hyponatremia may develop in patients hospitalized with chronic renal disease who are given quantities of hypotonic fluids which exceed the capacity of their kidneys to excrete free water. Serum sodium concentration, and urine volume and osmolality are usually guides to proper therapy.

Potassium Metabolism

Potassium depletion may occur because of malnutrition, nausea and vomiting, or diuretic use. Renal potassium excretion is generally conserved until late in the course of chronic renal disease, but may be limited by oliguria or marked diminution of GFR. Patients with renal diseases associated with the syndrome of hyporeninemic hypoaldosteronism, such as diabetic nephropathy or interstitial nephritis, may develop hyperkalemia with relatively mild diminution in renal function, or without concurrent oliguria. Volume depletion, sodium restriction, and oliguria can impair potassium excretion in such patients, as can the use of ACE inhibitors, NSAIDs, or potassium-sparing diuretics. Colonic potassium secretion plays a more important role in total body potassium homeostasis as renal function deteriorates. Preventing constipation may be important to the patient's overall potassium homeostasis. Dietary counseling regarding the potassium content of foods can be crucial in patients with hyporeninemic hypoaldosteronism and during late stages of chronic renal disease.

Acid–Base Metabolism

Metabolic acidosis develops because of the diseased kidneys' limitation in excreting hydrogen ions, secondary to disordered ammoniagenesis, decreased filtration of phosphate and sulfate compounds, and decreased maximal renal tubular hydrogen ion secretion. Acidemia may cause negative calcium balance and worsen bone disease. Factors predisposing to metabolic acidosis may be offset by forces engendering metabolic alkalosis such as vomiting and the use of base supplements or antacids. Bicarbonate supplementation is used to treat acidemia. Its use may be limited by sodium overload and hypertension. Sodium or potassium citrate are also base supplements. They should be used with caution because citrate increases the intestinal absorption of aluminum. This is a particular problem if aluminium hydroxide gels are prescribed to bind dietary phosphorus. In addition, potassium excretory capability may be limited. Calcium carbonate supplementation may be a useful alternative. Typically, alkali supplementation is indicated when the serum bicarbonate concentration drops below 20 mEq/L.

Divalent Ion and Calcitriol Metabolism

As renal function diminishes, hypocalcemia results from decreased renal $1,25\ (OH)_2D_3$ synthesis, hyperphosphatemia, and resistance to the peripheral action of PTH (see Chapters 14 and 69). Hyperphosphatemia may be directly involved in the pathogenesis of the progression of renal disease. Patients with a GFR less than $40\ mL \cdot min^{-1} \cdot 1.73\ m^{-2}$ may have already developed abnormal bone histology, indicative of renal osteodystrophy, because of diminished renal calcitriol synthesis and secondary hyperparathyroidism. Phosphorus-restricted diets increase calcitriol levels and may limit the development of secondary hyperparathyroidism in the early stages of renal disease. In later stages, hyperphosphatemia may be more difficult to manage with dietary restriction alone. The early use of low dose calcitriol supplementation, when monitored closely, may normalize serum calcium levels, and reduce biochemical features of secondary hyperparathyroidism and the development of renal osteodystrophy. Patients treated with calcitriol must be carefully monitored for the development of hypercalcemia, hyperphosphatemia, and worsened renal function. Newer vitamin D analogues currently under study may be useful for the treatment of such disorders with less associated hypercalcemia.

Anemia in Patients with Chronic Renal Failure

Anemia in patients with renal disease has been characterized as multifactorial; however, the most important mechanism involved in its pathogenesis is diminished renal synthesis of erythropoietin (see Chapter 72). Other possible causes of anemia should be considered and evaluated as appropriate. Treatment with synthetic erythropoietin is effective, resulting in a dose-dependent increase in hematocrit. This drug has improved exercise tolerance and quality of life in patients. Many symptoms previously attributed to uremia improve when patients with chronic renal disease are treated with erythropoietin.

Uremic Coagulopathy

Uremic coagulopathy may present a problem for patients with chronic renal disease undergoing surgical procedures. Although the platelet count and prothrombin and partial thromboplastin times are normal, the bleeding time is often prolonged. The lengthened bleeding time may correlate with a tendency to bleed during and after surgical procedures. The clinician must be aware of the possibility of the disorder, and check the patient's bleeding time preoperatively. Desamino-D-arginine-8-vasopressin (dDAVP), conjugated estrogens, and infusion of cryoprecipitate have been used successfully to treat such patients (see Chapter 72).

Lipid Metabolism

Patients with chronic renal failure may have several different disorders of lipid metabolism. The role of lipids in mediating the progression of renal disease is unclear, but is currently the subject of much research. Patients with the nephrotic syndrome often have hypercholesterolemia, specifically associated with high levels of low-density lipoprotein cholesterol. Such disorders may be involved in the pathogenesis of and lead to a higher incidence of cardiovascular disease in patients with chronic renal disease, although few well-designed clinical studies address these issues. Weight loss, dietary modification of cholesterol intake, and substituting foods low in saturated fats and cholesterol are probably the first steps in management. Low protein diets may decrease proteinuria, and therefore may improve cholesterol levels in patients with the nephrotic syndrome, although there have been few long-term studies performed in patients. HMG-CoA reductase inhibitors are effective in reducing low density lipoprotein (LDL)-cholesterol levels in patients with nephrotic syndrome. Treatment with probucol results in decreases in both LDL and high density lipoprotein (HDL) levels in patients with hypercholesterolemia. Patients with renal disease often have hypertriglyceridemia, associated with increased very-low-density and intermediate-density lipoprotein levels. Although proper diet and exercise may be recommended safely to any patient with hyperlipidemia, the optimum use of antihyperlidemic agents in these patients has not been determined.

Sleep Disorders

Day/night sleep reversal is a classic uremic symptom. Sleep apnea is an important problem in patients with chronic renal failure. The syndrome may be associated with cognitive defects, depressive affect, or hypertension. This disorder can be accurately diagnosed by polysomnography. Treatment with continuous positive airway pressure breathing may result in resolution of symptoms in patients with chronic renal disease.

Psychological Factors

Little is known about psychological adaptation in patients during early periods of the progression of renal disease. Depression as well as anxiety about the unknown, the prospect of starting ESRD therapy, sexual dysfunction, and loss of income, vocation, and social role may all be important in the development of depression. There have been few studies to delineate the diagnosis and treatment of depression in such patients.

DRUG THERAPY IN PATIENTS WITH CHRONIC RENAL FAILURE

Renal dysfunction makes the prescription of therapeutic agents more complicated. Renal disease may impair drug bioavailability and distribution because of changes in gastrointestinal function, the use of concurrent medications such as antacids, and changes in plasma protein binding and total body water levels. Intact hepatic drug metabolism associated with changed renal drug elimination may lead to the accumulation of pharmacologically active or inactive drug metabolites. This may interfere with attempts to monitor drug levels or may change therapeutic effects. In general, the loading dose of an administered drug is not altered by the presence of renal insufficiency. Antibiotic dosage, with the exception of aminoglycosides and vancomycin, may not need adjustment if more than 50% of the patient's renal function is preserved. However, impaired renal clearance and metabolism may dictate the use of lower maintenance drug dosages. One strategy is to lower the individual dose but maintain dosing intervals constant. This approach avoids wide fluctuations in plasma drug levels. Another strategy is to use regular maintenance doses but to extend the intervals between doses to achieve comparable blood or tissue drug levels. This approach may lead to higher peak and trough drug plasma levels. Free blood or plasma levels of drugs, especially when the therapeutic margin is low, should be monitored when feasible in patients with chronic renal disease. Drug dosing must be changed if renal function changes concurrently, and must be carefully instituted in elderly patients who may have markedly reduced levels of GFR despite normal or near-normal BUN and creatinine levels. Patients with chronic renal insufficiency should be cautioned to consult their physician before beginning any new medications or over the counter preparations. Drug dosing in renal failure is discussed in detail in Chapter 43.

SURGICAL CONSIDERATIONS IN PATIENTS WITH CHRONIC RENAL FAILURE

Care must be exercised in the preoperative evaluation of patients with chronic renal disease before they undergo surgical procedures, especially if general anesthesia is used. Attention must be paid to detecting and correcting any preoperative abnormalities of acid–base balance, potassium level, or coagulation. If a radiologic study employing contrast is contemplated, limiting the contrast osmolarity and dose, volume repletion with half-normal saline, and optimizing the patient's volume status and urine flow before contrast administration may decrease morbidity.

PREPARATION FOR ESRD THERAPY

As early as feasible, patients with progressive renal functional deterioration should be counseled regarding their options for treating ESRD. The risks and benefits, as well as the advantages and disadvantages of hemodialytic therapies, peritoneal dialytic methods, and renal transplantation should be clearly outlined. It is advantageous to arrange for a meeting with the patient and his or her family both to provide support during the first three stages of chronic renal disease and to inform the family so they can participate in planning for dialysis or transplantation. The team approach, including nurses, dietitians, social workers, psychologists, psychiatrists, and transplant surgeons and personnel has been successfully employed in such preparatory sessions. The social worker will often conduct a tour of the ESRD facilities, coordinate reviews of home-based therapies and transplantation, and investigate the financial and social resources the family brings to bear at the initiation of renal replacement therapy. The option of not starting ESRD therapy, or withdrawing it if therapy does not improve general well-being and quality of life should be discussed openly with the patient and family.

Access for dialysis should be considered and obtained as early as possible and practical. An arteriovenous (AV) fistula provides the longest lasting alternative and is least prone to infection. An AV fistula may take several months to mature, especially in elderly or diabetic patients, who comprise a large proportion of the incident population treated for ESRD. A peritoneal access catheter may be placed at the time therapy is initiated, although many physicians think a 10-to 14-day period before using the catheter is optimal. Psychological support may be advantageous, since denial of disease can be a powerful negative factor in the patient's care at this stage.

It may be difficult to determine when to start renal replacement therapy in an individual patient (Table 4). The goals of the patient and physician should, however, be clearly established during the stages of renal failure and incipient uremia: Whether to wait for the onset of uremic symptoms, using conservative management to maintain as long a time period as possible before starting dialysis, or

to employ early initiation of dialysis or transplantation. The former plan may be fraught with difficulty as uremic symptoms and complications multiply, and pharmacologic and dietary treatment becomes difficult. In consultation with the physician, however, individual patients may wish to accept the risks of such an approach. Early initiation of dialysis may avoid such complications as malnutrition, neuropathy, and possible progression of cardiovascular disease. Early dialysis and transplantation before the advent of uremic symptoms has been advocated in diabetic patients, as has early transplantation before initiation of dialytic therapy. In general, patients will start ESRD therapy when creatinine clearance ranges from 0 to 10 mL $\cdot$ min^{-1} $\cdot$ 1.73 m^{-2}, and when uremic complications and symptoms supervene. Time of initiation and modality of ESRD therapy should represent a well-formulated, jointly achieved patient–physician decision.

Bibliography

Attman PO, Samyuelsson O, Alaovic P: Lipoprotein metabolism and renal failure. *Am J Kidney Dis* 26:573–592, 1993.

Bourgoignie JJ, Jacob AI, Sallman AL, Pennell JP: Water, electrolyte and acid-base abnormalities in chronic renal failure. *Semin Nephrol* 1:91–111, 1981.

Delmez JA, Slatoplosky E: Hyperphosphatemia: Its consequences and treatment in patients with chronic renal disease. *Am J Kidney Dis* 19:303–317, 1992.

Felsenfeld AJ, Llach F: Parathyroid function in chronic renal failure. *Kidney Int* 43:771–789, 1993.

Goodman WG, Coburn JW: The use of 1,25-dihydroxyvitamin D3 in early renal failure. *Annu Rev Med* 43:227–237, 1992.

Grundy SM: Management of hyperlipidemia of kidney disease. *Kidney Int* 37:847–853, 1990.

Jacobson HR, Striker GE, for the workshop group. Report on a workshop to develop management recommendations for the prevention of progression in chronic renal failure. *Am J Kidney Dis* 25:103–106, 1995.

Klahr S: Chronic renal failure: Management. *Lancet* 338:423–427, 1991.

Levy AS, Adler S, Caggiula AW, et al.: Effects of dietary protein restriction on the progression of advanced renal disease in the Modification of Diet in Renal Disease Study. *Am J Kidney Dis* 27:652–663, 1996.

Livio M, Benigni A, Remuzzi G: Coagulation abnormalities in uremia. *Semin Nephrol* 5:82–90, 1985.

Llach F: Secondary hyperparathyroidism in renal failure: The trade-off hypothesis revisited. *Am J Kidney Dis* 25:663–679, 1995.

Ma JZ, Greene EL, Raij L: Cardiovascular risk factors in chronic renal failure and hemodialysis populations. *Am J Kidney Dis* 27:652–663, 1996.

Maki DD, Ma JZ, Louis TA, Kasiske BL: Long-term effects of antihypertensive agents on proteinuria and renal function. *Arch Intern Med* 155:1073–1080, 1995.

Malluche H, Faugere M-C: Renal bone disease 1990: An unmet challenge for the nephrologist. *Kidney Int* 38:193–211, 1990.

Maschio G, Alberti D, Janin G, et al.: Effect of the angiotensin-converting enzyme inhibitor benazepril on the progression of chronic renal insufficiency. *N Engl J Med* 334:939–945, 1996.

Massey ZA, Ma JZ, Louis TA, Kasiske BL: Lipid-lowering therapy in patients with renal disease. *Kidney Int* 48:188–198, 1995.

Pedrini MT, Levey AS, Lau J, Chalmers TC, Wang PH: The effect of dietary protein restriction on the progression of diabetic and

TABLE 4

Indications for Initiating ESRD Therapy

Uremic symptoms
Hyperkalemia[a]
Metabolic acidosis[a]
Cognestive heart failure[a]
Hypertension
Pericarditis
Neuropathy
Encephalopathy
Uremic coagulopathy

[a] Resistant to medical therapy.

non-diabetic renal diseases: a metaanalysis. *Ann Intern Med* 124:627–632, 1996.

Peterson JC, Adler S, Burkart JM, et al.: Blood pressure control, proteinuria and the progression of renal disease. The Modification of Diet in Renal Disease Study. *Ann Intern Med* 123:754–762, 1995.

Ratcliffe PJ: Molecular biology of erythropoietin. *Kidney Int* 44:887–904, 1993.

Ritz E, Stefanski A, Rambausek M: The role of the parathyroid glands in the uremic syndrome. *Am J Kidney Dis* 26:808–813, 1995.

Rudnick MR, Goldfarb S, Wexler L, et al., for the Iohexol Cooperative Study: Nephrotoxicity of ionic and non-ionic contrast media in 1196 patients: A randomized trial. *Kidney Int* 47:254–261, 1995.

Salem MM, Rosa RM, Battle DC: Extrarenal potassium tolerance in chronic renal failure: Implications for the treatment of acute hyperkalemia. *Am J Kidney Dis* 18:421–440, 1991.

ter Wee PM, De Micheli AG, Epstein M: Effects of calcium antagonists on renal hemodynamics and progression of non-diabetic chronic renal disease. *Arch Intern Med* 154:1185–1202, 1994.

Tsukamoto Y, Moriya R, Nagaba Y, Morishita T, Izumida I, Okubo M: Effect of administration of calcium carbonate to treat secondary hyperparathyroidism in nondialyzed patients with chronic renal failure. *Am J Kidney Dis* 25:879–886, 1995.

Wheeler DC, Bernard DB: Lipid abnormalities in the nephrotic syndrome: Causes, consequences and treatment. *Am J Kidney Dis* 23:331–346, 1994.

NUTRITION AND RENAL DISEASE

BRADLEY J. MARONI

INTRODUCTION

In contrast to carbohydrate and fat, excess protein is not stored, but degraded to form urea and other nitrogenous wastes eliminated by the kidney. Moreover, protein-rich foods contain phosphates, hydrogen ions, and other inorganic ions which are also excreted by the kidney (Fig. 1). Consequently, patients with chronic renal failure (CRF) who consume excessive dietary protein will accumulate nitrogenous wastes and inorganic ions, resulting in the clinical and metabolic disturbances characteristic of uremia. This is the basis for the observation that limiting dietary protein (and phosphorus) intake can ameliorate many uremic symptoms and some of the metabolic complications of CRF (e.g., secondary hyperparathyroidism, metabolic acidosis, etc.). Another less obvious relationship is also illustrated in Fig. 1. When protein intake is inadequate, waste products continue to accumulate due to the degradation of body protein stores.

Therefore, the goals of nutritional therapy in renal failure are to (1) ensure sufficient dietary intake to prevent malnutrition, (2) to limit the accumulation of nitrogenous wastes and metabolic disturbances characteristic of uremia, and (3) to possibly slow the rate of progression of CRF.

PROTEIN TURNOVER IN NORMAL PATIENTS AND CRF

Healthy Subjects

In healthy adults consuming adequate (but not excessive) energy and performing moderate physical activity, the average protein requirement is ~0.6 g of protein per kg per day. The "safe level of intake" (i.e., mean plus two standard deviations) is ~0.75 g of protein per kg per day, an amount that is adequate for ≥97.5% of the population. In Western societies, individuals typically ingest 1 to 2 g of protein per kg per day; i.e., an intake well above the daily protein requirement. Because excess dietary protein (and amino acids) is not stored, the principal response to a surplus of dietary protein is a marked increase in amino acid oxidation. The nitrogen resulting from amino acid catabolism is then converted to urea and other nitrogenous wastes which are eliminated primarily by the kidney. In contrast, the principal adaptive response to a reduction in dietary protein intake is a marked decrease in amino acid oxidation, resulting in more efficient utilization of dietary essential amino acids (EAA). Assuming protein intake meets (or exceeds) the minimum daily requirement, waste nitrogen excretion (principally urea) decreases, and nitrogen balance (i.e., nitrogen intake equals output) is achieved with the lower protein intake.

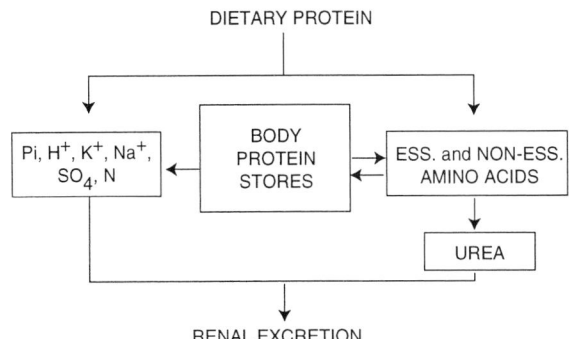

DIETARY PROTEIN

BODY PROTEIN STORES

Pi, H⁺, K⁺, Na⁺, SO₄, N

ESS. and NON-ESS. AMINO ACIDS

UREA

RENAL EXCRETION

FIGURE 1 Dietary protein yields essential and nonessential amino acids which can be used to synthesize body proteins. Protein-containing foods in excess of the daily requirement are degraded producing urea, nonurea nitrogen, and inorganic ions which must be excreted. Reprinted with permission from Mitch WE: In: Martinez-Maldonado M ed *Handbook of Renal Therapeutics*. Plenum, New York, pp. 349–373, 1983.

It should also be appreciated that protein turnover (i.e., protein synthesis and degradation) is a dynamic process resulting in the remodeling of ~1 kg of protein per day. During fasting, body protein stores (principally skeletal muscle) are degraded and the amino acids are utilized for hepatic gluconeogenesis. In response to feeding, anabolism (i.e., protein synthesis > protein degradation) occurs by suppressing whole-body protein degradation with or without an accompanying stimulation of protein synthesis. Assuming the diet is adequate, the net response over 24 hours is neutral nitrogen balance and preservation of lean body mass. In summary, successful adaptation to a low-protein diet includes: (1) feeding-induced suppression of whole-body protein degradation with or without stimulation of protein synthesis; and (2) marked suppression of EAA oxidation.

CRF Patients

Since avoiding malnutrition is a primary goal of nutritional therapy, it is important to recognize that low-protein diets can be used safely in CRF patients. Fortunately, even patients with advanced CRF (i.e., GFR ~10 to 15 mL/min) can maintain neutral nitrogen balance and preserve lean body mass when dietary protein intake is restricted. They activate the same adaptive responses to low-protein diets as healthy subjects; namely, a marked suppression of amino acid oxidation and feeding-induced inhibition of whole-body protein degradation. In addition, nitrogen balance, serum proteins, and anthropometrics remain normal during long-term protein restriction. In the Modification of Diet in Renal Disease (MDRD) study, minor, albeit statistically significant changes, did occur in some nutritional parameters in the low-protein diet groups, i.e., an *increase* in serum albumin and a *decrease* in serum transferrin and some anthropometric measures. However, abnormal values stabilized following the first few months of diet therapy, and the average values for the low-protein diet groups remained

within the normal range. Most importantly, a lower protein intake was not associated with a higher rate of hospitalizations or death.

Low-protein diets (LPD) can also be used safely in patients with the nephrotic syndrome. When nephrotic patients were fed a diet containing 0.8 protein (plus 1 g protein/g proteinuria) and 35 kcal per kg body wt per day, nitrogen balance was neutral; the principal compensatory response was a suppression of amino acid oxidation. Amino acid oxidation correlated inversely with urinary protein losses suggesting that proteinuria is also a stimulus to conserve dietary EAA. In conclusion, both nephrotic and *non-nephrotic* CRF patients can activate normal adaptive responses to dietary protein restriction allowing them to achieve neutral nitrogen balance and maintain lean body mass.

PROGRESSION OF CRF AND SPONTANEOUS PROTEIN INTAKE

Recently there has been concern that LPDs cause malnutrition and it has been suggested that these diets be used cautiously in patients with CRF. These fears arise principally from two observations: (1) evidence of a spontaneous decrease in protein intake and worsening of some indices of nutritional status in patients with progressive CRF consuming *unrestricted* diets; and (2) the association between hypoalbuminemia and mortality in hemodialysis patients. In fact, several lines of evidence suggest that LPDs can be used safely in CRF patients. First, the studies discussed above indicate that proper implementation of a LPD yields neutral nitrogen balance with maintenance of normal serum proteins and anthropometric indices during long-term therapy. Second, recent evidence suggests that hypoalbuminemia in hemodialysis patients is more closely related to inflammation than to dietary adequacy (vide infra). Without proper dietary education, CRF patients may inadvertently consume protein-rich meals resulting in the accumulation of nitrogenous wastes and uremic symptoms for several days. In this setting, satiety may actually represent anorexia and it is clear that protein intake and nutritional status can deteriorate if uremic symptoms persist, increasing the risk of malnutrition. In contrast, if the diet is planned so that sufficient protein is prescribed to maintain nitrogen balance while limiting the accumulation of nitrogenous wastes (Fig. 1), uremic symptoms will not develop and nutritional status will be maintained.

LPDS AND PROGRESSION OF RENAL DISEASE

An alarming feature of CRF is that once damage is established (serum creatinine ~2.5 to 3.0 mg/dL) the loss of renal function usually continues even when the initial disease process is no longer active. Evidence that an LPD slows renal progression in animals and the ability to assess changes in renal function in humans prompted investigators to examine whether restricting dietary protein might delay the loss of residual renal function in CRF patients.

Several prospective randomized trials involving small groups of CRF patients have concluded that an LPD can slow the loss of renal function in diabetic and nondiabetic renal disease. In contrast, the largest clinical trial—the MDRD Study—did not demonstrate a benefit of dietary protein restriction on renal progression, at least when an 'intention to treat" analysis was used (i.e., analysis of outcomes regardless of whether patients complied with the diet). When the MDRD results were analyzed according to the protein intake actually consumed, a $0.2 \text{ g} \cdot \text{kg}^{-1} \cdot \text{day}^{-1}$ reduction in protein intake was associated with a 29% slower rate of loss of GFR and a 41% prolongation in the time to dialysis ($P < 0.01$). Two meta-analyses (one including the MDRD study) have also concluded that an LPD was associated with a 33 to 46% risk of renal failure. In principle, an LPD could reduce the risk of renal failure by slowing the progression of renal disease or by ameliorating uremic symptoms. Interestingly, the authors of one of the meta-analyses estimated that a study would need to enroll at least 1000 patients to detect a 33% reduction in the risk of renal failure or death. Neither the MDRD study has any other clinical trial included this many patients.

In conclusion, despite many supportive observations, it has not been proved that dietary protein restriction will slow the progression of renal failure in humans. One approach to the treatment of patients with progressive CRF is initially to focus on treatment of hypertension, aiming for a blood pressure ≤125/75 mm Hg in patients with proteinuria exceeding 1 g/day, since more aggressive blood pressure control is associated with a slower rate of progression in proteinuric patients. Angiotensin converting enzyme inhibitors should be considered the firstline of therapy, since the rate of progression of renal disease is ~50% slower with these agents in both diabetic and nondiabetic patients. In motivated patients who are progressing despite hypertensive treatment, dietary protein restriction is recommended.

METHODS FOR ASSESSING NUTRITIONAL STATUS

The criteria for an ideal technique for assessing nutritional status in outpatients would be (1) readily available and easy to perform, (2) sensitive and reproducible, and (3) validated in patients with renal failure. Although a number of methods are available to assess the nutritional status and/or body composition of patients with renal failure, their utility is compromised in patients with renal disease due to: alterations in metabolism caused by renal disease independent of nutritional status (e.g., albumin, prealbumin, urinary creatinine excretion), lack of population-specific reference values (e.g., anthropometrics), changes in extracellular (or peritoneal) fluid volume (bioelectrical impedance); or, not widely available clinically (e.g., neutron activation analysis, dual X-ray photon absorptiometry, NMR spectroscopy). Presently, serial changes in anthropometrics (e.g., edema-free body weight), serum albumin, and transferrin are typically used to monitor nutritional status (vide infra).

MONITORING DIETARY ADEQUACY AND COMPLIANCE

When prescribing LPDs it is important to monitor dietary adequacy and compliance. Fortunately, a simple method is available for estimating protein intake in the outpatient setting (Table 1). To understand this technique and its limitations, it must be appreciated that waste nitrogen derived from degraded protein is excreted as urea and nonurea nitrogen (NUN). Whereas the urea nitrogen appearance rate (i.e., urea excretion plus accumulation) closely parallels protein intake, NUN excretion (i.e., nitrogen in feces and urinary ammonia, uric acid, creatinine, etc.) is relatively constant, averaging $0.031 \text{ g N} \cdot \text{kg}^{-1} \cdot \text{day}^{-1}$. If the patient is in neutral nitrogen balance (B_N), then nitrogen intake (I_N) equals urea nitrogen appearance (UNA) plus nonurea nitrogen (NUN) (Table 1, Formula 2). When the BUN is unchanging (i.e., steadystate), then urea nitrogen appearance (UNA) equals the 24-hour urinary urea nitrogen (UUN) excretion (Table 1 Formula 3). Thus, I_N equals UUN + 0.031 g N/kg body wt (Table 1, Formula 4).

In the example shown in Table 1, because the prescribed and estimated intake are similar, we can conclude that the patient is compliant with the protein prescription. If the estimated intake is less than prescribed, the patient should be instructed to increase protein intake to reach the goal. In contrast, if the estimated intake exceeds the prescription by more than 25% (i.e., the precision of the method), then the patient is noncompliant or a catabolic illness or condition (e.g., metabolic acidosis) is stimulating the breakdown of body protein and increasing waste nitrogen production. If a careful evaluation reveals no abnormality, the patient should be referred to the dietitian for assistance in achieving compliance.

Dietary recall or diaries are the only available methods for assessing energy intake in the outpatient setting. Al-

TABLE I
Estimating Protein Intake from the 24-Hour Urinary Urea Nitrogen Excretion

$B_N = I_N - (\text{UNA} + \text{NUN})$, where NUN = 0.031 g N/kg body wt

if $B_N = 0$, then I_N = UNA + 0.031 g N/kg body wt

when BUN unchanging, then UNA = UUN and,

I_N = UUN + 0.031 g N/kg body wt

Example: A 50-year-old man is seen in clinic 1 month following instruction on a diet providing 0.6 g of protein per kg per day (i.e., 70 kg × 0.6 protein/kg = 42 g protein).

Weight: 70 kg; UUN = 4.8 g/day; NUN = 0.031 g N × 70 kg = 2.17 g N/day

if $B_N = 0$, then I_N = UUN + NUN
= 4.8 + 2.17 = 6.97 g N
= 6.97 g N × 6.25 g protein/g N
= 43.6 g protein/day

Note: N, nitrogen; B_N, nitrogen balance (g N/day); I_N, nitrogen intake (g N/day); BUN, blood urea nitrogen; UNA, urea nitrogen appearance (g N/day); UUN 24-hour urinary urea nitrogen (g N/ day); NUN, nonurea nitrogen (g N/day).

though their limitations are well recognized, as a compromise between accuracy and compliance, three-day food diaries can be utilized to monitor energy intake. A skilled dietitian can facilitate menu planning and patient satisfaction while assisting with the monitoring of patient's compliance and nutritional status. Nutritional status is monitored by performing serial measurements of anthropometrics, serum albumin, and transferrin. Once patients are comfortable with the diet, they can be seen every 3 months while (1) estimating protein intake from the 24-hour UUN excretion; (2) estimating caloric intake from food diaries/recall; (3) monitoring anthropometrics, serum albumin and transferrin; and (4) using these measures to provide patient feedback.

The nutritional status of ESRD patients should also be monitored, because many individuals consume less than the recommended intake of protein and calories, and malnutrition is common in this population (vide infra). One frequently used method to estimate dietary protein intake is the protein catabolic rate (PCR). The PCR is analogous to the urea nitrogen appearance rate (UNA) described above and is calculated from equations relating the predialysis BUN, the normalized urea clearance (Kt), and volume of distribution of urea (V). In maintenance hemodialysis patients, urea kinetics are routinely measured to estimate the delivered dose of dialysis (i.e., Kt/V_{urea}; see Chapter 63); hence, the PCR is also calculated. In continuous ambulatory peritoneal dialysis (CAPD) patients, expended dialysate is collected during a 24-hour period and urea nitrogen and protein losses are measured. Dietary protein intake in clinically stable CAPD patients can then be estimated as: PCR (g protein/day) = 13 + 7.31 UNA (g N/day) + protein losses (g/day). Since protein requirements are determined primarily by lean body mass, PCR is typically normalized to body weight (i.e., nPCR, g protein $\cdot$ kg^{-1} $\cdot$ day^{-1}). As discussed previously, PCR will only reflect dietary protein intake only when patients are in neutral nitrogen balance; e.g., there are no superimposed catabolic illnesses. In addition to the nPCR, postdialysis weight ("dry weight") and serum albumin are also routinely monitored. In ESRD patients with low or declining values of body weight and serum albumin, or an nPCR <1.0, protein and calorie intake can be estimated from dietary recall or diaries.

FACTORS CONTRIBUTING TO MALNUTRITION AND INCREASED PROTEIN REQUIREMENTS IN DIALYSIS PATIENTS

Virtually all studies of nutrition in dialysis patients have found that these patients are frequently malnourished. Although the prevalence depends on the indices used to evaluate nutritional status, ~10% of ESRD patients suffer from severe malnutrition and another 33% from mild to moderate malnutrition. Factors which increase protein requirements and contribute to malnutrition include: (1) inadequate intake due to anorexia induced by uremia, comorbidity, medications, depression, etc.; (2) superimposed illnesses or catabolic states (e.g., acidosis); (3) increased requirements due to albumin and amino acid losses

into dialysate; and (4) catabolism induced by the hemodialysis procedure.

Several lines of evidence indicate that hemodialysis stimulates catabolism, at least when performed using bioincompatible membranes. For instance, cuprophane membranes activate complement and stimulate the release of interleukin 1 and other cytokines from monocytes. Hemodialysis with cuprophane membranes stimulates skeletal muscle catabolism, whereas the use of polyacrilonitrile membranes does not. Finally, with cuprophane membranes, *net* protein balance became more negative during the dialysis procedure due to a suppression of whole-body protein synthesis as well as dialysate amino acids losses.

NUTRITIONAL STATUS AND MORTALITY IN ESRD

A low serum albumin level is a powerful predictor of mortality in ESRD patients. Increased mortality is also associated with low values of BUN (suggesting a low-protein intake), cholesterol, and creatinine (index of muscle protein mass). Although these findings suggest that protein–calorie malnutrition increases mortality in dialysis patients, this is presently unproved. Other factor(s) besides nutritional status may result in abnormalities in these parameters. Albumin synthesis rates have been found to be decreased in hypoalbuminemic hemodialysis patients even with dietary protein intake similar to patients with normal serum albumin levels. Serum albumin (and albumin synthesis rates) correlated inversely with the serum levels of the acute-phase reactants, C-reactive protein (CRP) and α_2-macroglobulin. A preliminary report has confirmed the inverse relationship between serum albumin and CRP; in contrast to serum albumin, CRP was an independent predictor of survival in hemodialysis patients. Thus, serum albumin levels in hemodialysis patients are determined at least partly by nonnutritional factors (e.g., inflammation), and one should not necessarily equate hypoalbuminemia with malnutrition in this population.

Because laboratory surrogates of nutritional status may be influenced by nonnutritional factors, the relationship between other indices of nutrition and survival would be of great interest. Although it is well established that the prevalence of malnutrition is increased in the ESRD population (e.g., low anthropometric indices, decreased total body nitrogen), there is very little information relating nutritional status to patient outcomes (morbidity and mortality). Such studies have rarely been performed, because they are labor intensive, expensive, and require long-term follow-up of large numbers of patients with well-defined risk factors. Complex statistical models using multivariate analysis are required to evaluate which risk factors are independent determinants of mortality (or morbidity). Interpretation is also complicated by the difficulty in determining whether the risk factor (e.g., malnutrition) is the proximate cause of mortality or simply a complication of the underlying disease (e.g., cancer). Finally, statistical associations must be interpreted cautiously since they do not imply cause and effect.

DIETARY REQUIREMENTS IN RENAL FAILURE

Protein (Table 2)

As discussed earlier, the benefit of dietary protein restriction in slowing progression of renal failure remains controversial. Patients with mild renal insufficiency (i.e., GFR >60 to 70 mL/min) are usually asymptomatic, and there is no information regarding the utility of dietary protein restriction in this setting. Emphasis should focus on controlling hypertension and other coexisting problems such as hyperlipidemia.

In patients with GFRs between 25 and 60 mL/min, controversy remains, but LPDs may retard progression of renal failure and are safe when used properly. In motivated individuals, dietary therapy would begin with a conventional LPD providing 0.6 g of protein per kg per day, with twothirds provided as high-biologic value protein, i.e., the protein should have a high content of EAAs (usually animal proteins such as meat, fish, and eggs). In patients with advanced CRF (GFR 5 to 25 mL/min), in addition to a diet providing 0.6 g of protein per kg per day, a very-low protein diet containing ~0.3 g of protein per kg per day supplemented with a mixture of EAA or their nitrogen-free ketoanalogues has been used. In contrast to Europe and Japan, ketoacid supplements are not available in the US. Because patients with a GFR <10 mL/min are at the greatest risk for developing malnutrition, these individuals should be closely monitored to ensure adequate intake and maintenance of nutritional status. Dialysis is typically initiated when the GFR is <10 mL/min.

Because proteinuria is a risk factor for progressive renal insufficiency and LPDs reduce urinary protein losses and hypercholesterolemia in nephrosis, dietary protein restriction could be used as adjunctive therapy in nephrotic patients. A diet providing 0.8 g of protein per kg per day (plus 1 g protein/g proteinuria) yields neutral nitrogen balance in nephrotic patients. Moreover, there was no correlation between nitrogen balance and GFR (range: 19 to 120 mL/min). Finally, several long-term studies indicate that serum albumin levels remained stable or increased when nephrotic patients were prescribed diets providing 0.45 to 0.80 g of protein per kg per day. Taken together these studies suggest that dietary protein restriction is safe in the nephrotic syndrome, even in patients with advanced renal failure. However, the use of LPDs in nephrotic patients with very high levels of proteinuria (i.e., >15 g/day), or in patients with superimposed catabolic illnesses (e.g., systemic lupus) or receiving catabolic medications is not recommended.

The protein requirements of patients receiving hemodialysis or peritoneal dialysis are increased compared to healthy subjects or predialysis CRF patients (vide supra). It is recommended that maintenance hemodialysis patients consume ~1.1 to 1.2 g of protein per kg per day. Nitrogen balance studies performed in CAPD patients indicate that their requirements are at least 1.1 and preferably 1.2 to 1.4 g of protein per kg per day. It is commonly recommended that ~50% of the protein be high-biologic value, but with this level of protein intake it is unclear whether this is necessary. If the patient's dietary intake is marginal or the proposed diet severely limits food choices, it may be preferabe to relax restrictions on protein quality.

Energy (Table 2)

In both predialysis and dialysis patients, energy expenditure (and hence energy requirements) at rest and during

TABLE 2

Recommended Intakes of Protein, Energy, and Phosphorus for Patients with Chronic Renal Failure, Nephrotic Syndrome, and End Stage Renal Disease

	Protein (g · kg^{-1} · day^{-1})	Energy^a (kcal · kg^{-1} · day^{-1})	Phosphorus^b (mg · kg^{-1} · day^{-1})
Chronic renal failure			
GFR (mL/min)			
>60–70	Protein restriction not usually recommended	≥35	No restriction
25–60	0.60 g · kg^{-1} · day^{-1} including ≥0.35 g · kg^{-1} · day^{-1} of HBV	≥35	≤10
5–25	(1) 0.60 g · kg^{-1} · day^{-1} including ≥0.35 g · kg^{-1} · day^{-1} of HBV or	≥35	≤10
	(2) 0.28 g · kg^{-1} · day^{-1} supplemented with EAA or KA	≥35	≤9
Nephrotic syndrome			
GFR <60 mL/min	0.80 g · kg^{-1} · day^{-1} (plus 1 g protein/g proteinuria)	≥35	≤12
End stage renal failure			≤17
Hemodialysis	1.1–1.2 g · kg^{-1} · day^{-1}	≥35	
Peritoneal dialysis	1.2–1.4 g · kg^{-1} · day^{-1}	≥35	≤17

^{a} Energy intake may be cautiously decreased in obese individuals (>120% normal weight) or those who gain undesired adiposity with the recommended intake.

^{b} Phosphate binders are often needed to maintain normal serum phosphorus.

Note: HBV, high biologic value protein; EAA, essential amino acid supplement; KA, amino acid-ketoacid supplement.

exercise are similar to those in healthy subjects. An energy intake of ~35 kcal · kg^{-1} · day^{-1} is recommended because it maintains nitrogen balance, anthropometrics, and serum proteins in patients consuming the recommended intakes of protein (Table 2). In the elderly and obese individuals, or those gaining undesired weight, lower energy intakes may be cautiously prescribed (~30 kcal · kg^{-1} · day^{-1}).

Unfortunately, ESRD patients frequently consume less than the recommended intakes, e.g., daily average intakes of 0.95 to 1.01 g of protein and 23 to 32 kcal/kg body wt have been reported. Because malnutrition is common among ESRD patients, this decrease in energy intake cannot be an adjustment to a lower energy requirement, but must be considered maladaptive. To improve dietary intake, counseling sessions with the renal dietitian can be useful. If attempts to improve intake using conventional food sources are unsuccessful, a number of nutritional supplements are available which provide a high calorie or protein density, while limiting the fluid and electrolyte content. Examples include adding glucose polymers (Polycose) to beverages, or high-density oral supplements (Nepro; Suplena) and candy bars (Regain).

HYPERLIPIDEMIA IN RENAL DISEASE

Hyperlipidemia is common in renal failure, with a prevalence of 20 to 70% in predialysis and dialysis patients. The characteristic abnormality in *non*nephrotic predialysis as well as hemodialysis patients is hypertriglyceridemia with increased levels of very low-density lipoproteins (VLDL), decreased high-density lipoprotein cholesterol (HDL-C) and normal to low levels of low-density lipoprotein cholesterol (LDL-C). Although impaired catabolism of triglyceride-rich lipoproteins is the major cause of hypertriglyceridemia, increased production also contributes since hemodialysis patients with normal chylomicron clearance rates also have higher fasting serum triglyceride levels. In peritoneal dialysis patients, serum cholesterol frequently rises and then stabilizes during the first year of therapy; serum triglycerides are variable but hypertriglyceridemia has been attributed to absorption of glucose from the dialysate, and possibly to lipoprotein and apolipoprotein losses into the peritoneal fluid. In the nephrotic syndrome, plasma LDL-C is usually increased and HDL-C is normal or decreased; hypertriglyceridemia may also be present. Initially there is overproduction of VLDL, which are rapidly catabolized to form LDL. LDL clearance may also be impaired, especially in patients with severe nephrosis. The most likely explanation for hypertriglyceridemia in nephrosis is decreased clearance of triglyceride-rich VLDL particles.

In patients with renal disease, it is not known if hyperlipidemia increases the risk of atherosclerosis or if therapy designed to reduce lipid levels is beneficial. Proponents of therapy cite epidemiologic studies linking an elevated serum cholesterol with accelerated atherosclerosis and the reduction in coronary artery disease found in primary and secondary intervention trials of otherwise healthy subjects. Despite the lack of conclusive clinical data demonstrating a benefit of lipid-lowering therapy in patients with renal failure, some general guidelines are available.

As recommended for the general population, the National Cholesterol Education Program (NCEP) guidelines seem appropriate for hyperlipidemic renal patients. Specifically, adults with a total cholesterol >200 mg/dL on two occasions should be instructed in a Step I American Heart Association (AHA) diet providing <30% of total calories from fat (with <10% of calories from saturated fat) and <300 mg cholesterol daily. Attention should also be directed at eliminating other cardiovascular risk factors (e.g., smoking, obesity, and hypertension), avoiding excessive carbohydrate and alcohol intake, and improving glycemic control in diabetics. In patients with a total cholesterol >240 mg/dL or 200 to 239 mg/dL with two risk factors [i.e., documented coronary artery disease (CAD) or family history of CAD before age 55, cigarette smoking, male sex, hypertension, HDL-C <35 mg/dL, diabetes mellitus, history of cerebrovascular or peripheral vascular disease, or severe obesity] a lipoprotein profile should be performed. If the LDL-C remains greater than 190 mg/dL (or 160 mg/dL with two risk factors) following 6 months of dietary modification, drug therapy should be considered. Despite dietary modification, a number of patients (particularly nephrotic and transplant patients) are likely to have cholesterol levels above the desirable range (i.e., LDL-C <130 mg/dL). In view of their potency, once a day dosing, and favorable side-effect profile, HMG-CoA reductase inhibitors should be considered first-line therapy. In patients refractory to monotherapy, the combination of a HMG-CoA reductase inhibitor with either nicotinic acid or a bile acid sequestrant may be considered. Bile acid sequestrants interfere with cyclosporine absorption and cannot be used in transplant patients. The fibric acids, clofibrate and gemfibrozil, reduce serum triglycerides, but should be avoided in patients with renal failure because of the increased risk of myopathy.

MINERALS, TRACE ELEMENTS, AND VITAMINS IN RENAL FAILURE

Minerals and Trace Elements

Sodium intake is usually restricted to ~2 g/day to control hypertension and edema in CRF patients (see Chapters 15 and 79). In dialysis patients, sodium restriction will also reduce thirst, interdialytic weight gain, and the likelihood of intradialytic hypotension due to increased ultrafiltration requirements. Disorders of potassium metabolism are discussed in detail in Chapter 13. Hyperkalemia is uncommon until the CrCl <15 mL/min (and usually <5 mL/min), and it is usually not necessary to restrict potassium intake prior to initiating dialysis. Generally, potassium is restricted to ~2 g/day once dialysis is begun, although CAPD patients may tolerate or even require a more liberal intake.

Iron metabolism and the use of erythropoietin are discussed in Chapter 72. The impact of renal disease on calcium, phosphorus, vitamin D, and aluminum metabolism is reviewed in Chapters 14 and 69. However, several comments are warranted. First, because calcium absorption is impaired in CRF and protein-restricted diets are low in calcium, at least 1.0 to 1.5 g/day of elemental calcium should be provided to ensure neutral calcium balance; this is easily achieved with calcium-containing phosphate binders. Second, in view of the efficacy of calcium carbonate and acetate as phosphate binders, and the risk of augmenting aluminum absorption with citrate, the use of calcium citrate as a phosphate binder should be avoided. Magnesium-containing laxatives and antacids should be avoided in patients with renal insufficiency because the kidney is primarily responsible for magnesium excretion, and thus hypermagnesemia may result.

Although postmortem studies in uremic patients indicate that the tissue distribution of trace elements is abnormal, the clinical importance of these changes is unclear. Elevated serum nickel and chromium levels have been attributed to contaminated dialysate. Conversely, low plasma and red blood cell bromide levels have been reported in CAPD patients, perhaps due to dialysate losses. Plasma zinc is usually decreased, whereas tissue levels are generally increased. Zinc supplementation has been reported to increase B lymphocyte counts, granulocyte motility, and taste, and sexual dysfunction—although these findings have not been uniform. In conclusion, the dietary requirements for trace elements have not been well defined in renal failure. It would seem prudent to monitor closely dialysis water supplies and peritoneal dialysate for excessive concentrations of trace elements. Because the kidney is the principal route of excretion, supplementation is not recommended.

Vitamins

A water-soluble vitamin supplement is frequently prescribed for CRF patients based on studies indicating intakes below the recommended daily requirements (RDA), decreased intestinal absorption, impaired enzyme activity and the presence of circulating inhibitors (vitamins are cofactors), or losses into dialysate. Notably, diets which are restricted in protein, phosphorus, and potassium are often low in water-soluble vitamins. In CAPD patients, the net intake of folate, niacin, B_1, B_6, and B_{12} were below the RDA for healthy subjects. In contrast, one study found that after discontinuing a vitamin supplement most hemodialysis patients were able to maintain normal blood and erythrocyte water-soluble vitamin levels by diet alone; the blood levels of a few vitamins initially decreased but then stabilized within the normal range. Although further research is needed to quantify actual intakes and losses, renal patients should be given a water-soluble vitamin supplement formulated to meet their estimated requirements (e.g., Nephrocap, Nephrovite). However, "megavitamin" therapy should be discouraged, because severe peripheral neuropathy and hyperoxalemia have been reported with high-dose pyridoxine and vitamin C supplementation, respectively.

Treatment of vitamin D deficiency is discussed in Chapter 69. Vitamin A supplements should be avoided because plasma vitamin A (retinol) levels are increased in CRF patients. Vitamin A toxicity has been reported in CRF patients receiving parenteral nutrition containing a standard multivitamin supplement (providing 1500 μg vitamin A). Therefore, parenteral nutrition solutions should be screened for vitamin A before use in patients with renal failure. It has been suggested that oxidant stress may be in part responsible for increased erythrocyte turnover in uremia. However, Vitamin E supplementation is not recommended because plasma vitamin E levels are normal in patients with renal failure and it has not been demonstrated that vitamin E supplements increase erythrocyte survival in uremic patients.

NUTRITIONAL THERAPY IN ACUTE RENAL FAILURE

The goals of nutritional therapy in acute renal failure (ARF) are to: (1) avoid uremic symptoms and the need for dialysis prior to renal recovery; (2) maintain or improve functional and nutritional status, including host resistance and wound healing; and (3) promote recovery of the kidneys. Patients with ARF are frequently catabolic and it is likely that malnutrition is an important risk factor for morbidity and mortality in these patients. Factors contributing to wasting in ARF include: (1) superimposed catabolic conditions such as surgery, trauma, acidosis, and sepsis, (2) alterations in metabolism resulting from the loss of renal function; (3) preexisting malnutrition and inadequate nutrient intake; and (4) intradialytic losses and catabolism induced by the dialysis procedure.

Several caveats regarding nutritional therapy in ARF should be recognized. First, intuitively it would seem that the early institution of aggressive nutritional support in ARF is warranted, yet its impact on renal recovery, morbidity, and mortality remains unproved. Second, although nutritional intervention improves nitrogen balance in many catabolic states, it is unusual for these patients to become anabolic (i.e., positive nitrogen balance). Presumably, the metabolic defects responsible for protein (and amino acid) catabolism also impair utilization of dietary protein. Consequently, increasing protein intake above the daily requirement will not ameliorate wasting in patients with ARF; the excess protein is simply catabolized, increasing waste nitrogen production and the need for dialysis. Third, due to the limitations of nutritional intervention trials in ARF, the protein requirements of ARF patients are poorly defined. Consequently, protein requirements of ARF patients have been derived from clinical experience using nutritional support in acutely ill individuals with or without renal insufficiency and studies performed in CRF patients. When ARF is self-limited (e.g., radiocontrast nephropathy) and catabolism is modest, 0.6 g of protein per kg per day is usually recommended in order to minimize waste nitrogen accumulation and the need for dialysis while awaiting recovery of renal function. Patients requiring hemodialysis or peritoneal dialysis should receive 1.0 to 1.2 and 1.2 to 1.4 g of protein per kg per day, respectively. The protein requirements of patients receiving continuous renal replacement therapies (e.g., CAVHD, CVVHD, etc.) have not been carefully examined, although dialysate amino acid losses are increased compared to conventional hemodialysis. Intakes of 1.5 to 2.5 g of protein per kg per day have been recommended by some experts for patients receiving continuous dialysis therapies.

In the absence of sepsis, trauma, or burns, ARF patients are not hypermetabolic and their energy requirements are similar to normal subjects; 35 to 40 kcal · kg^{-1} · day^{-1} is commonly recommended. Alternatively, energy needs may be based on estimates of basal energy expenditure (BEE) derived from healthy populations using equations that take into account body weight, height, age, and sex; this value is then increased by 25% (i.e., 1.25 × BEE) to account for biologic variability and physical activity. Adjustment factors for patients with trauma, burns, and sepsis have been proposed (e.g., sepsis; 1.2 to 1.6 × BEE), although it should be appreciated that calculated and measured rates of energy expenditure may vary widely. When available, indirect calorimetry may help refine the energy prescription by directly measuring energy expenditure.

In ARF, water and mineral intake (e.g., sodium, potassium, phosphorus) must be restricted. Typically, fluid intake is limited to ~1 to 1.5 L/day, sodium and potassium is restricted to 2 g/day, and phosphorus is limited according to the level of protein intake (Table 2). A number of enteral formulas are available, including several products designed specifically for patients with renal failure (vide supra). These renal products are convenient and are also useful for individuals who can eat, but who would benefit from oral supplements. Tube-feeding mixtures taking into account the restrictions imposed by ARF can also be compounded by the pharmacy using other commercially available products. For individuals without a functioning gut, nutrition is given parenterally. Parenteral nutrition can be provided through a peripheral vein, but the solution must be diluted to minimize the risk of phlebitis, thus limiting its caloric content and increasing the volume administered. Consequently, most patients who require intravenous feedings receive total parenteral nutrition (TPN) through a central vein. The parenteral solution can be tailored according to the patient's dietary prescription and serum chemistries and usually delivered in a volume of 1.0 to 1.5 L, thus limiting the ultrafiltration requirement of patients receiving dialysis. Although the plasma amino acid profile is abnormal in ARF, the optimal composition of amino acid solutions for ARF patients is unknown, and a benefit of EAA solutions has not been proved. Therefore, conventional TPN amino acid solutions are typically used in patients with ARF. It should be emphasized that TPN is associated with many potential complications including mineral and electrolyte imbalances, acid–base disturbances, and catheter-related complications including sepsis. Therefore, whenever possible, the gut should be used for nutritional support. Besides reducing cost and the complications associated with parenteral nutrition, enteral nutrition also promotes mucosal growth and bowel integrity.

BIBLIOGRAPHY

Ahmed KR, Kopple JD: Nutrition in maintenance hemodialysis patients. In: Kopple JD, Massry SG, (eds) *Nutritional Management of Renal Disease.* William & Wilkins, Baltimore, MD, pp. 563–600, 1996.

Bergström J, Fürst P, Alvestrand A, et al.: Protein and energy intake, nitrogen balance and nitrogen losses in patients treated with continuous ambulatory peritoneal dialysis. *Kidney Int* 44: 1048–1057, 1993.

Blumenkrantz MJ, Kopple JD, Gutman RA, et al.: Methods for assessing nutritional status of patients with renal failure. *Am J Clin Nutr* 33: 1567–1585, 1980.

Blumenkrantz MJ, Kopple JD, Moran JK, et al.: Metabolic balance studies and dietary protein requirements in patients undergoing continuous ambulatory peritoneal dialysis. *Kidney Int* 21: 849–861, 1982.

Chertow GM, Lazarus JM: Malnutrition as a risk factor for morbidity and mortality in maintenance dialysis patients. In: Kopple JD, Massry SG (eds) *Nutritional Management of Renal Disease.* William & Wilkins, Baltimore, MD, pp. 257–276, 1996.

Coresh J, Walser M, Hill S:Survival on dialysis among chronic renal failure patients treated with a supplemented low-protein diet before dialysis. *J Am Soc Nephrol* 6: 1379–1385, 1996.

FAO/WHO/UNU: Energy and Protein Requirements. In Technical Report Series 724. World Health Organization, Geneva, pp. 206, 1985.

Ikizler TA, Greene JH, Wingard RL, et al.: Spontaneous dietary protein intake during progression of chronic renal failure. *J Am Soc Nephrol* 6:1386–1391, 1995.

Kaysen GA, Rathore V, Shearer GC, et al.: Mechanisms of hypoalbuminemia in hemodialysis patients. *Kidney Int* 48: 510–516, 1995.

Klahr S, Levey AS, Beck GJ, et al.: The effects of dietary protein restriction and blood pressure control on the progression of chronic renal disease. *N Engl J Med* 330: 877–884, 1994.

Kopple JD: Nutritional management of acute renal failure. In: Kopple JD, Massry SG (eds) Nutritional Management of Renal Disease. William & Wilkins, Baltimore, MD, pp. 713–753, 1996.

Maroni BJ: Requirements for protein, calories, and fat in the predialysis patient. In: Mitch WE, Klahr S (eds) Nutrition and the Kidney. Little, Brown, Boston, pp. 185–212, 1993.

Maroni BJ, Staffeld C, Tom K, et al.: Mechanism permitting nephrotic patients to achieve nitrogen equilibrium with a protein-restricted diet. *J Clin Invest* 99:2479–2487, 1997.

Maschio G, Alberti D, Janin G, et al.: Effect of the angiotensin-converting-enzyme inhibitor benazepril on the progression of chronic renal insufficiency. *N Engl J Med* 334:939–945, 1996.

Monteon FJ, Laidlaw SA, Shaib JK, et al.: Energy expenditure in patients with chronic renal failure. *Kidney Int* 30:741–747, 1986.

Owen WF Jr, Lew NL, Yan Liu SM, et al.: The urea reduction ratio and serum albumin concentration as predictors of mortality in patients undergoing hemodialysis. *N Engl J Med* 329: 1001–1006, 1993.

Tom K, Young V, Chapman T, et al.: Long-term adaptive responses to dietary protein restriction in chronic renal failure. *Am J Physiol* 4: E668–E677, 1994.

69

RENAL OSTEODYSTROPHY AND OTHER MUSCULOSKELETAL COMPLICATIONS OF CHRONIC RENAL FAILURE

JAMES A. DELMEZ

The term, renal osteodystrophy, is used in a generic sense to include all skeletal disorders that occur in patients with renal failure. These include osteitis fibrosa, osteomalacia, mixed and adynamic bone lesions, and dialysis-related amyloidosis. Because the kidney plays a major role in mineral homeostasis, by maintaining external balance for calcium, phosphorus, magnesium and pH, the occurrence of metabolic bone disease in patients with renal failure is predictable. For example, the kidneys are responsible for the excretion of phosphorus. When renal failure occurs, phosphorus accumulates causing a reciprocal fall in calcium levels and, therefore, stimulation of parathyroid hormone (PTH) secretion. Phosphorus retention also decreases the renal 1α hydroxylation of 25(OH)vitamin D to give $1,25(OH)_2D$ (calcitriol), the most potent metabolite of vitamin D. Calcitriol stimulates intestinal calcium absorption and mobilization of calcium from bone. It also directly suppresses PTH release, independent of its calcemic effect. Low levels of calcitriol may, therefore, cause malabsorption of calcium, hypocalcemia and further stimulation of PTH secretion. In addition, the kidney is the organ most responsible for the excretion of aluminum and β_2-microglobulin, substances implicated in the induction of dialysis-related osteomalacia and amyloidosis, respectively. The pathophysiology of renal osteodystrophy recently has been better defined, making possible a rational approach to its prevention and treatment.

The types of bone diseases seen in patients with renal failure are divided into those with accelerated rates of bone turnover (i.e., osteitis fibrosa and mixed lesions) due to persistently high levels of PTH and low bone turnover states (i.e., osteomalacia and adynamic lesions) due to aluminum toxicity or relatively low levels of PTH. Recent studies show that high turnover bone disease is the predominant lesion in patients treated with hemodialysis (50 to 60% of total) whereas low turnover is present in 60 to 70% of patients undergoing peritoneal dialysis.

OSTEITIS FIBROSA AND SECONDARY HYPERPARATHYROIDISM

High levels of PTH lead to the development of osteitis fibrosa. The histological features include increased number

and activity of osteoclasts, increased bone resorption, and marrow fibrosis. In addition, osteoblastic activity is increased with an abnormally large amount of the bone surface involved in bone formation. This state of high bone turnover is also characterized by an increased quantity of unmineralized bone matrix (osteoid). It differs from normal lamellar osteoid in that there is a haphazard arrangement of collagen fibers giving the appearance of a woven straw basket. Although woven osteoid can be mineralized, the calcium is deposited as amorphous calcium-phosphate instead of hydroxyapatite. These features are shown in Fig. 1 and contrast markedly with normal bone histology (Fig. 2).

Pathogenesis of Secondary Hyperparathyroidism

Although recent studies have shown that hyperparathyroidism may develop without hypocalcemia, it is well accepted that low levels of this cation stimulate PTH secretion. The factors that contribute to hypocalcemia and secondary hyperparathyroidism include phosphate retention, impaired vitamin D metabolism, skeletal resistance to the calcemic action of PTH, altered calcium-regulated PTH secretion, and decreased rates of degradation of PTH. The pathophysiological events are summarized in Fig. 3.

Phosphate Retention and Calcitriol Deficiency

The original explanation for the development of secondary hyperparathyroidism in patients with renal failure was the "trade-off hypothesis." As glomerular filtration rate (GFR) fell, it was reasoned that there would be a rise in serum phosphorus levels with a transient reciprocal fall in calcium concentrations. The latter would stimulate PTH secretion leading to a phosphaturia and a normalization of calcium and phosphorus levels. The trade-off was a normalization of phosphate levels at the cost of sustained PTH hypersecretion. Although hyperphosphatemia could not be consistently demonstrated in early renal failure, the hypothesis was supported by studies in animals and humans with mild renal failure showing that phosphate restriction

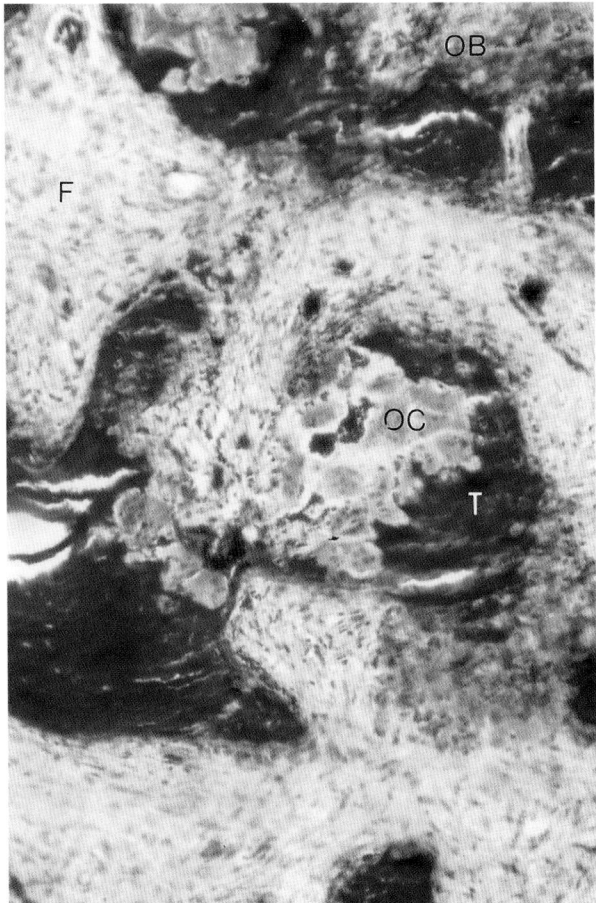

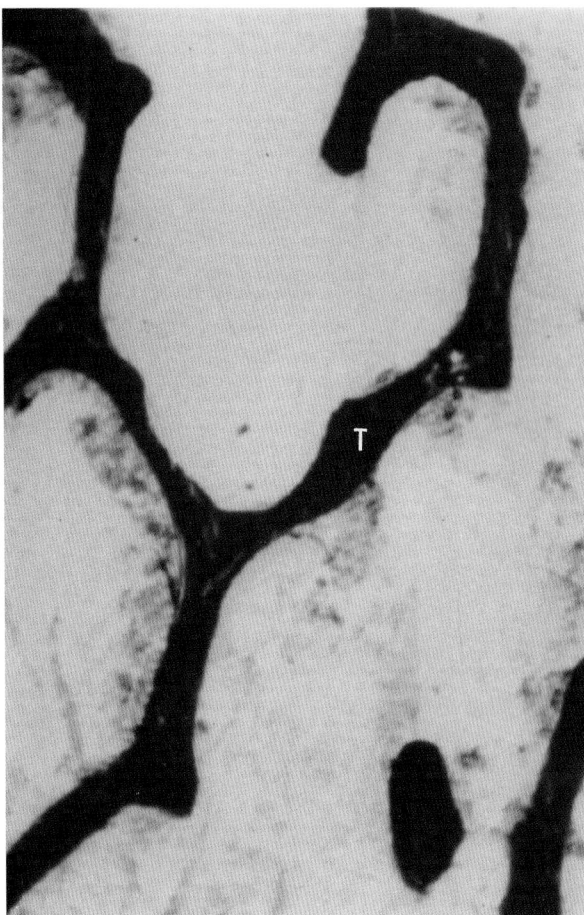

FIGURE 1 Histological features of severe osteitis fibrosa. Many multinucleated osteoclasts (OC) are actively resorbing trabecular bone (T), resulting in an irregular jagged surface. Osteoblasts (OB) are seen forming new bone surfaces. The marrow is replaced by fibrosis (F). (Courtesy of Steven L. Teitelbaum, M.D.; ×40, modified Masson stain.)

FIGURE 2 Normal bone histology. The trabecular bone (T) is fairly smooth without a prominence of osteoclasts or osteoblasts. No fibrosis or osteoid is seen. (Courtesy of Steven L. Teitelbaum, M.D.; ×40, modified Masson stain.)

in proportion to the decrease in GFR prevented or corrected the hyperparathyroid state.

Recent studies have shown that renal synthesis of calcitriol falls with worsening renal function, presumably because of declining renal mass. It is now appreciated that the principal effect of phosphorus restriction in early renal failure is to increase the renal production of calcitriol, resulting in near normal levels. However, as renal failure becomes advanced (GFR less than 20% of normal), hyperphosphatemia develops, leading to hypocalcemia and worsening hyperparathyroidism. Phosphate restriction no longer stimulates calcitriol synthesis, and thus calcitriol levels remain low. Presumably, this is due to the limited amount of residual renal mass available for synthesis. However, PTH levels may still decline with phosphorus restriction independent of changes in calcium or calcitriol levels. This suggests that phosphorus may directly affect PTH secretion. In vitro studies with parathyroid glands of normal rats have shown that high phosphorus levels in the media

stimulate PTH secretion in a process that requires protein synthesis.

Calcium Malabsorption

In patients with a moderate degree of renal failure, calcitriol levels are either normal or slightly low. Calcium absorption is usually normal. In advanced renal failure, calcitriol deficiency may lead to impaired gastrointestinal absorption of calcium and negative calcium balance. Hypocalcemia is a potent stimulus for PTH secretion that, in turn, raises calcium levels toward normal by increasing bone resorption.

Skeletal Resistance to the Calcemic Action of PTH

The calcemic response to an infusion of PTH extract is less in hypocalcemic patients with renal insufficiency than in normal subjects or in patients with hypoparathyroidism. In experimental animals, prior parathyroidectomy corrects the defect. This suggests that some form of downregulation

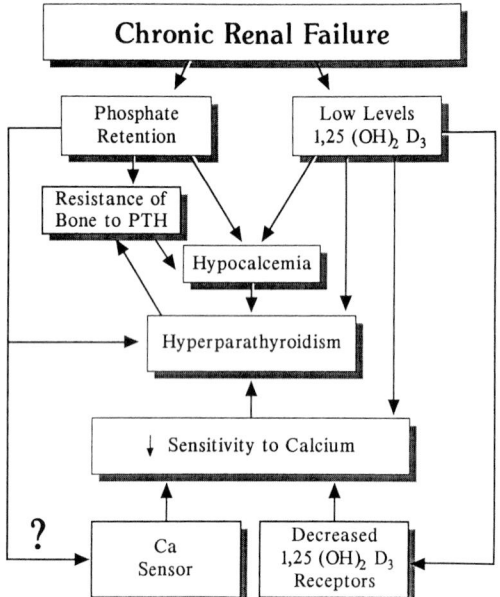

FIGURE 3 Pathogenesis of hyperparathyroidism in renal failure. From Slatopolsky E, Delmez J: *Miner Electrolyte Metab* 21:91–96, 1995. With permission from S. Karger AG Basel.

of the calcemic response to PTH occurs when the hormone is in excess. This would lead to a vicious cycle in renal failure where the impaired calcemic response leads to hypocalcemia, thus stimulating PTH secretion that would further impair the calcemic response of the bone. Phosphorus restriction improves the calcemic response to PTH via unknown mechanisms.

Altered Calcium-Regulated PTH Secretion

An insensitivity to the suppressive effects of calcium on PTH secretion has been shown in vitro in glands obtained from patients with chronic renal failure. The resistance to suppression by calcium may be overcome in a dose-dependent manner if the glands are incubated with calcitriol. Subsequent studies have shown that calcitriol reduces prepro-PTH messenger RNA levels by decreasing the rate of gene transcription. It has also been shown that there are a decreased number of calcitriol receptors in the uremic parathyroid gland that may promote a relative resistance to the steroid. Interestingly, the calcitriol receptor mRNA increases when the parathyroid gland is exposed to calcitriol. This suggests that calcitriol may upregulate its own receptor.

The low levels of calcitriol observed in patients with advanced renal failure could play a role in the abnormal secretion of PTH. Several studies have evaluated the PTH response to hypercalcemic suppression and hypocalcemic stimulation before and after intravenous calcitriol. Some, but not all investigators, have shown an increased sensitivity of the gland to ambient calcium levels following calcitriol.

Recently, a calcium receptor in parathyroid cell membranes has been cloned. By sensing extracellular calcium, the receptor regulates PTH secretion by changes in phosphoinositide turnover and cytosolic calcium levels. Decreased number of calcium receptors has been shown in glands of uremic patients. This may be another mechanism affecting the sensitivity of the parathyroid gland to calcium in renal failure.

Parathyroid Hyperplasia

Parathyroid hyperplasia is a prominent finding in uremic patients with severe secondary hyperparathyroidism. Little is known about the factors that lead to the cellular proliferation. Studies in vivo in uremic animals, however, suggest that calcitriol administration retards the development of parathyroid hyperplasia independent of changes in serum calcium levels. Hyperplasia, once established, is not reversed by short-term calcitriol treatment. Dietary phosphorus restriction also prevents parathyroid hyperplasia in uremia rats without affecting serum calcium or calcitriol concentrations. In uremic subjects with secondary hyperparathyroidism, monoclonal allelic losses on chromosome 11 have been demonstrated in the glands. This finding suggests that monoclonal transformation of previous hyperplastic parathyroid tissue often occurs.

Diagnosis of Uremic Hyperparathyroidism

The diagnosis of severe hyperparathyroidism is made by the findings of high levels of PTH and radiographic changes of osteitis fibrosa. Typically, these features include subperiosteal erosions of the phalanges (Fig. 4), and erosions at the proximal end of the tibia, the neck of the femur or humerus, and the inferior surface of the distal end of the clavicle. In the skull, there is a mottled and granular (salt

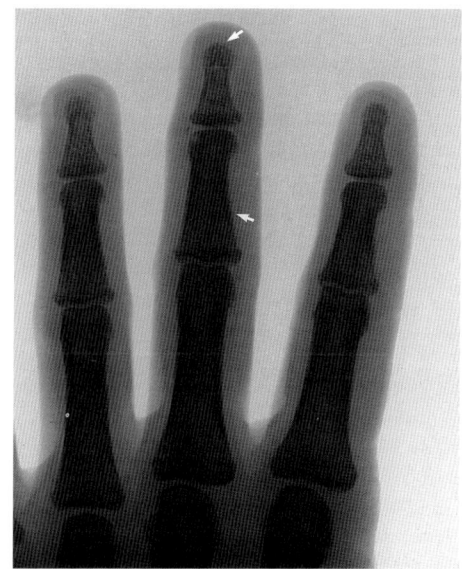

FIGURE 4 Radiographic changes of osteitis fibrosa. There are subperiosteal erosions of the phalanges and tuft (arrow).

and pepper) appearance with areas of resorption commonly associated with areas of osteosclerosis. Osteosclerosis is due to an increase in the thickness and number of trabeculae in spongy bone.

The correct interpretation of PTH levels in renal failure depends on an understanding of the metabolism of PTH and the specificity of the assay used to measure the hormone. PTH is primarily secreted as the intact hormone containing 84 amino acids. In the circulation, intact PTH undergoes degradation by the liver and kidneys, yielding biologically active amino-terminal and biologically inactive mid- and carboxyl-terminal fragments. The removal of the latter two depends primarily, if not exclusively, on glomerular filtration and subsequent reabsorption and degradation by the renal tubules. Therefore, in renal failure these fragments accumulate. This results in multiple forms of circulating PTH in which the concentration of biologically inactive fragments is about 100-fold greater than that of the biologically active amino-terminal fragments. To interpret PTH levels in renal failure, it is critical to know if the assay measures the intact, amino-terminal, mid-terminal, and/or carboxyl-terminal portions of the molecule. For example, if one uses an assay that measures the mid- and carboxyl-terminal regions, the values associated with severe hyperparathyroidism may be 100-fold greater than the upper limits of normal determined in subjects with normal renal function. By contrast, results of an assay specific for the amino-terminal portion or intact PTH may suggest severe osteitis fibrosa when the results are 10 times the upper limits of normal. Most clinical centers have now adapted the intact PTH assay, and its use is encouraged. Without liver disease, the serum alkaline phosphatase levels often correlate with PTH and may confirm the presence of hyperparathyroidism. A bone biopsy may be necessary when the diagnosis is uncertain.

Prevention and Treatment of Uremic Hyperparathyroidism

Phosphorus Control

In early renal failure, phosphorus accumulation may be avoided by restriction of a dietary phosphorus intake to 600 to 800 mg/day. This generally involves limiting meats and dairy products. More strict dietary phosphorus restriction is usually impractical. When the GFR falls to less than 20 to 30 mL/min, hyperphosphatemia develops and agents that bind phosphorus in the bowel are usually necessary. In the past, phosphorus binders containing aluminum were commonly used. It is now known that this metal may be absorbed and can cause substantial toxicity (see "Osteomalacia"). Calcium-containing phosphorus binders are now widely used. Agents such as calcium carbonate are most effective in binding phosphorus when given with meals in proportion to the usual phosphorus content of each meal. When calcium carbonate is ingested in the fasted state, less phosphorus is bound and more calcium is absorbed by the gastrointestinal tract. Because there is both patient-to-patient variability and variability from meal to meal in the same patient, a thorough dietary history and ongoing counseling are essential. Mismatching of the amount or timing of calcium carbonate and phosphorus ingested may lead to inadequate phosphorus control or hypercalcemia. The usual starting dose is 500 to 1000 mg/day of elemental calcium (1250 to 2500 mg calcium carbonate, 1 to 2 pills/day) with further titration based on the resultant changes in calcium, phosphorus, and PTH levels. Recently, much interest has focused on calcium acetate as a phosphorus binder. Short-term studies have shown that this compound binds about twice as much phosphorus per calcium absorbed compared with calcium carbonate. Compared with calcium carbonate, one half of the amount of elemental calcium is usually effective. Unfortunately the decreased dose does not result in a lower incidence of hypercalcemia. In addition, because calcium acetate pills contain only 167 mg of elemental calcium, patients taking this preparation often require greater number of pills per day. Thus, there may be no clinical advantage in using this preparation.

As patients begin dialysis therapy, the dietary protein requirements increase to more than $1 \text{ g} \cdot \text{kg}^{-1} \cdot \text{day}^{-1}$. This results in a requisite increase in dietary phosphorus to 800 to 1200 mg/day. Although hemodialysis removes approximately 1000 mg/treatment three times a week and continuous ambulatory peritoneal dialysis 300 mg/day, these effects are not sufficient to avoid the use of phosphorus binders in well-nourished patients. The physician may control the calcium fluxes during dialysis treatments by changing the concentration of calcium in the dialysate. A dialysate calcium concentration of 3.25 to 3.50 mEq/L (6.5 to 7.0 mg/dL, all ionized) causes a net influx of calcium to the patient. The use of phosphorus binders containing calcium also cavies a risk of developing hypercalcemia. If this occurs, the physician has the flexibility of decreasing the concentration of calcium in the dialysate to 2.0 or 2.5 mEq/L.

Control of Calcium

As the GFR falls below 50 mL/min, there is impaired absorption of calcium by the gastrointestinal tract. This is due partly to the decreased renal synthesis of calcitriol. Administration of sufficient amounts of calcium to bind phosphorus may suffice in reversing the negative calcium balance. In those patients with good control of phosphorus levels who nonetheless are hypocalcemic, calcium supplements may be added at night or between meals on an empty stomach. Alternatively, if the PTH levels are excessive (>200 to 400 pg/mL), calcitriol may be started. Calcium and phosphorus levels must be monitored closely because there is a tendency for hypercalcemia to develop after several months, often heralded by a fall in alkaline phosphatase to the normal range. A similar approach is appropriate for patients treated with dialysis. Increasing the dialysate calcium to 3.5 mEq/L is another option for increasing calcium levels.

Use of Vitamin D Sterols

Treatment with oral vitamin D, dihydrotachysterol, 25-hydroxyvitamin D, and calcitriol have all been shown to lessen symptoms of bone pain, improve bone histology, and lower PTH levels. All confer a risk of hypercalcemia. Vitamin D-induced hypercalcemia is particularly prolonged and may require weeks for resolution. The duration of hypercalcemia with calcitriol is usually 2 to 4 days. It is also the most potent metabolite of vitamin D in directly suppressing PTH secretion. Therefore, most investigator consider it the vitamin D sterol of choice for suppressing hyperparathyroidism in renal failure. Calcitriol should not be used when hyperphosphatemia is present because a calcium-phosphorus product of greater than 75 (with each concentration expressed in mg/dL) may lead to the development of soft tissue calcifications. In addition, calcitriol increases the gastrointestinal absorption of phosphorus and may require an increase in the dose of phosphorus binders. Analogues of calcitriol have been developed that suppress PTH secretion, yet are less active in raising calcium levels. Their efficacy is undergoing evaluation in clinical trials.

Many studies have demonstrated a marked suppression of PTH by administering 1.0 to 2.0 μg of calcitriol intravenously after each hemodialysis treatment three times a week. This suppression, which is greater than that observed with oral daily calcitriol, may be due to the very high serum levels achieved when the drug is given via this route. Pulse oral calcitriol (2 to 4 μg twice a week) also results in high levels and PTH suppression. This regimen is particular useful in patients treated with peritoneal dialysis wherein ready access to the circulation is not available. Some have advocated doses as high as 6 to 8 μg per treatment in refractory hyperparathyroidism. Whatever the route of administration and the dose, calcium and phosphorus levels should be carefully monitored during treatment with calcitriol. If PTH levels do not fall into an acceptable range after 1 year of treatment, a surgical parathyroidectomy should be considered.

OSTEOMALACIA

Osteomalacia is characterized by histological findings of impaired mineralization activity and an increase in the osteoid seam width (Fig. 5). Thus, in contrast to osteitis fibrosa, the rate of bone turnover is low. Patients often complain of bone and muscle pain, and spontaneous fractures occur in approximately 15% of those afflicted.

Pathogenesis

Although abnormalities of vitamin D metabolism and the presence of persistent metabolic acidosis may contribute to the development of osteomalacia, the most common cause in patients on dialysis is aluminum intoxication. Aluminum may accumulate due to contamination of the dialysate with this metal. With proper pretreatment of the tap water used to prepare dialysate, this route has diminished in relative importance. The main current source of aluminum accumulation is the ingestion of phosphorus binders containing aluminum. Because aluminum is normally excreted via urinary excretion, patients on dialysis are particularly prone to develop toxicity that, in its most severe state, encompasses dementia and premature death. Those with diabetes, prior parathyroidectomy, failed renal transplant, complete anuria, or a long history of consumption of large

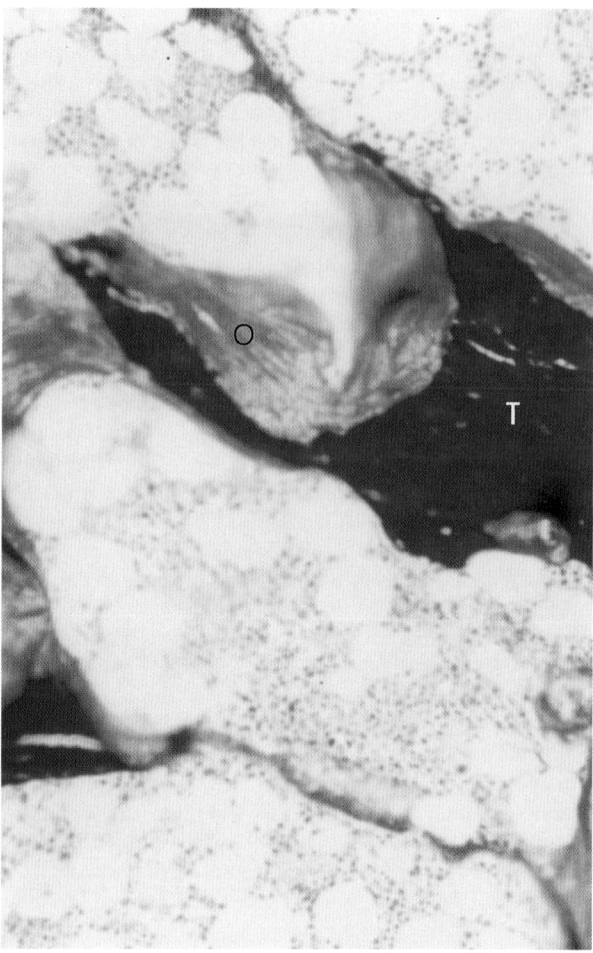

FIGURE 5 Histological features of osteomalacia. There are wide osteoid seams (O) surrounding trabecular bone (T). There is a paucity of osteoclasts and osteoblasts, thus reflecting a low rate of bone turnover. (Courtesy Steven L. Teitelbaum, M.D.; ×40, modified Masson stain.)

amounts of aluminum-containing phosphorus binders are at highest risk. Uremic patients prescribed medications containing citrate (calcium citrate, Shohl's solution), along with those medications containing aluminum (Basaljel, Amphogel, Carafate) are particularly prone to aluminum accumulation.

Diagnosis

The diagnosis of osteomalacia is often difficult. The clinical setting of a large exposure to aluminum and bone pain suggests the diagnosis. Aluminum directly suppresses PTH secretion, and a low PTH level is characteristic but not universal. The radiographic findings of osteomalacia are not distinctive. Some data suggest that a basal serum aluminum level of >100 μg/L and an increment in aluminum level of >150 μg/L following chelation with deferoxamine (DFO) in combination with a low PTH level has a high predictive power for the presence of aluminum bone disease. For the DFO challenge test, 20 mg/kg is administered intravenously at the end of dialysis and the serum aluminum is measured 24 to 48 hours later. The "gold standard" however remains the bone biopsy with appropriate staining for aluminum.

Prevention and Treatment of Osteomalacia Due to Aluminum

Prevention of osteomalacia is critical with attention given to dialysate purity and avoidance of phosphorus binders containing aluminum, if possible. Chronic chelation therapy with DFO cures the osteomalacia, and follow-up biopsies usually show the development of osteitis fibrosa of variable severity. The major mechanism for this is the removal of aluminum from the bone surface, associated with marked increases in osteoblast number and rate of bone formation. A major problem with DFO treatment is the risk of fatal mucormycosis infections, which occur in up to 5% of treated patients. DFO also binds iron and the DFO-iron chelate can function as a siderophore to stimulate the growth of mucormycosis. Thus, the use of DFO should be restricted to those who have severe symptoms of aluminum intoxication and histological evidence of aluminum accumulation in the bone. Patients with mild symptoms may be treated by eliminating all aluminum-containing phosphorus binders and substituting ones containing calcium. Over 1 to 2 years, the aluminum burden will decrease as will the symptoms.

Adynamic Bone Lesions

Adynamic (also termed aplastic) bone lesions are characterized by decreased bone mineralization, but normal amounts of osteoid. In approximately 50% of cases, the cause is aluminum deposition. The treatment is the same as osteomalacia due to aluminum. Little is known about the etiology in the remaining half of patients. However, this lesion may be more common in patients treated with peritoneal dialysis, in the elderly, and in patients with diabetes. The PTH levels are generally <3 times the upper limits of normal when measured with an intact PTH assay. It is likely that the lesion in some cases is the result of overzealous suppression of PTH. If so, allowing the PTH level to increase to four times the upper limits of normal may be advisable. It should be noted however that patients with adynamic bone lesions not due to aluminum overload report fewer symptoms of bone pain and myopathy and develop fewer fractures than those with either aluminum-related or osteitis fibrosa bone disease diagnosed by bone biopsy.

MIXED LESIONS

Some patients display histological evidence of both osteitis fibrosa and osteomalacia on bone biopsy. Such patients frequently have high PTH levels and impaired bone formation and mineralization. Mixed renal osteodystrophy may

be seen in patients with previously established osteitis fibrosa who are developing aluminum-related bone disease. The treatment is withdrawal of the aluminum exposure and aggressive treatment of the hyperparathyroidism.

Dialysis-Related Amyloidosis

It has long been known that there is an association between bone cysts, pathological fractures, arthritis, and carpal tunnel syndrome in patients treated with long-term dialysis. It is now clear that these are often due to the deposition of a form of amyloid unique to dialysis patients. This protein is composed of intact and modified β_2-microglobulin. This constant light chain of HLA class I antigens is excreted in the urine. Therefore, very high serum levels are uniformly seen in patients on dialysis. The amyloid is most frequently deposited in the flexor retinaculum of the wrist, entrapping the median nerve and causing carpal tunnel syndrome. The symptoms of hand pain can be relieved by a surgical release of the median nerve. The amyloid may also invade the synovium of joints causing pain, effusions and erosive arthritis. Periarticular radiolucent bone cysts (Fig. 6), the result of the replacement of bone by amyloid, may result in pathological fracture. Once established, there is no proven treatment for the amyloid arthropathy. High flux hemodialysis or hemodiafiltration removes some β_2-microglobulin and may delay the onset

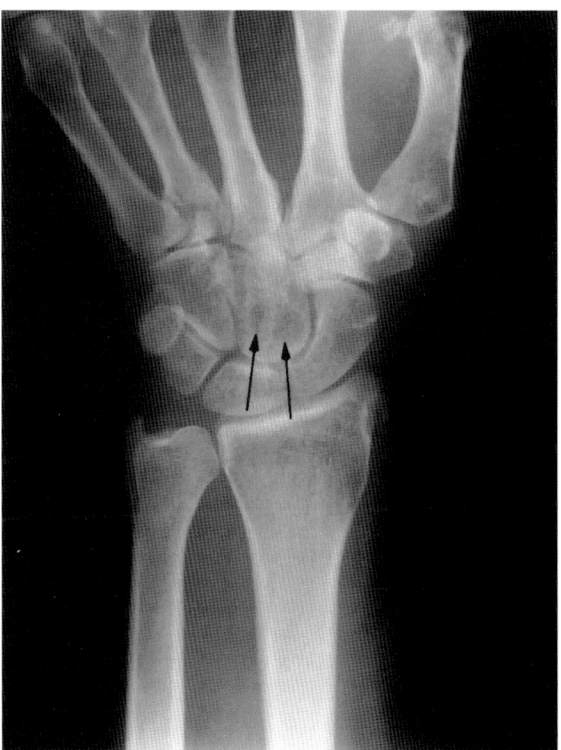

FIGURE 6 Bone cysts in a hemodialysis patient due to amyloid infiltration of bone.

of the clinical expression of the disease. Early renal transplantation completely prevents the disease.

Renal Osteodystrophy Following Renal Transplantation

Following a successful renal transplant, the histological abnormalities of mild to moderately severe osteitis fibrosa usually resolve within 1 year. However, bone density of the lumbar vertebrae decreases due to the effect of steroids in impairing bone formation. Severe hyperparathyroidism may not completely resolve and elevated PTH levels may persist for 5 to 10 years. In those patients with osteomalacia, return of renal function allows the removal of aluminum and, as a result, improvement in the bone histology. Unpublished data suggest that those with adynamic bone lesions are prone to avascular necrosis of the femoral head following transplant. The symptoms of amyloid deposition often improve dramatically following transplantation but the radiographic findings do not change. This suggests that the amyloid may be irreversibly bound to the tissue.

OVERALL APPROACH TO THE MANAGEMENT OF RENAL OSTEODYSTROPHY

Renal osteodystrophy is a dynamic process whose severity and even type of lesion may vary with time. In early renal failure, phosphorus restriction alone may suffice. With more severe renal failure (GFR less than 30 mL/min), calcium malabsorption should be countered by the administration of oral calcium with meals if the phosphorus level is high or at night if the phosphorus is normal. In the face of a calcium phosphorus product of greater than 75 mg^2/dL^2, the phosphorus should initially be lowered by use of aluminum-containing phosphorus binders to prevent soft tissue calcifications. When the product has decreased below this value, calcium carbonate with meals should be substituted for the long-term binding of phosphorus. The target calcium and phosphorus levels are 9.5 to 10.5 and 4.5 to 5.5 mg/dL, respectively. Frequent monitoring of these values is necessary to avoid iatrogenic complications such as hypercalcemia. In hemodialysis patients, calcium and phosphorus levels should be determined monthly and PTH concentrations quarterly. The target intact PTH levels should be three to four times the upper limits of normal. The dose of calcium carbonate should be adjusted in relation to the calcium, phosphorus, and PTH levels. For example, if the calcium is 8.5 mg/dL, the phosphorus level is acceptable, and the intact PTH concentration is normal to twice normal, one would consider doing nothing or lowering the dose of calcium carbonate. If, with the same levels of calcium and phosphorus, the PTH level is five times normal and progressively increasing, one would attempt a more aggressive approach. This may be achieved by increasing the dose of calcium given at night or by starting calcitriol therapy. When prescribing calcitriol, the calcium and phosphorus levels must be assessed more frequently. As with calcium carbonate, calcitriol should not be given in the presence of an elevated calcium-phosphorus product. This presents a problem in the patient with severe hyper-

parathyroidism. In this situation the patient's elevated serum calcium or phosphorus may be emanating from bone due to enhanced bone resorption. A surgical parathyroidectomy is often required. The other main indication for surgery is persistently high levels of PTH, corresponding to the presence of severe osteitis fibrosa and bone pain. A bone biopsy is usually not required to make the diagnosis. If, however, the patient is at risk for the development of aluminum accumulation (see above), a bone biopsy may be warranted to confirm the diagnosis and exclude aluminum-related osteomalacia as a cause for the bone pain or hypercalcemia. At time of surgery, all four glands should be identified. Some surgeons will do a $3\frac{1}{2}$ gland parathyroidectomy, whereas others will remove all glands and then implant small pieces of one gland into the forearm to avoid future neck surgery if hyperparathyroidism recurs.

Bibliography

Andress DL, Keith MD, Norris C, et al.: Intravenous calcitriol in the treatment of refractory osteitis fibrosa of chronic renal failure. N Engl J Med 321:274–279, 1989.

Boelaert JR, Fenves AZ, Coburn JW: Deferoxamine therapy and mucormycosis in dialysis patients; report of an international registry. Am J Kidney Dis 18:660–667, 1991.

Brown EM, Wilkson RE, Eastman RC, et al.: Abnormal regulation of parathyroid hormone release by calcium in secondary hyperparathyroidism due to chronic renal failure. J Clin Endocrinol Metab 54:172–179, 1982.

Delmez JA, Slatopolsky E: Hyperphosphatemia: Its consequences and treatment in patients with chronic renal disease. Am J Kidney Dis 19:303–317, 1992.

Delmez JA, Tindira C, Grooms P, et al.: Parathyroid hormone suppression by intravenous 1,25-dihydroxyvitamin D: A role for increased sensitivity to calcium. J Clin Invest 83:1349–1355, 1989.

Dunlay R, Rodriguez M, Felsenfeld AJ, et al.: Direct inhibitory effect of calcitriol on parathyroid function (sigmoidal curve) in dialysis. Kidney Int 36:1093–1098, 1989.

Fukuda N, Tanaka H, Tominaga Y, et al.: Decreased 1,25-dihydroxyvitamin D3 receptor density is associated with a more severe form of parathyroid hyperplasia in chronic uremic patients. J Clin Invest 92:1436–1443, 1993.

Goodman WG, Belin T, Gales B, et al.: Calcium-regulated parathyroid hormone release in patients with mild or advanced secondary hyperparathyroidism. Kidney Int 48:1553–1558, 1995.

Hruska KA, Teitlebaum SL: Renal osteodystrophy. N Engl J Med 333:166–174, 1995.

Julian BA, Laskow DA, Dubovsky J, et al.: Rapid loss of vertebral mineral density after renal transplantation. N Engl J Med 325:544–550, 1991.

Kifor O, Moore FD, Wang P, et al.: Reduced immunostaining for the extracellular Ca^{2+} sensing receptor in primary and uremic secondary hyperparathyroidism. J Clin Endocrinol Metab 81:1598–1606, 1996.

Llach F: Secondary hyperparathyroidism in renal failure: The trade-off hypothesis revisited. Am J Kidney Dis 25:663–679, 1995.

Malluche H, Faugere M: Renal bone disease 1990: An unmet challenge for nephrologist. Kidney Int 38:193–210, 1990.

Nebeker H, Andress D, Milliner D, et al.: Indirect methods for the diagnosis of aluminum bone disease: plasma aluminum, the desferrioxamine infusion test, and serum iPTH. Kidney Int 18:S96–S99, 1986.

Sheikh MS, Ramirez A, Emmett M, et al.: Role of vitamin D-dependent and vitamin D-independent mechanisms in absorption of food calcium. *J Clin Invest* 81:126–132, 1988.

Sherrard DJ, Hercz G, Pei Y, et al.: The spectrum of bone disease in end-stage renal failure—An evolving disorder. *Kidney Int* 43:436–442, 1993.

Slatopolsky E, Weerts C, Lopez-Hilker S, et al.: Calcium carbonate as a phosphate binder in patients with chronic renal failure undergoing dialysis. *N Engl J Med* 315:157–161, 1986.

Slatopolsky E, Weerts C, Norwood K, et al.: Long term effects of calcium carbonate and 2.5 mEq/L calcium dialysate on mineral metabolism. *Kidney Int* 36:897–903, 1989.

Slatopolsky E, Finch J, Denda M, et al.: Phosphorus restriction prevents parathyroid gland growth. *J Clin Invest* 97:2534–2540, 1996.

Szabo A, Merke J, Beier E, et al.: 1,25(OH)$_2$ vitamin D$_3$ inhibits parathyroid cell proliferation in experimental uremia. *Kidney Int* 35:1049–1056, 1989.

70

CARDIAC FUNCTION AND CARDIAC DISEASE IN RENAL FAILURE

ROBERT N. FOLEY AND PATRICK S. PARFREY

INTRODUCTION

Uremic pericarditis was a frequent cause of death in the predialysis era. Since the 1960s, cardiac disease has been shown repeatedly to be the major cause of death in end-stage renal disease (ESRD). This is still the case today, with older and sicker patients being accepted for renal replacement therapy. The excessive cardiac mortality of ESRD crosses the divides of nationality, race, gender, and cause of ESRD. Cardiac disease also accounts for a substantial degree of comorbidity. Most studies in industrialized nations show that symptomatic ischemic heart disease and cardiac failure are present prior to initiation of ESRD therapy in more than one third of patients. About 10% of patients will go on to develop each of these conditions every year after starting dialysis therapy. This chapter discusses the natural history, risk factors, and treatment of cardiomyopathy and ischemic heart disease in chronic uremia. The pericarditis seen in uremic patients will also be discussed.

EPIDEMIOLOGY

Prevalence

Echocardiographic left ventricular (LV) hypertrophy, coronary artery disease, and cardiac failure are conservatively estimated to be between two and five times more prevalent in ESRD patients compared to an age-matched general population.

Abnormalities of LV structure and function are very common in patients starting renal replacement therapy. Concentric LV hypertrophy (where wall thickening occurs in response to pressure overload) is present in 39% of patients starting dialysis programs for ESRD. Twenty-seven percent of patients had left ventricular dilatation (increase in cavity size in response to volume overload) and 18% had systolic dysfunction (inadequate contractility, defined on echocardiography as a fractional shortening less than 25%). A recent study of patients with chronic renal failure (not yet dialysis dependent) indicated that these abnormalities develop early in chronic renal failure and progress rapidly as renal function declines. Twenty-seven percent of patients with creatinine clearance greater than 50 mL/min had LV hypertrophy; this figure rose to 31% for clearances between 25 and 50 mL/min and 45% for clearances less than 25 mL/min.

Almost half of all hemodialysis patients in the US have had clinically defined ischemic heart disease. Silent coronary artery disease is also common in dialysis patients, especially in those with diabetes mellitus. The situation is confounded even more by the observation that over one quarter of dialysis patients with typical angina have normal coronary arteriograms.

Cardiac failure is also very common in dialysis patients; a recent report from the United States Renal Data System

Registry suggested that almost one half of all patients had a history of cardiac failure.

Risk Factors

Many of the traditional, Framingham-type parameters are also risk factors for cardiac disease in chronic uremia. Older age and diabetes mellitus have been consistently associated with mortality in ESRD patients.

In one study, even a moderate degree of hypertension was associated with progressive cardiac enlargement and subsequent cardiac failure. Hypertension was also associated with the development of new symptomatic ischemic heart disease. Two thirds of all deaths were preceded by an admission for cardiac failure. After development of cardiac failure, low blood pressure was the single greatest predictor of subsequent mortality. Low blood pressure and low serum cholesterol have been associated with mortality in large-scale epidemiological studies of dialysis patients as well. The basis for this apparent paradox is that low serum cholesterol levels reflect malnutrition, which has been shown to be the biggest predictor of mortality in most recent studies. High levels of lipoprotein (a) and apoB have been associated with an adverse outcome in patients with chronic uremia.

These data suggest that the association between low blood pressure and mortality reflects the very high frequency of advanced cardiomyopathy in dialysis patients. They also suggest that aggressive management of hypertension is needed in patients without clinically apparent cardiac disease. In predialysis patients with diabetic nephropathy, very aggressive control of blood pressure slows the progression of chronic renal failure; some have advocated targeting the lowest blood pressure that does not lead to symptoms—a practical target level is 120/80 mm Hg. There is emerging evidence that this may also be an appropriate target level in nondiabetics with chronic renal impairment. The target blood pressure that minimizes cardiac risk in chronic uremia is not yet clear.

The data linking smoking to cardiac disease in ESRD are inconsistent. Some studies suggest that smoking is an independent mortality factor in ESRD. Smoking and diabetes appears to be a particularly adverse combination of risk factors.

Recent epidemiological data suggest that many factors related to the uremic state may be associated with cardiac disease. As noted, hypertension contributes to development of concentric LV hypertrophy, LV dilatation, ischemic heart disease, and cardiac failure. Anemia promotes development of LV dilatation and cardiac failure. Hyperparathyroidism and inadequate dialysis may also play a role. Most of these factors are amenable to intervention.

Prognosis

Systolic dysfunction, concentric LV hypertrophy, and LV dilatation are all strong and independent predictors of future cardiac failure, ischemic heart disease, and death in dialysis patients. The adverse association between systolic

dysfunction and mortality is immediate. In contrast, the adverse impact of concentric LV hypertrophy and LV dilatation on survival is only apparent after a lag phase of approximately 2 years, suggesting a possible time window to target interventions. It is very likely that these echocardiographic abnormalities lead to death via the intermediate step of cardiac failure.

Coronary artery disease predicts mortality independently of age and diabetes. It predisposes to systolic dysfunction and cardiac failure, which seem to be the major mediators of its adverse impact in ESRD patients. Clinically defined cardiac failure is a rapidly lethal condition in ESRD patients, much the same as it is in the general population. In a prospective cohort study, cardiac failure preceded two thirds of all deaths of chronic dialysis patients with a median time interval of 13 months between admission for cardiac failure and death. It is often difficult to distinguish intrinsic cardiac dysfunction from salt and water excess in dialysis patients. It is thought that chronic salt and water excess can lead to progressive cardiac failure, which adds to the diagnostic confusion. Many dialysis patients can tolerate vast amounts of extracellular fluid (ECF) volume expansion without developing pulmonary edema. Although dialysis patients with normal hearts can develop pulmonary edema with the rapid accumulation of large amounts of salt and water, it is safer to assume cardiac dysfunction as opposed to simple ECF volume expansion in patients who develop pulmonary edema. Concurrently, patients like this should undergo further cardiac workup, initially by echocardiography. Noninvasive technology that can rapidly give an accurate assessment of ECF volume status should be routinely available in the near future. This technology should assist in distinguishing simple ECF volume expansion from intrinsic cardiac dysfunction.

Valvular dysfunction is common in dialysis patients. Some studies have noted abnormal mitral or aortic valvular abnormalities in half of all patients with chronic renal failure. Mild to moderate mitral regurgitation, usually secondary to LV dilatation, and calcification of the mitral valve are the most commonly reported abnormalities. The prevalence of hemodynamically important valvular dysfunction is not well described in the literature. In one study, about 10% of patients had hemodynamically important abnormalities of the mitral or aortic valves; the prognosis of these patients appears to be determined by the degree of associated cardiomyopathy. Figure 1 shows survival of ESRD patients with the major clinical and structural manifestation of cardiac disease.

DIAGNOSIS

Cardiomyopathy

Chest radiographs and electrocardiography are not sufficiently sensitive to detect cardiac enlargement. Echocardiography is noninvasive and relatively easy to perform. It gives information about cardiac dimensions, valve function, systolic function, and diastolic function. It is not clear how often echocardiography should be performed in chronic

Baseline Echocardiography

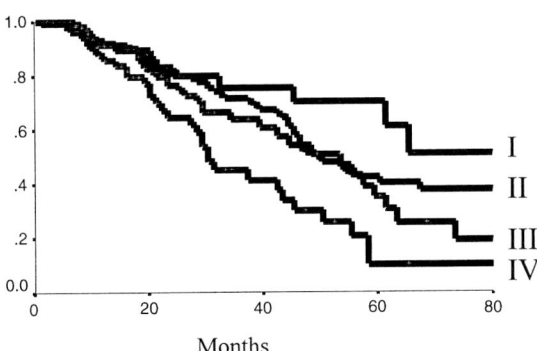

Baseline Clinical Status

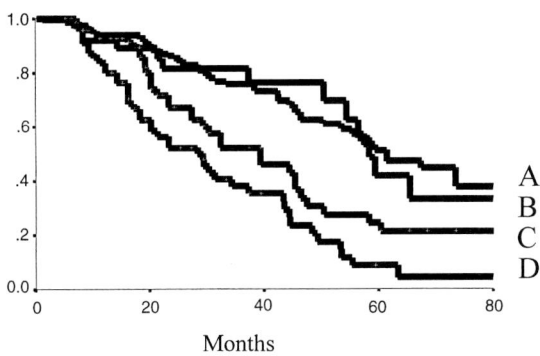

FIGURE 1 (*Top*) Survival according to baseline echocardiography in patients starting ESRD therapy. (I) Normal left ventricle. (II) Concentric LV hypertrophy. (III) LV dilatation. (IV) Systolic dysfunction. Data from Foley et al.: *J Am Soc Nephrol* 5:2024–2031, 1995; Parfrey et al.: *Nephrol Dial Transplant* 11:1277–1285, 1996. (*Bottom*) Survival according to presence or absence of ischemic heart disease and cardiac failure in patients starting ESRD therapy. (A) No ischemic heart disease, no cardiac failure. (B) Ischemic heart disease, no cardiac failure. (C) Cardiac failure, no ischemic heart disease. (D) Both ischemic heart disease and cardiac failure. Data from Harnett et al.: *Kidney Int* 47: 884–890, 1995, Parfrey et al.: *Kidney Int* 49:1428–1434, 1996. With permission.

ESRD. Cardiomyopathy often progresses rapidly in chronic uremia. Many of the causes of this rapid progression are treatable. There may be value in annual performance of echocardiography in chronic uremic patients. There are, however, no comparative studies available to tell us the optimum use of echocardiography in chronic uremic patients. It is important that echocardiography be carried out as close to dry weight as possible, preferably within 1 kg.

Ischemic Heart Disease

ESRD patients with symptoms of ischemic heart disease, diabetic patients, and older patients undergoing pretransplant assessment should be formally evaluated for the pres-

ence of coronary arterial narrowing. The role of noninvasive testing is still unclear. Exercise-based stress tests are often uninformative in ESRD patients, because most patients are unable to achieve an adequate level of exercise intensity. Of the other noninvasive screening tests available, adenosine [201]thallium, dipyridamole [201]thallium, and dobutamine stress echocardiography appear useful. Coronary arteriography, however, remains the gold standard. ESRD patients with symptomatic ischemic heart disease should be investigated with coronary arteriography if their physical state is such that revascularization would be seriously considered. The optimal approach to screening for coronary artery disease in asymptomatic prospective renal transplant patients is a matter of dispute (see Chapter 74) Our current approach is to perform noninvasive screening on the following subgroups: patients over 45 years, diabetics over 25 years, smokers, and those with ischemic changes on electrocardiography. Those who do not clearly have negative noninvasive screening tests should have arteriography.

TREATMENT

Risk Factor Management

There are no randomized trials to assess the efficacy of modification of Framingham-type risk factors in uremic patients without coronary disease and cardiomyopathy. The cardiac morbidity and mortality of these patients probably exceeds that of survivors of myocardial infarction in the general population. In the absence of high-quality data from randomized controlled trials, the following targets for all uremic patients, should minimize the risk of new cardiac disease and the progression of existing cardiac disease: nonsmoking, euglycemia, blood pressure <120 systolic and 80 diastolic in predialysis patients, <140 mm Hg systolic and 90 mm Hg diastolic in dialysis patients, total serum cholesterol less than 200 mg/dL, LDL cholesterol less than 140 mg/dL, hemoglobin 10 ± 0.5 g/dL, $Kt/V > 1.2$ in hemodialysis patients, weekly $Kt/V > 2$ in peritoneal dialysis patients, serum albumin >3.8 g/dL, serum calcium >2.2 mmol/L, PTH < 200 ng/L.

At present there is no good evidence pointing to the superiority of any antihypertensive or lipid lowering strategy in this overall picture. However, in predialysis patients, there is considerable evidence that angiotensin-converting enzyme (ACE) inhibitors may be the vasoactive agent of choice, because of their ability to retard the progression to ESRD. Malnutrition is a major killer in dialysis patients; as most dialysis patients are already on restricted diets, the threshold for using pharmacological treatment for hyperlipidemia should be low. HMG-CoA reductase inhibitors and fibrates are well tolerated and safe in patients with chronic renal failure. There is, as yet, no evidence that full correction of renal anemia is better than partial correction of anemia to hemoglobin levels of 10 g/dL. Erythropoietin (rHuEPO) is the agent of choice to treat renal anemia. Using rHuEPO in this manner will lead to an increase in blood pressure in about one third of patients; for most patients this increase in blood pressure is readily reversible with standard antihypertensive treatment. Using rHuEPO to increase hematocrit also increases the chance of arterio-venous graft loss; for most patients the benefits of partial correction of renal anemia outweigh the potential risks. The efficacy and risks of routine use of antiplatelet agents and anticoagulants in this patient group have not been satisfactorily resolved.

Management of Coronary Artery Disease

As in the general population, antiplatelet therapy should be used unless otherwise contraindicated. Calcium channel blockers, β-blockers, and nitrates are the cornerstone of symptomatic therapy. Risk factor management should be aggressive in this group. Patients should be encouraged to reach ideal body mass, stop smoking, and start a graded exercise program. Hypertension and hyperlipidemia should be aggressively managed. β blockers should be prescribed unless contraindicated. It is important that anemia be treated in this group; although full correction of anemia may ameliorate symptoms, such an approach has not been shown to increase longevity in this group, and has been associated with a clear excess of arteriovenous access loss; the target hemoglobin for these patients should be approximately 10 g/dL.

ESRD patients with symptoms of ischemic heart disease who do not have a very large burden of noncardiac comorbidity should have coronary arteriography. Dialysis patients fulfilling the anatomical and functional criteria used in the general population are likely to benefit from coronary revascularization. Generally accepted criteria are: (1) one, two, or three vessel disease with angina refractory to medical management, where the intent is symptom relief; (2) left main coronary artery disease where the intent is improved survival; and (3) triple-vessel disease associated with ventricular dysfunction or easily inducible ischemia, where the intent is also improved survival. There is some evidence that recurrence rates after coronary angioplasty are unacceptably high in dialysis patients. The perioperative morbidity and mortality rates associated with coronary artery bypass surgery are higher in dialysis patients than in the general population. Recent studies suggest that these rates are acceptable and justifiable on the basis of good subsequent survival rates.

Management of Cardiomyopathy

Eighty percent or more of dialysis patients have cardiomyopathy, which can progress rapidly. Because it is difficult to predict progression, and because there are many potentially reversible etiological factors (such as coronary artery disease, anemia, inadequate dialysis, uncontrolled hypertension, malnutrition, and hyperparathyroidism), we believe that all chronic renal failure patients should have regular echocardiography; our current recommendation is that they be done annually. All patients who develop cardiac failure should have echocardiography to try to distinguish systolic from diastolic dysfunction. ACE inhibitors,

calcium channel blockers, and β-blockers form the cornerstone of treatment in concentric LV hypertrophy. Based on data from the nonuremic population, we use ACE inhibitors as the first vasoactive agent in patients with LV dilatation, systolic dysfunction, and symptomatic cardiac failure. Digoxin may benefit patients with cardiac failure in the presence of systolic dysfunction, but is best avoided in patients with diastolic dysfunction. Recent studies in the general population suggest that β-blockers and calcium channel antagonists may have a role as primary therapy for cardiac failure associated with both diastolic and systolic dysfunction. Such an approach should be considered experimental at present, and is best done in consultation with a cardiologist. Nitrates are useful for symptomatic relief in frank cardiac failure, whether due to systolic or diastolic dysfunction.

PERICARDITIS IN UREMIC PATIENTS

Clinically important pericarditis is now an infrequent occurrence, although small pericardial effusions are very common on echocardiography. Some authors distinguish between uremic pericarditis, which occurs in uremic individuals who have never received dialysis therapy, and pericarditis in individuals already on dialysis. The uremic milieu is responsible for the former condition, although the specific culprits are unknown. About half of all patients who develop pericarditis while on dialysis therapy will respond to intensified dialysis therapy, suggesting that uremia is causative in only a proportion of these cases; it has been speculated that conditions such as viral pericarditis are responsible for the remainder.

Clinical Presentation

The major clinical findings are due to inflammation (precordial pain, dyspnea, fever, generalized ST changes on electrocardiography) and fluid in the pericardial sac leading to a restriction to ventricular filling (fluid overload and intolerance of ultrafiltration). With large effusions, frank cardiac tamponade and cardiogenic shock may occur. It is more likely that a given volume of pericardial fluid will lead to cardiac tamponade when this accumulates quickly.

Echocardiography should be performed to estimate the volume of fluid within the pericardium. Intensification of dialysis therapy (with avoidance of heparin) and analgesia form the cornerstone of management. The use of nonsteroidal antiinflammatory drugs is recommended by some but not all authors. In many centers, pericardiocentesis is used for management of large effusions (>250 mL), or where cardiac tamponade is present. The fluid is typically hemorrhagic and the pericardial sac may contain fibrin and clot. Surgical drainage with anterior pericardiectomy may thus be required.

Bibliography

Bloembergen WE, Stannard DC, Port FK, et al.: Relationship of dose of hemodialysis and cause-specific mortality. *Kidney Int* 50: 557–565, 1996.

Churchill DN, Taylor DW, Cook RJ, et al.: Canadian hemodialysis morbidity study. *Am J Kidney Dis* 19: 214–234, 1992.

Foley RN, Parfrey PS, Harnett JD, et al.: DC, Clinical and echocardiographic disease in end-stage renal disease: prevalence, associations and prognosis. *Kidney Int* 47: 186–192, 1995.

Foley RN, Parfrey PS, Harnett JD, Kent GM, Murray DC, Barre PE: The progostic importance of left ventricular geometry in uremic cardiomyopathy. *J Am Soc Nephrol* 5:2024–2031, 1995.

Harnett JD, Foley RN, Kent GM, Barre PE, Murray DC, Parfrey PS: Congestive heart failure in dialysis patients: Prevalence, incidence, prognosis and risk factors. *Kidney Int* 47: 884–890, 1995.

Levin A, Singer J, Thompson CR, Ross H, Lewis M: Prevalent left ventricular hypertrophy in the predialysis population: Identi-fying opportunities for intervention. *Am J Kidney Dis* 27: 347–354, 1996.

Murphy SW, Parfrey PS: Screening for cardiovascular disease in dialysis patients. *Curr Opin Nephrol Hypertens* 5: 532–540, 1996.

Owen SR, Lew NL, Yan Liu SM, Lowrie EG, Lazarus JM: The urea reduction ratio and serum albumin concentrations as predictors of mortality in patients undergoing hemodialysis. *N Engl J Med* 329: 1001–1006, 1993.

Parfrey PS, Foley RN, Harnett JD, Kent GM, Murray DC, Barre PE: Outcome and risk factors for left ventricular disorders in chronic uremia. *Nephrol Dial Transplant* 11: 1277–1285, 1996.

Parfrey PS, Foley RN, Harnett JD, Kent GM, Murray DC, Barre PE: Outcome and risk factors of ischemic heart disease in chronic uremia. *Kidney Int* 49: 1428–1434, 1996.

71

NEUROLOGICAL MANIFESTATIONS OF RENAL FAILURE

COSMO L. FRASER

Nervous system dysfunction is common among renal failure patients and contributes significantly to their overall morbidity and mortality. Patients with chronic renal failure who have not yet received dialysis may develop symptoms which could be as mild as sensorial clouding or as severe as coma and death. Even after the initiation of adequate maintenance dialysis, patients may continue to manifest subtle nervous system dysfunction such as impaired mentation, generalized weakness, sexual dysfunction, and peripheral neuropathy. Hemodialysis itself has been associated with distinct disorders of the central nervous system. Dialysis disequilibrium syndrome occurs in a small number of patients and is a consequence of the initiation of dialysis. Dialysis dementia is a progressive and generally fatal encephalopathy which can affect patients on chronic hemodialysis as well as children with chronic renal failure who have not yet started dialysis. Progressive intellectual dysfunction and peripheral neuropathy can occur in patients who are being treated with maintenance dialysis therapy.

UREMIC ENCEPHALOPATHY

The term uremic encephalopathy is used to denote the central neurological signs and symptoms that are mani-fested by patients with either an acute or chronic deterioration of their renal function. Symptoms are usually seen when glomerular filtration rate falls to a level below 10% of normal. In common with other organic brain syndromes, these patients display variable disorders of consciousness that can affect psychomotor behavior, thinking, memory, speech, perception, and emotion. The severity and rate of progression of symptoms varies directly with the rapidity with which renal failure develops. In patients with acute renal failure, uremic symptoms are generally more severe and progress more rapidly than in patients with chronic renal failure. In progressive chronic renal failure, the number and severity of symptoms in patients may be quite variable, and symptoms may also occur in a cyclic manner in that there are intervals of well-being in an otherwise inexorable downhill course (Table 1).

Differential Diagnosis

Uremic encephalopathy should be suspected in patients with renal failure if there are clinical signs and symptoms consistent with central nervous system deterioration. However, the presenting symptoms of uremic encephalopathy

TABLE I

Neurological Manifestations of Uremia

Predialysis	
Uremic encephalopathy	Acute CNS signs and symptoms of uremia
	Asterixis usually present
	Indication to initiate dialysis
Postdialysis	
Dialysis disequilibrium syndrome	Idiogenic osmoles result in brain-to-plasma osmolar gradient
	Caused by aggressive initial HD treatments
Dialysis dementia	Epidemic, endemic, and childhood forms
	Aluminum associated with epidemic form
	Frequently fatal
	Prevented by deionization of dialysis water and restriction of oral aluminum
	Avoid citrate and aluminum compounds
	Deferoxamine chelation therapy
Intellectual function	Generally impaired
Peripheral neuropathy	Motor and sensory impairment
Autonomic dysfunction	Postural hypotension, impaired sweating, gastrointestinal disturbances, impotence

may be similar to those of other metabolic encephalopathies so there is always a risk of misdiagnosis. The diagnosis may also be made difficult because patients with renal failure may also have other intercurrent illnesses which can induce encephalopathy. If a patient with renal insufficiency is taking a drug with potential central nervous system toxicity that is excreted or metabolized primarily by the kidney, the central nervous system symptoms could be due to achievement of toxic drug levels at ordinary dosage or uremia, or a combination of both factors. Also, in patients with both advanced liver and renal diseases, it is often difficult to determine whether the encephalopathy is due to hepatic or renal causes or both. In such patients the BUN and serum creatinine do not always adequately reflect the degree of renal function impairment. Because most alcoholics consume a diet inadequate in protein and calories, they are usually malnourished and have reduced muscle mass. Thus, their ability to generate creatinine from muscle is greatly impaired and there usually is not enough protein intake to produce amino acids and generate urea by the urea cycle. Apparently, normal blood urea nitrogen and creatinine levels may actually be indicative of a diminished capacity of the patient to generate urea and creatinine, rather than a normal glomerular filtration rate. Thus, when alcoholic patients have "normal" BUN and creatinine values, their GFR may be far below 30 mL/min.

Clinical Manifestations

Abnormalities of the mental state are early and sensitive indicators of the development of neurological disorders in patients with acute renal failure. The initial presentation of patients with acute renal failure may include signs of toxic psychosis, abnormal mental status, lassitude and lethargy, with disorientation and confusion occurring later. Physical findings may include cranial nerve signs, nystagmus, dysarthria, abnormal gait and abnormalities of skeletal muscles, manifested by weakness, fasciculations, and asymmetrical variation in deep tendon reflexes. These findings may progress to asterixis and hyperreflexia with unsustained clonus at the ankle. If uremia is left untreated and allowed to progress, seizures and coma often supervene.

Electroencephalograms (EEG) in patients with acute renal failure are generally grossly abnormal when the diagnosis of acute renal failure is first made. In most instances, the percentage of EEG frequency less than 7 Hz is 20 times greater than normal. The abnormal percentages of EEG frequencies both above 9 Hz and below 5 Hz are not usually improved by dialysis within the first few weeks of treatment, although they may return to normal with recovery of renal function. If renal failure continues, the EEG may transiently worsen both during and after hemodialysis and this pattern may continue for up to 6 months after starting dialytic therapy. In spite of these fairly characteristic EEG findings, patients who present with elevated BUN and creatinine and mental status changes do not require an EEG to make the diagnosis. The EEG is a tool which is not generally used in diagnosing uremic encephalopathy.

The neurological manifestations of chronic renal failure are also quite numerous. The EEG findings are usually not as severe as those reported in patients with acute renal failure. In general, there is good correlation between the percentage of EEG frequencies and power below 7 Hz and the decline of renal function as estimated by serum creatinine. After the initiation of dialysis, there may be an initial period of clinical stabilization during which the EEG continues to deteriorate. However, after approximately 6 months of dialysis treatment, the EEG tends to normalize. However, normal values may not be reached unless the patient receives a kidney transplant. In patients with chronic renal failure cognitive functions such as attention span, speed of decision making, short-term memory and mental manipulation of symbols are impaired.

Pathogenesis

Although many factors may contribute to uremic encephalopathy, no precise correlation exists between the degree of encephalopathy and any of the commonly measured blood chemistries associated with renal dysfunction (BUN, creatinine, bicarbonate, or pH). However, there is much evidence to suggest that parathyroid hormone (PTH) may be a uremic toxin.

In uremic animals, both the EEG and observed brain calcium abnormalities can be prevented by parathyroidectomy. Conversely, many of the CNS abnormalities observed in uremia can be reproduced by administration of PTH to normal animals. Parathyroid hormone has been shown to produce central nervous system effects in humans, even in the absence of impaired renal function. Patients with either primary or secondary hyperparathyroidism have EEG changes that are similar to those observed in patients with acute renal failure. In uremic patients, both the EEG changes and abnormalities of psychological testing are improved by either parathyroidectomy or medical suppression of PTH.

In early studies, the sodium potassium adenosine triphosphate enzyme activity in crude brain preparations was said to be normal to low in uremia. However, later studies with metabolically active brain synaptosomes have shown that both the sodium potassium adenosine triphosphate pump and several of the calcium pumps are altered in uremia. Alterations of the calcium pumps were thought to be due at least in part to PTH acting through monophosphate-independent pathways. The uremic environment also played a role as well. Since the calcium pumps at the nerve terminals mediate neurotransmitter release and information transfer, these abnormalities most likely have the potential to affect information processing in the uremic state.

PERIPHERAL NEUROPATHY

Two broad categories of peripheral neuropathy are associated with uremia. They are described in terms of their pattern of neuronal involvement and include: (1) bilaterally symmetrical disturbance of nerve function that can be designated as polyneuropathies (axonopathies). Polyneuropathy tends to be associated with toxic substances, metabolic disorders (uremia, diabetes, deficiency states) and certain immune reactions that diffusely affect the peripheral nervous system; and (2) isolated or multiple isolated lesions of the peripheral nerves designated as mononeuropathies. In severe symmetrical polyneuropathies, a generalized loss of peripheral nerve function may occur, and the impairment is usually maximal distally. This is characterized by a mixed motor and sensory polyneuropathy with a distal distribution which often results in weakness and wasting in the arms and legs. There may also be distal sensory changes of "glove and stocking" distribution. The motor nerve conduction velocity is frequently used to assess peripheral neuropathy. However, the test is somewhat unreliable in uremic subjects, because the procedure itself has a normal daily variation of up to 20%. Thus, motor nerve conduction velocity has very limited utility in detecting moderately impaired peripheral nerve function. Although sensory nerve conduction velocity is more sensitive than motor nerve conduction velocity, it is not widely employed because it is so painful.

Neuropathy of some degree is probably present in about 65% of patients with end stage renal disease who are undergoing dialysis. When the glomerular filtration rate is greater than about 10% of normal, peripheral neuropathy is uncommon. Abnormal nerve conduction may be present in the absence of symptoms or physical findings. However, many patients who volunteer no complaints have impotence or postural hypotension that may be detected with appropriate questioning or physical examination.

In summary, uremic neuropathy is a distal, symmetrical, mixed polyneuropathy that belongs to a group known as dying-back polyneuropathies or central peripheral axonopathies. Uremic neuropathy is also associated with a secondary demyelinating process in the posterior columns of the spinal cord and the central nervous system. Motor and sensory modalities are both generally affected and the lower extremities are more severely involved than are the upper extremities. Clinically, uremic neuropathy cannot easily be distinguished from the neuropathies associated with diabetes mellitus, chronic alcoholism, and other deficiency states. The occurrence of uremic neuropathy bears no relationship to the type of the underlying kidney disease. However, certain diseases which can lead to renal failure may simultaneously affect peripheral nerve function separately from the manifestations of uremia. Such diseases include amyloidosis, multiple myeloma, systemic lupus erythematosus, polyarteritis nodosa, diabetes mellitus, and hepatic failure.

Symptoms

The restless-leg syndrome is a common early manifestation of chronic renal failure. Clinically, patients experience sensations in their lower extremities such as crawling, prickling, and pruritus. The sensations are generally worse distally and are usually more prominent in the evening. The burning-foot syndrome, which is present in less than 10% of patients with chronic renal failure actually represents swelling and tenderness of the distal lower extremities. The physical signs of peripheral nerve dysfunction often begin with loss of deep tendon reflexes, particularly in the knee and ankle. There is also impaired vibratory sensation and loss of sensation in the lower leg in the form of "stocking glove" anesthesia. Sensory modalities which are lost include pain, light touch, vibration, and pressure.

Uremic Toxins as Causes of Neuropathy

A number of potential uremic toxins might lead to symptoms. Although any or all of these agents may play a role in the development of uremic neuropathy, the evidence that any of them are true "neurotoxins" is scant. For example, the "middle molecules" (MW 500 to 2500 Da), once thought to be uremic toxins, have not with stood the test of time. Several other potential "uremic toxins" have been suggested. One of these is PTH, which has received much of the attention. Suggestions that PTH may be a uremic neurotoxin are based on correlation between plasma PTH levels and motor nerve conduction velocity in patients and animals with chronic renal failure. However, in patients with hyperparathyroidism without uremia, there is no consistent observable effect of PTH on peripheral nerve function. Presently, no single uremic toxin has been shown to affect peripheral nerve function. Most of the evidence suggests that uremic neuropathy may be related to anatomical nerve damage of unknown etiology. It may also be related to cumulative effects of multiple toxic agents, and usually takes months to years to develop.

Autonomic and Cranial Nerve Dysfunction

Autonomic dysfunction is usually quite common in chronic renal failure, and is usually associated with postural hypotension, impaired sweating, impotence, gastrointestinal disturbances, abnormal Valsalva maneuver, and alterations in gastric motility. Dialysis-related hypotension is often associated with autonomic insufficiency particularly in patients with diabetes and amyloidosis. The autonomic nervous system function can be evaluated by the following means (1) the hand-grip dynamometer; (2) the heart rate response following Valsalva maneuver to determine the Valsalva ratio; and (3) the vascular response to norepinephrine infusion.

Cranial nerves are also often affected in uremic patients, and the nerve involvement is most often manifested as transient nystagmus, miosis, heterophoria, and facial asymmetry. Involvement of the eighth nerve affecting both auditory and vestibular divisions is most commonly seen. In such cases, it is important to distinguish deafness due to uremia from that associated with various hereditary interstitial nephropathies and ototoxicity of drugs such as the aminoglycosides.

Treatment

A number of treatments have been tried to alleviate symptoms of peripheral neuropathy. However, no one treatment appears to be effective in everyone, possibly because neuropathy in dialysis patients is of multifactorial etiology. For instance, a number of toxins such as alcoholism, arsenic, lead, and PTH can produce neuropathy. Systemic diseases such as diabetes, amyloidosis, and multiple myeloma can cause neuropathy independently of uremia. Additionally, vitamin deficiency such as beriberi and B_{12} can also cause neuropathy. As a result, it is often quite difficult to determine the precise etiology of the neuropathy. Nonetheless, a number of treatments have been tried, including analgesics, anticonvulsants, antidepressants, and antiarrythmics such as mexiletine which appears to have some benefit in diabetic neuropathy. In very severe cases, patients may only get relief from medical or surgical sympathectomy. There is presently no reliable evidence to suggest that the symptoms of neuropathy can be ameliorated by increasing the intensity of dialysis.

INTELLECTUAL FUNCTION IN DIALYSIS PATIENTS

Impairment of intellectual function is another frequently recognized complication in patients with chronic renal failure who are being treated with dialysis. However, this abnormality is not well characterized and there is no anatomical lesion that characterizes intellectual deterioration. Although some studies suggest that the overall intellectual ability in patients with chronic renal failure may not differ significantly from normal, others have suggested that the IQ in dialysis patients is below that of the general population. Based on psychological testing, the general consensus is that over time, chronic renal failure is associated with organic-like loss of intellectual function. Because patients on dialysis are susceptible to other conditions that can cause decline in intellectual function, it is often quite difficult to establish a clear etiology for this problem.

COMPLICATIONS OF DIALYSIS THERAPY

Dialysis Disequilibrium Syndrome

Several central nervous system disorders may occur as a consequence of dialytic therapy. One such disorder is dialysis disequilibrium syndrome (DDS), which can occur in patients who have recently initiated hemodialysis. The symptom complex is quite variable and may include muscle cramps, anorexia, restlessness, dizziness, headache, nausea, emesis, blurred vision, muscular twitching, disorientation, hypertension, tremors, and seizures. Although, it was originally thought that the EEG was abnormal in DDS, recent studies have indicated that the EEG may indeed be normal. DDS has been reported among patients of all age groups; however, it occurs most often in the elderly and in children. The syndrome is generally associated with rapid hemodialysis of patients who have just started hemodialysis, but it may also occur following routine maintenance hemodialysis in patients with chronic renal failure for as long as 6 months.

The pathogenesis of DDS has been extensively investigated in animal models. It was first postulated that DDS was probably due to the "reverse urea effect," where it was hypothesized that urea was cleared less rapidly from the brain than from the blood, and this resulted in an osmotic gradient between the blood and brain. It has since been shown that during dialysis, urea is cleared from brain at essentially the same rate as it is cleared from blood, so there is no significant blood-to-brain osmotic gradient based on the movement of urea alone. However, rapid hemodialysis of animals with renal failure does result in an increased brain-to-plasma osmolality often with resulting cerebral edema. It is now thought that the increased brain osmolality is due to the formation of organic acids, amino acids, methylamines, and polyols which are produced in the brain during the development of plasma hyperosmolality. These compounds act as effective osmolar agents and are called "idiogenic osmoles." Many of these solutes have now been identified (myoinositol, sorbitol, betaine, glycerophosphorylcholine, phosphocreatine, glutamate, glutamine, taurine), and are found not only in uremia but also in hyperglycemia and hypernatremia.

Idiogenic osmoles protect the brain from shrinkage during conditions of plasma hyperosmolality (uremia, hypernatremia, or hyperglycemia). In other words, the brain increases its osmolality to match that of plasma without losing water. A substantial decrease in brain volume could tear the brain from the skull and produce intracerebral hemorrhage. Thus, any treatment that acutely lowers plasma osmolality without allowing adequate time for the removal of idiogenic osmoles runs the risk of developing substantial brain-to-plasma osmolar gradient and cerebral edema. If the gradient is large enough (>25 mOsm/kg H_2O), the resulting cerebral edema may produce pressures that could result in brain herniation (brain damage or death). The complications of DDS are usually avoided in dialysis patients by decreasing both the length of dialysis and the blood flow rate through the dialyzer. These maneuvers generally necessitate more frequent dialysis treatments. As the plasma osmolality is gradually brought back closer to normal by this technique, idiogenic osmoles are removed and brain osmolality gradually returns to normal without any dramatic changes in brain volume.

Dialysis Dementia

Dialysis dementia is a progressive, frequently fatal neurologic disease which is seen almost exclusively in patients who are being treated with chronic hemodialysis. Although early studies focused on the distinctive neurological findings of this disorder, later reports have suggested that some forms of dialysis dementia may be part of a multisystem disease which includes dementia, osteomalacia, proximal myopathy, and anemia.

Although the etiology of dialysis dementia remains controversial, it most likely represents a symptom complex that is the final common pathway for a variety of processes. Dialysis dementia can be subdivided into three types: (1) an epidemic form; (2) dementia associated with childhood renal disease; and (3) an endemic form. The initial reports of dialysis dementia were all of the endemic form that occurred in patients who had been on chronic hemodialysis for more than 2 years. Initial symptoms of this disorder are dysarthria, apraxia, slurring of speech with stuttering, and hesitancy. Later in the course of the disease, symptoms progress to personality changes, psychosis, myoclonus, seizures, and eventually dementia and death within 6 months after the onset of symptoms.

Early in dialysis dementia, the EEG shows multifocal bursts of high amplitude delta activity with spikes and sharp waves, intermixed with runs of more normal appearing background activity. These EEG changes may precede overt clinical symptoms by up to 6 months. However, as the disease progresses, the normal background activity of the EEG will deteriorate to a predominance of slow frequencies. When accompanied by the appropriate clinical pictures, this EEG pattern is pathognomonic of dialysis dementia; however, these patterns may also be seen in other metabolic encephalopathies. Thus, the diagnosis of dialysis dementia depends on the presence of the typical clinical picture, the characteristic EEG findings, and, most importantly, exclusion of other causes of central nervous system dysfunction.

Finally, dialysis dementia has also been reported in children with renal failure, some of whom were neither on dialysis nor exposed to aluminum-containing compounds. Therefore, the cause of encephalopathy in such children cannot be ascribed to aluminum alone, and may represent developmental neurological defects resulting from exposure of the growing brain to uremia.

Role of Aluminum in Dialysis Dementia

Aluminum intoxication was probably first implicated in this disorder when it was observed that it was markedly elevated in brain gray matter in patients with dialysis dementia. Aluminum content in brain is also more than threefold greater in patients with dialysis dementia than in those on chronic hemodialysis without dementia. The reasons for the increase remain controversial although the actual source of the aluminum is evident. Aluminum is the second most common element in the earth's crust, and in the United States the typical dietary intake of aluminum is 10 to 100 mg/day. Aluminum intake is substantially greater in individuals taking aluminum-containing antacids. Normally, only a minimal amount of orally administered aluminum is absorbed, but for unknown reasons absorption appears to be increased in patients with renal failure. Prior to the routine deionization of the water used in hemodialysis, most of the aluminum in dialysis patients came from the water. It is estimated that a dialysate aluminum concentration of only 70 μg/L results in a minimum positive aluminum balance of 300 μg/day. Because aluminum is normally excreted by the kidney, renal failure leads to aluminum retention in such patients. Thus, the problem is not where the aluminum comes from, but rather how it enters the brain and how it causes dementia. In dialysis dementia, abnormalities of the blood brain barrier most likely play an important role.

Elevated brain aluminum levels are also present in several groups of patients who are not demented. These include patients with acute renal failure, hepatic encephalopathy, age greater than 60 years, and metastatic cancer. However, the levels are generally lower than that observed in dialysis dementia. In patients with dialysis dementia, aluminum appears to be important in the development of the epidemic form; however, whether aluminum plays an important role in the other types of dialysis dementia (endemic, childhood) is still unresolved. Deionization of the water used to prepare dialysate is now used as a preventive measure to reduce aluminum concentration in dialysate fluid. However, deionization not only removes aluminum but also cadmium, mercury, lead, manganese, copper, nickel, thallium, boron, and tin. Thus, not only aluminum, but several other trace elements might be involved in the pathogenesis of dialysis dementia.

Despite these unresolved questions, most outbreaks of the epidemic form of dialysis encephalopathy have been associated with high levels of aluminum in the dialysate. Thus, therapy has been directed toward removing aluminum both from dialysate and from the patients. Lowering the dialysate aluminum levels to below 20 μg/L by deionization and reverse osmosis appears to be quite beneficial for patients who are starting dialysis. In patients with overt disease, eliminating the source of aluminum has only rarely resulted in improvement in brain function. Diazepam or clonazepam appear to be useful in controlling initial seizure activity associated with the disease; however, they usually become ineffective later on and do not appear to alter the usually fatal outcome. Improvement in symptoms has been reported in several patients treated with deferioxamine, which chelates serum aluminum and reduces tissue burden of aluminum. However, some studies suggest that deferioxamine without diazepam may lead to worsening of symptoms because it promotes aluminum removal from other tissues but facilitates deposition in brain. Deferoxamine is also associated with a number of side effects that markedly limit it usefulness. These include fatal fungal mucormycosis in approximately 10% of treated dialysis patients, cataracts, retinal changes, and thrombocytopenia. Chelation therapy only appears to be effective if started early in the course of the disease. Thus, deferoxamine should be used early in all patients suspected of aluminum intoxication.

The best dose and route of administration of deferoxamine (DFO) is still in question. Symptomatic improvement has occurred as rapidly in inpatients receiving 0.5 g as in those receiving doses as high as 6 g/week. DFO can be given once a week or three times per week with dialysis. To avoid brain aluminum toxicity resulting from mobilization of aluminum from other sites; DFO should be given intramuscularly the evening prior to dialysis, so that much of the aluminum–DFO complex can be removed during dialysis on the following day.

Acute neurotoxicity from aluminum intoxication can develop in uremic patients who have received oral preparations of citrate and aluminum compounds simultaneously. It also appears that many nondialyzed children and adults with renal failure who develop dialysis dementia do so as a result of the oral administration of citrate solutions for acidosis and aluminum hydroxide as phosphate binder. The increased toxicity of aluminum under these circumstances occurs because of enhanced gastrointestinal absorption of aluminum when complexed with citrate. The elimination of aluminum from dialysate water mainly prevents the occurrence of dialysis dementia (epidemic form); however, removal of aluminum from patients with established dialysis dementia may not affect the course of their disease. Treatment of sporadic cases in which the etiology of the encephalopathy is unclear is more difficult. In this instance, it is most important to differentiate dialysis dementia from other metabolic encephalopathies and from structural lesions such as strokes and intracerebral hemorrhages.

Bibliography

Andreoli SP, Bergstein JM, Sherrard DJ: Aluminum intoxication from aluminum containing phosphate binders in children with azotemia not undergoing dialysis. *N EngL J Med* 310:1079–1084, 1984.

Arieff Al: Dialysis disequilibrium syndrome: Current concepts on pathogenesis and prevention. *Kidney Int* 45:629–635, 1994.

Arieff Al, Massry SG, Barrientos A, Kleeman CR: Brain water and electrolyte metabolism in uremia: Effects of slow and rapid hemodialysis. *Kidney Int* 4:177–187, 1973.

Arnaud CD: Hyperparathyroidism and renal failure. *Kidney Int* 4:89–95, 1973.

Bakir AA, Hryhorczuk DO, Berman E, et al.: Acute fatal hyperaluminemic encephalopathy in undialyzed and recently dialyzed uremin patients. *Trans Am Soc Aetif Organs* 32:171, 1986.

Fraser CL, Arieff Al: Nervous system complications in uremia. *Ann Intern Med* 109:143–153, 1988.

Fraser CL, Arieff Al: Nervous system manifestations of renal failure. In: Schrier RW, Gottschalk CW (eds) *Diseases of the Kidney,* 5th. Little, Brown and Co., Boston, pp. 2625–2646, 1997.

Fraser CL, Sarnacki P, Arieff Al: Abnormal sodium transport in synaptosomes from brain of uremic rats. *J Clin Invest* 75:2014–2023, 1985.

Lien Y-HH, Shapiro JI, Chan L: Effects of hypernatremia on organic brain osmoles. *J Clin Invest* 85:1427–1435, 1990.

Olivieri NF, Bungig RJ, Chew E, et al.: Visual and auditory neurotoxicity in patients receiving subcutaneous deferoxamine infusions. *N EngL J Med* 314:869–873, 1986.

Prior JC, Cameron EC, Knickerbocker WJ, Sweeney VP, Suchowersky O: Dialysls encephalopathy and osteomalacic bone disease. *Am J Med* 72:33–42, 1982.

Rotundo A, Nevins TE, Lipton M, Lockman LA, Mauer SM, Michael AF. Progressive encephalopathy in children with chronic renal insufficiency in infancy. *Kidney Int* 21:486–491, 1982.

Slatopolsky E, Martin K, Hruska K: Parathyroid hormone metabolism and its potential as a uremic toxin. *Am J Physiol* 238;F1–F12, 1980.

72

HEMATOLOGIC MANIFESTATIONS OF
RENAL FAILURE

JONATHAN HIMMELFARB

INTRODUCTION

The development of progressive chronic renal failure results in a number of adverse hematologic effects with significant clinical consequences. Uremia almost invariably results in profound changes in erythrocyte production and destruction resulting in anemia. The development of recombinant human erythropoietin to treat the anemia of renal disease has been one of the most significant advances associated with renal replacement therapy in the past decade. While patients with chronic renal failure generally have normal platelet and leukocyte counts, they often experience a qualitative change in platelet and granulocyte function. These changes are manifested clinically by an increased susceptibility to hemorrhage and infection. This chapter reviews the pathogenesis of the anemia of chronic renal failure, describe its clinical and laboratory manifestations, and provides an approach to its treatment. The pathogenesis, clinical manifestations, and treatment of platelet and granulocyte dysfunction in uremia will also be described.

ANEMIA OF CHRONIC RENEL FAILURE

Pathogenesis

Normal erythropoiesis is primarily regulated by circulating erythropoietin. When erythropoietin binds to specific receptors on bone marrow erythroid progenitor cells their proliferation, differentiation and development into mature erythrocytes is enhanced. Erythropoietin is now know to be a heavily glycosylated protein with a MW 30,400 Da comprised of 165 amino acids and four carbohydrate side chains. The gene for erythropoietin encompasses about 3000 base pairs and is located on chromosome 7.

The major site of erythropoietin production is the renal peritubular capillary endothelial cell. Renal interstitial fibroblasts may produce erythropoietin. The kidney produces up to 90% of circulating erythropoietin, accounting for its pivotal role in erythropoiesis. Most extra renal erythropoietin is produced in the liver by centrilobular hepatocytes. However, extrarenal erythropoietin production is rarely able to provide for sufficient erythropoiesis in an anephric state, suggesting that the liver is less sensitive than the kidney to hypoxic stimuli.

The precise mechanisms by which hypoxia stimulates renal erythropoietin secretion remain incompletely understood. Studies using a human hepatoma cell line suggest that the oxygen-sensing mechanism involves the locking of a heme protein in the deoxy conformation in response to low oxygen tension.

In normal subjects, erythropoietin circulates in minute quantities. In response to anemia, normal subjects have an exponential increase in plasma erythropoietin levels. In contrast, anemic patients with progressive renal failure have circulating plasma levels of erythropoietin similar to normal nonanemic subjects. In this patient population the relationship between the degree of anemia and plasma erythropoietin levels is also lost (Fig. 1).

The pathogenesis of anemia of chronic renal failure is multifactorial. Erythropoietin deficiency, shortened erythrocyte survival, the presence of uremic inhibitors of erythropoiesis, bleeding, and iron deficiency have all been proposed as major factors. However, with the advent of erythropoietin therapy, it has become clear that the principal cause of the anemia of chronic renal disease is a decrease in erythropoietin production due to the loss of functional renal tissue.

Support for the hypothesis that uremic toxins retained in the plasma inhibit bone marrow erythroid production comes from in vitro experiments where uremic human sera has been shown to blunt the growth of erythroid colony forming units (CFU-E). This in vivo erythroid inhibition has been thought to be due to polyamines such as spermine or putrescine as well as yet unidentified "middle molecules." Recent studies using human autologous cultured bone marrow cells have not demonstrated inhibition of erythroid progenitor cell growth by uremic serum. Furthermore, in vivo studies involving the infusion of recombinant erythropoietin into normal subjects and hemodialysis patients demonstrate that erythropoiesis, as quantitated by ferrokinetics and the reticulocyte response, are not blunted in subjects with chronic renal failure. Almost all patients with chronic renal failure, if iron replete and free of inflammation or infection, will have an appropriate erythropoietic response to erythropoietin. Thus, current evidence suggests that uremic inhibitors of erythropoiesis play a minimal role if any in the pathogenesis of the anemia of chronic renal failure.

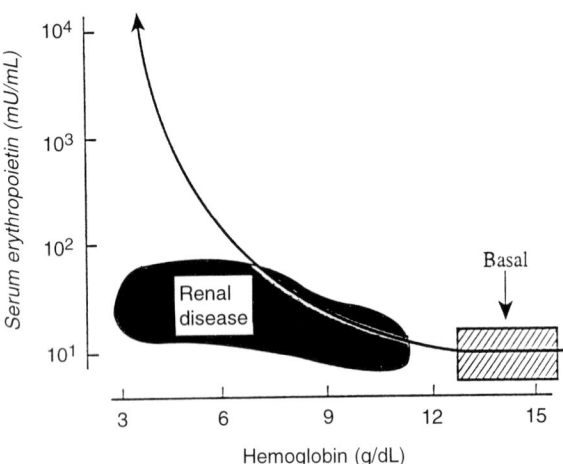

FIGURE I Erythropoietin levels in renal disease. The box entitled "basal" refers to serum erythropoietin levels in normal individuals. The upward arrow reflects the typical rise in serum erythropoietin levels in patients with anemia not due to chronic renal failure. From Hillman RS, Ault KA: *Hematology in Clinical Practice*. McGraw-Hill, New York, 1995. With permission.

TABLE I

Causes of Apparent Erythropoietin Resistance

Inadequate erythropoietin
Iron deficiency
Infection or inflammation
Osteitis fibrosa cystica
Aluminum intoxication
Folate deficiency
Multiple myeloma
Severe malnutrition
Hemolysis or blood loss

A decrease in erythrocyte survival has also been postulated to contribute to the anemia of chronic renal failure. The etiology of decreased erythrocyte survival in uremic patients is unclear but may be related to reduced resistance to oxidant stress. Erythrocyte survival generally does not improve with dialysis therapy. The degree of shortening of erythrocyte survival in uremia is generally mild (erythrocyte life span 60 to 90 days in uremic patients vs 120 days in normal individuals). There does not appear to be a correlation between the amount of erythropoietin required to maintain a stable hematocrit and erythrocyte survival suggesting that decreased erythrocyte survival is only a minor cause of the anemia of chronic renal disease. The use of erythropoietin may also extend erythrocyte survival.

Iron deficiency limits the erythroid response to erythropoietin and can contribute to the anemia of chronic renal failure. Patients may develop iron deficiency anemia because of occult gastrointestinal and other bleeding, the effects of routine phlebotomy, or because of occult blood losses in the dialysis tubing as part of the dialysis procedure. Other factors which can contribute to the reduction of the hematocrit level in some patients with chronic renal failure are shown in Table 1.

Clinical and Laboratory Manifestations

The anemia of chronic renal disease is normocytic and normochromic. Both the corrected reticulocyte count and serum erythropoietin levels are inappropriately low when compared to values seen in patients with similar degrees of anemia without renal failure. The bone marrow examination is usually normal in appearance and is not usually necessary for the hematologic evaluation. Measurement of serum erythropoietin levels is generally not required. An abnormal platelet count or white blood cell count may reflect a more generalized disturbance of bone marrow

function. Erythrocyte indices, reticulocyte count, and iron parameters are helpful in detecting many anemias which are not due to erythropoietin deficiency. Microcytosis can reflect iron deficiency, aluminum intoxication, and certain hemogloblinopathies. Macrocytosis may be associated with vitamin B_{12} or folate deficiency.

As renal failure progresses, there is an increased likelihood of developing anemia because diseased kidneys are unable to produce sufficient quantities of erythropoietin. Figure 2 indicates the relationship between the change in hematocrit and the serum creatinine in more than 900 patients. While the mean hematocrit drops below 30 at a serum creatinine of approximately 6 mg/dL, there is considerable interpatient variation. There is even less correlation between the BUN and hematocrit.

Many patients with polycystic kidney disease will have a higher hemoglobin level and hematocrit than would otherwise be expected for a comparable level of renal dysfunction. In contrast, patients who have undergone bilateral nephrectomies will generally have more severe anemia than other patients on chronic dialysis therapy. Even when kidneys are devoid of excretory function, they usually retain some capability for erythropoietin biosynthesis.

Patients with severe anemia display signs and symptoms attributable to tissue hypoxia. However, many of the symptoms usually attributable to anemia may be clinically difficult to distinguish from symptoms related to uremia. For most patients, symptoms develop when the hematocrit decreases to 30 or less. However, therapy is indicated at a higher level of hematocrit if angina pectoris or other significant symptoms develop. Younger patients often will adjust better to anemia. When anemia develops gradually, an intraerythrocytic increase in 2,3-DPG occurs, which shifts the oxygen dissociation curve to the right and allows oxygen to be unloaded at the tissue level more readily. Thus, many patients may not be as severely symptomatic as might be expected from the degree of anemia. Additional cardiovascular compensatory mechanisms may also develop over time, thereby limiting symptoms directly attributed to anemia.

The symptoms of anemia include weakness, fatigue, and dyspnea, particularly with exertion. Decreased exercise tolerance is common and many patients experience difficulty with concentration, attention span, and memory. Sexual

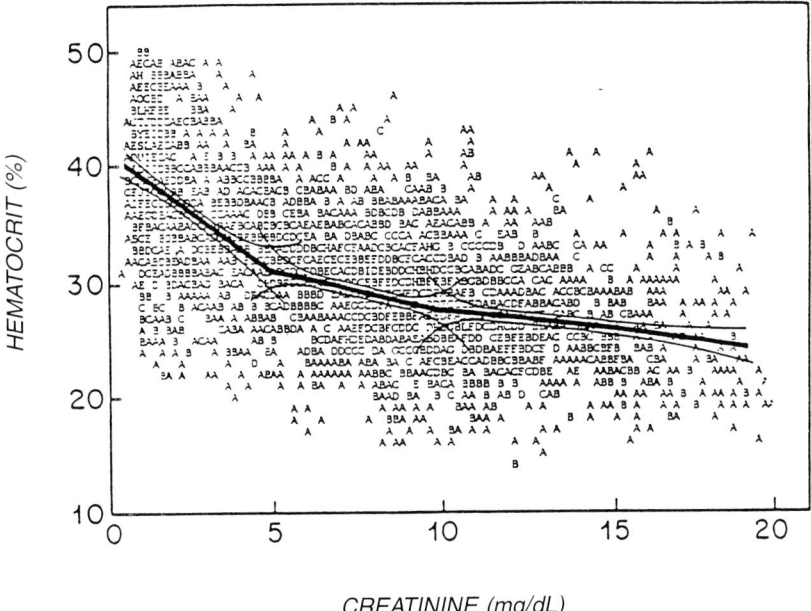

FIGURE 2 The change of hematocrit with creatinine in chronic renal failure. This figure represents approximately 4000 data points obtained from 911 patients followed at the Brigham & Women's outpatient renal clinic from 1977 to 1983. The 95% confidence limit of the slope is shown around each line. Each letter represents the number of data points at that value (e.g., A = 1 data point, B = 2 data points, etc.). From. Hakim RM, Lazarus JM: *Am J Kidney Dis* XI(3):238–247, 1988. With permission.

dysfunction, cold intolerance, and anorexia may also result from anemia.

The use of recombinant erythropoietin to treat the anemia of chronic renal failure has led to the recognition that the contribution of anemia to the morbidity of chronic renal failure is greater than formerly appreciated. The clinical benefits of improved tissue oxygenation have been quantitated to include improvements in exercise capacity, central nervous system function, and endocrine and cardiac function. Correction of the anemia of chronic renal failure has resulted in marked clinical improvement in exercise capacity. Recent data from both the United States Medicare ESRD Program as well as data from the Canadian Erythropoietin Study Group have demonstrated a reduction in hospital readmission in patients with end stage renal disease treated with erythropoietin. Chronic anemia and consequent tissue hypoxia results in a compensatory increase in cardiac contractility and heart rate in order to optimize tissue oxygenation. Over time, the cardiac response to anemia results in the development of left ventricular hypertrophy. Ultimately the development of left ventricular hypertrophy results in both diastolic dysfunction and an increased incidence of myocardial ischemia and cardiac arrhythmias. An inverse relationship between the degree of anemia and the extent of left ventricular end diastolic diameter has been demonstrated. Correction of the anemia of chronic renal failure with erythropoietin has generally but not always resulted in an improvement in left ventricular hypertrophy. The use of erythropoietin has resulted in a lower rate of hospitalization for myocardial infarction in

the United States Medicare population and a lower rate of hospitalization for cardiac disease in general in the Canadian dialysis population. A recent study has identified the degree of anemia as a risk factor for cardiovascular mortality in ESRD patients.

The use of erythropoietin to improve anemia in hemodialysis patients is also associated with improvement in cognitive function. This improvement has been quantitated both by documenting normalization of abnormal EEGs as well as improvement on neuropsychiatric testing. Normalization of cerebral blood flow has also been demonstrated with improvement in anemia. These improvements in cognitive changes have translated into a lessening of depression and improvements in quality of life indicators. Endocrine changes may also occur. Sexual function has improved in some men after an increase in hematocrit. Some but not all studies have demonstrated an increase in serum testosterone levels after erythropoietin therapy. Serum prolactin levels have decreased after erythropoietin in some but not all male hemodialysis patients. Some amenorrheic women experience a resumption in menstruation following the use of erythropoietin. Anemia may also play a role in growth retardation in pediatric patients. Impaired immune responsiveness and platelet function may also be partially related to anemia in this patient population.

Treatment

The therapeutic modalities available today for treatment of the anemia of renal disease include administration of recombinant erythropoietin, institution of renal replacement therapy including kidney transplantation, and packed red blood cell transfusions. Prior to the advent of erythropoietin therapy, approximately 75% of chronic dialysis patients had hematocrit values less than 30 while 15 to 25% required periodic red blood cell transfusions.

Phase I and II clinical trials demonstrated a clear-cut relationship between the dose of erythropoietin and the rate of rise in hematocrit (Fig. 3). Since these initial studies, patient variability in response to erythropoietin has been noted, and a bell-shaped distribution pattern of doses is required to maintain a stable hematocrit in iron replete stable dialysis patients. Erythropoietin response is dependent on dose, route, and frequency of parenteral administration. Although intravenous erythropoietin has 100% bioavailability, most of the administered intravenous dose is probably biologically ineffective once the relatively small number of erythropoietin receptors on erythroid progenitor cells are saturated. Subcutaneous erythropoietin administration results in a slower increase in serum erythropoietin levels with maintenance of a stable serum level for hours, and despite incomplete absorption, most studies indicate that there is on average a 20 to 40% reduction in erythropoietin requirements for subcutaneous compared to intravenous dosing. Erythropoietin can also be administered intraperitoneally, which may be preferable for children treated with peritoneal dialysis.

It is currently recommended that the initial administration of erythropoietin for treatment of anemia in predialysis, peritoneal dialysis, and hemodialysis patients be subcutaneous at a dose of 80 to 120 U · kg^{-1} · week^{-1} in two to three divided doses to achieve the target hematocrit.

Children less than 5 years of age frequently require higher doses than adults (300 U · kg^{-1} · week^{-1}). The site of erythropoietin injection should be rotated with each administration.

The appropriate target hematocrit for patients with chronic renal failure on recombinant erythropoietin therapy remains controversial. The target maintenance hematocrit for patients in the initial phase I to II clinical trial was 35 to 40% and was 35% for the phase III multicenter clinical trial. The target hematocrit recommended by the FDA in 1989 was 30 to 33%, which was subsequently widened to a target hematocrit range of 30 to 36% in June 1994. The most recent data from the United States Renal Data System (USRDS) 1996 Annual Data Report demonstrated that the mean hematocrit for erythropoietin treated dialysis patients in the United States was 30.2%, and that 43% of patients had values less than 30%. Preliminary analysis of a recent study involving more than 1200 hemodialysis patients with documented heart disease found that in the more than 600 patients randomized to have their hematocrit increased to normal (42 ± 3%) there was an increase in death or nonfatal myocardial infarctions compared to patients maintained at a hematocrit of 30%. Until further data are available, it seems prudent to exercise caution before attempting to raise the hematocrit above 36%.

A crucial aspect of erythropoietin therapy is the maintenance of adequate iron stores for the production of new erythrocytes. Normally three quarters of body iron is present in circulating erythrocytes and one quarter exists as storage iron primarily in the liver and bone marrow. Because the demands for iron by the erythroid marrow frequently exceed iron stores once erythropoietin therapy is initiated, iron supplementation is essential to ensure adequate response. In the pre-erythropoietin era, advanced renal failure and its associated hypoproliferative anemia were frequently accompanied by excess storage iron. However, since the widespread use of erythropoietin, iron overload is now uncommon, whereas iron deficiency has become quite common.

Iron status in patients receiving erythropoietin is monitored by measuring both the serum ferritin and the percent transferrin saturation. Serum ferritin and percent transferrin saturation are complementary tests because they measure different pools of body iron. The serum ferritin is proportional to storage iron and is also an acute phase reactant. It may be increased in the presence of acute or chronic inflammation. Thus, a low serum ferritin is a specific but not a sensitive marker for iron deficiency.

In contrast, the percent transferrin saturation (measured as the serum iron divided by the total iron binding capacity multiplied by 100) reflects iron that is readily available for erythropoiesis. The transferrin molecule contains two receptors for molecular iron transported from storage iron sites to erythroid progenitor cells. The percent transferrin saturation is decreased with either absolute or functional iron deficiency. Transferrin saturation appears to be a better predictor of iron responsiveness than the serum ferritin level. Other tests of iron status such as RBC ferritin or zinc protoporphyrin do not appear to increase diagnostic

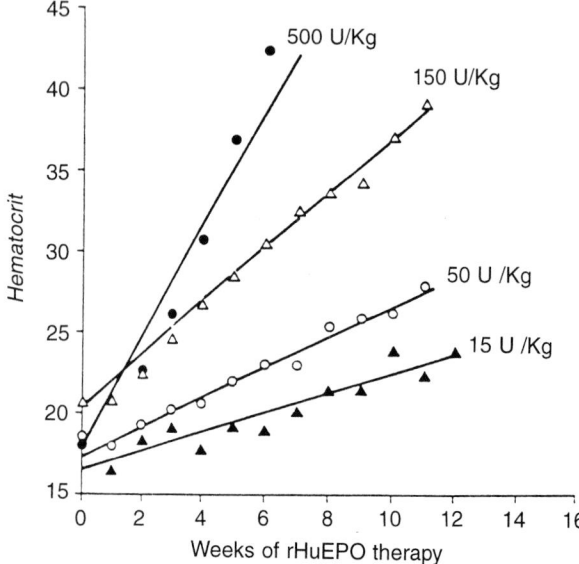

FIGURE 3 The response in hematocrit to erythropoietin therapy. Each line represents the response to the given dose of erythropoietin administered intravenously three times a week to hemodialysis patients. From Eschbach JW, Egrie JC, Downing MR, Brown JK, Adamson JW: *N Engl J Med* 316:73–78, 1987. With permission.

sensitivity or specificity. The definitive test for iron status, bone marrow stainable iron, is invasive and expensive and need not be used on a routine basis. For optimal responsiveness to erythropoietin, current recommendations are that the serum ferritin should be maintained at greater than 300 ng/mL and the percent transferrin saturation at greater than 30%.

Iron can be administered either as oral iron salts or intravenously. When oral iron is used it should be given as 200 mg of elemental iron per day in two to three divided doses. For optimal absorption, oral iron should be given more than 1 hour before meals or more than 2 hours after meals or ingestion of phosphate binders. When oral iron is insufficient to maintain adequate iron status, patients can receive intravenous iron. As of 1996, iron dextran is the only form of intravenous iron approved in the United States although intravenous ferric gluconate and ferrous saccharate are available in other countries. Anaphylactic reactions occur in 0.6% of intravenous iron dextran treated patients. Prior to initiating intravenous iron dextran therapy, a one time test dose of 25 mg must be given intravenously. However, anaphylactic reactions may occur in patients who have received any number of previous iron dextran injections. Iron dextran is frequently administered as a 100 mg dose with each hemodialysis treatment, with a total administered dose of 1000 mg. Some investigators now recommend that intravenous iron dextran be administered in 50 to 100 mg weekly doses continually in patients intolerant of oral iron salts or in patients who cannot maintain adequate iron status with oral iron.

True resistance to erythropoietin therapy for the treatment of chronic renal failure is rare (Table 1). In the largest clinical trial with erythropoietin, more than 96% of iron-replete dialysis patients responded when erythropoietin was given at 150 U/kg intravenously three times a week. The median dose of erythropoietin needed to maintain the target hematocrit was 75 U/kg intravenously three times a week. The most common cause of a poor response to erythropoietin is either an inadequate erythropoietin dose or the presence of iron deficiency. Other causes of erythropoietin resistance include the presence of inflammation or infection. Inflammation results in a deficient iron supply by blocking the release of iron from the reticuloendothelial system despite the presence of normal to increased iron stores. Iron absorption is also reduced in acute inflammatory states. Bone marrow fibrosis from osteitis fibrosa cystica as a consequence of hyperparathyroidism can cause true erythropoietin resistance. Hyperparathyroidism without osteitis fibrosa cystica does not blunt the effect of erythropoietin. The definitive diagnosis of osteitis fibrosa cystica requires a bone biopsy. Aluminum intoxication may be associated with a reduction in the response to erythropoietin. Aluminum intoxication can be suspected in the iron-replete patient who has a low erythrocyte mean corpuscular volume and can be confirmed by measuring an increased serum aluminum level after deferoxamine administration or by positive staining for aluminum in a bone biopsy. (see Chapter 69) Rarely, folate or vitamin B_{12} deficiency can be a cause erythropoietin resistance. Resistance to erythro-

poietin therapy has also been documented due to anti-N_{form} antibody-mediated hemolysis in patients with chronic formaldehyde exposure. Patients with multiple myeloma and those who are severely malnourished may also be resistant to erythropoietin therapy. Occult bleeding needs to be considered in erythropoietin-resistant patients.

Early experiences with erythropoietin therapy in hemodialysis patients suggested that accelerated hypertension, the development of seizures, and hyperkalemia were frequent accompaniments to erythropoietin therapy. However, recent clinical experience and the results of controlled trials have demonstrated that the adverse effects of erythropoietin therapy are infrequent and generally manageable. The most frequent adverse effect is aggravation of hypertension. Approximately 20 to 30% of erythropoietin-treated predialysis or dialysis patients developed hypertension or an increase in blood pressure during treatment of erythropoietin. An increase in blood pressure usually occurs in association with a rapid increase in hematocrit and/or at higher doses of erythropoietin. The development or worsening of hypertension is thought to be related to increased, vascular wall reactivity as well as hemodynamic changes that occur as a result of increasing red cell mass. Endothelial cells have now been demonstrated to possess erythropoietin receptors, and infusion of erythropoietin in vitro can result in release of endothelin and vasoconstriction. Worsening hypertension associated with erythropoietin therapy can be treated by initiating or increasing antihypertensive therapy, by intensifying ultrafiltration in dialysis patients with evidence of volume expansion, or by reducing erythropoietin dose.

The initial multicenter study with erythropoietin in the United States noted a higher incidence of seizures during the first 3 months of the study compared to historical controls. In subsequent studies, with the exception of patients with hypertensive encephalopathy, there is no evidence for an increased incidence of seizures in patients in whom appropriate dose and titration recommendations for erythropoietin therapy are followed. A prior history of seizures is not considered a contraindication to the use of erythropoietin. While serious hyperkalemia was observed during the early clinical experience with erythropoietin, recent studies have not confirmed this finding.

Whether the use of erythropoietin increases the likelihood of developing vascular access thrombosis in hemodialysis patients remains controversial. Most studies have not demonstrated an increase in the rate of either native fistulae or synthetic graft thrombosis when the hematocrit is kept at or below 36%. An exception is the Canadian multicenter trial which suggested that erythropoietin increased the rate of thrombosis in PTFE grafts. Preliminary analysis of a recent study in which hemodialysis patients with heart disease were randomized to a target hematocrit of 42 ± 3% did demonstrate a significant increase in thrombosis of both native fistulae and synthetic grafts in the higher hematocrit group.

ERYTHROCYTOSIS IN RENAL DISORDERS

Erythrocytosis is occasionally seen in previously anemic uremic patients who develop a renal cell carcinoma or large renal cyst, and is occasionally seen in patients with polycystic kidney disease. Erythrocytosis has also been reported to occur in up to 17% of renal transplant recipients. Recent observations indicate that angiotensin converting enzyme inhibition corrects renal transplant erythrocytosis. Treatment efficacy of angiotensin converting enzyme (ACE) inhibitors for posttransplant erythrocytosis has been demonstrated using captopril, enalapril, lisinopril, and fosinopril, suggesting that angiotensin II production is somehow related to the development of erythrocytosis. Studies of erythropoiesis after withdrawal of enalapril in posttransplant erythrocytosis have not demonstrated that high plasma levels of erythropoietin contribute to the development of posttransplant erythrocytosis. Thus, the pathogenesis of posttransplant erythrocytosis and mechanism underlying the beneficial effect of angiotensin converting enzyme inhibition remain undetermined. Phosphodiesterase inhibitors such as theophylline can also correct posttransplant erythrocytosis.

Because erythrocytosis of any etiology enhances the risks of thromboembolic disease, therapy for posttransplant erythrocytosis is recommended. Standard therapy includes discontinuation of cigarette smoking or diuretic use. While serial phlebotomy has been the recognized standard of care, most transplant centers now use low-dose ACE inhibitor therapy to successfully manage posttransplant erythrocytosis.

PLATELET DYSFUNCTION IN UREMIA

In the uremia patient, a bleeding diathesis is a major cause of morbidity and mortality. Both acute and chronic renal failure are associated with an increased frequency of bleeding complications, including gastrointestinal hemorrhage, bleeding from surgical sites, and mucocutaneous bleeding. Clinical bleeding in patients with uremia is due to an acquired qualitative platelet defect and has best been correlated with a prolonged bleeding time. At present, however, there is no single unifying pathogenetic mechanism to explain the acquired platelet dysfunction seen in patients with uremia.

Uremic platelet dysfunction is considered to be a multifactorial disorder. Defects in in vitro platelet aggregability, diminished thromboxane-A_2 production, abnormal intracellular calcium mobilization, and increased intracellular cAMP have all been described in uremic platelets. Several studies have emphasized a defect in platelet adhesion to vascular subendothelium in uremic patients. Platelet adhesion to vascular subendothelium is the initiating step in forming a platelet plug and thus is critical to achieving hemostasis. Platelet adhesiveness to subendothelium depends on the cooperative interactions of platelet glycoproteins with von Willebrand's factor in the vascular wall. Several studies have identified abnormal platelet glycoprotein function in hemodialysis patients. There is conflicting data as to whether patients with uremia have decreased von Willebrand factor activity. Several recent studies have emphasized that uremia may be associated with increased release of both prostacyclin and nitric oxide—both of which inhibit adhesion of platelets to endothelium.

The clinical bleeding tendency of patients with renal failure is generally improved by dialysis. Therefore, uremic toxins have been implicated as important mediators of the bleeding diathesis. However, the search for specific uremic toxins that interfere with primary hemostasis has not been conclusive. Furthermore, the general experience has been that dialysis only incompletely corrects the prolonged bleeding time, and, in some cases, may actually transiently worsen the bleeding diathesis.

The synthetic vasopressin derivative desmopressin (DDAVP) has been shown to shorten the bleeding time rapidly and improve clinical bleeding in uremia. The mechanism of action of DDAVP is thought to be related to release of large multimeric von Willebrand's factor complexes from endothelial cells and platelets, although this has not been conclusively demonstrated. A limitation to DDAVP therapy is the development of tachyphylaxis after two to three doses. Other therapeutic approaches have included the administration of cryoprecipitate or conjugated estrogens (Table 2). As with DDAVP, the mechanism of action of these agents is thought to be related either to release of large von Willebrand's factor multimers or to endothelial functional changes. Unfortunately, all of these agents have variable clinical efficacy in uremia.

In anemic patients, increasing the hematocrit to above 30, either via packed red blood cell transfusions or the use of high dose erythropoietin, has improved the bleeding time in most patients. While the primary pathogenetic mechanism of increasing the hematocrit in improving the bleeding time may be rheological, additional evidence suggests that increasing hemoglobin concentration may inactivate the platelet inhibiting effects of nitric oxide.

LEUKOCYTE DYSFUNCTION IN UREMIA

Infection remains a major cause of morbidity and mortality in the dialysis patient. Most infections in chronic hemodialysis patients are due to common catalase-producing bacteria rather than to opportunistic organisms. Vascular access infections, particularly with staphylococcus species, remain the leading source of serious infection in hemodialysis patients. The pattern of infectious organisms in chronic dialysis patients is similar to patients with chronic granulomatous disease who lack the phagocytic cell capability to produce reactive oxygen species.

The number and morphology of granulocytes in patients with uremia are normal except for a tendency toward hypersegmentation in some patients. Numerous studies in patients with uremia or on chronic dialysis have documented alterations in granulocyte function, including defects in chemotaxis, granulocyte adherence, phagocytic capability, and reactive oxygen species production.

In addition to the changes in granulocyte function associated with uremia, it is now well documented that hemodialysis with unmodified cellulosic membranes results in complement-mediated granulocyte activation and subsequent dysfunction. Changes in granulocyte function as a

TABLE 2
Treatment of Uremic Platelet Dysfunction

Therapy	Dose or goal	Onset	Duration	Comment
Increase hematocrit (EPO, RBC transfusion)	>30	Immediate	Prolonged	Highly effective
DDAVP	0.3 µg/kg iv	Immediate	4–8 hr	Rapid tachyphylaxis
Cryoprecipitate	10 U	1–4 hr	24 hr	Hepatitis, HIV risk
Conjugated estrogens	0.6 mg · kg^{-1} · day^{-1} × 5 days	6 hr	14 days	Hot flashes, HTN, abnormal LFTs

Note: HTN, hypertension; LFT, liver function test.

consequence of dialysis with cellulosic membranes include modulation of chemotactic receptors, changes in granulocyte reactive oxygen species production, alterations in granulocyte adherence and alterations in granulocyte expression of cell adhesion molecules. A recent cohort study using the USRDS database has demonstrated a correlation between the use of unmodified cellulosic dialysis membranes and the risk of mortality due to infection in chronic hemodialysis patients.

Changes in monocyte function as well as a reduction in number and function of lymphocytes in patients with uremia lead to altered immunity in this patient population. Evidence of altered immunity includes alterations in T cell-dependent humoral responses such as reduced responsiveness to vaccinations, diminished delayed hypersensitivity responses, and a dramatic attenuation of autoimmune disease activity with uremia. Recent data have suggested that the chronic use of unmodified cellulosic dialysis membranes may also exacerbate the underlying defect in immunity in patients with uremia.

Bibliography

Beusterien KM, Nissenson AR, Port FK, Kelly M, Steinwald B, Ware JE: The effects of recombinant human erythropoietin on functional health and well-being in chronic dialysis patients. *J Am Soc Nephrol* 7:763–773, 1996.

Cheung AK: Biocompatibility of hemodialysis membranes. *J Am Soc Nephrol* 1:150–161, 1990.

Churchill DN, Muirhead N, Goldstein M, et al.: Effect of recombinant human erythropoietin on hospitalization of hemodialysis patients. *Clin Nephrol* 43(3):184–188, 1995.

Erslev AJ: Erythropoietin. *N Engl J Med* 324(19):1339–1343, 1991.

Eschbach JW, Egrie JC, Downing MR, Browne JK, Adamson JW: Correction of the anemia of end-stage renal disease with recombinant human erythropoietin: Results of a combined phase I and II clinical trial. *N Engl J Med* 316:73-78, 1987.

Eschbach JW, Kelly MR, Haley NR, Abels RI, Adamson JW: Treatment of the anemia of progressive renal failure with recombinant human erythropoietin. *N Engl J Med* 321:158–163, 1989.

Eschbach JW: The anemia of chronic renal failure: Pathophysiology and the effects of recombinant erythropoietin. *Kidney Int* 35:134–148, 1989.

Eschbach JW, Haley NR, Egrie JC, Adamson JW: A comparison of the responses to recombinant human erythropoietin in normal and uremic subjects. *Kidney Int* 42:407–416, 1992.

Fishbane S, Frei GL, Maesaka J: Reduction in recombinant human erythropoietin doses by the use of chronic intravenous iron supplementation. *Am J Kidney Dis* 26(1):41–46, 1995.

Fishbane S, Maesaka JK: Iron management in end-stage renal disease. *Am J Kidney Dis* 29:319–333, 1997.

Foley RN, Parfrey PS, Harnett JD, Kent GM, Murray DC, Barre PE: The impact of anemia on cardiomyopathy, morbidity, and mortality in end-stage renal disease. *Am J Kidney Dis* 28(1):53–61, 1996.

Goldblum SE, Reed WP: Host defenses and immunologic alterations associated with chronic hemodialysis. *Ann Intern Med* 93:597–613, 1980.

Hakim RM, Lazarus JM: Biochemical parameters in chronic renal failure. *Am J Kidney Dis* XI(3):238–247, 1988.

Himmelfarb J, Hakim RM: Biocompatibility and risk of infection in haemodialysis patients. *Nephrol Dial Transplant* 9(Suppl 2):138–144, 1994.

Lewis SL, Van Epps DE: Neutrophil and monocyte alterations in chronic dialysis patients. *Am J Kidney Dis* 9:381-395, 1987.

Powe NR, Griffiths RI, Watson AJ, et al.: Effect of recombinant erythropoietin on hospital admissions, readmissions, length of stay, and costs of dialysis patients. *J Am Soc Nephrol* 4:1455–1465, 1994.

Ratcliffe PJ: Molecular biology of erythropoietin. *Kidney Int* 44:887–904, 1993.

Steiner RW, Coggins C, Carvalho CA: Bleeding time in uremia: A useful test to assess clinical bleeding. *Am J Hematol* 7:107–117, 1979

Vigano G, Remuzzi G: Bleeding time in uremia. *Semin Dialysis* 9(1):34–38, 1996.

73

ENDOCRINE MANIFESTATIONS OF RENAL FAILURE

EUGENE C. KOVALIK

Chronic renal failure (CRF), end stage renal disease (ESRD), and renal transplantation all have effects on the endocrine system. The effects are related to alterations in feedback mechanisms, hormone production, transport, metabolism, and elimination, hormone binding, and drug interactions (Tables 1 and 2). Diagnosis of endocrine disease in renal patients must take into account these effects in order to ensure proper treatment, when needed. Alterations of bone and mineral metabolism and erythropoiesis are discussed elsewhere and will not be covered in this chapter. Through a mechanism that is not understood, erythropoietin, ameliorates many of the endocrine abnormalities seen in CRF, as discussed below.

HYPOTHALAMIC-HYPOPHYSEAL AXES

Thyroid

Thyroid abnormalities have been well documented in renal patients. Up to 58% of uremic patients may have evidence of a goiter by palpation, thought to be due to some unknown circulating goitrogen when glomerular filtration rate (GFR) falls. Total thyroxine (T_4) is either normal or decreased and triiodothyronine (T_3) levels are depressed. Free T_4 levels may be low. The use of reverse T_3 (rT_3) to differentiate between hypothyroid states and so-called "euthyroid sick" state is not useful in patients with CRF. Although binding globulin levels are normal, circulating inhibitors result in decreased binding and interfere with the older resin uptake-based tests of thyroid function. These abnormalities tend to worsen the longer the patient is on dialysis. Thyroid stimulating hormone (TSH) tends to be normal despite the abnormalities in thyroid hormone levels, and is perhaps the best indicator of thyroid function, especially with the availability of ultrasensitive TSH assays. Basal metabolic rate is also normal. The differences in thyroid function between hemodialysis and patients on continuous ambulatory hemodialysis are inconsistent.

Although TSH levels are normal in patients with CRF, abnormalities exist in the hypothalamic-hypophyseal axes. Exogenous thyrotropin stimulating hormone (TRH) stimulation results in a blunted TSH response. The usual midnight TSH surge is absent. TSH administration results in

an increase in T_3 levels, but not in the expected increase in T_4. It has been postulated that two different problems occur in patients with CRF. First, there is an inappropriate response to decreased thyroid hormone levels due to a reset in the normal feedback loop with a lower level of TSH secretion for a given level of thyroid hormone. Second, thyroid gland resistance to TSH also occurs. The use of recombinant erythropoietin normalizes the TSH response to TRH but not the thyroid response to TSH.

Studies have suggested that the impaired thyroid axis may play a role in protecting the body by maintaining a positive nitrogen balance in the setting of the uremic state. After renal transplantation, thyroid function tests normalize, although some patients may still have an abnormal TSH response to TRH due to glucocorticoid suppression of TSH secretion.

Growth Hormone

Plasma growth hormone (GH) levels are elevated in patients with CRF. This is partly due to both increased secretion and impaired clearance of the hormone, although there seems to be no clinical significance. Insulin-like growth factor (IGF) levels are normal. Dynamic testing of the GH axis does show abnormalities. Oral glucose loading does not suppress GH levels, whereas intravenous glucose or glucagon or TRH paradoxically increase GH levels. Insulin-induced hypoglycemia does not stimulate GH secretion. Growth hormone releasing hormone (GHRH) and L-dopa infusions also cause a prolonged and exaggerated response in GH secretion. Correction of anemia with erythropoietin corrects the paradoxical response to TRH and insulin-induced hypoglycemia, although the prolonged GHRH response remains.

In children, uremia results in growth retardation despite normal or elevated GH and IGF levels. The cause is multifactorial and is thought to include protein malnutrition, chronic acidosis, recurrent infections, hyperparathyroidism, and decreased bioactive IGF. The assurance of adequate nutrition, dialysis, and correction of acidosis and hyperparathyroidism allows for improved growth. The use of recombinant human growth hormone has greatly improved the well-being of children with CRF, restoring growth velocity and increasing muscle mass without ad-

TABLE I

Pathogenetic Mechanisms of Endocrine Dysfunction in Chronic Renal Failure[a]

Increased circulating hormone levels
 Impaired renal or extrarenal clearance (e.g., insulin, glucagon, PTH, calcitonin, prolactin)
 Increased secretion (e.g., PTH, aldosterone?)
 Accumulation of immunoassayable hormone fractions that may lack bioactivity (e.g., glucagon, PTH, calcitonin, prolactin)
Decreased circulating hormone levels
 Decreased secretion by diseased kidney (e.g., erythropoietin, renin, 1,25-dihydroxyvitamin D_3)
 Decreased secretion by other endocrine glands (e.g., testosterone, estrogen, progesterone)
Decreased sensitivity to hormones
 Altered target tissue response (e.g., insulin, glucagon, 1,25-dihydroxyvitamin D_3, erythropoietin, PTH)

Note: PTH, parathyroid hormone.
[a] From Mooradian AD: In: Becker KL (ed) Principles and Practice of Endocrinology and Metabolism. Lippincott Company, Philadelphia, p. 1759, 1995. With permisssion

TABLE 2

Directional Changes of Hormones in CRF[a]

Hypothalamopituitary axis
 GH ↑ prolactin ↑
Thyroid
 TT_4 N or ↓, FT_4 N or ↓
 TT_3 ↓, FT_3 ↓, rT_3 N, TSH N
Gonads
 Testosterone ↓, spermatogenesis ↓
 Estrogen N or ↓, progesterone ↓
 LH N or ↑, FSH N
Pancreas
 Insulin ↑, glucagon ↑
Adrenals
 Aldosterone N or ↓, cortisol N or ↑, ACTH N or ↑
 Catecholamine N or ↑
Kidney
 EPO ↓, renin ↓, 1,25 Vit D_3 ↓

[a] From Lim VS: In: Greenberg A (ed) Primer on Kidney Diseases. Academic Press, San Diego, p. 315, 1994. With permission.

versely affecting bone age over chronological age. The fact that renal transplantation in children does not by itself reverse the abnormal growth patterns of the children is likely due to the effects of glucocorticoids. European data suggest return of growth after transplantation with the use of recombinant human growth hormone, although its use is not yet approved in the United States for pediatric patients post renal transplant.

Prolactin

Secretion normally is under inhibition via prolactin inhibitory factor (PIF), which in turn is controlled by catacholamines via dopaminergic fibers. Basal levels of prolactin are elevated up to six times normal in patients with CRF. Many medications that have antidopaminergic effects may contribute to the increased levels. The major effects of increased prolactin levels are reflected in the reproductive system of CRF patients with gynecomastia, impotence, and amenorrhea. Bromocriptine can reduce prolactin levels but its effectiveness in relieving symptoms has not been well proven, and side effects usually lead to discontinuation of therapy in one third of patients. Again, erythropoietin therapy can normalize prolactin levels and can improve sexual dysfunction in men and menstrual regularity in women, but it does not correct the abnormal hypophyseal response to TRH administration.

Any medications that can affect prolactin levels should be minimized or avoided if possible (i.e., α-methyldopa, phenothiazines, neuroleptics, metaclopramide, cisapride and H_2-blockers, and especially cimetidine), particularly if gynecomastia becomes painful or cosmetically displeasing for male patients, even though the pathogenesis of gynecomastia may be more related to an increased estrogen to androgen ratio as seen in pubertal gynecomastia in males.

Mammography should be performed since breast cancer does also occur in men. Alternative therapies for gynecomastia include subcutaneous mastectomies or breast bud irradiation.

Glucocorticoids

Patients with CRF exhibit normal to elevated levels of adrenocorticotropin hormone (ACTH). In various studies, ACTH response to corticotropin releasing hormone (CRH) has been observed to be blunted or normal. Correction of anemia with erythropoietin can lead to an exaggerated ACTH response to CRH. The standard ACTH stimulation test for diagnosing hypocortisolism is not affected by the uremic state.

Basal cortisol levels in CRF patients are normal although some assays may show elevated results. The reason for this discrepancy is that cortisol metabolites are primarily removed by glomerular filtration; the accumulation of glucoronidated metabolites can lead to cross-reactivity with the antibody in some assay kits. Assays which extract metabolites prior to the radioimmunoassay or chromatography can overcome the problem and consultation with the laboratory performing the test is important. Circadian rhythm of cortisol secretion remains intact. Because of the elevated levels of metabolites (conjugated 17-hydroxycorticosteroids), the negative feedback loop is altered. The usual low dose 1 mg overnight or 2 day dexamethasone suppression tests used to evaluate hypercortisolism do not suppress patients with CRF due in part to decreased oral absorption of the hormone and the altered set point of the axis. The 1 mg intravenous or 8 mg high dose overnight dexamethasone test will suppress cortisol levels in CRF patients. Although insulin-induced hypoglycemia fails to raise serum cortisol levels, the response to major stress, such as surgery, remains preserved.

Gonadotropins

Males

Loss of libido, impotence, testicular atrophy, gynecomastia, and infertility may occur in males with CRF. Testosterone is decreased, with elevated luteinizing hormone (LH) and follicle stimulating hormone (FSH) levels. Testosterone-binding globulin levels are normal. Testicular biopsy reveals abnormal sperm maturation. Prolonged stimulation with human chorionic gonadotropin (HCG) can result in increased testosterone levels, suggesting some testicular reserve. Administration of luteinizing hormone releasing hormone (LHRH) results in a normal, blunted, or an exaggerated, prolonged response. Thus it appears that both a central hypothalamic and peripheral testicular problem exist in men with CRF. Treatment with erythropoietin can improve symptomatology without actually affecting testosterone levels. Zinc deficiency has also been thought to contribute to the problem, although replacement therapy has yielded varying results. Transplantation reverses the problems; however, in some men, the hypogonadism may worsen due to the side effects of immunosuppressive therapy.

Impotence may also be related to neuropathies or vasculopathies. Drugs that may contribute (such as β-blockers) should be discontinued or their dose reduced. Unfortunately, many patients may have to resort to penile implants, cavernous injections (due to their vasoconstrictor effects, these drugs should be used with caution in severely hypertensive patients), or vacuum erector devices to resolve their problem. Table 3 outlines an approach to the male patient once medications have been modified. If testosterone levels are in the low normal range, a trial of replacement therapy can be undertaken.

Female

Women with CRF may also have impaired libido or inability to achieve orgasms. Approximately half of women on dialysis become amenorrheic, and those who still have menses find their periods progressively irregular and anovulatory as renal failure progresses. Only 10% or less of women on dialysis have regular menses. FSH levels are normal with mildly elevated LH, resulting in an increased LH : FSH ratio, similar to prepubertal patterns, with a defect in the positive hypothalamic feedback mechanism in response to estrogen. This lack of positive feedback results in the failure of the mid-cycle LH and FSH surge to occur and hence, anovulation. Estradiol, estrone, progesterone, and testosterone levels are normal to low. Unlike premenopausal women, postmenopausal women have the expected increases in both LH and FSH. Hyperprolactinemia may also contribute to some of the abnormalities. Despite these problems, women who have some residual renal function and who are well dialyzed can, on rare occasions, become pregnant and carry to term, although the fetus tends to be premature and small for gestational age (see Chapter 60).

TABLE 3

Management of Sexual Dysfunction in Patients with Chronic Renal Insufficiency[a]

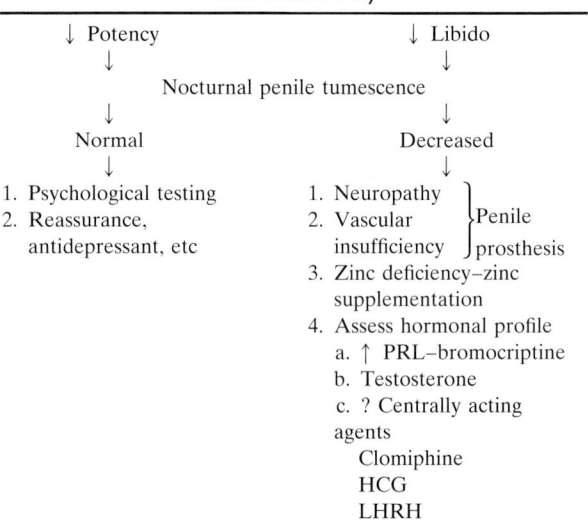

Note: PRL, serum prolactin; HCG, human chorionic gonadotropin; LHRH, luteinizing hormone releasing hormone.
[a] From Lim VS: *Am J Kidney Dis* 9(4):365, 1987. With permission.

The use of estrogen replacement therapy to decrease bone loss and cardiovascular risk in premenopausal CRF women has not been investigated.

Transplantation rapidly restores fertility to premenopausal women. Ovulation can start within 1 month of transplantation. Appropriate counseling should be undertaken to stress the need for contraception. Current guidelines call for women who wish to become pregnant to wait 2 years with stable graft function (creatinine under 1.8 mg/dL), to be on minimal immunosuppressant therapy, and to have easily controlled blood pressure. There are no good data on the use of oral contraceptives in the transplant patient group. Referral to a gynecologist should be made if this mode of contraception is considered, due to the possibility of thromboembolic disease. Blood pressure should be monitored carefully.

CARBOHYDRATE METABOLISM

Patients with CRF and uremia can develop what has been termed "pseudodiabetes." This condition results from a combination of peripheral resistance to insulin, circulating inhibitors, and abnormal islet cell release. The defect can be corrected with dialysis therapy. In contrast, diabetics with CRF often find that their need for oral hypoglycemic agents or insulin decreases due to reduced insulin clearance by the kidney. In the case of non–insulin-dependent diabetes mellitus (NIDDM), where the problem is mostly due to peripheral insulin resistance, endogenous insulin half life is prolonged, resulting in a decreased or eliminated need for medication. In addition, the decreased clearance of oral hypoglycemic agents (primarily first-generation sulfonylureas) can lead to prolonged hypoglycemia. Agents that are primarily hepatically metabolized such as second-generation sulfonylureas or insulin, should be used to treat NIDDM patients. Metformin is contraindicated in patients with CRF due to the increased risk of lactic acidosis. Patients with insulin-dependent diabetes mellitus (IDDM) may need their insulin dose reduced, but never discontinued since the underlying problem is a lack of endogenous insulin production. Glycemic control can worsen in peritoneal dialysis patients due to the glucose load absorbed from the peritoneal dialysis fluid. Intraperitoneal insulin administration, based on a sliding scale, may facilitate management.

Spontaneous hypoglycemia can occur in CRF patients due to malnutrition and impaired glycogenolysis. Although many CRF patients have glucose intolerance, fasting hyperglycemia with glucose values above 140 mg/dL suggests frank diabetes mellitus. Glycosylated hemoglobin values may underestimate the degree of hyperglycemia due to the shortened erythrocyte life span seen in uremia.

Transplantation often reveals an underlying abnormality of glucose metabolism in many patients due to the high doses of steroids used for immunosupression. Patients not previously thought to be diabetic can develop diabetes mellitus and require insulin therapy, whereas those already diabetic may require conversion from an oral hypoglycemic agent to insulin or large increases in their insulin doses due to steroid-induced peripheral resistance to insulin action.

MINERALOCORTICOIDS

Due to the progressive loss of renal tissue with CRF, renin production is decreased with either normal to low aldosterone levels. The renin-angiotensin-aldosterone response to volume contraction or hypotension is blunted. With low renin levels, hyperkalemia becomes the most important stimulus for aldosterone secretion. Aldosterone in turn stimulates colonic loss of potassium, an often overlooked means of potassium removal in CRF patients.

ADRENAL MEDULLA

Basal levels of catecholamines in CRF and dialysis patients are elevated. The cause is multi-factorial: decreased degradation, decreased neuronal uptake, and impaired renal clearance of metabolites. Hemodialysis treatments do remove catecholamines but this is not the reason for intradialytic hypotension. Because of the aforementioned problems, the diagnosis of pheochromocytoma is difficult in patients with CRF. Suppression testing has not been validated in this setting. The combination of high levels of catecholamines and appropriate radiologic studies should be used together to make the diagnosis.

LIPID ABNORMALITIES

Patients with CRF infrequently have hypercholesterolemia or elevated levels of low-density lipoprotein (LDL), but hypertriglyceridemia is observed in half of these pa-

tients. Low levels of high-density lipoprotein (HDL) are also common. Nephrotic patients are an exception; they have elevated levels of all lipid fractions. Heparin administration during hemodialysis causes release of both hepatic and lipoprotein lipase, resulting in a depletion of stores and worsening of triglyceride levels, particularly of triglyceride rich remnants that are highly atherogenic. Studies of lipoprotein a [Lp(a)] levels show variable results.

Until further data are available, treatment of lipid disorders in CRF and dialysis patients should follow general guidelines used in non renal failure patients. Patients with elevated LDL levels should be started on diet therapy and then advanced to pharmacologic therapy. Bile acid resins such as cholestyramine and cholestipol should be avoided since they can increase TG levels. Fibric acid derivatives such as gemfibrozil are relatively contraindicated in CRF patients because they are cleared primarily by the kidney and accumulation increases the risk of rhabdomyolysis. The safest agents are the HMG-CoA reductase inhibitors. They are particularly useful in nephrotic patients to decrease LDL levels and reduce cardiovascular risk. High doses may increase the risk of myalgias and rhabdomyolysis and require close patient follow-up. Because of its many side effects, nicotinic acid, is not a good lipid-lowering agent in the CRF population, and experience with its use is limited. Data on the use of probucol are lacking.

Recent studies have demonstrated the possible protective effects of vitamin E and folic acid in cardiac patients with normal renal function. Studies also suggest that elevated LDL levels, particularly oxidized LDL, can hasten the progression of CRF to ESRD. Since the mechanism of action of these agents is either to serve as antioxidants (in the case of the former) or to reduce homocysteine levels (in the case of the latter), they should be safe to use in the CRF population as a means to reduce cardiac risk and theoretically to slow the progression of renal disease. Although vitamin C also acts as an antioxidant, its clearance is reduced in CRF, because it can lead to hyperoxalemia or hyperoxaluria and renal calcification, it should not be used.

Renal transplant patients should be considered separately from other CRF patients when it come to lipid abnormalities. Since cardiovascular disease is the major cause of death in the transplant population (as is the case for dialysis patients), every effort should be made to reduce risk factors. Total cholesterol, TG, LDL, oxidized LDL, and Lp(a) levels are elevated, whereas HDL levels are variable. In addition to the increased cardiac risk of post-transplant lipid abnormalities, some evidence suggests that hyperlipidemia may also contribute to chronic graft rejection.

Treatment of lipid abnormalities in transplant patients is similar to that of CRF patients. Bile resin binders should be avoided because they interfere with cyclosporine absorption. Gemfibrozil use is associated with an increased risk of rhabdomyolysis. HMG-CoA reductase inhibitors (lovastatin, simvastatin, and pravastatin have been used successfully in studies on transplant patients). But again, higher doses should be used with caution. Simvastatin and pravastatin have been employed in several studies, without any major side effects. At least one study has shown a reduction in acute rejection episodes using pravastatin. The use of vitamin E, vitamin C, and folic acid has not been investigated.

Bibliography

Deck KA, Fischer B, Hillen H: Studies on cortisol metabolism during hemodialysis. *Eur J Clin Invest* 9:203–207, 1979.

Ferraris JR, Domene HM, Escobar ME, et al.: Hormonal profile in pubertal females with chronic renal failure: Before and under haemodialysis and after renal transplantation. *Acta Endocrinologica (Copenh)* 115:289–296, 1987.

Fine RN: Growth hormone and the kidney: The use of recombinant human growth hormone (rhGH) in growth-retarded children with chronic renal insufficiency. *Jo Am Soc Nephrol* 1:1136–1145, 1991.

Grundy SM: Management of hyperlipidemia of kidney disease. *Kidney Int* 37:847–853, 1990.

Holdsworth S, Atkins RC, Kretser DM: The pituitary-testicular axis in men with chronic renal failure. *N Engl J Med* 296(22):1245–1249, 1977.

Jones DC, Hayslett JP: Outcome of pregnancy in women with moderate or severe renal insufficiency. *N Engl J Med* 335(4):226–232, 1996.

Katznelson S, Wilkinson AH, Kobashigawa et al.: The effect of pravastatin on acute rejection after kidney transplantation—A pilot study. *Transplantation* 61(10):1469–1474, 1996.

Kokot F, Wiecek A, Grzeszczak W, et al.: Influence of erythropoietin treatment on function of the pituitary-adrenal axis and somatotropin secretion in hemodialyzed patients. *Clin Nephrol* 33(5):241–246, 1990.

Lim VS, Henriquez C, Sievertsen G, et al.: Ovarian function in chronic renal failure: Evidence suggesting hypothalamic anovulation. *Ann Intern Med* 93(Part 1):21–27, 1980.

Lim VS, Flanigan MJ, Zavala DC, et al.: Protective adaptation of low serum triiodothyronine in patients with chronic renal failure. *Kidney Int* 28:541–549, 1985.

Lim VS: Reproductive function in patients with renal insufficiency. *Am J Kidney Dis* 9(4):363–367, 1987.

Massey ZA, Kasiske BL: Post-transplant hyperlipidemia: Mechanisms and management. *J Am Soc Nephrol* 7:971–977, 1996.

Mooradian AD: Endocrine dysfunction due to renal disease. In: Becker KL (ed) *Principles and Practice of Endocrinology and Metabolism*. Lippincott, Philadelphia, pp. 1759–1762, 1995.

Ramirez G, Jubiz W, Gutch CF, et al.: Thyroid abnormalities in renal failure: A study of 53 patients on chronic hemodialysis. *Ann Intern Med* 79:500–504, 1973.

Ramirez G, O'Neill WM, Bloomer HA, et al.: Abnormalities in the regulation of Growth Hormone in Chronic Renal Failure. *Arch Intern Med* 138:267–271, 1978.

Ramirez G, Gomez-Sanchez C, Meikle WA, et al.: Evaluation of the hypothalamic hypophyseal adrenal axis in patients receiving long-term hemodialysis. *Arch Intern Med* 142:1448–1452, 1982.

Ramirez G, Butcher DE, Newton JL, et al.: Bromocriptine and the hypothalamic hypophyseal function in patients with chronic renal failure on chronic hemodialysis. *Am J Kidne Dis* 6(2):111–118, 1985.

Ramirez G: Abnormalities in the hypothalamic-hypophyseal axes in patients with chronic renal failure. *Semin Dialysis* 7(2):138–146, 1994.

Schaefer RM, Kokot F, Geiger H, et al.: Improved sexual function in hemodialysis patients on recombinant erythropoietin: A possible role for prolactin. *Clin Nephrol* 31(1):1–5, 1989.

Spitalewitz S, Porush JG, Cattran D, et al.: Treatment of hyperlipidemia in the nephrotic syndrome: The effects of pravastatin therapy. *Am J Kidney Dis* 22(1):143–150, 1993.

74

THE EVALUATION OF PROSPECTIVE RENAL TRANSPLANT RECIPIENTS

BERTRAM L. KASISKE

TIMING OF TRANSPLANTATION

Once it is certain that a patient has end stage renal disease (ESRD) and is likely to be a transplant candidate, consideration should be given to the optimal timing of transplantation. Although every attempt should be made to maximize the benefit that patients receive from their native kidneys, it is sometimes possible to perform preemptive transplantation before initiating maintenance dialysis. In such cases, the morbidity and expense of acquiring a permanent dialysis access and undergoing dialysis initiation may be avoided. Since the median waiting time for cadaveric kidneys in the United States is now 24 months, preemptive transplantation is usually only possible for recipients with living donors. Prior to acceptance for transplantation, a careful evaluation should determine if the patient is prepared not only for immunosuppression and its consequences, but also for the surgical procedure itself.

INITIAL ASSESSMENT

The evaluation should begin with a brief history and physical examination so that obvious contraindications to transplantation can obviate the need for other expensive or invasive tests. The history and physical examination should give the transplant team an indication of the overall well-being of the recipient. There is no absolute age that precludes transplantation, but physiologic age and overall health status should be carefully considered in individuals older than age 60. Patients should also be screened for severe pulmonary disease, which might greatly increase the risk of surgery. Obesity per se is rarely a contraindication to transplantation, but obesity increases morbidity and may increase the rate of graft failure. Therefore, weight reduction should be attempted prior to transplantation. Baseline laboratory evaluation should include a complete blood count with differential, routine serum chemistries, and a lipoprotein profile.

Patients with diabetes require special consideration. Cardiovascular complications are particularly common among diabetics, and may greatly increase the risk of transplant surgery (see below). In addition, some diabetic patients may be candidates for simultaneous pancreas-kidney (SPK) transplantation. There are no controlled clinical trials showing SPK to reduce the long-term complications of diabetes compared to kidney transplantation alone. Poor blood glucose control remains the sole indication for SPK. Patients should be informed that, compared to kidney transplantation alone, there is increased surgical morbidity and an increased risk of renal allograft rejection with SPK compared to kidney transplantation alone. Most agree that a diabetic with a potential living donor should undergo kidney transplantation without a pancreas.

SCREENING PROCEDURES

Cancer

It is generally accepted that immunosuppression may favor the growth of malignant tumors, and an active malignancy is usually an absolute contraindication to transplantation. Exceptions may be locally invasive basal or squamous cell skin carcinomas. All patients should undergo routine screening with a physical examination, chest radiograph, and stool hemoccult. Older individuals should also have flexible sigmoidoscopy. Women should have had recent mammography, a pelvic examination, and a pap smear.

Although immunosuppression may increase the risk of cancer recurrence, it is not justified to deny transplantation to a patient who has had a tumor that was cured. Data from registries, although imperfect, provide some guidance on the chances of recurrence of different malignant tumors. In general, registry data suggest that a patient who has been free from all evidence of malignancy for 2 years has about a 47% chance of recurrence after renal transplantation. Although a 5-year waiting period would reduce this to 13%, it is probably unreasonable to demand that all patients wait 5 years. Individual tumors behave differently, and guidelines address how different tumors in potential transplant candidates should be approached.

Infections

Immunosuppression greatly increases the risk for life-threatening infections. Immunizations for influenza, pneumococcus, and hepatitis B should be mandatory. Although the effectiveness of these vaccinations is not well documented in large numbers of patients with ESRD, potential benefits outweigh negligible risks. Patients should also be carefully screened for infections that may become problematic with immunosuppression. Sites of occult infection include the lung, urinary tract, and dialysis access catheters. Dialysis-related peritonitis within 3 to 4 weeks is a relative contraindication to transplantation. Patients should be screened for human immunodeficiency virus (HIV). Although occasional HIV patients may have a prolonged, disease-free interval after transplantation, an even greater number will die within 6 months of surgery. Therefore, the current practice in the United States is to avoid transplantations in HIV-positive patients.

Tuberculosis is common in the ESRD population, and may be asymptomatic. Screening should include a high index of suspicion, a chest radiograph, and a purified protein derivative (PPD) skin test (unless there is already a history of a positive skin test). High-risk individuals should receive prophylactic therapy. High-risk individuals are those: (1) with a past history of active disease; (2) from a high-risk population, and (3) with an abnormal chest radiograph consistent with active or inactive tuberculosis. It is less clear whether any PPD-positive individuals who have no evidence of tuberculosis or other risk factors should receive prophylaxis.

Although cytomegalovirus (CMV) infection is common and is commonly transmitted with the transplanted organ, the presence or absence of CMV antibodies in donors and recipients should not preclude transplantation. Some centers routinely use prophylactic therapy with hyperimmune globulin, ganciclovir, or acyclovir for recipients of kidneys from CMV-seropositive donors. Potential recipients who are seronegative for the varicella-zoster virus are at risk for disseminated infection, and should be identified before transplantation. Patients from tropical regions should be screened for *Strongyloides stercolaris*. Viral hepatitis should also be considered in the pretransplant evaluation (see below).

RECURRENT RENAL DISEASE RISK

Although renal disease frequently recurs in the transplant recipient, the threat of recurrent renal disease is rarely a contraindication to transplantation. Estimated rates of clinically evident renal disease recurrences are: systemic lupus erythematosus (1%), hemolytic uremic syndrome (10 to 25%), Henoch-Schönlein purpura (10%), mixed essential cryoglobulinemia (50%), Waldenström's macroglobulinemia (10 to 25%), light chain deposition disease and fibrillary glomerulonephritis (50%), amyloidosis (20 to 30%), antiglomerular basement membrane disease (25%), Wegener's granulomatosis (rare), scleroderma (20%), IgA nephropathy (10%), membranoproliferative glomerulonephritis (MPGN) type 1 (20 to 30%), MPGN type 2 (80%), membranous nephropathy (10 to 25%), and focal segmental glomerulosclerosis (FSGS; 10 to 30%). Patients who have already lost one allograft to recurrent FSGS have a 40 to 50% chance of losing another. Patients with primary oxalosis (once thought to be an absolute contraindication to transplantation) should be considered for preemptive transplantation with aggressive orthophosphate and pyridoxine therapy, and possibly liver transplantation to provide a source of the deficient enzyme. Although diabetic nephropathy often recurs in the allograft, the rate of progression is generally slow enough to make this an unusual cause of graft failure. One-year graft survival in patients with sickle cell nephropathy has been reported to be as low as 25% or as high as 67%. Finally, patients with Alport's syndrome have a small chance of developing antiglomerular basement membrane disease after transplantation, but this risk should not preclude transplantation.

LIVER DISEASE

Liver failure is a major cause of morbidity and mortality after renal transplantation, and transplant candidates should be carefully screened for liver disease. The A and E viruses are not known to cause chronic liver disease in transplant recipients, while hepatitis B virus (HBV) and hepatitis C virus (HCV) are common causes of chronic active hepatitis post-transplant. Transplant recipients who are hepatitis B surface antigen (HBsAg) positive are at increased risk of dying in the post-transplant period; however, HBsAg per se is not a contraindication to transplantation. Patients who are HBsAg positive and have serologic evidence of viral replication should probably forego transplantation. Likewise, HBsAg positive patients who also have hepatitis D (fortunately rare) develop severe liver disease and should not receive a transplant. Otherwise, HBsAg positive patients with elevated liver enzymes should probably undergo biopsy, and those with chronic active hepatitis may wish to stay on dialysis due to the increased risk of disease progression with immunosuppression. Fortunately, the incidence of HBV is declining in the ESRD population, mainly due to the use of an effective vaccination. Certainly, patients who do not have liver disease and who are HBsAg negative should receive vaccination for HBV, if not already immunized.

Although the natural history of HCV liver disease is less well defined, patients who are HCV antibody positive should probably undergo liver biopsy if enzymes are elevated. HCV positive patients with evidence of viral replication and/or chronic active hepatitis on biopsy are probably at increased risk for progressive liver disease after transplantation. Antiviral therapy (interferon-α) has been used in an attempt to induce a remission in ESRD patients with HBV or HCV viral hepatitis, and thereby allow renal transplantation. Although the long-term results of antiviral therapy in patients with ESRD are unclear, the number of patients who remain in remission after such therapy appears to be small.

CARDIOVASCULAR DISEASE

Ischemic heart disease (IHD) is a major cause of death after renal transplantation. All patients should be evaluated for possible IHD as part of the routine history and physical examination, chest radiography and electrocardiogram. Patients with a history of IHD, or with signs and symptoms suggestive of IHD, should undergo a more thorough evaluation with noninvasive stress testing and/or angiography. Asymptomatic patients with multiple risk factors for IHD should also have noninvasive stress testing. The best noninvasive stress test remains to be defined. However, thallium scintigraphy (with exercise or dipyridamole) and echocardiography (with exercise or dobutamine) may have reasonably high positive and negative predictive values in ESRD patients—a population which has a high prevalence of IHD. Because many ESRD patients may be unable to exercise to achieve the target heart rate needed for a valid exercise stress test, pharmacologic stress testing may be a better choice. Patients with critical coronary artery lesions should undergo revascularization prior to transplantation. All patients should be encouraged to reduce their risk of cardiovascular disease by managing known risk factors. In particular, patients should be encouraged to stop smoking.

CEREBROVASCULAR DISEASE

There is also an increased risk of atherosclerotic cerebral vascular disease complications after renal transplantation. Patients with a history of transient ischemic attacks or other cerebrovascular disease events should be evaluated by a neurologist for possible treatment and should be symptom-free for at least 6 months before surgery. Whether asymptomatic patients should undergo screening with a carotid ultrasound examination is unclear. In the general population, controlled clinical trials have shown that the success of prophylactic carotid endarterectomy is dependent on the center and on the selection of patients. Similarly, whether to treat patients who have asymptomatic carotid bruits with aspirin and risk factor intervention, or to use carotid ultrasound to select individuals for prophylactic endarterectomy is a decision that must be tailored to the patient and the center.

PSYCHOSOCIAL EVALUATION

Transplant candidates should be screened for cognitive or psychological impairments that may interfere with their ability to give informed consent. Failure to adhere to immunosuppressive therapy is a major cause of renal allograft failure, and the psychological assessment should also attempt to identify patients who are at risk. However, reliably identifying patients who will not adhere to therapy is difficult at best, and care should be exercised to avoid unjustifiably refusing transplantation. Most centers require patients with a history of substance abuse to undergo treatment and to demonstrate a period of abstinence prior to transplantation. Major psychiatric disorders are usually apparent during the routine pretransplant evaluation, and appropriate psychiatric care can be sought.

UROLOGIC EVALUATION

Evidence for possible chronic infection and/or incomplete bladder emptying should be sought on history and physical examination. In the absence of such evidence, a routine voiding cystourethrogram is probably not warranted. For patients with a ureteral diversion, every effort should be made to overcome the need for the diversion posttransplant. This can often be achieved surgically, but may sometimes require intermittent bladder self-catheterization. Indications for pretransplant nephrectomy include: (1) reflux associated with chronic infection, (2) polycystic kidneys that are too large to allow placement of the allograft or have infected cysts, (3) severe nephrotic syndrome, (4) nephrolithiasis associated with infection, and (5) renal carcinoma.

GASTROINTESTINAL EVALUATION

Patients with a history of cholecystitis should undergo cholecystectomy, because cholecystitis in an immunocompromised transplant recipient may be more severe, more difficult to diagnose, and more difficult to treat. However, it is less clear whether patients should be routinely screened with ultrasound, and subjected to cholecystectomy for asymptomatic cholelithiasis. Similarly, patients with symptomatic diverticulitis may be considered for partial colectomy; however, whether it is justified to conduct screening and surgery for asymptomatic diverticular disease is less clear, and most centers do not. Peptic ulcer disease is common in the posttransplant period, but can usually be managed medically. Pretransplant evaluation for peptic ulcer disease can probably be reserved for patients with appropriate signs and symptoms.

BLOOD AND TISSUE TYPING

The immunologic evaluation is designed to determine the compatibility of a donor kidney with the recipient. Three major immunologic barriers to transplantation are addressed.

1. Transplants should not cross ABO blood group barriers.
2. The degree of matching at the major histocompatibility (MHC) loci A, B, and particularly DR correlates with long-term graft survival and is used in the United Network for Organ Sharing (UNOS) point system for cadaveric organ allocation (see below).
3. The presence of preformed antibodies and how broadly they react to a random panel of antigens from the general population is directly correlated to the likelihood of a positive crossmatch when an organ becomes available, and is also used in the UNOS kidney allocation scheme.

As a final screen, the recipient's serum is tested against donor tissue, since a positive cross-match indicates the presence of preformed antibodies that can cause hyperacute rejection and is, therefore, a contraindication to transplantation.

ALLOCATION OF CADAVERIC ORGANS IN THE UNITED STATES

Once a patient has been found to be suitable for transplantation and is ready for transplant surgery, he or she can be placed on the UNOS waiting list to receive a cadaveric kidney. In general, a patient should not be placed on the waiting list until the glomerular filtration rate (most commonly estimated by creatinine clearance) is less than 15 mL/min. Kidneys are usually allocated based on the UNOS point system (Table 1). Occasionally, UNOS may allow a center to transplant kidneys outside of the UNOS point system (usually for research purposes). The UNOS point system is designed to balance equity with efficiency. Equity demands that all patients be given the same access to transplantable organs, regardless of race, ethnicity, gender, or socioeconomic status. Efficiency dictates that kidneys be given to the patients who are likely to benefit the most, which is usually patients in whom the longest graft survival can be expected. Unfortunately, the goals of equity and efficiency often conflict. Although the UNOS point system is designed to allocate organs, the final decision to accept a particular organ once it is offered by UNOS rests in the hands of the patient's physician.

Although the median waiting time for people listed in 1993 was 23.9 months (95% confidence interval 23.2 to 24.6 months), waiting time varies substantially according to a patient's ABO blood group. For patients who were listed in 1992 and were ABO blood group O, median waiting time was 25.0 (24.1 to 25.9) months, for A it was 13.2 (12.8 to 13.8) months, for B it was 32.6 (30.6 to 35.3) months, and for AB it was 6.2 (5.2 to 7.6) months. It would be relatively disadvantageous for patients who are ABO blood group O if A, B, and AB blood group patients could also compete for O kidneys, so UNOS has established that all ABO blood group O kidneys must go to O recipients (Table

1). In the UNOS scheme, points awarded for waiting time and points given for having preformed antibodies (preformed antibodies make it more difficult to find a cross-match negative kidney) are designed to make the system equitable (Table 1). On the other hand, points are also assigned for how well matched a kidney is according to MHC antigens, because grafts that are better matched are, on average, more likely to survive longer.

Usually, a kidney is first offered locally, then if there is no suitable donor, it is offered regionally, and thereafter nationally. This scheme is designed to minimize the time it takes to ship kidneys, because prolonged cold ischemia time may delay graft function and possibly decrease graft survival. On the other hand, the long-term survival of 0 antigen mismatched kidneys (there are 2 A, 2 B, and 2 DR MHC antigens) overrides concerns regarding increased cold ischemia time, and there is a mandatory policy that a kidney must be shipped anywhere in the United States if there is a cross-match negative, 0 antigen mismatched recipient. Thus, an 0 antigen mismatched recipient from another region may receive a kidney even if a potential local recipient has more points. The only exception to the 0 antigen mismatch rule is a recipient of a simultaneous kidney and nonrenal organ transplantation. Under the UNOS scheme, kidneys can voluntarily go to a recipient of a simultaneous kidney and nonrenal organ transplant with fewer points, although the receiving center must then "pay the kidney back" at a future date. Thus patients receiving simultaneous organ transplants take precedent over recipients of a kidney alone. Unfortunately, patients awaiting only a kidney may wait longer, not only because a kidney that may have gone to them went instead to a simultaneous nonrenal organ recipient, but also because another kidney that may have gone to them was shipped somewhere else as a payback.

MHC antigens influence waiting time. One reason why the waiting time for African-Americans is longer than for whites (median 29.6 vs 15.9 months) is that there are relatively fewer African-American donors combined with the fact that African-Americans have a different frequency distribution of MHC antigen types as compared with whites. One solution to this particular problem, and to the growing length of waiting times in general, is to increase the rate of organ donation. Indeed, one of the medical tragedies of our age is our increasingly frustrating inability to offer transplantation to all suitable recipients due to the growing organ shortage. Although increasing organ donation is one partial solution, this alone is probably not enough, and many centers are placing a greater emphasis on living donation.

TABLE I
Synopsis of the UNOS Point System
for Kidney Allocation

Criteria	Points
ABO blood group O kidneys to O recipients	NA
O antigen mismatch (mandatory sharing)	NA
Medical urgency (local arrangement only)	NA
Time waiting since listing	
Relative (least to most)	0–1
Each year	1
Number of B or DR antigen mismatches	
0	7
1	5
2	2
Panel reactive antibody level ≥80%	4
Pediatric age (yr):	
<11	4
≥11 and <18	3

Note: When information on a cadaveric kidney donor becomes available, all active patients on the UNOS list who have an ABO blood type that is compatible with that of the donor are assigned points as indicated in the table. Locally, the patient's physician can use "medical urgency" to give priority to a recipient who has fewer points if there is only one transplant center. If there is more than one center a cooperative medical decision is required. NA, not applicable.

LIVING DONORS

Kidneys from living donors generally survive longer than cadaveric kidneys. The duration of graft survival based on the source of the donor kidney is, on average, identical twin > 2-haplotype-matched sibling > 1-haplotype-matched sibling or parent > 0-haplotype-matched sibling = distantly related or unrelated (emotionally related) living donor > cadaveric kidney. Living donor kidneys have the added advantages of allowing preemptive transplantation and making more kidneys available for individuals who do not have suitable living donors.

Detailed guidelines have been developed for the evaluation of living donors. Potential living donors should be counseled regarding both the short- and long-term risks of donation. In a recent survey of transplant centers, mortality from donation was estimated to be 0.03%, while major morbidity was 0.23%. With regard to long-term risk, a recent meta-analysis of 48 studies including 3124 patients and 1703 controls found little evidence of progressive renal dysfunction among normal individuals with only one kidney. Although there was a small increase in blood pressure, this increase was not enough to raise the prevalence of hypertension in patients who had a single kidney. Although there was a statistically significant increase in proteinuria, it was probably too small to be of clinical relevance.

In general, proteinuria greater than 200 mg/24 hr should be considered a contraindication to donation. Microhematuria and pyuria should be investigated to rule out underlying renal disease that would preclude donation. Renal function should generally be normal, after adjusting for gender, age, and possible dietary influences on glomerular filtration rate.

Blood typing and cross-matching are often the first steps in evaluating a living donor. If a potential donor and recipient are blood group compatible and cross-match negative, further evaluation can then be carried out. This should include a psychological evaluation to ensure that the donation is truly voluntary and that the patient can give an informed consent. A complete medical evaluation should also be carried out to uncover conditions that would increase the risk of surgery. Potential donors should also be screened for conditions such as diabetes or hypertension that may worsen by having only one kidney. How diligently to test for possible incipient diabetes in donors with a positive family history or other risk factors for diabetes is unclear. This is because the effect of having one kidney on the rate of progression of diabetic nephropathy (if diabetes occurred), is uncertain. Consideration should be given to the risk of inherited renal diseases such as autosomal dominant polycystic kidney disease and hereditary nephritis. Finally, the medical evaluation should ensure that the donor is free of diseases that could be transmitted with the kidney, including malignancies, HIV, viral hepatitis, and tuberculosis.

If there is more than one potential living-related donor, selection should be based on both medical and nonmedical factors, and good matching need not be the only determinant of donor choice. Although the best donor is usually a member of the recipient's immediate family, most centers would consider an emotionally related donor. Once a potential donor has been selected and evaluated, the final step is usually arteriography to define the renal vasculature and to look for potential anatomic abnormalities.

TRANSPLANT PROCEDURE

The kidney is usually placed retroperitoneally in the iliac fossa. The renal artery is usually anastomosed (end-to-end) with the internal iliac artery. Different techniques are available for dealing with multiple renal arteries and atherosclerosis in the recipient's iliac artery. The renal vein is usually anastomosed (end-to-end) with the external iliac vein. The ureter is implanted via a long submucosal tunnel into the bladder. In general, this surgical approach has made the transplant procedure relatively routine; however great care must be taken because immunosuppression delays wound healing and increases the risk of postoperative infection.

Bibliography

1995 Annual Report of the U.S. Scientific Registry for Transplant Recipients and the Organ Procurement and Transplantation Network -- Transplant Data: 1988-1994. UNOS, Richmond, VA, and the Division of Transplantation, Bureau of Health Resources Development, Health Resources and Services Administration. Rockville, MD, 1995.

American Diabetes Association. Pancreas transplantation for patients with diabetes mellitus. *Diabetes Care* 16 (Suppl 2):21, 1993.

Bia MJ, Ramos EL, Danovitch GM, et al.: Evaluation of living renal donors. The current practice of US transplant centers. *Transplantation* 60:322–327, 1995

Kasiske BL, Ma JZ, Louis TA, Swan SK: Long-term effects of reduced renal mass in humans. *Kidney Int* 48:814–819, 1995

Kasiske BL, Ramos EL, Gaston RS, et al.: The evaluation of renal transplant candidates: Clinical practice guidelines. *J Am Soc Nephrol* 6:1–34, 1995

Kasiske BL, Ravenscraft M, Ramos EL, Gaston RS, Bia MJ, Danovitch GM: The evaluation of living renal transplant donors: Clinical practice guidelines. *J Am Soc Nephrol* 1996, 7:2288–2313.

Ramos EL, Kasiske BL, Alexander SR, et al.: The evaluation of candidates for renal transplantation: The current practice of U.S. transplant centers. *Transplantation* 57:490–497, 1994

United Network for Organ Sharing. UNOS Policies as of March 22, 1996, 1996 (UnPub).

75

RENAL TRANSPLANTATION: IMMUNOSUPPRESSION AND POSTOPERATIVE MANAGEMENT

DOUGLAS J. NORMAN

Renal transplantation is the preferred treatment for failed native kidneys. In 1995, 11,807 kidney transplants were performed in the United States. This is a small number compared to the 31,045 patients on waiting lists at the 251 transplant centers. The success of kidney transplantation has greatly lengthened the list of patients requesting to be transplanted. Survival is improving steadily because of a number of factors including the availability of potent drugs that better suppress the immune response. Expected clinical outcomes for renal transplantation in 1997 are substantially better than those of 15 years ago, before cyclosporine, OKT3, and globally improved patient care and donor management. Typical 1-year patient survivals are 97% and 93% for living-related donor and cadaveric donor transplants, respectively. One-year graft survivals are 91% for living-related donor transplants and 81% for cadaveric donor recipients.

RATIONALE FOR IMMUNOSUPPRESSION

To achieve these excellent survivals requires measures to counter the immune response engendered against a transplanted kidney. Antibodies produced by activated B lymphocytes and cytolytic cells derived from T lymphocytes are the key mediators of graft damage. B and T lymphocytes are dependent on accessory cells including tissue macrophages, monocytes, and endothelial cells, on cytokines, including a variety of growth and differentiation factors, and on adhesion molecules and receptors that promote specific or nonspecific cell-to-cell contacts and interactions. Immunosuppression strategies for organ transplantation are increasingly being directed against specific elements of the immune response cascade that develop in response to an allograft.

A natural way to diminish the strength of the immune reaction propagated against a kidney allograft is to match the major histocompatibility antigens. Human lymphocyte antigens, known as HLA, are coded by the short arm of the sixth chromosome. Both class I (HLA A, B, C) and class II (HLA DP, DQ, DR) antigens are major targets of the immune response. The longest graft survival, with a half life of 22 years, is achieved with an HLA identical, or two haplotype, match. HLA A, B, C, DP, DQ, and DR alleles on both haplotypes of the donor match those of the recipient. The next longest survival with a 12-year half life, is with a one haplotype match. The worst survival, with a 5-year half life, is with an organ from a cadaveric, unrelated donor with no matches for any of the six HLA A, B, and DR antigens. Among unrelated donor-recipient pairs, however, there is a step-wise increase in graft survival with increased matching.

The goal of clinical immunogenetics testing is to ensure that an adequate tissue match is achieved and that a pretransplant cross-match to rule out the presence of antidonor antibodies in the serum of a prospective recipient is negative. While a negative cross-match is required, a good antigen match is not and, unfortunately, only 10 to 20% of cadaver organs are transplanted into well-matched recipients.

CLASSIFICATION OF ALLOGRAFT REJECTION

Following transplantation of a kidney, episodes of renal dysfunction can occur for a variety of reasons. The most important of these is rejection. The three distinct syndromes of rejection have unique pathology, immunopathogenesis, and clinical presentations. Hyperacute rejection is caused by preformed antidonor antibodies present in the recipient's serum at the moment of transplantation. Hyperacute rejection leads to kidney failure almost immediately after transplantation (within 24 hours). Allografts, which must be removed from the recipient, demonstrate fibrin thrombi in the glomerular capillaries and small vessels, vasculitis, and necrosis. Acute rejections often occur in the first 3 months after transplantation. They are cell mediated, caused by T cells, via direct cytotoxicity, and by T cells and macrophages, via local cytokine release. The pathological appearance of acute rejection is a mononuclear interstitial cell infiltrate and with tubulitis, lymphocytes invading renal tubules, and sometimes with endothelial damage suggestive of a vascular rejection. Glomeruli are spared. These rejections are usually reversible by using a pulse of corticosteroids or anti-T cell antibody therapy. Chronic rejection, the most common cause of late graft loss, is generally progressive and refractory to immunosuppressive therapy. Its pathological appearance is a vasculopathy with intimal thickening and occlusion leading to ischemia and subsequent interstitial fibrosis and glomerulosclerosis. Chronic rejection is most likely triggered by endothelial cell damage and is mediated by various components of the immune system, that cause subsequent smooth muscle cell proliferation and fibrosis. Acute rejection episodes might begin this process; their occurrence correlates directly with long-term graft survival. A variant of chronic rejection, transplant glomerulopathy, is characterized by glomerular capillary loop thickening and significant proteinuria. It too is untreatable. However, when this condition is suspected, it may still be useful to perform a renal biopsy to distinguish this entity from recurrent or *de novo* glomerulonephritis.

OTHER CAUSES OF ALLOGRAFT LOSS

Other causes besides true chronic rejections are now known to contribute to the pathological process that is still commonly termed chronic rejection. Thus, other factors can contribute to chronic allograft failure. Hyperfiltration damage occurs in the remnants of kidneys of laboratory animals that have had one kidney and part of another removed (see Chapter 66.) It is therefore assumed that when the glomerular filtration rate of a renal allograft falls below 20% of normal that hyperfiltration might be an important cause of further damage to the allograft and subsequent loss of kidney function. Any factor that might reduce the number of functioning nephrons in a transplanted kidney can contribute to chronic allograft failure by shortening the time to the onset of hyperfiltration-induced kidney damage. Such factors include advanced age, female sex, African-American ancestry, and small size of the donor. Preexisting renal damage in the donor from hypertension, lipids, drugs or other illness may also contribute, as can complications occurring around the time of organ harvesting including the cause of death of the donor, hypotensive episodes, cardiac arrest, and the use of nephrotoxic drugs prior to the declaration of brain death. Still others include any nonrejection damage that can supervene in an allograft after transplantation due to hypertension, infections, nephrotoxic drugs, etc.

Some forms of glomerulonephritis, particularly focal glomerulosclerosis, may recur after retransplantation, and are a relative contraindication to retransplantation. IgA nephropathy recurs in a high percentage of allografts but rarely causes graft loss. Systemic lupus erythematosus may also recur. Anti-GBM disease will recur in patients with a high titer of anti-GBM antibodies. In general, glomerular diseases that have a rapid and malignant course have the highest potential for recurrence in an allograft.

GENERAL POSTTRANSPLANT CARE

Posttransplant in-hospital surgical management of a transplant patient begins with care of the wound, drains, urinary catheter, central venous line, gastrointestinal function, diet, and ambulation. Routine medical care includes dialysis if the allograft does not function at once, fluid–electrolyte management, blood pressure control, infection surveillance, renal function monitoring, and immunosuppression. The pharmacist and transplant coordinator play important roles in teaching the patient about drug use, drug interactions, and side effects, providing pivotal education about the post transplant routine, and preparing the patient for the outpatient follow-up. This team approach to transplant patient management combining physician, surgeon, nurses, social worker and pharmacist, is key to the success of transplantation.

Management of patients post transplantation requires special attention to renal function, side effects of the immunosuppressive drugs, and consequences of overimmunosuppression. Renal dysfunction episodes can occur due to a variety of causes. A careful history and physical and laboratory examination will often disclose the cause of dysfunction, but more detailed testing, including a kidney biopsy, renal scan, or sonogram may be required. The classic signs and symptoms of acute rejection include oliguria, graft swelling and tenderness, fever, hypertension, graft pain, anorexia, and progressive azotemia. With the the recent use of stronger immunosuppressive drugs, these finding seldom develop. When they do, only pyelonephritis needs to be ruled out before treatment with corticosteroids is begun. Rejection typically presents as only a minimal rise in the serum creatinine, without accompanying signs and symptoms. Other causes of renal dysfunction must be considered, including cyclosporine or tacrolimus nephrotoxicity, urinary tract infection, hypersensitivity reaction to a penicillin or other drug, volume depletion from diuretic use or hyperglycemia, or other drug effect such as that of trimethoprim or cimetidine to decrease creatinine secretion. If none of these can be documented by clinical or routine laboratory findings, anatomical abnormalities such as obstruction, urinary leak, and renal artery or vein thrombosis must be considered. The radionucleide renal scan is probably the most useful single diagnostic test because it can demonstrate each of these abnormalities. If other studies have not provided a diagnosis, a renal allograft biopsy is the definitive diagnostic tool. As the biopsy is generally performed under ultrasound guidance, additional information about obstruction and presence of an extrarenal fluid collection, such as a lymphocele, hematoma, or urinoma due to a urine leak is also provided. Some centers use fine needle aspiration of the allograft with cytologic examination in lieu of biopsies.

IMMUNOSUPPRESSIVE DRUGS

Immunosuppression is the cornerstone of a successful kidney transplantation. The evolution of immunosuppression during the past decade has been extraordinarily brisk and will likely continue at an accelerated pace during the next 10 years. Immunosuppressive drugs can be divided into a few broad categories. The monoclonal and polyclonal antibodies and other biological agents are antitarget recognition drugs that prevent cell–cell interaction and antigen recognition. Cyclosporine, cyclosporine Neoral, and tacrolimus are anticytokine synthesis drugs. They block IL-2 synthesis by preventing transcription of the IL-2 gene. Key steps are the binding of cyclosporine or tacrolimus to a specific immunophilin (cyclophilin or FK binding protein respectively), blockade of calcineurin (a phosphatase that promotes the activation and movement of transcription factor NFAT), and prevention of the transcription of cytokine genes, specifically IL-2. Rapamycin is the only known example of an anticytokine action drug. It prevents IL-2 driven cell activation via an unknown mechanism. Rapamycin binds to FK binding protein and antagonizes the effect of tacrolimus. Azathioprine, cyclophosphamide, mycophenolate mofetil, methotrexate, and brequinar sodium are anti-cell proliferation drugs. They block enzymes vital to purine or pyrimidine production and therefore to DNA replication. Finally, corticosteroids are both antiinflammatory and immunosuppressive. As a rule, immunosuppressive drugs are given in combination. Typically, an anticytokine synthesis drug (cyclosporine or tacrolimus), an antiproliferation drug (azathioprine or mycophenolate mofetil), and an antiinflammatory drug (corticosteroids) will be employed together. Whether such triple therapy is better than double therapy with a corticosteroid and anticytokine drug alone is uncertain despite the theoretical benefit of using agents with complementary modes of action. Different combinations of these drugs are currently being evaluated.

PHASES OF IMMUNOSUPPRESSION

Three distinct phases of immunosuppression follow kidney transplantation: (1) immunosuppression induction, (2) immunosuppression maintenance, and (3) antirejection treatment. Immunosuppression induction requires drugs that are powerful yet specific for cells that initiate and effect the allograft-directed immune response. The immune response is strongest when it encounters the allograft initially. Passenger leukocytes from the graft flow to regional lymph nodes and directly activate the immune response. Strong immunosuppression is required during this period, which is unfortunately also the time at which a patient is at greatest risk for bacterial wound, lung, and urinary tract infections. Therefore, drugs that promote delayed wound healing or broadly affect all leukocyte function are potentially dangerous. Moreover, during this period, exposure to potentially nephrotoxic drugs like cyclosporine or tacrolimus, which can exacerbate preservation-induced organ damage, must be limited or avoided. The antilymphocyte antibodies, in combination with corticosteroids, an antiproliferative drug, and the delayed use of an cytokine inhibitor drug, are widely used for induction. Several drugs are available. OKT3 is a murine, monoclonal anti-CD3 (pan T cell) antibody. Atgam is an equine, polyclonal, antithymocyte antibody. Thymoglobulin is a rabbit, polyclonal, antithymocyte globulin. All have been proven effective for induction, if given for 7 to 14 days. They prevent early rejection episodes that would otherwise require high doses of corti-costeroids, and also improve long-term graft survival. Induction of immunosuppression is accomplished at some centers with an intravenous cytokine inhibitor and corticosteroids, with or without an antiproliferative drug. Although this approach may be successful, it is associated with a higher incidence of early rejection as compared with antilymphocyte antibody induction.

Immunosuppression maintenance generally requires lower doses of the same drugs, except that antilymphocyte antibodies are never used for maintenance. The use of lower doses of the drugs is possible because the body adapts to the organ after the donor passenger leukocytes have been destroyed or dispersed. The maintenance phase begins after 1 to 3 months and extends for life. Immunosuppressive drugs can never be discontinued because of a very high risk of rejection without them, even years after transplant.

The third phase of immunosuppression is antirejection treatment. Acute cell-mediated rejections occur most frequently during the first 3 months after transplantation and after major sensitizing events such as infections, trauma, surgery, or noncompliance with medications. First-line treatment of acute rejections is usually with an increased dose of corticosteroids given either intravenously or orally. Treatment of steroid-resistant or steroid-dependent rejections requires one of the antilymphocyte antibody preparations. These are generally effective for 75 to 80% of steroid-resistant rejections when administered for 7 to 14 days. Some of the drugs used for maintenance have also been used for treating both mild rejections and steroid-resistant or recurrent rejections. Mild rejections have been treated by increasing the doses of cyclosporine and or azathioprine that a patient is already taking. Resistant rejections have been treated by switching from azathioprine to mycophenolate mofetil or tacrolimus.

Standard doses of the most commonly used drugs are as follows: azathioprine (1 to 2 $mg \cdot kg^{-1} \cdot day^{-1}$ once a day); mycophenolate mofetil (1g bid); cyclosporine (4 to 8 $mg \cdot kg^{-1} \cdot day^{-1}$ in one or two divided doses); tacrolimus (0.15 $mg \cdot kg^{-1} \cdot day^{-1}$ in two divided doses), and prednisone (0.10 $mg \cdot kg^{-1} \cdot day^{-1}$ or alternatively 0.2 mg/kg every other day for maintenance). Cyclosporine and tacrolimus therapy are monitored with drug levels. These desired levels vary according to assay used and frequency of dosing.

SIDE EFFECTS OF IMMUNOSUPPRESSIVE DRUGS

The drugs required for renal transplant patients have a variety of side effects, as summarized in Table 1. Corticosteroids have the most deleterious long-term effects, including osteopenia and osteonecrosis—neither of which has a satisfactory treatment. Steroids also cause a variety of cosmetic problems, including hirsutism, acne, and fat deposits in the face ("moon face"), neck (buffalo hump), and abdomen. In children, growth retardation can be a serious problem. Cyclosporine causes nephrotoxicity almost universally, although its severity is variable and dose related. Hepatotoxicity also occurs rarely and much more commonly with the intravenous use of cyclosporine. Hirsutism can be a

TABLE I

Individual Drug Toxicities

Corticosteroids	Suppress the adrenal gland, decrease intestinal absorption, and increase renal excretion of calcium
	Weight gain and redistribution of fat to the abdomen, face, and neck
	Osteoporosis, osteonecrosis
	Myopathy
	Delayed wound healing
	Hyperlipidemia accelerated atherosclerosis
	Diabetes mellitus
	Cataracts
Cyclosporine	Nephrotoxicity
	Hypertension
	Hirsutism
	Gingival hyperplasia
	Tremors, dysesthesias, seizures
	Hepatotoxicity
Azathioprine	Myelosuppression
	Pancreatitis, gastrointestinal hypersensitivity hepatotoxicity, venoocclusive disease of the liver
	Alopecia
Tacrolimus	Nephrotoxicity
	Tremors, dysesthesias
	Gastrointestinal hypersensitivity
	Diabetes mellitus
Mycophenolate Mofetil	Myelosuppression
	Gastrointestinal hypersensitivity
OKT3	Cytokine release syndrome with fever, chills, nausea, diarrhea encephalopathy, pulmonary edema and nephropathy
	Human antimouse antibody production (HAMA)
ATG (polyclonal)	Serum sickness
	Thrombocytopenia, leukopenia
	Mild cytokine release syndrome

problem among dark-haired individuals, and gum hypertrophy is occasionally severe enough to require surgical resection. Neurotoxicity manifests as tremor or paresthesias, is usually dose related, and can be controlled. Cyclosporine-induced hypertension and hyperuricemia with gout are common. Tacrolimus also causes nephrotoxicity and neurotoxicity, perhaps more severe than that due to cyclosporine. One of the most serious side effects of tacrolimus is insulin-dependent diabetes. Fortunately, this is dose related. However, in some cases it has not been reversible. Tacrolimus causes diarrhea in some patients. In contrast to cyclosporine, tacrolimus does not cause hirsutism, gingival hyperplasia, or hypercholesterolemia. Therefore, it is an excellent alternative for patients who develop any of these problems. Azathioprine causes myelosuppression, including leukopenia and anemia, which can also occur as an isolated effect. Hepatotoxicity occurs rarely, as does pan-

creatitis. The latter carries a high mortality in immunosuppressed patients, whether azathioprine associated or not. A severe form of hepatotoxicity, veno-occlusive disease, is generally progressive even if azathioprine is discontinued. Hair loss can occur, but it is reversible and does not preclude the reuse, or even continued use of azathioprine. Mycophenolate mofetil causes myelosuppression and gastrointestial toxicity.

OKT3 causes the "cytokine release syndrome" which is probably mediated by IL-2, tumor necrosis factor, interferon-γ, IL-6, other cytokines, and possibly complement activation products. Its features include fever, chills, nausea, diarrhea, headache, and photophobia. Pulmonary edema, due in part to a "capillary leak syndrome" and exacerbated by concurrent volume overload, hypotension, and encephalopathy are rare. Human antimouse antibody (HAMA) production occurs in approximately 75% of patients receiving OKT3, and occasionally (10 to 20%) prevents subsequent use of OKT3 when present in a titer greater than 1:1000. The polyclonal antilymphocyte antibody preparations are rarely associated with a cytokine release syndrome. Atgam, however, causes thrombocytopenia, which occasionally requires dosage adjustment. Approximately 75% of patients make antibodies to horse (Atgam) or rabbit (Thymoglobulin) antibodies and these rarely can cause a serum sickness syndrome with a petechial skin rash and fever. Table 2 lists the organ-specific abnormalities that occur in some transplant patients as a result of the drugs used for immunosuppression. When any of these occur the transplant physician must consider a drug toxicity as a cause.

POSTTRANSPLANT INFECTION

Infection may result from overimmunosuppression. In the immediate postoperative period, the most common infections are bacterial urinary tract, pulmonary, wound, and intravenous line-related infections. These can be avoided, or mitigated by careful anticipation and use of preventive measures. Opportunistic infections can occur at any time after transplantation, but generally they develop when immunosuppression is most intense, such as during the first few months after transplant and following treated episodes of rejection. Herpes simplex is commonly activated by immunosuppression but can be prevented by acyclovir prophylaxis. Cytomegalovirus (CMV) is a particular problem when a CMV seronegative recipient receives an organ from a seropositive donor. Approximately 80% of such patients will develop CMV disease ranging from fever alone to pneumonitis, hepatitis, and enteritis. Reactivation CMV disease also occasionally occurs in seropositive recipients with prior CMV infection but is generally much less severe than the primary form. It may be difficult to distinguish CMV shedding in the urine, saliva, or bronchoalveolar lavage fluid from true infection. CMV is most likely to occur between 1 and 6 months posttransplant. Treatment with ganciclovir is usually very effective and patients rarely die of CMV disease, although significant morbidity and expense can result. Active CMV may present during a

TABLE 2
Organ-Specific Drug Toxicity

General	Increased susceptibility to infections and malignancies
	Weight gain
Integument	Cancer
	Acne
	Fungal infection
	Warts
	Bruising
	Hirsutism
	Alopecia
Musculoskeletal System	Osteopenia
	Osteonecrosis
	Myopathy
Respiratory System	Pulmonary edema
Carciovascular System	Accelerated atherosclerosis
	Hypertension
Hemodynamic System	Myelosuppression
	Anemia
	Thrombocytopenia
	Thrombocytosis
	Hemolysis
Digestive System	Peptic ulcer disease
	Diarrhea
	Pancreatitis
	Hepatotoxicity
Urinary Tract	Nephrotoxicity
	Pyelonephritis
	Cystitis
Sexual Function	Impotence
	Loss of libido
Endocrine System	Diabetes mellitus
Nervous System	Dysesthesias
	Euphoria
	Depression
	Encephalopathy
	Seizures
	Tremors
Eyes	Cataracts

rejection; reduction of immunosuppression during active disease may promote rejection. Various preventive measures such as the use of high-dose acyclovir, CMV immune globulin, and ganciclovir are available but the only treatment that has proven to be highly successful is ganciclovir given for 3 months after transplant. The intravenous form of ganciclovir is effective for preventing CMV. An oral formulation is effective for both preventing and treating CMV retinitis in HIV-infected patients, and trials with this agent in transplant patients have begun. One of the most effective ways to prevent a primary CMV infection, which generally is more serious than reactivation disease, is by seromatching: the avoidance of transplanting a seronegative recipient with a kidney from a seropositive donor. However, most transplant centers view this as impractical.

The transplant physician must also be vigilant regarding the development of other rarer diseases such as pneumocystis carinii, listeria, legionella, toxoplasmosis, and cryptococcal meningitis. The incidence of pneumocystis and legionella infection has been reduced by the routine use of postoperative trimethoprim/sulfamethoxazole prophylaxis. Community-acquired infections such as the common cold, influenza, pneumococcal pneumonia, chlamydia, diarrheal syndromes, and sexually transmitted diseases can also affect transplant patients. All prospective transplant patients should be vaccinated against hepatitis A and B, tetanus, diphtheria, and pneumococcal disease. Like any other infectious diseases, these are potentially much more serious in immunosuppressed patients; the benefit of prevention is obvious.

POSTTRANSPLANT MALIGNANCIES

Neoplasia may also result from excessive immunosuppression. The incidence rates of most malignancies are probably increased among transplant patients, although lymphomas and skin cancers are the most significantly increased. Approximately 1% of kidney transplant patients develop lymphoma and approximately 5% develop skin cancer. B cell lymphomas are the most common, are often associated with Epstein-Barr virus and, if identified early, can sometimes be successfully treated by a drastic reduction in immunosuppression. An increased incidence of lymphoma has been linked to use of antilymphocyte antibodies in some centers but this relationship is not consistent. Prolonged or repeated courses of antilymphocyte antibodies, and in particular OKT3, as well as high doses of immunosuppression are generally thought to place a transplant patient at greater risk for developing lymphoma. Both squamous cell and basal cell carcinomas should be anticipated in transplant patients, and appropriate referrals made to a dermatologist for evaluation of suspicious skin lesions. Many solid tumors that become manifest clinically after a transplant were actually present before hand. Therefore, a careful evaluation for tumors in age-appropriate patients should be conducted during the pretransplant recipient evaluation (see Chapter 74). Rarely, tumors are inadvertently transplanted with the allograft. Their discovery should prompt immediate discontinuation of immunosuppression.

POSTTRANSPLANT HYPERTENSION

Hypertension posttransplant is common and often requires multiple drug therapy. While essential hypertension and cyclosporine are the usual causes, allograft renal artery stenosis and excessive renin production by the native kidneys should always be considered. Calcium channel blockers are usually the first-line therapy for hypertension for several reasons, including a demonstrated reversal of the reduction in renal plasma flow and GFR induced experimentally by cyclosporine and a possible direct immunosuppressive effect. Verapamil and diltiazem decrease the metabolism of cyclosporine and raise its blood levels.

Nifedipine can independently cause gingival hypertrophy. Angiotensin converting enzyme inhibitors, alpha- and beta-adrenergic blockers can also be used effectively in renal transplant patients.

POSTTRANSPLANT HYPERLIPIDEMIA

As the result of using prednisone and cyclosporine, many patients will develop hyperlipidemia following transplantation. Generally, transplant physicians delay the treatment of hyperlipidemia until the prednisone dose has been tapered to maintenance levels, because the problem often disappears or lessens. However, recent data from the heart transplant literature indicating that HMG-CoA reductase inhibitors improve outcome by reducing the incidence of both acute and chronic rejection suggest that these drugs should be used earlier. After the prednisone dose has been tapered to low levels (e.g., 0.1 mg $\cdot$ kg^{-1} $\cdot$ day^{-1}), further reductions or discontinuation of prednisone altogether have generally not had any additional effect on lowering lipid levels. Since tacrolimus does not cause hyperlipidemia, one must consider conversion from cyclosporine to this drug if posttransplant hyperlipidemia is severe. Finally, dietary maneuver should always be a part of any attempt to lower a patient's lipid levels.

POSTTRANSPLANT HYPERCALCEMIA

In patients who have had long-standing renal failure, the parathyroid glands are often quite hyperplastic and it may take months to years for them to regress to normal activity. The usual practice is to wait for this to happen, unless a patient is symptomatic from hyperparathyroidism. Occasionally a posttransplant patient will develop significant and symptomatic hypercalcemia. In this case, early surgery should be considered.

OTHER POSTTRANSPLANT COMPLICATIONS

Some patients develop diabetes mellitus after transplantation because of steroid use or tacrolimus. Many of these patients require insulin. Urinary tract infection and pneumocystis prophylaxis are generally prescribed for 3 to 4 months after transplant, and both goals can be accomplished with trimethoprim sulfamethoxazole, one double strength tablet every Monday, Wednesday, and Friday. Hypophosphatemia and hypomagnesemia are both very common following renal transplantation because of renal tubular abnormalities induced by cyclosporine, as well as hyperparathyroidism and other causes. These minerals should be replaced as needed. Calcium, alendronate, vitamin D, and calcium-sparing diuretics might reduce the severity of osteopenia. Erythrocytosis may result from excessive erythropoietin production by the allograft or native kidneys. Phlebotomy may be required; however, some patients respond to angiotensin converting enzyme inhibitors or theophylline.

POSTTRANSPLANT DRUG PRESCRIPTIONS

Numerous drugs may have adverse effects in transplant patients. Nonsteroidal antiflammatory drugs often cause precipitous and protracted declines in GFR, presumably because they block production of vasodilator prostaglandins that counter the renal vasoconstriction induced by cyclosporine. Allopurinol, a xanthine oxidase inhibitor, inhibits breakdown of 6-mercaptopurine, the active metabolite of azathioprine and increases the latter's marrow suppressive effect. Together, these effects complicate management of cyclosporine-induced gout. Intra-articular steroid injections, temporary increases in oral prednisone dosing, colchicine, and judicious coadministration of azathioprine and allopurinol may be necessary. Erythromycin, ketoconazole, fluconazole, itraconazole, diltiazem, nicardipine, verapamil, and methylprednisolone may interfere with cyclosporine degradation. Rifampin, phenytoin, phenobarbital, and carbamazepine accelerate cyclosporine metabolism. Cyclosporine levels should be closely monitored and a need for dosage adjustment anticipated when these agents are prescribed. Because transplant patients are typically receiving numerous medications, and because of the propensity for adverse interactions among them, the physician should be especially vigilant when altering the medication regimen of transplant patients.

MANAGEMENT OF A FAILED RENAL ALLOGRAFT

When a renal allograft fails and a patient returns to dialysis, a decision must be made regarding discontinuation of immunosuppression and removal of the allograft. A retained allograft that is uncovered by immunosuppression can become inflamed causing local and even systemic symptoms. A more serious consequence of a retained allograft is the development of anti-HLA antibodies. If a patient desires retransplantation, these antibodies can be devastating. In general, most allografts that are lost acutely to rejection are removed and immunosuppression is discontinued with a short taper of the prednisone. Allografts that are lost to chronic rejection can be retained if immunosuppression is continued (usually azathioprine and prednisone because they are inexpensive), if the patient is interested in being retransplanted, and if anti-HLA antibodies are absent so that it is likely that a kidney will be found within months. For sensitized patients in whom the wait for a subsequent transplant will be long, continuing the immunosuppression becomes too risky and it is wiser to remove the kidney and discontinue the drugs. If the patient is not a candidate for retransplantation and the allograft was lost to a chronic process, it is reasonable to discontinue immunosuppression and observe the patient. A spike in anti-HLA antibodies occurs in about 25% of patients after the removal of an allograft if immunosuppression is discontinued immediately. Therefore, if there is no major risk of continuing immunosuppression, the drugs can be continued for 1 month before tapering. It has not been proved that this prevents antibody formation.

OUTCOME OF RETRANSPLANTATION

The survival of second transplants is clearly inferior to that of first transplants. If a previous graft was lost to rejection within 3 months of transplant, the outcome of a retransplant is especially poor. However, patients who did well with a first transplant can do well with a second one and should not be denied that opportunity. The cause of a poorer survival with a retransplant is usually undetected sensitization. Patients receiving a second transplant are of high risk for failure and are usually given more potent immunosuppression. This makes them more susceptible to the adverse consequences of immunosuppression.

Bibliography

Almond PS, Matas A, Gillingham K, et al.: Risk factors for chronic rejection in renal allograft recipients. *Transplantation* 55:752–757, 1993.

Barbosa LM, Gauthier GJ, Davis CL: Bone pain that responds to calcium channel blockers: A retrospective and prospective study of transplant recipients. *Transplantation* 59:541–544, 1995.

Barret W, First MF, Orm BS, et al.: Clinical course of malignancies in renal transplant recipients. *Cancer* 72(7):2186–2189, 1993.

Bass NM, Ockner RK: Drug induced liver disease. In: *Hepatology: A Textbook of Liver Disease*. Saunders, Philadelphia, 1990.

Braun WE: Long-term complications of renal transplantation (Nephrology Forum: Clinical Conference). *Kidney Int* 37:1363–1378, 1990.

Curtis JJ: Hypertension following kidney transplantation. *Am J Kidney Dis* 23:471–475, 1994.

de Mattos AM, Olyaei AJ, Bennett WM: Pharmacology of immunosuppressive medications used in renal diseases and transplantation. *Am J Kidney Dis* 28(5):631–667, 1996.

Hricik DE, Almawi WY, Strom TB. Trends in the use of glucocorticoids in renal transplantation. *Transplantation* 57:979–989, 1994.

Kasiske BL: Risk factors for accelerated atherosclerosis in renal transplant recipients. *Am J Med* 84:985–992, 1988.

Kuo PC, Dafoe DC, Alfrey EJ, et al.: Post-transplant lymphoproliferative disorders and Epstein-Barr virus prophylaxis. *Transplantation* 59:135–138, 1995.

Luke RG: Pathophysiology and treatment of post-transplant hypertension. *J Am Soc Nephrol* 2:537–544, 1991.

Mahony JF: Long-term results and complications of transplantation: The kidney. *Transplant Proc* 21:1433–1434, 1989.

Penn I: The effect of immunosuppression on pre-existing cancers. *Transplantation* 55:742–747, 1993.

Pereira BJ: Hepatitis C in organ transplantation: Its significance and influence on transplantation policies. *Curr Opin Nephrol Hypertens* 2:912–922, 1993.

Rubin RH: Infection in transplantation. *Infect Dis Clin North Am* 9(December):811–1092, 1995.

Solez K, Axelsen RA, Benediktsson H, et al.: International standardization of criteria for the histologic diagnosis of renal allograft rejection: The Banft working classification of kidney transplant pathology. *Kidney Int* 44(2):411–422, 1993.

Watkins PB. Drug metabolism by cytochrome P450 in the liver and small bowel. *Gastroenteroly Clin North Am* 21(3):511–526, 1992.

SECTION 11

HYPERTENSION

76

PATHOGENESIS OF HYPERTENSION

STEPHEN C. TEXTOR

Blood pressure control and hypertension reflect forces governing systemic hemodynamic variables, specifically blood flow (cardiac output) and peripheral vascular resistance. Understanding these components will enable the reader to approach the complex and expanding list of proposed causes of the various forms of primary and secondary hypertension.

Hypertensive disorders are common and are of particular relevance for the nephrologist. Most diseases which impair kidney function ultimately lead to a rise in arterial pressure, usually accompanied by impaired urinary sodium excretion and volume regulation. This relationship is so uniform that many authors believe that any sustained rise in blood pressure *requires* the participation of the kidney. Conversely, hypertension is itself an important mechanism of kidney disease, which accelerates many forms of nephron injury when transmitted as increased hydraulic pressure to the glomerulus.

HEMODYNAMIC RELATIONSHIPS IN HYPERTENSION

The fundamental hemodynamic equation relating blood pressure to the product of cardiac output and total systemic vascular resistance is depicted in Fig. 1. Arterial pressure is determined by the diverse combination of factors that affects either (or both) of these variables. Hypertension therefore results from a relative imbalance of cardiac output and systemic vascular resistance.

Cardiac output and blood flow are affected by blood volume reaching the heart, often described as "cardiac filling volume." This expression reflects the general relationship, albeit imprecise, between total blood volume and arterial pressure. At the extremes of low volume, as produced by hypotensive hemorrhage or gastrointestinal fluid losses, arterial pressure falls. Conversely, conditions producing a rise in blood volume without other major organ abnormalities regularly lead to systemic hypertension. Sodium retention following acute glomerulonephritis is one example. However, it should be emphasized that large portions of the total blood volume are located in capillary networks, venous beds and the spleen, which are distensible capacitance compartments (Fig. 1). These are not in direct equilibrium with the arterial circuit.

Hence, blood volume alone does not directly determine blood pressure. In some situations, blood volume is dissociated from systemic arterial pressure altogether. This is the case in end stage liver failure, in which widespread systemic vasodilation produces low arterial pressures despite expansion of blood volume.

When measured in most essential hypertensive patients, cardiac filling volumes and cardiac output are normal. Although occasional instances of hypertension due to an increased cardiac output in patients with hyperkinetic circulatory states have been reported, these are unusual and often temporary. Even experimental models of hypertension induced by volume expansion ultimately return cardiac output to normal with a secondary rise in peripheral resistance.

Understanding hypertension, therefore, should be viewed as a problem of understanding the relative determinants of both blood volume and vascular resistance.

VOLUME CONTROL AND BLOOD PRESSURE REGULATION

Some of the major regulators of sodium and volume homeostasis are listed in Table 1. The importance of intravascular volume in blood pressure regulation is obvious when blood pressure is restored after administration of volume during hypotensive hemorrhage. At the other extreme, "refractory" hypertension in patients with end stage renal disease becomes manageable after removal of extracellular fluid volume with dialysis. However, the role of volume control is more subtle in patients with clinical hypertension and apparently normal renal function.

Guyton et al. have argued that *sustained* elevations in blood pressure require a disturbance in the kidney. This concept derives from well-established experimental observations of "pressure natriuresis," as depicted in Fig. 2. This model indicates that the kidney functions as a precise controller of arterial pressure. Changes in blood pressure, and therefore renal perfusion pressure, shown in the left curve, are translated into steep changes in sodium excretion. This scheme fits well with the clinical observation that sodium excretion falls with a drop in blood pressure and does not return to normal until pressure is restored. Conversely, a rise in arterial pressure leads to enhanced sodium excretion until the pressure again falls. In principle, sodium retention has no limit and can proceed until blood pressure is fully restored. For that reason, it has been described as a response system with "infinite gain."

Such a model would lead hypertensive subjects to undergo natriuresis and eventual volume depletion. Actually,

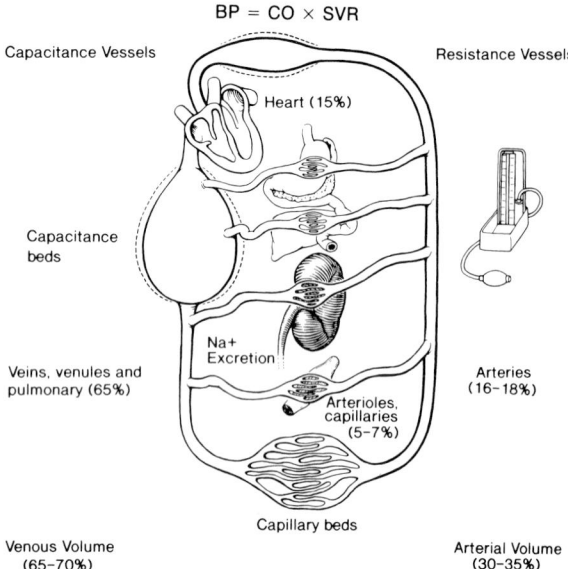

FIGURE 1 Systemic blood pressure is measured on the "resistance" side of the circulation. Organ perfusion is determined both by the pump capacity [cardiac output (CO)] and the systemic vascular resistance (SVR), which is the impedance to blood flow, primarily determined by the lumen diameters of resistance vessels. The blood volume within the arterial circuits is less than that sequestered in the venous portions of the circulation.

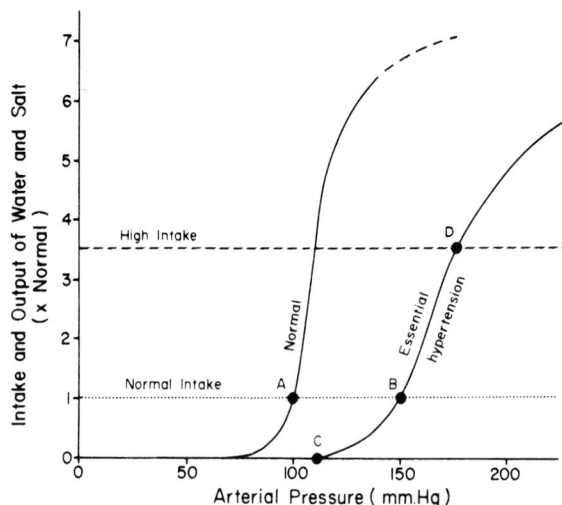

FIGURE 2. Schematic figure illustrating the ability of the normal kidney to adjust sodium excretion depending on renal perfusion pressure. Normally, a steep excretion curve provides precise control of sodium excretion around normal levels of pressure. Experimental data indicate that hypertensive models depend on a shift of this curve to the right, requiring higher pressures to achieve sodium balance (see text). From Guyton AC: In: Guyton AC (ed) *Textbook of Medical Physiology.* W. B. Saunders, Philadelphia, pp. 205–220, 1991.

TABLE I
Regulatory Mechanisms Affecting Cardiac Output and "Filling Volumes"

Systemic	Clinical examples
Sodium balance: dietary intake	"Salt-sensitive" hypertension
Aldosterone	Primary aldosteronism
Glucocorticoids	Cushing's syndrome
Atrial natriuretic factors	
Thyroid hormones	Hyper- and hypothyroidism
Local: Renal: "Pressure natriuresis"	Chronic renal failure
Adrenergic nerves	
Intrarenal hormones	
Prostanoids: prostacyclin	Loss of blood pressure control during NSAID use
Kallikrein	
Nitric oxide	Cyclosporine-induced hypertension
Renin-angiotensin system	Renovascular hypertension
Interstitial pressure	Obstructive uropathy
Distal tubular epithelial sodium channel	Liddle's syndrome

NSAID, Nonsteroidal anti-inflammatory drug; HTN, Hypertension.

measured intravascular volumes are reduced in essential hypertension, although an occasional patient with severe hypertension develops volume depletion, such that even a minor vasodilation leads to hypotension. An important corollary to this hypothesis is that any patient who maintains normal sodium and volume balance despite high blood pressures must have an "abnormal" kidney. This paradigm is illustrated in Fig. 2 as the curve on the right.

If progressive volume depletion does not occur, the argument follows that resetting of renal function must have occurred to allow pressure natriuresis to occur at higher renal perfusion pressures. While this model has some unproven elements, it nonetheless fits many clinical observations, some of which follow.

First, experimental and clinical studies have established that hypertension follows the kidney. Experimental models of "salt-sensitive" hypertension in which animals who are genetically susceptible to develop high blood pressure during high sodium intake lose this susceptibility when transplanted with a "salt-resistant" kidney. In humans, transplantation of kidneys from normotensive organ donors to patients that have lost their own kidneys from hypertensive nephrosclerosis can lead to reversal of hypertension. Second, disorders of sodium transport, either acquired (such as an aldosterone-producing adenoma) or genetic (such as an abnormal epithelial sodium transporter in Liddle's syndrome), can lead to hypertension by changing the pressure-sodium relationship, effectively shifting from point (A) to point (B) in Fig. 2. Third, the long-established role of diuretics in treating hypertension becomes comprehensible without postulating "volume depletion": One important effect of diuretic administration is to "reset" pressure natriuresis to lower pressures. Hence, hypertensive patients can maintain sodium balance despite lower arterial pressures than their "hypertensive" native kidneys would normally tolerate, thereby moving from point (B) to point (A). Fourth, efforts to lower blood pressure that do not "reset" pressure natriuresis typically induce sodium retention and eventually fail. Hence, antihypertensive therapy with alpha-methyldopa commonly was complicated by "pseudoresistance" during which blood pressure rose after a period of successful reduction. This was shown to reflect occult volume retention and could be reversed with diuretics.

Taken together, blood pressure and the integrity of circulatory perfusion depend on maintaining sodium balance and cardiac filling volumes. The other major element in the equation is systemic vascular resistance.

DETERMINANTS OF VASCULAR RESISTANCE

The major hemodynamic abnormality underlying hypertension is unquestionably elevated vascular resistance. With time, severely hypertensive patients develop hemodynamic profiles characterized by marked vasoconstriction and reduced cardiac outputs. Vascular resistance itself cannot be explained in simple terms, but reflects an expanding list of interrelated mechanisms that change vessel characteristics and lumen diameter.

Major mechanisms regulating the level of vasomotor tone are depicted in Fig. 3 and listed in Table 2. They may be viewed as representing different "levels" of cardiovascular control, depending than where they originate. They

TABLE 2
Regulatory Mechanisms Affecting Vascular Resistance

"Functional" Regulation	Clinical examples
Long range	
Neurogenic	
CNS adrenergic stimuli e.g., stress, pain, trauma	Posttraumatic hypertension
Regional adrenergic tone: renal nerves	
Baroceptor reflexes	Autonomic failure
Hormonal systems	
Renin-angiotensin	Renovascular hypertension
Aldosterone	Primary aldosteronism
Adrenal catecholamines	Pheochromocytoma
Thyroid hormone	Hyper- and hypothyroidism
Insulin	?Essential hypertension
Na,K-ATPase inhibitors	?Essential hypertension
Short range	
Paracrine systems	
Prostaglandins, e.g., Prostacyclin PGI$_2$/ Thromboxane	?Essential hypertension NSAID use/pregnancy/steroid administration
Endothelin	?Cyclosporine
Nitric oxide	?Cyclosporine
"Structural" regulation	
Vascular tissue	
Medial hypertrophy	?Essential hypertension
Calcium compartmentalization	?Essential hypertension

NSAID, nonsteroidal anti-inflammatory drug.

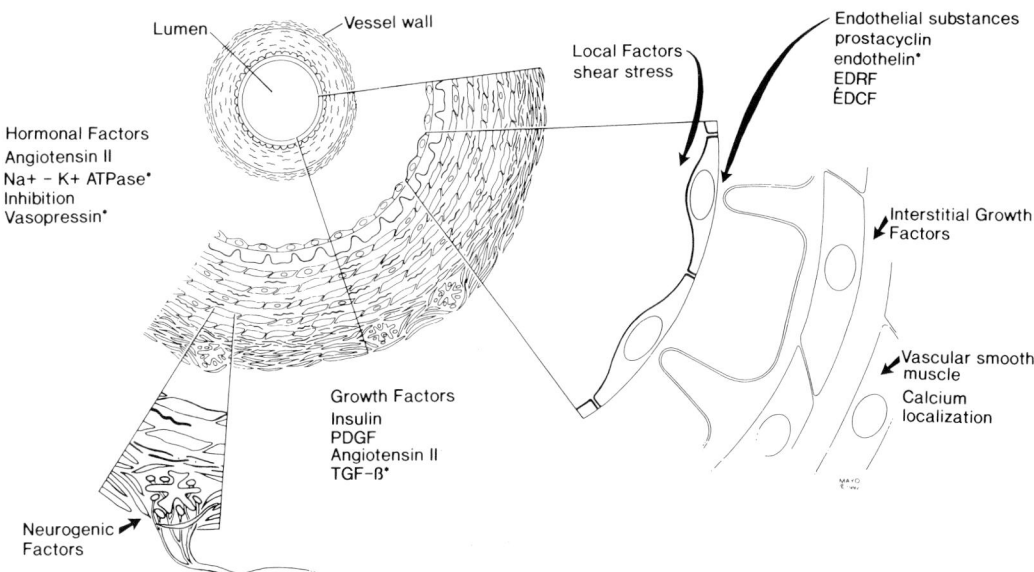

FIGURE 3 Schematic view of arterial resistance vessel, for which the lumen diameter and the resistance to blood flow are regulated by many levels of control. Systemic factors such as neurogenic and hormonal stimuli are combined with local systems including vascular-derived materials such as EDRF (nitric oxide) and medial hypertrophy. The rise in systemic vascular resistance which characterizes most hypertensive states results from an imbalance of these forces.

range from global mechanisms from distant sites, such as adrenergic vasomotor stimuli from the central nervous system, to local factors limited to the vessel wall itself. An example of the latter is nitric oxide (NO) [previously referred to as "endothelium-derived relaxing factor" (EDRF)] from the surface layer of endothelial cells diffusing to adjacent vascular smooth muscle cells.

Some general comments are warranted to place these mechanisms in a clinical perspective. Many of these systems provide "redundancy" and are activated under specific circumstances. The renin-angiotensin system, for example, is suppressed when patients ingest a surfeit of dietary sodium, i.e., more than 150 mEq/day. When dietary sodium is restricted, however, renin is released from the kidney as part of an integrated response that maintains blood pressure and retains sodium. This characteristic applies equally to normal subjects and patients with essential hypertension. It follows that pharmacologic blockade of the renin-angiotensin system has different effects depending on the pretreatment activation of the system.

Administering such an agent to patients depleted of sodium and therefore dependent on circulating angiotensin for vascular tone produces a profound fall in vascular resistance and blood pressure that would not occur if that individual is taking larger amounts of sodium. Renin is also released when perfusion pressures are reduced to the kidney. Hence, any condition with reduced renal perfusion pressure activates this potent pressor and sodium-retaining mechanism. The ability of these systems to change under various conditions cannot be overstated. Understanding these interactions is an important component of treating hypertensive diseases effectively.

Another reflex response activated during reduced aortic pressure is the adrenergic system, which compensates with increased sympathetically mediated vasoconstriction. Thus, adrenergic vasoconstriction and the renin-angiotensin system reinforce each other to protect the organism from hypotension and shock. Hypertension, therefore, appears as "inappropriate" activation of these mechanisms which normally "defend" blood pressure.

Regulators of vascular tone interact with one another at many levels, e.g., vasodilating prostaglandins, such as prostacyclin, and other vasodilators including nitric oxide "buffer" vasoconstricting forces, such as angiotensin II. The latter itself stimulates local prostacyclin and nitric oxide production. Hence, a vasoconstrictor's effect is limited by the vasodilators it induces. Such counteraction protects tissue microcireulations from extreme changes. The importance of these relationships becomes apparent clinically when one arm is pharmacologically disrupted. For example, during inhibition of prostaglandin synthesis by the administration of nonsteroidal antiinflammatory drugs, unopposed vasoconstriction due to removal of prostacyclin leads to deterioration of blood pressure control and renal function.

Excess activity of specific vasoconstrictor mechanisms may lead to hypertension as noted in Table 2. Many experimental models and clinical forms of "secondary" human hypertension reinforce this concept. Pheochromocytoma is an example of autonomous production of catecholamines,

usually norepinephrine, which leads to either sustained or paroxysmal hypertension. Both unilateral renovascular disease and renal infarction lead to overactivity of the renin-angiotensin system and hypertension characterized by angiotensin II-mediated vasoconstriction. Verification of this sequence depends, of course, on reversal of hypertension by removal of the offending mechanism, which, in fact, occurs after surgical removal of a pheochromocytoma or revascularization of the kidney.

The fundamental abnormalities underlying vascular regulation in essential hypertension are uncertain. Rare forms of hypertension appear to be the result of single gene mutations. An example is the familial form of Liddle's syndrome, for which a mutation in the gene coding for an epithelial sodium transporter leads to enhanced distal nephron sodium reabsorption. However, population studies indicate that arterial blood pressure generally is an inherited phenotypic trait of polygenic origin. Hence, no single gene plays a dominant role in essential hypertension. Rather, the interaction of many genes with each other and with environmental factors such as sodium intake, ultimately leads to a rise in pressure. Provocative data suggest that insulin "resistance" also is a trait commonly present in patients developing essential hypertension. Such insulin resistance is present in offspring of hypertensive parents prior to the onset of clinical hypertension in the children. Whether this trait and the potential for insulin to magnify vascular effects leading to medial hypertrophy participate in the development of essential hypertension are under study. Ouabain-like inhibitors of Na,K-dependent ATPase have long been suspected of circulating in humans. It has been proposed that such an inhibitor may offset a subtle defect in urinary sodium excretion. Hence, inhibition of Na,K-ATPase can restore sodium balance, but at the price of enhanced vasoconstriction in vascular smooth muscle. Taken together, insulin resistance and sodium pump inhibitors offer potential examples of how circulating factors may participate in abnormal vascular regulation that ultimately leads to hypertension. It is likely that the effects of genetically determined components of blood pressure in humans are modulated heavily by interaction with environmental factors, such as the level of dietary sodium intake and obesity.

Recent data suggest that vessel-derived vasoactive substances also modulate vascular resistance locally. The precise role of these substances in human disease states is only partly understood. Recent studies using inhibitors of No indicate that NO plays a tonic role in blood pressure control. Another local factor is endothelin, a potent vasoconstrictor peptide demonstrated first in endothelial cell cultures. This substance is released during conditions of vascular wall injury, such as with atherosclerosis or cyclosporine administration. Hence, control of vascular resistance and smooth muscle tone are subject to extensive local and systemic controls. The force of vascular smooth muscle contraction depends on intracellular calcium, and perhaps other cations such as magnesium. These ions are in continuous redistribution within cellular compartments and across the cell outer membrane, moving via complex transport mechanisms and ion "channels." Most vascular regulatory mechanisms exert effects by changing the rate or distribution sites of calcium, as do antihypertensive drugs. Whether essential hypertension depends also primarily on abnormalities of intracellular ion kinetics is not yet known.

Most of the aforementioned factors change vascular resistance by increasing smooth muscle contraction surrounding the blood vessel. It is likely also that *structural* alterations of the vessel wall contribute to changes in vascular geometry and resistance. Classic studies have demonstrated that hypertrophy of vascular tissue reduces lumen size. Whether these "structural" changes represent a permanent disease process or are in some way reversible is uncertain. Recent studies indicate that cellular growth and medial hypertrophy can be induced by altered local shear forces. Continuous remodeling of the vessel can be demonstrated. These changes in turn may be modified by growth-promoting factors including insulin, platelet-derived growth factors, and probably many others.

INTEGRATION OF VOLUME AND RESISTANCE ABNORMALITIES

Taken together, the determinants of circulatory volume and vascular resistance are complex and interrelated. Examination of Tables 1 and 2 indicates that many of the mechanisms that appear in both tables affect both parameters of the pressure equation. It should come as no surprise that a biologic variable as critical as organ perfusion pressure should be subject to multiple levels of regulation and redundant systems. This has sometimes been described as a "mosaic," from which elevated blood pressure derives from many permutations of affected systems. Hence, it is rare to encounter a "pure" form of hypertension in which only one parameter is deranged. Even reversible, secondary forms of hypertension are regulated by multiple mechanisms, as suggested in the right-hand columns of Tables 1 and 2. This "plasticity" of blood pressure control is sometimes not fully appreciated. Changing one element leads to other changes, which may finally return pressures to the original level, albeit sustained by a different balance of forces. A corollary of this observation is that effective treatment of hypertension requires intervening simultaneously at multiple levels.

The complexity of blood pressure control necessarily makes it difficult to identify the dominant factors in a specific patient. For the same reason, determining what primary pathogenic process (or processes) is responsible for "essential" hypertension is hard. Nonetheless, understanding the determinants of volume and vascular resistance provides a framework for approaching and intervening rationally in hypertensive disorders.

Bibliography

Cowley AW, Roman RJ: The role of the kidney in hypertension. *JAMA* 275:1581–1587, 1996.

Curtiss JJ, Luke RG, Dustan HP, et al.: Remission of essential hypertension after renal transplantation. *N Engl J Med* 309:1009–1015, 1983.

Dominiczak AF, Bohr DF: Nitric oxide and hypertension in 1995. *Curr Opin Nephrol Hypertens* 5:174–180, 1996.

Gavras H: The place of angiotensin-converting enzyme inhibition in the treatment of cardiovascular diseases. *N Engl J Med* 319:1541–1543, 1989.

Goldstein DS: Plasma catecholamines in essential hypertension: An analytical review. *Hypertension* 5:86–99, 1983.

Guyton AC: Dominant role of the kidneys in long-term regulation of arterial pressure and hypertension: The integrated system for pressure control. In: Guyton AC (ed) *Textbook of Medical Physiology*. W.B. Saunders, Philadelphia, pp. 205–220, 1991.

Heagerty AM, Bund SJ, Izzard AS: Long-term structural changes in human hypertensive vessels. *Basic Res Cardiol* 86 (Suppl 1):19–23, 1991.

Kuchel O: The autonomic nervous system and blood pressure regulation in human hypertension. In: Genest J, Kuchel O, Hamet P, Cantin M (eds) *Hypertension: Physiopathology* and *Treatment*. McGraw-Hill New York, pp. 140–160, 1983.

Levin ER: Mechanisms of disease: Endothelins. *N Engl J Med* 333:356–363, 1995.

Reaven GM: Role of insulin resistance in human disease. *Diabetes* 37:1595–1607, 1988.

Romero JC, Lahera V, Salom MG, Biondi ML: Role of the endothelium-dependent relaxing factor nitric oxide on renal function. *J Am Soc Nephrol* 2:1371–1387, 1992.

Tarazi RC: The hemodynamics of hypertension. In: Genest K, Kuchel O, Hamet P, Cantin M (eds) *Hypertension: Physiopathology and Treatment*. McGraw-Hill, New York, pp. 15–42, 1983.

Vane JR, Anggard EE, Botting RM: Regulatory functions of the vascular endothelium. *N Engl J Med* 323:27–36, 1990.

77

ESSENTIAL HYPERTENSION

JOSEPH V. NALLY, JR.

Hypertension is one of the most common problems in clinical medicine in the United States and is the leading indication for both physician office visits and prescription drugs. Essential or primary hypertension is the sustained elevation of systemic arterial pressure without a readily definable etiology. It is by far the most common form of hypertension, accounting for over 90% of the nearly 50 million Americans with hypertension. This increase in arterial pressure exists as a major rick factor for cardiovascular disease. Consequently, there has been a tremendously increased effort over the past two decades to identify and effectively treat patients with this "silent killer."

DEFINITION OF HYPERTENSION

There is no strict definition of hypertension, yet arbitrary limits have been proposed to identify increasing cardiovascular risk as a function of the elevation of systemic blood pressure. Initial efforts by the World Health Organization (WHO) suggested that blood pressure determinations greater than 160/95 mm Hg defined hypertension and increasing risk. In the United States, the 1984 report of the Joint National Committee on Detection, Evaluation, and Treatment of High Blood Pressure (JNC III) determined that cardiovascular risk increases at a lower threshold and established a limit of 140/90 mm Hg averaged over repeated measurements on three separate visits. Traditionally, elevation of blood pressure had been stratified based on the diastolic blood pressure. The Fifth Report of the JNC (JNC V) recognized the importance of systolic hypertension correlating with increased cardiovascular risk and proposed a definition of blood pressure determinations based upon both the systolic and diastolic readings. Table 1 summarizes these various levels of blood pressure determinations and the JNC V recommendations for patient follow-up or referral.

PREVALENCE AND CARDIOVASCULAR RISK

The most exhaustive source of data for the prevalence of hypertension, hypertension awareness and control in the US population emanates from the National Health and Nutrition Examination Survey (NHANES). Population surveys regarding hypertension were performed during four time periods (1960 to 1962, 1971 to 1975, 1976 to 1980, 1988 to 1991). For these studies, three blood pressure determinations were taken at a single visit and individuals were questioned about their blood pressure and/or antihypertensive therapy. NHANES employed the WHO definition of hypertension, i.e., systolic blood pressure >160 mm Hg, diastolic blood pressure >95 mm Hg, or currently taking antihypertensive medications. Using these criteria, 20 to 22% of the United States' population were deemed hypertensive. As seen in Table 2, there has been a gratifying increase in patient awareness, use of antihypertensive therapy, and control of blood pressure. Since the inception of the National High Blood Pressure Education Program (NHBPEP) in 1972, there has been a concomitant decrease in age-adjusted cardiovascular mortality rates, with a marked reduction in deaths from coronary heart disease (about 50%) and stroke (about 57%) over the past two decades. Since 1984, a lower threshold for defining hypertension (140/90) has been adopted by the JNC such that approximately 50 million Americans are deemed hypertensive.

Special subsets within a population have an increased risk of hypertension. Both age and race are important variables. Blood pressure, especially systolic blood pressure, increases with age such that hypertension is quite common in the elderly. Over 50% of adults older than 65 have a systolic blood pressure greater than 140 or diastolic blood pressure greater than 90. Isolated systolic hypertension, defined as systolic pressure >140 and diastolic pressure < 90, is particularly problematic in the elderly population. Isolated systolic hypertension confers the same cardiovascular risk of stroke, congestive heart failure, and coronary heart disease as does combined systolic/diastolic hypertension. During the Systolic Hypertension in the Elderly Program (SHEP) trial, active treatment with diuretics ± β-blocker significantly reduced stroke and coronary heart disease. Active treatment of systolic/diastolic hypertension in the elderly in the Swedish Trial in Old Patients with Hypertension (STOP-Hypertension) and the Medical Research Council (MRC) trial with a diuretic- and β-blocker-based regimen significantly reduced all cardiovascular mortality. Overall, the elderly have a greater prevalence of hypertension, yet they benefit from active antihypertensive therapy.

TABLE I

Classification of Blood Pressure and Recommendations for Follow-up for Adults Age 18 and Older[a]

Category	Systolic (mm Hg)	Diastolic (mm Hg)	Follow-up recommended
Normal	< 130	< 85	Recheck in 2 years
High normal	130–139	85–89	Recheck in 1 year
Hypertension			
Stage 1 (Mild)	140–159	90–99	Confirm within 2 months
Stage 2 (Moderate)	160–179	100–109	Evaluate or refer to source of care within 1 month
Stage 3 (Severe)	180–209	110–119	Evaluate or refer to source of care within 1 week
Stage 4 (Very severe)	≥ 210	≥ 120	Evaluate or refer to source of care immediately

[a] Not taking antihypertensive drugs and not acutely ill. When systolic and diastolic pressure fall into different categories, the higher category should be selected to classify the individual's blood pressure status.

From The Fifth Report of the Joint National Committee on Detection, Evaluation, and Treatment of High Blood Pressure.

Race is also an important variable regarding the prevalence and target organ effects of elevated systemic pressure. Hypertension (defined as blood pressure >160/95) is nearly twice as common in African-Americans and rates of more severe hypertension (diastolic blood pressure > 105) are several-fold higher than in their white counterparts. Furthermore, for a given level of hypertension, African-Americans tend to have more target organ damage with left ventricular hypertrophy (LVH), strokes, and renal insufficiency.

Overall, cardiovascular risk in the entire population increases with elevation of systemic pressure above an arbitrary "normal" of 120/80. Simply stated, "the higher the pressure . . . the higher the risk." For example, a sustained elevation of diastolic pressure of 5 to 6 mm Hg increases the risk of stroke by 34% and the risk of coronary heart disease by 21%. Conversely, reduction of blood pressure by a similar degree during large-scale antihypertensive studies has lowered the rate of stroke by approximately 40%; although it only reduced coronary heart disease by about 14%. Additional cardiovascular risk factors such as hyperlipidemia, diabetes mellitus, smoking, and LVH may coexist with hypertension in any given patient. The goal of antihypertensive therapy in the 1990s is both the reduction of systemic blood pressure and the simultaneous modification of other cardiovascular risk factors. Increasingly, LVH has been identified as an independent risk factor for coronary heart disease and congestive heart failure. A recent meta-analysis suggests that different classes of antihypertensive agents may reduce blood pressure equally well, but have a variable effect on the regression of LVH. Whether regression of LVH in the short term translates into reduced patient morbidity and mortality remains to be determined.

To date, the incidence of end stage renal disease (ESRD) attributed to hypertension and nephrosclerosis has not decreased and remains a leading cause of renal failure in the African-American community. The question of which antihypertensive agents could have a renal protective effect remains unclear. The Afro-American Study of Kidney Disease (AASKD) has been initiated to address this important issue.

CLASSIFICATION OF HYPERTENSION

Over 90% of all patients with high blood pressure presenting to their primary care physician will have essential hypertension as the cause of their hypertension is not readily definable. A classification of hypertension is outlined in Table 3, with the estimates of prevalence of the various forms of hypertension within the general population also listed. As seen in Table 3, approximately 5 to 10% of patients may have secondary forms of hypertension. Renal parenchymal disease is the most common medical condition associated with hypertension. Renovascular hypertension is the most common potentially remediable form of hypertension. Primary aldosteronism, pheochro-

TABLE 2

Hypertension[a] Awareness, Treatment, and Control Rates

	1971–1972	1974–1975	1976–1980	1988–1991
Aware: Percentage of hypertensives told by physician	51	64	(54) 73	(65) 84
Treated: Percentage of hypertensives on medication	36	34	(33) 56	(49) 73
Controlled: Percentage of hypertensives with blood pressure < 160/95 mm Hg on one occasion measurement and reported currently taking antihypertensive medications	16	20	(11) 34	(21) 55

Note: Numbers in parentheses are percentage at 140/90 mm Hg.

[a] Defined as ≥ 160/95 mm Hg on one occasion measurement or reported currently taking antihypertensive medication.

TABLE 3
Classification of Hypertension

	Prevalence
Systolic and diastolic hypertension	
Essential (primary) hypertension	90–95%
Secondary hypertension	5–10%
Renal	2.5–6.0%
Renal parenchymal disease	
Polycystic kidney disease	
Hydronephrosis	
Renin-producing tumors	
Renovascular hypertension or renal infarction	0.2–4.0%
Coarctation of the aorta	
Endocrine	1–2%
Oral contraceptives	
Adrenal	
Primary aldosteronism	
Cushing's syndrome	
Pheochromocytoma	
Congenital adrenal hyperplasia	
Liddle's syndrome	
Thyroid (hypo- and hyper-)	
Hypercalcemia	
Hyperparathyroidism	
Exogenous hormones—glucocorticoids, mineralocorticoids, sympathomimetics	
Pregnancy-induced hypertension	[a]
Neurogenic	[a]
Alcohol and drugs (cyclosporine A, erythropoietin)	[a]
Systolic hypertension	
Isolated systolic hypertension (especially elderly)	
Increased cardiac output	
Thyrotoxicosis	
AV fistula	
Aortic insufficiency	
Paget's disease	
Beriberi	

[a] Special circumstances.

mocytoma, and Cushing's disease are seen less frequently. Note that use of oral contraceptives and excesses of alcohol present potentially reversible causes of hypertension.

PATHOPHYSIOLOGY

Simply stated, blood pressure (BP) is the product of cardiac output (CO) and total peripheral resistance (TPR):

$$BP = CO \times \overline{TPR}$$

Nearly all forms of sustained clinical hypertension are due to an elevation of TPR in the face of a normal or mildly depressed cardiac output. This simple concept is important to grasp in order to appreciate the intricacies of pathophysiology and implications for therapeutic intervention. In over 90% of cases, the precise cause of hypertension is not readily definable and the patient is said to have idiopathic or essential hypertension. The etiology of essential hypertension is a heterogeneous mixture of complex interactions of heredity/environmental factors, sodium homeostasis, the renin-angiotensin system, sympathetic nervous system, and other factors which are incompletely understood. A detailed discussion of the pathophysiology of hypertension is found in Chapter 76.

CLINICAL PRESENTATION

Hypertension is often discovered in an asymptomatic individual as a result of a community screening program or during an evaluation for another clinical problem. As noted previously, the systemic pressure should be persistently elevated on at least three different occasions before labeling a patient as "hypertensive." The next important decision is the extent of the diagnostic evaluation required. Three key questions need to be addressed:

1. What is the cause of hypertension? Specifically, is there a potentially reversible form of secondary hypertension?
2. Is there evidence for target organ damage?
3. Are there coexistent cardiovascular risk factors?

All patients should undergo a thorough medical history and physical examination and have a selected laboratory evaluation to address these three important questions. The following evaluation is recommended by JNC V.

Medical History

A detailed medical history should include:

1. Known duration and level of blood pressure elevation

TABLE 4
Manifestations of Target Organ Disease

Organ system	Manifestations
Cardiac	Clinical, electrocardiographic, or radiologic evidence of coronary artery disease
	Left ventricular hypertrophy or "strain" by electrocardiography or left ventricular hypertrophy by echocardiography
	Left ventricular dysfunction or cardiac failure
Cerebrovascular	Transient ischemic attack or stroke
Peripheral vascular	Absence of one or more major pulses in the extremities (except for dorsalis pedis) with or without intermittent claudication; aneurysm
Renal	Serum creatinine (1.5 mg/dL) Proteinuria (1+ or greater) Microalbuminuria
Retinopathy	Hemorrhages or exudates, with or without papilledema

2. Antihypertensive therapy, results, and side effects
3. History of cardiovascular, cerebrovascular, or renal disease and knowledge of diabetes, hyperlipidemia, or gout.
4. Symptoms suggesting secondary hypertension
5. Family history of hypertension
6. Family history of premature atherosclerotic heart disease, stroke, diabetes, or hyperlipidemia
7. History of weight gain, smoking, physical activity, or mental stress
8. Dietary assessment including salt, fat, and alcohol use
9. Thorough medication history, especially oral contraceptives, steroids, NSAIDS, cold remedies, appetite suppressants, tricyclic antidepressants, MAO inhibitors, cyclosporine, erythropoietin.

Blood Pressure Measurements

The patient must refrain from smoking, caffeine use, and exogenous adrenergic stimulants for 30 to 60 minutes. The patient should be resting comfortably (seated or supine) in a quiet room for at least 5 minutes. Using the appropriate equipment and cuff size (15 cm wide cuff with bladder size 80% of arm circumference), two or more BP measurements separated by 2 minutes should be obtained and then repeated after standing for at least 2 minutes. During the initial exam, verify blood pressure in the contralateral arm (if different, the higher value should be used).

Physical Examination

A thorough examination is required to search for evidence of target organ damage (see Table 4) or a cause of secondary hypertension. The initial exam should include:

1. Height and weight
2. Fundoscopic exam (with pupil dilatation if necessary) for arteriolar narrowing, arteriovenous nicking, hemorrhages, exudates, or papilledema (see Table 5)
3. Examination of the neck for carotid bruits, jugular venous distension, thyroid gland enlargement
4. Examination of the heart for rhythm, displaced point maximal impulse, murmur, or congestive heart failure
5. Examination of the abdomen for bruits, large kidneys, masses, or abnormal aortic pulsations
6. Examination of the extremities for decreased or absent pulses, bruits, or edema
7. Neurological assessment

Routine Laboratory Evaluation

The JNC V has recommended that a few laboratory tests should be performed routinely prior to initiating therapy. These studies include: urinalysis, serum chemistry profile (fasting blood sugar, potassium, creatinine, calcium, uric acid), cholesterol/triglyceride profile, and electrocardiogram. The purpose of this testing is to screen for secondary causes of hypertension, cardiovascular risk factors, and existent cardiovascular disease. Although the echocardiogram is a more sensitive test than the ECG for detecting LVH, routine echocardiography is not recommended because of cost concerns. In the diabetic hypertensive population, the presence of microalbuminuria may be predictive of the increased risk of renal or cardiovascular disease. Additional laboratory testing for secondary forms of hypertension may be required if clinical suspicion exists.

Searching for Remediable Forms of Hypertension

In general, patients with essential hypertension present during mid-life (30 to 55 years of age) with mild to moderate hypertension, mild or no target organ damage, and often have a family history of hypertension. However, a common exception is the young African-American male with essential hypertension who may present with severe hypertension and significant renal impairment or LVH. Table 6 summarizes the clinical features that are "atypical" for essential hypertension and should alert the physician to possible secondary forms of hypertension. Five to ten percent of all hypertensive patients may have definable forms of secondary hypertension, as outlined in Table 3. For example, patients with edema and proteinuria may have renal parenchymal disease requiring further evaluation. Patients with a family history of renal disease and hypertension who have a normal urinalysis should undergo renal ultrasonography to screen for polycystic kidney disease. Others with severe or resistant hypertension and/or an abdominal bruit may be candidates to screen for renovascular hypertension (see Chapter 78). Coarctation of the aorta should be excluded by careful examination with blood pressures measured in the upper and lower extremities.

TABLE 5
Simplified Classification of Hypertensive Retinopathy

Group	Retinal arterioles		Hemorrhages	Exudates	Papilledema
	Sclerosis	Narrowing grade			
1	< 1	0–4	−	−	−
2	1 or more	0–4	±	−	−
3	0–4	0–4	±	+	−
4	0–4	0–4	±	±	+

TABLE 6

"Atypical" Features of Essential Hypertension

Age < 30 or > 55

Abrupt onset, severe hypertension ($\geq$ stage 3)

Hypertension resistant to effective medical therapy

Target organ damage
  Fundi with acute hemorrhages/exudates
  Renal dysfunction
Left ventricular hypertrophy

Features indicative of secondary hypertension
  Unprovoked hypokalemia
  Abdominal bruit or diffuse atherosclerosis
  ACE inhibitor-induced renal dysfunction
  Labile hypertension, sweats, tremor, headache
  Family history of renal disease

In selected cases, adrenal causes of hypertension should be considered as potentially remediable forms of hypertension. Patients with a symptom complex suggestive of pheochromocytoma (episodic hypertension, sweats, headaches, etc.) may be evaluated with plasma catecholamines, urinary vanillylmandelic acid/metanephrines, or a clonidine suppression test. Clinical clues suggesting Cushing's syndrome may be investigated with a dexamethasone suppression test and ACTH measurement. Alternatively, patients with unprovoked hypokalemia and metabolic alkalosis may be screened biochemically for aldosterone overproduction. If a biochemical abnormality is suggestive of adrenal hyperfunction in these three states, the adrenal glands should be imaged with thin-cut CT.

THERAPY

The overall goal of antihypertensive therapy for patients with essential hypertension is to reduce cardiovascular morbidity and mortality. The goal of therapy may be best met by both lowering elevated systemic pressure and favorably modifying other cardiovascular risk factors. Specifics of nonpharmacologic and pharmacologic therapy in the management of the hypertensive patient are detailed in Chapter 35.

Bibliography

Bravo EL: Evolving concepts in the pathophysiology, diagnosis, and treatment of pheochromocytoma. *Endocrinol Rev* 15(3): 356–368, 1994.

Bravo EL: Primary aldosteronism: Issues in diagnosis and management. *Endocrinol Metab Clin North Am* 23:271–283, 1994.

Breslin DJ, Gifford RW, Fairbairn JF, Kearns TP: Prognostic importance of ophthalmoscopic findings in essential hypertension. *JAMA* 195:335–338, 1996.

Dahlöf B, Lindholm LH, Hansson L, et al.: Morbidity and mortality in the Swedish Trial in Old Patients with Hypertension (STOP-Hypertension). *Lancet* 338:1281–1284, 1991.

The Fifth Report of the Joint National Committee on Detection, Evaluation, and Treatment of High Blood Pressure: *Arch Intern Med* 153:154–183, 1993.

Gifford RW Jr: Treatment of patients with systemic arterial hypertension. In: Schlant RC, Alexander RW (eds) *Hurst's The Heart* 8th ed. McGraw-Hill, New York, pp. 1427–1448, 1993.

Hypertension Detection and Follow-up Program Cooperative Group. Five-year findings of the Hypertension Detection and Follow-up Program: I. Reduction in mortality of persons with high blood pressure, including mild hypertension. *JAMA* 242:2562–2571, 1979.

Hypertension Detection and Follow-up Program Cooperative Group. Five-year findings of the Hypertension Detection and Follow-up Program. II. Mortality by race-sex and age. *JAMA* 242:2572–2577, 1979.

Hypertension Detection and Follow-up Program Cooperative Group. Five-year findings of the Hypertension Detection and Follow-up Program. III. Reduction in stroke incidence among persons with high blood pressure. *JAMA* 247:633–638, 1982.

Kannel W. Hypertension and global cardiovascular risk. In: Black H (ed) *Primer on Hypertension*. American Heart Association, Chicago, 1993.

Kaplan NM: Hypertension in the population at large. In: Kaplan NM, Lieberman E (eds). *Clinical Hypertension*, 5th ed. Williams and Wilkins, Baltimore, pp. 1–25, 1990.

MRC Working Party. Medical Research Council trial of treatment of hypertension in older adults: Principal results. *Br Med J* 304:405–412, 1992.

Multiple Risk Factor Intervention Trial Research Group: Risk factor changes and mortality results. *JAMA* 248:1465–1477, 1982.

Schmieder RE, Martus P, Klingbeil A: Reversal of left ventricular hypertrophy in essential hypertension. A meta-analysis of randomized double-blind studies. *JAMA* 275:1507–1513, 1996.

SHEP Cooperative Research Group: Prevention of stroke by antihypertensive drug treatment in older persons with isolated systolic hypertension. Final results of the Systolic Hypertension in the Elderly Program (SHEP). *JAMA* 265:3255–3264, 1991.

78

RENOVASCULAR HYPERTENSION

LAURA P. SVETKEY

Renovascular hypertension is a potentially curable form of high blood pressure. Its treatment, with angioplasty, stenting, or surgery, provides the opportunity to prevent cardiovascular morbidity and mortality due to hypertension and to avoid the expense and potential morbidity of lifelong pharmacotherapy for hypertension. Therefore, this condition should be identified and corrected whenever possible.

DEFINITION

Renovascular hypertension (RVH) is defined as high blood pressure secondary to renal artery stenosis. In clinical practice the diagnosis is made retrospectively, i.e., one says that a patient has RVH if hypertension improves after repair of a renal artery stenosis. Improvement in blood pressure, as defined by the Cooperative Study of Renovascular Hypertension, means that previously elevated blood pressure becomes normal without antihypertensive medication, or that less medication is required to control blood pressure. Hypertension does not have to be cured to make the diagnosis of RVH.

Any process that narrows a main renal artery can cause RVH. In this discussion, renal artery stenosis (RAS) will generally refer to narrowing of a main renal artery, although stenosis of a branch or accessory artery may occasionally be responsible for RVH. RAS is most commonly due to either fibromuscular dysplasia (particularly but not exclusively in young women) and atherosclerosis. Rarely, stenosis may be due to neurofibromatosis, radiation fibrosis, extrinsic compression, embolism, congenital anomaly, and Takayasu's disease.

It is unclear how severe a stenosis must be in order to cause RVH. Some authors consider 50% luminal narrowing to indicate significant stenosis of a renal artery, but perfusion pressure in large arteries may be preserved until the lumen is reduced by at least 70%. In addition, the obstruction to blood flow depends on the length and configuration of the stenosis, so that the two-dimensional view on arteriography may over- or underestimate the three-dimensional process of luminal narrowing. This problem may be particularly severe in the case of fibromuscular dysplasia (FMD), in which the lesion is often web-like across the lumen. The relevant information is the degree to which a stenosis interferes with perfusion and stimulates renin release, but this information is not obtainable clinically. In the absence of reliable hemodynamic information, a conservative approach would dictate that luminal narrowing of 50% or greater should be considered significant, particularly if there is poststenotic dilatation.

PATHOPHYSIOLOGY

When RAS is present, blood pressure increases because of activation of the renin-angiotensin-aldosterone axis (Fig. 1). Decreased perfusion to the affected kidney leads to renin release, which in turn promotes the conversion of angiotensinogen to angiotensin I. In the rate-limiting step, angiotensin converting enzyme converts angiotensin I to angiotensin II (A-II), which is a potent vasoconstrictor. A-II also leads to aldosterone release, which promotes salt and water retention. Vasoconstriction without the ability to compensate through increased salt and water excretion leads to sustained hypertension.

An animal model of renovascular hypertension, the two-kidney, one-clip Goldblatt rat, demonstrates the pathophysiology of RVH. In the Goldblatt rat, a metal clip is applied to one renal artery, decreasing perfusion to that kidney. Shortly thereafter, as indicated in Fig. 2, Phase I, plasma renin activity rises, leading to the generation of A-II, and blood pressure consequently rises. In Phase II, hypertension persists, despite the return of plasma renin levels toward normal. Although plasma renin activity is within the normal range, it should actually be considered elevated in the setting of elevated blood pressure. During this phase, the animals are volume expanded and may have increased vascular responsiveness to A-II. The persistence of hypertension in these rats without elevated renin activity may be analogous to RVH in humans with normal plasma renin levels.

Relieving the Goldblatt rat's stenosis by removing the clip helps us predict the response to intervention in humans with RAS. As demonstrated in Fig. 2, if the clip is removed during Phase I or II, and blood flow to the kidney is restored, blood pressure promptly returns to normal. In Phase III, however, removing the clip does not lead to decreased blood pressure. After a period of stenosis, hypertension is fixed, presumably due to alterations in the renin-angiotensin system acting locally (i.e., in renal or vascular smooth muscle cells), as well as irreversible vascular changes. One can extrapolate to humans and assume that when blood pressure does not improve after correction of a RAS either

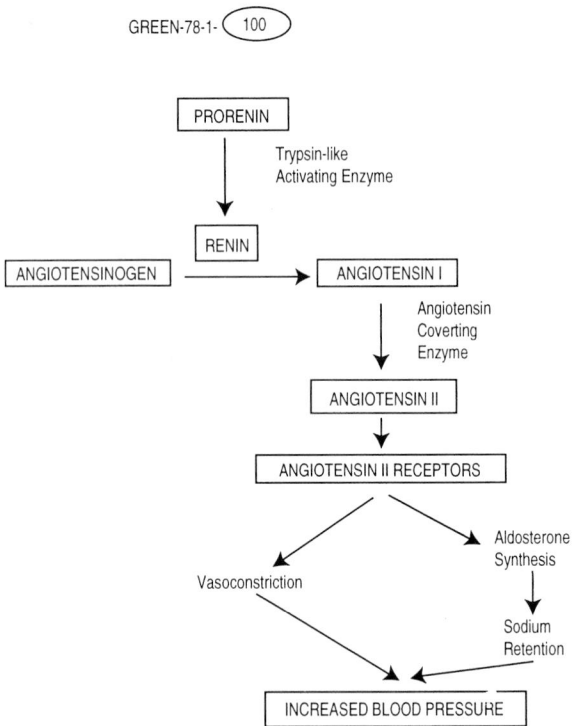

GREEN-78-1- (100)

FIGURE I Renin-angiotensin-aldosterone axis.

the stenosis was not hemodynamically significant (i.e., it didn't cause the elevated blood pressure to begin with) or the hypertension, originally due to the stenosis, is now irreversible.

EPIDEMIOLOGY

Estimates of the prevalence of RVH vary widely, depending primarily on the population studied. Overall, however, probably less than 5% of all hypertensives have this secondary form. Its occurrence is associated with several clinical features, discussed below. When clinically selected populations are evaluated, approximately 25 to 35% will

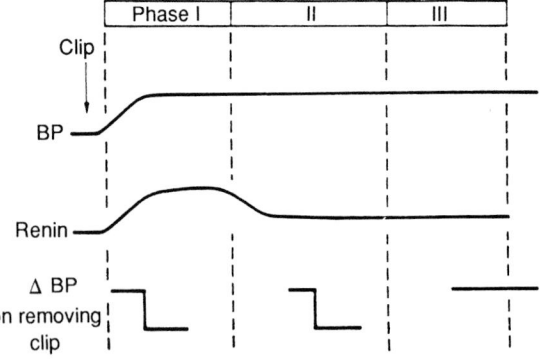

FIGURE 2 Phases of renovascular hypertension in the two-kidney, one-clip Goldblatt rat.

have RAS, and 10 to 20% (about 65% of those with RAS) will have reduction in blood pressure following correction of the stenosis.

Many clinicians assume that RVH is exceptionally rare in African-Americans. This idea persists because the prevalence of essential hypertension is so high among African-Americans that the subset of all hypertensives with RVH is small. However, in populations that are assessed carefully (i.e., with arteriography performed in all subjects), it is clear that clinically selected African-Americans have similar prevalence rates to clinically selected whites.

CLINICAL FEATURES

Table 1 lists clinical features that are associated with renovascular hypertension. RVH is found in up to 32% of patients with a history of malignant hypertension (severely elevated blood pressure with papilledema) or accelerated hypertension (severely elevated pressure with fresh retinal hemorrhage), and in almost 50% of patients with abdominal or flank bruit. Some authors specify that the bruit must persist into diastole, but similarly high prevalence of RVH may be found associated with systolic bruits. In fact, bruit may simply be a marker for severe and/or diffuse vascular disease.

The presence of either severe hypertension or bruit makes RVH likely, but their absence does not rule it out. RVH should also be considered in the other settings listed in Table 1. In addition, although cigarette smoking is too widely prevalent to be useful in distinguishing RVH from essential hypertension, tobacco use is associated with increased prevalence of both atherosclerotic and fibromuscular RAS.

Among patients (with or without hypertension) undergoing cardiac catheterization, 15% have significant RAS. Even when RAS exists without accompanying hypertension, it is associated with increased 5-year mortality. In a large prospective study, RAS was associated with severe coronary artery disease, congestive heart failure, and peripheral vascular disease. Therefore, the presence of these conditions should increase the clinical suspicion of RVH.

DIAGNOSTIC TESTS

As stated above, the diagnosis of RVH can be made with assurance only when blood pressure falls in response

TABLE I

Clinical Characteristics Associated with Renovascular Hypertension

Malignant or accelerated hypertension
Abdominal or flank bruit
Progression in the severity of chronic hypertension
Onset early (age < 25 yr) or late (age > 60 yr)
Hypotension or renal failure with ACE inhibitor
Severe or difficult to control hypertension
Recent onset of hypertension
Moderate hypertension and diffuse vascular disease
New onset of hypertension following renal
    transplantation

to interventional therapy—an assessment that can only be made retrospectively. In clinical practice, however, diagnostic tests are used to detect RAS, which is a necessary precondition for the diagnosis of RVH. The gold standard of diagnosis for RAS is conventional renal arteriography. Intravenous digital subtraction renal angiography (IVDSA) will detect most stenoses and will be normal in most patients without RAS. IVDSA has the advantage of venous rather than arterial access, with a comparable dose of contrast material. However, IVDSA requires subjective judgment in interpretation, and it becomes uninterpretable if there is overlying bowel gas or the patient is extremely obese. In addition, in many institutions, there may be no cost advantage to IVDSA over arteriography, and both procedures can be performed on an outpatient basis. If IVDSA is used instead of arteriography, a technically poor result should never be considered adequate to rule out RAS. In general, if the complication rate for arteriography at a particular institution is low, arteriography offers advantages over IVDSA in accuracy and clarity, and is the preferred method of diagnosing RAS. The ordinary intravenous pyelogram is insufficiently sensitive and specific for detection of RAS, and should not be used for this purpose.

It is frequently appropriate to proceed directly from clinical suspicion to angiography (see below). But in other cases, the expense and risk of this procedure may not be warranted. Several noninvasive techniques have been developed (Table 2), and may be useful in determining which patients should be evaluated more definitively. These screening tests are briefly summarized.

Peripheral Renin Activity

Many patients with RVH do not have elevated plasma renin activity (PRA), and 16% of patients with essential hypertension do. Therefore, PRA alone is not useful in determining which patients should be evaluated further for RVH. In order to improve the predictive value of PRA, two tests take advantage of the expected excessive increase with angiotensin converting enzyme (ACE) inhibition in the setting of RVH: elevation of PRA after a single oral dose of ACE inhibitor, or, alternatively, a measure of the degree to which PRA increases from baseline after ACE inhibitor (the Captopril Test). Unfortunately, these tests are most useful in unmedicated patients (often difficult to do safely in patients with severe hypertension), and in patients with normal renal function. Even when these

TABLE 2
Diagnostic and Screening Tests for Renovascular Hypertension

Conventional renal arteriography
Intravenous digital subtraction renal angiography
ACE inhibitor-stimulated peripheral renin activity
ACE inhibitor-stimulated renography
Duplex ultrasound
Magnetic resonance angiography

conditions are met, however, sensitivity and specificity may be as low as 75%. In addition, ACE inhibitor-stimulated plasma renin may be less useful in detecting RVH in African-Americans.

ACE Inhibitor-Stimulated Renography

In the setting of RVH, both glomerular filtration rate and renal plasma flow depend on angiotensin II-mediated constriction of the glomerular efferent arteriole. Treatment with an ACE inhibitor antagonizes this vasoconstriction and decreases renal uptake and excretion of radiopharmaceuticals. A renogram is considered abnormal at baseline if there is evidence of assymmetric function, or if uptake or excretion of the marker is delayed. RAS is suspected if the abnormalities are exacerbated by ACE inhibition (see Fig. 3). False positive results (due to ACE inhibitor-induced oliguria and consequent "hang-up" of radiopharmaceutical in the renal cortex) can be avoided by simultaneous injection of furosemide. The test's utility may be limited in bilateral disease since asymmetry may not occur and because renal dysfunction may further confound interpretation. Estimates of the sensitivity and specificity of ACE inhibitor-stimulated renography vary widely, but on average probably exceed 80% (somewhat lower in the setting of renal insufficiency). Patients should be well hydrated and must discontinue chronic ACE inhibitor therapy (they may continue taking other blood pressure medications). ACE inhibitor-stimulated renography is currently the most useful noninvasive screening test for RVH. However, this test must be interpreted cautiously since its interpretation

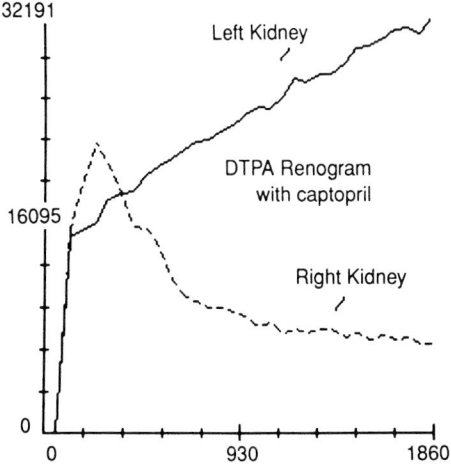

FIGURE 3 Captopril renography in renal artery stenosis. The figure shows accumulation of counts over the kidneys vs time after injection of ^{99m}Tc-DTPA—a GFR and renal perfusion marker. Before administration of captopril (not shown), both kidneys showed similar and normal prompt uptake and excretion. After captopril, the right kidney continues to show rapid uptake and excretion, but the left shows a marked delay in uptake and release of labeled marker. At arteriography, the patient was found to have an atherosclerotic lesion of the renal artery. Courtesy of Dr. A. N. Shah.

is somewhat subjective and its accuracy is reduced in the setting of renal disease or bilateral RAS.

Duplex Ultrasound

The use of color-flow doppler in the diagnosis of RVH is an attempt to combine anatomic information from ultrasound with hemodynamic information from doppler. This technique seems to be seriously limited by the fact that the proximal main renal artery is not visualized in 25% of cases. In addition, small accessory and secondary renal arteries are often not detected. Duplex ultrasound is highly operator-dependent, and requires over 1 hour to perform correctly. For these reasons, duplex ultrasound is not useful in screening for RVH.

Magnetic Resonance Angiography (MRA) and Computerized Tomographic Angiography

MRA is a noninvasive modality that can provide information about both anatomy and blood flow. Extensive data are not yet available, but small studies suggest that MRA detects RAS with a sensitivity of 70 to 90% and specificity of 78 to 94%. If the more favorable of these results are corroborated, MRA may offer a reasonable alternative to conventional arteriography in patients at high risk for contrast-related complications. Computerized tomographic angiography (CTA) require intravenous contrast but avoids the need for an arterial puncture. At some centers, it has shown promise in detecting RAS (see Chapter 6, Fig. 3).

DIAGNOSTIC STRATEGY

The utility of any given test for screening and diagnosis of RVH will depend on the prevalence of RVH in the population being evaluated (the pretest probability), and on the sensitivity and specificity of the test. Even an excellent screening test, for example one with 90% sensitivity and 90% specificity, will provide little help if the prior probability of RVH is low. If one assumes that unselected hypertensives have a 5% chance of having RVH, this hypothetical test will increase that likelihood to 32% if it is positive, leaving 68% of those with an abnormal test with a false positive result. A negative test will essentially rule out RVH (negative predictive value = 99%), but the likelihood that RVH was absent was 95% before the test.

Because of these limitations of diagnostic tests that perform well (and not all of the procedures in Table 2 have a sensitivity and specificity as high as 90%), Mann and Pickering have suggested a strategy, somewhat modified here, for selecting patients for further evaluation. This strategy involves the definition of subgroups, based on the clinical suspicion (pretest probability) of RVH.

If a patient has a history of malignant hypertension, history of renal failure following ACE inhibitor, or the presence of an abdominal or flank bruit, the likelihood of finding RAS is greater than 30%, and one should proceed directly to angiography. In addition, 'if the motivation to find RAS is extremely high, for instance if a patient has severe hypertension (JNC-5 Stage 3 or 4) that is difficult to control in the setting of progressive renal insufficiency, or if the patient has moderate hypertension (Stage 2) and is unable to tolerate any antihypertensive regimen, then it is reasonable to proceed directly to angiography. At the other end of the spectrum, if a patient has borderline or mild hypertension (Stage 1) that is easily controlled, and none of the clinical clues discussed above are present, then no further workup is indicated.

Diagnostic difficulties arise in patients with clinical clues that lead to an intermediate pretest probability of RVH. This group comprises, for example, those with severe hypertension without history of a malignant or accelerated phase, abrupt onset of hypertension very early or very late in life, sudden increase in the severity of chronic hypertension, and unexplained renal insufficiency, especially if there is evidence of vascular disease elsewhere. In this subgroup, a noninvasive test may be helpful. In most circumstances, the ACE inhibitor-stimulated renogram is the most useful screening test. With an intermediate pretest probability of RAS, renography is sufficiently sensitive and specific that a negative test will effectively rule out RVH, and obviate the need for further evaluation. A positive test will increase the likelihood of RVH sufficiently to warrant angiography. The decision to pursue this diagnosis in any individual patient should include consideration of the potential risks of arteriography and revascularization, risks which may be magnified by diffuse atherosclerosis and renal insufficiency.

HEMODYNAMIC SIGNIFICANCE

After RAS has been detected, it would be useful to predict blood pressure response to correction of the lesion. Traditionally, measurement of the renal vein renin ratio is used for this purpose. This test is based on the expectation that a hemodynamically significant lesion will stimulate renin release from the stenosed kidney and suppress its release from the contralateral kidney. The predictive value of this test is improved if renin release is stimulated with a single oral dose of ACE inhibitor, but nonetheless remains quite poor. In practice it is very difficult to predict blood pressure response to intervention. In addition, relieving a stenosis without lowering blood pressure may still be beneficial if it protects that kidney from progressive ischemia Therefore, if RAS is detected, and it is possible to intervene safely, this should be attempted, reserving conclusions about the hemodynamic significance of the stenosis for retrospective consideration.

TREATMENT

Renal vascular disease is occasionally treated medically unless blood pressure is difficult to control. However, the implication of this approach is that many individuals will be exposed to the expense and risk of lifelong antihypertensive medication unnecessarily. In addition, the presence of RAS may increase the risk of chronic renal disease, and reperfusion may preserve renal function. Therefore, RAS should be corrected whenever possible without undue risk.

Renal artery stenosis can be relieved by either surgical revascularization, percutaneous transluminal angioplasty (PTA), or renal artery stenting. When technically feasible, angioplasty is preferred since it can be performed without general anesthesia or lengthy hospitalization (see Kuhlmann et al., 1985). PTA is less likely to be technically successful if an ostial stenosis is present (because these lesions usually originate in the wall of the aorta and are thus not affected by a balloon catheter inflated in the renal artery). The recent introduction of stents has markedly improved success rates in relieving ostial RAS.

The main limitations of PTA are primary failure and subsequent restenosis. Primary failure occurs if the balloon catheter can not be passed beyond the lesion. In addition, even when the procedure can be performed, angiography performed immediately after dilatation occasionally demonstrates persistent stenosis. These problems will be detected at the time of the procedure, and should lead to alternative treatment (repeat PTA, stenting, or surgical revascularization). After successful angioplasty, restenosis will occur over the following year in approximately 20% of patients, with slightly higher rates in patients with atherosclerotic than FMD lesions. Stents markedly reduce restenosis rates. When restenosis occurs following PRA, a second angioplasty is often successful, but stenting or surgical revascularization may ultimately be necessary.

Bibliography

Davidson RA, Wilcox CS: Newer tests for the diagnosis of renovascular disease. *JAMA* 268:3353–3358, 1992.

Harding MB, Smith LR, Himmelstein SI, et al.: Renal artery stenosis: prevalence and associated risk factors in patients undergoing routine cardiac catheterization. *J Am Soc Nephrol* 2:1608–1616, 1992.

Hudspeth DA, Hansen KJ, Reavis SW, Starr SM, Appel RG, Dean RH: Renal duplex sonography after treatment of renovascular disease. *J Vasc Surg* 18:381–388, 1993.

Jacobson HR: Ischemic renal disease: an overlooked clinical entity? *Kidney Int* 34:729–743, 1988.

Kuhlmann, U, Greminger P, Gruntzig A, et al.: Long-term experience in percutaneous transluminal dilatation of renal artery stenosis. *Am J Med* 79:692–698, 1985.

Mann SJ, Pickering TG: Detection of renovascular hypertension: state of the art, 1992. *Ann Intern Med* 117:845–853, 1992.

Miller GA, Ford KK, Braun SD, et al.: Percutaneous transluminal angioplasty vs surgery for renovascular hypertension. *AJR* 144:447–450, 1985.

Martinez-Maldonado M: Pathophysiology of renovascular hypertension. *Hypertension* 17:707–719, 1991.

Olin JW, Piedmonte MR, Young JR, DeAnna S, Grubb M, Childs MB: The utility of duplex ultrasound scanning of the renal arteries for diagnosing significant renal artery stenosis. *Ann Intern Med* 122:833–838, 1995.

Plouin P-F, Darne B, Chatellier G, et al.: Restenosis after a first percutaneous transluminal angioplasty. *Hypertension* 21:89–96, 1993.

Rimmer JM, Gennari FJ: Atherosclerotic renovascular disease and progressive renal failure. *Ann Intern Med* 118:712–719, 1993.

Simon N, Franklin SS, Bleifer KH, et al.: Clinical characteristics of renovascular hypertension. *JAMA* 220:1209–1218, 1972.

Svetkey LP, Kadir S, Dunnick NR, et al.: Similar prevalence of renovascular hypertension in selected blacks and whites. *Hypertension* 17:678–683, 1991.

Working Group on Renovascular Hypertension: Detection, evaluation and treatment of renovascular hypertension. *Arch Intern Med* 147:820–829, 1987.

Ying CY, Tifft CP, Gavras H, Chobanian AV: Renal revascularization in the azotemic hypertensive patient resistant to therapy. *N Engl J Med* 311:1070–1075, 1984.

79

THERAPY OF HYPERTENSION

JOHN M. FLACK

By definition, hypertension is present when there is a persistent elevation of either systolic blood pressure ($\geq$140 mm Hg) or diastolic blood pressure ($\geq$90 mm Hg), or when a patient is taking antihypertensive medication (regardless of the blood pressure level). The blood pressure level correlates directly with the magnitude of risk for clinical sequelae such as premature death, stroke, myocardial infarction, congestive heart failure, renal insufficiency, dementia, and peripheral vascular disease. Table 1 in Chapter 77 displays the blood pressure classification from the fifth report of the Joint National Committee on the Detection Treatment and Evaluation of High Blood Pressure expert panel. This scheme determines hypertension stage according to the highest pressure—either systolic or diastolic. The preponderance of epidemiological data suggests that systolic, not diastolic, blood pressure is the primary determinant of pressure-related risk.

RATIONALE FOR TREATMENT

A compelling case can be made for pharmacological treatment of elevated blood pressure. Pharmacological blood pressure lowering reduces the risk of premature cardiovascular morbid and fatal events as well as all-cause mortality. Antihypertensive drug therapy has also been shown to prevent the gradual progression of mild hypertension to more severe elevations of blood pressure. The prevalence of pressure-related target-organ damage (i.e., elevated serum creatinine, left ventricular hypertrophy) is also greater at higher blood pressure levels. Hypertensives with pressure-related target-organ damage manifest a several-fold higher risk for pressure-related clinical complications at a given blood pressure level compared to hypertensives with similar levels of pressure without target-organ damage. Early treatment of hypertension favorably impacts long-term clinical risk, in part, by preventing the development of pressure-related target organ damage. It is not well appreciated that drug-treated hypertensive patients subjectively feel better (i.e., improved quality of life and fewer pressure-related symptoms) after successful blood

pressure lowering. The evidence in support of this thesis is compelling.

GENERAL THERAPEUTIC PRINCIPLES

Several important therapeutic principles should be consider in treating hypertensive patients. In most hypertensives there is little to be gained from the pursuit of rapid blood pressure control. The most important therapeutic goal for the vast majority is to prescribe a combination of appropriate lifestyle modifications (weight loss, salt and alcohol restriction, and increased physical activity) plus the lowest doses of drug(s) that allow blood pressure normalization over the long term. The erroneous clinical perception that diastolic blood pressure is the predominant pressure mediator of clinical risk contributes to physician hesitancy to intensify treatment to normalize systolic blood pressure once diastolic blood pressure has been lowered to <90 mm less than Hg. Many antihypertensive medications have dose-related side effects. Drug acquisition costs also usually increase at higher dose levels. In certain instances, cost is a major barrier to patient compliance with prescribed drug therapies. The clinician and nursing staff should routinely ask patients whether they can afford the prescribed medications. Drug acquisition costs are but one consideration, albeit an important one, in embarking on a hypertension disease management strategy.

Establish a Goal Blood Pressure

Establishing a goal blood pressure is an extremely important consideration prior to the initiation of antihypertensive drug therapy. In most uncomplicated hypertensive patients, the target blood pressure level will be <140/90 mm Hg. Nevertheless, in selected high-risk subgroups (i.e., renal insufficiency, diabetes), the target blood pressure may justifiably be lower (<130/85 mm Hg). The Treatment of Mild Hypertension Study [TOMHS] findings support a more stringent goal blood pressure (< 130/85 mm Hg) even for uncomplicated stage 1 diastolic hypertensives. In TOMHS, drug-treated hypertensives (also prescribed a multifactorial lifestyle intervention) had an average blood pressure of 140/91 mm Hg at baseline. After 4 years of treatment in this group, blood pressure averaged 127/

79 mm Hg vs 133/82 mm Hg in TOMHS participants receiving only the multifactorial lifestyle intervention. The incidence of major and minor clinical events was 11.1% in the drug-treatment group vs 16.2% in those receiving only lifestyle modification.

Clinical Implications of Drug Pharmacokinetics

Drug pharmacokinetic profiles influence both the time to onset of maximal blood pressure lowering and the degree of protection against loss of blood pressure control during the intervals between missed medication doses. The terminal drug half life in general, though not always, correlates directly with both the duration of blood pressure lowering as well as with the time to reach steady-state drug levels. Drugs with a longer duration of action have a delayed onset of maximal blood pressure lowering compared to drugs with a shorter duration of action. However, once steady-state drug levels have been achieved, long duration of action drugs provide superior blood pressure control throughout the 24-hour dosing interval and also have a slow offset of action which minimizes the loss of blood pressure control when medication doses are missed. Pharmacokinetic considerations are important, as only 60% of hypertensives who take antihypertensive medications over the long term do so without missing scheduled doses.

Frequency of Monitoring/Drug Titration

A reasonable time frame for attainment of normal blood pressure levels should be measured in months, not days or weeks. In most patients, it matters little over the long term if blood pressure control is achieved in 4 months as opposed to 4 weeks. Long-acting antihypertensive drugs usually take up to 3 to 6 weeks to fully manifest their maximal blood pressure lowering effect. Thus, in most hypertensives, dose increases or medication changes should be undertaken no more frequently than every 6 weeks. This strategy will facilitate attainment of goal blood pressure with a minimum of office visits and also will minimize the likelihood of precipitating symptoms attributable to rapid blood pressure lowering. Nevertheless, if a patient manifests insignificant blood pressure lowering during the first few weeks of therapy, the likelihood of a meaningful blood pressure response over the ensuing weeks is low. A reasonable strategy at this point is to titrate the dose upward, add another medication, or stop the current medication and switch to another drug. Potential problems with rapid blood pressure lowering are listed in Table 1.

Side Effects

Both the patient and physician usually attribute subjective side effects experienced by drug-treated hypertensives to antihypertensive medication, because hypertension has long been considered an asymptomatic condition. However, there is considerable evidence that hypertensive patients do indeed experience a constellation of symptoms (Table 2) that correlate with the blood pressure level. Even

TABLE I

The Potential Hazards of a Hypertension Disease Management Approach Utilizing Rapid Upward Titration of Antihypertensive Agents and Frequent Office Visits to Accomplish Rapid Blood Pressure Lowering

Subjective side effects
  Dose-related
  Correlate with rapidity of BP fall
Target organ ischemia
  Angina pectoris, MI, TIA, or stroke
Higher total cost of care
  Increased Drug doses
  Unnecessary office visits
  Excessive medication changes
  Excessive patient monitoring

though antihypertensive drugs can cause symptoms, they appear to alleviate more symptoms than they cause, as drug-treated hypertensives report fewer subjective side effects than placebo-treated individuals with higher blood pressure levels. Pressure-related symptoms such as weakness and fatigue not only relate to the blood pressure level, but may also occur in a time-limited manner when the blood pressure levels change rapidly in either direction. Hypertensive patients are most at risk for time-limited pressure-related symptoms during the transition from one medication to another as a consequence of a transient loss of blood pressure control. There is also an increased risk for pressure-related symptoms of limited time duration after rapid blood pressure lowering that correlates with the height of the pretreatment blood pressure. The symptomatic drug-treated hypertensive is not uncommon in clinical practice as fewer than 50% of drug-treated hypertensives attain blood pressure levels <140/90 mm Hg.

ANTIHYPERTENSIVE DRUG SELECTION

Monotherapy

The clinician must have reasonable expectations about the likelihood of blood pressure normalization with monotherapy. If expectations are unrealistic, then subsequent therapeutic decisions will be misguided and therefore unlikely to result in blood pressure normalization. The lack of therapeutic success will frustrate both the patient and physician. The probability of achieving blood pressure normalization with monotherapy in the overall hypertensive population ranges between 50 and 60%. Two or fewer drugs will control about 85 to 90% of all hypertensives, whereas three or more drugs will be required for blood pressure normalization in the remainder. The probability of blood pressure normalization with monotherapy is significantly influenced by the magnitude of the pretreatment blood pressure elevation. The Fifth Joint National Committee

TABLE 2

Constellation of Symptoms Reported More
Often in Hypertensives with Elevated Blood
Pressures Compared to Drug-Treated
Hypertensives with Lower Blood
Pressure Levels

Headache
Fatigue/weakness
Lack of stamina, poor exercise tolerance
Cardiac awareness
Dizziness
Nervousness
Sleep disturbance
Chest pain

blood pressure classification scheme can thus be quite useful in guiding therapeutic decisions (Table 3). A common clinical mistake is to expect monotherapy to normalize blood pressure levels in hypertensives with "high" Stage 2 or higher hypertension. If, however, an adequately dosed therapeutic trial of monotherapy of sufficient duration is undertaken, then it is a more effective strategy to add a second drug when monotherapy fails. However, if a second drug from an additional drug class is substituted, it is also likely that this agent will fail to normalize blood pressure. In this situation, drug substitution leads to extra office visits, excessive patient monitoring, and unnecessary changes in their therapeutic regimen, all of which contribute to a higher total cost of care. Conversely, in "high" Stage 2 or higher hypertension, initial monotherapy is a viable initial treatment strategy even though the probability of ultimately achieving blood pressure control with a single drug is low. Table 4 displays the advantages and disadvantages of the major antihypertensive drug classes.

Diuretics

Monotherapy with thiazide diuretics effectively lowers blood pressure with a similar degree of efficacy in both African-American and white hypertensives. Thiazides are, however, ineffective when the glomerular filtration rate is < 40 mL/min; a clinical rule of thumb is that thiazides should be avoided when serum creatinine levels are ≥ 2.3 mg/dL. Current recommendations are to prescribe 25 mg/day or less. Doses as low as 6.25 mg/day have been shown to effectively lower blood pressure. These agents are cheap, as drug acquisition costs can be as low as pennies per day. The absence of a diuretic is perhaps the most common cause of resistant hypertension in patients treated with complex [> 2] antihypertensive drug regimens. The relatively long drug half lives of thiazides (chlorthalidone > hydrochlorothiazide) is a favorable pharmacokinetic characteristic for long-term hypertension management. Thiazides have dose-related side effects such as hypokalemia (< 3.5 mEq/L), hypomagnesemia, and hyperuricemia. Hypokalemia is the most common meta-

bolic side effect, occurring in 30 to 35% of diuretic-treated hypertensives consuming an ad libitum sodium diet. The likelihood of hypokalemia can be reduced by these nonmutually exclusive strategies: (1) reduce the diuretic dose; (2) lower intake of dietary sodium; or (3) add a potassium-sparing diuretic or potassium supplement. Thiazides can impair free water clearance and thus their use occasionally results in hyponatremia in older hypertensives. These agents also cause modest lipid disturbances, as they raise cholesterol levels ~6% and triglyceride levels approximately 15%, while leaving high density lipoprotein levels unaffected. Thiazides can adversely affect glycemic control; however, this can be avoided by preventing potassium depletion. These agents are the worst offending drug class for causing sexual dysfunction in men. Loop diuretics, metolazone, and indapamide maintain their blood pressure lowering efficacy in patients with compromised renal function. Though loop diuretics are more potent diuretics than the thiazides, these agents lower blood pressure less effectively in individuals with normal renal function. Diuretics are especially useful in hypertensives with congestive heart failure.

β-Blockers

β-blockers are a heterogeneous group of drugs which can be subclassified according to their relative affinity for beta receptor subtypes, the presence or absence of intrinsic sympathomimetic activity, and their lipophilicity. β-blockers can be categorized as: (1) nonselective (β_1 and β_2) (i.e., nadolol, propranolol, timolol), (2) cardioselective (β_1) (i.e., atenolol, metoprolol), (3) cardioselective with intrinsic sympathomimetic activity (acebutolol), (4) nonselective with intrinsic sympathomimetic activity (i.e., pindolol), or (5) α-β blocker (labetalol). β_1 receptors are the predominant β receptor subtype in the heart while β_2 receptors predominate in the lung and peripheral blood vessels. Nevertheless, both receptor subtypes are found in target organs. Cardioselective (β_1) β-blockers have theoretical advantages in patients with bronchospastic lung disease as nonselective β blockers (β_1 and β_2) are more prone to incite bronchospasm. However, because target tissues are not populated by distinct β receptor subtypes, even cardioselective β blockers can cause bronchospasm and should be avoided in patients with lung disease. β blockers (without intrinsic sympathomimetic activity) should be a favored antihypertensive therapy in the postmyocardial infarction patient because of their proven cardioprotection and their ability to lower mortality. Likewise these nonintrinsic sympathomimetic activity β blockers are particularly useful in the hypertensive patient with either angina pectoris or migrane headaches. These agents are highly effective blood pressure lowering agents when used alone or in combination with diuretics. In the calcium antagonist group, only the dihydropyridines are suitable for combination therapy with β-blockers. β-blockers reduce cardiac output by approximately 20 to 25%; thus, these agents have been associated with low cardiac output symptoms such as weakness, fatigue, and poor exercise tolerance. β-blockers can also worsen symptomatic peripheral vascular disease, have been

TABLE 3
An Adaptation of the JNC V Blood Pressure Classification Scheme That Describes Therapeutic Options When Monotherapy
Fails to Lower Blood Pressure to <140/90 mm Hg According to Patients Initial Blood Pressure Level

	SBP (mm Hg)	DBP (mm Hg)	When monotherapy is unsuccessful
Stage 1	140–159	90–99	Switch drugs
Stage 2			
"low"	160–169	100–104	Switch drugs; however, consider adding a second drug
"high"	170–179	105–109	Add a second drug
Stage 3–4	≥180	≥110	Add a second drug; however, consider two drug treatment initially

linked to depression, and lower high density lipoprotein while raising triglycerides. The adverse lipid effects are less pronounced with intrinsic sympathomimetic activity β-blockers. Less lipophilic β blockers may cause less depression because they poorly traverse the blood brain barrier into the central nervous system. β-blockers should be used with caution in hypoglycemia-prone diabetics because they: (1) blunt the tachycardia accompanying hypoglycemia, and (2) delay the metabolic recovery from hypoglycemia. There are new data suggesting the benefit of low-dose β blockade in patients with congestive heart failure. Nevertheless, until more data are available, the clinician should avoid β-blockers in congestive heart failure patients unless there are contraindications to one or more of the standard congestive heart failure treatments (digitalis, diuretics, and angiotensin-converting enzyme inhibitors).

Angiotensin-Converting Enzyme Inhibitors

Angiotensin-converting enzyme inhibitors are particularly useful in diabetic hypertensives with proteinuria as well as in hypertensives with congestive heart failure and in those who have survived myocardial infarction. These agents are metabolically neutral, do not cause male erectile dysfunction, and have no effect on fasting glucose even though they modestly improve insulin sensitivity. The major side effect of this drug class is cough, which occurs in ~ 9% of hypertensives taking angiotensin-converting enzyme inhibitors. Angioedema is a potentially life-threatening side effect occuring in approximately 3/1000 angiotensin-converting enzyme inhibitor-treated patients. Angioedema can occur months after the initiation of angiotensin converting inhibitor therapy. The incidence of hyperkalemia in all angiotensin-converting enzyme inhibitor-treated hypertensives is less than 1%. However, those with renal insufficiency as well as those treated with nonsteroidal anti-inflammatory drugs, potassium-sparing diuretics, potassium supplements, and/or heparin have a higher risk. Angiotensin-converting enzyme inhibitors should be avoided in patients with bilateral renal artery stenosis and should be used cautiously in patients with unilateral renal artery stenosis because of the risk of iatrogenic renal failure. African-Americans, particularly those with high intake of dietary sodium, may require higher doses of these agents to achieve blood pressure control. The combined use of angiotensin-converting inhibitors

with either a diuretic or a calcium antagonist appears to be highly efficacious and well tolerated. Angiotensin-converting enzyme inhibitors also blunt thiazide-induced hypokalemia. These agents are potentially teratogenic and should be avoided in pregnancy. Women of child-bearing potential should be counseled to use contraceptives while taking angiotensin-converting enzyme inhibitors and should be changed to another agent if they are attempting to become pregnant.

Alpha₁ Antagonists

Alpha₁ antagonists improve insulin sensitivity and cause modest favorable changes in all blood lipoproteins making them desirable in hypertensives with either diabetes mellitus or dyslipidemia. These are preferred agents in older men with benign prostatic hyperplasia as they improve maximum urine flow rates in a dose-dependent manner. This drug class either does not affect or modestly improves erectile function in men. Doses required to achieve blood pressure control are slightly higher in African-American hypertensives than in white hypertensives. These agents can precipitate or worsen orthostatic hypotension. Thus the clinican should routinely take orthostatic blood pressure measurements in at-risk groups including older persons, diabetics, sedentary individuals, and hypertensives concurrently treated with diuretics, central adrenergic inhibitors, or combined α-β blockers.

Calcium Antagonists

Calcium antagonists are a heterogenous class of vasoactive compounds which effectively lower blood pressure in all racial, ethnic, and demographic groups. These agents have variable hemodynamic, inotropic, chronotropic, and neurohumoral effects. There is essentially no role for short-acting calcium antagonists in the long-term therapy of hypertension. Short-acting nifedipine can be useful for acute blood pressure lowering during legitimate hypertensive urgencies, although some recent evidence suggests caution when using this agent for this indication. Calcium antagonists also can be subclassified as either rate-limiting (verapamil, diltiazem) or dihydropyridine (i.e., nifedipine, amlodipine, felodipine). Rate-limiting calcium antagonists, in contrast to the dihydropyridines, have atrioventricular nodal blocking properties and usually should not be used in combination with β-blockers, nor should they be used

TABLE 4
Advantages and Disadvantages of Seven Commonly Used Antihypertensive Drug Classes

Advantages	Disadvantages
Angiotensin-Converting Enzyme (ACE) Inhibitors	
Renoprotective in type 1 diabetes	Cough ($\sim$ 9%)
Profoundly antiproteinuric	Rare angioedema ($\sim$ 3/1000)
↓ Morbidity and mortality and symptomatic improvement in CHF patients	Rare hyperkalemia
↓ Ventricular remodeling and mortality post-MI	Higher dose requirements in *some* African-Americans
Leftward shift of pressure-natriuresis curve	BP lowering effect very sensitive to level of dietary sodium intake
Safely combined with other anti-hypertensives, especially diuretics or calcium antagonists	
α_1 Antagonists	
Positive effect on all lipoprotein fractions	Orthostatic hypotension (particularly in the elderly, in
Positive effect on all lipoprotein fractions	combination with other vasodilators, in the setting of autonomic
Improved insulin sensitivity	dysfunction, and in volume depleted patients)
Unchanged to improved sexual function in men	Slightly higher doses needed in African-Americans
Blunts thiazide-induced rise in cholesterol	
Improves maximal urine flow in men with BPH	
Angiotensin II (AT_1) Receptor Antagonists	
Lesser peak BP lowering compared to ACEs	Relatively flat BP dose–response curve
Nearly complete blockage of A-II effect	No effect on bradykinin
No effect on bradykinin, enkephalins, or substance P	Limited data available in African-Americans
Uricosuric (losartan)	Absence of hard clinical endpoint (i.e., CHF, MI, renal) data
Profoundly antiproteinuric	Rare hyperkalemia
Metabolically neutral	
Rare angioedema	
No cough	
β Blockers	
Differential cardiac and hemodynamic effects	Can worsen CHF; however, at low doses may improve CHF
Proven to lower morbidity and mortality post-MI	Low cardiac output symptoms
Selected agents useful in patients with migraine or angina	Can worsen or precipitate depression
	Can aggravate PVD symptoms
	Lowers HDL and raises TGs
	Delays recovery from and masks symptoms of hypoglycemia
	Abrupt discontinuation can lead to rebound hypertension
Calcium Antagonists	
Unqualified efficacy profile (African-Americans, diabetics, elderly)	Immediatley post-MI or during unstable angina (short-acting dihydropyridines) may increase CHD risk
Heterogeneous electrophysiologic, inotropic, hemodynamic, and SNS effects	Rate-limiting CBs can worsen CHF and ↑ mortality in patients with systolic heart failure
Useful in diastolic dysfunction	Side effect profile varies (constipation-verapamil, pedal edema,
Metabolically neutral	and vasodilatory symptoms-dihydropyridines)
Minimal erectile dysfunction in men	Combination with β-blockers can result in profound bradycardia
BP lowering effect is robust in setting of high dietary sodium intake	and depression of myocardial contractility
BP lowering effect not attenuated by NSAIDs	
Central Adrenergic Inhibitors	
Relatively cheap	Sedation
Useful in hypertensive urgencies (clonidine)	Depression (high dose reserpine)
Methyldopa is drug of choice for pregnant women	Orthostatic hypotension
	Decreased heart rate (clonidine)
	Frequent skin irritation (clonidine patch), dry mouth
	Abrupt discontinuation can lead to rebound hypertension
	Positive Coombs test in ~15% (methyldopa)
Direct Vasodilators	
Relatively cheap	Best suited for adjunctive therapy
Effective in severe hypertension (minoxidil > hydralazine)	Salt and water retention necessitate use of loop diuretics
	Reflex tachydardia necessitates use of rate-limiting CCB or β-blocker
	Do not regress LVH

(continues)

TABLE 4 (*continued*)

Advantages	Disadvantages
	Lupus-like syndrome (>200 mg/day of hydralazine)
	Hirsutism (minoxidil)
	Edema (minoxidil)
Diuretics	
Cheap acquisition cost	Thiazides ineffective when GFR <40 mL/min
Highly effective and lowers BP similarly in all demographic groups	Dose-related hypokalemia
	Raises cholesterol and triglycerides
Proven to lower BP-related morbidity and mortality	Glucose intolerance especially in setting of K^+ depletion
Enhances the BP lowering effect of all other BP drugs	Increased uric acid
Thiazides and metolazone have relatively long half lives	Erectile dysfunction in men
	"Hidden" costs of metabolic monitoring

BP, blood pressure; BPH, benign prostatic hyperplasia; ACE, angiotensin-converting enzyme inhibitors; A-II, angiotensin II; CCBs, calcium channel blockers; CHD, coronary heart disease; CHF, congestive heart failure; HDL, high-density lipoprotein; PVD, peripheral vascular disease; TG, triglycerides, SNS, sympathetic nervous system; NSAIDs, nonsteroidal anti-inflammatory drugs.

in patients with impaired systolic heart function. Dihydropyridine calcium antagonists are more potent peripheral vasodilators and therefore do not depress myocardial contractility. Lower extremity edema can occur with any calcium antagonist but has been more closely associated with the dihydropyridines. Neither rate-limiting nor dihydropyridine calcium antagonists should be prescribed to patients with sick sinus syndrome unless a functioning ventricular pacemaker is in place.

Angiotensin Receptor Antagonists

Angiotensin receptor antagonists are the first new antihypertensive drug class introduced into clinical practice in over a decade. Losartan and valsartan are the only currently available agents in this class; however, irbersartan, telmisartan, seprosartan, and candesartan will likely soon be available. Angiotensin recep tor antagonists are well tolerated as monotherapy and have been most extensively studied in combination with diuretics. These agents are metabolically neutral and do not cause erectile dysfunction in men. Like the angiotensin-converting enzyme inhibitors, angiotensin receptor antagonists antagonize the renin-angiotensin-aldosterone system (though at a different site). Unlike the angiotensin-converting enzyme inhibitors, angiotensin receptor antagonists do not cause cough. Anecdotal reports of angioedema with angiotensin receptor antagonists have, however, now surfaced, though the incidence is probably lower than with the angiotensin converting enzyme inhibitors. Similar to the angiotensin-converting enzyme inhibitors, these agents should be avoided in individuals with bilateral renal artery stenosis and used cautiously in patients with unilateral renal artery stenosis. These agents should also be used with caution in hyperkalemia-prone individuals.

Central Adrenergic Inhibitors

Central adrenergic inhibitors (i.e., clonidine, methyldopa) are most useful for adjunctive antihypertensive therapy. These agents effectively lower blood pressure and also cause regression of left ventricular hypertrophy. However, sedation, dry mouth, and orthostatic hypotension limit patient acceptance of these agents. Abrupt discontinuation of these drugs can lead to rebound hypertension making these agents less than ideal therapeutic agents for patients with known noncompliance. The use of these agents in combination with β-blockers should be discouraged because of the risk of bradycardia. Methyldopa is the antihypertensive agent of choice in hypertensive pregnant women.

Direct Vasodilators

Direct vasodilators (i.e., minoxidil, hydralazine) are uncommonly used as monotherapy mostly because they evoke marked arterial vasodilatation and thus cause reflexive activation of the sympathetic nervous system. This leads to both salt and water retention as well as tachycardia. The latter raises myocardial oxygen consumption and therefore can precipitate new or worsen preexisting coronary ischemia in patients with coronary heart disease. These agents are most effectively used in combination with diuretics and β-blockers or a rate-limiting calcium antagonist. Lower extremity edema may complicate minoxidil therapy even when potent diuretics are simultaneously prescribed.

Combination Therapy

Almost 50% of all hypertensives and most Stage 2 or higher hypertensives will require more than a single antihypertensive agent to achieve blood pressure normalization. Thus, physicians should become familiar with the clinical scenarios when combination therapy will likely be needed. In "high" Stage 2 or higher hypertensives, it is reasonable for physicians to consider initiating antihypertensive therapy with two drugs. Dual drug therapy can be initiated either by prescription of two separate pills or by prescribing a single combination pill. The combined blood pressure lowering effect of two drugs at low-to-moderate doses usually exceeds the magnitude of blood pressure, lowering obtainable effect by upward titration of either drug alone

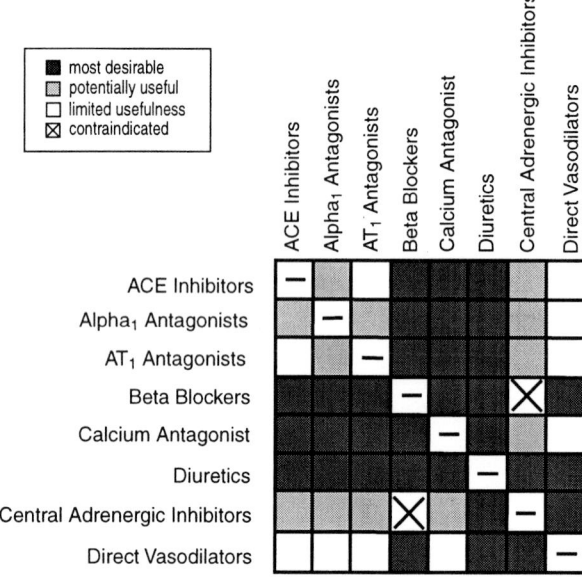

FIGURE 1 Two agent drug combinations for seven antihypertensive drug classes according to their relative clinical utility.

to its maximum dose and with fewer side effects. Figure 1 shows useful therapeutic combinations of antihypertensive drugs.

THERAPEUTIC CONSIDERATIONS FOR SPECIAL POPULATIONS

African-Americans

African-Americans have a premature onset of hypertension that is associated with a greater burden of pressure-related target organ damage (i.e., microalbuminuria, left ventricular hypertrophy, elevated serum creatinine) compared to whites. The clinician will not infrequently encounter severe hypertension (Stages 2 to 4) with concomitant diabetes mellitus and other cardiovascular conditions (i.e., stroke) in the hypertensive African-American. Obesity, particularly among African-American women, contributes to the high frequency of salt sensitivity, an intermediate blood pressure phenotype which correlates with higher antihypertensive drug requirements. Persuasive data indicate that even modest reductions in dietary sodium intake (<135 mmol/day] will augment the hypotensive effect of virtually all antihypertensive drugs in all hypertensives, though more so in African-Americans.

Diuretics will often be required to achieve blood pressure normalization given the higher prevalence of renal insufficiency and reduced natriuretic capacity in African-Americans. Nevertheless, African-Americans should be viewed as individuals for whom the most appropriate antihypertensive drug therapy is chosen based on considerations (i.e., concomitant diseases, drug synergy/interactions, renal function) unique to that individual. It is an outdated concept that race should be the primary consideration when selecting antihypertensive drug therapy for any individual.

Monotherapy with diuretics and calcium antagonists has, however, been shown to result in greater blood pressure lowering in African-Americans compared to other commonly used nondiuretic drug classes (i.e., angiotensin-converting enzyme inhibitors, α-antagonists, and β-blockers]. Nevertheless, the clinician should not generalize these data to an individual and therefore presume a lack of blood pressure lowering efficacy solely, or even mostly, because of their race or ethnicity. When an adequately dosed therapeutic trial of sufficient duration is undertaken, most African-Americans will have a meaningful blood pressure response to antihypertensive agents from any of the commonly used drugs classes. It also seems prudent to establish a lower therapeutic blood pressure goal [< 130/85 mm Hg] because of the exceedingly high risk of morbid and fatal pressure-related sequelae in hypertensive African-Americans.

Elderly

Although some clinicians have been hesitant to initiate antihypertensive therapy in older individuals (≥ 60 years), the totality of evidence from epidemiological studies and clinical trials documents that older patients have a higher risk for pressure-related clinical events than younger hypertensives at any given blood pressure level. Moreover, drug-treated older hypertensives take their antihypertensive medication and comply with lifestyle modifications (i.e., weight loss, salt and alcohol restrictions) as well or better than their younger counterparts. Elderly hypertensives actually manifest more impressive reductions in pressure-related complications within a shorter time frame compared to younger hypertensives. Concomitant cardiovascular conditions (i.e., diabetes mellitus, vascular disease, renal insufficiency), noncardiovascular chronic conditions, and poverty are more common in older compared to younger hypertensives. In part because of impaired baroreceptor reflexes, older hypertensives are prone to develop orthostatic hypotension and should therefore be checked for postural hypotension. If present, then the standing blood pressure should be used to guide therapeutic decisions. The clinician should have a heightened suspicion for the presence of orthostatic hypotension in older hypertensives treated with alpha$_1$ antagonists, diuretics, and/or central adrenergic inhibitors.

Renal Insufficiency

Hypertension is a risk factor for renal insufficiency, and in turn, renal insufficiency irrespective of etiology causes hypertension. Approximately 85% of individuals with renal insufficiency also have hypertension. Diabetes mellitus and hypertension account for over one half of all cases of end-stage renal disease. The major therapeutic goal for individuals with hypertension associated with renal impairment is to set and subsequently achieve an aggressive therapeutic blood pressure goal [< 130/85 mm Hg] over many weeks to months. The average number of drugs needed to achieve blood pressure control in this hypertensive subgroup is 4.3;

thus, therapeutic debates that focus on choices of a single agent are mostly superfluous given that complex drug regimens are the rule. Limited renal natriuretic capacity, routine utilization of complex drug regimens, and the frequent use of drugs (i.e., angiotensin-converting enzyme inhibitors), which can cause hyperkalemia, are important reasons to use diuretics (loop diuretics or metolazone) in hypertensive patients with compromised renal function. Potassium-sparing diuretics and potassium supplements should be used with considerable caution, if at all, in these patients, particularly when angiotensin-converting enzyme inhibitors, angiotensin receptor antagonists, or nonsteroidal anti-inflammatory drugs are concurrently prescribed. Angiotensin-converting enzyme inhibitors, and perhaps angiotensin receptor antagonists may be particularly useful because in addition to being antiproteinuric, they antagonize the renal renin-angiotensin system which appears to be pathophysiologically linked to the characteristic structural and functional renal abnormalities found in experimental models of renal injury (see Chapter 66). Because of the potentially serious risk for hyperkalemia, these agents should, however, be used with caution in patients taking potassium-sparing diuretics or potassium supplements. Nonsteroidal anti-inflammatory drugs also further augment the risk for hyperkalemia. In hypertensives with renal impairment, simply lowering blood pressure can lead to a rise in creatinine which, in most instances is followed by a fall in creatinine to lower than pretreatment levels. Angiotensin-converting enzyme inhibitors and perhaps angiotensin receptor antagonists can incite a precipitous decline in renal function as evidenced by a rise in creatinine in patients with critical bilateral renal stenosis or unilateral stenosis in a solitary kidney.

Diabetics

Over 50% of diabetics are hypertensive. Diabetic hypertensives usually manifest disproportionate elevations in systolic compared to diastolic blood pressure and more often than not will require complex multidrug regimens to achieve blood pressure normalization. The long-term target blood pressure should minimally be < 130/85 mm Hg in this high risk group. Roughly one third of diabetics have hyporeninemic hypoaldosteronsim (type IV renal tubular acidosis), a condition which attenuates renal potassium secretion. Thus, diabetic hypertensives should be regularly checked for hyperkalemia, particularly when potassium-sparing diuretics, potassium supplements, nonsteroidal anti-inflammatory drugs, angiotensin converting enzyme inhibitors, or angiotensin receptor antagonists are prescribed. If blood pressure normalization is to be achieved, diuretics will often be required in complex drug regimens [> 2 drugs]. Diuretics augment renal potassium secretion because the reduction in plasma volume causes secondary hyperaldosteronism. Several major hypertension drug treatment trials (Hypertension Detection and Follow-up Program and the Systolic Hypertension in the Elderly Program) have documented a similar reduction in risk for pressure-related clinical events in diabetics and nondiabet-

ics when treated with diuretic-based regimens. Angiotensin-converting enzyme inhibitors have proved to be renoprotective in type I diabetics with proteinuria and thus should be utilized in such patients even in the absence of established hypertension. Though the risk of end-stage renal disease is much lower in type II diabetics (lifetime risk ~8%) compared to type I diabetics, the former accounts for the overwhelming majority of diabetes-related end-stage renal disease cases. A reasonable clinical extrapolation is that angiotensin-converting enzyme inhibitors should also be preferred antihypertensive agents in type II diabetics with proteinuria. Angiotensin receptor antagonists, like the angiotensin-converting enzyme inhibitors, are antiproteinuric, although long-term clinical outcome studies are lacking with the former. α_1 antagonists, like the angiotensin-converting enzyme inhibitors, improve insulin sensitivity and additionally have a favorable impact on all blood lipoprotein fractions. (See Chapter 29 for an in-depth discusssion of treatment of the diabetic hypertensive.)

HYPERTENSIVE URGENCIES AND EMERGENCIES

Hypertensive Urgencies

A hypertensive urgency can be defined as a blood pressure elevation in the absence of ongoing major pressure-related symptoms that is high enough to engender concerns regarding the new onset or worsening of pressure-related target organ damage (i.e., congestive heart failure, new or progressive renal insufficiency, neurological symptoms) unless the blood pressure is lowered over the ensuing hours to days. Hypertensive urgencies represent the most common indication for which acute blood pressure lowering therapy is undertaken. In true hypertensive emergencies, blood pressure levels usually exceed 210 mm Hg systolic or 130 mm Hg diastolic. A sizable proportion of hypertensives treated acutely to lower blood pressure have only uncontrolled hypertension, not a legitimate hypertensive urgency. In minimally symptomatic hypertensives with less severe blood pressure elevations, the short-term risks of treatment (Table 1) clearly exceed the potential benefits of immediate blood pressure lowering. However, blood pressure levels higher than the aforementioned cutpoints do not automatically warrant therapeutic intervention. Treatment when indicated is usually via the oral route (Table 5). Oral therapy can be conveniently administered in a wide range of clinical settings. However, the blood pressure response to oral therapy is unpredictable. In special clinical situations (i.e., postoperative period, intractable epistaxis), hypertensive urgencies may be most appropriately treated with intravenous medications.

Malignant/Accelerated Hypertension

The incidence of both malignant and accelerated hypertension has steadily declined, mainly because of increasingly effective treatment of chronic hypertension. The clinical presentation of both entities can be quite dramatic, leading to devastating clinical consequences including death and serious long-term disability unless recognized

TABLE 5

Oral and Intravenous Antihypertensive Drugs Commonly Used to Treat Hypertensive Urgencies and Emergencies

Drug	Dose schedule	Duration	Comment
Oral			
Clonidine	0.1 mg initially then 0.1 mg every 2 hr until a maximum dose of 0.7 mg reached	3–12 hr	Onset of action is within 30–45 min; peak BP lowering 3 to 4 hr postdose; side effects include sedation, dry mouth, and orthostatic hypotension; can dramatically lower BP in volume-depleted and older patients; CBF, CO, pulse rate, and PVR all reduced; favor use when SNS tone is high (i.e., abrupt cessation of β-blockers, alcohol/drug withdrawal); avoid use in CHF or in setting of greater than first degree heart block.
Nifedipine	5–10 po or -5.1., repeat after 1 hr maximum total dose = 20 mg	4–6 hr	Onset of action is 10–15 min; peak BP lowering occurs 1–1.5 hr postdose; abrupt onset of action evokes SNS activation which can lead to reflex tachycardia thus increasing myocardial oxygen demand with precipitation or worsening of coronary ischemia; should be avoided in patients with unstable angina pectoris, MI or aortic stenosis; only short-acting formulation is useful in HTN urgencies.
Captopril	6.25–25 mg po or chewed. maximum total dose = 25 mg		Onset of BP lowering within 15–30 min after po dosing; peak BP lowering occurs 1–2 hr postdose; BP lowering effect will likely be blunted in setting of volume overload; however, rapid and excessive BP reductions can occur in volume-depleted patients; preload and afterload are decreased and CBF preserved; avoid use in bilateral renal artery stenosis and in patients with a history of ACE inhibitor-induced angioedema.
Intravenous			
Sodium nitroprusside	0.25 to 8 mg $\cdot$ kg^{-1} $\cdot$ min^{-1} with titration every 5 min	<5 min	Rapid onset (seconds) and offset of action allow precise titration of BP response; very potent; balanced preload and afterload reduction; increases CO thus desirable in CHF; may, however, cause a "coronary steal" syndrome and precipitate or worsen coronary ischemia; hypoxemia may result from intrapulmonary shunting; activates SNS, thus avoid in aortic dissection; raises ICP; thiocyanate and cyanide toxicity can occur.
Nitroglycerine	5–200 mg/min	<5 min	Onset and offset of action is within minutes; reduces preload and, at higher doses, afterload; shunts blood flow into the subendocardium, an ischemia-prone area; intravenous agent of choice for treating severe hypertension in setting of MI, unstable angina, or in individuals with known CHD; also desirable in setting of pulmonary edema and CHF; occasionally causes bradycardia; raises ICP; also may result in excessive BP lowering in setting of volume depletion; causes methemoglobinemia rarely.
Labetalol	Bolus: 20–40 mg every 20–30 min continuous infusion: 0.5–2.0 mg/min max dose = 200–300 mg/24 hr	2–6 hr	BP response is variable thus precise titration not possible; onset of action is rapid; however, offset of action takes hours; CBF is preserved; avoid use in setting of bronchospastic lung disese or CHF; excessive BP lowering can occur in setting of volume depletion; monitor for orthostatic hypotension.
Nicardipine	2–4 mg/hr with titration every 15 min; when goal BP attained lower infusion to 4 mg/hr	>4 hr	Onset of action is within 15 min; (offset of action takes hours; avoid in setting of ongoing coronary ischemia (MI, unstable angina pectoris) and in aortic dissection, unless combined with β-blockade; maintains or increases CO in CHF; potent dilatory effect on coronary arteries.
Enalapril	0.625–1.25 mg every 6 hr; reduce initial dose by 50% in patients on diuretics or if renally impaired	~6 hr	Onset of action is within 15 min; offset of action takes hours; reduces both preload and afterload and dilates coronary vessels; thus is a desirable agent in CHF and CHD patients with severe hypertension; CBF maintained; avoid in bilateral renal artery stenosis and in patients with a history of ACE inhibitor-induced angioedema; can result in excessive BP lowering in volume-depleted patients.
Furosemide	May initiate treatment with doses as low as 5–10 mg if renal function is normal; 20–40 mg in CHF; if renal function abnormal may need to dose much higher	~4.5 hr	Onset of action is within 15 min; initiates peripheral venous pooling resulting in preload reduction followed by a diuresis, the latter being maximal at 1.5 hr; favor when severe HTN is complicated by CHF, pulmonary edema, and/or renal insufficiency; avoid in setting of dehydration; use cautiously in conjunction with aminoglycosides because of ototoxicity; need to monitor glucose and electrolytes, especially potassium and magnesium. Can lower BP when used alone but mostly used to potentiate other agents.

ACE, angiotensin converting enzyme; BP, blood pressure; CBF, cerebral blood flow; CHD, coronary heart disease; CHF, congestive heart failure; CO, cardiac output; HTN, hypertensive; ICP, intracranial pressure; MI, myocardial infarction; PVR, peripheral vascular resistance; SNS, sympathetic nervous system.

Note: A brief description of the pharmacokinetic, hemodynamic, and clinical indications and contraindications is provided for each drug.

and treated appropriately. While these two hypertensive emergencies can be distinguished on clinical grounds, they portend a similar ominous prognosis. The 1-year survival rate in untreated accelerated or malignant hypertension is only 20%; however, 5-year survival rates are over 90% after successful treatment. Blood pressure is usually higher than 200/130 mm Hg. Patients typically present with one or more of the following: severe headaches, blurred vision, nystagmus, focal neurological symptoms, nystagmus, positive plantar reflexes, congestive heart failure, and/or renal failure. The fundoscopic examination routinely confirms severe retinopathy (bilateral hemorrhages and exudates). Papilledema is, however, required to make the diagnosis of malignant hypertension. Abrupt cessation of either β-blockers or central adrenergic inhibitors can also lead to a rebound in blood pressure to much higher than pretreatment levels and thus may present as a hypertensive emergency.

Patients with malignant or accelerated hypertension should always be treated with intravenous medications (Table 5) in a setting where close patient monitoring is feasible (i.e., intensive care unit). Intravenous sodium nitroprusside and nitroglycerin are the most commonly used effective therapies for hypertensive emergencies. The major advantage of these agents is that their onset and offset of action occurs within seconds to minutes, allowing for precise titration of the infusion according to the blood pressure response. The therapeutic goal for these patients is not blood pressure normalization but rather a gradual reduction of mean arterial pressure [((2 × diastolic blood pressure) + systolic blood pressure) /3] of no more than 15 to 20%. Systolic and diastolic blood pressure should not be lowered to < 170 and < 110 mm Hg, respectively. Gradual and cautious blood pressure lowering will minimize the probability of iatrogenic target organ ischemia as a consequence of vital organ hypoperfusion. In special situations such as unstable angina pectoris, congestive heart failure, pulmonary edema, or aortic dissection a lower target blood pressure may be justified. Secondary causes of hypertension such as critical renal artery stenosis, glomerulonephritis, Cushing's syndrome and pheochromocytoma should be sought in patients presenting with malignant or accelerated hypertension.

Chronic Hypertension in the Hospital Setting

The clinician should have a relatively high threshold for prescribing acute blood pressure lowering therapy, even via the oral route, in asymptomatic to minimally symptomatic hospitalized hypertensives with poorly controlled blood pressure. Potentially reversible causes for elevated blood pressure should be considered such as pain, hypoxia, hypercarbia, hypoglycemia, pulmonary edema, and status epilepticus. Withdrawal from alcohol or drugs or even rebound hypertension attributable to prior abrupt discontinuation of either β-blockers or central adrenergic inhibitors may underlie blood pressure elevations in hospitalized patients. Infusion of saline containing intravenous fluids should be minimized and

dietary sodium restricted to 2 (88 mmol) per day or less. If no reversible cause of elevated blood pressure is identified, and the blood pressure level is high enough, then the approach to treatment is virtually identical to that utilized in hypertensive urgencies. Hospitalized patients are prone to orthostatic hypotension because of prolonged bed rest. Thus, if feasible, blood pressure should be periodically measured in both the seated or supine and upright positions. Automated blood pressure measurement devices should be regularly calibrated against a mercury manometer to ensure their accuracy. Most hospitalized patients will be optimally treated simply with intensification of their ambulatory blood pressure medication regimen. The tendency to titrate drugs every day or so on hospital rounds can result in excessive blood pressure lowering leading to side effects and/or targetorgan ischemia. The ultimate therapeutic goal in hospitalized patients with poor blood pressure control is to keep blood pressure under levels that are likely to incite target organ damage over the short term. Thus, blood pressure normalization (< 140/90 mm Hg), per se, is not the usual therapeutic goal. In minimally symptomatic patients with elevated blood pressure, the pressure levels triggering physician notification should be stated in their admission orders. The blood pressure level should be high enough (210/120 mm Hg) to minimize the likelihood of unnecessary and potentially harmful therapy being prescribed for acute blood pressure lowering.

Bibliography

Abdelwahab W, Frishman W, Landau A: Management of hypertensive urgencies and emergencies. *Ther Rev* 35:747–762, 1995.

Calhoun DA, Oparil S: treatment of hypertensive crisis. *N Engl J Med* 323(17): 1177–1183, 1990

Flack JM, Neaton JD, Daniels B, et al.: Ethnicity and renal disease: Lesson from multiple Risk factor intervention trial and the treatment of mild hypertension study. *Am J Kidney Dis* 21 (4): 31–40, 1993.

Epstein M, Bakris G: Newer approaches to antihypertensive therapy. Use of fixed-dose combination therapy. *Arch Intern Med* 156:1969–1978, 1996.

Flack JM, McVeigh GE, Grimm RH Jr: Hypertension therapy in the elderly. *Curr Opin Nephrol* 2: 386–394, 1993.

Flack JM, Mensah, McVeigh GE, et al.: Diagnosis, evaluation and management of hypertension in an ambulatory clinic setting. *J Clin Outcome Manage* 2(5):1–21, 1995.

Flack JM, Cushman W: Evidence of the efficacy of low-dose diuretic monotherapy. *Am J Med* 101(Suppl. 3A):53S–60S, 1996.

Flack, JM, Neaton J, Grimm RH Jr, et al.: Blood pressure and mortality among men with prior myocardial infarction. *Circulation* 92:2437–2445, 1995.

Flack JM, Novikov SV, Ferrario CM: Benefits of adherence to anti-hypertensive drug therapy. *Eur Heart J* 17(a):16–20, 1996.

Grimm RH Jr, Flack JM, Grandits GA, et al.: Long-term Effects on plasma lipids of diet and drugs to treat hypertension. *JAMA* 275:1549–1556, 1996.

Joint National Committee. The fifth report of the Joint National Committee on Detection, Evaluation and Treatment of High Blood Pressure (JNC V). *Arch Intern Med* 153:154–183, 1993.

Lewis CE, Grandits GA, Flack JM, et al.: Efficacy and tolerance of antihypertensive treatment in men and women with stage 1 diastolic hypertension. *Arch Intern Med* 156:377–385, 1996.

Murphy C: Hypertensive emergencies. *Emerg Med Clin North Am* 13(4):973–1001, 1995.

Meredith PA. Therapeutic implications of drug holidays. *Eur Heart J* 17 (Suppl A):21–24, 1996.

National High Blood Pressure Education Program. 1995 Update of the Working Group Reports on Chronic Renal Failure and Renovascular Hypertension. *Arch Intern Med* 156:1928–1947, 1996.

Neaton JD, Grimm RH Jr, Prineas RJ, et al.: Treatment of mild Hypertension Study (TOMHS) final results. *Jo A M Ass* 270:713–724, 1993.

INDEX